Postgraduate Surgery

The candidate's guide

Postgraduate Surgery

The candidate's guide

Second Edition

Edited by

M.A.R. Al-Fallouji
PhD(Lond), FRCS(Ed), FRCS(Glas), FRCSI, LRCP&S(Ed&Glas), MB, ChB
Consultant Gastrointestinal Surgeon, Pilgrim Hospital, Boston, UK

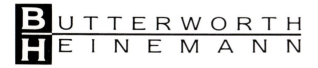
BUTTERWORTH
HEINEMANN

Butterworth-Heinemann
Linacre House, Jordan Hill, Oxford OX2 8DP
225 Wildwood Avenue, Woburn, MA 01801-2041
A division of Reed Educational and Professional Publishing Ltd

A member of the Reed Elsevier plc group

OXFORD AUCKLAND BOSTON
JOHANNESBURG MELBOURNE NEW DELHI

First published 1986
Reprinted 1988
Reprinted 1989
Reprinted 1990
Reprinted 1991
Reprinted 1993
Reprinted 1995
Second edition 1998
Reprinted 1999

British Library Cataloguing in Publication Data
Postgraduate surgery: the candidate's guide – 2nd ed.
1   Surgery
I   Al-Fallouji, M. A. R.
617

ISBN 0 7506 1591 5

Library of Congress Cataloguing in Publication Data
Postgraduate surgery: the candidate's guide/edited by M.A.R. Al-Fallouji – 2nd ed.
  p. cm.
  Rev. ed. of: Postgraduate surgery/M.A.R. Al-Fallouji and M.P. McBrien, 1986.
  Includes bibliographical references and index.
  ISBN 0 7506 1591 5
  1. Surgery – Examinations, questions, etc. 2. Surgery – Outlines, syllabi, etc. I. Al-Fallouji, M. A. R.
  [DNLM: 1. Surgery. 2. Surgery – examination questions. WO 100
  P8573
  RD37.2.P67
  617'.0076 – dc21   97–22534
                                                                    CIP

Composition by Genesis Typesetting, Rochester, Kent
Printed and bound in Great Britain by The Bath Press plc

Contents

Contributors

M.A.R. Al-Fallouji PhD(Lond), FRCS(Ed), FRCS(Glas), FRCSI, LRCP&S(Ed & Glas), MB, ChB Consultant Gastrointestinal Surgeon, Pilgrim Hospital, Boston, Lincs, UK (*Principal author and editor of the book except for contributions on topics provided by professional colleagues as indicated below*)

M.I. Aldoori PhD, FRCS(Glas), FRCS Consultant General and Vascular Surgeon, Huddersfield Royal Infirmary, West Yorkshire; Honorary Lecturer, University of Leeds (*Stroke – Surgical Prevention*)

N.K. Al-Quisi DA, DCH, FRCA(Eng) Consultant Anaesthetist, Huddersfield Royal Infirmary, West Yorkshire (*Artificial ventilation; Postoperative Analgesia*)

S.J. Becker FRCS(Ed) General Practitioner, Wakefield, West Yorkshire (*Critical Review of Abdominal Stoma; Common Surgical Conditions Affecting the Hip Joint*)

J.S.G. Blair OBE, ChM, FRCS(Ed) Consultant Surgeon, Perth Royal Infirmary, Scotland; President of the British Society for the History of Medicine; Examiner in Final FRCS(Ed), Senior Lecturer in History of Medicine, University of St Andrews; and Honorary Lecturer in Surgery, University of Dundee (*Urinary Diversion Procedures*)

M.F. Butler FRCS(Eng) Senior Consultant Surgeon, Thanet General Hospital, Margate, Kent (*Peripheral vascular disease; Aortic Aneurysm Surgery; Aortic Bypass; Arterial Embolectomy*)

P.W. Davis FRCS(Eng) Consultant Surgeon, Barnet General Hospital, Hertfordshire (*Solitary Thyroid Nodule*)

H. El Teraifi FRCPath Consultant Pathologist, Christie Hospital, Manchester (*Histopathology in Surgical Pathology*)

M.P. McBrien MS (London), FRCS(Eng) Senior Consultant Surgeon, West Suffolk Hospital (East Anglia); Hunterian Professor, Royal College of Surgeons of England; Lecturer and Demonstrator, St Thomas's Hospital and Cambridge Final FRCS Course; Clinical Teacher and Examiner in Surgery, Cambridge School of Clinical Medicine (part of *Clinical Radiology*).

J.A.K. Meikle FRCP, FRCR Consultant Radiologist and Postgraduate Clinical Tutor, Perth Royal Infirmary, Scotland (part of *Clinical Radiology*)

R.A. Mun'im MD Consultant Urologist, Al Ain Hospital, Al Ain, United Arab Emirates (*Surgery for Impotence*)

I.M.A. Salam FRCSI Consultant Surgeon, Al Ain Hospital, Al Ain, United Arab Emirates (*Tropical Surgery*)

R.E.B. Tagart ChM, FRCS(Eng) Senior Consultant Surgeon, West Suffolk Hospital, East Anglia; Hunterian Professor, Royal College of Surgeons of England (*Principles in Colonic Surgery*)

A.B. Woodyer ChM, FRCS, FRCS(Ed) Consultant General and Vascular Surgeon, Tameside General Hospital, Ashton-under-Lyne, Lancashire (*Peripheral Vascular Disease; Examination of Leg Ulcer*)

Foreword

This is a uniquely focused work, the aim of which is to guide the candidate for postgraduate surgical examinations in the United Kingdom and Ireland towards the successful achievement of their goal.

Surgery has changed rapidly in the last few years with an increasing tendency to specialization, and his had led to changes in the examination system with the realization that the traditional FRCS was failing to meet the needs of specialist disciplines. Coupled with these changes there has been the requirement for standardization of surgical training throughout the EEC, and modification of the career structure for surgical trainees to fit into European directives relating to hours of work. This book, like no other, gives a guide to the current career structures and examination systems in considerable depth which will be helpful for overseas surgeons, from the EEC or further afield, and UK and Irish graduates alike.

The book is very comprehensive and should form the surgical trainees 'bible' with a format specially designed to suit the needs of examination candidates. Excellent line drawings give up to the minute information on any newer techniques and help to clarify many of those more traditional areas of surgery which candidates have so often found confusing.

I wholeheartedly recommend this book to any surgical trainee in the United Kingdom and Ireland and it will also serve as a valuable guide to their trainers.

Michael J McMahon, FRCS, ChM, PhD, MD(Hon)
Professor of Surgery, University of Leeds,
Consultant Surgeon, Centre for Digestive Diseases,
The General Infirmary at Leeds,
Director Leeds Institute for Minimally Invasive Therapy

Preface to the First Edition

The FRCS has a reputation for being a difficult examination. Sound basic and updated knowledge coupled with good surgical practice and experience are essential in approaching this examination. Flexibility in substantiating your reasoning for choosing one operation rather than another and familiarity with the examination techniques (practised instinctively according to a well-planned methodical approach) are paramount.

The final FRCS is basically designed to test clinical wisdom, judgement, insight and practicality rather than an encyclopaedic knowledge. This book therefore, is not intended to replace or to be a substitute for a surgical reference textbook. It has two aims:

Surgery

Proper orientation of the candidate towards:
- Selective surgical topics (theoretical).
- Commonly presented cases (clinical).
- Popular surgical specimens (pathological).
- Commonly examined instruments, X-rays and bones (principles).
- Commonly discussed surgical procedures (operative).

Practical examples, succinct comments, reviews and discussion with the pros and cons of each approach are included (these aspects are common to all Colleges in the United Kingdom and Ireland). We present a well-balanced selection of material, with detailed discussion only when deemed essential.

Background

Familiarisation of candidates with the type of conduct, skills, techniques and approaches that have proved highly successful in the Colleges' examinations (stemming from our own experience as a candidate and an examiner). Historical background is also provided.

While we are aware of the increasing complexities of surgical approaches (e.g. there are six approaches to femoral hernia repair and many approaches to breast carcinoma management) we stress the importance of one approach (especially the one commonly used) with its substantiation. In the written part you can write about various approaches freely within the limits of the question asked but in the clinical part when you are face to face with the examiner you are very limited in your answer. You therefore have to talk from the most common to the rare and from the general to the specific and to adopt your personal surgical approach to a problem (one operation). Your presentation of the case history, methodical examination and personality all play a definite role in passing the FRCS.

This book is intended to serve not only as an essential theoretical and clinical review but also as a practical guide to the various examination parts in the Colleges. We believe that our combined effort, as an examiner (M.P. McBrien) and as a candidate and organiser of the clinical part of the final FRCS Edinburgh (M. Al-Fallouji) has enabled us to produce a comprehensive and unique guide.

In order to make the volume as compact as possible and to avoid distracting the reader from essential points, we have kept textual references to a minimum. Where important relevant statistics (e.g. 5 year survival rates in treated cancer cases) have been included in studies referred to, the source for these can be found in the appropriate section of the References and Further Reading. Where names and dates are mentioned (e.g. Cuschieri, 1984), these are not usually listed individually in the References and Further Reading, but can be found in one of the main sources listed in the appropriate section.

The book is written primarily for doctors preparing for their final FRCS. However, since the FRCS is historically reputed to be the first examination for surgical qualification and is therefore the prototype for most subsequent examinations, it should also be of benefit to all surgeons sitting similar high postgraduate surgical diplomas such as the Australasian, Canadian and South African Fellowships as well as the American and Arab Boards in Surgery. We feel that there is a great need for such a book not only because it will provide a pan British-Irish comprehensive course condensed in one volume but also because all written books in this field (however excellent they are) represent only one fraction of the final FRCS (written part only) which is probably suitable to one College but not another.

We also believe that examples and illustrated discussions, together with our evaluation of the 'causes of failure' and comments on 'what to read' and 'what to do', based on our experience and the experience of our colleagues, are more important than mere listing or enumeration of topics.

It is common sense, selective reading, proper orientation and clinical approaches together with the digestion and crystallisation of essential facts that really prove to be the safe ship in the sea of examination bewilderment in which the drowning rate is 80%.

M.A.R. Al-Fallouji
M.P. McBrien
London, 1986

Preface to the Second Edition

The success of this book, both in the UK and abroad, testifies that the book fulfils a need; the first edition was reprinted 6 times. The book was listed among the bestselling surgery titles by many publishing agencies (including the Medicine International group) and was widely read throughout the world. In the words of two surgeons (both now consultants) who read *Postgraduate Surgery* during their training:

> *. . . this book is a descrambler or decoder of the complex field of surgery and surgical examinations*

and

> [it] *is a demystifier of the difficult field of surgery often shrouded by a thick veil of mystery.*

I was contacted by candidates and examiners alike, all of whom expressed their satisfaction about the content and demanded an urgent expansion of the book in order to include the latest advances in surgery and to conform with the new regulations of the FRCS. Candidates have used the book as a main revision guide and as a preferred concise mini-textbook of reference in surgery, and I am overwhelmed by their positive feedback wherever I go.

The past decade has witnessed the explosive era of minimal access surgery and laparoscopy (key-hole surgery); restorative proctocolectomy and pouch surgery; the launch of surgical audit and the CEPOD national audit; the continuous challenge of AIDS to clinicians and its implications in surgery; the use of monoclonal antibodies in surgical diagnosis and treatment; and the increasing use of lasers in surgical practice. Advances have also been made in tumour immunobiology and oncogenesis (particularly the genetic aetiology of cancer). Care of critically ill patients has improved; nosocomial infections have reduced; and multi-system organ failure due to trauma and/or sepsis has decreased with better understanding of pathogenesis and aetiology. I have also included a section on military surgery in conventional warfare and mass destruction.

This book aims to reflect state-of-the-art medical education. The do-it-yourself system of postgraduate education is being replaced by well-taught courses of instruction and training; surgery now is not merely a matter of the skilful manual dexterity of surgeons performing major operations via long incisions, it is about the intellectual exercise of decision-making, patient selection through the identification of high-risk groups of patients (assessing and, if possible, correcting such risk prior to surgery), and about continuing medical education (CME), radiology tutorials, self-criticism and objective criticism (audits) to ensure the highest health care in surgery. Patients' expectations of excellent results and the psychological implications of surgery have influenced and changed our surgical practice immensely.

I have reviewed and updated the whole book, striving for perfection. I have contacted world colleges and boards in surgery for details of latest regulations and conduct of postgraduate examinations in surgery and included them in the book. I have collected sources and arduously collated the various subjects into one volume *only* to meet the highest expectations of both candidates and examiners, and to ensure the text maintains a standard that will carry it into the twenty-first century, before a third edition can be commenced.

Candidates are also advised to use the companion volume *Clinical Radiology in Postgraduate Surgery* by the author for self-assessment in the clinical and radiological challenges of the management of surgical disease.

M.A.R. Al-Fallouji
London, 1997

Acknowledgements

I wish to thank the Presidents of the Royal Colleges of Surgeons of England, Edinburgh, Glasgow, Ireland, Australasia and Canada, the College of Medicine of South Africa and the Arab Board for Medical Specialties (Damascus) for their kind cooperation in providing the historical data of their institutions and details of the conduct of their examination of surgery.

I am especially grateful to the Presidents of the Royal Colleges of Surgeons of England, Edinburgh and Glasgow for their kind permission to publish samples of written examination papers. I acknowledge the technical skill and expertise of the Medical Illustration Department of Ipswich Hospital (East Anglia) and Bridge of Earn Hospital (Tayside, Scotland).

I would like to thank all those who helped me with producing this book, whether candidates or consultants, and in particular Dr K. Sikora, PhD, MRCP, FRCR (Professor of Oncology, Royal Postgraduate Medical School, Hammersmith Hospital, London) for reviewing the chapters on oncology; Dr C. Swan (Consultant Physician, Stoke-on-Trent), from the British Society of Gastroenterology, for providing information for the chapter on endoscopy; Mr T.G. Brennan, FRCS (Consultant Surgeon, St James's Hospital, Leeds), for help in teaching me the minimal access therapy; Dr I.F. El Ramli, MSc, PhD (Consultant in Laser Applications) for help with the chapter on the use of lasers in surgery; Mr Sankaran-Kutty, FRCS (Associate Professor in Orthopaedic Surgery, UAE University, Al Ain, United Arab Emirates) for help with the chapter on low back pain.

I would also like to thank Miss E.A. Campling, BA, DipHSM for kind permission to publish relevant data from the report of the National Confidential Enquiry into Perioperative Deaths, 1990, and the General Medical Council for allowing reproduction of their document 'Tomorrow's Doctors' and their statement on ethical considerations in HIV and AIDS.

I am indebted to Susan Devlin (Senior Medical Editor at Butterworth–Heinemann) for her continued diligence and intelligent assistance during the preparation of this updated second edition. To the very many candidates who have updated me with pertinent topics over the years I offer my thanks, and my appreciation for their patience during the preparation of this long-awaited second edition. I am aware I have left unnamed a great number of people who directly or indirectly have contributed to the completion of this edition; to them all, I return my grateful thanks.

PART ONE

Surgical Training

The Shape of Surgical Training and Accreditation in General Surgery and its Sub-specialties

1 Legal Aspects

The European Specialist Medical Qualification Order of December 1995 No. 3208 (issued by the British Government and entitled 'Medical Profession', which came into force on 12 January 1996) makes new provision about training for specialist medical professionals, and the recognition in the UK of specialist medical qualifications awarded elsewhere. The Order implements European obligations relating to the training of specialist doctors and mutual recognition of their diplomas to facilitate the free movement of doctors of the European Economic Area (EEA) in line with the Protocol signed at Brussels in March 1993.

It states that the **Specialist Training Authority of the Medical Royal Colleges (STA)** is designated for purposes relating to training for those qualifications in the UK; it issues the Certificate of Completion of Specialist Training (CCST) to those who complete approved specialist training (and makes recommendations to the GMC that a doctor's name be added to the new Specialist Register), and provides also for the conditions which training must satisfy before it can be approved for this purpose. The STA is therefore empowered by the European Specialist Medical Order 1995 to be legally responsible for safeguarding the standards of postgraduate training in hospital practice in the UK and for ensuring that the training requirement stipulated in the European Council Directive 93/16/EEC are adhered to. The STA must also set up an appeal mechanism against its decision to refuse an award of CCST, and provides for removal and suspension from the specialist register. The order also states that the **General Medical Council (GMC)** is the supervisory body for the medical profession designated for registration and recognition of specialist medical qualifications. The GMC has to establish and publish a register of specialists, including not only those who have been awarded a CCST, but also European doctors with specialist qualifications awarded elsewhere in the EEA whose qualifications are entitled to automatic recognition, and doctors with qualifications from other countries which will be assessed by the STA before being recognised.

From 1 January 1997 entry in the **GMC Specialist Register** is a prerequisite for appointment as a consultant in the National Health Service. Doctors who are already consultants or accredited in such a specialty or have satisfied the STA (with UK training and qualifications awarded in the UK equivalent to CCST in that specialty) can be included in the specialist register provided they apply before 1 January 1998 (or in some circumstances, later).

There are therefore several ways in which doctors can be entered on to the Specialist Register. They can be included if they are:

- holders of CCST (holding only the old style CST would not allow a doctor's name to be included in the Specialist Register);
- holders of European Economic Area specialist certificates recognised under the EC Medical Directive 93/16/EEC;
- overseas trained specialists whose training is assessed by the STA as equivalent to CCST standards;
- those engaged in academic and research medicine but have not followed a traditional training pathway, provided their expertise is assessed by the STA as equivalent to CCST standards.

In making these CCST awards and recommendations, the STA will have received the advice of the relevant Royal College or Faculty, who will in turn have been advised by the appropriate Higher Training Committee.

2 Surgical Training for UK, European and Overseas Doctors

UK AND EUROPEAN DOCTORS

For a surgical trainee whose training is undertaken entirely in the UK (or in the European Union or EEA) and after completion of the pre-registration House Officer year, the candidate must spend an obligatory minimum of 2–3 years as a Senior House Officer in Basic Surgical Training (**BST**). After such a period he or she must pass the **MRCS** Examination (Member of the Royal College of Surgeons of England or Glasgow) or **AFRCS** Examination (Associate Fellow of the Royal College of Surgeons of Edinburgh or Ireland) in core surgery (clinical surgery in general), and applied basic sciences (including systematic surgery).

The candidate then has to enter Specialist Higher Surgical Training (**HST**). The current HST has been reshaped to be in line with European HST to provide a compact, planned, shorter and a more structured training programme with a well-defined career framework prior to an independent surgical practice. The new scheme of training has been introduced by Chief Medical Officer Sir Kenneth Calman and is popularly referred to as 'Calmanisation'.

The current HST aims to fulfil the following objectives:

- To provide a comprehensive and structured training programme in general surgery and its sub-specialties for those who have completed Basic Surgical Training.
- To enable trainees to reach standards of quality and, having passed the Intercollegiate Examination, to be awarded a Certificate of Completion of Specialist Training

(CCST) and enter independent practice in general surgery with one or two of its sub-specialties.

The great advantage of 'Calman' training is that trainees will be recruited at an early stage (within 2–3 years of qualifying) and will have a planned progressive programme.

Following BST (leading to the award of MRCS/AFRCS), the candidate has to apply for a **Specialist Registrar** post, to be enlisted for HST rotation with a National Training Number (NTN) for 6 years depending on the surgical specialty (minimum of 5 clinical years plus 1 flexible year for research or specialist training in one or two sub-specialties). Those wishing to undertake a longer period of research for degree by thesis will be encouraged to do so but only with approval of the Specialist Advisory Committee. The 5 clinical years may be extended to 6 or 7 years by the postgraduate dean in special circumstances.

At the end of fourth year of HST, the candidate must sit and pass the **Intercollegiate Examination** (regulations of which can be obtained from the Intercollegiate Board in General Surgery, see below); successful candidates will then be awarded the Full Fellowship of the Royal College of Surgeons in a specialty, e.g. FRCS England (General Surgery) or FRCSEd (Urology), as an exit degree to an independent practice. The candidate will then be allowed to finish the last 1–2 years of HST, at the conclusion of which, and on the recommendation of the appropriate College, the trainee will be awarded, by the STA, the **Certificate of Completion of Specialist Training** (CCST).

Award of the CCST will entitle the candidate to be enlisted in the GMC Specialist Register (usually within the last 3 months of HST); then and only then he or she may apply for an appointment as a **substantive NHS Consultant Surgeon in the United Kingdom** with specialist interest in one or occasionally two sub-specialties (see Figs. 1 and 2A).

Calmanised training has many loopholes:
– the SHO may not pass MRCS/AFRCS in time;
– delayed enlisting into SpR scheme due to bottle-neck competition or even stagnation at SHO level due to saturation of SpR training programme (the so-called **proximal shift effect of calmanisation**);
– absence of a traditional research period leading the surgeon to become a professional as well as a scientist (2 years in the old scheme taken prior to senior registrar rotation leading to a higher degree by thesis such as MS, MD, or occasionally a PhD with research expansion more than 2 years);
– inability of SpR to clear the intercollegiate examination in time with delay in completion of higher surgical training and CCST award; and
– possible delay in securing Calman Specialist posts due to limited slots and increased demands.

Professor I. Taylor *et al.* (Supplement to Annals of The Royal College of Surgeons of England 1997; **79**: 73–8) considered research activity in danger of being 'squeezed' out of Calmanised surgical training, and in view of the difficulties

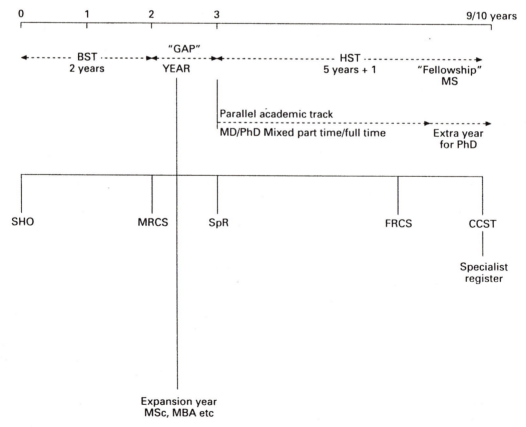

Fig. 1.   Incorporation of academic activity in a Surgical Training Programme (from a letter by Professor I. Taylor *et al.* in Supplement to the Annals of the RCS England 1997, **79**, 73–8)

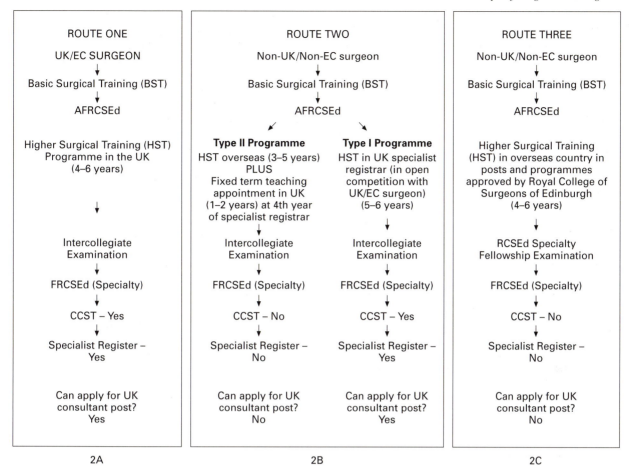

ROUTE ONE	ROUTE TWO		ROUTE THREE
UK/EC SURGEON	Non-UK/Non-EC surgeon		Non-UK/Non-EC surgeon
↓	↓		↓
Basic Surgical Training (BST)	Basic Surgical Training (BST)		Basic Surgical Training (BST)
↓	↓		↓
AFRCSEd	AFRCSEd		AFRCSEd
	↙	↘	
	Type II Programme	**Type I Programme**	
Higher Surgical Training (HST) Programme in the UK (4–6 years)	HST overseas (3–5 years) PLUS Fixed term teaching appointment in UK (1–2 years) at 4th year of specialist registrar	HST in UK specialist registrar (in open competition with UK/EC surgeon) (5–6 years)	Higher Surgical Training (HST) in overseas country in posts and programmes approved by Royal College of Surgeons of Edinburgh (4–6 years)
↓	↓	↓	↓
Intercollegiate Examination	Intercollegiate Examination	Intercollegiate Examination	RCSEd Specialty Fellowship Examination
↓	↓	↓	↓
FRCSEd (Specialty)	FRCSEd (Specialty)	FRCSEd (Specialty)	FRCSEd (Specialty)
↓	↓	↓	↓
CCST – Yes	CCST – No	CCST – Yes	CCST – No
↓	↓	↓	↓
Specialist Register – Yes	Specialist Register – No	Specialist Register – Yes	Specialist Register – No
Can apply for UK consultant post? Yes	Can apply for UK consultant post? No	Can apply for UK consultant post? Yes	Can apply for UK consultant post? No
2A	2B		2C

Fig. 2. Various routes of surgical training for UK/EC (EEA) surgeons and overseas surgeons (from Professor R. Shields, President's letter RCSEd Newsletter July 1996)

facing basic surgical trainees to enter higher surgical training scheme, he proposed that the SHO should pursue a period of research activity in a **'gap' year between BST and HST** (Fig. 1). Add to this, one flexible year of research at HST scheme leading to a thesis and research degree such as an MSc in Surgical Sciences. The 'gap' year, should it occur, may be viewed as an expansion research year to acquire e.g., an MD, an MBA in business management, qualifications in ethics, law or computing that may enrich the practice of surgery. If an additional 3rd research year is taken after obtaining intercollegiate examination and prior to the award of CCST it can be devoted for completion of a PhD degree or utilised in clinical 'Fellowship' abroad. A long term academic career as NHS consultant or as a Professor must also be re-emphasised for individuals recognised at an early stage of HST and must be encouraged to enable a higher degree by thesis (MD, MS, PhD) to be achieved during surgical training.

Specialisation: a surgeon is a specialist after
– training programme including surgical principles, steep learning curve, and prolonged practical maturation.
– declared interest
– future performance within that declared specialty

Specialisation recognition demands minimum requirements in terms of:
– minimum cases operated on by a trainee (Endocrine Surgery).
– minimum unit requirement of cases per year (Breast Surgery).
– both of the above (Vascular Surgery).
It is assumed that 'more is better' and that large series are the work of experts, but:
– How many cases are needed to become an expert?
– What about quality of experience?
– What about new operations?
– What about non-operative factors?
The obligatory volume must consider in coloproctology, for instance, cancer cases as well as inflammatory bowel diseases and anorectal diseases. Subspecialty training may also include a mandatory maximum of two specialties; a colomastologist may have to deal with large bowel cancers in addition to the breast unit load. Specialisation while concentrating on surgical training, should not ignore the following important facets of surgery:
– diagnosis
– staging

– perioperative care
– intensive care
– multi-modality treatment
– inter-disciplinary approach
– rehabilitation
– follow-up
– documentation
– research

Furthermore, specialisation may result in many problems, such as:

– de-skilling in other aspects of surgery
– boredom due to specialisation in a limited field (tunnel vision)
– undergraduate teaching may be affected
– emergency rota has to be arranged accordingly
– consultant number has to be increased with increased specialisation (e.g. coloproctologists, vascular surgeons, upper GI/HPB surgeons, surgical oncologists).

OVERSEAS DOCTORS

The NHS Executive on behalf of the Department of Health produced in 1996 *A guide to Specialist Registrar Training*, which defines overseas doctors as doctors who are not nationals of the European Economic Area (EEA) or who do not hold a primary qualification obtained in the EEA. They may either have a right of indefinite residence or settled status in the UK (as determined by immigration and nationality law, or benefit from European Union right), then such doctors may apply for Specialist Registrar posts in open competition with UK and EEA candidates; or these overseas doctors may have no right of indefinite residence and they will qualify for Visiting Specialist Registrar (VSpR) posts.

The annual report of The Royal College of Surgeons of Edinburgh for 1995/1996 revealed that the RCSEd had organised examinations in eight countries overseas. The total number of candidates examined was 4155 in that one year, and out of this number the candidates attending 'Clinical Surgery in General' examinations was 3101 (75% of total candidates). When the geographical area of origin was plotted it was apparent that only 19% of such candidates originated from the UK and only 6% from Europe, making a total of 25% from the UK and EEA, while 75% *of all candidates were from overseas*. Out of those overseas candidates, 35% originated from the Indian Sub-Continent, 16% from the Middle East, 16% from the Far East, 5% from Africa and 3% from the rest of the world.

Professor R. Shields, the President of the Royal College of Surgeons of Edinburgh, in the RCSEd newsletters No. 45/April 1996 and No. 46/July 1996, has led the way in highlighting various routes available for overseas surgical training in the UK (see Fig. 1).

The standards for overseas and UK trainees must not be different. Measures are needed to achieve such parity and to ensure that overseas doctors wishing a training in surgery – either in the UK or overseas – can take the examinations of the College, aspire to the full Fellowship and begin a lifetime association with the College.

Overseas equivalence to UK basic surgical training (AFRCS/MRCS) may be granted on the basis of acquisition of the MS or M Med (surgery) diploma after 3 years of overseas basic surgical training. The overseas doctor can then fulfil the requirements to sit for AFRCS/MRCS without the need to go through the United Kingdom BST.

Thereafter, there are three possibilities for higher surgical training of overseas doctors in the UK.

1. The overseas doctor may wish to enter a complete higher surgical training programme in the UK (**Type I programme**, see Fig. 2B.). The trainee has to apply in competition with the United Kingdom applicants for Specialist Registrar posts for 5 years. If the overseas doctor has a right of indefinite residence then such a doctor is qualified for a Specialist Registrar grade and a National Training Number (NTN) will be awarded (if successfully appointed), but if the overseas doctor has no right of indefinite residence then a Visiting National Training Number (VNTN) will be awarded. However, should a Visiting Specialist Registrar (VSpR), embarked on a Type I training programme leading to a CCST acquire an indefinite right of residence while in training, then he/she would become a Specialist Registrar and the 'V' suffix would be dropped. However, this change would not apply to those VSpRs on fixed-term training appointments (**Type II programme**, see below) whose immigration status altered in a similar way.

At the end of the fourth year the trainee can sit intercollegiate examination and complete training at the end of the fifth year; the trainee may be eligible to be awarded the Certificate of Completion of Specialist Training (CCST) and may be enrolled in the Specialist Register of the General Medical Council if he or she wishes to pursue this course. Whether they are able to stay in this country will, of course, depend upon Home Office regulations.

2. The trainee may wish to enter a higher surgical training programme in his or her own country for 3 years and to come to the UK on the fourth year of training in an approved post for a **Fixed-Term Training Appointment (FTTA)** (the so-called **Type II programme**, see Fig. 2B) as a Visiting Specialist Registrar (VSpR) for 1–2 years, following an agreement with one of the Royal Colleges. Such a trainee will be awarded a VNTN irrespective of his/her immigration status on the right of indefinite residence; short-term locum appointments do not attract a NTN or a VNTN.

The trainee can sit the intercollegiate examination and, if successful, receive the full Fellowship of one of the four Royal Colleges in a specialty. However, they will not be awarded a CCST, nor can they be admitted to the Specialist Register held by the GMC, so that they will not, on this basis, be able to apply for consultant posts within the UK. This course requires a programme of training in hospital posts mutually approved in the UK and abroad.

3. The trainee may wish to receive the entire higher surgical training programme in his or her own country (see Fig. 2C). Measures are needed to ensure parity with the UK training, and mutual hospital posts approval in the UK and abroad. After 4 years' training, the College would hold examinations in the host country, which would be identical in format and standards to the inter-collegiate examinations in the UK. The examining team would be drawn jointly, with at least 50% of the examiners being UK-based Fellows; all internal examiners from the host country or the UK will be Fellows of

the Royal College of Surgeons of Edinburgh (for instance). External examiners will be invited from other Colleges in the UK and from the American and Royal Australasian Colleges of Surgeons. At the completion of higher surgical training, the successful candidate would be awarded in this example the full FRCSEd in the specialty, and where applicable, the equivalent diploma of the trainee's own country. They will not be eligible for the award of a CCST, nor can they gain entry to the Specialist Register of the GMC, so that they will not, on this basis, be able to apply for consultant posts within the UK. The arrangements would obviously have to vary from one country to another because each country has different systems. Considerable flexibility would be required to set joint programmes for higher training and examinations.

The Colleges are also very much aware that there will be many doctors with overseas diplomas and/or overseas training who, while not eligible for the award of the CCST, will on the basis of training which they have received and their clinical experience in the UK, seek entry into the Specialist Register in order that they may apply for consultant posts in the UK. Considerable work will have to be undertaken by the Specialist Training Authority, and its constituent Colleges, to determine equivalence of training and standards.

There will be no specific quota for VSpRs for the grade or for individual specialties within the grade; instead it will be for each postgraduate dean to determine how many VSpRs may be accommodated within training programmes (including those appointed to fixed-term training appointments).

All overseas doctors are strongly advised to enlist in an approved programme in the UK; Colleges deprecate strongly overseas trainees arriving in the UK and spending several years working in posts which are not approved for training and indeed returning home without receiving a formal recognised training. Postgraduate deans are responsible for advising the Home Office on matters relating to the immigration status of doctors pursuing postgraduate training and in so doing will ordinarily consult the relevant College regional adviser. Inevitably the circumstances of individual overseas doctors may vary significantly.

It is therefore strongly recommended that all overseas doctors seek advice from the postgraduate dean in whose area they wish to train before applying for a placement in the grade and advise the dean of their intended training goal and the period of permit-free training that is available to them. Before the postgraduate dean confirms any placement for a sponsored overseas doctor, the sponsor or representative should contact the postgraduate dean.

3 MRCS/AFRCS Diploma

This award has been introduced to signify the successful completion of Basic Surgical Training. This replaces the two-part FRCS (Applied Basic Science and Clinical Surgery in General), and the FRCS will in future be awarded to signify the successful completion of the Intercollegiate Specialty Examination as an exit examination from HST into independent surgical practice.

The new MRCS Regulations for BST examinations came into effect from 1 August 1996 and apply to all those who started training on or after that date in surgical posts approved for entry to the examination.

In the transitional period, however, trainees who started training before 1 August 1996 and who do not opt to be trained and examined under the MRCS Regulations must comply with the current FRCS Regulations amended as follows by Council on 13 July 1995.

1. The Applied Basic Sciences (ABS) examination, the current Clinical Surgery in General (CSiG) examination and the opportunity to sit both parts of these examinations together will cease completely after MRCS examination held in January 1998.

2. Surgeons in training before 1 August 1996, but who have not passed ABS, must enter the new MRCS Diploma Examination.

3. After January 1998 trainees who have passed ABS will be required to sit a modified CSiG examination consisting of:
- a written paper on clinical topics;
- a clinical examination (short cases)
- 4 × 15 minutes viva voce examinations conducted in the college within 2 months of the clinical examination.

4. Trainees who have not passed CSiG by the time it ceases after the examination in October 2000 will not be allowed to enter the new MRCS examination.

The Colleges strongly advise those in training after February 1996 to enter under the new MRCS Regulations (obtained by writing to any of the four Royal Colleges of the UK and Ireland).

The candidate must spend an obligatory minimum of 2–3 years as a Senior House Officer in Basic Surgical Training, which includes:
- 6 months general surgery with general emergency work;
- 6 months orthopaedics with general musculoskeletal trauma;
- 2 × 6 months in other surgical specialties, e.g. accident/emergency medicine (casualties), urology, neurosurgery, cardiothoracic surgery, plastic surgery, paediatric surgery.

After such a period he or she must pass the MRCS Examination (Member of Royal College of Surgeons of England or Glasgow) or AFRCS Examination (Associate Fellow of Royal College of Surgeons of Edinburgh or Ireland). The MRCS/AFRCS Syllabus is based on Principles of Surgery in General (five core modules) and Systematic Surgery (five system modules) (see below). The new style programme includes a greater degree of continuous assessment than the previous system. However, the four Royal Colleges have retained their individuality in the structure of the examination.

The Examination consists of:
- MCQ section (after completion of 8 months' mandatory training).
- Clinical section (after completion of 20 months' mandatory training and a 'pass' in the MCQ section).
- *Viva voce* section (after completion of 22 months' mandatory training with a certificate of satisfactory training from a college tutor or consultant trainer with completion of the Basic Surgical Skills course, a 'pass' in the MCQ section and a 'pass' in Clinical section).

MRCS regulations can be obtained by writing to:

The Examinations Department
The Royal College of Surgeons of England
35–43 Lincoln's Inn Fields
London WC2A 3PN
Tel: 0171 405 3474   Fax: 0171 973 2179

Alternatively, **AFRCS** regulations can be obtained by writing to:

The Examinations Department
The Royal College of Surgeons of Edinburgh
Nicolson Street
Edinburgh EH8 9DW
Tel: 0131 556 6206   Fax: 0131 557 6406

The MRCS/AFRCS regulations and syllabus are detailed below. © Copyright of The Royal College of Surgeons of England. Reproduced with kind permission:

Educational approval

Posts recognised by council

Council has approved the following training posts.

England and Wales

(a) Posts that have been inspected by the Hospital Recognition Committee and approved by Council.
(b) Posts in Gynaecology (but not those combined with Obstetrics) recognised by the Royal College of Obstetricians and Gynaecologists for the MRCOG Diploma.
(c) Posts in Intensive Therapy recognised by the Royal Colleges of Physicians in the British Isles or by the Royal College of Anaesthetists.
(d) Full-time supernumerary (unpaid) appointments at hospitals in the UK with recognised posts if it is certified that the duties are identical to those of a full-time paid recognised post, and are completed under Full or Limited Registration.
(e) Posts in Oral and Maxillofacial Surgery recognised under MRCS regulations by the Faculty of Dental Surgery (which may be undertaken after dental but before medical qualification).

Other countries

(a) Posts in hospitals within their own country and elsewhere in the World inspected and approved by:
   the surgical Royal Colleges of England, Edinburgh and Ireland;
   the Royal Australasian College of Surgeons;
   the College of Medicine of South Africa;
   the Royal College of Physicians and Surgeons of Canada;
   the Royal College of Physicians and Surgeons of Glasgow.
(b) Residency appointments approved by the American Board of Surgery.

Posts not formally recognised by council

Council will consider accepting, as part of the two years of mandatory training, up to 12 months of training in non-recognised overseas posts if the candidate complies with the following provisions.

1. The candidate must have completed 12 months in recognised posts in the British Isles.
2. The overseas training for consideration must have been completed at Senior House Officer level and the quality of training must be verified by the production of authenticated trainee-assessment forms and log book or, when this is not possible, of signed statements by the trainee's Consultant trainers.
3. The request must be supported by a Consultant in the British Isles for applicants who already hold a post in the British Isles.
4. The request for such an assessment must be submitted to the Head of Examinations at least three months before the closing date for examination entries.

Syllabus

The UK Surgical Colleges and the Irish Surgical College have reached agreement in two documents entitled *'Outline Proposals for the Reform of Basic Surgical Training and Examinations* (July 1995)' and *'Integrated Syllabus for Basic Surgical Training* (May 1995)'. These are both available from the External Affairs Department.

The first document describes agreement on the nature of the syllabus.

There will be a common syllabus for the basic surgical training examinations of the four Colleges in which the basic sciences are integrated with clinical surgery-in-general. Each College may alter the presentation, but not the content, of this syllabus to correspond to the format of its own courses and examinations.

The second document describes agreement on how the syllabus will be delivered.

The Colleges will encourage the provision of education for basic surgical trainees through distance-learning courses and short courses in basic surgical skills and basic patient management skills.

The Royal College of Surgeons of England recommends, pursuant to these agreements, that trainees should follow its MRCS distance-learning course in parallel with the training posts. This 20-month course comprises five 10-week core modules and five 6-week systems modules and the content of the common syllabus detailed in the second document above has, accordingly, been presented in modular form. The scheduling of these modules is described in the context of the timetable for the MRCS examination.

Principles of Surgery-in-General

Core Module 1: perioperative management 1

(1) Preoperative management

● Assessment of fitness for anaesthesia and surgery.
● Tests of respiratory, cardiac and renal function.
● Management of associated medical conditions
   e.g. diabetes; respiratory disease; cardiovascular disease; psychiatric disorders; malnutrition; anaemia; steroid, anticoagulant, immunosuppressant and other drug therapy.

(2) Infection

- Pathophysiology of the body's response to infection.
- The sources of surgical infection – prevention and control.
- Surgically important micro-organisms.
- Principles of asepsis and antisepsis.
- Surgical sepsis and its prevention.
- Aseptic techniques.
- Skin preparation.
- Antibiotic prophylaxis.
- Sterilisation.

(3) Investigative and operative procedures

- Excision of cysts and benign tumours of skin and subcutaneous tissue.
- Principles of techniques of biopsy.
- Suture and ligature materials.
- Drainage of superficial abscesses.
- Basic principles of anastomosis.

(4) Anaesthesia

- Principles of anaesthesia.
- Premedication and sedation.
- Local and regional anaesthesia.
- Care and monitoring of the anaesthetised patient.

(5) Theatre problems

- Surgical technique and technology.
- Diathermy. Principles and precautions.
- Lasers. Principles and precautions.
- Explosion hazards relating to general anaesthesia and endoscopic surgery.
- Tourniquests. Uses and precautions.
- Prevention of nerve and other injuries in the anaesthetised patient. Surgery in hepatitis and HIV carriers (special precautions). Disorders of coagulation and haemostasis (prophylaxis of thromboembolic disease).

Core Module 2: perioperative management 2

(1) Skin and wounds

- Pathophysiology of wound healing.
- Classification of surgical wounds.
- Principles of wound management.
- Incisions and their closure.
- Suture and ligature materials.
- Scars and contracture.
- Wound dehiscence.
- Dressings.

(2) Fluid balance

- Assessment and maintenance of fluid and electrolyte balance.
- Techniques of venous access.
- Nutritional support. Indications, techniques, total parenteral nutrition.

(3) Blood

- Disorders of coagulation and haemostasis.
- Blood transfusion. Indications, hazards, complications, plasma substitutes.
- Haemolytic disorders of surgical importance.
- Haemorrhagic disorders; disorders of coagulation.

(4) Postoperative complications

- Postoperative complications – prevention, monitoring, recognition, management.
- Ventilatory Support – indications.

(5) Postoperative sequelae

- Pain control.
- Immune response to trauma, infections and tissue transplantation.
- Pathophysiology of the body's response to trauma.
- Surgery in the immunocompromised patient.

Core module 3: Trauma

(1) Initial assessment and resuscitation after trauma

- Clinical assessment of the injured patient.
- Maintenance of airway and ventilation.
- Haemorrhage and shock.

(2) Chest, abdomen and pelvis

- Cardiorespiratory physiology as applied to trauma.
- Penetrating chest injuries and pneumothorax.
- Rib fractures and flail chest.
- Abdominal and pelvic injuries.

(3) Central nervous system trauma

- Central nervous system: anatomy and physiology relevant to clinical examination of the central nervous system, the understanding of its functional disorders particularly those caused by cranial or spinal trauma and the interpretation of special investigations.
- Intracranial haemorrhage.
- Head injuries, general principles of management.
- Surgical aspects of meningitis.
- Spinal cord injury and compression.
- Paraplegia and quadriplegia. Principles of management.

(4) Special problems

- Pre-hospital care.
- Triage.
- Trauma scoring systems.
- Traumatic wounds – principles of management.
- Gunshot and blast wounds.
- Skin loss – grafts and flaps.
- Burns.
- Facial and orbital injuries.

(5) *Principles of limb injury*

- Peripheral nervous system: anatomy and physiology.
- Fractures – pathophysiology of fracture healing.
- Non-union, delayed union, complications.
- Principles of bone grafting.
- Traumatic oedema, compartment and crush syndrome, fat embolism.
- Brachial plexus injury.

Core module 4: intensive care

(1) *Cardiovascular*

- The surgical anatomy and applied physiology of the heart relevant to clinical cases.
- Physiology and pharmacological control of: cardiac output, blood flow, blood pressure, coronary circulation.
- Cardiac arrest, resuscitation.
- Monitoring of cardiac function in the critically ill patient, coma, central venous pressure, pulmonary wedge pressure, tamponade, cardiac O/P measurements.
- The interpretation of special investigations.
- The management of haemorrhage and shock.
- Pulmonary oedema.
- Cardiopulmonary bypass; general principles, cardiac support.

(2) *Respiratory*

- The surgical anatomy of the airways, chest wall, diaphragm and thoracic viscera.
- The mechanics and control of respiration.
- The interpretation of special investigations; lung function tests, arterial blood gases, radiology.
- The understanding of disorders of respiratory function caused by trauma, acute surgical illness and surgical intervention.
- Respiratory failure.
- Complications of thoracic operations.
- Adult respiratory distress syndrome.
- Endotracheal intubation, laryngotomy, tracheostomy.
- Artificial ventilation.

(3) *Multi-system failure*

- Multi-system failure.
- Renal failure: diagnosis of renal failure, complications of renal failure.
- GI tract, hepatic.
- Nutrition.

(4) *Problems in intensive care*

- Sepsis, predisposing factors, organisms causing septicaemia.
- Complications of thoracic operations.
- Localised sepsis, pneumonia, lung abscess, bronchiectasis, empyema, mediastinitis.

(5) *Principles of ICU*

- Indications for admission.
- Organisation and staffing.
- Scoring.
- Costs.

Core module 5: neoplasia – techniques and outcome of surgery

(1) *Principles of oncology*

- Epidemiology of common neoplasms and tumour-like conditions; role of cancer registries.
- Clinicopathological staging of cancer.
- Pathology; clinical features, diagnosis and principles of management of common cancers in each of the surgical specialties.
- Principles of cancer treatment by surgery; radiotherapy; chemotherapy; immunotherapy and hormone therapy.
- The principles of carcinogenesis and the pathogenesis of cancer relevant to the clinical features, special investigations, staging and the principles of treatment of the common cancers.
- Principles of molecular biology of cancer, carcinogenesis; genetic factors; mechanisms of metastasis.

(2) *Cancer screening and treatment*

- The surgical anatomy and applied physiology of the breast relevant to clinical examinations, the interpretation of special investigations, the understanding of disordered function and the principles of the surgical treatment of common disorders of the breast.
- The breast – acute infections; benign breast disorders; nipple discharge; mastalgia.
- Carcinoma of the breast; mammography; investigation and treatment.
- Screening programmes.

(3) *Techniques of management*

- Terminal care of cancer patients; pain relief.
- Rehabilitation.
- Psychological effects of surgery and bereavement.

(4) *Ethics and the law*

- Medical/legal ethics and medico-legal aspects of surgery.
- Communication with patients, relatives and colleagues.

(5) *Outcome of surgery*

- The evaluation of surgery and general topics.
- Decision-making in surgery.
- Clinical audit.
- Statistics and computing in surgery.
- Principles of research and design and analysis of clinical trials.
- Critical evaluation of innovations – technical and pharmaceutical.
- Health service management and economic aspects of surgical care.

Systematic Surgery

System module A: locomotor system

Musculoskeletal anatomy and physiology relevant to clinical examination of the locomotor system and to the understanding of disordered locomotor function, with emphasis on the effects of acute musculoskeletal trauma.

(1) Effects of trauma and lower limb

- Effects of acute musculoskeletal trauma.
- Common fractures and joint injuries.
- Degenerative and rheumatoid arthritis (including principles of joint replacement).
- Common disorders of the foot.
- Amputations.

(2) Infections and upper limb

- Common soft tissue injuries and disorders.
- Infections of bones and joints (including implants and prostheses).
- Pain in the neck, shoulder and arm.
- Common disorders of the hand, including hand injuries and infections.

(3) Bone disease and spine

- Common disorders of infancy and childhood.
- Low back pain and sciatica.
- Metabolic bone disease (osteoporosis, osteomalacia).
- Surgical aspects of paralytic disorders and nerve injuries.

System module B: vascular

The surgical anatomy and applied physiology of blood vessels relevant to clinical examination, the interpretation of special investigations and the understanding of the role of surgery in the management of cardiovascular disease.

(1) Arterial diseases

- Chronic obliterative arterial disease.
- Amputations.
- Carotid disease.
- Aneurysms.
- Special techniques used in the investigation of vascular disease
- Limb ischaemia – acute and chronic; clinical features; gangrene; amputations for vascular disease.
- Principles of reconstructive arterial surgery.

(2) Venous diseases

- Vascular trauma and peripheral veins.
- Varicose veins.
- Venous hypertension, post-phlebitic leg, venous ulceration.
- Disorders of the veins in the lower limb.
- Deep venous thrombosis and its complications.
- Chronic ulceration of the leg.
- Thrombosis and embolism.

(3) Lymphatics and spleen

- Thromboembolic disease.
- Spleen; splenectomy; hypersplenism.
- Lymph nodes; lymphoedema.
- Surgical aspects of autoimmune disease.
- The anatomy and physiology of the haemopoeitic and lymphoreticular systems.
- Surgical aspects of disordered haemopoiesis.

System module C: head, neck, endocrine and paediatric

The surgical anatomy and applied physiology of the head and neck relevant to clinical examination, the interpretation of special investigations, the understanding of disorders of function, and the treatment of disease and injury involving the head and neck.

(1) The head

- Laryngeal disease, maintenance of airway; tracheostomy.
- Acute and chronic inflammatory disorders of the ear, nose, sinuses and throat.
- Intracranial complications.
- Foreign bodies in ear, nose and throat.
- Epistaxis.
- Salivary gland disease.
- The eye – trauma, common infections.

(2) Neck and endocrine glands

- The surgical anatomy and applied physiology of the endocrine glands relevant to clinical examination, the interpretation of special investigations, the understanding of disordered function and the principles of the surgical treatment of common disorders of the endocrine glands.
- Common neck swellings.
- Thyroid. Role of surgery in diseases of the thyroid; complications of thyroidectomy; the solitary thyroid nodule.
- Parathyroid; hyperparathyroidism; hypercalcaemia.
- Secondary hypertension.

(3) Paediatric disorders

- Neonatal physiology – the special problems of anaesthesia and surgery in the newborn – the principles of neonatal fluid and electrolyte balance.
- Correctable congenital abnormalities.
- Common paediatric surgical disorders – cleft lip and palate; pyloric stenosis; intussusception; hernia; maldescent of testis; torsion; diseases of the foreskin.

System module D: abdomen

The surgical anatomy of the abdomen and its viscera and the applied physiology of the alimentary system relevant to clinical examination, the interpretation of common special investigations, the understanding of disorders of function, and the treatment of abdominal disease and injury.

(1) Abdominal wall

- Anatomy of the groin, groin hernias, acute and elective. Clinical features of hernias, complications of hernias.
- Anterior abdominal wall, anatomy, incisions, laparoscopic access.

(2) Acute abdominal conditions

- Peritonitis; intra-abdominal abscesses.
- Common acute abdominal emergencies.
- Intestinal obstruction; paralytic ileus.
- Intestinal fistulae.
- Investigation of abdominal pain.
- Investigation of abdominal masses.
- Gynaecological causes of acute abdominal pain.
- Pelvic inflammatory disease.
- Abdominal injury.

(3) Elective abdominal conditions

- Common anal and perianal disorders.
- Jaundice – differential diagnosis and management.
- Portal hypertension.
- Gallstones.
- Gastrostomy, ileostomy, colostomy and other stomata.

System module E: urinary system and renal transplantation

The surgical anatomy and applied physiology of the genito-urinary system relevant to clinical examination, special investigations, understanding of disordered function, and the principles of the surgical treatment of genito-urinary disease and injury.

(1) Urinary tract I

- Urinary tract infection.
- Haematuria.
- Trauma to the urinary tract.
- Urinary calculi.

(2) Urinary tract II

- Retention of urine.
- Disorders of prostate.
- Pain and swelling in the scrotum; torsion.

(3) Renal failure and transplantation

- Principles of transplantation.
- Renal failure; dialysis.

---

4 Final FRCS/Intercollegiate Examination

The examination is set by the Intercollegiate Board in General Surgery of the four Royal Colleges of the UK and Ireland.

Regulations and application forms are provided by writing to:

The Secretariat
The Intercollegiate Board in General Surgery
3 Hill Square
Edinburgh EH8 9DR
Scotland
Tel: 0131 662 9222 Fax: 0131 662 9444

The candidate must show an evidence of:

- recognised medical qualification;
- completion of BST with MRCS/AFRCS;
- being a Specialist Registrar (with a Number) who has already been enlisted in an HST rotation for 5–6 years depending on the surgical specialty;
- completion of 3 years (out of the total 5–6 years of HST) in the specialty acceptable to the relevant Board and a record of operative experience throughout this period.

At the end of fourth year of HST, the candidate must sit and pass the Intercollegiate Examination; successful candidate will then be awarded the Full Fellowship of the Royal College of Surgeons in a specialty as an exit degree to an independent practice. The candidate will then be allowed to finish the last 1–2 years of HST at the conclusion of which he or she will be awarded a Certificate of Completion of Specialist Training (CCST) after a successful application to the Specialist Training Authority (STA) under the auspices of the medical Royal Colleges.

The format of the Intercollegiate Examination is based on clinical and oral examinations (see below).

Guide to scope and format of the examination

The format consists of clinical and oral examinations in all aspects of general surgery. This includes the relevant aspects of anatomy, physiology and pathology.

The Examination consists of the following:

1. Clinical examination

This has two sections, namely a Long Case and Short Cases, each section lasting for half an hour. In the Long Case the history will be provided to the candidates and the results of investigations will be available. These form the basis for further discussions regarding the management of the patient.

2. Oral examination

There are three oral examinations, each lasting for half an hour.

(i) *Critical care* This covers the subject of emergency and trauma surgery and the management of the critically ill; relevant pathology investigations and operative surgery are included.

(ii) *General surgery* Part of this oral is directed towards the candidate's major subspecialty interest, if such an interest is declared.

(iii) *Academic* This oral is designed to enquire into the critical abilities of the candidate. Candidates will be sent references to published papers which must be reviewed in advance of the examination. Discussion of one or more of these papers forms the first part of this oral. **Candidates** ***must*** **provide, in advance of the examination, three** abstracts (**each *not* exceeding 300 words**) **of their own published or presented work** (e.g. to a local clinical meeting). These abstracts should be specially prepared for the examination and should not be photocopies of a summary of a published paper. This work is discussed in the oral.

(iv) *Log books*   Log books, together with a summary of the operative experience, should be brought to the oral examination.

5 Curriculum of HST in General Surgery

The Joint Committee on Higher Surgical Training (JCHST)/ Specialist Advisory Committee (SAC) (representing the Royal Colleges of Surgeons, the Association of Professors of Surgery and the Specialist Surgical Associations in Great Britain and Ireland) has produced a most comprehensive document on HST in General Surgery entitled: *A Curriculum and Organisation for Higher Surgical Training in General Surgery and its Sub-specialties*. This important document contains useful information on the levels of training and also offers a person specification for a Specialist Registrar in Surgery. All trainees, therefore, are strongly advised to read it through carefully and refer to it from time to time. Full copies of the curriculum document may be obtained by writing to:

The Secretary of JCHST/SAC in General Surgery Joint Committee on Higher Surgical Training
The Royal College of Surgeons of England
35–43 Lincoln's Inn Fields
London WC2A 3PN
Tel: 0171 405 3474   Fax: 0171 973 2133

The HST curriculum released in June 1996 is reproduced below.

© Copyright of The Joint Committee on Higher Surgical Training. Reproduced with kind permission.

A Curriculum and organisation for higher surgical training (HST) in general surgery and its sub-specialties

Organisation

Objectives

● To provide a comprehensive and structured training programme in General Surgery and one or more of its sub-specialties for those who have completed Basic Surgical Training.

● To enable trainees to achieve the experience and training necessary for independent practice and, having passed the Intercollegiate Examination, to be awarded a Certificate of Completion of Specialist Training and entry on to the Specialist Register of the GMC.

Entry criteria

Completion of basic surgical training (or equivalent) and possession of MRCS/AFRCS (or equivalent), such equivalence being jointly agreed by the Surgical Royal Colleges of Great Britain and Ireland.

Duration

The duration of HST will be for 6 years with a minimum of 5 clinical years plus one flexible year for research or further specialist experience.

Organisation

1. **The Training Programme Director** for each training scheme will have overall responsibility for all trainees, for their enrolment, the weekly programmes of training, annual rotation, regular formal assessment, problem solving and feedback of progress.

2. **The Training Posts** will be monitored regularly by the Regional (Deanery) Higher Surgical Training Committee and the Programme Director.

3. **The SAC** will formally inspect the Regional Training Programmes at 5 yearly intervals and, in addition, individual hospitals and posts where significant changes have occurred or problems with training have been identified.

4. **The SAC Liaison Officer** from outside the region, appointed by the SAC, acts as an independent observer/adviser to the trainees and the training scheme, attends annual formal assessments, may attend appointments committees for SpR, and participates in problem solving and Stage 1 of the Appeal Mechanism against assessment of progress.

5. **The Educational Supervisor**, who is the College approved consultant trainer in day-to-day contact with the trainee, has responsibility for regular appraisal and discussion with the trainee.

6. In some hospitals there may be a **Director of Surgical Training** – often the College appointed **surgical tutor** who can advise and help the trainee where local problems with education or training exist.

Assessment

The continuous appraisal and regular assessment of trainees, especially in the early part of HST is an essential element of the programme. Regional Assessments will take place after the first 6 months, at the end of the first year, and then annually.

Research

One year of structured and supervised research is strongly encouraged for those who have not undertaken research prior to taking up their SpR post. This period will be flexible and may lead to an MSc, MPhil or M Med Sci. Those wishing to undertake a longer period of research for degree by thesis will be encouraged to do so. Training numbers will be retained for up to 2 years in an approved research post or longer with the approval of the SAC and Postgraduate Medical Dean.

Rotation date

It is agreed that SpR Training Schemes in General Surgery will rotate on 1 October each year.

Levels of training

Specialist Registrar Training in General Surgery is designed to reconcile the need for a broad training in general surgery to ensure the safe management of emergency cases, with the provision of subspecialty expertise in a limited field. Three levels of training will be recognised.

Training in general surgery (Level 1) Training that all general surgeons will be expected to have achieved by completion of HST. The trainee will need to be proficient to perform the listed procedures unsupervised, and others he or she will be expected to be familiar with or have assisted at.

Sub-specialty training

Mandatory (level 2): Training that a surgeon with a sub-specialty interest will be expected to have achieved by the completion of HST. A maximum of two sub-specialties is allowable.

Advanced (level 3): Sub-specialty training that would be required of a consultant who might practise almost exclusively in this field and which, whilst not essential, is desirable for a general surgeon with a sub-specialty interest. This level of training lends itself to specific modules. Some may only be achievable after CCST. Only one sub-specialty is allowable within HST.

Content Details of the operative skill required for each level of training and for each sub-specialty are described in the sub-specialty summary tables. The skill is matched by the theoretical basic science and knowledge relevant to each operation or procedure. This curriculum will constantly be revised by the SAC on the advice from the relevant sub-specialty associations.

A model job description*

Operating lists	**2–3 sessions** (NHDs) all supervised to an extent depending on the level of training.
Out-patients	**1 session** (minimum) new and old patients. The Consultant will be available for advice.
Ward work	**2 sessions** daily business round + at least one Consultant round/week.
Specialist interest	**1 Session**, e.g. endoscopy, sub-specialist outpatients, investigation etc.
Academic	**2 sessions**, e.g. education, research, teaching and audit.
Emergencies	**1 session**.

Content of training

1. **Sub-specialty requirements**. Schedules 1–8 which follow are a summary of the requirements for each sub-specialty. Fuller details of sub-specialty requirements will be available from the SAC and sub-specialty associations.
2. **Operative skill**. The procedures in which competence is required by the completion of training are detailed in each sub-specialty (1–8) for each stage of training. All trainees in general surgery will be required to have achieved general training in each sub-specialty by the completion of training (see summary, p. 15). Responsibility for the assessment and feedback of operative skill lies with the Educational Supervisor.
3. **Logbook**. The trainee's logbook will detail the number of procedures carried out, the extent of personal operative experience and the degree of supervision for each case. The logbook will form part of the Training Record†.
4. **Minimum requirements for units and number of procedures**. Some sub-specialties require a minimum number of cases operated on by the trainee (Endocrine), some require sub-specialty training to be undertaken in a unit with certain minimum requirements (Breast) and some sub-specialties stipulate both requirements (Vascular).
5. **Expected basic science and knowledge**. The content of the expected basic science and knowledge is detailed in the sub-specialty schedules 1–8. Trainees will be expected to know the surgical anatomy and physiology of each procedure skill acquired in Basic Surgical Training (BST) and in general surgical aspects of each sub-specialty. The examination of basic science and knowledge will be a component of the Intercollegiate Specialty Examination.
6. **Emergency general surgery**. Specialist Registrars, working in highly specialised units, may participate in the emergency rota for that sub-specialty in lieu of involvement in the general surgical rota for up to one year of their training. For the remaining four clinical years, trainees must be involved in the general surgical rota no less frequently than 1 in 6.
7. **Recommended courses**. Attendance at educational and surgical skills courses organised by the Royal Colleges of Surgeons and both clinical and NHS management courses is strongly recommended. Although not yet agreed as mandatory, a limited number of subspecialty courses may be recommended for sub-specialty training.

Introduction to sub-specialty requirement

1. The sub-specialty bodies have been consulted but are constantly updating their recommendations. The SAC Working Party will be seeking further guidance to be included in future revisions of this curriculum. There is no agreement that stated minimum numbers of operative procedures should be stipulated, although they may be included in future.
2. It is envisaged that over the next few years an increasing proportion of patients will be seen in dedicated specialty-specific clinics where they can be seen and treated by a surgeon with a special interest, e.g. breast or rectal clinics. It is desirable

---

*The job description should be based on training requirements and not on service needs.

†A Training Record to match the curriculum is being prepared by a Working Party of the SAC.

BODIES CONSULTED ON SUB-SPECIALTY TRAINING REQUIREMENTS

1. Breast	British Association of Surgical Oncology
2. Endocrine and Salivary Gland	The British Association of Endocrine Surgeons
3. Vascular	Vascular Surgical Society of Great Britain and Ireland
4. Coloproctology	The Association of Coloproctology of Great Britain and Ireland
5. Upper GI/HPB	The Surgical Gastroenterology Group (representing a-h below)
6. Trauma/Military Surgery	The Armed Forces
7. Paediatrics	British Association of Paediatric Surgeons
8. Transplant	The British Transplantation Society
9. All sub-specialties	The Specialties Board of the Association of Surgeons of Great Britain and Ireland:

(a) The Association of Surgeons of Great Britain and Ireland
(b) The Surgical Section of the British Society of Gastroenterology
(c) The Association of Coloproctology of Great Britain and Ireland
(d) Association of Endoscopic Surgeons of Great Britain and Ireland
(e) Pancreatic Society of Great Britain and Ireland
(f) The Oesophageal Group
(g) The Gastric Group
(h) The Hepatobiliary Group

SUB-SPECIALTY SUMMARY SCHEDULES

1. Sub-specialty: Breast

	Higher Surgical Training	
Training in General Surgery	**Sub-specialty** Mandatory	Advanced
Operative skill: to be proficient unsupervised		
Treatment of breast abscess	Wide excision breast tumors	**Reconstruction module**
Trucut biopsy	Needle localisation	Myocutaneous flaps
Excision of breast lump	Mammary duct fistula	Tissue expanders
Mastectomy	Microdochectomy	Complications and re-operations
FNA	Block dissection of axilla	Reduction
Operative skill: to be familiar with (to have assisted at)		
(As per sub-specialty: mandatory)	(As per sub-specialty: advanced)	
Expected basic science and knowledge		
The anatomy and physiology relevant to each operation or procedure		
Anatomy and physiology of breast	Chemotherapy: adjuvant/advanced	Genetics
Hormone therapy for benign and malignant disease	Radiotherapy	Immunocytochemistry
	Histo/cytopathology	Clinical trials
	Radiology u/s	
	Counselling	
	Hospice care	
	Epidemiology	
	Breast screening programme	
	Stereotaxis	
	Breast training course	

2. Sub-specialty: Endocrine

Higher Surgical Training

Training in General Surgery	Sub-specialty	
	Mandatory	Advanced
Operative skill: to be proficient unsupervised		
Cervical node biopsy	Thyroidectomy – toxic goitre	Re-do
Branchial cyst	Parathyroidectomy	Parathyroidectomy
	Total thyroidectomy	(Pituitary surgery)
	Retrosternal goitre	Endocrine pancreatic tumour
		Adrenalectomy
		Block disection of neck
		Salivary gland module (advanced)
Operative skill: to be familiar with (to have assisted at)		
(As per sub-specialty: mandatory)	(As per sub-specialty: advanced)	
Thyroidectomy – solitary nodule		
Thyroglossal cystectomy		
Expected basic science and knowledge		
The anatomy and physiology relevant to each operation or procedure		
Patho-physiology of : thyroid, parathyroid, pituitary, adrenal cortex, adrenal medulla, the gut as endocrine organ	Patho-physiology as per BST in much greater depth	Pituitary and adrenal Pathophysiology in detail
Management of thyrotoxicosis	Counselling and screening in familial disease	
Adrenal insufficiency	Anaesthetic/pharmacol. problems	
Hyper/Hypo calcaemia	Radioimmuno assays	
Carcinoid syndrome	Imaging techniques	
	Histo-cytopathology	

3. Sub-specialty: Vascular

Higher Surgical Training

Training in General Surgery	Sub-specialty	
	Mandatory	Advanced
Operative skill: to be proficient unsupervised		
Varicose veins	Re-do varicose veins	Upper limb vascular reconstruction
Vascular anastomosis and approach to major vessels	Aortic aneurysm	Thoracic outlet syndrome
	Axillofemoral carotid endarterectomy	Renal artery stenosis
Amputations	Ilio-femoral, femoro-femoral, femoro-popliteal and femoro-crural grafts	Supra-coeliac aneurysm
Fasciotomy		Infected intra-abdominal grafts
Embolectomy	On-table angiography	Percutaneous angioplasty
	Vascular access for dialysis	Insertion of stents
	Thoraco/laparoscopic sympathectomy	Angioscopy
Operative skill: to be familiar with (to have assisted at)		
Aortic aneurysm leaking and elective	Thrombolytic management	
(As per sub-specialty: mandatory)	(As per sub-specialty: advanced)	
Expected basic science and knowledge		
The anatomy and physiology relevant to each operation or procedure		
DVT and coagulation	Hand-held Doppler, duplex	A/v malformations
The ischaemic leg	Thrombolysis	Paediatric vascular
The diabetic foot	Graft technology	Lymphoedema
Graded compression		Cerebral and carotid vascular imaging
Management of arterial trauma		Imunological vascular diseases
Rehab. of amputees		
Post-phlebitic syndrome		
Anastomosis workshop		
Indications for arterial reconstruction and other techniques		
Claudication		

4. Sub-specialty: Coloproctology

Higher Surgical Training

Training in General Surgery	Sub-specialty	
	Mandatory	Advanced

Operative skill: to be proficient unsupervised

Proctoscopy/rigid sigmoidoscopy	Diagnostic and therapeutic colonoscopy	Incontinence surgery
Flexible sigmoidoscopy	Low fistula-in-ano	Sphincter repair
O/P haemorrhoid treatment	Ant. and A/P resecton of rectum	Recto-vaginal fistula
Haemorrhoidectomy	Colonic obstruction/perforation	Ileo-anal and colonic pouch
Fissure-in-ano	Ileorectal anastomosis	Colo-anal anastomosis
Perianal abscess	Panproctocolectomy	Re-op.pelvic malignancy
Management of abdom. injuries	Closure of Hartmann's	Re-op.inflammatory bowel disease
Segmental resections of large bowel i.e.	Prolapse surgery	Intestinal fistula
right and left hemicolectomy	Diverticular disease/fistula	Complex fistula-in-ano
Small bowel resection	Colostomy complications	Posterior approach to rectum (Kraske–
Hartmann's procedure	Block dissection of groin	York–Mason)
Colostomy	**Laparoscopy**: therapeutic	Transanal microsurgery
Ileostomy		Posterior pelvic clearance
Abdominal wall hernias		**Laparoscopy**: advanced
Appendicectomy		
Cystoscopy		
Laparoscopy: diagnostic		

Operative skill: to be familiar with (to have assisted at)

(As per sub-specialty: mandatory)   (As per sub-specialty: advanced)

Expected basic science and knowledge

The anatomy and physiology relevant to each operation or procedure

Patient counselling. Audit	Pelvic autonomic nerves
Care of critically ill. Nutrition	Anal tumours
Appropriate use of diagnostic radiology	Colonic bleeding
Microbiology and infection	Screening for colorectal cancer
Irritable bowel syndrome	Place of radiotherapy and chemotherapy in
Management of inflammatory bowel	treatment
disease	Anorectal manometry
Radiation injury and other enterocolitis	Incontinence
Management of colorectal tumours and	Constipation
colonic obstruction	Genetics
Pseudo-obstruction	Management of intestinal fistula
Postoperative peritonitis	
Use of staplers	

5. Sub-specialty: Upper GI/HPB

Higher Surgical Training

Training in General Surgery	Sub-specialty	
	Mandatory	Advanced

Operative skill: to be proficient unsupervised

Groin and incisional/parastomal hernia: elective and strangulated	Upper GI endoscopy	**Upper GI**
Appendicectomy	Upper GI bleeding	Oesophagectomy
Perforated ulcer	Oesophageal dilatation	Radical gastrectomy
Ileostomy	Gastrectomy	Re-do gastric and hiatus hernia
Small bowel resection	Peptic ulcer surgery	Radiation enteritis
Use of staplers	Biliary by-pass	Laser
Cholecystectomy – open	Exploration of bile duct	**Laparoscopy**: advanced
Laparoscopy: diagnostic	Hiatus hernia repair	
	Small bowel stricturoplasty	**HPB**
	Splenectomy elective	ERCP
	Drainage of pancreatic pseudocyst.	Biliary stricture repair
	Laparoscopy: therapeutic, e.g. cholecystectomy and conversion	Whipple's operation
		Pancreatectomy
		Drainage of infected pancreatitis
		Liver injuries
		Liver resection
		Hydatid disease
		Liver transplant
		Portosystemic shunt

Operative skill: to be familiar with (to have assisted at)

(As per sub-specialty: mandatory)	(As per sub-specialty: advanced)	

Expected basic science and knowledge

The anatomy and physiology relevant to each operation or procedure

Gastrointestinal physiology	Radiation enteritis	**Upper GI**
Pathophysiology of intestinal obstruction	Chronic pancreatitis	Oesophageal manometry & pH
Nutrition re. fistula	Screening for GI and liver tumours	Motility disorders
Microbiology. Non-ulcer dyspepsia	Oesophageal and gastric pathophysiology	
Management of: GI bleeding, perforation, obstruction, malignancy, Crohn's disease, acute pancreatitis		**HPB**
		Transplant
		Portal hypertension

---

6. Sub-specialty: Trauma/Military Surgery

Higher Surgical Training

Training in General Surgery	Sub-specialty	
	Mandatory	Advanced

Operative skill: to be proficient unsupervised

Penetrating and blunt abdominal trauma	Renal injuries	Military: penetrating missile injuries
Splenectomy for trauma	Thoracotomy/sternotomy	
Simple liver injury	Pericardiocentesis	
Bowel injury	Burr holes	
Skin grafts	Osteoplastic flaps	
Suprapubic cystotomy	Arterial injuries	
Haemo/pneumothorax	Limb injuries	
	Z-plasty – skin flaps	

Operative skill: to be familiar with (to have assisted at)

(As per sub-specialty: mandatory)	(Rectal injuries and pelvic floor injuries)

Expected basic science and knowledge
The anatomy and physiology relevant to each operation or procedure

Head injuries*	Triage: major accidents	Military: battle triage
Burns	Spinal injuries	Field hospitals
Flail chest/tamponade	Facial fractures	Diploma in Disaster Medicine and Surgery
Splenic conservation	CT/MRI interpretation	
Prophylaxis for asplenia	Multiple/critical injuries	
Pancreatic injury	BATLS	
Ruptured diaphragm		
Renal injury and conservation		
Management of urethral injury		
Pelvic fractures		

*A proportion of general surgeons will be required to take primary responsibility for the initial management of head injuries. Appropriate training should be available for the trainees who will have this responsibility.

7. Sub-specialty: Paediatric

Higher Surgical Training

Training in General Surgery	Sub-specialty	
	Mandatory	Advanced

Operative skill: to be proficient unsupervised

Appendicectomy	Infant pyloric stenosis	**Neonatal and complicated cases**
Herniotomy	Unreduced intussusception	Should be transferred to a Specialist
Paraphimosis/circumcision	Orchidopexy	Paediatric Unit
Torsion of testis	Thyroglossal cyst	

Operative skill: to be familiar with (to have assisted at)

(As per sub-specialty: mandatory)

Expected basic science and knowledge
The anatomy and physiology relevant to each operation or procedure

Tracheo-oesophageal fistula/atresia	Spina bifida
Diaphragmatic hernia	Hirschprung's disease
Intestinal atresia	Burns in children
Duplication cysts	Meconium ileus
Other congenital abnormalities	Exomphalos, gastroschisis

8. Sub-specialty: Transplant

	Higher Surgical Training	
Training in General Surgery	**Sub-specialty**	
	Mandatory	Advanced

Operative skill: to be proficient unsupervised

Insertion peritoneal dialysis catheter	Organ harvesting	Transplant renal artery stenosis
Central venous access	Renal transplantation	Pancreatic transplantation*
	Vascular access for haemodialysis	Liver transplantation*
	Secondary vascular access procedures	
	Renal transplant biopsy	
	Renal transplant nephrectomy	
	Native nephrectomy	

Operative skill: to be familiar with (to have assisted at)

(As per sub-specialty: mandatory)	(As per sub-specialty: advanced)	
	Parathyroid surgery	
	Ureteric and bladder reconstruction	

Expected basic science and knowledge

The anatomy and physiology relevant to each operation or procedure

Peritoneal dialysis	Immunosuppression	Liver pathophysiology
Haemodialysis	Opportunistic infection	Bladder dysfunction and reconstruction
Electrolyte balance	HLA system and tissue typing	
Pathology of rejection	Preservation of organs	
Brain stem death	Graft versus host disease	
Transplant co-ordination	Renal pathology	
Management of diabetes	Angioplasty	

*Requires sub-specialty training in a specialist unit.

SUMMARY OF GENERAL SURGICAL OPERATIVE SKILL TO BE ACHIEVED BY COMPLETION OF HST

Operative Skills	
To be proficient unsupervised	**To be familiar with/have assisted at**

Breast

Treatment of breast abscess	Wide excision breast tumours
Excision of breast lump	Needle localization
Mastectomy	Mammary duct fistula
Trucut biopsy	Michrodochectomy
FNA	Block dissection of axilla

Endocrine and Salivary Gland

Cervical node biopsy	Thyroidectomy
Branchial cyst	Parathyroidectomy
Submandibular duct stone	Thyroglossal cystectomy
	Retrosternal goitre

Vascular

Varicose veins	Re-do varicose veins
Vascular anastomosis and approach to major vessels	Aortic aneurysm: leaking and elective
Endarterectomy	Vascular by-pass: axillo-femoral cartoid
Amputations	Ileo-femoral, femoro-femoral and femoro-crural grafts
Fasciotomy	On-table angiography
Embolectomy	Thoraco/laparoscopic sympathectomy
	Vascular access for dialysis

To be proficient unsupervised	To be familiar with/have assisted at

Coloproctology

Proctoscopy	Colonoscopy, diagnostic and therapeutic
Rigid sigmoidoscopy	Low fistula-in-ano
Flexible sigmoidoscopy	Anterior and A/P resection of rectum
Outpt. treatment of haemorrhoids	Colonic obstruction/perforation
Haemorrhoidectomy	Ileorectal anastomosis
Fissure-in-ano	Panproctocoletomy
Perianal abscess	Closure of Hartman's
Management of abdominal injuries	Diverticular disease/fistula
Segmental resections of large bowel	Colostomy complications
(Right and left hemicolectomy)	Block dissection of groin
Small bowel resection	
Hartmann's procedure	Laparoscopy: therapeutic
Colostomy	
Ileostomy	
Appendicectomy	
Cystoscopy	
Abdominal wall hernias	
Laparoscopy: diagnostic	

Upper GI/HPB

Hernia: groin, incisional and parastomal: elective, recurrent and strangulated	Upper GI endoscopy
Appendicectomy	Upper GI bleeding
Perforated ulcer	Oesophageal dilatation
Use of staplers	Peptic ulcer surgery
Cholecystectomy – open	Gastrectomy
Ileostomy	Biliary bypass
Small bowel resection	Cholecystectomy and conversion – laparoscopic
	Exploration of bile duct
	Hiatus hernia
	Small bowel stricturoplasty
	Splenectomy elective
	Drainage of pancreatic pseudo-cyst

Trauma/Military Surgery

Splenectomy for trauma	Renal injuries
Penetrating and blunt abdominal trauma	Thoracotomy/sternotomy
Simple liver injury	Pericardiocentesis
Bowel injury	Burr holes
Skin grafts	Osteoplastic flaps
Suprapubic cystotomy	Limb injuries
Haemo/pneumothroax	Z-plasty – skin flaps
	Rectal and pelvic floor injuries
	Arterial injuries

Paediatric

Appendicectomy in childhood	Infant pyloric stenosis
Herniotomy	Unreduced intussusception
Paraphimosis/circumcision	Orchidopexy
Torsion of testis	Thyroglossal cyst

Transplant

Insertion peritoneal dialysis catheter	Organ harvesting
Central venous access	Renal transplantation
	Vascular access for haemodialysis
	Secondary vascular access procedures
	Renal transplant biopsy
	Renal transplant nephrectomy
	Native nephrectomy

Person specification for a specialist registrar in surgery

Requirements	Essential	Desirable
1. Qualifications and academic achievements	● Qualified medical practitioner* ● Registered with GMC ● CSIG/FRCS (AFRCS/MRCS after 1998) or approved overseas equivalent†	● Distinctions, prizes, awards, scholarships, other degrees, higher degrees ● Presentations ● Publications
2. Training	● Completed BST in posts approved by the surgical Royal Colleges or approved overseas equivalent ● Validated logbook indicating appropriate operative experience	● Competence in preoperative and postoperative management ● Computer skills ● Evidence of participation and understanding of the principles of audit
3. Personal attributes‡	● Caring attitudes ● Honest and trustworthy ● Reliability	● Ability to work in a team
4. Personal skills and attitude	● Organisational ability ● Potential to cope with stressful situations and undertake responsibility ● Understand and communicate intelligibly with patients ● Trustworthy and reliable ● Behave in a manner which establishes professional relationships with patients	● Initiative ● A critical enquiring approach to the acquisition of knowledge
5. Practical requirements	● Be physically and mentally fit and capable of conducting operative procedures, which may be demanding of a number of hours of close attention ● Manual dexterity as confirmed by referees	● Outside interests

Note: It is appreciated that requirements 3 to 5 all require a degree of subjective assessment. It is these requirements which will need to be assessed by Consultant Supervisors or colleagues and detailed in the written references in support of the applicant. It is advised that applicants discuss these details of the person specification with the referees from whom they seek support.

* Qualified medical practitioner and qualified dental practitioner, registered with GMC (and GDC) for Oral and Maxillofacial Surgery.

† And FDSRCS or equivalent for Oral and Maxillofacial Surgery.

‡ See also 'Tomorrow's Doctors' below.

that trainees should also be taught general surgical sub-specialty procedures in this environment.

3. The distinction between mandatory and advanced training in the sub-specialties is sometimes related to the depth and volume of the experience in the sub-specialty rather than the complexity of the surgery. For example, not all breast surgeons will wish to do reconstructive surgery.

4. Advanced sub-specialty training will only be achievable in units with a significant case load of the procedures concerned. The threshold workload for such designation is currently being established by sub-specialty associations. This may be in regional or supra-regional centres and may, in some training schemes, necessitate experience to be gained after CCST.

5. Some of the schedules do not refer to recognised sub-specialties, e.g. Endocrine and Salivary Gland, Trauma/Military and Paediatric.

6. Endoscopic (laparoscopic) surgery is becoming established for certain procedures. Trainees are strongly advised to attend formal courses in these developing techniques, in addition to gaining apprenticeship training with their Consultant Super-

visor. (Laparoscopic surgery has been recognised in April 1997 at the Association of Surgeons of Great Britain and Ireland as a specialty, not as a stand-alone specialty but to be practised along with one or two other sub-specialties.)

7. Further sub-specialty advice will be incorporated in the next edition, to be published for use from 1 January 1998.

General Medical Council: 'Tomorrow's Doctors – Recommendations on Undergraduate Medical Education' (December 1993)*

Attributes of the independent practitioner

1. The ability to solve clinical and other problems in medical practice, which involves or requires:

(a) an intellectual and temperamental ability to change, to face the unfamiliar and to adapt to change;

*© General Medical Council, 1993.

(b) a capacity for individual, self-directed learning; and

(c) reasoning and judgement in the application of knowledge to the analysis and interpretation of data, in defining the nature of a problem, and in planning and implementing a strategy to resolve it.

2. Possession of adequate knowledge and understanding of the general structure and function of the human body and workings of the mind, in health and disease, of their interaction and of the interaction between man and his physical and social environment. This requires:

(a) knowledge of the physical, behavioural, epidemiological and clinical sciences upon which medicine depends;

(b) understanding of the aetiology and natural history of diseases;

(c) understanding of the impact of both psychological factors upon illness and of illness upon the patient and the patient's family;

(d) understanding of the effects of childhood growth and of later ageing upon the individual, the family and the community; and

(e) understanding of the social, cultural and environmental factors which contribute to health or illness, and the capacity of medicine to influence them.

3. Possession of consultation skills, which include:

(a) skills in sensitive and effective communication with patients and their families, professional colleagues and local agencies, and the keeping of good medical records;

(b) the clinical skills necessary to examine the patient's physical and mental state and to investigate appropriately;

(c) the ability to exercise sound clinical judgement to analyse symptoms and physical signs in pathophysiological terms, to establish diagnoses, and to offer advice to the patient taking account of physical, psychological, social and cultural factors; and

(d) understanding of the special needs of terminal care.

4. Acquisition of a high standard of knowledge and skills in the doctor's specialty, which include:

(a) understanding of acute illness and of disabling and chronic diseases within that specialty, including their physical, mental and social implications, rehabilitation, pain relief, and the need for support and encouragement; and

(b) relevant manual, biochemical, pharmacological, psychological, social and other interventions in acute and chronic illness.

5. Willingness and ability to deal with common medical emergencies and with other illness in an emergency.

6. The ability to contribute appropriately to the prevention of illness and the promotion of health, which involves:

(a) understanding of the principles, methods and limitations of preventive medicine and health promotion;

(b) understanding the doctor's role in educating patients, families and communities, and in generally promoting good health; and

(c) the ability to identify individuals at risk and to take appropriate action.

7. The ability to recognise and analyse ethical problems so as to enable patients, their families, society and the doctor to have proper regard to such problems in reaching decisions; this comprehends:

(a) knowledge of the ethical standards and legal responsibilities of the medical profession;

(b) understanding of the impact of medico-social legislation on medical practice; and

(c) recognition of the influence upon his or her approach to ethical problems of the doctor's own personality and values.

8. The maintenance of attitudes and conduct appropriate to a high level of professional practice, which includes:

(a) recognition that a blend of scientific and humanitarian approaches is required, involving a critical approach to learning, open-mindedness, compassion and concern for the dignity of the patient and, where relevant, of the patient's family;

(b) recognition that good medical practice depends on partnership between doctor and patient, based upon mutual understanding and trust; the doctor may give advice, but the patient must decide whether or not to accept it;

(c) commitment to providing high quality care; awareness of the limitations of the doctor's own knowledge and of existing medical knowledge; recognition of the duty to keep up to date in the doctor's own specialist field and to be aware of developments in others; and

(d) willingness to accept review, including self-audit, of the doctor's performance.

9. Mastery of the skills required to work within a team and, where appropriate, assume the responsibilities of team leader, which requires:

(a) recognition of the need for the doctor to collaborate in prevention, diagnosis, treatment and management with other health care professionals and with patients themselves;

(b) understanding and appreciation of the roles, responsibilities and skills of nurses and other health care workers; and

(c) the ability to lead, guide and coordinate the work of others.

10. Acquisition of experience in administration and planning, including:

(a) efficient management of the doctor's own time and professional activities;

(b) appropriate use of diagnostic and therapeutic resources, and appreciation of the economic and practical constraints affecting the provision of health care; and

(c) willingness to participate, as required, in the work of bodies which advise, plan and assist the development and administration of medical services, such as NHS authorities and trusts, Royal Colleges and Faculties, and professional associations.

11. Recognition of the opportunities and acceptance of the duty to contribute, when possible, to the advancement of medical knowledge and skill, which entails:

(a) understanding of the contribution of research methods, and interpretation and application of others' research in the doctor's own specialty; and

(b) willingness, when appropriate, to contribute to research in the doctor's specialist field, both personally and through encouraging participation by junior colleagues.

12. Recognition of the obligation to teach others, particularly doctors in training, which requires:

(a) acceptance of responsibility for training junior colleagues in the specialty, and for teaching other doctors, medical students, and other health care professionals, when required;

(b) recognition that teaching skills are not necessarily innate but can be learned, and willingness to acquire them; and

(c) recognition that the example of the teacher is the most powerful influence upon the standards of conduct and practice of every trainee.

PART TWO

Surgery

SECTION 1
The Written Examination
(Clinical Surgery-in-General)

Introduction

The written papers are an essential part of the examination. *You have to pass* the written and the clinical parts *individually* in order to pass. (Borderline marking in some parts could be compensated for by others.) Some people know enough about the subject but are unable to organise their thoughts and write clearly within the time available. Others can write fluently but often do not answer the question asked, through misinterpretation. The following points and hints provide a useful guide on writing answers.

Planning

1. Read the instructions at the top of the paper carefully, and divide the time equally between the questions, allowing 10 minutes for revision. Candidates often answer too many or too few questions, or leave no time for the last one. *The marking system makes it impossible to recover from an unanswered question or even to compensate for a half answered question.*
2. Read the question through several times slowly, noting exactly what is asked for and underline the key words. *The examiners take great care in phrasing each question, but candidates often answer them entirely differently.*
3. Spend about 5 minutes (for planning), jotting down all your relevant thoughts and notes on the scrap paper provided and referring back to the question from time to time.
4. Rearrange and refine your ideas in a logical sequential practical order (for clarity) with common things first, resisting the temptation to dwell on rarities, and avoid repetition. All clinical answers are best considered under the headings:

History   *Examination*   *Special tests*

(History and physical examination are clinical investigation; special tests are mainly laboratory, radiological and other investigations.)

Layout (introduction and body)

The capacity to earn marks is highest at the start of an answer and you should therefore impress the examiner by your introduction. It is easy to get bogged down here, and if you are not sure where to start always revert to the basic principles.
   The following hints are helpful.
1. Imagine that you are writing for a tired, bored examiner, who only wants to see if you are fit to become a safe surgeon.

2. Examiners get their first impression of an answer from its physical appearance and the opening of your introduction, so make your answer *legible and concise* (legibility pleases the examiner and conciseness saves your time in writing).
3. Use well-spaced, underlined, and numbered headings and subheadings and start a new paragraph for each new idea you wish to record. (Leave the page margin free and avoid crowding.)
4. Illustrate your answer wherever necessary. Good figures and simple line diagrams are an extra bonus and facilitate interpretation of the answer.
5. Avoid jargon (i.e. unintelligible words and debased language) and unfamiliar incorrect abused terms. Short and common phrases with basic simple English are best.
6. Avoid lists (without further explanation and elaboration).

Revision

Spend about 10 minutes on reading over what has been written for punctuation, correct spelling, sequence of phrases and checking the illustrations.

Special terms

The use of some of the terms used in examination questions needs to be explained.

Describe   Write in details. Usually forms an introduction to a question involving a pathological process and commonly leads to a second part about management (each part of the question should be allotted equal time).

Give an account of   Give a comprehensive account of that particular condition including: incidence; pathology; aetiology; symptoms and signs; and treatment.

Discuss   Select the most important and controversial aspects of the subject (compare and contrast) and discuss pros and cons; if you are in favour of a particular feature you must give the reasons clearly.

Symptomatology
Clinical findings } Symptoms and signs.

Diagnosis   How would you prove what it is? Anatomically – what structure is involved? Pathologically – what is wrong with it? The answer is considered under the headings *History, Examination, Special tests*. Differential diagnosis is only referred to incidentally.

Differential diagnosis   What else could it be and how would you exclude the other possibilities? This usually calls for a list of the various alternatives that might cause the disease or symptom, with notes on the means of excluding them, by *History, Examination, Special tests*. The various possibilities may be thought of in the following way.

● Anatomical structures
● The pathological conditions (e.g. swelling): congenital or acquired
  – Congenital (since birth ± family history)
  – Traumatic (history)
  – Inflammatory
    Acute (days): infective (bacterial, viral, parasitic)
    Subacute (weeks)
    Chronic (months): non-specific or specific (leprosy, tuberculosis, syphilis, actinomycosis)
  – Neoplastic (months or years): benign or malignant
  – Allergic (minutes)
  – Miscellaneous (metabolic, vascular, rheumatic)

Pathology   One's first thought is 'What on earth can I write about for 55 minutes?' but this topic includes:
  Incidence (age, sex, race, geography)
  All relevant *investigations* that can be done
  Natural history of the disease (including aetiology, pathogenesis, course, spread and final outcome)
  Morbid anatomy (macroscopy)
  Histology (microscopy)
  Pathological physiology (complications and prognosis).

Pathogenesis   Underlying mechanisms (of causation and clinical presentation), including predisposing factors (and in cancers, the precancerous conditions).

Aetiology   Causes

Treatment   This calls for a technical account of the various methods of treatment of the condition and the indications for each:

Prophylaxis
Non-operative conservative measures
Interventional radiology measures
Operative measures
Rehabilitation

Operation   In describing an operation, it is convenient to use the headings:
  Preoperative preparation
  Anaesthetic
  Position
  Skin preparation, draping (special draping, e.g. thyroid surgery should be mentioned)
  Access (including incision)
  Procedure
  Postoperative instruction (if any)

Management   This describes the handling of the patient from first presentation in casualty or Outpatients to return to normal health (i.e. diagnosis and treatment), including rehabilitation and follow-up. Thus the field is large and *the review correspondingly superficial*. If the question concerns a symptom (e.g. diarrhoea) the diagnostic procedures must be described, but if it concerns a diagnosis (e.g. carcinoma of the rectum) this may be assumed to have been established already.

Final points

Write clearly and tidily (erase or delete your mistakes unambiguously) and do not abbreviate.

If your handwriting is poor, print your answers (preferably in capital letters) and save your time by writing the basic principles in a concise, summarised manner. Use a good quality biro (fine point) or fountain pen (with a good nib such as an italic nib). Black ink is preferable. It is also useful to have various coloured pens for illustration purposes whenever necessary. Pack everything in a small case – you may also place your admission card in the case so that you will not forget it.

PRINCIPLES OF SURGERY-IN-GENERAL

APPLIED PATHOPHYSIOLOGY

1.1 Endocrine and Metabolic Response to Trauma

Injury, surgical operation, burn and sepsis produce profound endocrine and metabolic responses, which parallel the magnitude of the trauma. Surgery evokes a wide variety of metabolic changes, including increased thermogenesis, hyperglycaemia, loss of muscle protein, acute phase protein synthesis, a decrease in plasma divalent cations: iron and zinc and increased white cell count.

MECHANISM OF NEUROENDOCRINE RESPONSE

The most likely explanation is that the injury induces an afferent neuronal input from the operative site, both autonomic and somatic, and release of cytokines from damaged tissue resulting from surgical trauma. The local mediators include interleukin-6, bradykinin, histamine, serotonin, prostaglandins, leukotrienes, anaerobic metabolites and cellular enzymes which via cutaneous nocireceptors send afferent nerve impulses from the traumatic or operative site to the brain stem, activating the afferent autonomic fibres, and leading to endocrine and metabolic changes. This reflex is also initiated by pain, apprehension (pain and fear affect cerebral cortex which in turn affects hypothalamus/pituitary axis), fasting, dehydration and haemorrhage (hypovolaemia affects brain stem via baro-receptors). In the postoperative period, infection (sepsis affects hypothalamus/pituitary axis), prolonged bed rest, arterial hypoxaemia (hypoxia affects brain stem via chemoreceptors) and even alterations in the usual day–night physiologic cycles can all contribute to the endocrine changes.

The role of interleukin-6

The mediator role of cytokines in the causation of metabolic, immunological, haematological and possibly hormonal respon-ses to surgery deserves attention. Cytokines are a large, and rapidly expanding group of polypeptides; the group includes interleukins (IL-1 to 12 so far), tumour necrosis factor (TNF α and β) and the interferons. Cytokines have numerous effects on a wide variety of tissues, particularly immunological cells. Major sites of cytokines synthesis are macrophages and monocyte cells as well as fibroblasts and glial cells. Both TNF and IL-1 have been implicated as mediators of the 'sepsis syndrome'. IL-6, however, is the main cytokine released after routine surgery; the increase in concentration of circulating IL-6 is approximately proportional to the severity of the surgery. However, circulating TNF and IL-1 values remain unincreased. The IL-6 not only stimulates acute phase protein synthesis in the liver (serum C-reactive protein CRP is increased), but also has effects on the immune system and haemopoiesis. These include B cell proliferation and T differentiation, T cell co-stimulation and plasmocyte proliferation, with a possible role in anterior pituitary hormone secretion. In a Belgian study comparing the hormonal and metabolic responses to cholecystectomy con-ducted by either conventional laparotomy or laparoscopy, the duration of hospital stay was reduced by nearly 50% in patients operated on laparoscopically (2.75 days versus 5.0 days), although the duration of surgery was longer (121 min versus 96 min). The improved recovery in the laparoscopy group was associated with a decreased duration of postoperative fasting, an improvement in simple respiratory function tests and a decrease in analgesic consumption (although pain scores were similar in the two groups, probably because analgesics were readily available). The IL-6 results showed a significantly decreased response in the laparoscopy group and this was associated with a decrease in circulating concentrations of CRP and white blood count. The improvement in the IL-6 response confirms the original observation by others that tissue damage is a major determinant of the circulating value of this cytokine. Changes in plasma adrenaline, noradrenaline and blood cortisol concentra-tions were comparable in the two groups and this emphasises the importance of the IL-6 related changes in determining the rate of recovery from surgery. These findings suggest that visceral afferent stimulation is the main factor in stimulating the neuroendocrine response to surgery.

ENDOCRINE AND METABOLIC CHANGES AFTER SURGERY

The efferent hormonal secretions represent the outputs of two neuroendocrine sites:

1. Pituitary hormones: increased ACTH, ADH (vasopressin), endorphins and enkephalins, growth hormone, and prolactin.
2. Brain stem outflow of autonomic fibres leading to increased catecholamines, activation of renin–angiotensin–aldosterone system and increased glucagon. Catecholamines (adrenaline mainly) themselves act on the pancreas leading to increased catabolic glucagon secretion and decreased insulin secretion (relative hypoinsulinaemia despite hyperglycaemia, *see below*). Furthermore, the action of insulin in muscles is suppressed by catecholamines, growth hormone, and cortisol, thus limiting substrate (glucose) peripheral tissue utilisation. The ratio of insulin/glucagon is the critical determinant of the balance of anabolism and catabolism.

There are two phases: the initial catabolic phase is characterised by protein and fat mobilisation with increased urinary nitrogen excretion and weight loss, and **usually lasts 2–7 days; this is followed by the anabolic recovery phase, lasting some weeks**, during which protein and fat stores are restored, and weight is regained.

Initial endocrine response (within 48 h) is characterised by an increase in circulating concentrations of catabolic hor-mones, including catecholamines, glucagon, cortisol (they increase gluconeogenesis from muscle amino acids), ADH (vasopressin) and aldosterone (causing salt and water reten-tion) (Fig. 1.1.1). At the same time, there are decreases in plasma concentrations of the anabolic hormones, insulin (despite co-existing hyperglycaemia), luteinising hormone, follicular stimulating hormone and testosterone. Thyroid hor-mones and thyroid stimulating hormone are unaffected by injury or surgery. *Insulin is the only hypoglycaemic hormone* (all other hormones are hyperglycaemic); thus the normal regulation of blood glucose is suppressed in response to surgical stimulation. In fact, increased blood glucose levels during anaesthesia and surgery are predictable. As a result, excessive amounts of glucose delivered i.v. via maintenance fluids can result in intraoperative hyperglycaemia. The most likely mechanism for decreased insulin release and associated

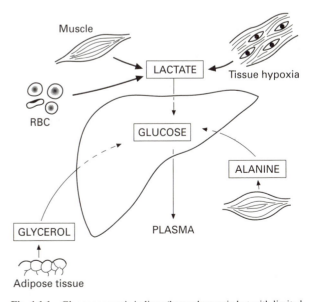

Fig. 1.1.1 Gluconeogenesis in liver (hyperglycaemia but with limited tissue utilisation)

hyperglycaemia during general anaesthesia is non-specific response to stress, mediated by increased sympathetic nervous system activity and adrenaline secretion. Adrenaline produces hyperglycaemia by stimulation of glycogenolysis and gluconeogenesis, as well as by directly inhibiting release of insulin from the pancreas. Most tissues depend on insulin to increase glucose peripheral utilisation; however, *brain, both kidneys, bowel and blood cells (RBC) utilise glucose directly without the need for insulin.*

Increases in protein degradation are a major metabolic response of the body to surgical trauma. *Catabolic glucagon accounts for most of the increased muscle catabolism as well as the increased urinary secretion of nitrogen for 4–6 days after abdominal surgery.* A man with average body build can lose 0.5 kg of lean tissue each day after a major abdominal operation. The main effect of protein degradation is release of amino acids, particularly alanine. Alanine is transported to the liver for conversion to glucose by gluconeogenesis. In addition, surgical stimulation often activates the renin–angio-

tensin–aldosterone system and results in release of antidiuretic hormone, as evidenced by *sodium and water retention and urinary excretion of potassium.* Angiotensin is a potent vasoconstrictor and with catecholamines has direct chronotropic and inotropic effects on the myocardium. Angiotensin 2 is a major stimulus to aldosterone secretion from zona glomerularis; aldosterone acts on the renal tubule, the colon, the terminal ileum, salivary glands and sweat glands to retain sodium. *Inappropriate secretion of antidiuretic hormone in the postoperative period combined with i.v. infusion of sodium-deficient solutions may result in life-threatening hyponatraemia* (Figs 1.1.2 and 1.1.3).

MODIFICATION OF ENDOCRINE AND METABOLIC RESPONSES

These neuroendocrine responses to injury are essential to the immediate short-term survival of the patient. Nevertheless,

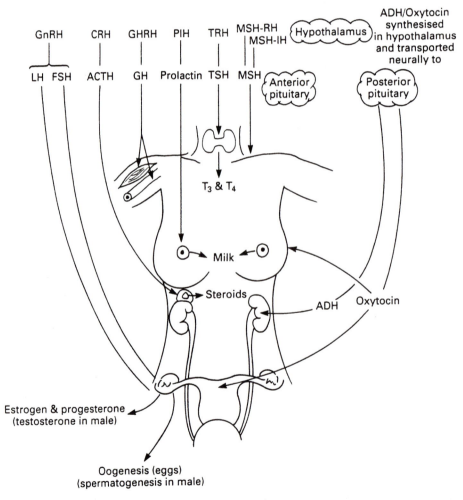

Fig. 1.1.2 Hypothalamus and pituitary hormones. GnRH = godadotrophin-releasing hormone; LH = luteinising hormone; FSH = follicle-stimulating hormone; CRH = corticotropin-releasing hormone; ACTH = adrenocorticotropic hormone; GHRH = growth hormone releasing hormone; GH = growth hormone; PIH = prolactin inhibiting hormone; TRH = thyrotropin-releasing hormone; TSH = thyroid-stimulating hormone, T4 = thyroxine; T3 = triiodothyronine; MSH = melanocyte-stimulating hormone; MSH-RH and MSH-IH = MSH releasing and inhibiting hormones; ADH = anti-diuretic hormone (vasopressin). All hypothalamic hormones are transported to the anterior pituitary by hypothalamo-hypophyseal portal venous blood, but to the posterior pituitary by the neural tract

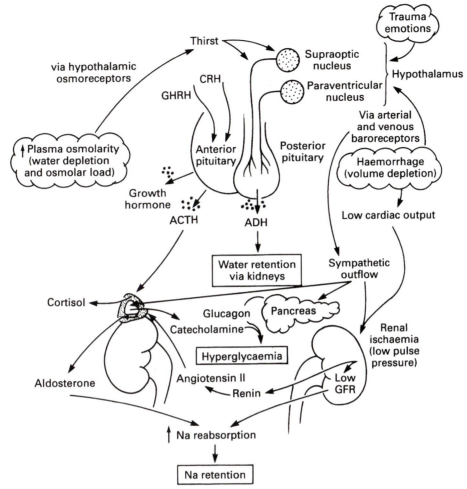

Fig. 1.1.3   Endocrine response to trauma

these physiological adjustments possess some detrimental changes, such as the following.

- Increased protein catabolism (presents a particular problem in patients who are already cachectic and emaciated prior to surgery).
- Poor substrate utilisation, e.g. glucose despite hyperglycaemia (presents a particular problem in diabetic patients).
- Persistent water/sodium retention and dilutional hyponatraemia (presents a particular problem in patients with co-existing poor cardiopulmonary reserve).
- Inadequate clearance of metabolic byproducts leading to acidosis (presents a particular problem in elderly patients or patients with renal impairment).

Therefore, modification of these endocrine and metabolic responses may be desirable at some stages following the trauma.

The early response to trauma can be blocked by section of the nerves to the traumatised area, although conscious perception of pain is not necessary for the neuroendocrine response; however, hypovolaemia, hypoxia and acidosis may all play overriding roles in the early responses.

Inhaled or injected drugs used to produce anaesthesia result in minimal effects on hormone secretion in the absence of surgical stimulation. However, endocrine responses following surgical trauma can be modified via afferent neuronal blockade, as with regional anaesthesia, or by inhibition of hypothalamic function with large doses of opioids. For example, epidural analgesia (T4 sensory level) reduces or abolishes the increases in blood glucose, cortisol and catecholamine concentrations induced by lower abdominal surgery; it is likely that extradural analgesia merely postpones hyperglycaemia and adrenocorticol responses until the postoperative period. Complete neuronal block can be achieved only for surgery of the eye, limbs and pelvic organs (via extradural block from T4–S5 dermatomes for pelvic surgery). While hyperglycaemia can be prevented, acute phase protein synthesis remains unaltered. Even when abolition of neuroendocrine response has been achieved, little benefit in postoperative morbidity (according to one study) has been shown, in spite of occasional claims (by another study) to the contrary.

Large doses of morphine (4 mg/kg), and fentanyl (75 µg/kg) have also been shown to inhibit endocrine and metabolic responses to surgery. Large doses of opioids, however, are not sufficient to prevent the endocrine response evoked by institution of cardiopulmonary bypass. Increases in plasma adrenaline concentrations and stimulation of the CVS associated with surgical skin incision are prevented in 50% of adults by administration of 60% nitrous oxide and a volatile anaesthetic (halothane, enflurane) or morphine (1.13 mg/kg). Furthermore, a subarachnoid block sufficient to prevent the pain of skin incision eliminates both adrenergic and CVS responses to surgical stimulation in all patients.

Although it is difficult to quantify total adverse effects produced by endocrine and metabolic responses to surgical stimulation, it would seem prudent to minimise the magnitude and duration of these changes whenever possible. This is ideally achieved by rapid correction of adverse physiological disturbances, and assurance of adequate depths of anaesthesia relative to the magnitude of surgical stimulation. Indeed, the concept that administration of the lowest possible amount of anaesthetic is best may not be valid during periods of acute surgical stimulation.

It should be appreciated that exogenous glucose administered to critically ill patients undergoing major surgery makes little or no difference in the magnitude of protein catabolism. Indeed, there is no basis for the recommendation that administration of 100 g/day of exogenous glucose will provide optimal sparing of body proteins.

1.2 Pain in Surgery

INTRODUCTION

Pain is a subjective experience usually due to an underlying organic lesion. It varies from person to person and within any given individual as a result of the interplay of biological, psychological and environmental factors. There are three basic theories about pain mechanisms.

Specificity theory Maintains that pain is a specific stimulus received by special receptors (free nerve endings discovered by Von Frey, different from touch discovered by Meissner, pressure by Pacini, heat by Ruffini and cold by Krause) that make special connections in the CNS. Pain travels along thick, myelinated, fast-conducting A fibres and along thin, unmyelinated, slow-conducting C fibres, producing respectively immediate short and delayed persistent responses. These fibres synapse with the neurons of the substantia gelatinosa in the dorsal horn of the spinal cord. The second-order neurons cross the midline in the white commissure and ascend in the lateral spinothalamic tract to reach the posterolateral ventral nucleus of the thalamus, whence they are relayed via third-order neurons to the postcentral gyrus of the cerebral cortex (Fig. 1.2.1).

Pattern theory Suggests that afferent nerves carry all kinds of impulses impartially and that the patterns of impulses are programmed in the spinal cord and interpreted by the brain. Certain spatiotemporal patterns are perceived as pain after intense stimulation of non-specific receptors.

Modulation (gate) theory Melzack and Wall (1965) proposed the existence of input control in the substantia gelatinosa, which operates as a gate (Fig. 1.2.1). Persistent intense high

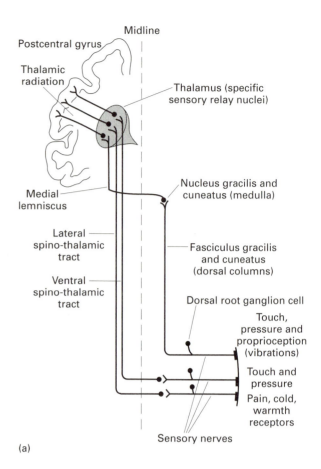

(a)

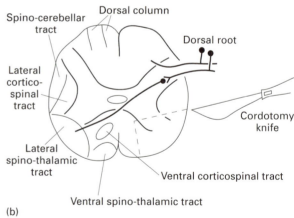

(b)

Fig. 1.2.1 Major spinal pathways in pain, temperature and proprioceptive sensations: (a) shows the pathways in profile while (b) shows them in cross-section of the cord

threshold impulses carried by the C fibres (perceived as severe pain) can be blocked if a 'gate mechanism' in the dorsal horn is first closed by faster low-threshold pain impulses carried by A fibres or by modifying impulses descending from the brain, e.g. initiated by stress or emotion. This theory explained 'combat analgesia': a soldier in the heat of battle can be oblivious to the pain from a serious wound. It also explains intractable post-herpetic neuralgia where selective degeneration of the peripheral thick A fibres is said to leave the gate

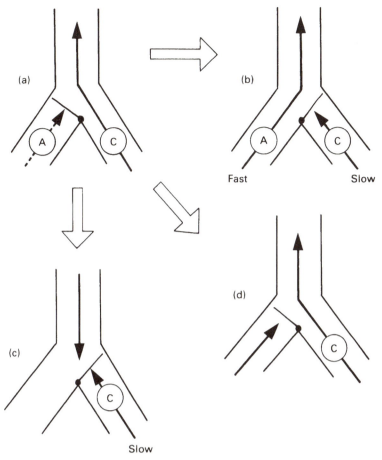

Fig. 1.2.2 Gate theory of pain. (a) Persistent severe pain via C fibres after cessation of A fibre impulses. (b) acupuncture and transcutaneous nerve stimulation. (c) Stress, emotion and stored experience (combat analgesia). (d) Post-herpetic neuralgia (degeneration of A fibres)

open to the more persistent C fibre impulses. The gate theory can also explain why pain is relieved (after a painful blow) by rubbing the skin, topical application of counter-irritants (such as liniments), transcutaneous nerve stimulation with an electrode applied to the trigger zone (dermatome), or needles inserted into the meridians in acupuncture. In all these situations peripheral A fibres are stimulated, thus closing the gate against the C fibres.

Enkephalins and endorphins

These represent the brain's own opiates (or endogenous naturally occurring morphines) and were discovered in the 1970s. Enkephalins are pentapeptides and it was found that methionine, or metenkephalin, consisted of the same amino acid sequence as the terminal five amino acids of a much larger peptide, β-lipotrophin. Furthermore, the terminal 31 amino acids of β-lipotrophin are called β-endorphin. It is now certain that the lipotrophin-related peptides and ACTH have a common precursor, 'pro-opiocortin', which codes for the formation of β-endorphin, met- and leu-enkephalins via a special messenger RNA. These opiate peptides are hydrolysed by enkephalinase enzyme, and like morphine their effects are antagonised by naloxone. Enkephalins are distributed in the limbic system, thalamus and substantia gelatinosa as well as in the gastro-

intestinal tract and adrenal medulla. Endorphin distribution is more restricted, being found abundantly in the pituitary which is devoid of enkephalin. These natural peptides together with their synthetic analogues as well as most narcotic analgesics (notably opiate alkaloids) occupy special receptors (opioid receptors) in the CNS of which μ, κ, σ, δ, and ε were found, the last being specific for β-endorphin only. These endogenous opiates act as neurotransmitters. Morphine and enkephalins inhibit noradrenergic firing of locus ceruleus. Withdrawal of opiates leads to massive neuronal discharges which are associated with the 'opiate abstinence syndrome'. Clonidine acting as an α_2 agonist at these neurons slows the discharge and reverses or prevents the withdrawal syndrome. It was also found that acupuncture-induced analgesia is reversed by naloxone (narcotic antagonist) and conversely, the analgesia is potentiated by giving the enkephalinase-inhibitor D-phenylalanine with electroacupuncture; this suggests that acupuncture is associated with the release of enkephalins and endorphins into CSF. These opiates act only intrathecally or intraventricularly since they cannot cross the blood–brain barrier by parenteral administration. Disappointingly all these opiate peptides produce tolerance and dependence. Their role in psychiatric disorders is not proven yet and it is uncertain whether they have any endocrine function. Therefore, their actual therapeutic use is still not fully explored.

Types of pain

Pain itself can be acute or chronic. *Acute pain* (e.g. post-operative pain, myocardial infarction and colics, whether intestinal, ureteric or biliary) is commonly of less than 1 month's duration and is due to a known and treatable cause. The pain may cause anxiety but treatment is logical and effective with good results and normal life expectancy. *Chronic pain*, on the other hand, is comparatively uncommon (often neglected), of several months' duration and due to an uncertain cause that is difficult to treat, leading to depression. Treatment is empirical, often only partly effective with sometimes disappointing results and possibly short life expectancy (as in malignancy). The causes of chronic pain include:

Traumatic
● Neuromuscular injuries (e.g. neuroma and tendon injuries)
● Fractures
● Painful scars
● Amputation stump and phantom pain

Degenerative
● Disc protrusion, sciatica and low back pain
● Osteoarthritis
● Ankylosing spondylitis and Paget's disease

Inflammatory
● Post-herpetic neuralgia
● Chronic peptic ulcer
● Chronic pancreatitis

Neoplastic

Vascular
● Lower limb ischaemia
● Sympathetic dystrophy syndrome (Sudeck's atrophy and shoulder–hand syndrome)
● Raynaud's disease

Neurological
● Nerve lesions, entrapment and neuralgias
● Trigeminal (facial) neuralgia
● Headache (migraine)
● Causalgia

GENERAL PRINCIPLES OF MANAGEMENT

The management of pain involves three aspects: physical, emotional and rational.

The physical aspect

1 Removal of noxious stimuli

For example, partial gastrectomy to remove hydrochloric acid content in cases of chronic peptic ulcer, or removal of mechanical obstruction in nerve entrapment.

2 Prevention of neural integration of pain

(a) Natural mechanisms

By counterstimulation which includes rubbing, manipulation, percussion, heating, cooling, acupuncture, electrical stimulation and application of counter-irritants.

(b) Analgesic drugs

The mild non-narcotic analgesics act peripherally by inhibiting prostaglandin synthesis while the narcotics exert their effect on opiate receptors in the CNS. For *mild pain* aspirin (may cause gastrointestinal bleeding) or paracetamol may be used, while for *moderate pain* codeine, dihydrocodeine (may cause constipation), pentazocine (causes dysphoria) and dextropropoxyphene in combination with paracetamol (Distalgesic) are preferred (banned in USA). Pyrazole and indole derivatives have strong anti-inflammatory action and are indicated in chronic painful inflammatory conditions of the joints. As gastric ulcers and serious blood disorders are side-effects, their use is monitored with laboratory tests. Mefenamic acid causes less gastrointestinal bleeding but can cause diarrhoea. For severe and intractable pain, potent analgesics (narcotics) should be considered. Narcotic analgesics fall within the spectrum between pure agonists such as fentanyl and pure antagonists such as naloxone. The following are clinical remarks about some of them.

Morphine   Is the most commonly used; it sets the standard by which all the others are judged. It produces CNS depression (which promotes analgesia, tranquillisation, sleep, respiratory depression and suppression of cough) as well as excitation (vomiting, anxiety and restlessness). It acts directly on smooth muscles, increasing sphincteric tone and decreasing peristalsis (hence constipation, increase in intrabiliary and pancreatic pressure) and is therefore contraindicated in colonic diverticular disease, irritable colon, pancreatitis and biliary colic (unless preceded by an antispasmodic such as atropine and anticholinergic drugs). It may cause euphoria and addiction. Dose 10–20 mg i.m., i.v. or orally.

Diamorphine (heroin)   More powerful analgesic than morphine with more euphoria and less sedation; thus associated with considerable risk of addiction. Its duration of action is half that of morphine, i.e. 2 h, but is otherwise similar to morphine. Dose 5–10 mg i.m. or i.v. on regular basis in terminal care cases.

Methadone   Is effective orally with fewer side-effects; thus used in ambulant patients with intractable pain. It does not cause euphoria and is less addictive. Indeed, morphine addiction is treated by gradual replacement with high doses of methadone which can be terminated eventually without causing morphine withdrawal symptoms. Dose 5–10 mg orally or i.m. *Dextromoramide* and *dipipanone* are similarly used orally for ambulant patients with severe chronic pain.

Pethidine   Is not well absorbed from the gastrointestinal tract. It has short action, causes dry mouth, tachycardia (atropine-like action), hypotension and dysphoria, and it is painful on injection. Phenoperidine and fentanyl similarly have no place in the treatment of chronic pain but are used in general anaesthesia and intensive postoperative cases. Dose 50–100 mg i.m. or i.v.

Pentazocine (Fortal) Shorter in duration, it causes slight respiratory depression but recently it was found that the CO_2 response curve can be depressed as much by pentazocine 60 mg/70 kg as by morphine 10 mg/70 kg. There appears to be a ceiling effect in the anaesthetic action so that increasing the dose produces no further increase in analgesia. Gastric absorption is good but slow. It causes dysphoria and hallucination with less sedation. Pentazocine is less addictive and has minimal effects on smooth muscle (can therefore be given in irritable colon, diverticular disease, biliary and pancreatic disease). It is a narcotic antagonist and 1 mg/kg has been used to reverse respiratory depression produced by fentanyl leaving adequate analgesia for a prolonged period. Dose 30–60 mg orally, i.m. or i.v.

Buprenorphine (Temgesic) Has powerful agonist and partial antagonist actions with low addiction. There is a ceiling effect for its respiratory depression which could well be the case for its analgesic action. Vomiting is troublesome, especially with ambulant patients. The prolonged action (twice that of morphine), availability of the sublingual route and absence of serious side-effects (except for vomiting) makes this drug a considerable advance in the treatment of postoperative pain. Dose 0.3–0.4 mg sublingually.

Butorphanol Is a narcotic antagonist analgesic. It is seven times as potent as morphine and 40–50 times as potent as pethidine and has a similar duration of action. Ceiling effect in its respiratory depression has been reported. Successfully used postoperatively but drowsiness is a common side-effect.

Meptazinol Narcotic antagonist analgesic with potency equal to pethidine in postoperative patients. It produces minimal respiratory depression and sedation.

Nefopam Antihistamine derivative with less anticholinergic and antihistaminic activity. Its non-narcotic analgesic potency in postoperative pain is in the region of 20 mg neforpam, equivalent to 7.5 mg morphine (i.m.). Intravenous injection has ceiling analgesic effect at about 60 mg so that increasing the dose will only increase its side-effects (tachycardia, nausea, sweating and restlessness).

3 Nerve blocks

Using local anaesthetics can be diagnostic (pain relief confirms the selected responsible nerve pathway), prognostic (if no pain relief, no need for neurolytic block as the case is difficult to treat), palliative, and even curative. This can be performed either directly via a needle or for prolonged use via a catheter. Because local anaesthetics selectively affect amyelinated and thin myelinated fibres, motor function is spared. Blocking sites are:

Local infiltration to: tender spots
                        trigger areas

Regional blocks to: brachial plexus
                     cranial nerves
                     peripheral nerves (i.v. and tourniquet – Bier's block)
Sympathetic blocks to: stellate ganglion
                        lumbar ganglion
                        coeliac plexus
Axial blocks to: paravertebral somatic nerves (epidural or intrathecal)

Note: epidural and intrathecal routes can be used for narcotic injection to block pain receptors only (pure analgesia) and for local anaesthetics to block sensory (anaesthesia) and/or motor fibres depending on injected dose.

4 Destructive blocks

(a) Chemical blocks

In this, the commonest form of block, intrathecal injection of alcohol or phenol (in glycerine) as neurolytic agents is employed (extrathecal injection should not be used). Intrathecal injection of hypertonic or iced saline is also used. They take effect in 2–5 days and pain relief lasts for 1–3 months. These blocks should bathe only the required dorsal roots with the agent and must be kept away from ventral roots to avoid motor loss (chemical posterior rhizotomy). Sympathetic ganglia blocks using alcohol or phenol can also be used (chemical sympathectomy).

(b) Physical means

Barbotage is repeated (15 ×) aspiration and replacement of CSF via a wide-bore needle. It damages the dorsal root and offers pain relief for up to 3 months in cancer cases. Cooling CSF before replacement may be painful and requires general anaesthesia.

5 Neurosurgery

Usually needs general anaesthesia. Possible procedures are the following.

- Nerve section or surgical posterior rhizotomy.
- Anterolateral cordotomy on the side opposite the pain. If it is done bilaterally bladder and bowel problems occur and if done bilaterally at the cervical level then the patient may die of sleep apnoea (Ondine's curse) (Fig. 1.2.1).
- Radiofrequency percutaneous cervical cordotomy selectively destroys the lateral spinothalamic tract. It should be done unilaterally.
- Dorsal column stimulation with an electrode implanted intrathecally at laminectomy.
- Stereotactic thalamotomy.
- Cingulotomy.
- Prefrontal leucotomy.
- Pituitary ablation (under image intensifier taking 30 min) by transethmoidal surgery or transnasal radioactive pellets, implantation or alcohol injection or cryoprobe ablation can relieve pain of advanced cancer with secondary deposits (whether hormone-dependent, like breast and prostatic carcinomas, or not).

6 Other modalities

- Specific treatment of underlying disease, e.g. local resection of tumour.
- Endocrine therapy, e.g. calcitonin in Paget's disease, hormones in breast and prostatic carcinomas.
- Radiotherapy, e.g. for bony deposits.
- Chemotherapy, e.g. for Hodgkin's lymphoma.
- Cryosurgery, e.g. in palliation of residual or recurrent malignancy of the oral cavity.
- In trigeminal neuralgia, where the pain is a specific entity rather than a symptom of underlying lesion (as in malignancy), carbamazepine (Tegretol) should be tried first before destructive means.
- Rarely superadded infection (e.g. in malignancy) can be painful and can be treated symptomatically with antibiotics.
- Steroids although not analgesic can lessen the inflammation, improve appetite and elevate mood.

The emotional aspect

Depends on severity, duration and significance of the pain. Its control involves:

- Psychological support: by good doctor–patient relationship and explanation.
- Drug therapy: since morphine suppresses the limbic system it has an adverse emotional effect. Diazepam (anxiolytic) or even chlorpromazine can be used. For depression, imipramine may be used. Psychotropic drugs are being used more and more for analgesia in chronic pain, apart from their psychological effect.
- Psychosurgery: selective operation on the limbic system (emotion centre) such as cingulotomy, is preferred to extensive prefrontal leucotomy.

The rational aspect (paramedical modulation)

The patient can be helped to learn to live with the pain by:
- Good doctor–patient relationship.
- Occupational therapy (a form of distraction).
- Group therapy (to counteract the psychological and social isolation).
- Mental relaxation: by autohypnosis.

REFLEXES

Reflex is an involuntary response to a stimulus. The response can either be a muscle contraction, glandular secretion, or conductive alteration in pulse rate and rhythm; the stimulus can either be external (e.g. pin prick) or internal (e.g. altered blood pH).

The reflex has many important characteristics:
1. Reflex is involuntary.
2. Reflex is purposeful, aiming at protection from noxious stimuli and maintaining the internal homeostasis.
3. Reflex is a stereotyped and specific response to the specific stimulus.
4. Reflex can be prolonged in response to a strong stimulus due to repeated firing of motor neurons (after-discharge).

5. Reflex pattern varies with the part of body stimulated (local sign).
6. Reflexes can be summated to produce greater response (fractionation and final common path).
7. Reflexes can be excited or inhibited by polysynapses via excitatory (with reverberating circuits) or inhibitory interneurons; mild noxious stimulus in marked central excitation in chronic paraplegia may cause prolonged withdrawal of four limbs as well as urination, defecation, sweating and blood pressure changes (mass reflex).

There are three groups of reflexes, depending on the anatomical level.

- *Spinal reflexes* (at the level of spinal cord) are somatic reflexes which can be *monosynaptic*, with one synapse between afferent and efferent neurons, e.g. stretch reflex (elicited in knee jerk, triceps reflex, ankle jerk and other somatic reflexes), which is the only monosynaptic reflex in the body; or *polysynaptic*, which has two to many hundreds of synapses with one or more interneurons interposed between afferent and efferent neurons in the reflex arc, e.g. withdrawal reflex following noxious and usually painful stimuli, abdominal reflex, cremasteric reflex (also temperature, touch, and vibration reflexes). The components of the simplest monosynaptic reflex arc include:
  1. Stimulus
  2. Receptor
  3. Afferent neuron
  4. Synapse with junctional transmission via chemical mediators
  5. Efferent neuron
  6. Effector such as myoneural junction
  7. Response
- *Midbrain reflexes* (at the level of midbrain) are visceral autonomic reflexes following internal alteration in blood pressure and blood gases conducted via baroreceptors and chemoreceptors; they are responsible for maintaining the internal homeostasis.
- *Conditioned reflexes* (at the subcortical level of the brain) are acquired learning reflexes. A conditioned reflex is a reflex to a stimulus which did not previously elicit the response, acquired by repeatedly pairing the stimulus with another stimulus that normally does produce the response, e.g. Pavlov's reflex in dogs: salivation is induced by placing meat in a dog's mouth, but if a bell was rung just before placing meat in a dog's mouth, and this was repeated many times, then the animal would salivate when the bell was rung even though no meat was placed in its mouth; the meat in the mouth produces an *unconditioned* stimulus, as it normally produces an innate response, bell-ringing is the new *conditioned stimulus*, which on frequent pairing with an unconditioned stimulus will produce a response. These reflexes are the basis for training circus animals; an immense number of somatic, visceral and other neural phenomena can be made to occur as conditioned reflex responses. These reflexes are essential for man's acquired learning, memory, instinctual and emotional behaviour after reinforcement by pairing the new conditioned stimulus from time to time with the unconditioned stimulus so that the newly created reflex can persist indefinitely.

1.3 Acid–Base Disturbances in Surgery

Normal hydrogen ion concentrations in arterial blood and extracellular fluid are 36–44 nmol/l. This concentration is expressed as pH, the negative logarithm of hydrogen ion concentrations, and corresponds to a pH of 7.44 to 7.36, respectively.

$$pH = -\log [H]$$

Maintenance of pH over a narrow range despite continued generation of acids during metabolism is accomplished by neutralisation of hydrogen ions with endogenous buffers. Important buffers in plasma are proteins, bicarbonate and reduced haemoglobin. Lungs are important for removal of excess acid as CO_2. In addition, kidneys are important for excretion of acids (see below).

An *acid* is any compound capable of donating H ions to a base. a *base* is any substance which accept H ions. Thus, HCl, H_2SO_4, H_2CO_3 and H_3PO_4 all are acids, while H_2O, NH_3 and anions of salts of weak acids are bases.

Maintenance of arterial pH over a narrow range is necessary to:

1. Ensure optimal functions of enzymes.
2. Maintain proper distribution of electrolytes.
3. Prevent reductions in myocardial contractility.

When pH falls below 7.2, acidosis induces catecholamine release yet with decreased cardiac responsiveness to catecholamines and diminished inotropic effect. Cardiac arrhythmias in the presence of alkalosis may be accentuated by hypokalaemia.

4. Minimise alterations in systemic and pulmonary vascular resistance. For example, alkalosis produces cerebral and coronary artery vasoconstriction.
5. Maintain optimal saturation of haemoglobin with oxygen at prevailing PaO_2. Alkalosis shifts the sigmoid oxyhaemoglobin dissociation curve to the left, thus impairing tissue oxygenation.

Oxygen-haemoglobin dissociation curve The three important conditions that affect the O_2-haemoglobin dissociation curve are blood pH, temperature and concentration of 2, 3-DPG (produced by glycolysis in red blood cells via the Embden-Meyerhof pathway). Acidosis (low pH), fever (increased temperature) and increased 3, 3-DPG contents of red blood cells all shift the curve to the right, thus facilitating tissue oxygenation by decreasing O_2 affinity of haemoglobin (loosening the bound O_2). This decrease in O_2 affinity of haemoglobin when blood pH falls is called 'Bohr effect'. While acidosis directly shifts the curve to right, it also decreases 2, 3-DPG (acidosis inhibits red cells glycolysis) and so indirectly shifts the curve to left; this however, is superseded by its direct effect (resultant shift to the right). For changes in 2, 3-DPG see *Blood transfusion*.

6. Provide a chemical control in the regulation of respiratory centre activity. Hydrogen ion concentration can stimulate the respiratory centre directly via central brain stem chemoreceptors, through cerebrospinal fluid hydrogen ion concentration (which parallels hypercapnoea of arterial PCO_2) and/or indirectly via peripheral chemoreceptors located in the two carotid bodies (one near the carotid bifurcation on each side) and two or more aortic arch bodies through arterial hypoxia or acidosis (low blood pH).

Regulation and control of respiration Spontaneous respiration is under separate voluntary and automatic control. The voluntary system is located in the cerebral cortex, sending impulses down to the respiratory muscles and diaphragm via corticospinal tracts; breathing stops if the spinal cord is transected above the origin of the phrenic nerves.

Automatic respiratory centres are located in the pons and medulla (close to the 4th ventricle) sending impulses via lateral and ventral portions of the spinal cord. Expiratory muscles are inhibited when inspiratory muscles are active, and vice versa (reciprocal innervation). Chemical drive for respiratory stimulation includes mainly arterial hypoxia and acidosis (via carotid and aortic bodies' chemoceptors), and to a certain extent arterial hypercapnoea (via brain stem chemoceptors); conversely, metabolic alkalosis, e.g. after protracted vomiting, depresses ventilation.

Non-chemical stimuli of respiratory centres include afferents from proprioceptors (joint movement stimulates respiration), afferents for sneezing, coughing, swallowing, yawning and Hering-Breuer reflex (expiratory and inspiratory reflex responses to lung inflation and deflation, respectively).

Afferents from higher centres, such as consciousness, and from the limbic system and hypothalamus, such as emotion and pain feeling, can also stimulate respiration; in Ondine's curse, seen clinically in compression of the medulla, bulbar poliomyelitis, or bilateral anterolateral cervical cordotomy for pain, the automatic control of respiration is disrupted without loss of voluntary control, so that the patient can stay alive only by staying awake and remembering to breathe (Ondine is a water nymph in German mythology, who punished her unfaithful lover by casting this curse upon him and taking away all his automatic functions; her lover had to stay awake in order to survive, but eventually fell asleep after sheer exhaustion and his respiration stopped).

BODY BUFFERS

Blood pH is regulated by chemical and physiological buffering mechanisms.

Chemical buffers

- Proteins of plasma, extracellular fluid and cells including haemoglobin. All can act as either base binding H (change into weak acid), or as weak acid giving H to neutralise the added base.
- Plasma bicarbonate (H_2CO_3), while not normally a strong buffer, is present in high concentration in extracellular fluid (24–32 mmol/l), and on buffering strong acids, volatile acid is formed and removed from the lungs as CO_2, and therefore the buffering capacity of plasma bicarbonate is greatly enhanced, making HCO_3/H_2CO_3 the major and most effective buffer. Each litre of extracellular fluid contains 24–32 mmol of HCO_3 and 1.2–1.7 mmol of H_2CO_3, the base/acid ratio is 20/1. The log of 20 is 1.3, which when added to pK of HCO_3 (6.1) = pH of 7.4 (see below).

According to the Henderson–Hasselbalch equation, which determines the pH of a solution containing a weak acid or base:

pH = pK + log base/acid

Example:

pH = pK + log HCO_3/H_2CO_3
pH = 6.1 + log 24/1.2
pH = 6.1 + log 20
pH = 6.1 + 1.3
pH = 7.4

Addition of a strong acid, base/acid ratio would decrease with corresponding decrease in pH. Compensation begins at once by breathing stimulation and alveolar ventilation to remove excess acid (H_2CO_3) as CO_2 through the lungs, thus making this poor chemical buffer a remarkably effective physiological one.

Physiological buffers

- Respiratory system – regulates HCO_3/H_2CO_3 ratio by removing CO_2.
- Kidneys – regulate extracellular bicarbonate and acid excretion by three mechanisms:
  - Reabsorption of 99.9% of filtered HCO_3 normally (mainly in proximal tubules with minimal reabsorption in distal tubules) to keep plasma concentration at 24–32 mmol/l. Any increase in plasma HCO_3 above renal threshold of 28–32 mmol/l leads to appearance of HCO_3 in urine. HCO_3 reabsorption increases if $Paco_2$ increases, if K ion concentration decreases, if Cl ion concentration decreases. (Fig. 1.3.1).

- Excretion of titrable acids via dibasic phosphate to acidic monobasic (H + $NaHPO_4$ → NaH_2PO_4).
- Excretion of ammonia salts (H + NH_3 from deaminated glutamine → NH_4).

The first line of defence therefore is the chemical buffers of cells and extracellular fluid, absorbing the immediate shock of acid or base liberated in the body. In metabolic acidosis, 57% of buffering will be cellular (36% exchange H for Na, 15% H–K exchange, and 6% H–Cl exchange), while 43% of buffering is extracellular, mainly via bicarbonate mechanism in 42% (H + HCO_3 → H_2CO_3 → H_2O + CO_2 removed by lung) with protein in 1%. Respiratory compensation is the second line of defence. Alkalis are poorly compensated by lungs by increasing hypoxia, so concentration of alkali will depend upon HCO_3 excretion by kidneys. The third and final correction of acid–base imbalance depends on renal compensation by excretion of acid or base.

DIFFERENTIAL DIAGNOSIS OF ACID–BASE DISTURBANCES (Fig. 1.3.2)

This is based on direct measurements of arterial pH, $Paco_2$ and plasma bicarbonate concentration. Arterial pH differ-

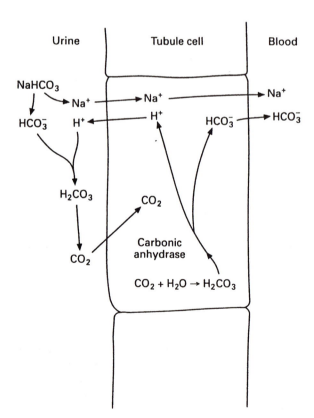

Fig 1.3.1   Reabsorption of filtered bicarbonate

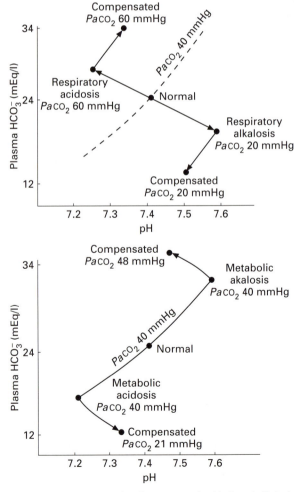

Fig. 1.3.2   Uncompensated and compensated acidosis and alkalosis

entiates between acidosis and alkalosis, while Pa_{CO_2} and plasma bicarbonate concentrations will help distinguish respiratory and metabolic causes of acidosis or alkalosis. Arterial blood is in normal acid–base balance when the:
1. pH is 7.36–7.44
2. Pa_{CO_2} is 40 ± 4 mmHg
3. Plasma bicarbonate concentration is 24 ± 2 mEq/l.
Acidosis is present when arterial pH is less than 7.36; alkalosis is present when arterial pH is greater than 7.44.

By definition, Pa_{CO_2} greater than 44 mmHg represents hypoventilation; hyperventilation is present when Pa_{CO_2} is less than 36 mmHg. Hypoventilation is a synonym with *respiratory acidosis*, and hyperventilation is a synonym with *respiratory alkalosis*. Acidosis and alkalosis not related to alterations in Pa_{CO_2} are considered to be primary metabolic disturbances.

Acid–base disturbances due to respiratory acidosis or alkalosis are compensated for by renal-induced changes in plasma bicarbonates returning the ratio of bicarbonate concentration/CO_2 concentration to 20/1 and thus restoring a normal pH in chronic respiratory acidosis or alkalosis.

Acid–base disturbances due to metabolic acidosis or alkalosis are compensated for by ventilation-induced changes in Pa_{CO_2} leading to hyperventilation or hypoventilation respectively. In metabolic alkaosis, hypoventilatory compensation leads to acute increase in Pa_{CO_2}, which on hydration becomes carbonic acid, thus restoring a normal pH in chronic metabolic acidosis.

Respiratory acidosis (Fig. 1.3.3)

This occurs because of increased Pa_{CO_2} due to hypoventilation resulting from:
1. CNS depression by drugs (barbiturates and opiates) or acute hypoventilation during anaesthesia resulting in depression of the respiratory centre.
2. Neuromuscular diseases, such as myasthenia gravis, poliomyositis, Guillian-Barre syndrome (acute post-infective polyneuritis), diphtheria, poliomyelitis or neuromuscular depression by drugs.
3. Intrinsic pulmonary diseases, such as acute airway obstruction (asthmatic bronchospasm or plugging with mucus secretion or inhaled foreign bodies) and chronic obstructive airway diseases (emphysema and chronic bronchitis).

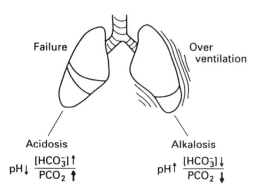

Fig. 1.3.3 Respiratory acidosis and alkalosis

The initial increase in Pa_{CO_2} results in increased carbonic acid (after hydration) which on dissociation increases the concentration of hydrogen ions.

$$CO_2 + H2_O \rightarrow H_2CO_3 \rightarrow HCO_3 + H$$

Since CO_2 readily crosses lipid membranes, such as blood–brain barrier, low pH produced by hydration of CO_2 occurs to similar extents in arterial blood and cerebrospinal fluid (CSF). This low pH results in stimulation of ventilation (to a lesser extent) via carotid bodies, and (to a great extent or 85% of response) via medullary chemoreceptors located on the ventrolateral surface of the 4th ventricle of the brain. With time, CSF pH is restored to normal by active transport of bicarbonate into CSF, and thus removing the stimulus to ventilation.

There is also compensation by secondary increase of bicarbonate produced by hydration of CO_2, of about 1 mEq/l for every 10 mmHg increase in Pa_{CO_2} above 40 mmHg.

Kidneys also compensate by increased excretion of hydrogen ions, resulting in increased reabsorption of bicarbonate by about 2 mEq/l for every 10 mmHg rise in Pa_{CO_2}; thus the total increase in arterial concentration of bicarbonate is 3 mEq/l for every 10 mmHg increase in Pa_{CO_2} above 40 mmHg. With bicarbonate reabsorption, chloride is being excreted with ammonium, resulting in characteristic *hypochloraemia* of chronic respiratory acidosis. Treatment of hypoventilation by artificial mechanical ventilation is necessary in markedly increased Pa_{CO_2}. *Correction must be slow*, otherwise neuromuscular irritability and CNS excitation may occur resulting in seizures. Antibiotics and bronchodilators may also help. It must be realised that O_2 therapy may worsen chronic respiratory acidosis, because this may diminish the sensitivity of the respiratory centre to CO_2 as hypoxia is the major stimulant of the respiratory centre. *If hypoxia is partly or totally corrected, ventilation may deteriorate further, with the patient passing into coma then death.* Oxygen must therefore be given in low concentration under direct supervision.

In the presence of respiratory acidosis complicated or associated with metabolic alkalosis due to pre-existing hypochloraemia (facilitates renal reabsorption of bicarbonate) and hypokalaemia (stimulates renal tubules to excrete hydrogen ions), treatment is mechanical ventilation and i.v. administration of potassium choride.

Respiratory alkalosis (Fig. 1.3.3)

This is always due to hyperventilation, reducing Pa_{CO_2}, and thus decreasing the drive (CO_2 is the main respiratory stimulant) or the stimulus to breathe normally by carotid bodies and medullary chemoreceptors.

$$CO_2 + H_2O \rightarrow H_2CO_3 \rightarrow HCO_3 + H$$

Active bicarbonate transport out of CNS subsequently restores pH of CSF to normal despite persistent hypocarbia (low Pa_{CO_2}). Similarly, hyperventilation during anaesthesia to 20 mmHg for 2 hours results in spontaneous ventilation at lower Pa_{CO_2} than before. Likewise, continued hyperventilation, upon returning to sea level from high altitude, reflects maintenance of ventilation by medullary chemoreceptors exposed to normal CSF pH.

The causes of hyperventilation are:

1. Iatrogenic – mechanical or self-induced (hysteria and anxiety)
2. Decreased barometric pressure as in high altitude
3. CNS injury
4. Arterial hypoxaemia
5. Pulmonary vascular diseases with diffusion defect (alveolar capillary block) resulting in hypoxaemia and hyperventilation.
6. Hepatic disease and hepatic coma
7. Sepsis
8. Fever
9. Pregnancy
10. Salicylate overdose

During hyperventilation, three mechanisms for compensation occur. First, as the arterial pH increases, CO_2 is produced from bicarbonate. Secondly, compensation is by generation of lactic acid from glycolysis. Both mechanisms operate rapidly to reduce bicarbonate by 1 mEq/l for every 10 mmHg decrease in Pa_{CO_2}. The third mechanism is increased renal tubular reabsorption of hydrogen ions reducing bicarbonate by 3 mEq/l for every 10 mmHg reduction in Pa_{CO_2}. Thus, reduction of plasma bicarbonate by these three mechanisms is 5 mEq/l for every 10 mmHg decrease in Pa_{CO_2}, which is sufficient to return pH to normal in chronic hypocarbia. Chloride is retained in the process, and thus mild *hyperchloraemia* and *hypokalaemia* characterise respiratory alkalosis. Treatment is required to correct the underlying disorders. During anaesthesia this can be adjusted by rebreathing the exhaled gases containing excess CO_2. In hysteria and anxiety hyperventilation, rebreathing in a paper bag may help, and if this fails, sedation may be required.

Metabolic acidosis (Fig. 1.3.4)

The decreased pH here is due to accumulation of non-volatile acids following major organ failures. *Plasma bicarbonate is decreased* as a result of acid accumulation or alkali loss. Lungs try to maintain normal pH by hyperventilation to remove excessive acid as CO_2. Metabolic acidosis is dangerous as it depresses cardiac contractility and predisposes to cardiac arrhythmia which is enhanced by the associated *hyperkalaemia* due to H–K ion exchange across cellular buffers in acidosis. Acidosis may also lead to lethargy and coma with clinical manifestations of the underlying diseases (uraemia and diabetic ketoacidosis).

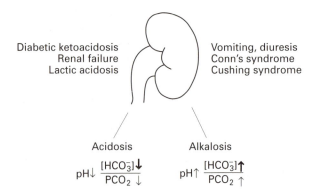

Fig. 1.3.4 Metabolic acidosis and alkalosis

Once metabolic acidosis is documented, the exact cause must be determined; the 'anion gap' or concentration of unmeasured anions is of particular help. Anions in blood and extracellular fluid are Cl (105 mmol/l) and HCO_3 (24 mmol/l) = 129 mmol/l of anions. The cations are Na (140 mmol/l) and K (4 mmol/l) = 144 mmol/l of cations. So the anion gap = 15 mmol/l, due to anions that we do not measure in the laboratory as sulphate and phosphate.

Normally the anion gap = 10–15 mmol/l, but in metabolic acidosis, reduction of HCO_3 may or may not be accompanied by an increase in the anion gap.

Causes of metabolic acidosis with increase in the anion gap are always associated with hyperkalaemia (or occasionally, normal K concentration). If the gap is increased, one can conclude that H ions have been added with some ions other than Cl.

Causes of metabolic acidosis with increased anion gap include:

1. *Diabetic ketoacidosis* due to imbalance between excessive production and poor utilisation of acetoacetic acids, most of which will be converted into beta-hydroxybutyric acid, while some is decarboxylated to acetone resulting in accumulation of these *ketone bodies* in extracellular fluids with metabolic acidosis.
2. *Renal failure*. The kidneys cannot excrete the normal dietary acid load resulting in acid accumulation in extracellular fluid.
3. *Lactic acidosis* due to circulatory insufficiency and poor tissue perfusion seen in shock states and also in liver cirrhosis with decreased removal of lactate. There is a shift from aerobic to anaerobic gycolysis due to decreased delivery of oxygenated blood to tissues. Hypotension and hypoxaemia can predispose to *spontaneous lactic acidosis* with unknown aetiology and fatal outcome; such a condition is associated with diabetes mellitus, hepatic failure, subacute bacterial endocarditis, leukaemia and diabetic patients on phenformine therapy.
4. If a patient with metabolic acidosis and an increase in the anion gap shows no evidence of diabetes or lactic acidosis and is not in failure, serious drug or chemical poisoning must be considered, such as salicylate intoxication, ethylene glycol poisoning, or methyl alcohol poisoning.

Metabolic acidosis with no increase in the anionic gap results in acidosis, due either to reduced bicarbonate or accumulation of H ions with Cl; these conditions therefore are always associated with hypokalaemia and hyperchloraemia, also called *hyperchloraemic metabolic acidosis*. Causes of metabolic acidosis with no increased anion gap include:

1. Diarrhoea – the most common cause, due to loss of bicarbonate in the stool.
2. Drainage of pancreatic juice.
3. Uretero-sigmoidostomy.
4. Renal tubular acidosis (RTA).

Type 1 (distal) RTA results from inability of the distal tubules to secrete H ions in exchange for Na with increase in Na–K exchange; the urine is alkaline in face of systemic acidosis. The urine pH cannot go below 6 despite severe acidosis. This rare condition is commonly idiopathic and transmitted genetically and results in osteomalacia, nephrocalcinosis and hypokalaemia. However, it can be acquired as a result of renal disease, such as pyelonephritis, or as a consequence of myelomatosis, hyperparathyroidism, hyperthyroidism, Wilson's disease, use of degraded tetracycline and increased gamma-globulins in chronic active hepatitis, Sjögren's syndrome (rheumatoid arthritis with keratoconjunctivitis sicca and xerostomia), systemic lupus erythematosus, sarcoidosis, tuberculosis, Hodgkin's disease and liver cirrhosis.

Type 2 (proximal) RTA is due to inability of proximal tubules to reabsorb HCO_3 (normally amounts to 90% of HCO_3) from glomerular filtrate, resulting in delivery of large amounts of HCO_3 to distal tubules which have limited ability of HCO_3 absorption (15%), leading to alkaline urine despite systemic acidosis. However, when metabolic acidosis becomes severe and plasma HCO_3 drops below 12–14 mmol/l, the filtered HCO_3 will be less than capacity of the proximal and distal tubules, and all that is filtered is reabsorbed, resulting in acidic urine with a pH below 5.5 in contrast to distal RTA in which urine pH is always above 6 regardless of how severe the acidosis is. This disease occurs as primary genetically transmitted disease; it is also acquired in many diseases, such as multiple myeloma, Sjögren's syndrome and amyloidosis. Treatment is directed toward the underlying disease. However, if acidosis is life-threatening, HCO_3 therapy is necessary (see below).

Kidneys compensate, first, by increased excretion via the renal tubules of hydrogen ions in the form of ammonium, secondly by hyperventilation induced by low pH stimulation of carotid bodies and active transport of bicarbonate into CNS leading to reduced Pa_{CO_2} in CSF in order to restore CSF pH (there thus will be inhibition of medullary chemoreceptors and blunting hyperventilation induced by carotid bodies) and thirdly by the use of bone buffers to neutralise non-volatile acids in circulation (chronic metabolic acidosis is commonly associated with loss of bone mass).

Metabolic acidosis will reduce Pa_{CO_2} by 1 mmHg for every 1 mEq/l reduction in plasma bicarbonate. Patients with lactic acidosis hyperventilate to a greater degree than ketoacidosis. This is because in lactic acidosis, brain medullary chemoreceptors are exposed to acid produced partly in CNS, while ketoacids produced by diabetics are synthesised in the liver and must be transported across the blood–brain barrier for stimulation of ventilation to occur.

Treatment is by removing the causes for the accumulation of acids in the circulation. Sodium bicarbonate i.v. is indicated when metabolic acidosis is associated with myocardial depression or arrhythmias according to the following formula:

$$\frac{Sodium}{bicarbonate} = \frac{Body}{weight} \times \frac{Plasma}{bicarbonate} \times \frac{\text{Extracellular fluid volume as a fraction of body}}{\text{mass (20\% or 0.2)}}$$

About one-half the calculated dose of sodium bicarbonate should be administered i.v., followed by a repeat measurement of pH to evaluate the impact of therapy. Acute correction of chronic metabolic acidosis is not recommended. In diabetic ketoacidosis, HCO_3 therapy is not required unless it is below 7 mmol/l, since insulin therapy allows rapid oxidation of ketone bodies generating HCO_3.

Metabolic alkalosis Fig 1.3.4)

This is characterised by loss of acids from extracellular fluid (or retention of alkali) resulting in *high plasma bicarbonate*

concentration. Both hypochloraemia and hypokalaemia are usually present in patients with metabolic alkalosis.

Causes of metabolic alkalosis include:

1. Vomiting and nasogastric suction resulting in loss of hydrochloric acid from the stomach, particularly in pyloric stenosis and obstruction, and Zollinger–Ellison syndrome.
2. Diuretic therapy (frusemide and thiazides) inhibiting Na reabsorption in exchange for K by proximal tubules, and thus resulting in increased excretion of K and H ions, leading to metabolic alkalosis.
3. Primary hyperaldosteronism (Conn's syndrome), Cushing's syndrome and exogenous steroid therapy.
4. Bartter's syndrome (hyperplasia of juxtaglomerular apparatus resulting in high renin–angiotensin–aldosterone concentrations leading to hypokalaemia and metabolic alkalosis. Despite these changes, patients are characteristically normotensive, due to surprisingly decreased vascular reactivity to vasopressor actions of angiotensin II and noradrenaline. Another cardinal feature of this syndrome is overproduction of prostaglandins.
5. Milk alkali syndrome in patients with compulsive milk drinking, particularly in patients with neurosis or with peptic ulcer (pain is relieved on drinking an alkaline milk). Excess calcium is absorbed from the bowel leading to hypercalcaemia and resulting in nephrocalcinosis. The ensuing alkalosis aggravates nephrocalcinosis which may result in renal failure.
6. Colorectal villous adenoma (hypokalaemia) and chloride-wasting diarrhoea.
7. Post-hypercapnoeic metabolic alkalosis develops in patients with respiratory failure with high Pa_{CO_2}; the body responds to high Pa_{CO_2} by increasing HCO_3 to maintain the ratio of HCO_3/H_2CO_3 of 20/1.

Another cause of metabolic alkalosis is overzealous i.v. administration of sodium bicarbonate to treat metabolic acidosis; conversion of lactate present in *i.v.* fluid solutions (e.g. Ringer's lactate) to bicarbonate by the liver can also contribute to metabolic alkalosis.

The first line of defence by tissue buffers is the movement of H ions from cells to extracellular fluid in exchange for Na and K. Compensation evoked by metabolic alkalosis includes pulmonary and renal correction; the lungs compensate immediately by hypoventilation increasing Pa_{CO_2} (increased H_2CO_3 to restore HCO_3/H_2CO_3 ratio of 20/1). The final, and third, correction is decreased renal tubular excretion of hydrogen ions and increased excretion of HCO_3 excess; renal threshold is 28–32 mmol/l (see also below).

Increases in Pa_{CO_2} will initially stimulate medullary chemoreceptors, and thus offset the compensatory hypoventilation. With time, CSF pH is normalised despite increased Pa_{CO_2}.

Depletion of intravascular fluid volume is the most important factor in the maintenance of metabolic alkalosis. Indeed, hypovolaemia should be considered in postoperative patients who develop metabolic alkalosis. Hypokalaemia (with skeletal muscle weakness) often complicates metabolic alkalosis.

An abnormally high renal threshold may account for frequent cases of metabolic alkalosis (plasma HCO_3 40–50 mmol/l) seen in patients who are neither receiving HCO_3 nor losing gastric juice; this is supported by their typically acidic urine (low pH) with no HCO_3 (*paradoxical aciduria*) despite systemic alkalosis. Such paradoxical aciduria is seen in advanced pyloric stenosis after loss of HCl acid (metabolic alkalosis), renal response by excreting alkaline urine with Na and K excretion (until K is depleted and not available for Na exchange), followed by exchange of H ions for Na reabsorption leading to acidic urine. This may be accentuated by hypokalaemic damage to the kidneys (hypokalaemic nephropathy).

Treatment is directed at correction of the underlying causes, plus appropriate replacement of electrolytes (replacement therapy of Cl and K by normal saline and KCl) and correction of dehydration (following vomiting). Diuretic therapy may be supplemented by KCl or changed into K-sparing diuretics. Infusion i.v. of hydrogen ions in the form of ammonium chloride or 0.1 N hydrochloric acid is used to facilitate the return of arterial pH to near normal; this requires insertion of a central venous catheter, as peripheral injections can cause sclerosis of veins and haemolysis. Tumours (Conn's syndrome, Cushing's syndrome and Bartter's syndrome) may require surgical excision.

1.4 Fluid and Electrolyte Disorders in Surgery

Alterations of water and electrolytes content and distribution can produce multi-system dysfunction in the perioperative period. Impairment of CNS, cardiac and neuromuscular function are likely in the presence of water and electrolyte (sodium, potassium, calcium, magnesium) disorders. Furthermore, these disorders often accompany events associated with the perioperative period.

Body mass = Body fat + Fat-free body mass

The body fat is the storage fat, mainly in subcutaneous tissues, but nearly half of it is in less visible sites, such as the abdominal cavity. Body fat constitutes a major energy store of the body. Thus for two patients of equal weight, the fatter patient has less fluid, electrolytes and metabolic requirements.

The fat-free body mass is composed of:

Water + Minerals + Protein + Glycogen

In healthy subjects 70% of the fat-free body mass is water (in emaciated, very ill surgical patient it may increase to over 80%).

Total body water content is greatest at birth (70% of body weight in kilogrammes). With increasing age, total body water decreases, constituting 60% in adult man and 50% in adult woman; this difference is due to greater fat content of women. Since fat is essentially anhydrous, it contributes to body weight without a proportionate increase in the volume of total body water.

Constant total body water content is important for viability of cells and for being the medium for all metabolic reactions; all nutrients and solutes of the body are dissolved or suspended in water.

Body water comprises intracellular (55%) and extracellular water (45%).

About 55% of body protein is intracellular, 45% being intravascular solute plasma proteins and extracellular connective tissue protein and skeletal protein.

Most of the minerals are contained in the skeleton; the remainder, less than 0.5 kg in weight, play a more crucial role in water distribution.

Glycogen stores weigh less than 0.5 kg and provide an emergency energy source.

BODY WATER (Figs 1.4.1, 1.4.2)

The total body water is distributed into:
● Intracellular compartment (55%)
● Extracellular compartment (45%), subdivided into:
   – interstitial fluid (37%)
   – intravascular fluid or plasma (8%)

Transcellular fluid represents the natural secretions of the body (not a transudate of plasma or lymph) with continuous movement across the barriers within the extracellular compartment; it mainly includes intraluminal gastrointestinal fluids as well as secretions of the exocrine glands, liver, biliary tree, kidneys and eyes, cerebrospinal, pleural, pericardial and peritoneal fluid and synovial fluid contained within the joints and synovial sheaths. Thus in patients with distal intestinal obstruction, the transcellular fluid may be 5–10 times that of normal GIT secretions and will be at the expense of other extracellular water. In severe sepsis, peritonitis, and extensive burns, large fluid translocations occur. In ascites, pericardial and pleural effusion, the fluid loss is referred to as invisible loss which must be considered in fluid replacement therapy.

In soft-tissue injuries or after extensive dissection in major surgery, extracellular fluid accumulates around the area of injury (*3rd space phenomenon*).

Almost all illness results in a redistribution of body water. ECW tends to be maintained as wasting proceeds. The ECW, including plasma and interstitial water, maintains volume while cell mass shrinks. The practical implication of this is that very wasted surgical patients who are not clinically sodium-and water-depleted are intolerant of excessive salt and water loads; there is a tendency to oedema, hypoproteinaemia and hypotonicity.

Acute reductions in intravascular fluid volume (hypovolaemia), as occur with fluid deprivation in the preoperative period, blood loss, or surgical trauma that results in tissue oedema (*3rd space loss*), elicit the release of antidiuretic hormone and renin acting on renal tubules and leading to restoration of intravascular fluid volume. The interstitial fluid is in dynamic equilibrium with intravascular fluid, serving as a reservoir from which water and electrolytes can be mobilised into circulation. Conversely, interstitial fluid spaces can accept water and electrolytes if these substances are present in excess in intravascular fluid spaces; peripheral oedema is a manifestation of excess water in interstitial fluid spaces. Water moves freely across cell and capillary membranes depending on osmotic, hydrostatic and oncotic pressures.

Osmotic pressure is the pressure necessary to prevent movement of solvent (water) to another fluid space across cell

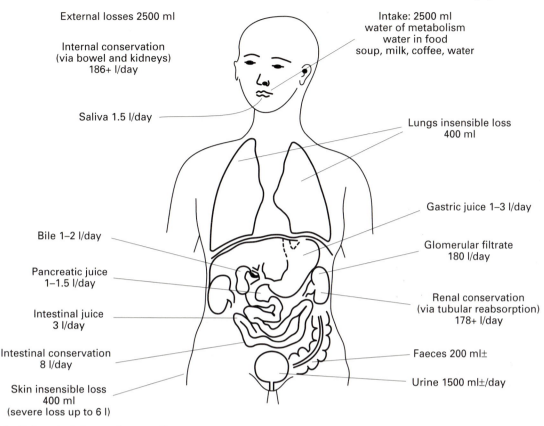

Fig. 1.4.1 Daily water balance and conservation

membrane; it depends on the number of molecules or ions (osmoles) present in the solvent. Osmolarity denotes the concentration of solute (osmoles) present in 1 litre of water. Sodium is the most important cation for determining plasma osmolarity. Indeed, plasma osmolarity can be predicted clini-

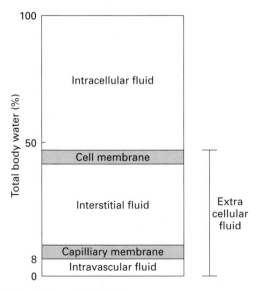

Fig. 1.4.2 Body water distribution

cally by doubling the plasma sodium concentration. Low plasma osmolarity (below 285 mosmol/l) means a high concentration of water; a high osmolarity (above 295 mosmol/l) means a low water concentration. Intravenous solutions are considered isotonic, hypotonic, or hypertonic according to their effective osmotic pressures relative to plasma. Normal saline and 5% glucose in water has an osmolarity similar to body fluids (isotonic). However, cellular uptake of glucose present in 5% glucose in water results in hypotonic solutions; the resulting free water can distribute itself among all fluid compartments with less than 10% remaining intravascular. Lactated Ringer's solution, containing 5% glucose, is initially hypertonic (527 mosmol/l), but the hypertonicity diminishes as glucose is metabolised and taken up by cells.

Movement of water across cell membranes is influenced by osmotic pressure and not by hydrostatic pressure, since the transmembrane pressures exerted by the latter are low. Conversely, the pressure produced by the heart results in a hydrostatic pressure gradient of approximately 20 mmHg across capillary membranes. If this pressure gradient is not counterbalanced, it tends to force intravascular water into the interstitial fluid compartment. Indeed, were it not for large protein molecules (principally albumin), which cannot freely cross capillary membranes, there would be continuous loss of intravascular fluid volume. The concentrations of these proteins are just sufficient to balance the hydrostatic pressure difference of 20 mmHg that exists between the intravascular and interstitial fluid compartments. This osmotic effect produced by proteins maintains the circulating plasma volume and is called 'the colloid osmotic' or 'oncotic pressure'. An important way to increase circulating plasma volume is to infuse albumin, which draws water from the interstitial into the intravascular fluid space.

DISTRIBUTION OF ELECTROLYTES

The major cation in intravascular fluid is sodium, plus small amounts of potassium, calcium, and magnesium. In contrast, the major cation in intracellular fluid is potassium. The net effect is a concentration of total cation that is esentially equal throughout body water. These positive charges are balanced by anions such as chloride, bicarbonate, phosphate and the negative charged sites on proteins.

Changes in sodium concentrations in extracellular fluid are usually due to changes in the volume of solvent (water) and not changes in total body content of sodium. Therefore, changes in plasma sodium concentrations must be interpreted with respect to total body water content. Indeed, acute changes in plasma sodium concentrations usually reflect alterations in total body water content and not sodium content.

Electrophysiology of excitable cells (nerve and muscle)
(Fig. 1.4.3)

This is dependent on intracellular and extracellular concentrations of sodium, potassium and calcium. The interior of cells is negative relative to exterior; at rest this resting membrane potential (RMP) is –90 mV with respect to the outside of cells. The stimulus (electrical, chemical, or mechanical) results in altered permeability of cell membranes, such that sodium enters and potassium leaves the cells, resulting in spontaneous depolarisation (so that the RMP becomes less negative), until the threshold potential is reached at about –70 mV. When the threshold potential is reached, there are sudden increases in permeability of cell membrane to sodium influx that produces an action potential starting with rapid depolarisation. After this propagation of the action potential with maximum depolarisa-

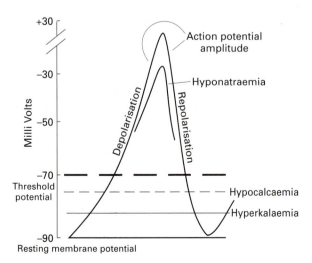

Fig. 1.4.3   Electrophysiology of automatic pacemaker cell

tion, the permeability of cell membranes is restored; sodium is pumped out of the cells and repolarisation ensues. Automatic cardiac pacemaker cells differ from the contractile cells in that the RMP is not stable but undergoes spontaneous depolarisation until the threshold potential is reached.

This electrophysiology is altered by changes in electrolyte concentrations. Sodium is essential for cellular depolarisation and generation of action potential; the amplitude of action potential is decreased in hyponatraemia. Potassium gradients across cell membranes are the most important determinants of RMP; hyperkalaemia results in less negative RMP that are closer to threshold potential, i.e. the excitability of cells is increased so that a smaller impulse can elicit an action potential. Conversely, hypokalaemia results in more negative RMP. Calcium is also necessary for maintenance of threshold potential; hypocalcaemia results in more negative threshold potential.

Renal regulation of sodium excretion and water volume
(Fig. 1.4.4)

Sodium excretion and therefore volume may be regarded as the result of interplay of three factors: glomerular filtration rate (GFR), aldosterone and 'third factor'.

- *GFR*   Na excreted in urine = Na filtered (Na load) – Na reabsorbed. Increased filtered Na (via glomerulus) leads to increased Na reabsorption (via tubules) and vice versa. This proportional glomerulotubular balance occurs predominantly in proximal tubules and is *not* under hormonal control.
- *Aldosterone*   This hormone is secreted from zona glomerulosa of the cortex of the adrenal gland. In normal man, output of aldosterone is increased during dietary salt restriction and is decreased during high salt intake. Its secretion is also controlled by renin–angiotensin (see below). Aldosterone acts on a variety of epithelial tissue including distal renal tubules, where it stimulates Na-K and Na-H exchange (cation exchange) leading to Na retention (reabsorption) with K and H ions excretion. Distal renal tubules are also the site of another hormonal control i.e. ADH leading to water reabsorption (retention) (Fig. 1.4.5).
- Third Factor (GFR is the first factor and aldosterone the second). This is an unknown factor that influences Na excretion by the kidneys.

GFR, plasma creatinine and plasma urea

In clinical practice, plasma concentrations of creatinine and urea provide a guide to GFR; their clearance usually parallels GFR, but if GFR falls their plasma concentrations rise. Due to problems in measurement of inulin clearance, the renal clearance of endogenous creatinine is widely used clinically to estimate GFR. Plasma creatinine (normally 50–100 µmol/l or 0.05–0.1 mmol/l) is the best single guide to renal function. It depends on muscle bulk and is thus lower in children, women and the elderly, but tends to be reasonably constant in that particular person. It is relatively independent of diet, unlike plasma urea. Plasma urea (normally 2.5–8 mmol/l) is the principal breakdown product of protein metabolism; it reflects diet and protein intake, starvation (paradoxically due to

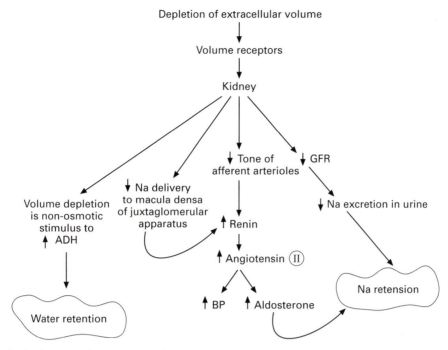

Fig. 1.4.4   Net result of volume depletion is Na and H₂O retention

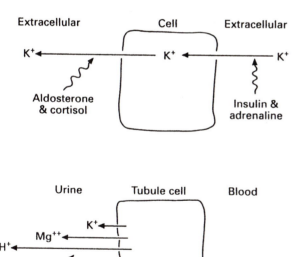

Fig. 1.4.5   Actions of aldosterone as compared with other hormones

associated acceleration of endogenous protein catabolism), catabolic state and hydration. In clinical practice urea concentration correlates with uraemic symptoms. For instance, a patient with severe renal failure and a plasma creatinine of 1000 μmol/l may be nauseated, anorexic and lethargic with urea of 40 mmol/l but may feel well following low protein diet with same creatinine but urea of 20 mmol/l.

The ratio of plasma urea (mmol/l) to creatinine (μmol/l) provides further useful information. The ratio is normal in normal renal function (7/100), moderate chronic renal failure, and severe chronic renal failure. If ratio is high, diuretic therapy, dehydration, fever, profound catabolism, steroid therapy, GIT bleeding or obstruction should be considered. A low ratio is associated with a low protein diet or severe liver disease. GFR increases in pregnancy so that both plasma creatinine and urea are normally low. Notice that both plasma creatinine and urea concentrations:

– show little changes until a functional loss of one kidney.

– lag behind changes in GFR e.g. during first few days of acute renal failure there may be gross reduction in GFR with initially a relatively small rise in plasma urea or creatinine.

– may change unproportionately following a small reduction of a pre-existing low GFR e.g. patient with moderate renal failure and plasma urea of 10 mmol/l may develop heart failure or GIT haemorrhage with a rise in plasma urea to 30 mmol/l due to a superimposed decrease in GFR of only 10 ml/min.

Renin–Angiotensin–Aldosterone System (Fig. 1.4.6)

The afferent arteriole, just before entering Bowman's capsule (to form the glomerulus), becomes closely applied to the distal convoluted tubule of the same nephron. Cells of media and adventitia of the afferent arteriole become more numerous and modified in form and histological staining forming a thickened cuff known as Polkissen cells or polar-cushion cells or juxtaglomerular cells of the afferent arteriole; the opposing specialised segment of distal convoluted tubule is called macula densa. Together the two structures are termed juxtaglomerular apparatus, which serves an important endocrine function. Granular cells of Polkissen secrete renin, while macula densa acts as a sensor organ responding to Na concentration of distal tubular urine and controls renin output

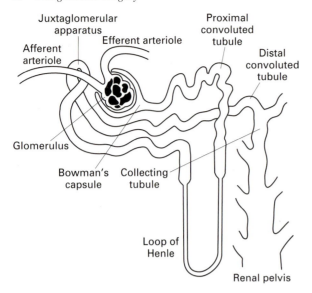

Fig. 1.4.6   Anatomy of a nephron

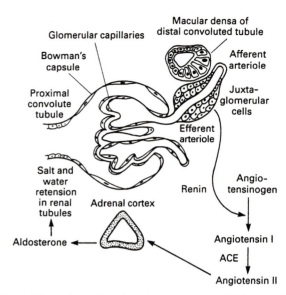

Fig. 1.4.7   Renin–angiotensin–aldosterone system. ACE = angiotensin-converting enzyme

from its associated Polkissen. The juxtaglomerular apparatus secretes renin in response to:

- Beta-adrenergic stimulation. That is why beta-adrenergic blockers (e.g. propranolol) may be effective in decreasing renin release.
- Decreased perfusion pressure or tone in afferent arterioles. This can be seen in volume depletion or renal ischaemia.
- Reductions in Na load delivered to distal convoluted tubules.

Renin is a proteolytic enzyme that acts on angiotensinogen (alpha-2 globulin synthesised in the liver) to form angiotensin I. Angiotensin I in the blood is then split by converting enzyme in lungs to form Angiotensin II which has two actions: stimulation of aldosterone secretion from adrenal cortex (zona glomerulosa), and potent renal artery vasoconstriction (with subsequent decreases in renal blood flow and GFR and inhibition of renal tubular reabsorption of Na) (Fig. 1.4.7).

Total body water excess

The hallmark here is hyponatraemia in the presence of normal or increased intravascular fluid volume. Because kidneys have an extraordinary ability to excrete increased amounts of body water, patients here are likely to have impaired renal function due to associated congestive heart failure, nephrosis and cirrhosis of the liver. Peripheral oedema is a manifestation of excess body water. Excess body water can also be due to inappropriate secretion of antidiuretic hormone, but oedema does not occur. Intravascular absorption of large volumes of water, as during transurethral resection of the prostate, can result in iatrogenic water intoxication. Regardless of aetiology, excess body water results in reduction of plasma sodium and plasma osmolarity. Clinically, the picture is that of hyponatraemia; it depends on the absolute plasma sodium concentrations and the rate of its decline. Below 120 mEq/l, CNS symptoms of confusion and drowsiness occur. Below 110 mEq/L, seizures and coma occur. These CNS abnormalities reflect

cerebral oedema and increased intracranial pressure. Below 100 mEq/L, cardiac arrhythmias, including ventricular fibrillation, may occur.

The **emergency treatment** aims at reduction of cerebral oedema by hypertonic saline or mannitol. Every 1 ml of 5% saline will increase sodium concentrations of a litre of body water by 1 mEq. So, to increase plasma sodium concentrations from 130 mEq/l to 140 mEq/l in a 70 kg adult male (predicted total body water content = 70 × 60/100 = 42 l) would require about 420 ml of 5% saline (1 ml × 140 – 130 mEq × 42 l). The rate of sodium administration varies from 30 minutes to several hours, depending on the urgency of the situation and should stop once seizures cease or cardiac arrhythmias are corrected. In contrast to saline, mannitol not only removes water from cells, but also results in an osmotic diuresis. Both saline and mannitol will initially expand the extracellular fluid volume.

Inappropriate secretion of antidiuretic hormone (ISADH)

ISADH was first described in 1957 in a patient with bronchogenic cancer secreting ADH-like substances continuously and autonomously causing severe water retention and hypotonicity which failed to suppress the release of ADH.

ISADH therefore, results in water retention (hypo-osmolality similar to water intoxication), low output of a highly concentrated urine and dilutional hyponatraemia. Urinary excretion of sodium is increased, which further lowers plasma sodium. Despite excessive sodium loss, hypovolaemia does not occur, since the concomitant water retention has expanded the intravascular fluid volume. The secretion is inappropriate because there is no physiological stimulus or body demand for ADH. Physiologically, ADH is released from posterior pituitary in response to hyperosmolality (high osmotic pressure via brain osmoreceptors), or after non-osmotic stimuli, such as hypotension (secondary to vascular or extracellular volume contraction via carotid and aortic baroreceptors), emotional stress (pain and fear), trauma and surgery and drugs (morphine, barbiturates and nicotine).

ISADH has been described in the following situations:
1. Postoperative period (though ADH secretion is considered appropriate postoperatively by many physiologists)
2. Positive pressure ventilation
3. Endocrine disorders
– Myxoedema
– Adrenal cortical insufficiency
– Anterior pituitary damage
4. Tumours, such as bronchogenic carcinoma, pancreatic carcinoma and lymphosarcoma
5. Infections, such as pneumonia, pulmonary tuberculosis and lung abscess
6. CNS dysfunction
– Haemorrhage
– Trauma (head injury)
– Brain tumours
7. Drugs
– Chlorpropamide
– Opioids
– Diuretics
– Antimetabolites
8. Acute intermittent porphyria

The possible occurrence of ISADH in the postoperative period should be carefully observed; a consistent metabolic response to surgery is the release of ADH for up to 96 hours postoperatively. Indeed, acute hyponatraemia is the most common acute biochemical disorder found after surgery. The most likely mechanism for this hyponatraemia is acute expansion of intravascular fluid volume secondary to hormone-induced reabsorption of water by renal tubules. This excessive hormone secretion (ADH and also aldosterone) may be an exaggerated response to decreases in intravascular fluid volume occurring during invasive operations. Abrupt reduction in plasma sodium (especially below 110 mmEq/l) can lead to cerebral oedema and seizures. *Indeed, i.v. administration of sodium-deficient solutions to oliguric postoperative patients has led to hyponatraemia, seizures and permanent brain damage.*

Inappropriately elevated urinary sodium and osmolarity in the presence of hyponatraemia and decreased plasma osmolarity (less than 280 mosmol/l) is virtually diagnostic of ISADH.

Treatment is initially with restriction of water intake to 500 ml/day. Establishment of a negative water balance leads to spontaneous decreases in the release of ADH and often is the only treatment necessary in postoperative patients in whom ISADH is transient. Demeclocycline may be administered to antagonise effects of ADH on renal tubules. However, these measures are not immediately effective for the management of the clinical manifestations of hyponatraemia. In these patients, i.v. infusion of hypertonic saline sufficient to elevate plasma sodium concentration by 0.5 mEq/h is a useful practice. Overly rapid correction of symptomatic hyponatraemia has been associated with a fatal neurological disorder known as 'central pontine myelinolysis'.

Iatrogenic water intoxication

The most likely cause is the intravascular absorption of large volumes of non-electrolyte solutions used for irrigation during transurethral resection of the prostate. The volume of water absorbed during this procedure has been estimated to be 10–30 ml for every minute of resection time. Dilution of plasma sodium due to absorption of non-electrolyte solutions can occur precipitously, leading to grand mal seizures, particularly if plasma sodium is below 120 mEq/l. Visual disturbances may accompany cerebral oedema. Hypertension, bradycardia, increased CVP, agitation and pulmonary oedema may all occur. Plasma osmolarity and haematocrit are predictably decreased. A high index of suspicion is important in early detection and recognition of iatrogenic water intoxication.

Treatment of water intoxication is with saline, guided by repeated measurements of plasma sodium. Congestive heart failure may require administration of diuretics (frusemide) and digitalis.

Total body water deficits

The hallmark is plasma sodium above 145 mEq/l. Pure water deficits are rare, as most conditions leading to water loss are also accompanied by loss of electrolytes. Causes of pure water loss include deficiencies or absence of ADH (diabetes insipidus) or resistance of renal tubules to the effects of this hormone, e.g. in hypercalcaemia, hypokalemia and chronic nephritis. Pure water deficits can also occur in elderly or confused patients who do not respond to the sensation of thirst. Prolonged mechanical ventilation with unhumidified gases can also lead to substantial water loss.

Clinically, mucous membranes are dry and skin less turgid; when dehydration is severe, blood pressure, central venous pressure and urine output are reduced while the heart rate is increased. Postural hypotension may also be present. Peripheral cyanosis reflects a sluggish peripheral circulation with maked venous desaturation. CNS dysfunction, e.g. drowsiness and coma, may also occur. Haematocrit (PCV) will not rise significantly because intracellular and extracellular compartments are both reduced. Blood urea nitrogen and serum creatinine concentrations will increase, as hypovolaemia produces decreases in blood pressure and cardiac output leading to reduced renal blood flow and GFR. Urine osmolarity will be high (above 800 mOsmol/l) and specific gravity will be high too (above 1.030). Peripheral oedema is absent.

Treatment consists of administering free water or 5% dextrose in water guided by changes in blood pressure, CVP, urine output and repeated determinations of plasma sodium concentration. Rapid correction may lead to cerebral oedema.

Anaesthesia (while operating on such patients) may induce hypotension with exaggerated barbiturate action due to the patient's increased sensitivity to muscle relaxants.

Hypernatraemia (plasma sodium above 145 mEq/l)

The kidneys closely regulate total body sodium content, such that sodium excess is almost impossible unless there is altered renal function. Impairment of sodium excretion by kidneys often occurs in patients with congestive heart failure, nephrotic syndrome and liver cirrhosis with ascites due to secondary hyperaldosteronism; this, however, is counterbalanced by dilutional hyponatraemia due to inadequate circulation (despite expanded extracellular volume) leading to ADH secretion.

Hypernatraemia predominates in primary aldosteronism, yet with little expansion of the interstitial fluid volume. However, the most common cause of hypernatraemia is not an excess of total body sodium, but rather a decrease in the total body water. A hemiplegic patient with cerebrovascular accident (CVA) with aphasia can neither walk nor move to drink water, nor can ask for it. Diabetes insipidus patients with polydipsia and polyuria are usually in balance, but if they stop drinking (due to coma, head injury with damage to thirst centre) negative water balance occurs and they become hypernatraemic. A head injury, therefore, may either produce ISADH resulting in hyponatraemia, or may damage the posterior pituitary causing diabetes insipidus which, with coma, may cause hypernatraemia; however, the majority of head injuries are not associated with Na alterations.

Tube hyperosmotic enteral feeding without adequate water may result in hypernatraemia too.

Clinically, peripheral oedema is the hallmark of hypernatraemia (see Fig. 2.4.1); interstitial fluid spaces, however, can be expanded by as much as 5 L in normal adults before oedema is detectable. Other clinical features include ascites, pleural effusion and expanded intravascular compartment manifested as hypertension.

Treatment is by enhancing sodium excretion via kidneys by the administration of diuretics that prevent reabsorption of sodium by renal tubules.

Hyponatraemia (plasma sodium below 135 mEq/l)
(Fig 1.4.8)

Excessive sodium loss occurs in volume depletion resulting from combined GIT losses (vomiting, nasogastric suction, diarrhoea, pancreatobiliary fistula, ileostomy), Kidney losses (chronic renal failure, diuretic phase of acute renal tubular necrosis, administration of thiazide diuretics and adrenal insufficiency – Addison's disease), and/or skin losses (diaphoresis or perspiration, third-degree burns). However, the most common cause of hyponatraemia is not the deficiency of total

body sodium, but rather an excess of total body water. Clinically, sodium deficit is evidenced by decreased intravascular fluid volume and cardiac output. Conversely, hyponatraemia due to excess of total body water is associated with an increased intravascular fluid volume, such as heart failure, liver cirrhosis, nephrotic syndrome (oedematous patients with circulatory insufficiency) and ISADH (no circulatory insufficiency). Furthermore, hyperglycaemia in uncontrolled diabetics may expand extracellular volume by hyperosmolarity leading to hyponatraemia; this can be corrected by insulin therapy to distribute free glucose into cells. In *sick-cell syndrome* seen in malnutrition and chronic diseases, osmoreceptors are set at a lower level and can eventually lead to hyponatraemia.

Manifestations of reduced intravascular fluid volume include decreased blood pressure, venous pressure and GFR with increased heart rate. Haematocrit (PCV) is typically increased, reflecting reductions in intravascular fluid volume without concomitant loss of erythrocytes. Hyponatraemia with reduced interstitial fluid volume is reflected by decreases in skin turgor. Because underlying fat can also affect skin elasticity, a useful site to look for decreased skin turgor is the forehead. Loss of skin elasticity in limbs can not be distinguished from poor skin turgor of the ageing process.

Failure of sodium pump mechanisms (*sick cell syndrome*) results in passage of sodium into cells. As a result, other ions leave cells, and hyponatraemia is not associated with expected decrease in plasma osmolarity.

Treatment is difficult because of the associated loss of body water. The deficit can be calculated according to this formula:

$$Sodium\ deficit = 140 - Plasma\ sodium \times Total\ body\ water$$

For example: the predicted sodium deficit in 80 kg male (total body water is 60%) with plasma sodium concentration of 120 mEq/l would be calculated as:

$$= (140 - 120) \times (weight\ in\ kg \times 0.6)$$
$$= (140 - 120) \times (80 \times 0.6)$$
$$= 20 \times 48$$
$$= 960\ mEq$$

Despite calculation of the deficit, use of hypertonic saline is usually reversed for symptomatic hyponatraemia when sodium concentration is below 110 mEq/l.

Hyperkalaemia (plasma potassium above 5.5 mEq/l)

This can be due either to increased total body potassium content or alterations in potassium distribution between intracellular and extracellular sites.

Increased total body potassium content

Kidneys are unable to excrete sufficient potassium cations to maintain plasma concentration below 5.5 mEq/l. Patients with severe renal disease (but not requiring haemodialysis), may be vulnerable to hyperkalemia if they are challenged with potassium loads; such potential hazard must be considered when penicillin (1.7 mEq/l of potassium for every 1 million units of penicillin) or banked whole blood (1 mEq/l/day of

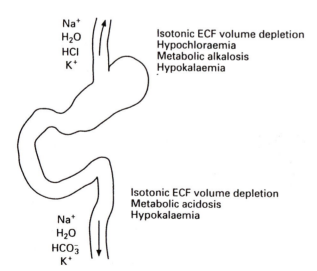

Na⁺
H₂O
HCl
K⁺

Isotonic ECF volume depletion
Hypochloraemia
Metabolic alkalosis
Hypokalaemia

Isotonic ECF volume depletion
Metabolic acidosis
Hypokalaemia

Na⁺
H₂O
HCO₃⁻
K⁺

Fig. 1.4.8 Effects of vomiting and diarrhoea. Vomiting can be due to cicatrised peptic ulcer, pyloric carcinoma and congenital pyloric stenosis

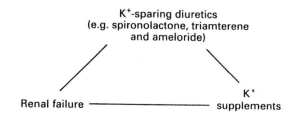

Fig. 1.4.9   The dangerous triad in hyperkalaemia

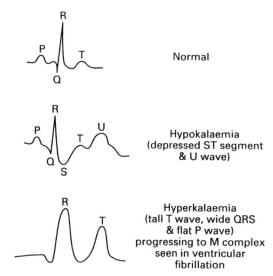

Fig. 1.4.10   ECG changes in hypo- and hyperkalaemia

storage) is administered to patients with chronic renal disease (Fig 1.4.9).

Thus the underlying conditions are renal and adrenal diseases:
– acute oliguric renal failure
– chronic renal disease usually in terminal stages (GFR less than 15 ml/min)
– decreased aldosterone secretion:
    adrenal cortex disease (Addison's disease)
    potassium-sparing diuretics (spironolactone and triamterene acting as aldosterone antagonists)

Altered potassium distribution between intracellular and extracellular sites

● Respiratory or metabolic acidosis enhances passage of potassium from intracellular to extracellular locations. Specifically a 0.1 unit decrease in arterial pH, as produced by a 10 mmHg increase of $Paco_2$, can increase plasma potassium concentrations by 0.5 mEq/l.
● Chemotherapy can lead to tumour lysis and release of intracellular constituents, including potassium. This response is most likely to occur in patients receiving cancer chemotherapeutic drugs for treatment of leukaemia or lymphoma.
● Iatrogenic (exogenous) i.v. bolus administration due to poor mixing of potassium chloride in plastic fluid containers. However, the likelihood of inadequate mixing is minimal when potassium chloride is added, with the plastic bags held in the vertical position with the injection port uppermost.
● Patients with diabetes mellitus can have increased potassium concentrations due to impaired glucose transfer into cells due to the absence of insulin.
● Succinylcholine administration to patients with burns, spinal cord transection or muscle trauma may lead to release of intracellular potassium and subsequent hyperkalaemia.

Clinically, acute hyperkalaemia is usually symptomatic while chronic hyperkalaemia is often asymptomatic due to normalisation of gradients between extracellular and intracellular concentrations of potassium and return of the resting membrane potentials of excitable cells to near normal.

The most detrimental effect of hyperkalaemia is on the cardiac conduction. Characteristic ECG changes include: prolonged P–R interval with ultimate loss of P waves, broadening QRS complexes, ST segment elevation, and peaking of T-waves (atrial standstill with intraventricular block, sometimes indistinguishable from idioventricular rhythm or acute myocardial infarction). Peaking T-waves (tented T-waves), although diagnostic, occurs in less than 25% of patients with hyperkalaemia (Fig 1.4.10). ECG changes depend on the absolute levels of plasma potassium and on the rapidity with which plasma potassium concentrations have increased. Thus, cardiac conduction abnormalities are frequently present when plasma potassium concentration exceed 6.5 mEq/l, although these changes can occur at even lower plasma potassium concentration if the increase has been acute. Peaked T-waves and ventricular arrhythmia seem to be most likely when plasma potassium concentrations approach 7 mEq/l, and although ventricular fibrillation can occur, the more likely event in the presence of hyperkalaemia is *cardiac standstill in diastole*. Furthermore, hyperkalaemia is often accompanied by skeletal muscle weakness of obscure mechanism. Treatment of acute hyperkalaemia is designed to move potassium from plasma into cells and to antagonise effects of potassium on the heart. If plasma potassium concentrations are less than 6.5 mEq/l and there are no indications of cardiac toxicity on the ECG, the treatment of hyperkalaemia may be conservative, being directed at correction of the underlying condition.
● The exogenous potassium chloride administration (if any) must be stopped immediately.
● The quickest way for reversal of the cardiac effects of hyperkalaemia is i.v. administration of calcium (rapid onset with a duration of action of 15–30 min). This is given i.v. as 20 ml of 10% calcium gluconate over 10 min. every 2–4 h.
● Potassium can be shifted into cells by production of systemic alkalosis (hyperventilation of lungs or administration of sodium bicarbonate). The onset starts after 15–30 min with a duration of action of 3–6 h, or:
● i.v. injection of glucose combined with regular insulin, providing 1 unit insulin for every 2 g glucose; a common approach is the i.v. infusion of 25 g of glucose combined with 10–15 units of insulin (10–15 units insulin in 500 ml of 5% glucose). Insulin is given to ensure that glucose enters cells and carries potassium with it. Onset and duration of action are similar to sodium bicarbonate regimen (Fig 1.4.11).

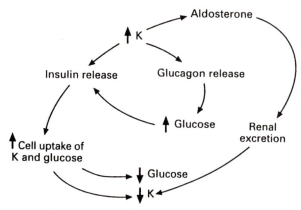

Fig. 1.4.11 Pancreatic hormones in hyperkalaemia which also stimulate aldosterone to increase potassium excretion and maintain normal level

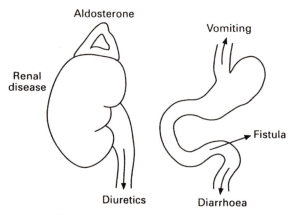

Fig. 1.4.12 Causes of hypokalaemia

All these treatments are temporary measures leading to potassium redistribution, until elimination of excess potassium from the body can be accomplished. The latter goal can be achieved through:
● Potassium binding resins (Kayexalate) used as enemas 100 g in 200 ml water; the onset starts after 1–3 h, or Calcium Resonium enema, or:
● Institution of peritoneal dialysis (onset after 1–3 h) or haemodialysis (rapid onset).
Ideally, plasma potassium concentrations should be below 5.5 mEq/l before subjecting patients to elective surgery. However, in emergency surgery, the anaesthetist must monitor the heart with ECG and proper ventilation must be assured to prevent CO_2 accumulation (respiratory acidosis). Metabolic acidosis due to unrecognised arterial hypoxaemia must be prevented; mild hyperventilation during surgery may even be recommended since a 10 mmHg decrease in $Paco_2$ reduces plasma potassium concentration about 0.5 mEq/l. Arterial blood gases and pH must be measured frequently. Responses to muscle relaxants must be considered since succinylcholine administration can lead to hyperkalaemia itself. Presence of preoperative muscle weakness may indicate decreased muscle relaxant requirements intraoperatively. Perioperative i.v. fluids must be selected with the understanding that most solutions contain potassium, e.g. Ringer lactate solution contains 4 mEq/l. Calcium and glucose-insulin must be readily available. Unlike alterations in plasma sodium, hyperkalaemia is not associated with alterations in requirements for volatile anaesthetics.

Hypokalaemia (plasma potassium below 3.5 mEq/l)

This can be due either to decreased total body potassium content or alterations in potassium distribution between intracellular and extracellular sites. Chronic hypokalaemia is likely to be associated with decreased total body potassium content as well as reductions in plasma potassium concentrations. In contrast, acute hypokalaemia is usually due to intracellular translocation of potassium, without a change in total body content.

While measuring plasma potassium concentrations is the only practical means of assessing hypokalaemia, 98% of total body potassium is intracellular; enormous potassium deficits can be present with only a small decrease in plasma potassium concentrations, for example it is estimated that chronic reductions of 1 mEq/l in plasma potassium concentrations can reflect total body deficit of 600 mEq to 800 mEq of potassium.

Decreased total body potassium content (Fig 1.4.12)

● Extra-renal causes include: GIT losses, such as vomiting, diarrhoea, nasogastric suction (commonly seen in postoperative patients), laxative abuse (inducing diarrhoea), and villous adenomas of the rectum secreting excessive mucus with potassium loss.
● Renal losses occur in response to:
  – increased aldosteron secretion in zona glomerulosa overactivity seen in primary hyperaldosteronism (Conn's syndrome) and secondary hyperaldosteronism (liver cirrhosis with ascites, nephrotic syndrome, congestive heart failure and unilateral renal artery ischaemia) (Fig. 1.4.13). Also, Cushing's syndrome (overactivity of zona fasciculata/reticularis) and steroid therapy may result in hypokalaemia (endogenous or exogenous cortisol) (Fig. 1.4.14).
  – diuretics (loop diuretics such as frusemide and thiazide diuretics). Also, osmotic diuresis of hyperglycaemia may also result in hypokalaemia.
  – trauma. Trauma as produced by surgery results in loss of potassium 50 mEq/day for the first 2 days postoperatively via the kidneys. Inadequate oral potassium intake is an uncommon cause of hypokalaemia unless the patient's only source of nutrition is potassium-free parenteral fluids.
  – renal diseases, such as renal tubular acidosis with inability to secrete H by tubules. Na is reabsorbed in exchange for K (alkaline urine despite systemic acidosis). Fanconi syndrome, the diuretic phase of renal failure, and chronic pyelonephritis may also lead to hypokalaemia.
Urinary potassium concentration is used to differentiate hypokalaemia due to GIT losses from that due to renal losses.

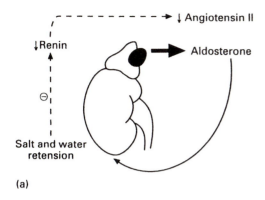

(a)

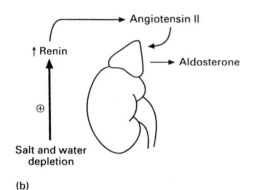

(b)

Fig. 1.4.13 Primary (a) and secondary (b) hyperaldosteronism

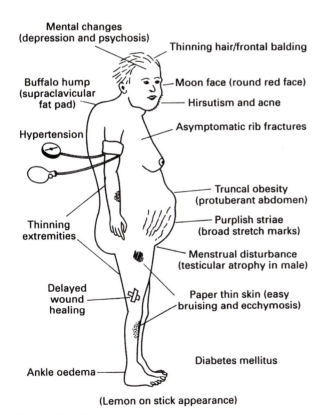

(Lemon on stick appearance)

Fig. 1.4.14 Clinical features of Cushing's syndrome

If the GIT is the source of loss, the kidneys will respond by reducing urinary excretion of potassium to less than 10 mEq/l. Conversely, if the kidneys are the source, urine potassium content is likely to exceed 40 mEq/l.

Altered potassium distribution between intracellular and extracellular sites

This occurs when potassium is acutely shifted from the extracellular fluid into cells to replace hydrogen ions in respiratory or metabolic alkalosis. Plasma potassium concentration is decreased by 0.5 mEq/l for every 10 mmHg reduction in $Paco_2$. Thus, hyperventilation during anaesthesia is the most frequent cause of acute hypokalaemia. Other causes include the following.

- Glucose-insulin infusions drive potassium into cells without altering the total body content of potassium.
- Hypokalaemic familial periodic paralysis.
- Sympathetic stimulation through the use of β_2 agonist sympathomimetic caused by adrenaline causes reduction in plasma potassium concentration due to catecholamine-induced intracellular redistribution of potassium. The use of terbutaline and ritodrine in premature labour may cause hypokalaemia.

Clinically, hypokalaemia produces adverse effects on heart, neuromuscular junction, GIT, and kidneys.

- Heart: chronic rather than acute hypokalaemia is associated with poor myocardial contractility. Sudden decreases in plasma potassium concentrations exert more profound effects on electrochemical gradients for potassium in chronically hypokalaemic patients. Orthostatic hypotension in the presence of hypokalaemia may reflect autonomic nervous system dysfunction. ECG hypokalaemic changes reflect impaired conduction; the P–R intervals and Q–T intervals are prolonged, ST segments are depressed, T waves flat and prominent U waves are present. Ventricular fibrillation is a common terminal arrhythmia in the presence of hypokalaemia.
- Neuromuscular junction: hypokalaemia is associated with skeletal muscle weakness (legs usually) and rarely muscles innervated by cranial nerves.
- GIT: paralytic ileus (particularly after abdominal surgery).
- Kidneys (hypokalaemic nephropathy): polyuria is due to impaired urine concentrating ability. However, hypokalaemia is associated with decreased GFR and renal blood flow.

Treatment in acute hypokalaemia (when total body potassium content is normal) begins with correction of the underlying cause, such as excessive intraoperative hyperventilation. Chronic hypokalaemia is treated with supplemental potassium chloride. Chloride is important, since hypochloraemic metabolic alkalosis is frequently associated with hypokalaemia. However, 50% of patients fail to attain normal plasma concentrations of potassium. Potassium salts are preferably given as a liquid (or effervescent) preparation rather than slow-release tablets which may cause nausea and vomiting; where appropriate, potassium-sparing diuretics are preferable. In chronic hypokalaemia, the potassium deficits exceed 500 mEq or even 1000 mEq, emphasising that potassium content cannot be totally corrected in the 12–24 hours preceding elective surgery. Nevertheless, i.v. infusion of potassium chloride

(0.2 mEq/kg/h) in the few hours preceding surgery is beneficial, even in severely depleted patients. Correction should be slow and ECG monitoring, plasma potassium measurements, and measurements of arterial blood gases and pH are essential. Hypokalaemia enhances digitalis toxicity, thus when digitalis toxicity is suspected, potassium chloride can be administered as 0.5–1 mEq i.v. boluses every 3–5 minutes until the ECG reverts to normal. However, the incidence of intraoperative cardiac arrhythmias is not increased in asymptomatic patients with chronic hypokalaemia. It is imperative to administer potassium in glucose-free solutions; hyperglycaemia would favour potassium entrance into cells, thus further exaggerating the degree of hypokalaemia. Use of adrenaline or any β_2 agonist should be discouraged. Similarly, hyperventilation must be rigorously avoided.

CALCIUM (*see also* 1.86 Primary Hyperthyrodism)

Practical points

The plasma calcium normally is about 5 mEq/l or 2.5 mmol/l or 10 mg/100 ml because:

    each 1 mEq of ion   = 1 mmol/valency
    1 mEq of calcium   = 1/2 mmol
                           (calcium ion has two positive
                           charges)
So

    5 mEq/l plasma calcium   = 2.5 mmol/l

Also because:

    each 1 mmol of ion   = mg molecular weight
    1 mmol of calcium   = 40 mg
                           (molecular weight of calcium
                           is 40)
So

    2.5 mmol/l plasma calcium   = 2.5 × 40
                                 = 1000 mg/l
                                 = 100 mg/100 ml
                                    (1 litre = 1000 ml)

Total plasma calcium concentrations are maintained between 4.5 and 5.5 mEq/l by the action of parathyroid hormone. Plasma calcium is partly bound to protein (albumin mainly) and partly ionised. The albumin-bound calcium is physiologically inactive and is probably purely a transport form or carrier (comparable to iron bound to transferrin and to unconjugated bilirubin bound to albumin to be transported to liver). It is the free ionised calcium which constitutes 45% of the total plasma calcium that is physiologically active and essential for blood coagulation, normal cardiac and skeletal muscle contraction, and nerve conduction (compared to thyroxine and to cortisol). Therefore symptoms due to altered calcium concentration reflect changes in plasma level of ionised calcium. Ideally, ionised rather than total calcium should be measured, but techniques for this are not available in routine laboratories. The concentration of ionised calcium is dependent on many factors; surgeons should therefore beware of *sources of error in estimating and interpreting levels of plasma calcium.* They include:

- Factors increasing plasma calcium
  - arterial pH (acidosis increases ionised calcium while alkalosis decreases it). In conditions with prolonged acidosis, e.g. uretero-sigmoidostomy and in renal tubular acidosis, the tendency to increase ionised calcium leads to bone resorption (increased solubility of bone salts) with the ultimate result of osteomalacia, even in the presence of good calcium intake and normal parathyroid function;
  - recent meal;
  - upright posture and exercise;
  - venous occlusion by tourniquet (causes local acidosis);
  - plasma albumin must be considered; in hypoalbuminaemia there will be less calcium bound to albumin and the excess non-ionised calcium is free to return to storage sites like bones, and therefore total plasma calcium concentration will be reduced but with normal ionised calcium concentration and no symptoms of hypocalcaemia (it is a relative or pseudo-hypocalcaemia). Likewise, hyperalbuminaemia is associated with hypercalcaemia, but the ionised calcium can again be normal.
- Factors decreasing plasma calcium
  - recumbency (supine position) due to the effect of posture on plasma protein concentration;
  - precipitation of proteins in the blood sample (e.g. by delay in performing the calcium estimations);
  - low plasma proteins, especially hypoalbuminaemia (see above);
  - alkalosis may cause tetany because of the reduction of ionised calcium fraction in the presence of normal total plasma calcium concentration.

For practical purposes, therefore, the *blood sample for plasma calcium estimation must be taken in the morning while the patient is fasting* (apart from hypercalcaemia caused by the ingested food, absorbed lipids in the blood sample may also interfere with the spectrophotometrical analysis), *in a sitting position, without the application of a tourniquet, and must be sent without delay to the laboratory.* If the sample reaches the laboratory reasonably quickly and the plasma calcium is reported as being in the normal range (particularly if it is at the lower end), one can be pretty certain that hypercalcaemia is not present.

Hypercalcaemia (plasma calcium above 5.5 mEq/l)

The most common causes are hyperparathyroidism and malignant diseases with skeletal metastases. Less common causes include sarcoidosis, vitamin D intoxication and immobilisation.

Clinically, hypercalcaemia affects CNS, GIT, kidneys and heart. Early findings include sedation and vomiting. Persistently high calcium (7–8 mEq/l) can interfere with urinary concentration leading to polyuria; it can also lead to renal stone formation and oliguric renal failure. When plasma calcium exceeds 8 mEq/l, cardiac conduction is disturbed with characteristic ECG changes of prolonged P–R interval, wide QRS complexes, and shortened Q–T interval leading ultimately to *cardiac standstill in systole.*

The cornerstone of treatment of hypercalcaemia is hydration with normal saline. Hydration lowers plasma calcium concentration by dilution, and sodium acts to inhibit the renal reabsorption of calcium. Frusemide produces diuresis which will minimise the risk of overhydration and further facilitates renal elimination of calcium. Ambulation reduces calcium release from the bone (associated with immobilisation). Hypercalcaemia due to myeloproliferative disorders can be lowered by mithramycin, as a means of cancer chemotherapy; however, it acts slowly and is not helpful in acute hypercalcaemia.

During surgery on patients with hypercalcaemia, hydration and good urine output must be maintained with i.v. fluids containing sodium; ECG monitoring must also be used. Hyperventilation may be beneficial by inducing respiratory alkalosis which reduces ionised calcium thus lowering total plasma calcium (though it will also reduce plasma potassium).

Hypocalcaemia (plasma calcium below 4.5 mEq/l)

The commonest cause is hypoalbuminaemia in critically ill patients (though ionised calcium is normal). However, normal plasma calcium in the presence of hypoalbuminaemia may indicate increased ionised calcium concentration.

Other causes of hypocalcaemia are acute pancreatitis, hypoparathyroidism, particularly after thyroid surgery, hypomagnesaemia (malnutrition, sepsis, aminoglycoside administration), vitamin D deficiencies and renal failure. Radiographic contrast media containing calcium chelators (edetate and citrate) may acutely lower plasma calcium concentrations. Hyperventilation by inducing respiratory alkalosis increases calcium binding to proteins and thus lowers ionised calcium. Giving sodium bicarbonate to control metabolic acidosis can also cause acute ionised hypocalcaemia. Increased plasma free fatty acids, as in total parenteral nutrition, may lower plasma ionised calcium without altering total plasma calcium concentration. Hypocalcaemia and hyperphosphataemia due to use of hypertonic phosphate enemas (Fleet enema) has been associated with cardiac arrest during induction of anaesthesia.

Clinically, hypocalcaemia affects CNS, heart and neuromuscular junction.
- CNS: numbness, circumoral paraesthesia can progress to confusion and occasionally seizures.
- Heart: acute reduction in ionised calcium may induce hypotension with non-specific prolonged Q–T intervals.
- Neuromuscular junction: skeletal muscle weakness and fatigue though acute hypocalcaemia after total parathyroidectomy (below 3.5 mEq/l), can produce skeletal muscle spasm or tetany, manifested by laryngospasm.

Treatment is by correction of any coexisting respiratory or metabolic alkalosis. In symptomatic hypocalcaemia (tetany hypotension) or when plasma calcium decreases below 3.5 mEq/l, infusion i.v. of 10 ml 10% calcium chloride (1.36 mEq/ml) or calcium gluconate (0.45 mEq/L) is given. Calcium should be repeated until plasma calcium approaches 4 mEq/l or the ECG returns to normal.

During surgery and anaesthesia, it is imperative to appreciate that respiratory or metabolic alkalosis can rapidly decrease plasma ionised calcium concentrations. This can occur during ventilation or after i.v. administration of sodium bicarbonate for treatment of metabolic acidosis. Administration of whole blood containing citrate preservative usually does not reduce plasma calcium because calcium is rapidly mobilised from body stores. Ionised calcium, however, can be decreased with rapid infusions of blood (500 ml every 5–10 minutes) or when citrate elimination is limited by hypothermia, liver cirrhosis, or renal impairment (leading to possible citrate intoxication). Intraoperative monitoring of ECG and hypotension are essential since cardiac depression may be produced by anaesthetic drugs. Arterial blood gases, pH and plasma calcium measurements are valuable in guiding intraoperative management. Plasma protein assessment and replacement must be considered with fluid replacement; administration of colloid solutions may be important because of intravascular fluid loss into tissues operated on. Postoperatively, laryngospasm may follow any sudden reduction in plasma calcium.

MAGNESIUM (see Fig. 1.4.5)

Total body magnesium stores are about 2000 mEq, most of which is located intracellularly. It is excreted by the GIT and kidneys. Magnesium-deficient diet makes the kidneys conserve magnesium, excreting less than 1 mEq/day. The most important physiologic effect of magnesium is regulation of presynaptic release of acetylcholine from nerve endings. Magnesium is an essential constituent of many enzyme systems.

Hypermagnesaemia (plasma magnesium above 2.5 mEq/l)

The commonest cause of hypermagnesaemia is iatrogenic, i.e. administration of magnesium sulphate to treat toxaemia of pregnancy and excessive individual use of antacids or laxatives. Patients with chronic renal dysfunction are at increased risks for development of hypermagnesaemia, since magnesium elimination is dependent on GFR (particularly if GFR is below 30 ml/min.) Clinically, hypermagnesaemia affects CNS, heart and neuromuscular junction:
- CNS depression manifested by hyporeflexia and sedation, which may progress to coma.
- Cardiac depression.
- Skeletal muscle weakness due to reduced acetylcholine release secondary to hypermagnesaemia, can be so severe as to impair ventilation. Indeed, the commonest cause of death from hypermagnesaemia is cardiac and respiratory arrest.

Symptomatic cases can be temporarily reversed with the i.v. administration of calcium. Magnesium elimination can be facilitated by fluid loading and diuresis produced by frusemide. However, definitive therapy for persistent and life-threateneing hypermagnesaemia requires either peritoneal dialysis or haemodialysis.

During surgery on patients with hypermagnesaemia, acidosis and dehydration must be prevented intraoperatively, as they lead to hypermagnesaemia. So hyperventilation-induced respiratory acidosis must be avoided. Arterial blood gases, and pH determinations are valuable in the management. Fluid maintenance and replacement should be adjusted to maintain urine output. Hypermagnesaemia potentiates the action of muscle relaxants; initial doses of muscle relaxants therefore must be reduced. Hypermagnesaemia also can potentiate cardiac depression induced by anaesthetic agents and can produce peripheral vasodilatation.

Hypomagnesaemia (plasma magnesium below 1.5 mEq/l)

Hypomagnesaemia is associated with chronic alcoholism, malabsorption syndromes, hyperalimentation therapy without added magnesium, protracted vomiting, and diarrhoea.

Clinically, hypomagnesaemia is similar to hypocalcaemia. Indeed, losses from stomas and fistulas both frequently are combined electrolyte disorders. Clinical manifestations of hypomagnesaemia include CNS irritability reflected by hyper-reflexia and seizures, skeletal muscle spasm and cardiac irritability. Hypomagnesaemia can also potentiate digitalis-induced cardiac arrhythmias.

Treatment with magnesium sulphate 1 g administered i.v. for 15–20 minutes, is indicated when seizure activity or skeletal muscle spasm is present. Blood pressure, heart rate and patellar reflexes should be monitored. Depression or disappearance of patellar reflexes is an indication to stop magnesium replacement. During surgery on patients with hypomagnesaemia, anaesthetic management is primarily related to associated disorders such as alcoholism, malnutrition and hypovolaemia.

SURGICAL APPLICATIONS IN POSTOPERATIVE PATIENTS

Requirements for water and electrolytes may be considered as maintenance and replacement.

Maintenance is water and electrolytes required daily for the maintenance of *milieu interieur* in all human beings. This applies to *uncomplicated non-febrile postoperative patients* who are not allowed oral fluids. This includes basic metabolic requirement (fluid for internal body reaction), insensible fluid loss (lung and skin), water in urine and stool.

Replacement involves water and electrolytes required to replace previous deficits and on-going losses (GIT) and fluid loss because of fever. For each 1 °C increase in body temperature, losses via sweating can increase by 250 ml/24 h, requiring replacement with 250 ml normal saline. All abnormal losses must be replaced in addition to maintenance requirements.

Maintenance fluids of 3 litres of water, 140 mmol Na, and 70 mmol of K are daily required for a 70 kg man. This can be given as 3 litres (2 litres of 5% dextrose and 1 litre of normal saline) at a rate of 1 litre 8-hourly, providing 3 litres of water, 154 mmol Na to which 20–30 mmol K is added to each 1 litre bag.

A 40 kg elderly woman requires only 2 litres of water a day, 80 mmol Na and 40 mmol K. This can be given as 1500 ml of 5% dextrose and 500 ml of normal saline at a rate of 500 ml 6 hourly, to which 27 mmol K is added to every other 500 ml of fluid (total of 54 mmol K).

Replacement fluids must be added daily to any maintenance fluids; '*replace like with like*' is an important rule. Mild to moderate dehydration of up to 5% total body weight (3.5 l in 70 kg man) shows as a loss of skin turgor (on pinching gently), sunken eyes and dry tongue. This extracellular interstitial fluid loss is usually without haemodynamic compromise. Severe dehydration of 10% total body weight or more results in intravascular loss as well as interstitial loss; patients present with signs of circulatory impairment, with cool peripheries,

poor capillary filling, tachycardia, postural hypotension, and later supine hypotension. The acutely shocked patient has often lost 10–15% or more of circulating volume and presents with cool peripheries, tachycardia and hypotension. History is different in shock.

Adequacy of fluid replacement can be monitored by measurement of urine output, clinical assessment, electrolytes estimation, CVP measurement and peripheral/core temperature difference.

Using the big toe as a peripheral site, peripheral and core temperature difference is a useful indicator of peripheral perfusion. Following major surgery with good fluid replacement, peripheral temperature should rapidly come to be only slightly less than core temperature. A drop in peripheral temperature may indicate fluid loss from circulation and poor tissue perfusion. This technique is less satisfactory in patients with peripheral vascular disease.

GIT losses (Table 1.4.1)

Prolonged paralytic ileus after surgery may lead to high volume nasogastric loss. This must be replaced with normal saline containing adequate potassium (hypokalaemia accentuates paralytic ileus). Estimation of K loss may be made by measurement of K concentration in aspirate and plasma.

In biliary fistula after common bile duct (CBD) exploration, T-tube may lead to a loss of 500–800 ml H_2O/day, together with considerable Na and K loss. This should be replaced with normal saline with added K.

Small bowel fistula may be anatomically high or low, internal or external, and of low or high output (< 1 litre, or > 1 litre/24 h respectively). An estimate of content of effluent can be made from electrolyte content of secretions at the level of the fistula. A high duodenal or jejunal fistula may lose 5–6 L daily. The fluid should be collected in a stoma bag and measured, losses being replaced with equivalent amounts of normal saline and K. The daily estimation of plasma electrolytes is essential. Parenteral nutrition is an adjunct to management.

In intestinal obstruction clinical, radiological and biochemical investigations help determine whether obstruction is:

– complete or incomplete;
– intermittent or continuous;
– high or low;
– mechanical or functional (paralytic ileus).

Table 1.4.1 Volume and composition of gastrointestinal secretions

	Volume (ml/24 h)	Na⁺ (mmol/l)	K⁺ (mmol/l)	Cl⁻ (mmol/l)	HCO₃ (mmol/l)
Salivary	1500	10	25	10	30
Stomach	2500	60	10	130	–
Duodenum	Variable	140	5	80	–
Ileum	3000	140	5	104	–
Colon	Minimal	60	30	40	–
Pancreas	250	140	5	75	115
Bile	750	145	5	100	35

Patients with a short history and minimal abdominal distension require smaller fluid volume replacement than patients vomiting for many days with distended abdomen.

Despite gaseous distension, large amounts of H_2O and electrolytes are lost (sequestrated) into the bowel lumen; such sequestration is greater in low ileal obstruction than high jejunal obstruction. Low ileal obstruction is characterised by colicky abdominal pain followed hours or days later by bilious (and later faeculent) vomiting. High jejunal obstruction is characterised by early profuse bilious vomiting with minimal abdominal distension and a paucity of bowel loops on abdominal X-rays. Large bowel obstruction leads to distension and total constipation preceding vomiting and pain by several days unless decompressed by patent incompetent ileocaecal valve or a closed loop obstruction occurs with volvulus or with distal left colon obstruction and competent ileocaecal valve (obstruction). Closed loop obstruction results in ischaemia and perforation.

Because fluid lost is isotonic, plasma concentration of electrolytes is initially preserved, but within hours, electrolyte concentrations change with increased plasma urea and increased PCV (haematocrit), combined with oliguria and high urine specific gravity (reflecting fluid volume deficit). Hypokalaemia occurs with prolonged vomiting, distension, diarrhoea, or taking K-losing diuretics. Care is taken to prepare the obstructed patient for theatre; fluid replacement (with normal saline to which K is later added) is essential because anaesthetic induction results in loss of vasomotor tone with profound hypotension. A deficit of 3–4 L may present in high small bowel obstruction, while 7–10 L may be required for long-standing low small bowel obstruction.

Duodenal or high jejunal obstruction results in hypokalaemic hypochloraemic alkalosis with normal plasma Na; this is primarily due to loss of acidic gastric fluid, Na and chloride. Such alkalosis is also seen in infantile pyloric stenosis, and alkalosis is paradoxically worsened by renal compensation. Replacement with normal saline and K allows kidneys to correct acid–base deficit. Low small bowel obstruction or colonic obstruction results in vomiting of large volumes of alkaline intestinal fluid, resulting in metabolic acidosis which is accentuated by ketosis of starvation. Again normal saline should be used as replacement fluid. Patients with limited cardiac reserve must not be overloaded.

Electrolyte-free solutions (e.g. 5% dextrose) should not be used alone because they will lead to dilutional hyponatraemia. Intestinal fluid recovery usually occurs between the second and fifth postoperative day and is reflected by increased urine output.

Diarrhoea, nasogastric suction and ileostomy abnormal intestinal losses lead to H_2O, Na and K deficits with acid–base disturbances.

Diarrhoea results in high electrolyte loss; normal saline with K should be used for replacement. Prolonged nasogastric suction may average 3 litres or more per day, and requires replacement with normal saline.

Patients with ileostomies experience episodes of diarrhoea, possibly due to infection, dietary indiscretion or partial small bowel obstruction. If this exceeds 1 litre a day, the patient is prone to H_2O and electrolyte depletion (and excoriation of peristomal skin). Oral electrolyte solutions may be sufficient in mild cases, but in more severe cases i.v. normal saline and K are required.

Newly fashioned ileostomies tend to produce a high volume effluent. It may be tempting to remove the i.v. drip and encourage oral fluids; however, it is advisable to maintain the drip, replacing ileostomy loss with normal saline and K, while administering daily maintenance fluids. This is continued until ileostomy output has reduced and thickened.

Postoperative fluids after major GIT surgery

Following laparotomies with handling or resection of bowel, GIT motility ceases for a variable length of time resulting in a state of ileus (this does not usually continue for more than 48 hours postoperatively). The bowel then fails to conduct fluid and absorption is also impaired, resulting in fluid accumulation and bowel dilatation (which may also compromise any anastomosis). Nasogastric suction is used to remove fluid and decompress gaseous distension of stomach to prevent gastric dilatation; the patient may be allowed 30 ml H_2O/h while the nasogastric tube is in situ to moisten the oral cavity.

Reappearance of audible bowel sounds signifies some GIT activity, and when combined with the passage of flatus suggests the return of normal motility; this is associated with fall of nasogastric aspirate volume. The tube may then be removed and oral fluid intake is increased. Once the patient tolerates this, the i.v. drip is removed.

1.5 Nutrition in Surgery

As a general rule, the gastrointestinal tract should be used as frequently and as completely as possible. However, repeated attempts to feed enterally patients who have intermittent episodes of ileus or intolerance to the feedings are ill-advised and parenteral nutrition is a better choice. It may be necessary to use more than one type of enteral nutrition or a combination of enteral and parenteral feedings.

Enteral nutrition is used in patients with a normally functioning gastrointestinal tract who cannot eat enough. It may be given:

● Orally
● Via nasoenteric soft Silastic fine-bore tube (e.g. 8 Fr), cooled in the refrigerator before use (to harden it and facilitate its passage), with continuous slow infusion. Such tubes are tolerated well even for 2 months with few complications. The large-bore nasogastric tube should be avoided since it is badly tolerated and associated with aspiration pneumonia (residual gastric volume should be checked frequently and if it is 150 ml or over the feeding should be stopped) and other complications, e.g. oesophageal erosion with subsequent reflux oesophagitis, haemorrhage, perforation or tracheo-oesophageal fistulation.
● Via tube enterostomies, e.g. pharyngostomy, cervical oeso-phagostomy, gastrostomy, jejunostomy to bypass a proximal lesion.

If the bleeding source is still unknown then visceral angiography is performed to identify the site and possibly the cause of bleeding, e.g. angiodysplasia, to be followed by elective surgery. However, if there is still continuous bleeding of unknown origin, emergency surgery should be performed with or without repeated angiography preoperatively and with or without on-table colonoscopy. Angiography can visualise bleeding only if it is flowing in a rate of 0.5 m/min (30 ml/h) or more.

In bleeding of unknown origin, a blind subtotal colectomy is performed, bringing up the proximal end as an ileostomy and the distal end as a separate colostomy. Postoperative monitoring is carried out. If there is no bleeding then bowel continuity is restored once the patient has recovered. If the distal end starts bleeding through the colostomy then excision of the rectum, completed as for abdominoperineal resection, is recommended, keeping the ileostomy as a permanent stoma. However, if the ileostomy starts bleeding then the patient should be reinvestigated, as initial misdiagnosis is possible. The underlying cause may be in the upper gastrointestinal tract and one should proceed with upper gastrointestinal tract endoscopy with barium meal and repeated angiography.

Haemobilia

Haemobilia is a rare cause of acute or chronic blood loss from the GIT (diagnosed after exclusion of common causes). It can lead to biliary colic and obstructive jaundice.

Diagnosis is easy in operated patient if the T-tube is already in situ, when clots can be flushed out and bleeding may stop spontaneously. However, in the unoperated patient diagnosis is suspected in GIT bleeding with biliary colic and jaundice and necessitates upper GIT endoscopy and ERCP, where blood may be seen emerging from the sphincter of Oddi. Ultrasound, CT scan, Tc^{99} scan and selective hepatic arteriogram can locate the bleeding site within the liver; treatment may include therapeutic embolisation or ligation of the feeding vessel as close as possible to the angiographic leak. Occasionally, partial hepatectomy is needed in heavy post-traumatic haemobilia arising deep in the liver substance.

Causes of haemobilia are:
- Traumatic liver and inferior vena cava injury due to arteriobiliary communication.
- Iatrogenic, in difficult and traumatic exploration of common bile duct.
- Gallstone disease, whether spontaneous or operated on.
- Neoplastic in cholangiocarcinoma and liver tumours communicating with bile ducts.
- Parasitic hepatobiliary infestation (Oriental parasites such as Ascariasis).
- Vascular disorders.

1.7 Shock in Surgery

Shock is defined as: acute haemodynamic disturbance causing a reduction in capillary blood flow with decreased tissue perfusion and anoxia.

Shock is a clinical syndrome manifested by (in addition to apprehension and irritability) changes in:
1. blood pressure and pulse rate – indicative of cardiac output;
2. skin temperature and colour – indicative of peripheral resistance;
3. state of venous filling and colour of nail beds – indicative of blood flow;
4. urinary output – indicative of tissue perfusion.

The feature that appears to be common to all types of shock is inadequate tissue perfusion. The cardiac output may be inadequate because the heart is damaged or the volume of circulating blood may be less than the capacity of the circulation either because the blood volume is reduced or the capacity is increased (Fig. 1.7.1).

On this basis, three general types of shock can be delineated (Table 1.7.1).

I. HYPOVOLAEMIC SHOCK

Hypovolaemic shock is also called 'cold shock' and is manifested typically by hypotension, rapid thready pulse, cold, pale, clammy skin, intense thirst, rapid respiration, restlessness and reduced CVP. This type includes traumatic shock, crush syndrome, surgical shock, wound shock and burn shock. The fluid lost in hypovolaemic shock is one of the following.

Blood

- Externally – haemorrhage and gastrointestinal bleeding.
- Internally into the tissues – fractures; pancreatitis; haemothorax; haemoperitoneum; ruptured spleen; ectopic gestation.

Plasma

- Burns – major problem.
- Inflammation – minor problem, i.e. the exudate.

Extracellular fluid

Loss of extracellular fluid occurs as a consequence of:
- Deviation of normal exchange mechanisms at transcellular level. These losses include: gastrointestinal losses via vomiting (as in pyloric stenosis and intestinal obstruction) and fistulae; and renal losses via urine (as in diabetes mellitus, diabetes insipidus and excessive use of diuretics).
- Increased extracellular fluid loss along a normal pathway as in excessive sweating – insensible water loss without replacement.
- The 'third space phenomenon':
  - Increased capillary permeability as in an inflamed area.
  - Loss of biochemical integrity of cell membrane (due to hypoxia) which increases the level of cellular sodium and decreases the level of cellular potassium. This is presumably related to increased permeability of cell membrane or damage to the sodium/potassium pump mechanism. The effective extracellular fluid volume is thus reduced.

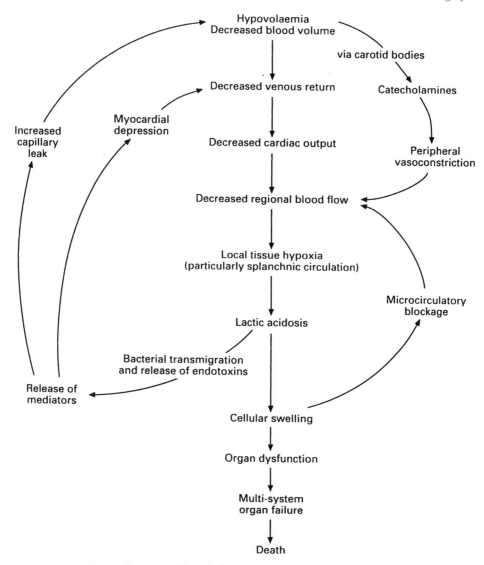

Fig. 1.7.1   Pathophysiology of shock revealing many vicious circles

For **treatment**, see Table 1.7.1. In restlessness and anxiety, narcotics (e.g. morphine) should be given i.v. for reliable immediate action, but also because i.m. injection results in accumulation and when circulation improves, sudden release causes respiratory depression.

Classes of haemorrhage: based on percentage of acute blood loss, physiological and clinical manifestations, there are 4 classes:

Class I = up to 15% blood volume loss (blood donor): no clinical findings apart from minimal tachycardia (heart rate still below 100/min) with normal blood pressure, urine output (> 30 ml/hr), and respiratory rate (14–20/min). Compensatory mechanisms restore blood volume within 24 h.

Class II = 15–30% blood volume loss (uncomplicated shock): in a 70-kg man, this loss represents 750–1500 ml of blood. Clinical findings are: anxiety, a drop in urine output (20–30 ml/hr) tachycardia (heart rate > 100/min), tachypnoea (respiratory rate 20–30/min), and decreased pulse pressure (difference between systolic and diastolic pressures) due to a rise in diastolic pressure following release of catecholamines causing increased peripheral resistance (systolic pressure however, changes minimally). Blood pressure however, is normal.

Class III = 30–40% blood volume loss (complicated shock): an estimated loss of 1500–2000 ml of blood can be devastating. Clinical findings are: anxiety (with confusion), sharp drop in urine output (5–15 ml/hr), marked tachycardia (heart rate > 120/min), tachypnoea (30–40/min), and a measurable fall in systolic pressure with decreased pulse pressure, and hypotension.

Class IV = more than 40% blood volume loss (preterminal shock): a loss of more than 2000 ml of blood is life-threatening. Clinical findings are: confusion (and lethargy), negligible urine

Table 1.7.1   Differentiation of major shock states

	Hypovolaemic	*Septic*	*Cardiogenic*
Place of shock	Street (rarely hospital)	Hospital	Home
Triggering factor	RTA (or cold operation)	Peritonitis or emergency operation	Exercise
Presentation	Bleeding	Fever and rigor (shaking chill)	Chest pain
History	? Alcoholic intake (in RTA)	Steroid or insulin (diabetes)	Glyceryl trinitrate (no external trauma)
Mental status	Restlessness	Confusion	In pain
Appearance of limbs	Cold/pale	Warm → Pink → Cyanosis	Cold/cyanosis
Pulse rate	Tachycardia and tachypnoea	Tachycardia	Tachycardia
Other remarks	Rarely pure. Usually with element of septicaemia	Jaundice and splenomegaly Element of hypovolaemia	Basal crepitation (bilateral); 3rd heart sound ± arrhythmia (Gallop rhythm)
CVP	Decreased	Increased or decreased	Increased (Distended neck veins)
Special investigation	PCV, Hb, Blood Group and crossmatch	Peripheral smear (toxic granulation in WBC and Dohle bodies in RBC), Blood culture, gas chromatography, limulus test	ECG may show myocardial infarction
Basic treatment	Fluid replacement Arrest bleeding Surgery with fixation of fractures	Antibiotics Blood transfusion Surgical drainage	Intropic drug, e.g. dopamine ? Intra-aortic balloon

RTA = road traffic accident; CVP = central venous pressure; PCV = packed cell volume (haematocrit); Hb = haemoglobin; WBC = white blood cells; RBC = red blood cells

output (0 ml/hr), marked tachycardia (heart rate > 140/min), tachypnoea (> 35/min), and significant depression in systolic pressure with a very narrow pulse pressure (or unobtainable diastolic pressure), and severe hypotension. Skin is cold and pale. Loss of more than 50% of patient's blood volume results in total loss of consciousness, pulse, and blood pressure.

Most patients respond rapidly to initial fluid therapy and become haemodynamically stable indicating minimal blood loss (of less than 20% – Class II), and no further treatment is needed. A small group of patients with poor perfusion respond slowly to initial fluid therapy indicating an ongoing bleeding and have lost about 20–40% of their blood volume already. Continued fluid and blood administration (roughly at a ratio of 3 crystalloid to 1 blood or 3:1 rule) are indicated; the resonse to blood transfusion should identify patients who are still bleeding and require surgical intervention in cases such as bleeding peptic ulcer, ruptured ectopic gestation, ruptured spleen, and leaking aortic aneurysm.

II. CARDIOGENIC SHOCK

This type of shock is caused by failure of the heart pump action, which takes two forms.

Pump failure proper The commonest cause is sudden myocardial infarction; other less common causes are arrhythmia (as in electrocution), severe congestive heart failure with low cardiac output, following open heart surgery; and acute septal perforation.

Mechanical vascular obstruction as in massive pulmonary embolus, tension pneumothorax, cardiac tamponade, dissecting aortic aneurysm, intracardiac lesions (e.g. ball valve thrombus, atrial myxoma), regurgitation caused by a ruptured cusp, papillary muscle dysfunction and valve damage. The picture of pulmonary embolism is well known. Effects vary from immediate death to the almost symptomless and late development of cor pulmonale.

The symptoms of cardiogenic shock are those of shock plus congestion of the lungs and viscera due to failure of the heart to pump out all the venous blood returned to it and is therefore called 'congestive shock'. It occurs in 10% of myocardial infarction patients (when at least 45% of the left ventricular myocardium has been damaged).

Cardiogenic shock is differentiated from hypovolaemic shock by:
- No history and no signs of blood loss.
- Raised rather than lowered CVP.
- ECG evidence.

For treatment, see Table 1.7.1.

III. LOW RESISTANCE SHOCK

Includes a number of entities in which the circulatory volume is normal while the capacity of the circulation is increased by massive vasodilatation; it is therefore called 'warm shock'.

1. Vasovagal syncope or fainting (neurogenic shock)

Neurogenic shock occurs in response to strong emotion, such as overwhelming fear and grief. It is also seen in spinal cord injury, in drug-induced shock (anaesthesia, ganglion-blockers and other antihypertensive drugs, overdose of barbiturates, glutethimide, phenothiazines) and in orthostatic hypotension (primary autonomic insufficiency and peripheral neuropathies). Valsalva's manoeuvre occurring during defaecation, vomiting or labour may reduce the venous return to the heart and produce fainting. Micturition syncope due to the reflex bradycardia induced by voiding, carotid sinus syncope due to tight collars, cough syncope and effort syncope are all types of fainting. Severe pain (e.g. a blow to the testes) can also cause fainting. The physiological chain of events in neurogenic shock is: hypotension – adrenaline secretion – muscular vasodilatation – bradycardia – cerebral hypoxia – fainting. Note the combination of hypotension and bradycardia in this type of shock.

2. Septic shock

Due to endotoxaemia (endotoxin is a complex lipopolysaccharide bound to cell wall protein of dead microorganisms); rather than bacteraemia (transient bacteraemia, invariably of no consequence, is a common event in minor surgical procedures such as urinary catheterisation, sigmoidoscopy and biopsy, percutaneous liver biopsy and even barium enema).

Exposure of mammalian cells to endotoxin results in cell injury by several mechanisms:
- Direct cell membrane damage by endotoxin.
- Extracellular release of lysosomal enzymes from leucocytes.
- Activation of the complement cascade.
- Metabolic injury due to tissue anoxia.

The majority of patients with septic shock become infected while in hospital.

Surgical causes

Septic shock occurs in strangulated intestine (strangulated hernia, mesenteric thrombosis) or peritonitis, after gas gangrene and often following operations on the gastrointestinal tract especially the large bowel and rectum or genitourinary tract, particularly when surgery is performed under emergency or semi-elective conditions. Patients with major trauma, burns and transplantations are more susceptible.

Septic shock may also result from manipulation or instrumentation in the presence of obstruction of the urinary tract (e.g. cystoscopy and catheterisation), gastrointestinal tract (e.g. oesophagogastroduodenoscopy and ERCP) or genital tract (e.g. septic abortion after retained placenta; and following the birth of premature and full-term infants).

Parenteral feeding and blood transfusion are sometimes complicated by septic shock.

Non-surgical causes

These causes include pneumonia, endocarditis, meningitis and dermatological infections as well as hospital infection due to misuse and overuse of antibiotics. Advanced age, diabetes, malnutrition, uraemia, malignancy, immunological defects or treatment with chemotherapeutic and corticosteroid drugs (immunosuppression) are risk factors and common associated findings.

The responsible bacteria in order of frequency are: *Escherichia coli*, Proteus species, *Pseudomonas aeruginosa*, Klebsiella, *Bacteroides fragilis, Clostridium perfringens*.

The clinical features of infection, e.g. fever, tachycardia, hyperventilation (respiratory alkalosis) and warm extremities (dry, pink or suffused), together with a degree of hypotension, low peripheral resistance, and increased CVP, cardiac index and pulse rate predominate in the early stages (the hyperdynamic phase). Later features are cyanosis, vasoconstriction and increased peripheral resistance, oliguria and confusion with more marked degrees of hypotension as well as decreased CVP and cardiac index. This hypodynamic phase is more common than the hyperdynamic phase (Fig. 1.7.2).

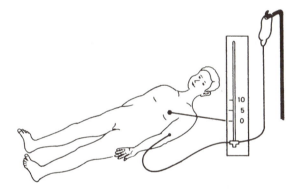

Fig. 1.7.2 Central venous pressure (CVP)

In the hyperdynamic phase cardiac output is usually high but nevertheless still inadequate to satisfy the metabolic requirements. Also, maldistribution of blood alone (due to constriction, dilatation, shunting) can be sufficient to produce shock even in the presence of high cardiac output and arterial blood pressure.

Jaundice, minor splenic enlargement, septicaemic rash or splinter haemorrhages under the nails are valuable confirmatory signs of toxaemia but their absence does not exclude septicaemia.

Hypovolaemia is almost invariably present in septic shock because of:
- Inadequate fluid intake postoperatively.
- Pyrexia.
- Hyperventilation.
- Gastrointestinal bleeding due to stress ulceration occurring in up to 15% of cases.

- Bleeding diathesis due to thrombocytopenia resulting from:
  - Disseminated intravascular coagulation.
  - Haemodilution.
  - Direct action of endotoxin on platelets.
  - Indirect action via immune complexes.

The treatment of a patient suffering from shock associated with sepsis can be summarised as follows (*see also* Table 1.7.1).

1. Assess adequacy of ventilation. Give oxygen and, if necessary, use mechanical ventilation (monitor blood gases).
2. Assess electrolyte and acid–base status. Insert a CVP line. Restore circulating blood volume and, if possible, correct metabolic imbalance.
3. Insert urinary catheter and assess renal function. Be prepared to treat acute renal failure.
4. Take blood and other cultures. Start appropriate antibiotic therapy. Give antibiotics intravenously. Consider hyperbaric oxygen therapy.
5. Assess haematological status. Should there be evidence of disseminated intravascular coagulation treat accordingly. Use fresh frozen plasma, check fibrinogen level – if this falls or there is bleeding from multiple sites then give heparin 100 units/kg immediately followed by 10 units/kg hourly. If bleeding does not stop use platelets especially when platelet count is less than 40×10^9/l.
6. Should there be a poor response to (2) and (4), give massive doses of methylprednisolone sodium succinate intravenously.
7. Consider digitalis.
8. Should the condition remain critical consider monitoring cardiac output and the use of drugs affecting the haemodynamic state.
9. Consider surgery.

(See also 5.1.11, Monoclonal antibodies).

Antibiotic choice

There is no perfect regimen for all patients with septic shock and the choice will be dictated by the suspected site of infection and host factors such as age, immunosuppression and hospitalisation. A reasonable approach to some of the commoner underlying infections would be as follows:

- Pneumonia or urinary tract
  community-acquired: co-amoxiclav or cefotaxime + erythromycin
  hospital-acquired: ceftazidime or piperacillin + gentamicin
- Intra-abdominal
  cefotaxime + metronidazole or piperacillin + gentamicin
- Biliary tract
  piperacillin + gentamicin
- Skin and soft tissue
  community-acquired: penicillin + flucloxacillin
  hospital-acquired: cefotaxime + flucloxacillin

3. Anaphylactic shock

This is a rapidly developing, severe allergic reaction that sometimes occurs when a sensitised individual is exposed to antigen, e.g. from injection of antitetanus serum or penicillin i.m., injection or iodine contrast medium i.v., or ruptured hydatid cyst fluid intraperitoneally.

The resultant Ag–Ab reaction releases large amounts of histamine leading to increased capillary permeability and widespread dilatation of arterioles and capillaries (splanchnic pooling) with a consequent fall in venous return and cardiac output. It is also associated with bronchospasm. It is treated with 0.5 ml of 1:10 000 adrenaline subcutaneously, i.v. steroids and antihistamine.

4. Endocrine failure (including Addison's disease and myxoedema)

Adrenocortical shock is mixed septic and haemorrhagic shock following the Waterhouse–Friderichsen syndrome (named after Danish and British physicians) in which intramedullary adrenal haemorrhage increases shock in children suffering from overwhelming infection. Adrenals treated with steroid drugs may be inhibited for up to 2 years after stopping treatment and then may become shocked following minor trauma or operations. The longer the duration of therapy the slower must be the withdrawal. Adrenocortical shock may occur following steroid withdrawal even without sepsis or bleeding. It is treated by prevention through adequate steroid administration i.m. or i.v. in the perioperative period then tailing it down.

5. Toxic shock syndrome

This is a potentially fatal multi-system illness due to *Staphylococcus aureus* infection and its toxins; exotoxin 1 and cytokines IL-1 and TNF are involved in the pathogenesis. It was initially reported in children, and later was reported in women using tampons during menstruation, or using vaginal contraceptive sponges. However, toxic shock syndrome may be a complication of staphylococcal pneumonia that follows an influenza-like illness (postinfluenza toxic shock syndrome); other non-menstrual causes are related to nasal packing, childbirth and abortion, surgical wound infections and vaginal infections.

It is diagnosed by the following criteria:

1. Temperature > 38.9 °C.
2. Macular erythematous rash: desquamation 2 weeks later is a characteristic feature of this syndrome.
3. Shock with hypotension < 90 mmHg and peripheral circulatory failure.
4. At least Three-system organ failure (including mucous membrane ulceration). Evidence of multi-system involvement may include diarrhoea, skeletal muscle myalgia (elevated plasma creatine kinase), renal dysfunction (elevated plasma creatinine), hepatic dysfunction (high plasma transaminases and bilirubin), disseminated intravascular coagulation and thrombocytopenia. Treatment is similar to that of septic shock.
5. Culture of toxin-producing *S. aureus* from ulcers/wounds/nasopharynx or secretions of the affected patient confirms the diagnosis. There is also a rise in TSST-1 antibody titre.

MONITORING OF SHOCK PATIENTS is defined as the use of noninvasive and invasive technology to acquire and interpret physiological data. Noninvasive or less invasive indirect clinical monitoring, though simple, usually (but not always) does not provide a continuous readout and has to be repeated by the same person. Adequacy of tissue perfusion can clinically be observed through following **noninvasive** or **less invasive measures:**

– **mental status** is a sensitive indicator of adequacy of perfusion, particularly in early septic shock.
– **blood pressure (standard cuff measurement) and pulse rate** (provided that the patient is not on beta-blocker) are good clinical indices. In shock states, hypotension is associated with tachycardia, except in neurogenic shock where bradycardia and hypotension characterise this condition. Neurogenic shock results from damage of descending sympathetic spinal outflow pathways causing loss of vasomotor tone (vasodilatation and hypotension) and loss of sympathetic innervation to the heart (bradycardia); fluid replacement therefore, is not advisable, because hypotension is not due to hypovolaemia and may result in fluid overload. Blood pressure can be restored by judicious use of vasopressors (this is an exception to general rule of not using pressors for shock treatment); atropine may be used to counteract bradycardia.
– **skin colour and feel** e.g. pink warm skin in normal person, pale cool skin in hypovolaemic shock, dry warm skin (either pink or cyanotic) in septic shock, and cold cyanotic skin in cardiogenic shock.
– **urine output** (usually via urinary catheter) is the most important single measurement in a patient with shock, particularly hypovolaemic or cardiogenic shock. If a patient is making 0.5 ml/kg/hr (e.g. 35 ml/hr in a 70 kg adult), then tissue perfusion is at least minimally adequate. An important caveat is that this does not apply in early sepsis; septic patients may have normal or even supernormal urine output while still having significantly underperfused peripheral circulation.
– **Core temperature** as measured via rectal, oesophageal, or tympanic membrane thermometer (central body) in relation to skin temperature (peripheral body) is a good indirect index of systemic vascular resistance. Oral temperature is not reliable as patient may have taken hot or cold drinks or be a mouth breather (false cold temperature). If patient's core temperature is normal and distal extremities are cool to the touch, there is a strong possibility that the patient is vasoconstricted and that inadequate tissue perfusion is already present.
– **ECG** is a useful noninvasive monitoring of heart rhythm, particularly in cardiogenic shock e.g. due to myocardial infarction.
– **Arterial blood sample for pH (blood gases) and serum lactate levels** being excellent biochemical markers of the adequacy of tissue perfusion. Metabolic acidosis with high lactate level is almost always caused by inadequate oxygen delivery to tissues with resultant tissue hypoxia. However, such measurements are intermittent with no continuous readout. Muscle surface pH though continuous does not reflect the state of perfusion because local circulation in muscles is independent of total body perfusion.
– **pulse oximetry** provides a continuous yet noninvasive measurement of transcutaneous oxygen saturation (of functional haemoglobin of arterial blood but not oxygen partial pressure (PaO_2) and pulse rate that are updated with each heart beat; it therefore monitors perfusion indirectly. The device combines the principles of spectrophotometric oximetry and plethysmography. A warmed electro-optical sensor is placed on skin and the area under the electrode becomes vasodilated; the light absorbed is conveyed audibly and visually into pulse rate and percent arterial haemoglobin oxygen saturation. With each heart beat, a pulse of oxygenated arterial blood flows to the sensor site. The relative amount of light absorbed by oxygenated haemoglobin differs from deoxygenated haemoglobin and the pulse oximeter uses these measurements to determine oxygen saturation percentage. A measured saturation of 95% or greater by pulse oximetry is strong corroborating evidence of adequate peripheral arterial oxygenation ($PaO_2 > 70$ mmHg). Pulse oximetry requires intact peripheral perfusion and cannot distinguish oxyhaemoglobin from carboxyhaemoglobin or methemoglobin, which limits its usefulness in the severely vasoconstricted patient and in the patient with carbon monoxide poisoning. Profound anaemia (haemoglobin < 5 gm) and hypothermia (< 30°C) impede the reliability of the technique. However, in most trauma patients pulse oximetry is not only useful, but continuous monitoring of oxygen saturation provides an immediate assessment of therapeutic interventions particularly when difficulties in intubation or ventilation are anticipated. This is more successful than muscle surface pH measurements, but again depends on local blood flow and often does not reflect total body circulation.

Indications for invasive monitoring: Arterial line, central venous pressure (CVP) line, and Swan–Ganz pulmonary artery catheters are needed in special patients constituting 15% of patients in a surgical ICU, indicating that most patients can be monitored with less-invasive technology.

1. High risk surgery
This is however not synonymous with high-tech surgery; risk of above-knee amputation in a patient with peripheral vascular disease is many times higher than the risk to a patient undergoing a coronary artery bypass graft. The risk should be estimated by careful history taking and physical examination.

2. Following surgery or trauma to patients with **preexisting organ dysfunction**, particularly:
    cardiac,
    pulmonary,
    renal,
    hepatic,
    hypertensive disease,
because haemodynamic instability is more likely to occur in these patients and may result from causes other than hypovolaemia e.g. cardiac failure which can be detected by a pulmonary artery catheter.

3. Haemodynamic instability unresponsive to initial management in:
    elderly patient
    multiple-trauma patient
    suspicion of sepsis

4. Use of high levels (10 cm H_2O) of PEEP. Patients on a high level of positive end-expiratory pressure (PEEP) for ARDS frequently require invasive monitoring, since application of PEEP can significantly and adversely affect cardiac output to the point where inadequate perfusion of peripheral tissues can occur.

– **Arterial line:** this is most frequently placed in the radial artery and is easily inserted percutaneously. It is crucially important to perform the Allen test beforehand to ensure the functional integrity of the palmar arch: the patient must make a fist actively or passively to expel as much blood from skin and subcutaneous tissue as possible, thereby blanching the skin; radial and ulnar arteries are then forcibly compressed by digital pressure and the hand relaxed. While maintaining pressure on radial artery, the pressure is removed from ulnar artery allowing blood to reenter the hand; if thenar eminence regains its normal pink colour within 1 or 2 seconds, this is evidence of patency of the palmar arch, and the line can be safely placed in the radial artery with minimal fear of distal ischaemia (should the radial arterial lumen become obliterated after inserting arterial line). Benefits of arterial line are:

  ● blood pressure measurements are more accurate in a low-flow state than those obtained by standard blood pressure cuffs.
  ● continuous measurement of blood pressure, rather than intermittent measurements with standard cuffs.

– **CVP line:** measures the right atrial pressure of the heart. It is important in the differentiation of shock states with a reduced CVP in hypovolaemic shock and an elevated CVP in cardiogenic shock.

– **Swan–Ganz pulmonary artery catheter:** measures (in addition to CVP) the pulmonary wedge pressure which is reflection of the left atrial pressure of the heart. Cardiac output and peripheral resistance can be processed (via the attached computer) and displayed on screen instantly. In general, the right and left sides of the heart work together; however, in discrepancy between right and left sides of the heart e.g. hypovolaemia but with increased CVP (due to tricuspid valve disease) with hypotension, the doctor is reluctant to give i.v. fluids for the fear of pulmonary oedema. Here the Swan–Ganz catheter is vital to indicate that such CVP is falsely high (through determining accurately right and left atrial pressures) resulting in fluid therapy. Also high cardiac output of sepsis can be differentiated from normal hypermetabolic states through the use of the Swan–Ganz catheter and the use of oxygen extraction ratio (normally is 25% of oxygen delivered to tissues, increased to 40% in hypermetabolic demands, and suppressed to below 20% in sepsis).

1.8 Blood Transfusion in Surgery

Blood storage

Until recently, ACD (citric Acid, trisodium Citrate and Dextrose) was used as both an anticoagulant and red cell preservative. This was superseded in the 1970s by CPD (Citrate Phosphate Dextrose), in which addition of sodium dihydrogen phosphate raised pH (less acidic than ACD) and improved red cell survival *ex vivo* (*in vitro*) because it preserved red cell

2,3-DPG better than ACD. However, red cell survival is dependent on ATP cellular level, and addition of adenine to CPD improves anticoagulant–preservative (CPD–A); it preserves its ATP and 2,3-DPG levels for up to 2 weeks with a slow fall thereafter, and thus enables shelf life of stored blood to increase to 28–35 days compared with 21 days for ACD and standard CPD. Saline adenine glucose mannitol (SAG–M) also preserves red cells for 35 days.

Red cells last well in bank refrigerated stored blood (2–6 °C); they die at a rate of 1% per day. Resort to domestic refrigerators may be hazardous because of risk of inadequate thermostatic control leading to freezing and lysis of red cells on warming in case of equipment failure. At such temperature, bacterial replication in blood is inhibited, red cell glycolysis is slowed with preservation of 2,3-DPG levels, and thus red cell survival *ex vivo* is preserved. Duration of storage considered suitable with anticoagulant is such that on the last day of storage, more than 70% of red cells survive in circulation 24 hours after transfusion. Red cells can be washed, suspended in glycerol and stored frozen in liquid nitrogen for many years. Only 2 hours are needed for thawing and washing to remove glycerol. They then should be used within 6 hours with mainly military applications.

The prime function of red cells is delivery of oxygen to tissues, and this is dependent on red cell level of 2,3-DPG. Stored red cells have increased affinity to oxygen, and are less ready to release oxygen than are fresh cells; this affinity increases with age of banked blood. It is 2,3-DPG which lowers this oxygen affinity. In ACD, red cells lose 40% and 90% of 2,3-DPG at 1 and 2 weeks respectively, with a resulting shift of oxygen dissociation curve to the left.

In CPD, 2,3-DPG is better maintained (20% loss at 2 weeks), but slightly less so in CPD-A. Whatever the storage medium, however, levels of 2,3-DPG return to normal in 6–24 h after transfusion. *In vivo* levels of 2,3-DPG are increased after exercise, ascent to high altitude, high hormone concentration (thyroid hormone, growth hormone, and androgen), and in hypoxia as in heart failure and chronic lung disease and anaemia, making oxygen more readily available to tissues. Acidosis and fetal haemoglobin reduces 2,3-DPG and increases haemoglobin affinity to oxygen.

Clotting factors, however, deteriorate progressively after 24 h storage. CPD blood contains no functioning platelets after 48 h; factor V has decreased to 50% after 14 days; factor VIII has decreased to 50% after 24 h and to 6% after 21 days; factor XI is only stable for 7 days. Other clotting factors (prothrombin and factors VII, IX, X) are stable and do not begin to fall before 21 days. Factors V and VIII, though unstable in blood, are stable in fresh frozen plasma.

White blood cells have a very short life; they are not viable in stored blood. White cell transfusions are available in specialised centres only.

Each unit contains 450 ml of blood and 60–68 ml of CPD or ACD solution; transfusion of 1 unit raises haemoglobin concentration by 1 g per 100 ml. The pH may be 6.7 and potassium content about 20 mmol/l after 3 weeks, but some of this is reabsorbed into red cells after warming and infusion. Each unit contains 10 g albumin, 2 g globulin and 0.7 g fibrinogen.

Indications for blood transfusion in surgical practice

1. Haemorrhage with reduction in blood volume of over 20–30%. This can be corrected after considering preoperative haemoglobin, cardiopulmonary status of recipient, and probability of continuing blood loss.
2. Severe anaemia.
3. Blood-clotting disorders.
4. Extracorporeal circulation.
5. Exchange transfusion.
6. Bleeding during major operations (*see* above).

However, blood conservation in elective surgery can be promoted by:
1. Induced hypotension.
2. Local infiltration with adrenaline and saline.
3. Use of tourniquet.
4. Haemodilution.
5. Autotransfusion.

Complications of blood transfusion

1. Acute haemolysis (immediate or delayed) immune reactions

Acute haemolysis is due to destruction of donor's red cells by antibodies in recipient's plasma, mainly anti-A, anti-B, and anti-D. ABO incompatibility usually causes more immediate and severe reaction than one due to Rhesus factor. Clinically incompatible transfusion in conscious patients is manifested by headache, precordial or lumbar pain, urticaria or pruritus, burning in limbs, bronchospasm, dyspnoea, tachycardia and restlessness, suffused face, nausea and vomiting, pyrexia and rigors, circulatory collapse and later haemoglobinaemia, haemoglobinuria and oliguria.

However, incompatible transfusion under general anaesthesia may not be obvious, because anaesthesia and sedation mask signs; there are hypotension, tachycardia, generalised oozing (bleeding) from surgical wound, urticarial rash and later jaundice and oliguria (in 5–10% of patients). Therefore, the anaesthetist must check blood pressure and pulse rate every 5 minutes for the first quarter-hour with each new unit of blood; if any red rash, hypotension, tachycardia, or cyanosis for which no other cause can be found, the transfusion should be stopped. The incidence of incompatible transfusions under general anaesthesia is between 1 in 3000 and 1 in 15 000 transfusions.

Acute haemolysis is largely mediated by histamine released from mast cells in response to C3a and C5a complement activation by antigen-antibody reaction. It is also mediated by anti-A or anti-B or both (IgM antibodies) causing red cell disruption, releasing phospholipid procoagulant (e.g. erythrocytin) and disseminated intravascular coagulation. Combination of intravascular fibrin deposition and vasospasm leads to acute cortical necrosis of kidneys.

In treatment of acute haemolytic reaction, blood transfusion must be stopped, i.v. colloids or crystalloids may be given to support blood pressure, oxygen may be given to overcome effects of intrapulmonary shunting, diuresis treated with mannitol 50 g or frusemide 100 mg, high doses of steroids and antihistamines may also be given; in disseminated intravascular coagulation, clotting factors and platelets must be replaced.

Delayed haemolytic reaction 4–10 days after transfusion can cause anaemia, jaundice and later renal failure.

Other immune reactions to leucocytes, platelets and plasma protein antigens may occur resulting in mild urticaria or fever; such reactions rarely result in acute anaphylaxis.

2. Transmission of infectious diseases

Many infectious diseases are transmitted by blood transfusion; they require proper medical history, strict criteria for donor selection and the use of laboratory screening tests for prevention.

Viruses

- Human T lymphotropic virus III or human immunodeficiency virus (HIV) can rarely be transmitted by transfusion. Blood should not be taken from those suspected of being at high risk and laboratory screening tests must be carried out on all donated blood.
- All hepatitis viruses (B virus, non-A non-B virus and A virus transmitting both serum and infective hepatitis). No specific screening tests are currently available for routine use in transfusion centres. A history of jaundice or hepatitis is not a reliable indicator of possible carriage of hepatitis viruses.
- Cytomegalovirus.
- Parvovirus.
- Post-perfusion or post-transfusion syndrome similar to infectious mononucleosis but with Epstein–Barr (EB) virus.

Bacteria

- *Staphylococci*.
- *Pseudomonas* and coliforms (Gram-negative septicaemia and shock).
- *Brucellus abortus* (brucellosis).
- *Treponema pallidum* (syphilis d'emblée, i.e. without primary chancre) from patients known to have sexually transmitted diseases.

Protozoa

- *Plasmodium* species transmitted by red cells (malaria). Prevention depends on careful questioning of donors about foreign travel, postponement of donation by those who have recently visited areas in which the disease is endemic, blood films demonstrating plasmodia within red cells and, in some cases, immunological tests for malarial antibodies.
- *Trypanosoma cruzi* (Chagas' disease).
- *Toxoplasma gondii* (toxoplasmosis).

Drugs and malignant diseases

Drugs in the donor's bloodstream may adversely affect a recipient. The taking of any drug could indicate underlying illness, which in itself is reason to exclude the donor. Patients with chronic diseases of unknown aetiology and malignancy should not give blood. Treated locally invasive tumours are exceptions (rodent ulcers or carcinoma *in situ* of the cervix).

3. Circulatory overload

This is a particular danger in heart disease or anaemia, and in elderly patients. The JVP should be watched, and CVP or pulmonary wedge pressure monitored if needed. Frusemide 20–40 mg i.v. can be given at the start of transfusion to prevent overload. Clinically, early signs of pulmonary oedema include cough, dyspnoea, tachycardia, basal crepitations and cyanosis. Blood transfusion must be stopped, the patient must sit up and oxygen is given with frusemide. Tourniquet or venesection may be required.

4. Immunosuppression

Blood transfusion is a potent immunosuppressive agent. It has been observed that haemodialysed patients receiving blood transfusion have less incidence of rejection to renal transplants than patients who have not received blood transfusion prior to transplantation. Similarly, patients who had been transfused because of previous heart surgery (on cardiopulmonary bypass) develop less rejection to heart transplantation than those with no history of cardiac surgery in the past. It is not humane nowadays to subject a patient to transplant surgery without prior blood transfusion in order to lower immunity and to accept the organ graft with less rejection (host versus graft reaction).

It has also been shown that blood transfusion results in reduced ability to clear bacterial load with enhanced morbidity and mortality because of increased incidence of infections. Enhanced sepsis was observed to be significantly more in patients receiving perioperative blood transfusion for penetrating abdominal trauma, Crohn's disease, compound limb fracture, cardiothoracic surgery and in colon cancer, than non-transfused patients in the same diseases mentioned.

It was also noted that perioperative blood transfusion was second only to Dukes' stage as a determinant of tumour recurrence in colorectal cancer. It was reported that while 9% of non-transfused patients undergoing colorectal cancer surgery developed recurrent disease, 43% of transfused patients developed recurrence. This rekindled an interest in the effect of transfusion on recurrence of breast cancer, lung cancer, gastric cancer, renal cancer, sarcomas and following excision of solitary hepatic metastases. Though opinion remains divided, the majority (two-thirds) of retrospective studies confirmed an association between transfusion and enhanced recurrence of human cancer.

Blood transfusion is associated with depression of cell-mediated immunity, including cell-mediated cytolysis, depressed mixed lymphocyte reactivity and depressed mitogen responsiveness due to general non-specific downgrading of immune responses. There are also reduced suppressor/helper T cell ratio, reduced IL-2 and anti-idiotype antibodies (antibodies in recipient directed against his own T cells, probably cytotoxic T cells). In fact addition of exogenous IL-2 may reverse transfusion effect. Transfusion is associated, therefore, with depletion of cytotoxic T cell precursors. The IL-2 may explain effects seen in transplantation, oncology and infection.

5. Hypothermia

Anaesthetised patients, especially children, are vulnerable to hypothermia. Oxygen consumption increases, and cardiac arrest may occur. Prevention is by using a thermostatically controlled blood warmer. The temperature should never exceed 40°C. Furthermore, hypothermia interfers with clotting cascade (enzyme-dependent process requiring heat) and results in bleeding in injured patients.

6. Embolism

Blood micropore filters (20–40 μm pore size) remove micro-aggregates of more than 20 μm diameter during transfusion. Three structures are in common use: (a) surface filters; (b) depth filters; and (c) combination filters. Various materials have been used in their construction, such as woven polyester screen, nylon screen, dacron wool and polyester sponge. They must be fully primed with blood before use. They may prevent lung damage caused by micro-aggregates, but a consensus has not been reached. Problems and dangers of these filters include: slowing of rate of transfusion, complete blockage after 4–10 units of blood, embolism of particles from the filter, haemolysis and massive activation of the clotting process if fresh frozen plasma is infused through a filter. The ordinary micropore infusion set filter pore size is about 170 μm, is more practical in whole blood transfusion and is more useful than micropore filters.

7. Potassium intoxication

Stored blood may contain up to 30 mmol/l of potassium by its expiry date. Potassium intoxication may cause cardiac arrest during transfusion of whole blood. Children and patients with acidosis, hypothermia or renal failure are particularly at risk.

Signs of potassium intoxication include elevation of the T wave on the ECG and widening of the QRS complex. In emergency, slow i.v. injection of 5–10 ml of calcium chloride 10% will temporarily counteract the effects on the heart.

8. Citrate intoxication and hypocalcaemia

A warm oxygenated adult can metabolise the citrate content of 1 unit of CPD blood in 5 min. If the transfusion is faster than this, citrate intoxication may cause tremors, arrhythmias, acidosis and hypocalcaemia. Calcium gluconate 10% 10 ml (2.3 mmol Ca^{2+}) may be required. This complication is most likely in cold or cyanosed patients, or those with severe hepatic disease.

In open-heart surgery and in renal dialysis, heparinised blood may be preferred (5 units/ml). Any haemorrhagic tendency can be controlled by protamine sulphate. Heparinisation does not interfere with calcium stores in the body and citrate intoxication does not arise, but its shelf-life is less than 2 days.

9. pH changes

The pH of stored blood varies between 6.6 and 7.2 due to an accumulation of lactic acid, pyruvic acid, citric acid and raised P_{CO_2}. This may be important in massive transfusion, although metabolism of citrate is likely to result in metabolic alkalosis.

10. Hypomagnesaemia

This is possible during massive transfusion, with particular loss from the myocardium.

11. Transfusion-related acute lung injury

This results from transfusion of the donor's leucocyte aggluti-nating antibodies. It is rare, but causes damage to the lung microvasculature. Washed red cells only should be used from donors who cause this problem.

Massive blood transfusion

Defined as total blood volume replacement by stored blood in under 24 h. It can be regarded as an organ transplant. A bleeding diathesis is common, due mainly to lack of platelets and fibrinogen, and to a lesser extent factors V and VIII. Platelets and fresh frozen plasma should be given as indicated by measurements of platelet count, fibrinogen levels and clotting times.

Precautions during blood donation

Selection of donors

All fresh blood components and manufactured blood products originate with blood donors, so the safety of blood transfusion begins with careful selection of donors. Donors must be:
- in good health,
- unpaid volunteers, as payment could encourage concealment of relevant medical history or personal behaviour.

The good health is assessed in terms of the following.

1. Age. The lower limit is 18 years to take account of the high iron requirements of adolescence, and the medicolegal age of consent. The upper limit is arbitrarily set at 65 years because of the high incidence of cardiovascular and cerebrovascular diseases above this age which make the removal of 450 ml of blood dangerous. However, first time donors are not accepted after the age of 60 due to increased incidence of ill effects; established donors may now be permitted to continue beyond 65.

2. Frequency of donations. This is normally two to three times a year. Women of childbearing age are especially liable to iron depletion. Pregnancy, mother with a baby under 12 months old, and anaemia are contraindications for donation. The minimum acceptable haemoglobin concentrations before donation are 13.5 g/dl for men and 12.5 g/dl for women.

3. Volume of donation. The donated volume should not be more than 13% of the estimated blood volume to protect against vasovagal attacks. The average bag accommodates 450 ml of blood.

4. Likelihood of ill effects during or after donation. Some first time donors faint. Contributory factors are anxiety, hot weather and a previous history of fainting which should be taken into account. A severe faint is a contraindication to future donation.

Questionnaire

Blood must not be accepted from the following donors:

1. AIDS high risk groups:
- Men and women who know they are infected with AIDS virus or who have AIDS.
- Men who have had sex with another man at any time since 1977.
- Men and women who have injected themselves with drugs at any time since 1977.
- Men and women who have had sex at any time since 1977 with men or women living in African countries, except those on the Mediterranean.
- Men and women who have had sex with anyone in these groups. Sexual partners of haemophiliacs.
- Men and women who are prostitutes.

2. Donor under the age of 18 or over 65.

3. Pregnant donor or with a baby under 12 months old.

4. Donors who have had ears pierced or been tattooed or received acupuncture or electrolysis in the last 6 months.

5. Donors who have returned from a malarial area in the last 3 months.

6. Donors who have had glandular fever in the last 2 years.

In addition, donors must be asked directly:

1. Are you taking any medicine or tablets including aspirin?

2. Have you been ill during the last month?

3. Have you received any injections or vaccinations during the last 3 months?

4. Have you had two or more pregnancies in the last 10 years?

5. Are you under 7.5 stone in weight?

6. Have you travelled or lived abroad within the last 2 years (Europe, North America, Australia and New Zealand in the last 3 months or lived in Africa since 1977?)

7. Do you have any of the following conditions: Anaemia, asthma, brucellosis (undulant fever), cancer, diabetes, epilepsy, glandular fever, goitre, hay fever, heart disease, high blood pressure, jaundice or hepatitis (including contact with a case during the past 6 months), kidney disease, malaria, major surgery, nettle rash, pregnancy, miscarriage or abortion (in the last year), stroke, syphilis, tuberculosis.

Screening tests

The blood should routinely be screened for:
- ABC typing.
- Rh D typing, Rh C and E typing. Only donations negative for C, D and E may be labelled Rh negative; those tested only for the D antigen and found negative should be labelled Rh (D) negative.
- Screen for antibodies to red cell antigens. Any donation found to have a high antibody titre should not be used therapeutically, though it may be a valuable source of red cell typing serum. Group O should be tested for high titre of haemolytic anti-A and anti-B and should not be given to patients of other groups except in an emergency.
- HLA histocompatibility for platelet matching.

In addition, all donations must be screened routinely for:
- HBs Ag
- Antibodies to HIV
- *Treponema pallidum.*

Selective microbiological screening, however, is carried out for antibodies to cytomegalovirus (to avoid such donation) and for high titre antitetanus antibodies (to act as a source of antitetanic immunoglobulins).

Quality assurance testing must be carried out on each donation to prevent deterioration during storage; this must be carried out in terms of volume of various blood components, package, sterility and meticulous monitoring of storage and transport with visual check for leakage (splits or pinholes), haemolysis, discoloration, or clotting.

Jehovah's Witnesses

It is important to know that Jehovah's Witnesses refuse blood transfusion on religious grounds; they may be transfused with plasma expanders or other colloid solutions.

There are said to be 3 750 000 Jehovah's Witnesses worldwide, 140 000 of whom live in the UK. They refuse to receive whole blood, packed red blood cells, plasma or platelets. The extracorporeal circulation of an individual's own blood is permitted, providing it does not lose contact with that individual's circulation. For elective surgery, bleeding in excess of 500 ml increases perioperative mortality. However, surgery is generally safe for Jehovah's Witnesses whose haemoglobin is as low as 6 g/dl so long as blood loss is kept below 500 ml.

Controlled preoperative hypotension, haemodilution and regional anaesthesia may be employed to minimise blood loss. Recently, recombinant erythropoietin, which is acceptable to Jehovah's Witnesses, has been used to increase red cell production in anaemic patients pre- and postoperatively. The search for a useful synthetic alternative to blood continues.

GENERAL PRINCIPLES AND PRACTICE IN SURGERY

1.9 Genetic Factors in Surgery and Genetic Diseases of Surgical Importance

Genetic factors can be an important underlying cause in the pathogenesis of the surgical disease. Indeed, some surgical conditions can be inherited from one generation to another within the same family, e.g. familial adenomatous polyposis (known previously as familial polyposis coli). Cancer can be considered a genetic disease; it now seems possible that up to half of colorectal cancer has an underlying genetic background.

Genetic diseases may have diagnostic implications in surgery. Sickle cell disease may cause acute abdominal pain, while hereditary spherocytosis may cause jaundice, and both must be considered in the differential diagnosis of abdominal pain and jaundice respectively.

Genetic diseases may have therapeutic implications too. In haemophiliacs, bleeding imposes a particular problem during surgical procedures, e.g. circumcision. Furthermore, surgery on patients with unrecognised inherited immunologically deficient diseases, such as Bruton's congenital agammaglobulinaemia, and Di George's thymic aplasia, may lead to infection and bleeding due to the congenital immunosuppression; specific surgical precautions must be taken (see sections 1.10, 1.13).

More importantly, many genetic diseases are either associated with visceral anomalies (e.g. congenital heart disease in Down's syndrome) or can themselves lead to complications (e.g. pathological fractures in osteogenesis imperfecta, gallstones in hereditary spherocytosis, mesenteric infarction in sickle cell disease) that require surgical treatment.

Furthermore, patients with familial and genetically determined diseases may face anaesthetic problems. These diseases must be enquired about by anesthetists in the preoperative assessment of a patient's fitness for surgery: e.g., porphyria, malignant hyperpyrexia, hypertension, haemophilia, myotonic dystrophy and familial hyperlipoproteinaemia.

While there is no effective treatment for most genetic diseases, surgery may occasionally provide the primary therapeutic option, e.g. prophylactic proctocolectomy in familial adenomatous polyposis, repair of hypospadias, spinal correction of scoliosis and orthopaedic correction of congenital dislocation of the hip and congenital club foot.

Genetic diseases can be classified into:
- Chromosomal disorders due to numerical or structural abnormalities of autosomes or sex chromosomes.
- Unifactorial disorders due to defects of a single gene of the chromosome (DNA coding); the inheritance and risks of recurrence can be predicted from Mendelian laws.
- Multifactorial disorders due to familial predisposition; the inheritance and risks of recurrence cannot be predicted from Mendelian laws. Empiric risks can be determined from the frequency of the disease among the relatives of affected individuals.

Oncogenes are genes (present in normal cells) which promote cell growth and proliferation. Tumour suppressor genes or antioncogenes have the opposite function. Cellular (c-) oncogenes are normal genes which code for proteins (oncoproteins) that are implicated in normal cellular proliferation, and are dominant oncogenes or recessive/suppressor oncogenes. Oncogenes become implicated in carcinogenesis when their encoded proteins become overexpressed, turncated (mutated), or modified. Retinoblastoma (Rb) dominant oncogene occurs only when the normal gene 13q14 undergoes spontaneous mutation in the eye. Similarly, P53 oncogene normally prevents malignant transformation by suppressing cell division preventing entry into cell cycle S-phase; mutated P53 inactivate suppressor P53 and 50% of tumours of breast, colon, lung, bladder and hepatomas are associated with mutated P53.

The chromosome has a short arm or p (from petite) and a long arm termed q (q comes after p and is therefore longer). Familial adenomatous polyposis (FAP) is an autosomal dominant and FAP gene is situated on the long arm of chromosome 5 (termed 5q21). Similarly, retinoblastoma, neurofibromatosis, Wilms' tumour, breast ovarian cancer syndrome, and hereditary non-polyposis colon cancer are all autosomal dominant diseases. The affected genes are 13q14 (with susceptibility to retinoblastoma and osteogenic sarcoma tumours); 17q11 and 22q13 (with susceptibility to schwanomas and optic neuroma/ acoustic neuroma/meningioma/glioma tumours); 11p13 (with susceptibility to nephroblastoma); BRCA1 – 17Q21 and BRCA2 – 13Q21 (with susceptibility to breast, ovarian, and pancreatic cancers); hMSH2 – 2p12, hMLH1 – 3p21, hPMS1 – 2q31, hPMS – 7p22 (with susceptibility to colorectal, endometrial, ovarian cancers) respectively.

CHROMOSOMAL DISORDERS

Gross abnormalities of chromosome number or structure are not compatible with survival in man, particularly if they affect more than one chromosome; both polyploidy (gaining a set of chromosomes) and monosomy (losing a whole autosome) were found to be lethal. They constitute a common cause of intrauterine death, associated with over 50% of spontaneous abortions and miscarriages. Trisomy however, results in less severe effects (see below).

Autosomal abnormalities

Trisomy-21 (addition of an extra chromosome resulting in three chromosomes instead of two at chromosomal set number 21) is the commonest autosomal disorder; it has a significant relationship to an increased maternal age.

Trisomy-21 results in Down's syndrome, which is associated with congenital visceral anomalies, particularly congenital heart disease, duodenal atresia and imperforate anus. Many of these cases, therefore, are referred to cardiac surgeons, and/or paediatric surgeons and/or general surgeons. It is also associated with acute leukaemia. Those who survive the first year of life may survive into adulthood and may marry; 50% of their offspring are normal and 50% will have Down's syndrome.

Sex-linked chromosome abnormalities

Numerical abnormalities here are more common than with autosomes and with less severe effects.

Klinefelter's syndrome XXY is sex chromosome aneuploidy in males (aneuploidy is numerical abnormality arising when one or more chromosomes are either lost or gained). Like Down's syndrome, klinefelter's syndrome affects the sons of elderly mothers. Clinically, the patient is sterile (azoospermia), with hypogonadism, gynaecomastia and often mental retardation. The patient may consult infertility clinics run by urologists, or may be referred to plastic surgeons for the reduction of gynaecomastia.

Turner's syndrome XO is sex chromosome aneuploidy in females. It does not show a relationship with increased maternal age. Clinically, the patient is short and mentally retarded; she lacks secondary sex characters and has primary amenorrhoea. The congenital anomalies may be a reason for referral to surgery; webbing of the neck may be referred to plastic surgeons, cubitus valgus (increased carrying-angle of the forearm) to orthopaedic surgeons, and coarctation of the aorta to cardiac surgeons.

UNIFACTORIAL DISORDERS

Autosomal dominant diseases

A dominant trait is manifested in the heterozygote, i.e. a person possessing both the abnormal (mutant) gene and the normal gene, the presence of only one mutant gene (single dose) being adequate for the trait to be manifested in the carrier. If the condition is common, then affected persons could be homozygotes (having a double dose of mutant gene), but if the condition is rare (as is usually the case), then affected persons are almost always heterozygotes.

In severe diseases such as orthopaedically crippled patients with **achondroplasia**, affected persons seldom have children because they are either infertile or do not survive to reach reproductive age. The disease will eventually become extinct in affected families; it can only be maintained by fresh new mutations.

In less severe diseases, such as **polycystic disease of kidneys** (followed up in urology clinics), and **familial adenomatous polyposis** (FAP, previously called familial polyposis coli) (followed up in clinics of colorectal surgery), the surgeon can trace the disease through many generations of the family tree. Although affected individuals may eventually die from renal failure and malignant intestinal obstruction respectively, they often remain asymptomatic until early adulthood or middle age.

Occasionally, a carrier of the mutant gene may not always express its effects. Those who do not exhibit any of of the gene effects are called *non-penetrant*, a phenomenon where the dominant trait has skipped generations in the family tree, thus imposing problems in genetic counselling and in assessing risks of recurrence. It is caused by the modifying influence of other genes and environmental factors. For a gene to be fully *penetrant*, its effects must be manifested in the carrier of that gene. Furthermore, severity of the clinical manifestations or expressivity may be variable. Patients with **osteogenesis imperfecta** seen in the orthopaedic department may express only blue sclerae, whereas others may express the full spectrum of the disease, i.e. blue sclerae, deafness and multiple fractures.

COLORECTAL CARCINOGENESIS – THE GENETIC BASIS

Cancer can be considered a genetic disease, in which increased expression of certain genes (oncogenes) and decreased expression of tumour-suppressor genes (TSG) give rise to loss of normal cellular control mechanisms resulting in neoplastic change. TSG exert most influence over tumour development. Although mutations in many TSG are needed for development of a tumour, replacement of any lost TSG not only causes reversion to a non-neoplastic phenotype, but prevents subsequent tumour growth in animal studies. These findings have considerable implications in cancer therapy. TSG have been identified by three different methods of study:

- Somatic cell hybridisation, where a neoplastic cell and a normal cell are combined to produce a non-neoplastic hybrid cell line with unstable subsequent mitoses resulting in loss of some chromosomes and a return to neoplastic phenotype when a TSG is lost.
- Loss of heterozygosity where tumour DNA is combined with genomic DNA from the same individual in order to identify regions in the genome in which mutations have occurred.
- Family studies in autosomal dominantly inherited conditions, such as FAP in order to localise the underlying single defective gene.

Geneticians were able to identify three TSG as being commonly mutated in colorectal cancer. These are:

- APC gene on the long arm of chromosome 5, mutations in which give rise to FAP.
- p53 gene on chromosome 17, which is mutated in over two-thirds of all human solid tumours.
- DCC gene on chromosome 18.

One oncogene, KRAS, is also commonly mutated in colorectal cancer; it is activated in over 40% of colorectal carcinomas.

Studies of adenomas of varying sizes and degrees of differentiation have shown that mutations in APC gene occur very early in adenoma formation and are likely to be the causative mutation in these tumours. Mutations in KRAS and p53 genes are only commonly seen in larger adenomas and so are likely to be involved in malignant change. Mutations in DCC are most commonly seen in malignant tumours and so are implicated in tumour progression.

There are two features of colorectal cancer which have greatly facilitated its molecular analysis. First, the existence of a clearly described autosomal dominant condition, FAP, enabled the causative agent to be identified and studied in colorectal cancer cases. Secondly, the fact that carcinoma can usually develop from premalignant adenomas enabled genetic steps to be traced from early adenomas through to metastatic carcinoma.

The two documented genetically inherited colorectal cancerous conditions are FAP and hereditary non-polyposis colon cancer (HNPCC). However, inherited predisposition to colorectal cancer is not limited to these rare conditions. Studies revealed that family members of patients affected by colorectal cancer were at 3–5 times higher risk of colorectal cancer than the general population, due to genetic predisposition; it now seems possible that up to half of colorectal cancer has an underlying genetic cause. There is considerable evidence to support prospective colonoscopic surveillance of family members at increased risk of colorectal cancer in order to reduce associated morbidity and mortality.

FAP and HNPCC are of genetic surgical importance and deserve elaborated discussion.

1. Familial adenomatous polyposis (FAP) (previously called familial polyposis coli)

The most widely recognised form of inherited colorectal cancer, FAP is easily recognised because of autosomal dominant inheritance facilitating rapid diagnosis and early treatment for affected members. However, it accounts for only 1% of all colorectal cancers. The condition is not confined to the colorectal region and documentation of extracolonic manifestations required the condition name (polyposis coli) to be changed to familial adenomatous polyposis.

About 80% of patients presenting with FAP will have a family history of a mother or father with the condition. About 20% of patients therefore, will not have any family history or relatives with the condition. Endoscopic examination of large intestine is important in parents of such a patient to be absolutely certain that they are not affected. These patients without family history are labelled as spontaneous mutation cases, i.e. they just happen to have developed the genetic make-up of FAP without inheriting it, though it may be difficult to be certain about spontaneous mutation, because a father that died in car accident at a young age, for example, could have had the disease without its being documented. However, the offspring of such patients with spontaneous mutation continue to transmit the autosomal dominant disease at the usual 50% risk level.

The majority of patients with FAP (80%) will show evidence of adenomatous polyps (predominantly tubular) in the rectum and sigmoid: by the age of 20 years, although occasionally some develop adenomas in the 20–30 year age group, and rarely after 30 years (the condition is extremely rare below the age of 10). It used to be thought that 100 polyps would be required for diagnosis of FAP; however, this is unrealistic because polyps grow in small numbers and increase in number over years so that early diagnosis could easily be made on a much lower number than a 100, particularly if it is known that the child's parent has the condition or is recorded in the FAP registry. The risk of malignant transformation in colorectal polyps would seem to be 100%, and cancers have been reported below the age of 20 and, more commonly, in the 20–30 and 30–40 age groups. Proctosigmoidoscopy should be performed from the age of 10 on all children from kindreds at risk, on an annual basis.

Extracolonic manifestations of FAP may be benign or malignant. These include epidermoid cysts and osteomas of jaws and skull bones which may occur prior to adenoma. FAP patients may have other jaw abnormalities, such as unerupted teeth and dentigerous cysts on occasions; a peroral X-ray of the jaw is a must for FAP patients and children at risk. They may also have abnormal pigmentation of the retina, which is called congenital hypertrophy of the retinal pigment epithelium (CHRPE), a characteristic ophthalmoscopic finding in FAP patients, affecting 70% of kindred. In fact, when a patient demonstrates CHRPE, all members of that kindred that have FAP will demonstrate the eye changes. CHRPE has been seen at 3 month of age; it is of great value as a screening tool in at-risk children (before the age of polyp formation) as a means of early diagnosis. CHRPE may be a heralding extracolonic sign for subsequent colonic polyp formation; members of kindred without CHRPE will be the group that do not develop adenomas. These pigmentation changes (CHRPE) do not seem to be disease-related and do not have disease potential; they are more of a birthmark of FAP. CHRPE must affect both eyes to be clinically predictive in FAP kindred.

Other extracolonic manifestations include ileal polyps and malignancies in either a continent ileostomy or an ileoanal reservoir as well as upper small intestinal polyps. Fundal gland type non-adenomatous polyps may develop in the stomach too, but with less malignant potential. However, duodenal polyps of tubular-villous and villous adenomatous nature may develop with strong malignant potential; in fact, in patients undergoing colectomy to avoid death from colon cancer, duodenal cancer is the next most common cause of death. Endoscopically these polyps are multiple sessile carpeting type, situated in the second part of doudenum; adenoma can also develop around papilla. About 10% of FAP patients will develop duodenal carcinoma. It is impossible to destroy duodenal polyps endoscopically; endoscopic surveillance with duodenal biopsies followed by surgical intervention at pre-malignant stage will be required.

Desmoid tumours are common in FAP patients, wrongly called fibrosarcoma. They are more likely to be excessive areas of scar tissue or fibromatosis resulting in excessive adhesions in the abdominal cavity and distinct masses, particularly small bowel mesentery, and usually arising following operations such as prophylactic colectomy. They may also arise on the back, buttocks, lumbar area and groin. They are of variable growth potential, some lying dormant for years, while others are aggressive. Their growth is hormonally controlled; drugs like tamoxifen, sulindac, indomethacin and progesterone have all been thought to create a shrinkage of desmoid tumour. Aggressive tumours may obstruct intestine and ureter. Recurrence is very high and can even follow massive resection of small intestine en bloc with the desmoid; they are better left for hormonal manipulation. Rapid response to medical therapy may create necrosis, and possibly abscess formation in desmoids with small bowel fistulas as well as Gram-Negative septicaemia.

Other rare tumours in FAP patients include childhood hepatoblastoma, medulloblastoma and gliomas in teenagers and adult thyroid cancer, ovarian cancer and adrenal cancer.

Management of FAP involves documentation of the disease, identification of kindred and of individuals at risk within that kindred, genetic counselling and education of family members as to that risk and recommendations for on-going clinical and endoscopic surveillance to detect disease in a presymptomatic and precancerous stage, offering prophylactic colectomy to prevent inevitable colorectal carcinoma.

Development of a FAP registry (data collection of reported cases with identified families and kindreds) helps. It can:
- provide early identification of patients at risk within families;
- maintain contact with families;
- offer genetic counselling to explain the condition by providing information and leaflets and alleviating the family's questions and anxieties;
- refer for screening at an appropriate age;
- document extracolonic manifestations by ensuring continuing surveillance of those at risk;
- provide tissue and blood samples for clinical studies and DNA chromosomal investigation;
- update families about new developments;
- offer support to families, including through formation of family support groups.

Diagnosis of FAP is established on the basis of age, family history, ophthalmoscopy (CHRPE), proctosigmoidoscopy and biopsy, and blood for chromosomal and DNA studies.

The most frequent cause of death in FAP is colorectal cancer, and if left untreated there is a 100% risk of malignancy occurring in the large bowel. In the past, prophylactic proctocolectomy and ileostomy was thought initially to cure the disease. Many of these patients are asymptomatic and young and it is difficult to persuade them, or their parents, of the necessity to have an ileostomy. However, colectomy with ileorectal anastomosis solved the problem of ileostomy but left a calculated risk in the residual rectal mucosa with potential for polyp formation and malignant transformation in the rectum. The ileoanal reservoir procedure has now become the popular option for FAP patients. The colon is removed, the rectum and lower rectal mucosa excised but leaving the anal sphincter. A new rectum is then created from the ileum as an ileal reservoir and this is anastomosed or stapled to the anus. This does remove large intestinal mucosa but preserves anal sphincter function, therefore avoiding a permanent ileostomy. The procedure is usually (though not always) performed in two stages with temporary loop ileostomy for a few weeks following the creation of a new rectum with ileal reservoir. Recent modifications of this operation have improved the functional results; stool frequency, incontinence and faecal and mucous leakage have been reduced considerably in the past few years.

The risk of cancer in the rectum and colon is obviated by this procedure. The real question is whether the complexity of this operation is warranted with a comparatively low risk of rectal cancer, with proponents for and against. Neither of these operations cures FAP disease, because extracolonic manifestations, which may also be malignant, cannot obviously be cured by excision of the colon and rectum. There is a possibility also that the ileoanal reservoir procedure may not be possible in FAP patients, because of desmoid tumours, or that the procedure may precipitate growth of desmoid tumours. This is of particular importance in patients who have already had ileorectal anastomosis, who develop large number of polyps and who are considered for conversion to ileoanal reservoir.

The most appropriate prophylactic colectomy has still to be defined. Young children with only a few rectal polyps may safely be handled by colectomy with ileorectal anastomosis, but with on-going surveillance of rectal mucosa. Those with more florid polyposis at diagnosis, particularly in the rectum, may well be appropriate candidates for ileoanal reservoir. It is possible in most cases to convert ileorectal anastomosis into ileoanal reservoir if rectal polyp deteriorates. It is seldom if ever necessary to perform proctocolectomy and ileostomy in FAP patients, except for those who develop cancer in the lower rectum at time of presentation. It is imperative to discuss the surgical options with patients so that they and their family members are fully aware of the consequences of their decision-making. Better education and avoidance of ileostomy offers compliance with follow-up of other family members.

Related polyposis syndromes may all result in polyps arising in the large intestine, indicating a genetic predisposition to adenoma and therefore colorectal cancers.
- FAP – the most significantly related to cancer.
- Peutz–Jegher's syndrome – with hamartomas developing predominantly in the stomach and small intestine resulting in periodic intussusception and small bowel obstruction. While small bowel malignancy can be a long-term compli-

cation, colonic hamartomatous polyps can arise in this condition.

- Gardner's syndrome (GS) – Dr Eldon John Gardner, an American geneticist, described in 1962 a family with FAP that demonstrated epidermoid cysts, osteomas and, added later, desmoid tumours. He initially thought GS was a distinctly separate syndrome, but it is apparent now that GS has crossover with FAP with extracolonic manifestations.
- Turcot's syndrome – described in patients with large bowel adenomas (of hereditary nature) associated with brain tumours, predominantly medulloblastoma. These are now thought to be FAP patients (at puberty age) with medulloblastoma as an extracolonic manifestation preceding colonic polyp formation.
- Cronkite Canada syndrome with colonic inflammatory adenomatous polyps at an older age than FAP patients. Polyps are commonly multiple, but in small number (fewer than a 100), with malignant transformation of polyps in older age groups.
- There are other inherited syndromes associated with colorectal cancer, including hereditary hyperplastic polyposis, juvenile polyps and syndromes described by Gorlin, Cowden and Muir–Torre.
- Inflammatory non-adenomatous pseudopolyposis, seen in colorectal ulcerative colitis, is also precancerous.

2. Hereditary non-polyposis colon cancer (HNPCC)

This is the second form of autosomal dominant inheritant colorectal cancer; it is more common than FAP, accounting for 5–10% of all colorectal cancers, but has a less characteristic phenotype. Consequently, it can only reliably be identified through family pedigree studies. Unlike FAP, which is diagnosed on pathology, HNPCC can only be diagnosed once further information is available from other affected family members. It is characterised by development of cancer at an early age, and by the excess of multiple primary cancers, with predominant proximal colonic cancers. It is therefore, divided into:

- Lynch syndrome type I, site-specific (colonic cancer).
- Lynch syndrome type II, HNPCC with other forms of cancer, e.g. endometrial carcinoma in female patients.

Diagnosis cannot be made in individual patients. The minimum criteria for diagnosing HNPCC (Amsterdam criteria) are:

1. At least three relatives with histologically proven colorectal cancer. One of them should be a first-degree relative. FAP should be excluded.

2. At least two successive generations should be affected.

3. In one of the affected relatives colorectal cancer should be diagnosed under 50 years.

Clinically, HNPCC usually starts 20 years earlier than in the general population. Peak age of onset is 30–50 years in both men and women. About 60% of tumours affect the proximal colon, while 40% of tumours are sporadic. Multiple (synchronous and metachronous) colorectal cancers are found in 25% of cases. In practice, however, many cancer families do not conform to the rules and need to be considered on a case-by-case basis. A regional registry is required, as for FAP families.

OTHER AUTOSOMAL DOMINANT DISEASES ENCOUNTERED BY SURGEONS

Hereditary spherocytosis

Hereditary spherocytosis may present with haemolytic anaemia, cholelithiasis (pigment stone formation) and cholecystitis, jaundice, splenomegaly and leg ulcers. It is, therefore, important in the differential diagnosis of jaundice; patients may be referred for cholecystectomy and splenectomy.

Haemoglobinopathies

Among all haemoglobinopathies, **sickle cell anaemia** (haemoglobin S) in negroes has a special impact on all surgeons, because of the excessive haemolysis, tissue infarction and vulnerability to infection. The haemolytic crises and sickling of red blood corpuscles (RBCs) result in obstruction of the blood flow at the level of terminal arterioles/capillaries; thrombosis may follow, resulting in tissue infarction and severe pain (commonly in bones and spleen). Furthermore, distorted cells are phagocytosed by the reticuloendothelial system leading to its enlargement and shortening RBC life span. Sickling is precipitated by dehydration, chilling, hypoxia (altitude or flying in an aeroplane) and infection, but sometimes the crisis occurs spontaneously.

Patients may be referred to orthopaedic surgeons because of bone pain/tenderness and fusiform swellings of fingers and toes (dactylitis), bone cysts, bone abscesses, aseptic necrosis of the head of the femur, leg ulcers, salmonella osteomyelitis and possible pathological fractures; these complications may all shorten bones and delay the growth.

General surgeons may be consulted for acute abdominal emergencies induced by the acute non-specific abdominal pain, or even mesenteric infarction. Excessive haemolysis, too, results in rapid enlargement of the spleen and liver and cholelithiasis/cholecystitis; with the patient's predisposition to salmonella infection, splenectomy and cholecystectomy may occasionally be required. Leg ulcers (due to avascular necrosis) may either be referred to general, orthopaedic or vascular surgeons.

Urologists may be called for painless haematuria resulting from an infarction of the renal papillae. Pregnancy is hazardous unless careful antenatal care is provided. Infarctive crises in bones may result in fat embolism, causing diffuse pulmonary microembolism, infarction, cor pulmonale and even death.

Patients with sickle cell anaemia are resistant to *Plasmodium falciparum* malaria (but not other types of malaria). Patients must be screened for sickling prior to surgery. Infections such as salmonellosis and malaria (malaria is a form of haemolytic anaemia and results in excessive haemolysis of RBCs) must be eliminated preoperatively with antibiotics and antimalarials respectively; 5 mg daily folic acid supplements must be prescribed (to activate erythropoiesis). Hypoxia, dehydration and chilling must all be avoided during anaesthetic induction and operation.

Bloodless field surgery should never be employed, because infarction of the entire limb below the tourniquet may occur. Blood transfusion is indicated only when the haemoglobin level drops below 5 g/dl (patients are habituated to low haemoglobin level, i.e. around 8 g/dl). Due to the recurrent nature of the disease, narcotic analgesia may lead to addiction; simple non-addictive analgesics, e.g. aspirin, paracetamol and codeine, are used instead.

Marfan's syndrome

Patients are tall with blue sclerae; they may be referred to vascular surgeons for elective repair of abdominal aortic aneurysms. Rarely, leaking aneurysms may require an emergency repair.

Neurofibromatosis

Excision of skin masses by general surgeons may be required when they become symptomatic due to pressure symptoms.

Hyperlipoproteinaemia type II

Occasionally these patients may be referred to general surgeons for resection of terminal ileum (main site for fatty acids reabsorption).

Porphyria

Patients undergoing surgery are associated with anaesthetic problems, due to drug interactions and labile blood pressure during perioperative monitoring.

Multiple endocrine neoplasms MEN (see s. 1.40, Skin markers of internal cancers)

Malignant hyperpyrexia

This is either familial (multifactorial disorder) or inherited as an autosomal dominant trait. The condition is a rare but lethal complication of anaesthesia. *In vitro* malignant hyperpyrexia susceptibility can be diagnosed by electrical stimulation of contracture response to caffeine and halothane.

Patients develop a rapid rise in temperature under general anaesthesia with halothane or suxamethonium; increased muscle rigidity (and excessively high Pa_{CO_2}), tachypnoea, tahycardia, hypotension, cyanosis and metabolic lactic acidosis develop with pyrexia in a very accelerated manner. Death may occur from arrhythmias or cardiac arrest quickly, sometimes even before the surgeon closes the patient's wound. In the majority of cases, skeletal muscles display increased tone and fasciculation; it may be a form of myopathy since high serum creatine phosphokinase (CPK) and aldolase are detected. Dantrolene (dantrium) acts on skeletal muscle by interfering with calcium efflux in muscle cell and stopping contractile process; a rapid i.v. injection of 1 mg/kg may be repeated as required to a cumulative maximum of 10 mg/kg.

Following fatality, a muscle biopsy from quadriceps femoris muscle (preferably vastus intermedialis) without formalin is required for histochemical analysis. Once the patient is labelled with this condition, other family members may undergo only necessary surgery in future, but with full anaestheic precautions, namely avoiding halothane or suxamethonium.

Autosomal dominant inheritance is, theoretically, the simplest form of inheritance, but in practice it can be very complicated. Because of its particular importance as a mode of inheritance in many diseases of surgical interest, the inheritance characteristics are worth considering:
1. Heterozygotes manifest the disease.
2. Males and females are affected equally.
3. Fifty per cent offspring of affected individuals will inherit the disease.
4. Variable expression: the disorder is expressed in individuals to a different degree, e.g. age of onset, extracolonic manifestation in FAP patients.
5. Penetrance: in some dominantly inherited disorders, some individuals known to possess the gene may show no sign of disease.
6. New mutation: apparently isolated cases may represent new mutations.
7. Germinal mosaicism: there may be a mutation in a clone of cells in one of the gonads, resulting in a normal parent having more than one affected child.
8. Locus heterogeneity: mutations in different genes may give rise to similar phenotypes.
9. Intragenic heterogeneity: different mutations in the same gene may account for some variation in phenotype.

Autosomal recessive diseases

Unlike dominant traits, recessive traits are manifest only in the homozygous state, i.e. manifestation requires double dose of mutant gene; heterozygotes are usually healthy. Offspring of the affected person are usually normal, because most recessive diseases are so rare that it would be most unlikely that an affected person would marry a heterozygous person. So one cannot trace the disease from one generation to another. Consanguineous mating is therefore not advisable (may be difficult in Britain because 1 in 200 marriages is between first cousins).

Autosomal recessive disorders include most inborn errors of metabolism, notably galactosaemia. However, xeroderma pigmentosum (premalignant skin disease), cystic fibrosis, congenital adrenal hyperplasia (female pseudohermaphroditism) and congenital goitrous cretinism may be of occasional surgical interest.

Sex-linked dominant diseases

With the exception of hairy ears, there are no proven examples of Y-linked single gene disorders in man.

Vitamin D resistant rickets is the notable representation of X-linked dominant disorders, which is manifested both in males and females who are heterozygous for the mutant gene; males carry the mutant gene on their single X chromosome.

Sex-linked recessive diseases

X-linked recessive diseases include haemophilia and Christmas disease, which are of great interest to surgeons. They are caused by a gene carried on the X chromosome and are manifested in females only when the gene is in the homozygous state, a rare predicament because she would have to inherit the gene from both parents; she will probably die of bleeding with the onset of her menstrual period. In males, a mutant gene on the single X chromosome is always manifest, because it is unopposed by modifying effect of a normal gene on the second X chromosome, as happens in females. An affected father (on marriage with a normal woman) transmits the gene to his daughters only (who become carriers later); an X-linked trait is never transmitted from father to son. On marriage with an affected son, the apparently healthy heterozygous mother acts as a carrier transmitting disease to her affected son and to her daughter who will become another carrier.

Other X-linked recessive disorders include **glucose-6-phosphate dehydrogenase deficiency** in RBCs, a common cause of haemolytic anaemia among negroes; haemolytic crises occur after eating broad beans or *Vicia faba* (favism), or following infections particularly if the patient is taking sulphonamides, antimalarials, acetylsalicylic acid, chloramphenicol, chloroquine and phenacetin.

Other X-linked recessive diseases include Duchenne muscular dystrophy, Lesch–Nyhan syndrome with gout and mental deficiency due to overproduction of uric acid (of interest to orthopaedic surgeons), and nephrogenic diabetes insipidus with excessive urine output and constant thirst (of importance in perioperative fluid and electrolyte correction).

MULTIFACTORIAL DISORDERS OR CONGENITAL AND FAMILIAL DISEASES

These are due to the interplay of many genes with the effects of environment. Many common disorders are inherited in this way. The developing fetus is sensitive to the action of acquired external factors (physical, chemical, living organisms and dietary deficiencies) influencing the mother. Intrauterine events may produce defects which are present at birth (congenital) but which are not inherited through a single known genetic mechanism. The liability is related to genetic predisposition facilitated by environmental factors. The threshold of liability among affected persons is different from the liability threshold of healthy persons. Relatives of affected individuals have a higher liability than the population (familial incidence is higher than population incidence).

Familial incidence varies with many factors: it is greater among relatives of more severely affected individuals. Thus, in hare lip with or without cleft palate, familial incidence of affected sibs (brothers and sisters) and children is 6% (hare lip and cleft palate), but it is only 2.5% (hare lip only). Familial incidence is also increased with subsequent pregnancies; in spina bifida, and related anencephaly, familial incidence among sibs born after one affected child is 5%, but it rises to 10% after the birth of two affected children. This is different from unifactorial inheritance where the risk to subsequent sibs remains constant irrespective of the number of affected persons in the family (in two heterozygous parents, it is 1 in 4 for autosomal recessive disorders). Finally, the relatives of the less frequently affected sex would be more often affected. Thus in congenital pyloric stenosis, which is five times more common in boys than girls, the affected relatives of a male patient are 5.5% for sons and 2.4% for daughters, but for a female patient it is 19.4% for sons and 7.3% for daughters.

Table 1.9.1 Multifactorial disorders

Disease	Incidence (%)	Sex ratio (M/F)	Heritability (%)
General surgery			
Peptic ulcer	4	M mainly	37
Congenital pyloric stenosis	0.3	5/1	75
Hirschsprung's disease	0.02	4/1	–
Orthopaedic surgery			
Congenital club foot	0.1	2/1	68
Congenital dislocation of hip	0.1	1/6	60
Scoliosis	0.22	1/6	–
Ankylosing spondylitis	0.2	M mainly	70
Neurosurgery			
Anencephaly	0.2	1/2	60
Spina bifida	0.3	2/3	60
Maxillofacial surgery			
Cleft lip = cleft palate	0.1	3/2	76
Cardiac surgery			
Congenital heart disease	0.5	–	35
Coronary artery disease	3	M mainly	65
Essential hypertension	5	–	62
Urology			
Hypospadias	0.2	M only	–

Heritability can be calculated from knowing the incidence of disease in the general population and among relatives; it estimates how much of the aetiology can be ascribed to genetic factors as opposed to environmental factors.

Important multifactorial diseases of surgical interest are shown in Table 1.9.1, with known population incidence, male/female sex ratio and heritability.

PREVENTION OF GENETIC DISEASES

There is no effective treatment for most genetic disorders, and the role of the doctor lies in the prevention of such conditions through genetic counselling.

Diagnosis of the disease and its genetic nature must first be established; the relatives must then be screened for the disease before genetic counselling is undertaken.

Genetic-counselling involves providing advice on the chances of recurrence, risks and consequences of disorder inheritance in children of either healthy parents who already have an affected child, or when one of the parents or a near relative is affected with an inherited disease, as well as discussion on possible prevention and amelioration. It may dissuade high-risk couples from procreation, but once conception has occurred, the only course open may be the induction of abortion. Genetic counselling is also important in planning appropriate screening for presymptomatic early diagnosis.

Antenatal diagnosis by amniocentesis (aspiration of 5–10 ml of amniotic fluid around the 16th week of gestation) with selective abortion of the affected fetuses (before the 20th week) is currently a viable option open to parents. The sex of the fetus, cytogenic abnormalities, some inborn errors of metabolism, Down's syndrome, anencephaly and open spina bifida (the latter two have high alpha-fetoprotein in amniotic fluid) can all be diagnosed in utero after the biochemical analysis of the supernatant of the amniotic fluid after centrifugation.

GENE THERAPY

In 1992/3, the National Institutes of Health at Bethesda (USA) devised an ingenious strategy for selectively killing tumour cells while sparing healthy ones by using a retrovirus to slip into the tumour cells of the gene for herpes simplex thymidine kinase, thereby rendering the cells targets for destruction by the antiviral drug ganciclovir. Retroviruses will insert their genes only into dividing cells and although ineffective for quiescent brain cells, are ideal for antitumour therapy. The retroviruses used are genetically altered so that they can infect a cell once and deliver their genes to the nucleus, but they cannot replicate. One drawback is the short survival – a few hours – of retroviruses after injection into brain tumour; this can be overcome by injection of engineered mouse cells (infected with retroviruses) surviving for 2–3 weeks inside the tumour and serving as a virus factory by continuously releasing the virus. The viruses then infect neighbouring tumour cells and plant thymidine kinase gene in their nuclei; if an infected tumour cell divides, the deadly gene is passed on to daughter cells as well. Mouse cells are delivered to the tumour using a stereotactic device guided by CT or MRI. Cells are not rejected because few immune cells circulate inside the brain. Seven days later, i.v. ganciclovir is administered and continued for 2 weeks. Patients stay in the hospital about 1 month and those who show an initial response are considered for repeated treatments.

1.10 Immunology in Surgical Practice

NON-SPECIFIC IMMUNE MECHANISMS

Host defences

1. Local superficial defences (mechanical barriers)

● **Skin** is provided with:
  – stratified epithelium (squamous)
  – fatty acids (make pH unfavourable to bacteria);
  – increased salt concentration with sweating providing mechanical flushing away from the skin due to sweating;
  – dryness;
  – normal flora themselves keep a natural balance with other organisms, so flora suppression leads to superadded infection.
● **Urinary tract** is provided with:
  – mechanical flushing of micturition;
  – dilution by urine.

● **Respiratory tract** is provided with:
  – nasal hair to filter foreign bodies and bacteria;
  – ciliated columnar epithelium pushing bacteria and foreign bodies upwards and away;
  – mucus, trapping bacteria;
  – cough reflex.
● **Female genital tract** is provided with:
  – mucus;
  – acidic pH by lactobacilli.
However, the patent fimbrial end of the Fallopian tube is connected to the peritoneal cavity under normal circumstances, i.e. the female peritoneal cavity is not a closed cavity as in males; a woman skiing on water may develop peritonitis (if she is unprotected with a vaginal pad).
● **Gastrointestinal tract** (GIT) is provided with:
  – acidic pH;
  – bile salts;
  – mucus;
  – normal flora in a balance with each other.
The GIT, however, is a highly specialised immunological apparatus, separate from systemic immunity. Prominent features in the normal mucosa include IgA-containing plasma cells and T-cells (present both in lamina propria and between epithelium). This concept has important implications in inflammatory bowel disease, since mucosal immune pattern is altered in inflammatory bowel disease (with more representation of IgG and IgM plasma cells with increased T-cell infiltrate), indicating the possibility of being either an autoimmune reaction directed against GIT epithelium, or a sensitisation of local mucosa (GIT immunological system) to GIT contents. Inflammatory mediators (such as cytokines) may also play a part in the aetiology of inflammatory bowel disease. Immunosuppressors are therefore used in inflammatory bowel disease; steroids are needed for acute or chronic active mucosal inflammatory disease or Crohn's disease; azathioprine and possibly 6-mercaptopurine or Cyclosporin A are second line of treatment. Sulphasalazine is effective in active Crohn's ileocolitis.

2. Humoral defences

These include mainly:
  – immunoglobulins (antibodies);
  – complement plasma proteins;
  – trace elements or metals such as iron, zinc and copper are important for resisting infection;
  – vitamins A, B and C, deficiency of which can lead to denuded respiratory mucous membranes, predisposing host to infection,
  – nutritional factors, since the malnourished are immunocompromised and more vulnerable to infections, so that AIDS patients are more vulnerable to *Pneumocystis carinii* infection than others.

3. Cellular defences

These include mainly:
  – phagocytosis,
  – cell-mediated immunity.

Table 1.10.1   Immune mechanisms

Cells and factors	Innate natural immunity (constantly active/non-specific)	Adaptive immunity (learned-specific)
Cells	Macrophages, monocytes neutrophils, eosinophils mast cells, platelets, 'natural killer cells'	T-(thymus-processed) and B-(bursa of Fabricius) lymphocytes, antigen-presenting cells (APC) of mononuclear phagocytic system (tissue macrophages, blood monocytes, and dendritic cells)
Soluble factors	Complement, cytokines, lysozymes, interferons, acute phase proteins	Antibodies (or immunoglobulins): IgM, IgG, IgA, IgD, IgE Lymphokines
Other factors	Physical and mechanical barriers, genetic-species susceptibilities	Immunogenetics

SPECIFIC IMMUNE MECHANISMS

Both cells and soluble factors involved in innate and adaptive immune mechanisms interact to destroy foreign antigens. These can be summarised as shown in Table 1.10.1.

Mammals do not posses the bursa (of Fabricius, near the cloaca of birds), but bone marrow (acting throughout life), and to some extent the fetal liver (acting during a limited period of life), are bursa-equivalent tissues and subserve a similar function.

The role of T-and B-lymphocytes (adaptive specific immunity)

T-lymphocytes

T-lymphocytes can be helper T-cells, killer cells, or suppressor T cells. T-lymphocytes are responsible for cell-mediated immunity (CMI) (Fig. 1.10.1).

CMI responses include:
- Resistance to infections with intracellular microbes
- Rejection of transplant grafts (acute)
- Graft vs host reaction
- Delayed type IV hypersensitivity
- Help for antibody production
- Contact dermatitis
- Resistance to some tumours (tumour immunity)
- Autoimmune diseases

B-lymphocytes

B-lymphocytes (and derived plasma cells) are responsible for humoral immunity (antibodies).

Antibodies responses include:
- Neutralisation
- Cell lysis of microbes
- Opsonisation
- Hyperacute graft rejection
- Type I–III and V hypersensitivity

Effects of lymphocyte loss

In the intact animal without lymphocyte loss, both CMI and humoral immunity are present. However, in T-lymphocyte loss, as in thymectomy or in Di George syndrome (congenital thymic aplasia), CMI is totally lost while the humoral immunity is preserved, though to a lesser extent than in the intact animal.

Conversely, in B-lymphocyte loss, as in bursectomy or in hypogammaglobulinaemia, CMI is intact while humoral immunity is lost.

Protein energy malnutrition and immune response

In protein energy malnutrition and iron deficiency, all immunological components are generally depressed.

In CMI, the following components are decreased.
- T-lymphocyte activity
- Lymphoid tissue T-lymphocyte count (in thymus, spleen and lymph nodes)
- Cytotoxic activity (killer cells, natural killer cells, killer lymphocytes)
- Phagocytic activity
- Cytokine production (interleukins IL-1 and IL-2)

In humoral immunity:
- B-lymphocyte count remains normal.
- Immunoglobulins are either normal or increased.
- Viral antibody titres are either normal or decreased.
- Complement system is either normal or decreased.
- Secretory IgA is decreased.

Trauma and immune response

Studies have highlighted the complex nature and the tremendous surge of hormone and catecholamine output from the pituitary–adrenal axis following trauma, which may be mediated through spinal cord along afferent neurons from the site of tissue destruction. Also, an immediate and generalised depression of immune system exists and this continues to be an ongoing area of research.

Virtually all components of immune response have been found to be depressed following injury including:
- macrophages, lymphocytes and neutrophil function;
- delayed type hypersensitivity;
- immunoglobulins;
- interferon production;
- serum opsonic capacity: opsonised bacteria become more palatable to phagocytes and themselves activate phagocytosis. Complement, antibodies, fibronectin and probably other proteins all contribute to opsonic capacity of serum.

Serum peptides suppressing lymphocyte proliferation *in vitro* have been defined, and the immunosuppressive role of excessive complement activation has also been recognised.

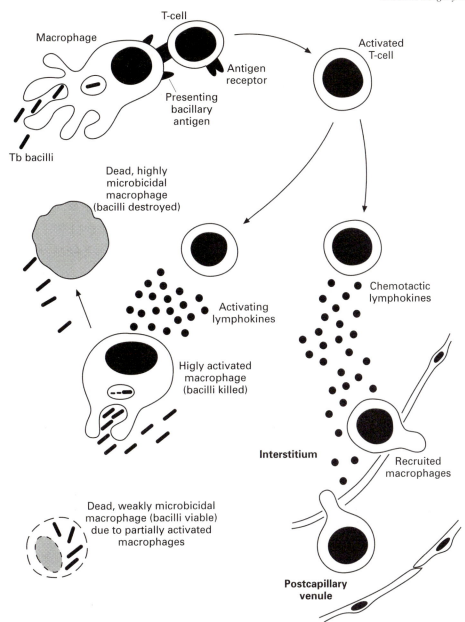

Fig. 1.10.1 Cell-mediated immunity in tuberculosis. The antigen presenting macrophage cells (APC) initiate the immunological cascade

Multisystem organ failure (MOF), depresses CMI (monocytes, lymphocytes and neutrophils) with development of monoclonal antibodies. However, there is a decrease in circulating stable complement components (C1, C3–5) in trauma and MOF. In septic shock too, there is massive complement activation.

Failure of host defences following trauma is a multifactorial and complex process, also involving decreased monocyte HLA-DR, and serum opsonic capacity, decreased endogenous interferon and IL-2 production, with increased PGE$_2$ production.

Anaesthesia

Anaesthesia is not usually a sole factor, but associated with surgery (see below). Anaesthesia initiates neutrophil leucocytosis for a few days. Halothane produces lymphopenia and inhibits neutrophil migration to sites of inflammation (*in vitro* nitrous oxide and thiopentone inhibit neutrophil chemotaxis). Patients may experience allergic reactions (anaphylactic or anaphylactoid) to drugs administered during anaesthesia (see below). Anaesthetic drugs may alter resistance to infection or malignancy. Chronic exposure to trace concentrations of anaesthetic gases may influence the function of the immune system.

Anaphylaxis, an immune-mediated type 1 hypersensitivity, is possible when prior exposure to an antigen (drug) has evoked the production of antigen-specific IgE antibodies and has thus sensitised the host. Most IgE antibodies attach to receptor sites on cell membranes of mast cells in tissues and basophils in plasma. Subsequent exposure of sensitised host to the same drug (antigen) results in an antigen–antibody interaction that initiates degranulation of mast cells and basophils. Degranulation releases histamine and vasoactive substances responsible for anaphylactic signs and symptoms.

Anaphylactoid reaction reflects massive histamine release from mast cells and basophils in response to drugs, independent of antigen–antibody interaction, though its manifestations are indistinguishable from those of anaphylaxis. Anaphylactoid reaction may occur with the first exposure to a drug in contrast to anaphylaxis, which requires previous sensitisation. Magnitude of histamine released on re-exposure to a drug (that previously resulted in anaphylactoid reaction) can be reduced by decreasing drug dose and slowing the rate of i.v. infusion. Opioids and long-acting muscle relaxants can all displace histamine molecules directly from cells resulting in histamine release. Treatment of anaphylactoid reaction is identical to that for anaphylaxis (adrenalin and anti-histamine mainly, and steroid occasionally).

Surgery

Pain and emotional arousal associated with anaesthesia and surgery as well as stimuli emanating from volume, temperature, chemoreceptors, glucose and amino acid alterations induce a complex neuroendocrine and metabolic response. Catecholamines, cortisol/ACTH, endogenous opiates and ADH (vasopressin) are all increased. Tissue damage as well as hypoxia and enhanced hormone output result in increased cytokines (IL-1), increased biological enhancers of inflammation (leukotriens), and release of prostaglandins. Despite postoperative leucocytosis, there is lymphopenia with decreased CMI (T-lymphocytes and T-helper cells).

Post-splenectomy infection

The rate of sepsis varies from 2.7% to 39%; sepsis includes septicaemia, meningitis, or pneumonia (usually fatal). More than 50% of infections occur within 2 years of splenectomy. Splenectomy in paediatric patients causes selective immunosuppression. Over 50% of cases of sepsis are caused by Pneumococci, then *Haemophilus influenzae*, *Neisseria meningitidis*, Streptococci of the β-haemolytic group, *Escherichia coli* and Pseudomonas species.

Splenectomy lowers IgM, inhibits IgM response and leads to poor opsonisation, and consequently reduces clearance of organisms because the liver can only remove well-opsonised bacteria from the blood. Post-splenectomy pneumococcal infection can be prevented by antibiotic prophylaxis with phenoxymethylpenicillin 500 mg orally (there are 250 mg in each 5 ml solution) given every 12 h; for children under 5 years, 125 mg every 12 h; children 6–12 years need 250 mg (i.e. 5 ml) every 12 h.

A pneumococcal vaccine (pneumovax) 0.5 ml by s.c. or i.m. injection, is preferable given 2 weeks prior to splenectomy with advice about increased risk of pneumococcal infection. The vaccine should not be given to children under 2 years, in pregnancy, or when there is infection.

Postoperative sepsis and immune response

Preoperatively, surgical patients may have immunosuppression due to the underlying surgical diseases such as cancer, severe malnutrition, burns, trauma, or shock. Sometimes, preoperative immunodepression is iatrogenic, related to drugs or radiotherapy; such preoperative immunodepression increases the risk of infection following surgery.

Postoperatively, immunodepression occurs very frequently. It occurs in surgical procedures under general anaesthesia with significant tissue manipulation and trauma; such procedures are accompanied by a transient state of immunodepression due to many factors:
1. Anaesthetic drugs.
2. Perioperative administration of blood components.
3. Release of acute phase proteins with immunosuppressive effects.
4. Humoral mediators induced by sepsis.
5. Immunosuppressive factors released by surgically induced wound.
6. Not infrequently, surgical patients are immunocompromised as a result of combined effects of pre- and postoperative immunosuppressing factors.
7. Splenectomy is an operation that especially adds to the risk of postoperative infection, particularly in infants and children due to loss of splenic defence mechanisms in combating infections e.g. pneumococcal infection.

Sepsis

Sepsis is a spectrum of conditions: it encompasses localised infections, bacteraemia, endotoxaemia, septicaemia (commonly due to endotoxaemia), septic shock and multi-system organ failure (MOF) (see s. 1.34).

Immunology also plays an important role in other fields of surgical practice. Other subjects of immunological importance for surgeons include:
- Tumour immunobiology and immunotherapy for cancers (s. 1.36).
- Transplantation immunology (s. 1.90).
- Complications of immunosuppression (s. 1.90).
- AIDS and surgery (s. 1.13).
- Monoclonal antibodies in surgical practice (s. 1.11).
- Sepsis, septic syndrome and MOF (s. 1.34).

1.11 Monoclonal Antibodies in Surgical Practice

Potential clinical applications of monoclonal antibodies include diagnosis of cancer and infection as well as treatment of cancer, sepsis, transplant rejection, autoimmune diseases and viral infections. Monoclonal antibodies can target various substances via their antigens; thus they neutralise toxins, block the interaction of growth factors, hormones, intercellular adhesion molecules or viruses with their cognate cellular receptors; they coat bacteria, viruses or cells, marking them for phagocytosis, for antibody-dependent cellular cytotoxicity and for complement-mediated lysis. The Centre for Exploitation of Science and Technology has estimated that the total world market for monoclonal antibodies will reach $6000 million by the year 2000.

Monoclonal antibodies were discovered by Kohler and Milstein in 1976 by fusing antibody-secreting B-lymphocytes with non-secreting immortal myeloma cells to produce a 'hybridoma' with continuous growth in culture. The first step involves immunisation of a rodent with a crude antigen extract, and then obtaining B-lymphocytes from its spleen. A suspension of lymphocytes is fused with a myeloma cell line (with capacity for indefinite replication). Fusion is facilitated by polyethylene glycol (reduces surface tension of the cell membrane) resulting in a hybridoma with antibody production (from immortalised B-lymphocytes). Only a proportion of cells fuse and antibody secreted by each hybridoma cell is different. Unfused B cells die out in culture. Clones producing antibodies are grown in wells of microtitre plates, subcultured and expanded either in rodent peritoneal cavity or in flasks of tissue medium. Antibodies then are purified by column chromatography.

Purity, stability and safety of monoclonal antibodies must be considered. Hybridoma cell grown in large-scale culture or in ascitic fluid needs to be screened for contamination by murine bacteria and retroviruses. Human or humanised monoclonal antibodies are preferable to rodent ones. Cocktails of monoclonal antibodies should be more effective than single antibodies; production of such cocktails can be helped by the advent of human phage antibody libraries. Enhancement of an antibody's affinity to improve therapeutic value is also possible by phage technology.

DIAGNOSTIC APPLICATIONS

Cancers

Detection of tumour markers (see Table 1.11.1)

Most tumour antigens are not truly tumour-specific products, but substances secreted in excess or inappropriately by tumour, e.g. ectopic hormones, and oncofetal products (normally found in embryonic tissues). Many tumour-associated antigens were first identified by polyclonal antisera. Now, monoclonal antibodies raised after immunisation with tumour cells or extract have identified new and clinically useful tumour markers.

CA125 marker is one such example discovered by a monoclonal antibody (OC125) raised against ovarian cell line; CA125 is an oncofetal glycoprotein secreted by coelomic epithelium during embryonic development and expressed in 80% of non-mucinous ovarian carcinomas. Raised serum level, however, was also found in non-maliganant ovarian diseases, non-gynaecological tumours and in a few healthy people. Measurement of CA125 is frequently used to monitor treatment and follow-up of patients with ovarian cancer; elevated CA125 usually antedates a clinical relapse.

Immunohistochemistry (see Table 1.11.2)

Immunohistochemistry gives information about biochemical characteristics of a tumour. Many tumour antigens can be

Table 1.11.1 Clinically useful circulating tumour-associated products and their tumour origin

Hormones	
Human chorionic gonadotrophin	Trophoblastic tumours
Insulin	Insulinoma
Adrenocorticotrophic hormone	Pituitary adenoma, small cell lung cancer
Antidiuretic hormone	Small cell lung cancer
Calcitonin	Medullary carcinoma of thyroid
Enzymes	
Prostatic acid phosphatase	Prostatic cancer
Placental alkaline phosphatase	Seminoma
Lactate dehydrogenase	Reflects cell turnover, e.g. testis, lymphoma
Neurone-specific enolase	Small cell lung cancer, neuroblastoma
Oncofetal proteins	
Carcinoembryonic antigen	Colorectal, pancreas, gastric, breast, lung
Alphafetoprotein	Yolk sac, hepatoma
CA125	Ovary (non-mucinous), cervix, breast
Cellular proteins and lipids	
CA50 (ganglioside or sialylated protein)	Breast, gastrointestinal, uterus, cervix, prostate, lung
CA15–3 (glycoprotein)	Breast
CA19–9 (sialylated Lewis hapten)	Colon, gastric, pancreas
Paraproteins: immunoglubulin, light and heavy chain	Myeloma, lymphoma
Beta-$_2$ microglobulin	Myeloma
Prostate specific antigen	Prostate cancer
TA-4 (squamous cell carcinoma antigen)	Cervix, head and neck squamous cell tumours

From Miles; X. Monoclonal antibodies. In A.V. Pollock and M. Evans (eds), *Immunology in Surgical Practice*. London: Edward Arnold, 1992

detected by immunohistochemical methods; some antigens can only be detected in fresh specimens, while others can still be detected in tissue fixed in formalin and embedded in paraffin. Approximately 5% of patients with malignant disease have metastatic tumours of unknown primary sites. Immunohistochemical staining using a panel of monoclonal antibodies can be valuable in identifying tumours that are curable or responsive to chemotherapy.

Radioimmunolocalisation (see Table 1.11.3)

Accurate staging of a tumour can greatly assist surgeons and physicians who treat patients with cancer. The potential usefulness of monoclonal anti-tumour antibodies to identify tumour deposits is enormous. It is now possible to inject radiolabelled antibody i.v. and detect where it localises by gamma camera imaging. The abdomen and pelvis are two areas

Table 1.11.2   Diagnosis of carcinoma of unknown primary by immunocytochemistry

Disease	Diagnostic method
Curable	
Non-Hodgkin lymphoma	Leucocyte antigens
Hodgkin's disease	Leucocyte antigens
Germ cell tumours	Human chorionic gonadotrophin, alphafetoprotein, placental alkaline phosphatase
Choriocarcinoma	Human chorionic gonadotrophin
Neuroblastoma	Neurone-specific enolase
Rhabdomyosarcoma	Myoglobulin
High response rate	
Small cell lung cancer	Neurone-specific enolase
Ovarian cancer	CA125
Breast cancer	Human milk fat globulin, CA15–3
Prostatic cancer	Prostate-specific antigen, acid phosphatase
Myeloma	Immunoglobulin

From Pollock and Evans (1992), see Table 1.11.1

Table 1.11.3   Radioimmunolocalisation of tumours

Tumour	Antigen
Colon	Carcinoembryonic antigen, tumour-associated glycoprotein, 791T
Germ cell tumour	Human chorionic gonadotrophin, alphafetoprotein, placental alkaline phosphatase
Choriocarcinoma	Human chorionic gonadotrophin
Ovary	CA125, human milk fat globulin, AUA*
Breast	Carcinoembyronic antigen, human milk fat globulin
Thyroid	Thyroglobulin
Melanoma	High molecular weight antigen
Lung	Human milk fat globulin
Lymphoma	Anti-T cell, anti-B cell antibody

*AUA, Arklie's unknown antigen.
From Pollock and Evans (1992), see Table 1.11.1

where radioimmunolocalisation may be useful as these regions are often difficult to image by conventional radiological and sonographic methods; it enables the detection of functioning tissue and this may help differentiate active tumour from other radiographic shadows. The first successful imaging of human colonic cancer used a polyclonal antibody to CEA conjugated with ^{131}I. Radioactivity in normal tissues and the circulation reduces the sensitivity of imaging, but techniques have been developed to reduce background effect and enhance the ratio of gamma emission by tumour to that by normal tissues. Although ^{131}I is most commonly used, it is not an ideal imaging agent.

^{123}I and ^{99m}Tc radioimmunoconjugates have shorter half-lives than ^{131}I. Indium-111 has a longer half-life but conjugation to antibody is more complex, and again less satisfactory than iodine.

Several types of tumour can be imaged with radiolabelled antibodies. Lesions with diameters of 5 mm have been visualised with radiolabelled antibodies; however, the value of radioimmunolocalisation depends not only on the specificity and sensitivity of the technique, but also on the way in which results alter clinical management. In patients with colorectal cancer, the presence of tumour markers such as CEA in the serum does not appear to interfere with tumour imaging. In a study, 93% of radioimmunolocalisation scans were positive; the tumour presence was confirmed by operation, or by conventional imaging with CT scan or ultrasound. Conventional imaging was negative in five positive radioimmunolocalisation scans of tumours confirmed at laparotomy. The technique appears to be most successful in management of drug-resistant trophoblastic tumours that can be successfully treated by surgery; in some cases radiolabelled antibodies to hCG have identified disease, aiding resection of tumours and prolonging patient survival.

The technique of **intraoperative radioimmuno-guided surgery** has emerged. Most experience has been gained in patients with colorectal cancer who are injected with monoclonal antibodies to CEA labelled with ^{125}I before operation. The antibody is allowed to clear from normal tissues before operation and a hand-held gamma probe is used to identify the limits of the tumour and sites of metastases.

Infections

Pneumonia

Severe nosocomial (community or hospital-acquired) pneumonia is a most important infection in ICU and major contributor to mortality in ICU; it is commonly caused by *Streptococcus pneumoniae*. Diagnosis can be made rapidly by Gram stain of sputum, when numerous Gram-positive diplococci can be seen. However, if sputum is not available, bronchoscopic material (either bronchoalveolar lavage or protected brush specimen) can be less contaminated (with upper respiratory tract flora). In pretreatment with antibiotics, pneumococcal antigen detection in sputum, serum, or urine may aid the diagnosis; the latex agglutination sensitive test for pneumococcal antigen can be performed within 30 minutes of receiving a sample.

However, the immunofluorescence technique using monoclonal antibodies, is rapid and highly sensitive; the technique can be used directly on sputum or bronchoscopic secretions for diagnosis of pneumonia with results available within a few hours. It is of most value in the rapid detection of microorganisms which are fastidious or slow-growing, such as the agents that cause atypical pneumonia.

Atypical Pneumonia

Diagnosis of Legionnaire's disease and psittacosis has traditionally relied on detection of rising serum antibody titre, which may not occur until after an acute episode. *Legionella pneumophila* can be detected in respiratory material by means of a direct immunofluorescence stain using monoclonal antibodies with results available within a few hours. There is also a highly specific antibody to *Chlamydia psittaci* for diagnosis of psittacosis by means of immunofluorescence or by enzyme-linked immunosorbent assay (ELISA) using respiratory material.

Viruses are less common causes of pneumonia, except in epidemics of influenza A, when it can lead to severe primary influenzal pneumonia. Respiratory syncytial virus is commonly associated with bronchitis in children, but may cause pneumonia in elderly or immunocompromised patients. A direct immunofluorescence method for detection of these viruses has been in use for some time, and is the main means of diagnosis.

Pneumocystis carinii pneumonia in immunocompromised patients is increasingly diagnosed in ICU. The diagnosis can now be made rapidly on induced sputum or bronchoscopy samples by using monoclonal antibodies and immunofluorescence stain; this method has been shown to be more sensitive and technically more practical than Giemsa stain and with no false-positive results.

However, nosocomial pneumonia in ICU can also be caused by Gram-negative bacilli; the time-honoured Gram stain of respiratory secretions is usually sufficient for diagnosis.

Septicaemia

This is a frequent problem in ICU, and is generally either a blood line-associated infection or Gram-negative septicaemia originating from a focal infection from respiratory, gastrointestinal or urinary tract. Sepsis is diagnosed clinically by fever, tachycardia and tachypnoea, and by non-microbiological tests, such as C-reactive protein. Other circulating acute phase proteins such as interleukins and tumour necrosis factor play a part in pathogenesis of septic shock, as does bacterial endotoxin. The classical method for detection of circulating endotoxins is by gelation of Limulus lysate assay; lysates from haemolymph of two horseshoe crabs, *Limulus polyphemus* and *Tachypleus tridentatus*, are commercially available for endotoxin testing. Limulus lysate assay, however, can be an unreliable test for the relatively low human endotoxin concentration causing incomplete gelation; hence the need for the modified chromogenic limulus test assessed spectrophotometrically. Monoclonal antibodies to endotoxin and to cytokines on the other hand can provide rapid and reliable results. However, bacteriological confirmation of septicaemia relies on blood cultures by sampling bottles at intervals (twice a day, usually taken during fever spikes), using BACTEC radiometric systems, which latterly were replaced by non-radiometric (Becton Dickinson Instrument) systems, and more recently by using the BacT/Alert colorimetric system. There is still no more rapid method than a time-honoured Gram stain for distinguishing various genera of bacteria.

Other diagnostic applications of monoclonal antibodies

Monoclonal antibodies are being developed for imaging of infarcted myocardium (antimyosin), deep venous or arterial thrombosis (antifibrin), and foci of infection of inflammation.

THERAPEUTIC APPLICATIONS AND CLINICAL USES

Monoclonal antibodies in the treatment of cancer

The identification of tumour antigens in tissues not only helps in the diagnosis of tumours but provides a target to attack the cancer cells. Monoclonal antibodies given alone or conjugated with radioisotopes, drugs, or toxins are being used to treat patients. Most experience has been gained from the use of radiolabelled antibodies.

In solid tumours, treatment with monoclonal antibodies has so far been disappointing; an important limiting factor is the inability of infused monoclonal antibodies to reach target cells, because they can reach surface blood vessels of a tumour deposit (relatively leaky to macromolecules), but cannot reach deep tumour vessels (not leaky). Monoclonal antibody treatment for haematological malignancies has been more successful in bone marrow and spleen (leukaemias and lymphomas), with nodal disease responding less readily.

Immunisation with tumour extracts leads to the formation of clones of antibody-forming cells; these antibodies have broad activity and many react with cellular components of both normal and tumour cells. The antisera can be purified to contain only anti-tumour antibodies. These polyclonal antibodies have variable immune responses and their supply is limited. Monoclonal antibodies react with a single epitope and the supply of antibodies is potentially limitless. There are two methods for their use, as follows.

1. Serotherapy

Here, anti-tumour antibodies stimulate cytotoxic activity in the host's immune system. A patient with cutaneous T-cell lymphoma responded to treatment with anti-T-cell antibodies, and another shows complete clinical remission of B-cell non-Hodgkin lymphoma following treatment with anti-idiotype antibodies. However, results of other studies in which anti-tumour anti-idiotype antibodies were used to treat patients with lymphoproliferative disorders, melanoma and GIT cancer have been disappointing. This cytotoxicity can be improved by combining antibodies with cytokines such as interferon or interleukins.

2. Immunoconjugate therapy

Here, noxious agents are conjugated with antibodies to destroy tumour cells. There are 3 classes of immunoconjugates:
- radionuclides (radioimmunotherapy) such as:
  - iodine-131 (beta- and gamma-emitter);
  - yttrium-90 (beta-emitter);
  - copper-67 (beta- and gamma-emitter);
  - bismuth-212 (alpha-emitter);
  - astatine-211 (alpha-emitter).
- toxins (immunotoxins): clinical experience is limited; ricin A chain immunotoxins were used in melanoma and colorectal cancer with 50% of melanoma patients reported responding with rare clinical remission.
- drugs: such as doxorubicin, daunomycin, methotrexate, or vinca alkaloids.

Treatment with radiolabelled antibody has an advantage over toxins and drugs, namely that delivery of the conjugate to every tumour cell is not essential, since poorly vascularised areas of tumour or cells that do not express tumour antigens can be destroyed if they are within the radiation field. Furthermore, the use of gamma-emitting isotope such as ^{131}I enables the distribution of antibody to be monitored by external scintigraphy, and the external radiation dose can be accurately assessed. Also, the lesions can become resectable after radioimmunotherapy. Radiolabelled antibodies have also been given i.v. to treat melanoma, lymphoma and colorectal cancer. Using external imaging has shown that the tumour receives five times more radiation than the blood. Improvements might be achieved using isotopes with higher beta energy or alpha emission; alternatively, acceleration of removal of therapeutic antibody from blood using 'second antibody' may lead to a greater therapeutic value.

In order to try to increase the delivery of antibody to tumours many have injected radioimmunoconjugates into the pleural or peritoneal cavities or into CSF. In ovarian cancer, preferential binding of antibody to tumour cells in ascitic fluid is observed, but it is unclear whether intraperitoneal injection increases the proportion of radiolabelled antibody taken up by fixed deposits of tumour. *Ex vivo* therapy with monoclonal antibodies has been confined to treating bone marrow before infusion into the recipient; neuroblastoma cells contaminating bone marrow can be removed using antibody conjugated to a magnetic bead. The incidence of graft versus host disease following bone marrow transplantation for leukaemia or lymphoma can be reduced by purging donor marrow of T lymphocytes by incubating with a monoclonal antibody and complement.

Antibody-dependent enzyme prodrug therapy (ADEPT) is promising. With this technique, an antibody-enzyme conjugate is administered to localise tumour deposits, and after a few days (during which non-specifically bound monoclonal antibody is cleared), an inactive prodrug is administered; the prodrug is converted by monoclonal antibody-linked enzyme in tumour deposits to an active, tumoricidal drug that is small enough to permeate deep in the tumour. A cocktail of humanised monoclonal antibodies is better than single antibodies.

Human response to anti-tumour monoclonal antibodies

Single administration of a large dose of monoclonal mouse antibody is well tolerated, but presence of foreign protein can result in immune response by the host. However, toxicity of cancer monoclonal antibodies is variable; with unmodified murine monoclonal antibodies, fever, rigors, nausea and vomiting are common after initial doses, immune hypersensitivity reaction can occur, and symptoms secondary to immune complexes are seen after prolonged treatment. Radioimmunoconjugates usually cause appreciable toxicity to normal bone marrow, and immunotoxins can cause the vascular leak syndrome.

An anti-antibody response is seen in about 50% of patients receiving single injection of a diagnostic or therapeutic dose of monoclonal antibody. Further administration of antibody is ineffective and may be hazardous. Intradermal skin testing for IgE anti-antibodies is carried out routinely, though less

sensitive. Formation of such human anti-idiotypic antibody increases the response to antibody serotherapy.

For successful immunoconjugate therapy, however, prevention of human immune response is required, as treatment must be repeated; this can be achieved by cyclosporin A immunosuppression or chimeric antibodies, so that the human antibody is encoded by mouse genes. Chimerism is referred to when one animal contains viable cells of another animal which is genetically different; chimerism arises naturally in binovular twins sharing a common placenta, but immunological enhancement or irradiation can also lead to chimerism. (Chimera is a mythical monster with many different heads).

Monoclonal antibodies in the treatment of sepsis

Multi-system organ failure (MOF) is a major cause of mortality among critically ill patients; the majority of deaths appear to be due to sepsis syndrome. Clinical observations have shown that there is a close relationship between sepsis syndrome and infection. However, the treatment of infection alone does not appear to be effective in resolving pathophysiological effects of sepsis syndrome; both sepsis syndrome and MOF are due to uncontrolled activation of macrophages resulting in uncontrolled stimulation of normal cytokine and prostaglandin mediators of inflammation. One of the major sources of macrophage stimulation in the critically ill patient is the bacterial endotoxin; this substance is a major component of the outer cell wall of Gram-negative aerobic bacteria (GNAB). Evidence suggests that endotoxin is absorbed from the GIT of the critically ill patient due to a combination of factors, namely:

- direct damage to the GIT at the initial onset of illness;
- ischaemic injury suffered during episodes of circulatory shock;
- gut malnutrition caused by prolonged fasting and parenteral nutrition.

Rational treatment must prevent macrophage stimulation and control deleterious effects of cytokine overproduction.

Monoclonal antibodies active against endotoxin can be produced; they must inactivate endotoxin before it stimulates macrophages. Monoclonal antibodies may also be produced to inactivate cytokines produced by macrophages such as antibodies active against tumour necrosis factor (TNFα).

Anti-endoxin antibodies

Polyclonal antibodies

Polyclonal anti-endoxin antibodies were discovered in California and used for treatment of septic shock caused by GNAB. Endotoxin is released from GNAB mostly when the cell wall breaks up at cell death; it is a complex, ampiphyllic, lipopolysaccharide molecule (composed of lipid and sugars) which consists of three parts: inner core, outer core and Lipid A hydrophobic end. Lipid A is responsible for toxic effects of endoxin. Monoclonal antibodies development must be specific for antigens common to endoxins derived from a range of GNAB. Lipid A and inner core structures are very similar in all endotoxins. Salmonella species share the same core structures; occasionally there are minor differences in core structure, e.g.

E. coli species share five different core structures. However, the major antigenic determinants of Lipid A appear to be a number of phosphate radicals attached to glucosamine rings which are constant in all Lipid A structures.

Antiserum to rough mutant J5 of Escherichia coli 0111 Human polyclonal anti-endoxin antibody was prepared in 1982 by inoculating human volunteers with heat-killed rough mutant J5 of *E. coli* 0111 to prepare the antiserum; endotoxin from this mutant expressed the Lipid A and inner core only. It was used in a controlled study of patients suffering from serious infection or bacteraemia caused by GNAB, with a good result in those classified as being seriously shocked with mortality reduction from 77% to 44%. In another study the anti-endoxin antibodies were given prophylactically to patients at risk of developing Gram-negative bacteraemia with reduced systemic manifestations of Gram-negative infection in the treated group though with no difference in the incidence of Gram-negative infection between the treated and the control group; the relative risk of developing septic shock was 2.3 times greater in the control group.

IgG anti-endotoxin core antibody This polyclonal antibody was procured in South Africa by screening normal blood donors for the high titre of anti-endoxin core activity, and by preparing IgG fraction of their plasma. It was used in a small study of septic gynaecological conditions; the mortality was reduced from 9 (out of 19 control patients) to 1 (out of 14 treated patients).

Monoclonal antibodies

HA-1A monoclonal antibodies Monoclonal antibodies were developed specific for antigens on the inner core of endotoxin. They were IgM antibodies raised by fusing B cells of mice immunised with J5 *E. coli* mutant with myeloma cell lines. The more successful monoclonal antibodies are HA-1A humanised IgM monoclonal antibodies specific for the Lipid A portion of endoxin (bind non-specifically to a wide range of GNAB). In tests on 105 patients suffering from sepsis syndrome, there was a 39% reduction in mortality (increased to 42% mortality in cardiovascular shocked patients with bacteraemia). The results were similar to those achieved by immunisation with J5 polyclonal anti-endoxin core antibody. HA-A1 therefore is beneficial in Gram-negative bacteraemia with or without shock, but not useful for focal Gram-negative infection.

E5 monoclonal antibodies The second antibody was a murine monoclonal antibody designated as E5 specific for Lipid A fraction of endotoxin. It was used in a trial with improvement in mortality among patients with Gram-negative infections only, whether bacteraemic or focal, but patients must not be in shock (no evidence of improvement in patients with refractory septic shock).

Experimentally, both were found to protect against i.v. injection of endotoxin or bacteria, but neither has been shown to protect in models of septic shock induced by focal bacterial infections (closer to clinical situations seen in patients). So far, clinical results have not shown irrefutable evidence to support the clinical use of monoclonal anti-endoxin antibodies in septic patients. Furthermore, these new biotechnologies are very expensive and it is likely that the cost problem will soon become a major issue; it is also difficult to design protocols that avoid treating large numbers of patients who subsequently prove not to have had Gram-negative bacteraemia (trials must be placebo controlled). However, a new generation of monoclonal antibodies may be produced with specificity for the more accessible binding of the core rather than Lipid A portion of endotoxin.

Anti-TNF antibodies

Inactivating cytokine mediators released by macrophages, mainly TNF, using monoclonal antibodies can block the TNF signal preventing production of secondary mediators; this line of therapy has been successful experimentally. In 1987, a first generation of anti-TNF monoclonal antibodies was produced to protect against systemic effects of both Gram-negative bacterial infection and endotoxin in experimental animals. There are some potential drawbacks to the clinical use of anti-TNF antibodies:

- there is *ex vivo* (better term than *in vitro*) evidence that other mediators are manufactured by the macrophage at the same time as TNF is produced in response to endoxin; IL-1 and PGE$_1$ can, on their own, initiate all sequential reactions of septic response;
- there is evidence that endotoxin can elicit a response directly from a target cell without requiring TNF intermediation; thus TNF therapeutic block may be bypassed (see below).

TNF is a normal mediator of inflammation present among higher and lower animals, indicating its crucial importance in the suvival of species. Its main role in cellular biology is the mediation of inflammation; however, its role in wound healing and in prevention of malignancy is poorly understood. By completely blocking TNF in an uncontrolled manner, it might be possible to raise other (as yet unseen) problems in relation to wound healing, block a physiological response to trauma and infection, or unmask latent malignancy.

Immunotherapy after improving monoclonal antibodies may become the sole therapy of sepsis in the future; the aim is to break the vicious circle of endotoxaemia being released from a site of infection or absorbed from the bowel, which then causes systemic upset and leads to further GIT ischaemic mucosal damage, allowing further endoxin absorption.

However, other therapeutic modalities can be used, along with immunotherapy, in order to break this vicious cycle and to correct its effects, including:

● Endotoxin blockage by the use of competitive inhibitors, such as non-toxic Lipid A analogues.
● Recombinant IL-1 receptor antagonists to downregulate the inflammatory cascade for septic shock by blocking the action of cytokine mediator IL-1.
● Use of n-3 polyunsaturated fatty acids administered later in the process to control the activated macrophages (in case therapeutic block of TNF is bypassed).
● Adequate resuscitation and restoration of splanchnic perfusion, and the use of agents, such as free radical scavengers, to prevent perfusion mucosal injury of the gut, and the use of white cell anti-adherence antibodies administered prior to and during resuscitation to prevent endothelial damage.

- Metabolic support by improved parenteral nutrition to support enterocyte function, promoting bowel peristalsis and bile secretion, as well as IgA secretion to reinforce gut barrier to endoxins.
- Selective decontamination of gut (SDG) is a radical technique to prevent overgrowth of endotoxin-producing Gram-negative aerobic bacteria within the bowel lumen.

Beside obvious examples of tetanus and diphtheria, other toxic states which may be amenable to monoclonal antibody therapy include drug overdosage, chemical poisoning and snake or spider bites. Already digoxin Fab fragments are well established for the treatment of digoxin overdose and monoclonal antibodies are being developed for neutralising tricyclic antidepressants.

Monoclonal antibodies in immunosuppression

Antibodies that target lymphocyte antigens offer less toxic immunosuppressive treatment than the currently available drugs; indeed, the first approved human use of monoclonal antibodies is an immunosuppressive agent for treating rejection of renal transplants. Immune responses to self or foreign antigens can lead to autoimmune destruction of tissues or rejection of transplanted organs, respectively.

Immunosuppressive therapies include corticosteroids, cyclosporin, cytotoxic drugs and polyclonal anti-lymphocyte antisera, all of which have high toxicity and are sometimes ineffective. Monoclonal antibodies offer a realistic alternative to these immunosuppressive drugs, and this is perhaps their most useful current application. Potential targets for immunosuppressive monoclonal antibodies include lymphocyte differentiation antigens, cytokines, cytokine receptors and cell adhesion molecules.

OKT3 monoclonal antibodies The first monoclonal antibody to be approved for human therapy is OKT3, an immunosuppressive murine reagent which binds to T-lymphocytes and is useful for treating rejection of renal transplants. These immunosuppressive monoclonal antibodies do not stimulate a strong antimouse response. The toxicity of OKT3 is worst with the first dose, which triggers release of cytokines from targeted cells and leads sometimes to hypotension, weight gain and breathlessness, progressing occasionally to pulmonary oedema. Other immunosuppressive monoclonal antibodies include antibodies against lymphocyte antigens CD4, and Tac (all of which have now been humanised by CDR grafting) as well as monoclonal antibodies that block adhesion of immune and inflammatory cells.

Monoclonal antibodies against CD4 These antibodies inhibit helper T-lymphocyte function and have been used with varying success to treat acute rejection of renal allografts, inflammatory bowel disease, rheumatoid arthritis, systemic lupus erythematosus, psoriasis, relapsing polychondritis, systemic vasculitis and mycosis fungoides.

Tac monoclonal antibodies These have high affinity to IL-2 receptors of activated lymphocytes and do not bind to resting (non-activated) lymphocytes. They can, therefore, block ongoing antigen-specific immune responses highly specifically without damaging resting lymphocytes. Murine Tac monoclonal antibodies can prevent early rejection of renal allografts, but antimouse responses were detected in 81% of patients after one month's treatment. Humanised Tac antibody (Tac-H) was compared with murine antibody in cardiac allografts; Tac-H had a longer circulating half-life. (103 versus 38 hours), was less immunogenic (0% versus 100% antiantibody responses before day 33), and produced a longer graft survival than murine antibody.

Monoclonal antibodies in the treatment of viral infections

Patients with agammaglobulinaemia suffer from recurrent bacterial sinopulmonary infection, meningitis and bacteraemia. However, viral infections are no more severe in such patients than in healthy people, suggesting that T-cells are the most important initial defence, but long-life immunity is lacking so multiple bouts of chickenpox and measles may occur (because no antibodies are formed). These data suggest that antibodies should be able to prevent bacterial and viral infections. Indeed, passive immunisation with purified human antibodies provides good protection for patients with agammaglobulinaemia, hypogammaglobulinaemia and dysgammaglobulinaemia.

Polyclonal human immunoglobulins (antibodies) have been used for many years to treat and prevent several viral diseases, including viral hepatitis A and B, chickenpox, measles and cytomegalovirus infection. It is surprising that antibacterial and antiviral monoclonal antibodies have rarely been used in clinical practice. However, many antiviral and antibacterial monoclonal antibodies are being developed, e.g. humanised versions of monoclonal antibodies to herpes simplex virus, to respiratory syncytial virus, to HIV. Antiviral antibodies can block attachment and penetration of viruses, opsonise virus and virus infected cells for phagocytosis, for antibody-dependent cellular cytotoxicity and for complement-mediated lysis of enveloped virus particles or infected cells. A cocktail of monoclonal antibodies will probably give greater benefit than single reagents.

However, it can be argued that antibodies are unlikely to be useful in treating these conditions, since it is T-cells and not antibodies that are essential for eradicating established viral infections.

Other therapeutic applications of monoclonal antibodies

Anti-rhesus monoclonal antibodies have been made for treating rhesus haemolytic disease, and platelet monoclonal antibodies for prevention of intravascular thrombosis. Monoclonal antibody enzyme conjugates targeted at blood clots are novel fibrinolytic reagents.

1.12 Antimicrobials in Surgery

Antimicrobials are drugs that damage microorganisms without harming the host tissue cells; they are either -cidal or -static. This is in contrast to antineoplastic drugs which harm both tumour and host cells and are always -cidal. Antimicrobials fall into two groups:

Synthetic Includes sulphonamides, nitrofurantoin, 4-quinolones (ciprofloxacin and nalidixic acid), para-aminosalicylic acid (PASA), isonicotinic acid hydrazide (INH) and cotrimoxazole (Septrin). Most are bacteriostatic (and work by inhibition of folate metabolism). However, INH and co-trimoxazole are bactericidal.

Antibiotics (natural products of one microorganism affecting another microorganism)
- Bactericidal, including mainly the following groups: penicillins, aminoglycosides, cephalosporins and other Beta-lactam antibiotics (imipenem and meropenem) and glycopeptides (vancomycin and teicoplanin).
- Bacteriostatic, e.g. chloramphenicol, tetracyclines and macrolides (erythromycin, azithromycin and clarithromycin).

Antibiotic combinations

A combination of bacteriostatic and bactericidal drugs is pharmacologically poor: the bactericidal drug is effective only in killing growing bacteria and once growth is arrested by the bacteriostatic drug, the bactericidal agent is useless. A combination of two bacteriostatic agents yields a bacteriostatic agent except for trimethoprim and sulphamethoxazole (both are folate metabolism inhibitors) which yield a synergistic bactericidal drug, cotrimoxazole. A combination of two bactericidal agents always yields a bactericidal agent. The combination effect may be antagonistic (less than each drug used alone), agonistic (more than each drug used alone), additive (equal to the algebraic sum of the effects of both drugs) or synergistic (more than the algebraic sum of the effects).

Indications for antibiotic combinations

Mixed bacterial infections in which the organisms are not susceptible to a common agent

- Intra-abdominal sepsis secondary to intestinal perforation and postoperative sepsis secondary to gastrointestinal operation. Here the anaerobes (particularly *Bacteroides fragilis*) and the aerobic Gram-negative bacilli, the Enterobacteriaceae (particularly *Escherichia coli*), predominate. The combination of aerobes and anaerobes is synergistic. Elimination of one or other of the organisms reduces the overall infectivity of the inoculum. Antibiotics with anaerobic coverage are metronidazole, clindamycin, lincomycin, chloramphenicol, or semi-synthetic penicillins (carbenicillin or ticarcillin). Antibiotics with aerobic coverage are aminoglycoside (with ampicillin to cover the anaerobic *Streptococcus faecalis*) or cephalosporins such as cefuroxime. Triple chemotherapy of metronidazole/gentamicin/ampicillin was originally used. This was largely replaced with double chemotherapy of metronidazole/cefuroxime and now a single agent is used – mezlocillin (semi-synthetic penicillin) or latamoxef (third-generation cephalosporins). Any of the above regimens, however, may be used prophylactically or therapeutically.

- Polymicrobial bacteraemia in a febrile, neutropenic patient. A bactericidal combination should be used such as semi-synthetic penicillin (carbenicillin or ticarcillin) with aminoglycoside *or* cephalosporin with aminoglycoside *or* semi-synthetic penicillin with a cephalosporin. These regimens have been shown to decrease the mortality of these infections.
- Endometritis and post-hysterectomy infections caused by aerobic and anaerobic vaginocervical flora.

To achieve synergistic antimicrobial activity against a single organism

Synergism occurs when a combination of drugs produces at least a fourfold decrease in the minimal inhibitory concentration of *each* drug, e.g.
- Penicillin and aminoglycoside (streptomycin) in enterococcal endocarditis are replaced by penicillin and gentamicin to cover possible *Pseudomonas aeruginosa*.
- Trimethoprim and sulphamethoxazole (co-trimoxazole, Septrin, Bactrim). Each drug has only bacteriostatic activity when used alone while their combination is bactericidal.

To overcome bacterial tolerance

Tolerance (*in vitro* phenomenon) is the resistance of an organism to the lethal action of an otherwise bactericidal agent. Tolerance to penicillins, cephalosporins and vancomycin have been described in *Staphylococcus aureus*, *Staphylococcus pneumoniae*, *Streptococcus viridans* and Group G streptococci infections. The goal of *in vitro* tests is to obtain the best single or combined regimen that will assure bactericidal activity against the causative organism.
- Co-amoxiclav (augmentin 375 mg tablets given 8 hourly or 1.2 gm i.v. given 8 hourly) consists of amoxycillin with beta-lactamase inhibitor clavulanic acid; the latter has no significant antibacterial activity but by inactivating penicillinases, it makes the combination active against penicillinase-producing bacteria that are resistant to amoxycillin. These include most staphylococcus aureus, 50% of *E. Coli* strains, and up to 15% of *H. influenzae* strains as well as many Bacteroides and *Klebsiella spp*.

To prevent the development of bacterial antibiotic resistance

Bacteria can become resistant to drugs by various mechanisms e.g. chromosomal mutation, recombination and acquisition of plasmids, e.g.
- Treatment of active tuberculosis particularly with cavitary pulmonary disease. To treat an intrinsically drug-resistant subpopulation as well as to prevent the development of a totally drug-resistant subpopulation of *Mycobacterium tuberculosis*, more than one effective antituberculosis agent must be used.
- Amoxycillin (derivative of ampicillin but with only one hydroxyl group with better absorption) 500 mg tds daily plus metronidazole 400 mg tds daily plus omeprazole 20 mg bd daily for one week is the triple therapy of duodenal ulcer to eradicate Helicobacter pylori infection.

- Co-Fluampicil (mixture of flucloxacillin and ampicillin) or magnapen is used for mixed infections involving penicillinase-producing staphylococci.
- Aminoglycoside with semisynthetic penicillins (carbenicillin or ticarcillin) to treat infections due to *P. aeruginosa*. These β-lactam antibiotics are excellent antipseudomonal drugs. Rapid development of bacterial resistance to the β-lactam drug caused by β-lactamase inactivating enzymes can be suppressed by the drug synergistic combination and by β-lactamase inhibitors (the prototype of this class of drugs is clavulanic acid).
- Rifampicin incorporation with antistaphylococcal regimen. Rifampicin is the most effective antimicrobial agent against both *S. aureus* and *Staphylococcus epidermidis* (on the basis of minimal inhibitory concentration). However, studies reveal that if staphylococci are exposed to rifampicin alone, they develop total resistance to this drug within 24 h but if a good second antistaphylococcal agent is combined with rifampicin, e.g. aminoglycoside or vancomycin, the totally rifampicin-resistant population is aborted. *S. epidermidis* is the most common organism responsible for endocarditis associated with prosthetic valves and infections associated with ventricular shunt devices and prosthetic joints, and since such regimens have been effective in eradicating this organism the prosthesis does not have to be removed.

To decrease the toxicity of the most effective agent

For example, by treating meningitis due to *Cryptococcus neoformans* with amphotericin B (effective and toxic) and 5-fluorocytocine the duration of the drug administration can be shortened.

Principles of chemoprophylaxis in surgery

- Not a substitute or alternative to aseptic practice and good surgical technique.
- Necessary only in high-risk cases of bacterial contamination.
- Timing is vital. It should start with premedication, aiming at a saturated tissue concentration at the time of surgical manipulation and throughout the operation. Thus administration for 24–48 h is as effective as administration for 7 postoperative days.
- Route of administration should be intravenous since the oral route is not suitable in all patients and may have undesirable side-effects, e.g. pseudomembranous enterocolitis. The topical route is limited although tetracycline lavage has been shown to reduce mortality in faecal peritonitis; kanamycin lavage proved to be toxic and lavage with normal saline alone actually increased the risk of sepsis (by spreading infection). Topical ampicillin is known to reduce wound sepsis but does not provide protection against intra-abdominal abscesses and septicaemia. The intramuscular preoperative route leads to a delayed peak level.
- Chemoprophylaxis should be employed only when scientific evidence shows that it has advantages. However it is logical to adopt a policy of selective use of antibiotics in general surgery in the knowledge that infection is more likely to

occur in some situations than others (Fig. 1.12.1). It must be remembered, nevertheless, that since *in vitro* sensitivity may be different from *in vivo* sensitivity, culture is far more informative (e.g. biliary and urinary organisms require not only an effective drug but an effective drug that can concentrate in the biliary tree or urinary system in adequate therapeutic concentrations).

- Choice of agent (preferably bactericidal) should be made on the basis of activity against the *pathogens* most commonly encountered. Most of these are endogenous (exogenous *S. aureus* is responsible for only 5% of postoperative sepsis). In the healthy person only a few body fluids, such as cerebrospinal fluid, seem to be permanently sterile, while all other fluids and cavities contain at least a few organisms per millilitre from time to time. The distribution of pathogens does not, however, always mirror their prevalence in infections. There are more Bifidobacteria than Bacteroides in faeces and of the latter, *Bacteroides fragilis* accounts for less than 5% but in clinical sepsis *B. fragilis* is the dominant pathogen.

Indications for antibacterial prophylaxis

Endogenous contamination

Endogenous bacteria are important in the pathogenesis of infections after gastrointestinal tract surgery.

- Surgery for oesophagogastric carcinoma or gastric ulcer, patients on cimetidine and those undergoing revisional gastric surgery and in emergency surgery. Bacteria are normally destroyed rapidly by gastric acid and when intragastric pH is > 4, microorganisms are almost invariably present. Cephalosporins (cefuroxime) with or without metronidazole are effective in such conditions.
- Biliary tract surgery, especially with high-risk factors: emergency surgery, age over 70 years, jaundice, obesity, exploration of common bile duct, concomitant alimentary procedures. Biliary instrumentation without surgery such as percutaneous transhepatic cholangiography and endoscopic retrograde cholangiopancreatography also requires prophylaxis. Cephalosporins (ceftriaxone or cefazolin), mezlocillin or aminoglycoside (gentamicin) are all effective in reducing the infection from 20% to 2–4%.
- Colorectal surgery is associated with a high rate of sepsis which may be primary (initiated at the time of surgery) or secondary (occurring postoperatively as a result of anastomotic dehiscence). Prophylaxis is mainly effective in preventing primary sepsis (secondary sepsis due to anastomotic leak is affected by other factors). Without prophylaxis, the incidence of wound sepsis has been 35–50%, that of abscesses 4–11% and that of septicaemia 4–35%. Metronidazole/cefuroxime is an appropriate prophylactic regimen, reducing the sepsis rate to less than 10%. For emergency operations (when infection is established), a stoma should be raised and contaminated wounds left open (closing the abdominal wall only, leaving skin and subcutaneous tissues to heal by second intention). For these patients antibiotic therapy should be prolonged (therapeutic not prophylactic).

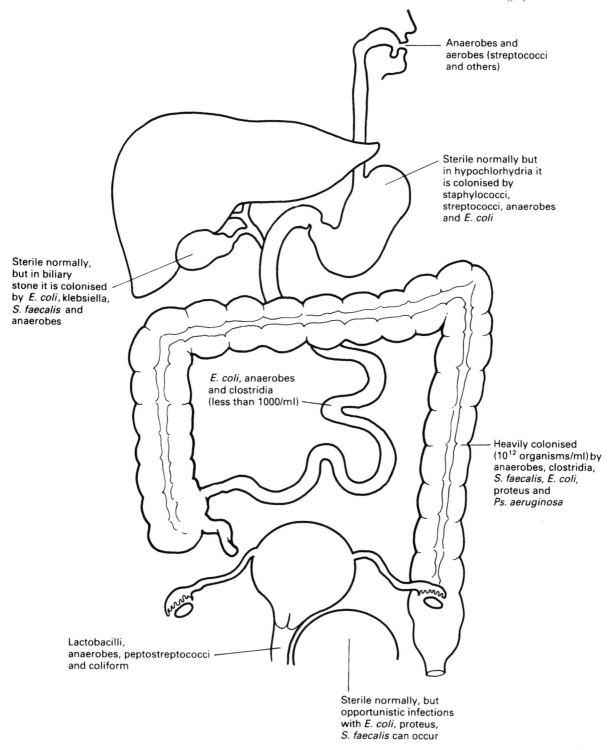

Anaerobes and
aerobes (streptococci
and others)

Sterile normally but
in hypochlorhydria it
is colonised by
staphylococci,
streptococci, anaerobes
and *E. coli*

Sterile normally,
but in biliary
stone it is colonised
by *E. coli*, klebsiella,
S. faecalis and
anaerobes

E. coli, anaerobes
and clostridia
(less than 1000/ml)

Heavily colonised
(10^{12} organisms/ml) by
anaerobes, clostridia,
S. faecalis, *E. coli*,
proteus and
Ps. aeruginosa

Lactobacilli,
anaerobes, peptostreptococci
and coliform

Sterile normally, but
opportunistic infections
with *E. coli*, proteus,
S. faecalis can occur

Fig. 1.12.1 Bacterial flora

- In appendicectomy the presence of perforation or local peritonitis justifies prophylaxis but because these complications cannot be identified preoperatively, it is reasonable to give metronidazole to all patients preoperatively and to continue it for 2 days only in those with obvious sepsis (Fig. 1.12.2).

- Vaginal or abdominal hysterectomy is associated with infection in 25–35%. Metronidazole is very effective.
- Sepsis is rarely a serious problem in urinary tract procedures and inappropriate prophylaxis can produce a population of drug-resistant bacteria which pose a potentially serious threat. There is no evidence that chemoprophylaxis prevents

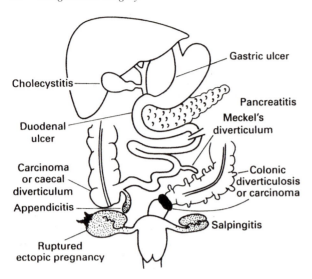

Fig. 1.12.2   Sites of origin of diseases which may lead to peritonitis

postoperative chest infections or that it is effective in preventing chest infections in tracheostomies or endotracheal intubation.

Exogenous contamination

● Lower limb surgery in the presence of peripheral vascular disease carries a small, but important, risk of gas gangrene (e.g. above-knee amputation stump) which is eliminated by perioperative benzylpenicillin.
● Prosthetic joint replacement, e.g. hip and knee: introduction of any prosthesis may be followed by infection (in less than 5% of cases). Because of the potentially disastrous consequences antibiotic prophylaxis is justified and effective. Joint replacements develop sepsis in 3.4% of untreated cases compared to 0.8% of those with prophylaxis. The antibiotic of choice is a β-lactamase-stable penicillin such as flucloxacillin. In all cases of prosthesis, staphylococci are the major pathogens (in heart surgery as well as neurosurgery).
● Prosthetic heart valves, e.g. Starr–Edward, Björk–Shilly and Porcine valves, and aortic grafts.
● Neurological shunts, e.g. Pudenz–Heyer and Hirtz–Holter valves.
● Extensive trauma and burns.
● Surgical procedures and instrumentations in rheumatic and valvular heart diseases and patients with pacemakers to avoid subacute bacterial endocarditis. The prophylactic antibiotic of choice depends on the site of operation and its prevalent organisms (*see* Fig. 1.12.1).
● Insertion of Marlex mesh in hernia repair and pacemakers in heart blocks.

Host immune system suppression

Such as in diabetes mellitus, chronic renal failure, leukaemia, aplastic anaemia, severe malnourishment, carcinomatosis, obstructive jaundice, steroid therapy and chemotherapy, e.g. azathioprine (Imuran) and cytotoxics.

Management of infected foreign bodies

Supportive devices are foreign bodies inserted via the skin; they can become infected with skin flora, mainly *S. epidermidis* (formerly *albus*), and occasionally *S. aureus* (formerly *pyogenes*); however fungi and Gram-negative organisms can occasionally be attracted to intravascular foreign bodies. They soon become a focus of infection showering bacteria into the bloodstream; foreign body infection is persistent despite intensive and prolonged therapy. It has been shown that host proteins (fibronectin, fibrinogen and laminin) can promote bacterial adhesion to foreign materials promoting initial bacterial colonisation; once bacteria become adherent to foreign material they behave differently and become tolerant or resistant to antibiotics that are otherwise bactericidal. This will lead to altered host defence in the vicinity of foreign material by weakening neutrophil activity of phagocytosis.

Clinically, there is fever with occasional pain due to thrombophlebitis; *S. epidermidis* infections of prosthetic heart valves can be extremely difficult to diagnose (due to their subacute course), and to treat (due to their resistance to many available antibiotics). Decision must be taken to remove or leave the device in situ. Certain facts emerge from clinical practice:

● Fungal disease or infection by resistant bacteria cannot be cured by chemotherapy alone without the removal of foreign body.
● Patients with prosthetic valves may develop endocarditis and heart failure and must, therefore, be considered for valve replacement.
● Antibiotic failure in treating foreign device-associated persistent bacteraemia or recurrent metastatic infection generally necessitates removal of the device.

Indications for keeping or removing infected devices

● Maintenance of device possible:
  – implantable i.v. subcutaneous catheters;
  – catheters for chronic ambulatory peritoneal dialysis;
  – cardiac pacemakers;
  – heart valve prosthesis.
● Removal of device recommended:
  – ventriculo-atrial or ventriculo-peritoneal CNS shunt.
● Removal of device mandatory:
  – central venous catheters causing bacteraemia;
  – orthopaedic prosthesis;
  – vascular grafts.

Diagnostic predicaments

In **febrile patient with central venous catheter**:

1. Search for infective focus unrelated to device (urinary infection, pneumonia, wound infection).
2. Do quantitative blood cultures percutaneously and via suspected catheter. Compare number of organisms to see if the catheter is the source of infection.
3. If blood cultures remain negative and transcutaneous puncture is not suspect, catheter may be left in place. Replacement of catheter is recommended if patient remains febrile despite antibiotic therapy, and no other source is detected.

4. Positive blood cultures and/or a suspect site indicate rapid removal of catheter. Insert a new catheter in a different site under adequate antibiotic cover.

Catheters with subcutaneous Dacron cuff (Hickman/Broviac catheters) are not necessarily removed even if causing bacteraemia; they can be treated successfully in 40%–70% of cases, probably due to high concentration achieved locally. However, catheters with signs of infection of the subcutaneous tunnel, or septic thrombosis of a central vein, or persistence of fever after several days of antibiotic therapy, should be removed.

In **infection of a joint prosthesis** (e.g. of the hip):

- In a majority of cases complete removal of the metallic prosthesis with cement and large debridement of infected bone and soft tissues will be necessary.
- Many surgeons believe that removal of an infected prosthesis must be followed by several weeks of i.v. therapy and that only after an interval of 3–6 months can a new prosthesis be implanted in order to decrease the likelihood of reinfection of the new prosthesis. This policy, however, necessitates the patient's immobilisation and severe disability of the extremity.
- In exceptional circumstances, in the presence of highly susceptible bacteria to antibiotics, such as streptococci to penicillin, the prosthesis may be left in situ with continuation of antibiotics for a relatively longer period.

Antibiotic therapy

Initial antibiotic therapy is based on direct microscopy of specimen stained with Gram stain. Culture and sensitivity results may dictate subsequent modification of antibiotics. The antibiotic must be bactericidal, and possibly in combination, and be administered i.v. and for a relatively long period (sometimes for 6 weeks).

In **bacteraemia with an i.v. device**, catheter removal is followed by vancomycin 2.1 g/day (since many staphylococci are resistant to methicillin), until culture and sensitivity results are obtained. If causative bacteria are methicillin-resistant staphylococci, vancomycin can be continued. However, if causative bacteria are staphylococci sensitive to penicillins, the treatment of choice is flucloxacillin 4.2 g/day.

Staphylococcus epidermidis bacteraemia in an immunocompetent host may only require 1–2 weeks of i.v. antibiotic therapy. In contrast, *Staphylococcus aureus* bacteraemia carries a considerable risk of metastatic osteomyelitis or endocarditis, and therefore requires at least 2 weeks of i.v. antibiotic therapy. In prolonged bacteraemia or signs of endocarditis or osteomyelitis, 4–6 weeks of i.v. therapy are required.

In **infection of a joint prosthesis** staphylococci as well as Gram-negative bacteria can be responsible, and therefore initial antibiotic therapy should include flucloxacillin with either aminoglycoside or third-generation cephalosporin. If causative organisms on blood culture are staphylococci, aminoglycoside may be continued for the first 2 weeks. Methicillin-resistant staphylococci require vancomycin which can be combined with aminoglycoside and rifampicin. Monitoring vancomycin is necessary, particularly in renal failure.

Anaerobic bacteria (Fig. 1.12.3)

Anaerobic bacteria may lead to serious infections in humans and various animals; they can involve virtually any organ when conditions are suitable. Most deep-seated abscesses and necrotising lesions involving anaerobes are polymicrobial and may include obligate aerobes, facultative anaerobes, or microaerophiles as concomitant microorganisms. These microorganisms, acting in concert with trauma, vascular stasis or tissue necrosis, lower the oxygen tension and provide favourable conditions for obligatory anaerobes to multiply. Anaerobic infection is commonly endogenous, e.g. brain abscess, gingivitis, dental and periodontal infection, meningitis, sinusitis, otitis media (head and neck); endocarditis, aspiration pneumonia, necrotising pneumonia, lung abscess, empyema (thoracic), antibiotic-associated diarrhoea and colitis (*Clostridium difficile* colitis), peritonitis, intra-abdominal abscesses, complications of appendicitis or cholecystitis (gastrointestinal); osteomyelitis, septic arthritis, gas gangrene, tetanus, decubitus and diabetic foot ulcer (musculoskeletal); tubo-ovarian abscess, salpingitis, vaginitis, endometritis, Bartholin's abscess (female genital tract). Anaerobic infection is less commonly exogenous in origin (some infections are of historical interest, e.g. food-borne botulism/infant botulism/wound botulism, gas gangrene, tetanus/tetanus neonatorum, human and animal bites, and septic abortion). Anaerobic bacteria must be identified because anaerobic infections are associated with high morbidity and mortality; also, the treatment of infection varies with the bacterial species involved, demanding proper antimicrobial cover and life-saving surgical interventions, such as debridement of necrotic tissue or amputation of a limb.

Anaerobic bacteria include:

- Spore-forming Gram-positive bacilli, e.g. *Clostridium botulinum* (botulism), *Clostridium welchii* (gas gangrene) and *Clostridium tetani* (tetanus).
- Non-spore-forming bacteria, which include:
  - Bacilli (rods), which can be either Gram-negative, e.g. Bacteroides and Fusobacteria, or Gram-positive, e.g. Actinomyces and Lactobacilli.
  - Cocci, which can be either Gram-positive, e.g. peptococci (anaerobic staphylococci) and peptostreptococci (anaerobic streptococci), or Gram-negative, e.g. Acidaminococci.

Practical points

Pseudomonas aeruginosa infection is difficult to eradicate because of three defence mechanisms – a barrier preventing antibiotic access, plasmid-mediated β-lactamases and inducible β-lactamases. Its main habitat is the large bowel and it likes moist surfaces, e.g. burns, urinary tract and tracheostomy wounds (intensive care organism). The main antimicrobials are:

- Semi-synthetic penicillins (e.g. carbenicillin in large doses, ticarcillin, carfecillin, azlocillin and mezlocillin).
- Aminoglycosides, e.g. gentamicin, netilmicin (less otonephrotoxic) and tobramycin. Both ticarcillin and carbenicillin can be given with gentamicin as the combination is synergistic.
- Colistin (polymyxin antibiotic).

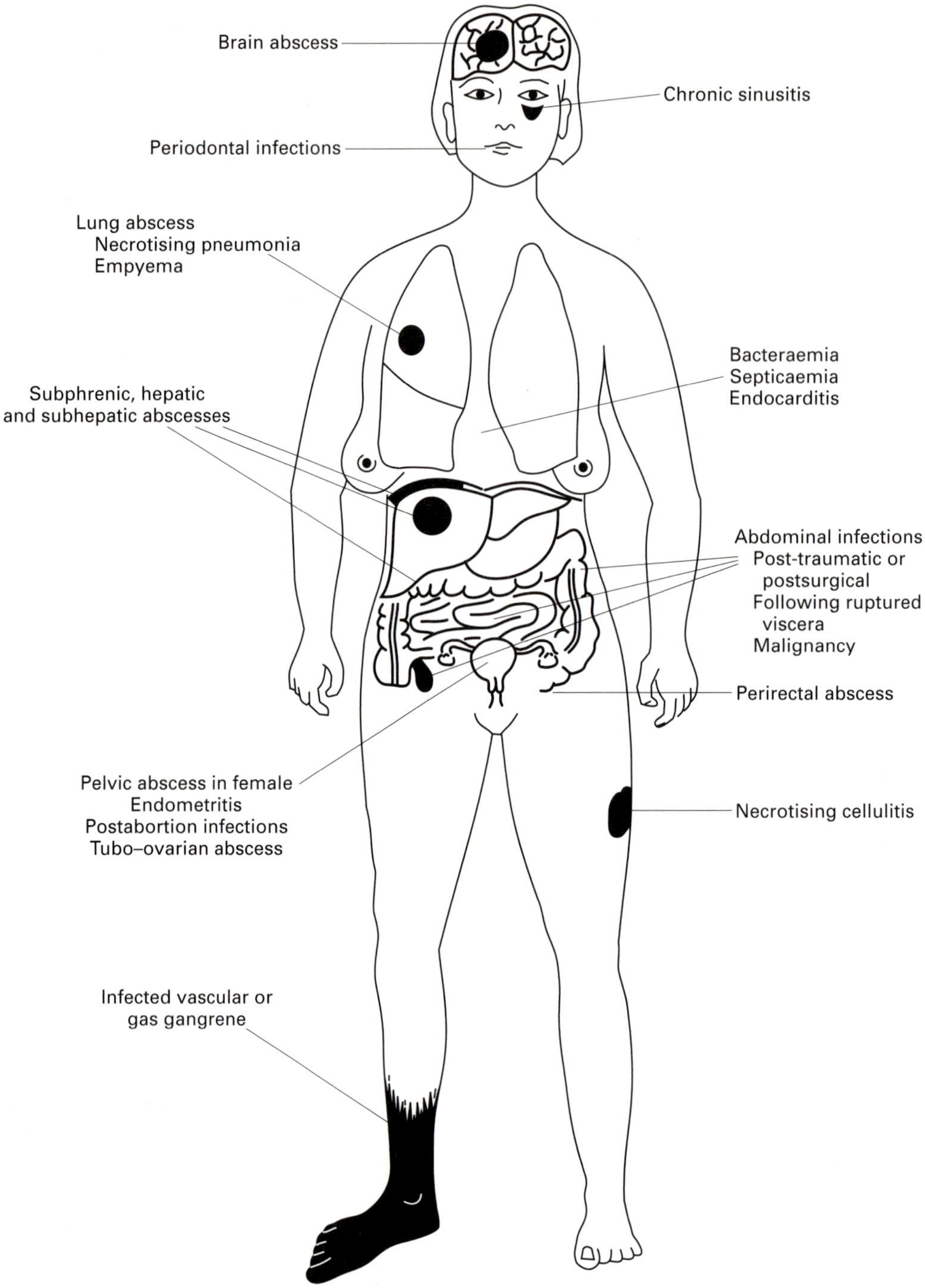

Fig. 1.12.3   Common anaerobic infections

- Some of the third-generation cephalosporins, e.g. cefsulodin.
- Povidone-iodine (Betidine) solution, with its remarkable bactericidal effect. This solution can be used freely since it does not cause burning or allergy. It can be used for skin preparation, intraperitoneal lavage, interparietal spray, intracolonic washout and even as an intraurethral ointment.

In gastrointestinal tract surgery the currently used common double prophylactic is cefuroxime/metronidazole combination. Single chemotherapy with mezlocillin or moxalactam can be used. However, the latter may produce clinically important bleedings in vitamin K store deficiency, e.g. in the elderly and in chemical sterilisation of the bowel.

- Avoid clindamycin and lincomycin as they cause pseudomembranous colitis which may be fatal. It is due to toxin produced by *Clostridium difficile*, which is sensitive to oral vancomycin.
- Food poisoning must always be remembered in meat eaters; the fatal outbreak of *E. Coli* 157 in Scotland spread in meat prepared unhygienically (1996/1997).

1.13 AIDS and Viral Hepatitis in Surgery

AIDS

It is probable that no other disease has been so rapidly, accurately and efficiently defined in the history of medicine, and no other disease has the potential for such major deleterious medical, social and financial effects on the health care systems of almost every country worldwide. By September 1991, a total of 418 404 cases which met the clinical definition of AIDS had been reported to WHO and, in addition, there were about 1.5 million adults with HIV infection in Western industrialised countries (with a twelve-fold increase in the USA and a nine-fold increase in Western Europe), 6 million in sub-Saharan Africa. 1 million in Latin America (Central and South America showing a forty-fold increase over 5 years from 1987 to 1992) and over 1 million in South and South-East Asia. This may be the tip of the iceberg, because of the lack of proper diagnosis or even disclosure of AIDS and HIV infection in many countries. It is thought that the future incidence of AIDS will be highest in India and South-East Asia. As a consequence of the high incidence of adult AIDS, WHO estimates that about 0.5 million children worldwide have AIDS (with a four-fold increase of infected babies in the USA and a five-fold increase in Europe).

Global HIV has spread from an estimated 100 000 people infected worldwide in 1980 to nearly 20 million by early 1993 due to enormous movement of people, the universality of sexual exchange, an international traffic in blood products and the international epidemic of drug misuse. WHO has estimated that the worldwide death toll of patients with AIDS will be 6 millions more by the year 2000. HIV vaccine is still in a primitive experimental stage and many years aways from clinical use for protection of doctors and staff as well as patients. AIDS, therefore, is the pandemic disease of this century and the coming one, just as plague was the pandemic disease of the Middle Ages.

AIDS was first recognised as an epidemic in Spring 1981 in the USA and as affecting the 4 Hs, i.e. Homosexuals, Haemophiliacs, Heroin and intravenous drug addicts and Haitian immigrants. AIDS can occur also in women after artificial insemination by donor. (AIDS has been found in normal heterosexuals in some parts of Africa.) AIDS is associated with a decrease in helper T-lymphocytes and a high incidence of cytomegalovirus (CMV) infection. It is thought that CMV or another virus (homosexuals usually harbour many viruses, e.g. hepatitis B virus, Epstein–Barr virus and CMV) may possibly cause the cellular immunodeficiency. However, a human retrovirus which was isolated and called human T-cell leukaemia–lymphoma virus (HTLV-3) is thought to be the causative agent in AIDS. This virus infection has a mean incubation period of 2 years and is thought to be responsible for persistent generalised lymphadenopathy (PGL) and Kaposi's sarcoma (a multifocal malignancy composed of new blood vessels and large spindle cells; it presents as firm, bluish-brown nodules in the skin usually on the limbs). However not everyone who becomes infected with HTLV-3 will develop AIDS. HTLV-3 is detected by antibody test, using immuno-fluorescence, radioimmunoassay and enzyme-linked immunoassay.

Clinically there is often a prodromal illness characterised by fever, weight loss, oral thrush (due to candidiasis and possible oesophageal extension and dysphagia), diarrhoea and PGL. The syndrome is frequently complicated by opportunistic infections, mainly *Pneumocystis carinii* and CMV pneumonia, bowel infestations with Giardia lamblia, Entamoeba histolytica, Shigella, Salmonella and campylobacter, CMV chorioretinitis and *Toxoplasma gondii* encephalopathy. AIDS is also often complicated by malignancies, e.g. Kaposi's sarcoma. The treatment is that of opportunistic infections. Radiotherapy and chemotherapy may be needed for skin malignancies. Neutralising antibodies, interferons, interleukin, thymic hormone, suramin and phosphonoformate drugs have all been tried with no dramatic improvement. The mortality is 40% but rises even higher in the presence of Kaposi's sarcoma of the skin.

Staging of HIV infection

According to the US Centers for Disease Control (CDC), patients with HIV infection are grouped as follows.

I Group 1
Acute HIV infection: a mononucleosis-like syndrome associated with seroconversion for HIV antibody.

II Group 2
Asymptomatic HIV infection: absence of any signs that cause patients to be classified as group 3 or 4.

III Group 3
Persistent generalised lymphadenopathy: lymph-node enlargement of 1 cm or more at two or more extrainguinal sites persisting for more than 3 months with no other explanation.

IVa Subgroup 4A
One or more of fever persisting for more than 1 month, involuntary weight loss of more than 10%, diarrhoea persisting for more than 1 month in the absence of an explanation other than HIV infection.

IVb Subgroup 4B
Neurological disease: one or more of dementia, myelopathy, peripheral neuropathy in the absence of an explanation other than HIV infection.

IVc 1 Category 4C1
Patients with *Pneumocystis carinii* pneumonia, chronic cryptosporidiosis, toxoplasmosis, extraintestinal strongyloidiasis, isosporiasis, candidiasis (oesophageal, bronchial or pulmonary), cryptococcosis, histoplasmosis, mycobacterial infection with *Mycobacterium avium* or *M. kansasii*, cytomegalovirus infection, chronic mucocutaneous or disseminated herpes simplex infection and progressive multifocal leucoencephalopathy.

IVc 2 Category 4C2
Symptomatic or invasive diseases with hairy oral leucoplakia, multidermatomal herpes zoster, recurrent Salmonella bacteraemia, nocardiosis, tuberculosis or oral candidiasis.

IVd Subgroup 4D
Secondary cancers: one or more cancers known to be associated with HIV infection, including Kaposi's sarcoma, non-Hodgkin's lymphoma or primary lymphoma of the brain.

IVe Subgroup 4E
Other conditions of HIV infection: other clinical findings or diseases not in other groups that may be attributed to HIV infection or are indicative of defective cell mediated immunity; examples include patients with constitutional symptoms not meeting the criteria for subgroup 4A, patients with infectious diseases not listed in subgroup 4C and patients with neoplasms not listed in subgroup 4D.

Gastrointestinal problems in AIDS

- Oral candidiasis, hairy leucoplakia of tongue and Kaposi's sarcoma of palate (50% of such cases have visceral involvement elsewhere).
- Oesophageal ulceration due to candidiasis and cytomegalovirus infection and occasional herpes virus infection.
- Weight loss in itself may markedly worsen the immune status of the patient. It is due to a variety of causes: anorexia, inability to eat due to emotional reactions, malabsorption of xylose and fat with mucosal abnormalities on jejunal biopsies and, finally, diarrhoea.
- Diarrhoea is a common event in AIDS patients. Diarrhoea in homosexuals is termed 'gay bowel syndrome' which is not necessarily related to AIDS, since other sexually transmitted diseases may cause diarrhoea. The causes of diarrhoea are:
  – Bacteria: Shigella, Salmonella, Campylobacter and *Salmonella typhimurium*.
  – Protozoa: *Giardia lamblia*, *Entamoeba histolytica* and Cryptosporidium.
  – Viral: Cytomegalovirus (CMV)
  – Rickettsial: Chlamydia.

Salmonella typhimurium, an intracellular parasite, produces a devastating typhoid-like illness in patients with AIDS. The commonest opportunistic bacterium in AIDS is *Mycobacterium avium intracellulare* which produces severe anaemia and occasional diarrhoea; it is found in a high proportion of patients dying of AIDS and is frequently first found in stool culture or on rectal biopsy. *Cryptosporidium* can cause profuse diarrhoea of 10 litres per day and the patient requires intravenous fluids.

Large bowel ulceration and diarrhoea due to CMV infection mimic inflammatory bowel disease. CMV can induce colonic arteritis and toxic megacolon which resolve spontaneously.

Anal carcinoma incidence is high in homosexuals because of venereal transfer of the polyoma/papilloma viruses. Body lice are a cause of pruritus ani. Other sexually transmitted diseases affect the anus; more than 80% of primary syphilis seen today occurs in the anus, and the condylomas of the secondary syphilis are easy to miss. Gonorrhoeal proctitis, *Chlamydia* proctitis and lymphogranuloma venereum may extend to the anus too.

Opportunistic infections in AIDS

- *Candida albicans* in AIDS patients can cause extensive colonisation and ulceration of the oesophagus or bronchi. It may present as dysphagia.

- *Cryptococcus neoformans* most commonly causes meningitis but can also present as disseminated fungal infection.
- *Cryptosporidiosis* affects the whole of the intestinal tract and causes chronic watery diarrhoea. This is particularly difficult to treat, as reservoirs of infection can persist in the small bowel or the biliary tree.
- *Cytomegalovirus (CMV)* can cause a disseminated infection of many organs. Classically it affects the retina (causing progressive blindness), the lung, (causing interstitial pneumonitis and resulting in progressive deterioration of lung function), the gastrointestinal tract (causing abdominal pain, bloody diarrhoea and rarely, toxic dilatation of the colon), and the pancreas (causing acute pancreatitis). It can also cause acute hepatitis and has been implicated in the development of HIV dementia.
- *Herpes simplex* infection can cause extensive ulceration of the mouth, oesophagus, rectum, anal canal and perianal skin.
- *Histoplasmosis* is a rare fungal infection which causes alveolitis and skin nodules.
- *Mycobacterium avium intracellulare* is responsible for 80% of atypical mycobacterial infections. It causes low grade fever, lethargy and anaemia, and the organisms are found in blood, bone marrow, lung, liver, and gastrointestinal tract.
- *Mycobacterium tuberculosis* infection constitutes a diagnosis of AIDS if it affects two extrapulmonary sites.
- *Pneumocystis carinii* pneumonia is an interstitial pneumonitis characterised by fever, dry cough and increasing shortness of breath on exertion. The accumulation of pneumocytes within the alveolar spaces causes progressive deterioration of respiratory function and if untreated is invariably fatal.
- *Progressive multifocal leucoencephalopathy* is a virally induced degeneration of the white matter of the central nervous system. It leads to progressive neurological dysfunction and is thought to be caused by papovavirus.
- *Strongyloidiasis* and *isosporiasis* are seen in the USA but are extremely rare in the UK. They cause diarrhoeal illness and other gastrointestinal disease.
- *Toxoplasmosis* can cause multifocal brain abscesses. These present as space-occupying lesions with headache, fever, focal neurological deficits and increased intracranial pressure.

Precautions during surgery

Precautions that the surgeon must take while operating on patients who are at 'high risk' for HTLV-3 or hepatitis virus are the same and will be listed together here.

1. All appropriate staff must be made aware of the patient's 'high risk' status. Health workers caring for patients with HIV infection may also be at increased risk of tuberculosis and should be offered protection (Table 1.13.1).
2. The anaesthetist must use a disposable endotracheal tube and anaesthetic circuit.
3. Disposable clothes, aprons, gowns and over-shoes should be used and impermeable footwear. A slow and careful surgical technique will help to safeguard the surgeon and other operating staff from scalpel and needle-stick injuries.

Table 1.13.1 HIV infection-risk factors and recommended precautions in operating theatres

Risk factors for HIV infection	Recommended precautions
Personal risk factors	
1 Homosexual or bisexual males	Full precautions are
2 Intravenous drug abusers	indicated where risk is
3 Persons who have had penetrative	known or suspected
sexual contact with others from areas	
of high HIV prevalence	
4 Persons who have received	
unscreened blood transfusions in	
areas of high HIV prevalence	
5 Haemophilic patients who have	
received untreated blood products	
6 Known HIV positive patients	
7 Sexual partners of any of the above	
8 Children born to seropositive	
mothers	
Geographical factors	
1 Local – where prevalence of HIV	Local 'high' prevalence
infection is known to be high	should be defined by
2 International – sub-Saharan Africa;	individual hospitals but
other countries with known high	greater than 5% should
prevalence of HIV	justify full precautions
Surgical factors	
1 Emergency operations – major	Full precautions should be
abdominal and orthopaedic	taken
operations; burns	
2 'High risk' elective operations –	Full precautions should be
major abdominal, gynaecological, and	taken except in areas of
cardiovascular operations; orthopaedic	low HIV prevalence
operations involving use of power	
tools	

4. The use of two pairs of gloves may afford greater protection (see below).

5. Eye protection with goggles should be used if there is a possibility of splash from body fluids.

6. Adoption of techniques that minimise the vulnerability to stab injuries; these techniques demand more care and are more time-consuming, such as:

- cutting needle(s) from suturing threads before tying the knot, using kidney dish or even magnetic mat for passing surgical instruments from sister to surgeon and vice versa;
- abstaining from the use of hand needles;
- making a habit of using forceps and non-touch techniques;
- preferring the use of staplers (whenever available) to needles for skin closure or visceral anastomosis whenever feasible;
- preferring laparoscopic surgery to open conventional operations whenever possible, e.g. laparoscopic cholecystectomy, appendicectomy and hernia repair.

7. Successful vaccination will provide protection against hepatitis B (homosexuals often harbour many viruses), and all staff coming into regular contact with HB-positive patients should consider being immunised.

8. Accidents resulting in needle pricks, minor cuts and bleeding must be washed immediately and copiously with soap and water and dressed if needed. Nursing staff often report such accidents in order to test the blood of both the patient and the injured staff for hepatitis and HIV viruses.

(While AIDS is a notifiable disease, many surgeons and hospital doctors resent sending their blood sample for hepatitis or HIV virus testing if they are punctured with a needle, because if the result is positive, it will ruin their career for ever as they have to stop practising medicine.)

Other measures

Contaminated tables and floors must be cleaned liberally with household bleach, freshly diluted 1:10 in water and applied for at least 30 min. All disposable sheets, clothes, and gloves must be discarded and incinerated. Surgical instruments must be cleaned with hot soapy water and then sterilised thoroughly in the autoclave.

In the wards, too, general hygiene principles must be applied; sanitary towels and infected toothbrushes and razors must be discarded and incinerated. Spillages of blood and vomitus should be cleaned up with hot household bleach 1:10 dilution poured and left for 30 min. It is essential to do no (or the fewest possible) invasive tests and techniques on the patient postoperatively.

Injuries occur during approximately 10% of surgical procedures and glove puncture occurs in up to 30% of operations. However, it is thought that there is an approximately 0.4% chance of being infected after a single inoculation injury.

There are many reports describing how gloves fail to protect individuals from contamination with body fluids. As many as 1 in 8 (12.7%) gloves are perforated at the time of surgical procedures in as many as 1 in every 3 (34.5%) operations. Double gloving, which results in an inner glove perforation rate of 2%, at the expense of decreasing sensitivity, is sometimes used to reduce the risk.

Precautions during sexual intercourse

The male condom remains an effective barrier against sexually transmitted diseases – including AIDS. A condom for women, called Femidon (shaped like a male condom but designed to line the vagina) is also available; it is made of soft pliable polyurethane and is the first disposable barrier method of protection under the control of women against infection with AIDS or other sexually transmitted diseases. It provides as effective a method of contraception as the male condom.

Symptomatic treatment

Pneumonitis due to the opportunistic protozoal infection of *Pneumocystis carinii* must be confirmed and treated. Diagnosis is based on sputum direct smear, culture and sensitivity, bronchoscopy and bronchial wash-out. It is treated with pentamidine isothionate or co-trimoxazole. As pulmonary disease due to tuberculosis cannot be distinguished from disease associated with opportunistic mycobacteria, all patients with suspected acid-fast bacilli in sputum should be given multiple anti-tuberculosis drug chemotherapy until the results of mycobacterial culture are known.

A tuberculin test is not recommended in people infected with HIV who have not had BCG vaccination (as it may lead to tuberculous flare-up), neither is it advisable to offer prophylaxis to those patients sensitive to tuberculin (since disseminated BCG infection may follow BCG vaccination after contracting HIV infection). Oxygen therapy and symptomatic treatment of any dry cough with antitussives may be useful.

It is important to provide symptomatic treatment of diarrhoea with oral rehydration and intravenous fluid replacement as well as specific therapy for the specific superinfection; for instance, systemic candidiasis needs Flagyl (metronidazole) or 5-fluorocytosine, oesophageal candidiasis needs a new effective antifungal ketoconazole at the expense of a small risk of inducing liver abnormalities. *Cryptosporidium* diarrhoea needs symptomatic treatment with macrolide antibiotics (erythromycin, clindamycin and spiramycin) which produce transient improvement. Fungal infections are best dealt with by stopping all antibiotic treatment and giving specific chemotherapy. Most viral diseases are self-limiting provided that the immunosuppression is reduced. CMV infection may be treated with one of two effective anti-CMV agents, namely foscarnet or the guanine-derivative DHPG (dihydropropoxy guanosine).

The patient's consent for blood testing for HTLV-3 immunoassay and, if positive, his approval to notify the nursing staff must be sought. Even if the patient has not agreed, he must be labelled as a 'high risk' patient on the basis of medical history so that full precautions are taken to protect medical and nursing staff from contracting AIDS.

Most viral diseases are self-limiting provided that the immunosuppression is reduced. However, it is worthwhile treating the opportunistic viral pneumonitis with a course of Septrin (trimethoprim-sulphamethoxazole) or erythromycin or tetracycline. Two new effective anti-CMV agents may be helpful: foscarnet or the guanine derivative DHPG (dihydropropoxy guanosine). As pulmonary disease due to tuberculosis cannot be distinguished from disease associated with opportunistic mycobacteria, all patients with suspected acid-fast bacilli in sputum should be given antituberculosis multiple drug chemotherapy until the results of mycobacterial culture are known. Oxygen is essential for all patients who are seriously ill with pneumonia, and is delivered via facemask to maintain PaO_2 above 8 kPa (60 mmHg). If this cannot be maintained with the patient breathing 60% oxygen, then the patient should be transferred to an intensive care unit with facilities for intermittent positive pressure ventilation (IPPV). Most patients who require IPPV do so within 4 days of admission.

Symptomatic treatment with antitussives (for dry cough) and antipyretics (for fever and headache) may also be required.

It is agreed that in an AIDS patient the minimum or no invasive techniques must be performed.

● See Appendix 2, HIV Infection and AIDS: The Ethical Considerations (pp. 629–631)

Therapeutic principles of HIV-1 infection

HIV exists in two forms: HIV-1 which causes most HIV disease worldwide and HIV-2 which is confined mainly to West Africa. The virus infects its key target, the CD4-positive T lymphocyte by attaching to the CD4 receptor and cell membrane molecules and then introducing its RNA into the cell. The viral enzyme reverse transcriptase uses this RNA as a template to generate DNA, which is then incorporated into host's DNA and in turn transcribed to produce viral RNA. This RNA serves to provide genetic material of, and polyproteins for, new virus particles. As these new particles mature, the enzyme viral protease cleaves the precursor polyproteins to generate essential viral structural proteins and enzymes. The mature particles then bud from the host cell and can infect other cells. HIV replicates rapidly and continuously. This process destroys and eventually depletes patient's CD4 T lymphocyte cells resulting in immunodeficiency which renders the patient susceptible to opportunistic infections and malignancies that characterise acquired immunodeficiency syndrome (AIDS). The **CD4 T cells count** in the blood correlates with the likelihood of progression to AIDS and death, and is used as a surrogate marker of the stage of HIV infection. The normal count is around 600–1500 cells/μL. In patients with symptomatic advanced HIV disease, counts below 200 cells/μL are typical. The concentration of HIV RNA in patient's plasma (a measure of ongoing viral replication) can be assayed and is termed the **viral load**. Patients with the highest viral loads are at greatest risk of rapid disease progression; reduction in viral load correlates with improved clinical outcome. Ideally, viral load assays and CD4 T cell counts should be used together in management with measurements every 3 months.

During HIV replication, mutations occur in DNA copies incorporated into host's DNA; these may confer resistance to single drugs, and sometimes, cross-resistance to drugs sharing the same mechanism of action, resulting in therapeutic failure.

Prophylaxis

1. Perinatal transmission of HIV In pregnant women with HIV infection, ZDV (*see* below) (taken by mouth antepartum, given i.v. during delivery, and then given by mouth to the newborn for 6 weeks) reduces the risk of perinatal transmission of the infection from 26% to 8%. This treatment is effective regardless of the mother's viral load and should be offered to all pregnant women who have HIV infection.

2. Needlestick injury and HIV The risk of HIV transmission following needlestick injury involving contaminated blood is 0.4%. Factors which increase the risk are deep injury, visible blood on injuring device, a procedure involving a device (e.g. hollow bore needle) being placed directly into a blood vessel and a terminally ill patient. ZDV prophylaxis (1000 mg daily for 3–4 weeks following exposure) reduces the transmission by about 80%. USA guidelines recommend combination therapy (*see* below) based on ZDV (200 mg tds daily) plus 3TC (lamivuine 150 mg twice daily) and possibly, indinavir (800 mg tds daily) for 4 weeks to health care professionals at risk of acquiring infection following occupational exposure; ideally treatment should start within 1–2 hours of such exposure. None of these drugs are licensed in UK for this indication.

3. Unprotected sexual intercourse and HIV As yet there is no agreement on whether to attempt prophylaxis where there is a risk of transmission of HIV infection following unprotected sexual intercourse.

Combination therapies for HIV infection

Anti-retroviral agents and immunomodulators include:
- Nucleoside analogues, e.g. ZDV, ddl, ddC, 3TC, with ZDV being the most effective single agent.
- Protease inhibitors, e.g. ritonavir, indinavir and saquinavir.
- Non-nucleoside reverse transcriptase inhibitors (NNRTI).
- Interleukins/cytokines.

Treatment of **symptomatic HIV infection** with zidovuridine (ZDV) monotherapy for six months results in improved survival, delayed disease progression and improved quality of life. Clinical trials show that ZDV is more effective as *initial monotherapy* than either didanosine (ddl) or zalcitabine (ddC). This can be followed by switching between nucleoside analogues – so-called *sequential monotherapy* – which may provide additional clinical benefit compared with simply continuing ZDV long-term monotherapy. Such sequential monotherapy between ddl and ddC appears to offer greatest benefit in patients who have not progressed to AIDS and who have CD4 cell counts greater than 150 cell/µl.

ZDV monotherapy in **asymptomatic HIV infection** suggests that this agent is well tolerated; at one-year follow-up the early intervention with ZDV delays both disease progression and immunological decline as compared with patients who did not start ZDV until clinical manifestations have appeared. At 3-year follow-up, however, there is no additional survival benefit. ZDV may suppress bone marrow (dose dependent).

Patients who become intolerant to ZDV or experience disease progression while receiving ZDV, a change to ddC or ddl may at least provide benefits anticipated from continued ZDV. However, ddC should be avoided in patients with peripheral neuropathy; ddl main obstacles are inconvenient administration and GIT side-effects, particularly life-threatening pancreatitis.

Massive viral turnover (increasing viral load), coupled with inaccuracy of HIV reverse transcriptase, lead to rapid genomic diversity during viral swarming of chronically ill patients with HIV. Resistance to anti-retroviral agents is an inevitable consequence of this genetic diversity. Appearance of resistant strains is more rapid in patients with low CD4 counts and with the clinical progression and diagnosis of AIDS, which may explain the limited response to anti-retroviral agents; appearance of ZDV resistance is a negative prognostic indicator even in patients who have switched to ddl therapy, suggesting that an aggressive combination may be useful.

Learning from combination therapy in tuberculosis and some neoplasms, it has been suggested that HIV treatment can be improved by combining two or more of these agents. Most anti-retroviral combinations are based on ZDV due to its proven clinical value and its ability to cross the blood–brain barrier.

Combination therapy in established HIV infection (before CD4 T cell count falls below 350 cells/µL and certainly while it is greater than 200 cells/µL) has shown considerable promise in clinical studies. Nucleoside combinations include ZDV with ddC, ddl or 3TC; they all appear to produce similar rises in CD4 count and reductions in viral load superior in both magnitude and duration to those with ZDV monotherapy, and are particularly well tolerated by healthier patients. Adverse reactions with 3TC include GIT disorders, hair loss, myelosuppression and exacerbation of pre-existing peripheral neuropathy.

ZDV–ddC or ZDV–3TC or ZDV–saquinavir are so far the best combinations. The effects have been apparent in patients previously untreated with anti-retroviral agents. Many physicians are choosing nucleoside analogue combinations as their first line therapy; 10–15% of seroconversions are possible, even with viruses resistant to ZDV.

The protease inhibitor saquinavir appear to have therapeutic efficacy both as a single agent and in combination regimens (synergistic with ZDV), as well as showing excellent safety profiles even in current doses of 600 mg tds and even when used in triple combination (with ZDV and ddC).

Identification of substantial viral replication from the time of acquisition of HIV suggests the need for early institution of anti-retroviral therapy. However, early introduction of currently available therapies has not been shown to provide additional benefit compared with treatment beginning at the onset of symptoms, but both single-agent and combination regimens appear to be best tolerated as early therapies and the appearance of resistance is much slower in people with great immunocompetence. Recently, measures of viral load, such as RNA PCR (polymerase chain reaction) have been shown to provide a monitoring tool for baseline diagnosis as well as a dynamic marker of anti-retroviral treatment effect.

VIRAL HEPATITIS

Causative organisms responsible for viral hepatitis mainly include type A, type B, non-A non-B viruses; occasionally Epstein–Barr virus and cytomegalovirus are implicated in aetiology. Many patients undergoing surgery are unrecognised, either because they are in the asymptomatic prodromal phase, or they remain subclinical and anicteric. The onset of viral hepatitis can be gradual or sudden; early symptoms occur in 90% of patients and include dark urine, fatigue and anorexia. Nausea, fever and abdominal pain occur in 50%. High plasma transaminases occur 7–14 days prior to the onset of jaundice. Plasma bilirubin does not usually exceed 20 mg/dl unless liver disease is severe or haemolysis is also present. Mild anaemia and lymphocytosis are common. Severe and potentially fatal hepatitis can be predicted by plasma albumin below 2.5 g/dl, or markedly prolonged prothrombin time. Failure of vitamin K to correct prothrombin time emphasises the severity of underlying hepatocellular disease. Nevertheless, in most patients, the clinical course of viral hepatitis is uneventful and recovery of liver function is complete.

Hepatitis A (infectious hepatitis or short incubation hepatitis)

- Causative agent is 27 nm picorna RNA virus; it is highly infectious with common cross-infection within families.
- Virus transmission is by the faecal–oral route or by ingestion of food contaminated with sewage. Viraemia occurs 1–25 days before onset of symptoms, but transmission by plasma or blood products rarely occurs.
- Very common in developing countries with poor sanitation; most preschool children acquire infection (faecal–oral) by serial passage from one individual to another.
- Incubation period is short, ranging from 2 to 6 weeks.

- Period of potential infectivity of patients harbouring type A virus is 2–3 weeks before and after onset of clinical symptoms; this corresponds to maximum duration of virus excretion in faeces. During this time, strict attention to stool isolation and appropriate hand washing (with soap and water) by all attending personnel is mandatory.
- Antibodies of immunoglobulin M or G (IgM and IgG) appear during early acute illness and persist in most patients for 3–4 months; this is diagnostic of recent infection with type A virus. Patients with hepatitis A antibodies are probably immune to the disease on re-exposure (nearly 50% of the adult population of the USA has high plasma antibodies against type A virus).
- Prophylaxis is by good hygiene and passive immunity. Pooled gammaglobulins (0.02 ml/kg) greatly reduce the severity of A hepatitis when given during the incubation period, and will provide protection against the disease for 6 months.
- Prognosis is good with symptoms disappearing and transaminases decreasing in 3–4 weeks. Chronic liver disease does not develop and chronic carrier state does not occur.

Hepatitis B (serum hepatitis or post-transfusion hepatitis)

- Causative agent is 42 nm DNA with surface and core components (Dane particle). Hepatitis B is probably the most common type of viral hepatitis.
- Transmission is usually via parenteral routes such as blood transfusion or percutaneous inoculation. Nevertheless, it has become increasingly apparent that non-parentral routes (oral-to-oral and sexual) can also be responsible.
- It is common in developed countries, Western Europe and North America; sporadic cases are often transmitted from carriers, and infusion of pooled blood products carries risk of hepatitis B virus transmission. Principal risk factors include: male homosexuality, low socioeconomic status, i.v. drug misuse, ethnic group, sexual promiscuity, residence in institutions for mental handicap, and employment in health professions.
- Incubation period ranges from 4 to 24 weeks.
- Electron microscopy and immunology techniques have identified several viral particles associated with B hepatitis. Of these materials, Dane particle may be synonymous with type B virus. Dane particle consists of hepatitis B surface antigen (HBsAg) and hepatitis B core antigen (HBcAg) and E antigen (HBeAg). Antibodies (anti-HBs, anti-HBc) may develop against these antigens. Plasma titre of these antigens and antibodies may help in:
  - follow-up of the course of hepatitis;
  - determining immunity;
  - assessing state of infectivity of patients;
  - screening of blood, e.g. HBsAg is detectable in plasma (by radioimmunoassay) of nearly all patients with hepatitis B several weeks before onset of symptoms. However, about 25% of infected adults develop clinical hepatitis.
- Period of infectivity is during HBsAg positivity. Since HBsAg titres decrease by the time of onset of clinical symptoms and are negligible by 6 weeks, presence of HBsAg in plasma indicates the potential for infectivity. Anti-HBs antibodies appear in 90% of patients during convalescence, and remain high as long as HBsAg persists in plasma. The incidence of anti-HBs antibodies in the general population is 10%, indicating that hepatitis B is self-limited in most patients. Anti-HBc antibodies become detectable soon after the onset of symptoms and persist for months to years, serving as a marker for previous or chronic hepatitis B infections. HBeAg are found only in nuclei of hepatocytes; anti-HBe antibodies can serve as markers of previous infections. HBeAg may also reflect patient's potential for infectivity and/or development of chronic disease states.

- Prognosis. The persistence of HBsAg for longer than 6 months in the absence of antibodies indicates that the patient is a chronic carrier and potentially infective to others. Approximately 1 in every 200 adults in the USA is classified as a chronic carrier. Carriers, however, are not susceptible to virus reactivation when subjected to anaesthesia and operation. Furthermore, HBsAg is rarely present in plasma of patients with unexplained jaundice in the postoperative period. However, some carriers may develop chronic active hepatitis, which often progresses to liver cirrhosis with oesophageal varices and ascites. Primary hepatocellular carcinoma is also 220 times more likely to develop in chronic carriers than in normal people.
- Prophylaxis includes good hygiene, vaccination and hepatitis B immunoglobulins. Prevention of hepatitis B infection is desirable, considering potential risks associated with this infection. Personnel administering anaesthesia and those exposed to patient's blood or body fluids, such as oral secretions, deserve prophylaxis, because they are five times more likely to show serological evidence of previous or current hepatitis B infection than the general population. Avoiding exposure to infected patients is not reliable prophylaxis, because many infective patients are asymptomatic and unrecognised, but more importantly, hepatitis B virus can survive on contaminated surfaces at room temperature for as long as 6 months. Heating to 60 °C for 4 h, steam sterilisation, or 2% glutaraldehyde destroy hepatitis virus. Immunisation with inactivated hepatitis B vaccine is a highly effective means of establishing an active immunity (protective antibody response in over 90% of vaccinated individuals) and protecting personnel at risk. Postoperative prophylaxis with hepatitis B immunoglobulins to establish passive immunity is recommended for non-immunised personnel exposed to patients known to be infective for hepatitis.

High-risk patients presenting to anaesthesia and surgery with a likelihood for harbouring HBsAg include patients on haemodialysis, immunosuppressed patients, drug addicts and male homosexuals. Proper perioperative management of potentially infective patients includes wearing of gloves by all those involved in caring for these patients, use of disposable equipment and clear labelling of blood specimens as possibly coming from patients with hepatitis (see also discussion of surgical precautions in AIDS patients above).

Non-A non-B hepatitis or hepatitis C

- The causative virus is similar to type B virus but this hepatitis may include several as yet undetected viruses.

- Route of transmission seems to be by inoculation, though oral-to-oral and perinatal transmission is possible. About 80–90% of hepatitis due to blood transfusion is felt to be due to this virus.
- Individuals at risk include i.v. drug misusers, haemophiliacs, haemodialysis patients, thalassaemiacs, hypogammaglobulinaemic patients, alcoholics, sexually promiscuous individuals, health care workers and transplant recipients of bone-marrow, kidney or liver.
- Incubation period is 2–20 weeks.
- Period of infectivity is unknown.
- It is not known if immunity develops to this type of hepatitis, but pooled gammaglobulins reduce the incidence of clinical disease. Good hygiene is imperative.
- Diagnosis is by exclusion, since serological markers are not available.
- Prognosis is similar to hepatitis B; chronic liver disease is not uncommon complication and chronic carriers are frequent. The mortality rate has not been well defined, but it may be similar to that of hepatitis B.

Other types of hepatitis

Hepatitis D

Hepatitis D is caused by defective virus or virusoid, hepatitis D RNA virus particle (36 nm encapsulated by coat protein, i.e. HBsAg). Transmission is by the parenteral route. Infection occurs mainly in i.v. misusers, haemophiliacs and institutionalised patients; areas of high incidence of infection are developing countries of the Amazon basin, Equatorial Africa, the Middle East, Asiatic areas of Russia and the Mediterranean basin.

Hepatitis E

Hepatitis E was first recongnised following epidemics of hepatitis in India; it is caused by RNA virus-like particles (27–34 nm long). Epidemics of hepatitis E have been observed in South-East and Central Asia, in Africa and in Mexico (developing countries). Spaoradic cases were observed in developed countries among migrant labourers and travellers.

OTHER VIRAL INFECTIONS

Ebola virus

Ebola virus is a great scientific enigma. It was first discovered in 1967 in a laboratory technician working on blood samples in Marburg (Germany). Zaire (Central Africa) has had two outbreaks: in 1976, 400 died and in 1995, 244 died. In 1989 an outbreak struck North Virginia (USA). When experimental monkeys in a laboratory began dying suddenly the infected monkeys were exterminated by military personnel, but the infection spread via the ventilation system of the building. In response, military personnel were finally authorised to kill all 400 monkeys at the laboratory to end the outbreak.

Human infection with Ebola virus is contracted from experimenting on monkeys or eating monkey brains (a delicacy in certain parts of Africa). The virus spreads via blood and attacks body organs such as the liver (resulting in severe coagulopathy), kidneys (renal shut-down) and brain (encephalopathy) in days, resulting in quick death in less than 10 days. Tears and blood act as vehicles for viral transmission. The patient initially develops fever, skin rash and looks helpless.

The most recent epidemic struck the town of Kikwit in Zaire, which had no sewage system, no news media and a lack of health education. Here illiterate people eat roasted monkey brains, rats, bats and insects (all creatures of the rain-forest suspected to be sources of Ebola virus). The infection is transmitted to attending relatives, nurses and doctors and lingers on after death; it can still be transmitted to people attending funeral and physically touching the corpse prior to burial, which is a part of African ritual. This is the so-called 'chain of death', when the patient dies followed by their children and then the carer, all one after another.

Prevention includes cleanliness, fostering health habits and education to change eating habits, non-touching of dead bodies and deep burial. Individuals must be warned to change their behaviour or risk death.

Initially, there were 9 deaths among every 10 infected patients. Those who survive Ebola virus infection in Africa because of their good immune system develop anti-viral antibodies in their blood; their blood can be used for transfusing infected patients, with a successful result. Out of 316 infected patients in the Kikwit outbreak, 244 died; those who survived were the source of biological immunisation for treating other infected patients. Out of every 8 transfused patients, 7 survived the infection, resulting in the end of the outbreak.

1.14 Minimal Access Therapy (MAT)

The introduction of laparoscopic cholecystectomy has been a major breakthrough in endoscopic microsurgery, and an important milestone in the history of surgery; it has rekindled the interest in laparoscopy, marking the beginning of a new era of minimally invasive surgery (MIS). MIS implies a reduction of (invasive) trauma inflicted by surgery, but without compromise of the exposure of the operating field, which is indeed magnified. MIS carries the connotation of increased safety which is incorrect, becuase there is no correlation between invasiveness and risk, and hence it may be better called minimal access surgery (MAS) or therapy (MAT).

The use of light in performing internal examination of the human body has been an investigation of great medical antiquity. The Arabian surgeon Albucasis or Abulkasim Al-Zahrawi of Andalusia (936–1013) is credited with being the first surgeon to use reflected light to inspect an internal organ, the cervix. In 1901, Kelling (Germany) inserted a cystoscope into the peritoneal cavity of a dog after air insufflation; he called the procedure 'coelioscopy'. The first procedure in man, however, was reported in 1910 by Jacobaeus (Sweden). Circa 1940, Goetz (Germany) and then Veress (France) developed the insufflation needle for safe gas introduction into the abdomen. These early procedures were entirely diagnostic in nature. The first laparoscopic appendicectomy, however, was performed in 1982 by Kurt Semm, a gynaecologist from Kiel (Germany). Ironically, the appendix was not inflamed, and Semm did not recommend the procedure in acute appendicitis; though it was introduced in France in 1983 by P. Mouret (whose name is also coined with the first laparoscopic cholecystectomy). However, laparoscopic surgery has gained momentum from the first laparoscopic appendicectomy for acute appendicitis (Schrieber, Germany, 1987), to the first laparoscopic cholecystectomy for diseased gallbladder (Eric Muhe, Germany, 1986, and Phillipe Mouret *et al.*, Lyons, France, 1987 – both based on verbal reporting), and with the first reported case in the English literature from François Dubois *et al.* (France, 1989), a new era of of minimal invasive surgery has started. Indeed, the progress has been so explosive, and the introduction of new procedures has profoundly influenced surgical training and work schedules, particularly the operating times and the length of hospital stay.

When ERCP and endoscopic sphincterotomy (papillotomy) were initially introduced, they were taken over by gastroenterologists mainly because of the lack of interest for the new technology among surgeons. Regrettably, the mistake was repeated with the introduction of interventional radiology, when many vascular surgeons and urologists were indifferent to new techniques of percutaneous balloon angioplasty and percutaneous nephroscopic stone retrieval, respectively; they were taken over by radiologists. Laparoscopy was initially practised by gynaecologists, and when it was extended to laparoscopic cholecystectomy, surgeons were again inflexible before they had even explored it to discover its merits. They took it over reluctantly, only because of the medicolegal consequences incurred by surgically untrained, though very interested, physicians, radiologists and gynaecologists. Then and only then did they come to appreciate its merits and embrace it fully.

There is a lesson here to be learned by surgeons, who must ensure that the future advances in endoscopic surgery and minimally invasive surgery are taken up by surgeons, and not left to those who are surgically untrained. MAS is the surgery of the future; it is here to stay.

MAS has now probably reached a plateau and the feasibility of an operation being done laparaoscopically does not always justify that that operation must be done routinely that way; operative time and other factors must be considered. MAS by no means supplants open surgery, but will become an essential part of our practice and one which patients will expect and perhaps demand. In fact, the future for laparoscopic surgery is as bright as the light source we rely on to visualise the field, and the only limiting factor is the imagination of surgeons! No matter what resistance and dislike some surgeons may display, the new generation of surgeons as well as older senior surgeons must learn it; the old dogs must learn new tricks.

Laparoscopic surgery became possible with the development of optics, particularly the Hopkins' rod-lens system and the introduction of the microchip endotelevision camera. The currently two-dimensional television image requires hand–eye coordination and depth perception. The surgery is performed from a distance using purpose-designed long fine (micro) instruments introduced into the peritoneal cavity through 5–12 mm cannulae after creation of a pneumoperitoneum using an electronic high flow insufflator (allowing preselection of intra-abdominal pressure at 12–15 mmHg) under the visual control of a television monitor with no compromise of the operating field, which is indeed magnified. In a study, over 95% of patients with symptomatic gallstones underwent laparoscopic cholecystectomy with no mortality and morbidity of 1.5%; conversion rate to open surgery is about 1.5% (around 1–2%). (In many large series, conversion rate is found to range between 15% and 30%.) Patients spent a mean hospital stay of 3 days, and returned to work or full activity within 11 days of discharge. Laparoscopic cholecystectomy does, however, take longer to conduct, but there is no correlation between the duration of laparoscopic surgery and postoperative course and recovery rate.

Advantages of MAT

The trauma of open surgery is multifactorial; the wound, the exposure of contents, cooling, drying and handling of viscera (ileus), tissue damage caused by prolonged metallic retraction, handling and direct trauma by instruments aggravate postoperative catabolic response resulting in more postoperative pain, postoperative complications (lung atelectasis and deep venous thrombosis). The psychological trauma is less after abdominal surgery without large painful wounds, and thus the patient may fare better in terms of metabolic response to surgical trauma inflicted laparoscopically than in response to open surgery.

Minimally invasive surgery minimises the trauma of access not only by virtual abolition of the wound, but also by permitting execution of complex operative procedures within a closed physiological environment with a magnified operative field, in a delicate fashion with the use of microinstruments and abolition of large retractors to achieve exposure.

Clinically, the accelerated recovery and rapid convalesence have substantial cost savings to the health service (less hospital stay with less nursing) and to the patient's employer by allowing the patient an early return to full activity or work. There is virtual abolition of wound infections; early ambulation is expected to be accompanied by less incidence of common postoperative complications, such as atelectasis and deep vein thrombosis, and perhaps less adhesion formation too. Furthermore, obese patients can benefit from MIS better than surgery, since deep fatty abdominal wall is simply 'left behind' after introduction of optics. The drastically reduced contact with patient's blood can result in a reduced risk of transmission of viral disease, particularly in AIDS patients. (MAT offers the necessary precautions and should represent a mainstay of surgical treatment in patients with AIDS.)

Disadvantages of MAT

Disadvantages include the following:
- There is a lack of direct handling of tissues with loss of tactile feedback, which is so important for evaluation of local pathology and orientation.
- MIS requires more technical expertise and is slower to perform, especially when one takes into consideration the setting-up time. The longer operative time relates to the execution of difficult cases (cholecystectomy for difficult

gallbladder takes twice as long to complete laparoscopically when compared to the standard open operation). This time-consuming exercise has an important impact on routine operative lists. Within the UK National Health Service performing less cases clashes with NHS drive for effective management of operative time (generating money and fulfilling the agreed number of contracted FCEs or Finished Consultant Episodes within the notional half-day operative session).

- Intra-arterial bleeding is a disadvantage, as haemostasis is difficult to achieve endoscopically because the bleeding point often retracts and bleeding obscures the visual field (due to light absorption by the extravasated blood). In an audit, bleeding was found to be the most common cause for elective conversion to open procedure during laparoscopic cholecystectomy. Other causes for conversion include extensive local inflammation (making recognition of vascular and biliary components difficult), uncertainty regarding the exact anatomy of biliary components, devices failure, such as poor-quality imaging, and unstable pneumoperitoneum should lead the surgeon, without losing face, to convert to traditional open surgery (the surgeon relies heavily on the equipment).

- With difficult laparoscopic operations, the incidence of bile duct damage has risen to four to six-fold higher than that following open cholecystectomy. This is due to lack of training, poor clinical judgement and the use of inappropriate technology, such as the laser to cut cystic duct and to dissect gallbladder. Conversion must not be regarded as 'failure', but as an indication that open surgery is the appropriate safe treatment in that particular patient. The stout refusal to compromise surgical principles, even at the expense of ego erosion, is fundamental to safe laparoscopic surgery. Medicolegally, the surgeon is protected if he or she converts in difficult cases; persistence to do such difficult cases laparoscopically may result in structural damage that is indefensible medicolegally.

- Organ extraction may demand 'morcellation, mincing, or liquidisation' of the organ to enable removal; this will interfere with histological examination, grading and staging assessment. However, occasionally the organ is extracted via natural pathways such as mediastinum for the oesophagus and rectum for the colon.

- Capnoperitoneum (pneumoperitoneum) causes perturbation of cardiac and respiratory function (see Gasless laparoscopy).

- Port site recurrence following laparoscopic surgery for malignancy, particularly colonic tumours, has been considerable, at least 11 trocar site recurrences were reported in laparoscopic surgery for colorectal cancer. Other cancers include: cholangiocarcinoma, ovarian malignancy, gastric and pancreatic cancer. The exact cause of this bizarre phenomenon is still obscure, but must be related to laparoscopic technique since incisional recurrence after curative abdominal cancer excision is virtually unpublished (wound recurrence accounts for 1% of cases in open colorectal surgery). A proposed mechanism for port site recurrence is the direct handling of the tumour surface causing exposure of cancer cells to pneumoperitoneum. Shedding of single cells or clumps of cells could also account for deposits found on sites of surgical trauma within the abdomen, and with the outward flow of gas and fluid via the ports, the sites of puncture could easily become points of implantation. The high level of carbon dioxide throughout the operation might favour the survival of clumps of tumour cells with predominantly anaerobic respiration. There is evidence that tumour cells are more proliferative in healing tissues such as wounds and anastomoses. A prudent surgeon will ensure that extraction is easy and will avoid the use of any force; for a readily palpable tumour, an incision of at least 5 cm in length would usually be required. There is clearly a need for a secure retrieval system in colorectal surgery.

This unexpected alarming complication of laparoscopic surgery in malignant disease is particularly concerning because, first, not all the recurrences were noted in the ports through which the specimen was removed and therefore may not be related to malignant cell contamination and thus cannot be prevented by using specimen retrieval bags. Secondly, the phenomenon is not limited to advanced lesions, as localised curable lesions have also implanted tumour cells at port sites. Laparoscopic colorectal surgery is feasible but not justified routinely in malignant disease, but rather in the management of benign colorectal disorders and *palliative* resection for cancer.

The expanding field of MIS

MIS encompasses many endoscopic procedures and minimal or no-scar surgery and spans a wide spectrum of many existing surgical specialties, namely general surgery, vascular surgery, urology, interventional radiology and orthopaedics. Endoscopic surgery involves several approaches:

1. Laparoscopic.
2. Thoracoscopic.
3. Endoluminal, e.g. flexible and rigid GIT telescopy and transanal endoscopic microsurgery (TEM).
4. Perivisceral endoscopic, e.g. retroperitoneal surgery (lumbar sympathectomy and nephrectomy) and dissection of oesophagus.
5. Intra-articular joint surgery.
6. Combined approaches, e.g. laparoscopically assisted colonic resection and thoracoscopically assisted oesophagectomy with open abdominal mobilisation and cervical anastomosis.

The MAT (or MAS or MIS) spectrum of procedures includes:

- All upper GIT endoscopic therapeutic procedures, including laser internal applications, e.g. photocoagulation of bleeding ulcer.
- Laparoscopic surgery whether diagnostic, semi-therapeutic or therapeutic (see below).
- Non-surgical treatment of gallstones, including extracorporeal shock wave lithotripsy.
- ERCP and endoscopic papillotomy with all related procedures of nasobiliary drainage, stenting and Dormia basket stone retrieval as well as interventional radiology for retrieval of residual biliary stone after surgery and insertion of endoprostheses and stents for obstructive jaundice.
- Percutaneous transhepatic dilatation, drainage and insertion of endoprosthesis in obstructive jaundice.

- All lower GIT endoscopic therapeutic procedures (therapeutic colonoscopy). Colonoscopy can be used with laparoscopy in limited colonic resection/anastomosis for malignant polyp or early carcinoma which can be marked preoperatively by colonoscopic injection by methylene blue dye.
- Transanal endoscopic microsurgery for resection of rectal adenomas and small rectal carcinomas.
- Percutaneous nephroscopy, drainage and renal stone removal.
- Extracorporeal shock wave lithotripsy of renal stones.
- Transuretheral resection of prostate – TUR (P) – and bladder tumour – TUR (BT).
- Percutaneous closed biopsies from lung lesions, liver, abdominal and retroperitoneal masses, and pelvic viscera under X-ray control.
- All interventional radiological procedures (see section 1.20 Medical imaging and interventional radiology), like drainage of intraperitoneal abscesses, chemical lumbar sympathectomy and removal of foreign bodies as well as many other procedures carried out by interventional radiologists under image intensifier.
- Non-surgical treatment of skin cancers (cryosurgery or radiotherapy) and haemorrhoids (cryosurgery). Also all laser external applications in surgery, e.g. for congenital naevi.
- Arthroscopic procedures for diagnosis and treatment, such as removal of torn meniscus (meniscectomy), removal of loose and foreign bodies, debridement of chondral flaps, drilling and abrasion of chondral lesions, patellar shaving, lateral release of the extensor mechanism, synovial biobsy, synovectomy, excision of osteophytes, excision of ganglia, screwing osteochondritis dissecans fragments, release of adhesions and arthrolysis, and removal of tumours. Arthroscopy is performed under general anaesthesia with tourniquet (should not be applied in local anaesthesia), and distension of the joint with saline or CO_2 to facilitate the use of the arthroscope, modified cystoscope (30° fore-oblique usually but 70° is useful for examining posterior compartments). The arthroscope is introduced commonly via an anterolateral approach, but lateral suprapatellar and anteromedial approaches may also be used, assisted by intra-articular probing and joint manipulation (applying valgus or varus stresses), and video-TV monitoring.
- Percutaneous vascular access procedures, whether diagnostic or therapeutic, and whether used via the venous, arterial, or rarely lymphatic vessels. The venous route can be utilised in venous sampling for assessment of blood picture and electrolyte concentrations; i.v. drip for fluid replacement, drug administration and blood transfusion; central vein catheterisation for central venous pressure (CVP) monitoring; ascending venography in deep venous thrombosis; parenteral nutrition; administration of anti-cancer chemotherapy drugs (Hickman's line); Swan–Ganz pulmonary artery floatation catheterisation (passing through the right atrium, right ventricle and pulmonary artery) to obtain a blood sample and to measure the pulmonary capillary wedge pressure (a reflection of left atrial pressure); transvenous insertion of pace-makers in heart block; ventriculo-atrial neurological shunts, e.g. Pudenz–Heyer and Hirtz–Holter valves in hydrocephalus (one end in the cerebral ventricle and the other through internal jugular vein into the right atrium); peritoneovenous shunts in ascites; as well as introduction of venous filters in ascending high deep venous (femoropopliteal segment) thrombosis, e.g. Mobin–Uddin umbrella in a capsule introduced via the internal jugular vein under X-ray control. Moreover, arteriovenous fistula is used for haemodialysis in renal failure; haemoperfusion and electrophoresis are used to rid the body of toxins; and exchange transfusion is used in haemolytic disease of (jaundiced) newborn babies.

The arterial route can be used for percutaneous translumbar aortography; arterial line for continuous blood pressure monitoring; for blood gases analysis; percutaneous transfemoral angiography; arterial embolisation; transluminal balloon angioplasty; and laser angioplasty (see S. 1.20 Medical imaging and interventional radiology). Cytotoxic chemotherapy can also be administered intra-arterially or regionally to the organ with cancer via its arterial blood supply.

The lymphatic vessels are used for diagnostic lymphangiography, and rarely for therapeutic endolymphatic injection of cytotoxic drug in malignant melanoma.

LAPAROSCOPY PROCEDURES

Laparoscopy can either be diagnostic, semi-therapeutic (laparoscopically aided operations), or totally therapeutic.

Diagnostic laparoscopy may be used in elective surgical conditions, such as needle biopsy in intraabdominal metastases (to assess staging and operability in oncology), liver biopsy, in ascites (preferably not in portal hypertension due to bleeding risk), abdominal masses, and pyrexia of unknown origin. In acute abdominal emergencies, such as stab wound, blunt abdominal trauma, diagnostic dilemma and ischaemic bowel, laparoscopy can avoid unnecessary abdominal exploration, particularly in the elderly high-risk patient with poor history and minimal physical signs; it can properly diagnose the condition whether due to acute appendicitis, perforated viscus, or haemoperitoneum due to injury.

In the past, it was erroneously thought that in generalised peritonitis (with intra-abdominal pus, increased peritoneal vascularity and fibrinous adhesions), emergency laparoscopy (whether diagnostic or therapeutic) may spread infection, cause bleeding and was likely to injure abdomen due to adhesions, respectively. In a study, emergency laparoscopy was found to be a safe and quick diagnostic procedure (lasts less than 10 minutes); it confirmed provisional clinical diagnosis of acute abdomen in 70% of cases (clinical accuracy of 70%), obviating the need for unnecessary laparotomy in 30%. Emergency laparoscopy therefore was recommended in surgical abdominal emergencies, particularly in acute abdominal pain of equivocal aetiology, lower abdominal pain in females, unsettled non-specific abdominal pain and in abdominal trauma with haemodynamic stability (instability usually requires laparotomy).

Laparoscopic evaluation of infected pancreatic necrosis has been performed via an open operation through gastrocolic omentum, following preoperative confirmation of pancreatic necrosis with CT-guided needle aspiration of the pancreas.

Laparoscopically aided operations, such as laparoscopically aided colectomy, start by making holes for initial laparoscopic mobilisation of the colon followed by a 10 cm transverse abdominal incision to deliver mobilised colon for extracorporeal resection/end-to-end anastomosis (using a stapler usually) on the skin which is then pushed inside, and followed by abdominal closure (see below).

A range of **therapeutic procedures** may be performed.

● *Laparoscopic surgical procedures* performed in man include:
  – Adhesiolysis using hook coagulation, scissors and blunt dissection.
  – Appendicectomy.
  – Cholecystectomy.
  – Complete truncal vagotomy.
  – Highly selective vagotomy.
  – Posterior truncal vagotomy and anterior seromyotomy.
  – Cardiomyotomy for achalasia of cardia.
  – Nissen fundoplication.
  – Ligamentum teres cardiopexy.
  – Stamm gastrostomy with gastropexy.
  – Suture closure/toilet of perforated peptic ulcer.
  – Closure of ulcer perforation with glue/balloon.
  – Nephrectomy (after delivering the kidney into a siliconised bag followed by morsellation to cut it into small pieces to assist bag removal via the port site).
  – Splenectomy (after delivering the spleen into a siliconised bag followed by morsellation to cut it into small pieces to assist bag removal via the port site).
  – Right hemicolectomy (laparoscopically assisted).
  – Left hemicolectomy (laparoscopically assisted sigmoid resection).
  – Laparoscopic colectomy.
  – Anterior restorative resection of recto-sigmoid carcinoma.
  – APE of rectum (laparoscopic colostomy with a perineal surgeon).
  – Laparoscopic fixation of sigmoid volvulus.
  – Reversal of Hartmann's operation.
  – Rectopexy.

  – Hernia repair (usually inguinal mesh implantation hernioplasty).
  – Varicocele.
  – Aspiration/deroofing of hepatic cysts.
  – Laparoscopic management of bile peritonitis after liver biopsy.
  – Repositioning of malfunctioning peritoneal dialysis catheters.
  – Biliary-enteric and entero-enteric anastomoses – possible with advances in suturing techniques and surgical stapling.
  – Gynaecological operations via pelviscopy allowing application of tubal rings, coagulation of endometriosis,

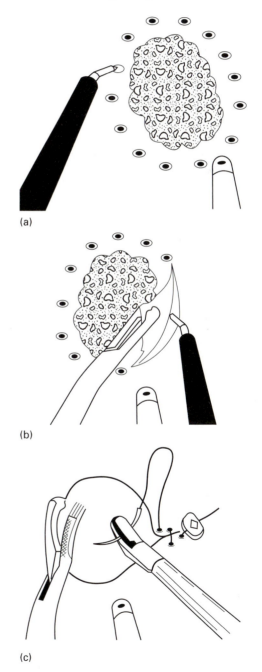

(a)

(b)

(c)

Fig. 1.14.2 Excision of rectal adenoma by TEM

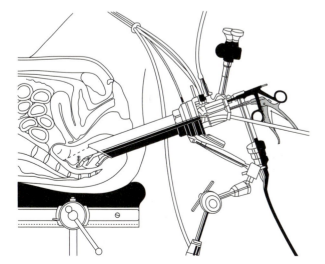

Fig. 1.14.1 Transanal endoscopic microsurgery (TEM)

salpingostomy, uterus fixation, salpingoopherectomy and occasionally myomectomy.

- *Thoracic operations* (using laparoscopic equipment) performed in the human include:
  - Cervical sympathectomy.
  - Parasympathetic denervation of the bronchial tree.
  - Truncal vagotomy.
  - Ligature of bullae/pleurodesis (pleurectomy for recurrent pneumothorax).
  - Oesophagectomy (laparoscopically-assisted or -aided operation).
- *Endoluminal surgical procedures* include:
  - Endoscopic sphincterotomy and related procedures (see S. 1.56 Non-Surgical Treatment of gallstones).
  - Endoluminal transanal endoscopic microsurgery (TEM) pioneered by Buess *et al.* has allowed excision of broad-based (sessile) large rectal adenomas and early small rectal carcinomas (pT1 and pT2) with minimum morbidity and inconvenience to the patient.
  - Endoscopic mucosectomy for early gastric cancer in Japan.

DIAGNOSTIC LAPAROSCOPY

(Contraindications are discussed in patient selection in laparoscopic cholecystectomy see p. 108.)

Under general anaesthesia, the patient is laid supine. In therapeutic laparoscopy, a lithotomy position is preferable to accommodate the second assistant between the patient's legs (see below). A nasogastric tube and urinary catheter are inserted to decompress the peritoneal cavity. The abdomen is shaved, prepared with sterilisation solution, and the operative field is delineated by drapes and secured by sutures.

The infra-umbilical skin fold is grasped with two towel clips, and incised with a size 11 blade, through which incision a Veress needle is inserted intraperitoneally. The incision must be small, because gas will be lost via a large incision while inducing pneumoperitoneum. The Veress is grasped between the finger and thumb of the right hand and is passed swiftly through the abdominal wall. This can be followed by insufflation of 3–4 litres of carbon dioxide at a preset pressure of 13–15 mmHg prior to introduction of the laparoscope. Once the preset pressure is reached, sufflation can be turned off to an automatic maintenence pressure of 10–12 mmHg; the incision of the infraumbilical fold can be increased, the Veress needle is withdrawn and the most important step in the procedure may start, namely the insertion of a 10 mm trocar held with the left hand and its top in the fist of the right hand, keeping the stylet within the trocar (two-hand procedure to control entry inside the abdomen).

After penetrating abdominal wall, a hissing sound of escaping gas is heard indicating that the trocar tip is within the peritoneal cavity. The left hand should be used as a brake to prevent the trocar accidentally being introduced too far, as this may injure major vessels resulting in the patient's exsanguination. It is wise to aim the trocar to one side rather than aiming it directly backwards at the aorta.

Once the trocar is in position, the stylet is removed and the insufflation tube is connected to the stopcock of the trocar.

When the preset pressure is reached again, insufflation flow rate may be turned up to maximum (8–10 l/min) when using multiple trocars.

During this time, the laparoscope (0 or 30° inclination) should have been prepared in hot water prior to introduction. If a 30° telescope is used, it is important to keep the orientation correct, i.e. light cable at the top and camera cable at the bottom, so that moving the telescope to the left will view the left side of abdomen, and moving it up to the right will view the anterior abdominal wall.

Occasionally, small vertical infraumbilical open laparoscopy may be used in difficult cases, particularly in obesity or abdomens with scars and adhesion, using the **Hasson** technique (described in 1974) of inserting a conical metallic rod followed by a sliding 10 mm trocar sheath mounted on the rod. An additional 5 mm right iliac fossa trocar (to introduce a manipulator) is inserted under scope direct vision, as seen on the video screen, after indenting the abdominal wall for site selection. In therapeutic laparoscopy an additional 10 mm subxiphoid (epigastric) site is usually used for dissection by the operating surgeon, with another 5 mm right hypochondrial trocar for introduction of various instruments (usually graspers).

The gas tube is better transferred from the telescope port to any other ports to prevent a foggy telescope. All trocars and instruments, therefore, must be passed under direct vision, not only to prevent visceral damage, but also to prevent the introduced instrument from fighting with the telescope ('fighting swords') by keeping an appropriate distance from the organ under consideration.

The patient's position can be manoeuvred to give better vision of the viscus under examination; reverse Trendelenburg position with rotation to the left is recommended in gallbladder visualisation by allowing the colon and stomach to fall away, while in appendicitis the head can be tilted down (Trendelenburg position) and the right side rotated upwards to the left in order to free and see the caecum better.

At the end of the procedure the pneumoperitoneum should be released through the trocar. To leave gas within the peritoneal cavity will cause the patient postoperative discomfort (particularly shoulder pain). Intraperitoneal or wound infiltration of bupivacaine is recommended so that the patient wakes up free of pain. Laparoscopy also results in postoperative nausea, and an anti-emetic injection before waking the patient is useful.

Important points in the technique

1. Site of election for insertion of Veress needle depends on whether the patient was operated previously or not. The inverted Y of the abdomen is the most dangerous area for Veress needle insertion for fear of vascular injury (indefensible medicolegally), since it overlies the aorta/inferior vena cava and bifurcation. (Each patient in laparoscopy must be assumed to have an abdominal aortic aneurysm.)

In a virgin abdomen the infraumbilical fold is the recommended site (with the needle directed towards the pelvis). If the patient has had pelvic surgery through a Pfannenstiel or lower midline incision, one can still use the infraumbilical fold because there are rarely adhesions this high. However, if the patient has had an upper midline incision, one can still go through the infraumbilical fold, though either of the hypochondrial sites may be preferred (the liver and spleen are under the ribs so there is no chance of puncturing them). For a left subcostal incision, the right iliac fossa is chosen and vice versa. The bowel puncture is defensible medicolegally, provided you recognise it and do something about it, i.e. suturing it laparoscopically or converting to open surgery to suture it.

Ports should not be too close (or worse still parallel) to each other. The instruments should not be too near the optic, and not too close to the operating field.

2. Tests confirming the intraperitoneal insertion of Veress needle are:
– When the needle passes through the abdominal wall one sees, feels and hears the click (needle passes through three areas of resistance: sheath, muscle and peritoneum).
– intra-abdominal pressure remaining 0 or low despite continuous flow of gas indicates free intraperitoneal location of the needle (any high pressure indicates Veress needle obstructed by tissues). 'A Good Flow while Pressure is Low' indicates a safe intraperitoneal insufflation.
– 'Hanging drop' is another technique to ensure that the needle is within the peritoneal cavity; a drop of saline is placed into the lumen of the needle and the tap is opened. The negative pressure inside the peritoneal cavity will draw fluid in when the patient breathes.
– A 10 ml syringe containing 5 ml of sterile saline can be attached. This is aspirated and injected twice; if there is no returned fluid and no resistance to injection, intraperitoneal location is confirmed.
– Alternatively, one may simply withdraw the plunger from the syringe while still attached to the Veress needle, and the fluid will flow into the abdominal cavity and should disappear.

3. If one retrieves blood (during aspiration), the needle should be withdrawn and reinserted because to insufflate gas into a major blood vessel (aorta, inferior vena cava, or common iliac vessels) can lead to serious complications or even a fatal outcome. Should intestinal content be retrieved, one should reposition the needle, continue with laparoscopy and assess the injury. If the injury is minor, the patient may well be treated with antibiotics and i.v. fluids, kept nil by mouth, preferably with nasogastric suction, and observed in hospital. However, if the injury is major, or involves the colon, the surgeon may explore and repair the damage. Catheterised urinary bladder is unlikely to be injured unless the patient has had cystosuspension or pelvic surgery. However, one should always check to ensure that Foley's catheter is draining prior to starting the laparoscopy.

4. When the insufflation tube is connected to the Veress needle, one can set the flow rate at 1.5 l/min and preset the abdominal pressure at 15 mmHg (above which insufflation will be automatically cut off). Insufflation at a rate higher than 1.5 l/min is to be decried as it runs the risk of rapidly stretching the diaphragm or inducing cardiac arrhythmias.

5. Normally, when an insufflation tube is connected to the Veress needle the pressure initially reads 4 mmHg, which represents the resistance of the line and needle at the preset flow rate (1.3 or 1.4 l/min), indicating no impedance to flow from contact with intraabdominal organs. If saline instillation techniques have indicated the needle is in the cavity but the

pressure is high and flow rate is low, then one should do following manoeuvres:
– One may twist the needle circumferentially in order for any omentum adherent to the needle to fall away.
– If this does not work, one may try changing the position of the needle without altering its depth (otherwise one may injure major blood vessels with dire consequences).
– Should all of these manoeuvres fail, the needle must be withdrawn and reintroduced and all of the above confirmatory tests must be performed again.

6. During insufflation to induce pneumoperitoneum, the surgeon must confirm that abdominal distension is uniform, and without subcutaneous emphysema. The anaesthetist must verify the stable clinical condition of the patient, checking blood pressure, pulse, ventilatory pressure and oxygen saturation. If any of these is abnormal or a cause for concern, the pneumoperitoneum should be released so that the anaesthetist can stabilise the patient. Carbon dioxide pneumoperitoneum may cause hypercapnia, and the anaesthetist may need to increase ventilatory rate.

7. The light cable must properly join the telescope, because a faulty connection may lead to massive light loss, interfering with image perception. The TV camera is attached to the telescope and the zoom lens should be set to minimal focal length, and 'white balanced' (set to see white swab).

The professional tricks used to solve telescope fogging include:
– The gas tube is better transferred from the telescopic sheath to any other port (preferably 10 mm port rather than 5 mm port to provide a smooth and quick insufflation) to prevent a direct fogging of the telescope.
– The light should be turned down and the telescope warmed in hot water to prevent fogging of optics when it is introduced into the peritoneal cavity because of the temperature difference between the warm peritoneal cavity (37°C) and the cold CO_2, laparoscope and camera unit set at room temperature of 19°C. However, the fog inside the peritoneal cavity is not only due to temperature difference; it is also due to the use of diathermy (smoke is less with laser).
– Wipe the blood from the inside of the trocar sheath by a swab.
– Alternatively, antifogging (demist) agent based on isopropyl alcohol may be used, e.g. Fred solution produced by R. Wolf.
– Saline injection via the port for clot removal.
– Occasionally, wiping the lens with betadine (povidone-iodine), which can serve as an antifogging demist solution.
– One can decrease fogging by opening the port valve (desufflation).
– The practice of wiping the telescope by touching intrabdominal organs (liver or bowel usually) inside the peritoneal cavity may be practised though is not to be recommended, because considerable heat is generated at the tip of the telescope which may result in burning of the organ (therefore the term of 'cold light source' of the telescope is a misnomer).
– It may sometimes be better to take the telescope out and clean it by immersion in hot water followed by wiping with a betadine swab. It is important when withdrawing the telescope from the abdomen *always* to turn the telescope

down, because this prevents blinding one's assistant with a bright scope light, rarely setting fire to the drapes and damaging the TV camera with light feedback.

8. Each patient undergoing laparoscopic surgery will have five lines (cables and tubes) – namely, insufflation gas tube, light cable (for light source), camera cable, suction tube and irrigation tube. The surgeon must, therefore, organise the layout in a standard way to have consistency in laparoscopic operations (light and camera cables in a drape fold on one side and other lines in a drape fold on the other side).

LAPAROSCOPIC SURGERY

Laparoscopic cholecystectomy (Fig. 1.14.3)

Patient selection is imperative. The procedure is indicated in chronic obstructive cholecystitis and acute acalculous cholecystitis, hereditary spherocytosis, poorly controlled diabetes, immunosuppressed patient and acute non-perforated cholecystitis in the elderly or those with cardiorespiratory disease where open surgery is better avoided.

General contraindications include asymptomatic gallstones, patients unfit for general anaesthesia for any reason, such as increased cardiac risk and respiratory insufficiency; they are better not subjected to laparoscopic cholecystectomy.

Local contraindications can be *absolute*, such as:
- Perforated cholecystitis with local or generalised peritonitis.
- Emphysematous cholecystitis (lethal anaerobic gas-forming mixed infection encountered in elderly diabetics and associated with cystic artery thrombosis).
- Jaundice (for the fear of underlying malignancy).
- Cholecystoenteric fistula.
- Any doubt of gallbladder malignancy.
- Intestinal obstruction with distended abdomen (distended bowel can easily be injured during laparoscopy resulting in faecal peritonitis). Also frozen abdomen due to dense adhesions.
- Current pregnancy.

- Mirizzi syndrome (rare obstruction of common hepatic duct from gallstone impaction in cystic duct or gallbladder neck with bilio-biliary fistula formation).

Relative contraindications include: gallstone pancreatitis, gallbladder empyema, gangrenous acute obstructive cholecystitis (without localised perforation), acute-on-chronic cholecystitis with walls greater than 4 mm thick on preoperative ultrasound (grossly thickened leathery walls making it impossible to grasp the fundus even after attempted decompression), asymptomatic common bile duct (CBD) stone, previous abdominal surgery, sepsis and portal hypertension (with cirrhosis resulting in bleeding disorder). Many surgeons now gain enough confidence to tackle most of the above conditions laparoscopically. ERCP can be performed preoperatively in CBD stone; ERCP can be also be done in residual stone following laparoscopic cholecystectomy.

Preoperative preparations are as in diagnostic laparoscopy, but with four surgiports or sites for trocars. Prophylactic cefuroxime 1 g and metronidazole 500 mg/100 ml are given i.v. 3 times daily, starting with premedication and continued for 48 hours.

Under general anaesthesia, the patient is laid supine in the lithotomy position (to accommodate the second assistant or the *cameraman* between the patient's legs); a nasogastric tube and urinary catheter are inserted to decompress the peritoneal cavity. The operative field is delineated by drapes and secured by sutures. The telescope is introduced via a subumbilical trocar (10 mm diameter), and dissection is performed via another 10 mm subxiphisternal (epigastric) trocar; the two lateral trocars (right iliac fossa and right hypochondrial) are used for grasping the gallbladder and Hartmann's pouch, positioning it on cephalic and caudal stretch, thereby displaying the anatomy of Calot's triangle (Fig. 1.14.4). McMahon's Endoflex retractor (manufactured by Stryker) can be introduced via the right iliac fossa 5 mm port to retract the liver; it can be fixed in place with a Martin arm to the side of the table (this step can obviate the need for a third assistant). Reverse Trendelenburg position with rotation to the left assists by allowing the colon and stomach to fall away.

Dissection may be performed by scissors, electrocautery or either contact laser (Nd: YAG) or free beam laser (KTP: YAG). Suction and irrigation may be delivered through an electrocautery hook device (Storz). A similar device with a spatula tip is useful for coagulation. In difficult cases, a sucker can be used for dissection. Always **hook, look and cook**. Using this method, the junction of the cystic duct and Hartmann's pouch is identified and a clip is placed on the cystic duct very close to the gallbladder. A small incision is made with microscissors into the duct and a cholangiogram is routinely performed through an Fr. 4 ureteric catheter using a special clamp (many surgeons now do laparoscopic cholecystectomy without performing intraoperative cholangiograms, others prefer doing selective intraoperative cholangiograms). Cholangiogram can detect unsuspected common duct stones in 5–9% of patients, and define the length of the cystic duct and the anatomy of the biliary tree, so that inadvertent iatrogenic injuries to the ductal system may be avoided. It is claimed that routine cholangiography can reduce 50% of postoperative ERCPs; also ductal injuries without cholangiography can be indefensible medicolegally (Fig. 1.14.5). After cholangiogram completion, the

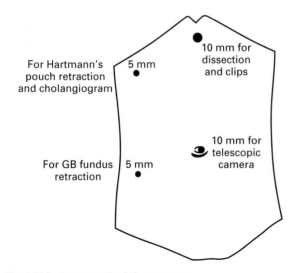

Fig. 1.14.3   Laparoscopic cholecystectomy

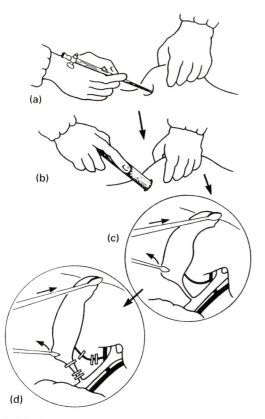

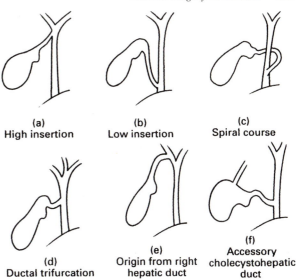

Fig. 1.14.5 Congenital varieties of cystic duct that may be encountered laparoscopically

Fig. 1.14.4 Laparoscopic cholecystectomy. Veress needle insertion followed by saline injection test (a) followed by trocar insertion with index finger (b); the gallbladder fundus is grasped and pushed cephalad while Hartmann's pouch is pushed caudally (c); the cystic duct and artery are clipped (twice proximally and once distally) and cut in-between using a micro-scissor (d) but the cut should never be made with a hook diathermy or diathermy scissor (see Section 4)

cystic duct is secured with either clips or preformed 'Endoloop' (Ethicon) applied after cystic duct transection.

The cystic artery is then identified as it enters the gallbladder and is similarly secured with clips and divided. Dissection of the cystic duct from front and behind, the so-called flag (drapeau) or flagging technique, is useful. The gallbladder is dissected free of the liver bed and withdrawn across the abdomen to the umbilical or right iliac port (if 10 mm trocar is inserted). The neck is grasped and withdrawn above the skin of the abdominal wall. Once the neck is outside it may be incised; bile is aspirated, it is irrigated and then aspirated again. Stones are removed or even crushed until the organ is small enough to pass through the abdominal incision. Finally, a 10 FG tube can be introduced via the right iliac fossa port for occasional intraperitoneal injection of 0.5% bupivacaine (Marcain) in a 10 ml ampoule; the tube then can be left in situ as a drain. The pneumoperitoneum must be completely deflated, trocars removed and puncture holes are closed (with McMahon's Endoclaw) and infiltrated with local anaesthetic.

Should **common duct stones** be found unexpectedly, the surgeon has the following options: either convert to open cholecystectomy and choledocholithotomy, which in patients under age of 60 has zero mortality (this is probably the safest approach); or, if the stones are small, the surgeon can choose to

do nothing and hope the stones will pass; however, there is a risk of complications ensuing. Another possibility is to refer the patient for postoperative endoscopic papillotomy/ERCP, but this may be anatomically impossible in a percentage of patients and has an attendant morbidity and mortality. However, if the cystic duct is dilated, the surgeon can pass a flexible ureteroscope or 3 mm choledochoscope laparoscopically into the common bile duct and retrieve the stone with a Dormia basket. Another approach is to pass a basket, Fogarty balloon catheter, angioplasty balloon catheter through the cystic duct under fluoroscopic control in an attempt to retrieve stones or try to flush them into the duodenum via a catheter. Choledochotomy may be done laparoscopically to pass a 5 mm choledochoscope to irrigate and flush ductal stones and to pass a Dormia basket to retrive ductal stones; intracorporeal suturing skills are necessary here to close the duct opening.

In **acute cholecystitis** with adhesions and inflammation it may be wise to resort to open emergency cholecystectomy. However, in extremely sick patients the surgeon may perform diagnostic laparoscopy to confirm the diagnosis of acute cholecystitis, empyema or mucocele, and pass a catheter into the gallbladder and secure it to the abdominal wall with some sutures (laparoscopic cholecystostomy). The procedure buys the surgeon time and saves the morbidity of a large abdominal incision.

Complications of laparoscopic cholecystectomy

1. General include veress needle and trocar injuries such as perforated bowel, major vascular injury, abdominal wall vessel injury (port bleeding), and urinary bladder injury. Instruments (including sucker) may result in diaphragm injury (and pneumothorax), liver or gastric injury, omental injury (usually minor) and duodenal injury (with late leak).

2. Anaesthesia-related complications include poor muscle relaxation (with narrow peritoneal cavity) predisposing to injuries, and aspiration.

3. Pneumoperitoneum-related complications include subcutaneous emphysema, pneumothorax (but related to diaphragm injury), decreased venous return (patient must have DVT prophylaxis and inflatable boots), and CO_2 embolism. Postoperative shoulder pain 24 h after surgery is due to diaphragmatic stretch and patient must be warned preoperatively; it usually settles within 2–3 days.

4. Diathermy complications include skin burn, bowel injury, direct coupling, pedicle burn, capacitative coupling, and faulty insulation (*see* Section 4).

5. Patient-specific complications are related to obesity (requires longer needles, trocars, and ports pushed cephalad, also poor vision due to hypertrophic omentum, large falciform ligament), elderly patient, organomegaly, abdominal hernias, diabetes, clotting disorders, cirrhosis and portal hypertension, abdominal scars and adhesions (keep needle away from scars, watch for asymmetrical abdominal expansion, open laparoscopy is preferred).

6. Operation specific complications include:
– Port hole bleeding (avoid vessels in anterior abdominal wall, inspect sites at the end of procedure, enlarge incision and control bleeding, through and through stitch, Foley's catheter ballon pressure for 24 h, or convert to to open).
– Intraoperative bleeding due to cystic artery or hepatic artery avulsion (Don't panic, Don't use blind clips or diathermy, apply pressure with an instrument, identify bleeding points and use bipolar diathermy or clip if vessel identified, or convert to open if bleeding is uncontrollable).
– Bleeding from gallbladder bed (adequate suction of blood and irrigation, apply pressure, and application of non-contact diathermy).
– Peritoneal contamination due to bile spillage (biloma) or stones spillage (use suction, spoons or bags and irrigate/suck until sucked fluid is clear, clear port hole of stones, attempt closure of gallbladder with endoloop and use endoscopic bag (or pouch) to remove lacerated gallbladder and/or spilled stones, enlarge port by incising over a fistula grooved director, and continue antibiotics therapeutically). Drain may be left behind to vent the remaining gas and fluid; if no drainage seen, drain can be removed within hours, however drainage dictates leaving drain tube for 24 h. Continued blood/bile loss from a drain is an indication for re-exploring the abdomen; if there is continued biliary leak, and ERCP may be indicated to check the continuity of bile duct.
– Bile duct injury due to thermal injury, clipped common bile duct, division of common bile duct (CBD), congenital anomalies, and avulsion of cystic duct–CBD junction, surgeon persistence to do laparoscopic surgery in unclear anatomy without conversion, leaked or spilled bile is a good conductor of electricity (it contains salts: bile salts). Always be careful in dissection of Calot triangle and avoid using diathermy, always identify gallbladder–cystic duct junction as a reference point in laparoscopic surgery (as opposed to cystic duct–CBD junction in open surgery), use superior and lateral traction, and adopt the six clips rule (three on cystic duct and three on cystic artery), do intraoperative cholangiogram, and if in doubt convert to open. **To err is human, but to try to prevent recurrence of error is science.** Ductal injuries may present early (0–2 days) or late (weeks to months); ultrasound and ERCP may give the answer. Patient requires a recon-

structive procedure depending on the type of injury. Classification for laparoscopic bile duct injury has been proposed by Dr L. W. Way and reported by Schol *et al.* (1994):

Class I   A minor defect resulting from an erroneous tangential incision
Class II   Clipping of the bile duct
Class IIIa   Complete transection of the bile duct without tissue loss
Class IIIb   Transection of the bile duct with tissue loss
Class IV   Injuries to the right or left hepatic duct

7. Port hole complications include:
– Port hole bleeding
– Hernias (close all ports of larger than 5 mm and avoid rapid desufflation with a loop of bowel out)
– Sinus formation
– Port hole metastases in gallbladder cancer (must convert to open if you know it is cancer on ultrasound evidence, and be away from tumour during dissection, and use bag for retrieval).

When to convert?

Conversion of laparoscopic into open cholecystectomy is not a sign of failure; we always do open surgery and safety of the patient comes first. Conversion should be contemplated earlier in the procedure. The rate of conversion varies with experience, it may be a part of learning curve, is less important than safety, can be less than 5% with safety, and should be discussed with patient prior to surgery as part of informed consent. Indications for conversion include:
– Unclear anatomy (inadequate access to Calot triangle, cystic duct cannot be identified with certainty, operative cholangiogram here is of limited value).
– No tissue planes (gallbladder mass, large stone in Hartmann's pouch, fibrosis of Calot triangle, or Mirizzi syndrome).
– Bleeding may look worse than it is with danger of obscuring anatomy (control with pressure with good suction irrigation).
– Dense adhesion may be easier than it looks (awkward angle requiring patience, instruments/laparoscope relocations, and may necessitate a conversion to mini-cholecystectomy)
– Accidental damage.
– Equipment failure.
– Lack of safe progress (length of operation, logistics of theatre time, predicting difficulty with consideration for safety are paramount). Conversion should be attempted after setting target time but without progress.

Laparoscopic appendicectomy (Figs. 1.14.6–1.14.7)

As an alternative method to open appendicectomy, endoscopic appendicectomy has gained popularity only recently with the advent of minimally invasive surgery in the past few years.

Following diagnostic laparoscopy, laparoscopic appendicectomy can be performed selectively in free anatomical appendices with mild or severe inflammation, but non-perforated appendicitis. It is ideal for chronic recurrent appendicitis.

Sub-serosal or high retrocaecal and perforated cases (peritonitis) may not be suitable for laparoscopic surgery (though practised by some surgeons). However, the release of adhesions

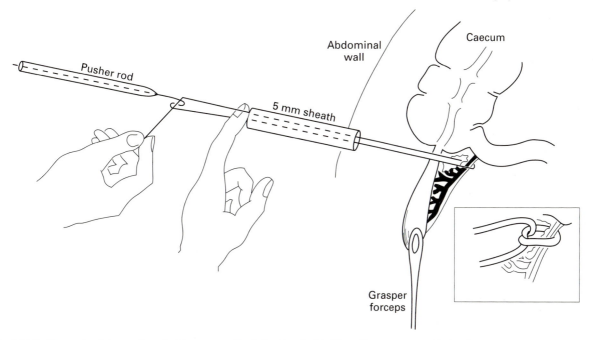

Fig. 1.14.6 Conventional throw of surgical knot, externally tied and pushed inside to ligate mesoappendix (see inset)

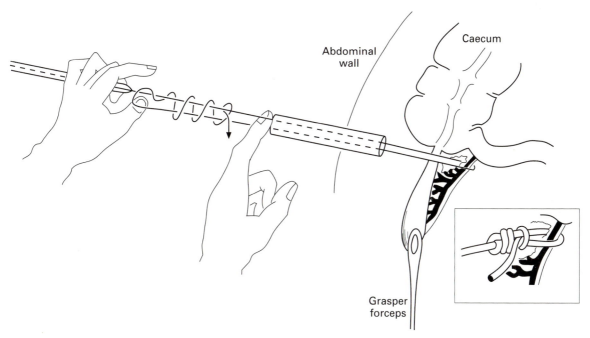

Fig. 1.14.7 Roeder slip knot, a modification of the fisherman's knot (see inset for knot details)

(adhesiolysis), parietal peritoneal mobilisation to free subserosal appendix and the suction of pus in perforated cases can technically aid open appendicectomy and shorten operation time (*laparoscopically-aided appendicectomy*).

Prophylactic cefuroxime 1 g and metronidazole 500 mg/ 100 ml are given i.v. 3 times daily, with premedication, and continued for 48 hours. Under general anaesthesia, the patient is laid supine in the lithotomy position (to accommodate the second assistant between the patient's legs); a nasogastric tube and urinary catheter are inserted to decompress the peritoneal cavity. The operative field is delineated by drapes and secured by sutures. The laparoscope is introduced through the umbilicus and a second 10 mm trocar is introduced through the right iliac fossa site under visual control. The patient's head can be tilted down and the right side tilted upwards to the left in order to free and see the caecum and the acutely inflamed appendix better.

The tip of the appendix is grasped with a forceps introduced via a suprapubic port; the mesoappendix is partly diathermised with diathermy forceps introduced via the epigastric surgiport. The mesoappendix can thus be skeletonised, and vessels are

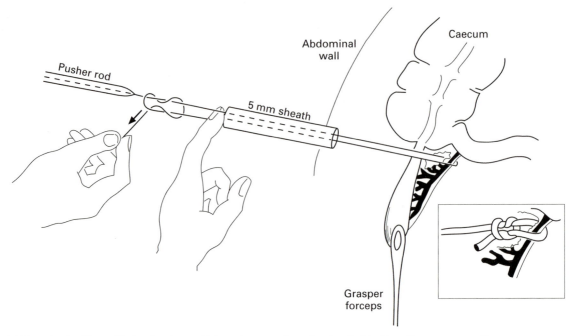

Fig. 1.14.8   Al-Fallouji's modified reef-on-loop, which can be externally tied and pushed inside to ligate mesoappendix

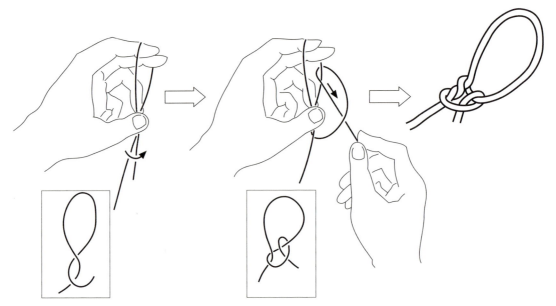

Fig. 1.14.9   Author's modification of ENT tonsillectomy knot into an endoloop

either dealt with using bipolar coagulation or the application of clips. Alternatively, the hole in the mesoappendix can be used to negotiate 00/chromic catgut or 0/silk thread introduced on a forceps via the right iliac fossa trocar through which both ends of the thread can be tied externally and pushed down with a pusher rod to ligate the mesoappendix. The thread is then cut off with a scissor introduced via the surgeon's epigastric port. This externally tied modified reef-on-loop (Fallouji's loop 1993) can be repeated and the mesoappendix is then divided in between (see below).

The base of the appendix is ligated with the pre-knotted ready-made Roeder loop (Endoloop, Ethicon) and the appendix is divided by coagulation. Alternatively, if the preformed knot is not available, an ENT loop (Fallouji's hand-made loop which is easy to make, equally effective, cheap and always available) can be made extracorporeally, held on a forceps, and introduced inside. It is then guided to loop around the crushed appendicular base, and tightened by pusher rod; the short arm of the knot can tightened by a grasper introduced via the epigastric port. The latter hand-made loop can be repeated thrice so that the appendicular base is divided between the proximal two and the distal loops. The excised appendix can be manoeuvred to be grasped by its base; it is then removed via the 10 mm right iliac fossa trocar. There is no need for the stump to be oversewn (may be difficult and time-consuming).

Finally, a 20 FG tube is introduced via the same port for sterile saline irrigation, followed by intraperitoneal injection of 0.5% bupivacaine (Marcain) in a 10 ml ampoule; the tube is then left in situ as a drain. The pneumoperitoneum must be completely deflated, trocars removed and puncture holes are closed and occasionally infiltrated with local anaesthetic.

Extracorporeal loop-making and knot-tying

The popularity of laparoscopic cholecystectomy and appendicectomy has led to the introduction of the pre-made endoloops as a corollary tool in surgical laparoscopy; Endoloop chromic gut ligature is a trade mark of Ethicon (1991), while Surgitie ligating loop is the Autosuture equivalent (1992). The technique commonly employed by the industry for making endoloops is derived from either the Hangman's knot or fisherman's knot tied outside and then pushed inside the abdomen by pusher rod (knot tightener). The Roeder slip knot recommended by Autosuture and Ethicon is basically a modification of the fisherman's knot.

Endoloops and Surgities used in laparoscopic surgery are not always available; hand-made knots or loops are equally effective, simpler, cheaper and readily available. Many surgeons prefer hand-made knots and loops to multi-fire, disposable clip appliers (such as autosuture Endoclip applier) and mechanical endostaplers (such as multifire Endo GIA 30), which require a 12 mm surgiport and also because of the high cost, unavailability and frequent technical failure. Furthermore, metallic clips can slip off large vessels, may cause accidental entrapment of adjacent structures, can distort any future CT scan and interfere with NMR. Some surgeons prefer many throws of a conventional reef knot fashioned externally, and then pushed and tightened inside the peritoneal cavity, one after another. Al Fallouji (1993) reviewed extracorporeal loop-making and the indications in laparoscopic surgery; he described 13 versions of hand-made loops and knots (many innovated by him) and recommended them as alternatives to the ready-made loops (Figs 1.14.6–1.14.9).

Laparoscopic inguinal hernia repair

Indicated in direct and small indirect inguinal hernias in non-obese patients for the beginners. Recurrent, obstructed, strangulated and large irreducible indirect inguinal hernias are better repaired by the open method (Lichtenstein tension-free mesh repair).

A pneumoperitoneum is induced and via an immediate supraumbilical incision a 10 mm port telescope is inserted; under direct vision two more 12 mm ports are created lateral to linea semilunaris at the level of umbilicus for introduction of an Endo Hernia Stapler (Autosuture) (only three ports are required for laparoscopic hernia repair). The surgeon stands on the left side of the patient when repairing the right inguinal hernia and vice versa.

The indirect inguinal hernia is located lateral to the lateral umbilical fold (raised by inferior epigastric vessels) and assisted by external digital pressure over internal ring. The hernial orifice appears larger than expected due to dilatation by pneumoperitoneum and laparoscopic magnification. Hernial contents, such as omentum, is reduced by traction or division; the surgeon uses the two lateral ports for grasping peritoneum over the hernia and uses a diathermy scissor for dissection to create a peritoneal pouch prior to mesh implantation. Then 10 × 15 cm polypropylene mesh is rolled up like a cigar and introduced into the pouch where it is spread and positioned extraperitoneally to cover the hernial defect adequately (better than 6 × 11 cm mesh which is not large enough to cover the defect and prevent recurrence). The mesh is then stapled with the Endo Hernia stapler on to pubic bone and to the inside of the anterior abdominal wall aided by the assistant's external hand pressure on the abdominal wall. The peritoneum is then drooped and overlapped edges are stapled to cover the mesh (TransAbdominal PrePeritoneal Stapled hernia or TAPPS).

About 10 staples on average are used. Care is taken not to damage the inferior epigastric vessels and spermatic cord (vas deferens); the latter moves longitudinally with assisstant's traction on the testicle.

Then gas is evacuated and instruments and trocars are removed (gas spreading through mesh pores into the hernia may make it bulge temporarily until absorption of gas is complete).

Laparoscopic surgery of duodenal peptic ulcers

Under general anaesthesia the patient is placed in the Trendelenburg position, laid supine in the lithotomy position (to allow the surgeon to operate comfortably between the patient's legs).

A nasogastric tube and urinary catheter are inserted to decompress the peritoneal cavity. A fibreoptic gastroscope is passed via the nasogastric tube (in difficulties, a paediatric endoscope is used), not only to distend the oesophagus, but to transilluminate and identify important anatomical landmarks, such as the gastro-oesophageal junction. The operative field is delineated by drapes and secured by sutures. Each assistant is stationed on one side of the patient. The forward-viewing laparoscope is introduced 5 cm above the umbilicus through a 10 mm trocar. Then, under direct vision, three trocars are inserted via 5 mm ports in the subxiphoid (epigastric), right hypochondrial and left hypochondrial (along mammary lines) sites. The fifth 10 mm trocar is introduced to the left of the laparoscope, through the left rectus muscle; this is the operating port through which hook coagulator, scissors, collagen applicator and haemostatic clip appliers are later introduced. A full survey of the hiatal region is performed by retracting the left lobe of the liver with a fan-like retractor or endoflex retractor. Then one can perform one of three procedures for treating duodenal peptic ulcer.

1. Complete truncal vagotomy (with balloon dilatation of pylorus)

The lesser sac is entered through an opening (in pars flaccida and pars nervosa), which allows the surgeon to dissect in cephalad fashion the lesser curvature to the hiatal region. The left gastric vein is encountered and divided between clips or sutures as necessary. Right crus of diaphragm is the landmark and has to be retracted to the left, while a coagulator/dissector hook is used to open the pre-oesophageal peritoneum to visualise the meso-oesophagus where the posterior vagus nerve can be found. The oesophaqus is retracted to the left with a probe, and the inferior margin of the hiatus is dissected with a hook probe to identify the nerve. Gentle traction is exerted on the nerve while it is dissected free from the surrounding tissues. The nerve is then transected between two surgical clips and a small fragment retrieved for histology (vagectomy).

Then the anterior vagus must be divided; it can be identified after incising the pre-oesophageal peritoneum with a hook-coagulator near the left crus of diaphragm. The anterior vagus can be divided between two clips. Vagotomy is complete once Grassi's criminal branch is identified and divided, as well as any other aberrant branches along the left oesophageal margin. The entire circumference of the oesophagus may be examined by retracting it to the left, then to the right.

To prevent postoperative pyloric contraction, a 16 mm pyloric balloon is inserted via the working channel of the endoscope and inflated within the pylorus to partially rupture oblique and circular muscles of pylorus resulting in a widely patent channel. The laparoscope can be left within the abdomen to confirm intrapyloric position of the balloon and to ensure that dilatation-induced perforation has not occurred.

Haemostasis must be confirmed and additional clips may be applied if necessary. A suction drain can be left near the hiatus if necessary. Sterile saline irrigation may be required, followed by intraperitoneal injection of 0.5% bupivacaine (Marcain) in a 10 ml ampoule. The pneumoperitoneum must be completely deflated, trocars removed and puncture holes are closed and occasionally infiltrated with local anaesthetics.

2. Posterior truncal vagotomy and anterior seromyotomy (Taylor's procedure)

The posterior vagus nerve is dissected free from the posterior aspect of the oesophagus and divided between surgical clips. The anterior lesser curve seromyotomy is then performed starting at the cardia and extending to within 6 cm of the pylorus, where the branching of the nerve of Latarget commences (crow's foot). Seromyotomy is maintained at a distance of 1.5 cm from the lesser curve. Care is taken not to penetrate the gastric mucosa; magnification by video laparoscopy minimises this risk. A monopolar cautery hook is used to perform seromyotomy followed by running overlap suturing using 3/0 or 2/0 monofilament to approximate the seromuscular defect to minimise risk of postoperative bleeding and tissue adhesions. A fibrin sealant (e.g. Tissucol) is applied over the suture line to further ensure haemostasis.

3. Posterior truncal vagotomy and anterior highly selective vagotomy

Surgical pioneers used five sites as before, but the operator trocar is not to the left of the umbilicus but through the right mid-abdomen. A 48 Fr dilator is used to distend the oesophagus and place the stomach on tension. This results in pushing the greater curvature of the stomach laterally to the left and posteriorly. The lesser curvature is pulled medially and anteriorly, thus facilitating exposure of anterior vagal nerve fibres. The oesophagus is retracted to the left with a blunt probe and the lesser omentum opened. The posterior vagus is dealt with as before. The anterior vagus nerve is identified near the anterior aspect of the oesophagus and placed on tension with a blunt probe inserted via the subxiphoid trocar. The serosa is carefully opened with Semm hook scissors along the lesser curvature. Individual branches of the anterior vagus nerve are then easily displayed as they enter the stomach. Clips are applied to each branch and then divided using Semm hook scissors. Laparoscopic magnification often enables the nerve to be dissected separate from adjacent blood vessels. Branches of the nerve of Latarget innervating the gastric antrum are easily identified and preserved 7–8 cm from the pylorus.

4. Closure of perforated duodenal ulcer

Suture closure/toilet of perforated peptic ulcer can be performed laparoscopically. The perforation can be closed in either of two ways. Simple closure with 2–3 sutures can be done using a laparoscopic needle holder with a 20 mm straight needle attached to 15 cm long thread, to approximate omentum over the site of perforation with each suture (collagen/fibrinogen may be sprayed over operative site). Alternatively, the perforation can be closed by using combined endoscopic and laparoscopic approach: a grasping instrument is inserted via the biopsy channel of a flexible gastroscope and out through the duodenal opening to pull and secure the omentum in place as before using sutures laparoscopically. A drain placed via the right hypochondrial trocar is maintained under 30 mmH$_2$O negative pressure (closed suction drainage). Pneumoperitoneum is then desufflated and abdominal punctures are closed as previously described.

Laparoscopic anti-reflux surgery

The operation is indicated if medical treatment has failed to control symptoms and is indicated to prevent complications. Weight reduction in obese patients is highly desirable since surgery in such patients is difficult (though not impossible).

Preparations, position and ports are as in duodenal ulcer surgery.

1. The abdominal oesophagus is dissected from all sides with blunt dissection using pedget and spatula:
- dividing the peritoneum over hiatal margins anterior to the oesophagus;
- cutting through lesser omentum with its hepatic branch of vagus nerve and accessory hepatic vessels away from the left gastric vessels on the right side of the oesophagus; and
- teasing through the peritoneal lining and phreno-oesophageal membrane and dividing the gastrophrenic peritoneal reflection on the left side of the oesophagus and fundus.
- The upper part of the fundus is mobilised; division of upper short gastric vessels is unnecessary. However, if needed, electrocoagulation together with application clips can be used. Even better is to use a Harmonic Scalpel machine to coagulate and divide vessels and tissues using ultrasonic frequencies (Harmonic Scalpel is ideal for vasa brevia

division and splenic hilum separation in laparoscopic splenectomy).

- A sling or fine catheter can be introduced via the 5 mm port and applied around the abdominal oesophagus and grasped with forceps as a traction for oesophageal dissection.

2. Fundoplication is performed by pulling and wrapping the fundus posterior to the oesophagus and then suturing it anterior to the oesophagus.

- The fundus is pulled through posterior to the oesophagus with a flexible atraumatic grasper; then
- The fundus is sutured with 00 vicryl or silk after checking that an oesophgeal dilator size 50 Fr can pass easily.
- In Nissen fundoplication, fundus is sutured to fundus anchoring it to the anterior oesophageal wall with the first stitch (a total of three stitches are applied along 2 cm length).

This is the standard and conventional anti-reflux procedure.

3. The surgeon can choose one of four anti-reflux procedures (including the conventional Nissen fundoplication).

- Ligamentum teres cardiopexy (of Narbona-Arnau *et al.*) consists of mobilisation of a round ligament with vascular supply from the falciform ligament after creating a peritoneal window above the liver, and then mobilising the abdominal oesophagus from all sides with blunt dissection using pedget and spatula, followed by suture fixation of a round ligament sling to the oesophagogastric junction and anterior wall of the stomach.

Fundoplication, however, can take one of three forms:

- Total (Nissen–fundal wrap posterior to oesophagus followed by fundus-to-fundus suturing anchoring it to the anterior oesophageal wall with the first of three stitches – see above)
- Partial (Toupet–fundal wrap posterior to the oesophagus and fundus sutured to each side of the oesophagus).
- Watson fundoplication without a fundal wrap around the oesophagus but suturing fundus to the diaphragm and side of oesophagus on the same left side.

4. Crural repair (continuous or interrupted suturing) and fundopexy (fixing fundus or plicated fundus to diaphragm) can be added to any of the above-mentioned procedures.

Laparoscopic rectopexy for rectal prolapse

This is performed under general anaesthesia with nasogastric suction and urinary catheterisation for intraperitoneal decompression, and with the patient in the Lloyd-Davies position. Pneumoperitoneum is created using a closed Veress needle. Via an infraumbilical 10 mm port a 0° or 30° telescope is inserted and under direct vision two 12 mm ports are created in the right and left iliac fossae to facilitate the use of a laparoscopic stapling or tacking instrument (Endo-Hernia, Autosuture; Tacker, Origin Medsystems). A further 10 mm port is inserted suprapubically. The laparoscope is inserted into the right iliac fossa port, freeing both infraumbilical and left iliac fossa ports for dissecting and grasping instruments. The operator stands on the left side of the patient and a video screen is positioned to the right of the right foot.

Initially the patient is placed in a steep Trendelenburg position allowing the small bowel to drop into the peritoneal cavity (critical angle). To facilitate exposure in the pelvis, both round ligaments are elevated and stapled to the peritoneum overlying the public ramus exposing the pouch of Douglas. Similarly, the uterus is also stapled or sutured to the peritoneum overlying the pubis symphysis. A Babcock grasping instrument is passed via the left iliac fossa port holding the rectosigmoid junction anteriorly and to the left. A second Babcock instrument is passed via a suprapubic port to elevate the middle third of the rectum. This provides tension on the peritoneal reflection on the right side of the rectosigmoid junction.

A small incision is made in the peritoneal reflection just to the right of the rectum overlying the sacral promontory away from the right ureter. This allows carbon dioxide gas into the post-rectal space and assists in identification of the avascular post-rectal plane. By careful dissection, the avascular plane between the fascial capsule of the rectum anteriorly and the fascia of Waldeyer posteriorly is dissected under direct vision.

Identification of both ureters is established early in the dissection and the use of diathermy is restricted until ureters are identified in order to reduce the risk of thermal injury.

Division of the lateral ligaments is easily performed under direct vision. Posteriorly, pelvic nerves are identified and preserved. Close and magnified views of the mesorectum ensure that dissection continues within the correct planes with minimal bleeding. In a female, retraction of the pouch of Douglas is facilitated by holding the cervix upwards with a blunt Hulka cervical forceps held per vagina by an assistant. This elevates the cervix and body of the uterus, facilitating completion of anterior dissection. The assistant may pock and indent the perineal skin to indicate to the surgeon (from outside) the depth and completion of dissection.

Having mobilised the rectum down to the pelvic floor, the surgeon introduces polypropylene mesh 15 × 15 cm (marked with a pen for orientation) via the subumbilical port for placement in the presacral space. An endoscopic stapler is then introduced via the umbilical port, and the mesh is stapled to the sacrococcygeal area. On average 3–4 staples or 2 tacks are then inserted in a vertical line to fix the mesh to the sacrum and presacral fascia. After mesh fixation to the sacrum, the rectum is held on light tension using laparoscopic Babcock forceps and the right wing of the mesh is sutured to the serosa of the rectum using 00 silk on a curved needle. Around 3 staples could also be employed to staple the mesh on the side wall of the rectum. The rectum is then retracted to the right, and the left wing of the mesh is brought around the rectum and secured to the rectal wall in a similar fashion at the upper and lower mesh edges. Alternatively, intracorporeal suturing may be employed using 2–3 stitches on each side.

A Szabo–Berci needle holder and Flamingo (Storz Ltd, Germany) or in-line needle holder (KeyMed) are used to facilitate suture and knot-tying. The surgeon uses right iliac fossa and left iliac fossa ports for suturing while the telescope is repositioned in between, through the infraumbilical port. The stapler is then used to reapproximate the peritoneal edges before the operation is completed. The laparoscopic ports are then removed, followed by closure of fascial defects with interrupted sutures using Endoclaw. Perioperative antibiotics are employed in all cases.

TRAINING IN LAPAROSCOPIC SURGERY

With the introduction of minimal access therapy in surgical practice, not only surgeons in training but also established surgeons face the problem of familiarisation with completely new techniques and organisation. New to the general surgeon are:

– Trocar access through the abdominal wall.
– Insufflation of the peritoneum with gas.
– Manipulation of miniaturised long-handled instruments.
– Loss of tactile sense because of the inability to handle organs directly.
– Working without direct vision and 3-dimensional orientation.
– Inability to insert large retractors.
– Loss of direct hand manipulation.

Trainees must be taught never to compromise surgical principles (applied in open surgery) while performing laparoscopic surgery; this is the fundamental basis for safety of these procedures.

Surgeons must attend well-structured training courses. Initial experience on animals and/or phantom models for acquisition of new manual skills is recommended. Courses should include didactic sessions on diagnostic laparoscopy and practical hands-on experience concentrating on safety issues. Surgeons must also acquire the necessary skills of equipment/instrument handling, manipulation and extracorporeal loop-making and knot-tying. They may then preferably start by assisting and then by doing diagnostic laparoscopy on human subjects under direct supervision of a trained surgeon (or they can perform a guided surgery on experimental animals) before performing laparoscopic surgery independently on human subjects. The trainee may perform an independent laparoscopic cholecystectomy after undertaking each of the following under supervision on **two** occasions:

● Veress needle insertion/intra-abdominal insufflation
● port insertion
● cameraman role
● assistant role in gallbladder retraction
● dissection of cystic artery/duct and clip application
● gallbladder dissection and removal via port

Improvements in suturing techniques with curved needles and advanced technology of surgical stapling will allow senior surgeons to perform many of the procedures they are more familiar with in open surgery. Trainees must master the open conventional surgery prior to training on the equivalent laparoscopic procedure. Due to expansion of laparoscopic surgery, open surgery may theoretically become one day in the future a limited field for adequate training of junior surgeons (particularly, if conversion of laparoscopic cases into open surgery is required). Junior surgeons in developed countries may be advised therefore to spend a period of their surgical training on open surgery in developing countries.

Furthermore, the learning curve for either laparoscopic colorectal surgery or fundoplication is more prolonged than that for laparoscopic cholecystectomy, hernia repair or appendicectomy. There are several reasons for this.

● The more complex anatomy in such operations and the skill required to perform these operations. Whereas cholecystectomy is accomplished in a very limited anatomical zone that is nearly 2-dimensional, colorectal operations are performed throughout much of the abdominal cavity within a complex 3-dimensional environment which is also required for perception and conduct of fundoplication. This challenges the surgeon's sense of orientation on the 2-dimensional video monitor.

● Also the movement of instruments during a cholecystectomy is very limited and the operation can be performed with a one-hand technique. During a laparoscopic colorectal operation, the surgeon must move instruments throughout the abdomen with relocation of instruments, monitors and even personnel. Moreover, the surgeon must operate with two instruments, one in each hand.

● Removing a small organ such as the gallbladder or appendix through a small port or stapling a defect without organ removal allows the entire procedure to be performed through small (5–12 mm) ports. Most colorectal operations require specimen retrieval and therefore require the use of larger-calibre trocars or incisions.

● While the requisite skills to remove a gallbladder or repair a hernia defect are no doubt formidable, once the organ is extirpated or the defect is repaired the procedure is concluded. However, at this point in a laparoscopic colectomy the challenging part begins: a well-vascularised tension-free circumferentially intact anastomosis must be fashioned.

● Vascular control at cholecystectomy and appendicectomy is quick, easy and inexpensive. Ensuring safe vascular control of the entire colonic mesentery is a more challenging and time-consuming procedure and vascular stapling achieves the goal but only at a high financial cost.

● Cholecystectomy, hernia repair and appendicectomy are operations surgeons learn early in their training, whereas colectomy is saved until the registrar has accumulated years of experience with easier operations.

FUTURE DEVELOPMENTS AND INNOVATIONS

Possible innovations and techniques (some have already been developed) are on their way to improve the effective use of laparoscopic surgery. They include:

● Stereoscopic (3-dimensional) scopes to overcome the current 2-dimensional vision.
● Powerful insufflators that overcome any leak (available now from Stryker, model NuMo insufflator).
● Gasless laparoscopy (see below).
● Electronic simulators and reality systems/robotics to facilitate training through simulated exercises, like airline pilots.
● Miniaturised optical systems in the Veress needle (optical Veress needle) (available).
● Ultrasound probe (available).
● Articulating instrumentation (retractors).
● Use of biological glue.
● Improved suturing techniques and intra/extracorporeal knot-tying and hand-made loop-making.
● Re-usage and recycling of disposable instruments.

Gasless laparoscopy

Apart from anaesthetic effects, laparoscopic surgery has marked measurable effects upon human physiology. The so-called pneumoperitoneum is in fact a capnoperitoneum. Major alterations in CVP, cardiac output, cardiac rhythm, mesenteric blood flow, arterial $Paco_2$ arterial pH and hormonal responses have been identified; the blood pressure and CVP are increased. Laparoscopic cholecystectomy performed at capnoperitoneum of 15 mmHg CO_2 (the insufflation pressure most commonly used in laparoscopic surgery) was found to produce a reduction in cardiac output of much as 30%.

Many of these changes are due to the reverse Trendelenburg position often used during laparoscopic cholecystectomy; however, a significant proportion are due to the capnoperitoneum itself. Capnoperitoneum causes perturbation of cardiac and respiratory function by many mechanisms, such as direct pressure of insufflated gas upon blood vessels, especially inferior vena cava and pelvic veins which are squeezed by increased abdominal pressure resulting in pooling of blood in the legs.

The concern over port site recurrence following laparoscopic surgery for malignancy, particularly colonic tumours, has been considerable; in many centres this phenomenon has killed laparoscopic surgery for malignant disease. One of the proposed tumour seeding mechanisms is the effect of positive pressure of CO_2 and an unstable pneumoperitoneum forcing tumour cells along port sites. Additionally, there are the physiological effects of raised $Paco_2$ and decreased arterial pH resulting from absorption of carbon dioxide from the peritoneal cavity. Laparoscopic surgery during pregnancy was associated with a decrease in fetal pH and fetal tachycardia, probably as a direct response to changes in maternal physiology.

Other gases, such as nitrous oxide and argon, have been used to lessen physiological consequences of abdominal insufflation, but they are:

– neither ideal nor practical;
– still associated with mechanical effects upon blood vessels;
– associated with a small but real risk of gas embolism.

There are two alternatives to standard pneumoperitoneum.

1. An **entirely gasless laparoscopic surgery** using a U-shaped retractor and/or subcutaneous wires to lift the skin and subcutaneous tissues, or a wire system with winch mechanism to elevate the anterior abdominal wall, or fan-shaped retractor and mechanical arm to provide planar elevation of the anterior abdominal wall (the most widely used is the Laprolift system by Origin Medsystems). All systems provide tenting of abdominal wall to facilitate a space in which to perform laparoscopic surgery.

Advantages of gasless systems include:

● avoidance of physiological effects of capnoperitoneum;
● avoidance of the risk of gas embolism;
● avoidance of problems of gas leak and maintenance of capnoperitoneum;
● ability to circumvent port site recurrence in malignant colonic resectional surgery;
● ability to use conventional instruments during laparoscopic surgery.

However, the main disadvantage of all systems is that overall exposure is usually inferior to that obtained with capnoperitoneum.

2. **Hybrid systems**, using low pressure (6–8 mmHg) capnoperitoneum together with an abdominal wall-lifting device provides the advantages of both systems using a sling or T-bar retractor introduced via a laparoscopic cannula to retract the abdominal wall.

In performing laparoscopic cholecystectomy, a pneumoperitoneum at pressure of 15 mmHg was found to be associated with a 26% reduction in stroke volume and a 28% reduction in cardiac output while such changes were not seen at a pneumoperitoneum of 7 mmHg CO_2, thus confirming that such composite systems enable laparoscopic surgery to be carried out at a low intra-abdominal pressure. Laparoscopic cholecystectomy has been carried out at a pressure of 6–8 mmHg without the use of an abdominal lifting device, reserving the use of a T-bar retractor for high-risk obese patients in whom exposure at low pressure of 3 mmHg was adequate (M. J. McMahon *et al.*, 1996).

Gasless laparoscopy and the hybrid system of low-pressure capnoperitoneum with mechanical augmentation are novel developments in MAT and are highly recommended for high-risk patients. Gasless laparoscopy has been used for laparoscopic cholecystectomy, during pregnancy, gastric surgery, colonic resectional surgery for malignancy, gynaecological surgery, trauma, hernia repair and appendicectomy.

TELEPRESENCE SURGERY

It is reckoned that by the end of year 2000 telepresence surgery may well be an integral component of national telemedicine systems and a fixture in modern operating theatres. Telemedicine has been limited to diagnostic imaging and remote clinical consultation.

Remote handling of dangerous isotopes using robot technologies has long been in use in the atomic energy industry. Teleoperation is the manipulation of objects in remote locations by human operators who maintain direct and continuous control; this can safely be performed by technicians monitoring hazardous environment on TV screens. This level of control requires approximate positioning of procedures of minimal complexity, owing to the lack of sensory cues needed for fine motor skills.

Telepresence is not virtual reality, in which the remote environment is created by computer software and is completely simulated. Nor does telepresence surgery involve robot-assisted operations in which a robot responds to a pre-programmed sequence of instructions generated by a computer, as in automated laparoscopic positioning. In telepresence surgery, an operation is performed on a patient physically remote from the surgeon who manipulates real tissues at a different location, to which he or she is linked only by electronics.

A prototype telepresence surgery system has been developed at the Stanford Research Institute (USA). The system consists of a surgeon's workstation and a remote surgical unit. The workstation provides a colour high resolution stereo (3-dimensional) imaging screen of the operative field which can be magnified as desired. Beneath the screen are conventional surgical instrument handles, which are grasped by the surgeon. The remote surgical unit is positioned over the operative field and has two high resolution digital video cameras oriented to provide stereoscopic images for the surgeon; beneath the cameras are servo-controlled manipulator arms with interchangeable surgical instrument tips on the ends. Hand motions at the surgeon's workstation are translated precisely and immediately to the remote manipulator arms via a computer controller. The system provides tactile feedback to the surgeon allowing accurate feeling of tissue resistance and natural eye–hand coordination. When grasping or retracting tissues, the surgeon instantly feels the sense of resistance to stretch.

Experimental cholecystectomy, nephrectomy, repair of arterial laceration, small bowel anastomosis, gastrostomy closure and enterotomy were all performed on live pigs.

Telepresence surgery futuristic applications include:

- Extending surgical services to locations where specialist care is unavailable, such as rural hospitals, military battlefield casualties and casualties isolated from contaminated or hazardous environments (minimising risks to the operating team). Telepresence surgery (surgeon carrying out operation from a nearby room) may be the only method of dealing with high-risk patients (highly infective such as Ebola virus) who also require emergency surgery.
- Laparoscopic surgery, in which the manipulator arms could be introduced through 10–12 mm cannulas, allowing surgeons to regain the natural eye–hand coordination, fulcrum and tactile feedback lost in current systems.
- Enhancement of manual dexterity and better tactile sensation in microscopic and endoscopic surgery owing to scaling down or up of surgeon's hand motions, e.g. a 10 mm hand excursion can be scaled to 1 mm or even 0.1 mm at tissue level, dampening hand tremor electronically.

1.15 Day Case Surgery

A surgical day case is a patient who is admitted for investigation or operation on a planned non-resident basis and who none the less requires facilities for recovery. Concept of 'admission' is retained here to emphasise the need to observe proper admission procedures and records. This definition excludes minor operative procedures undertaken in outpatients (e.g. FNABC of breast masses or Baron's rubber band ligation of haemorrhoids) or emergency departments (e.g. incision and drainage of abscesses).

Day surgery is not a subspecialty of surgery, it is appropriate surgery performed on a day basis in dedicated day units. It therefore requires similar facilities to those available for ordinary inpatient surgery, with modifications to promote efficient performance in an appropriate environment. Adequate facilities for day surgery should be given a high priority in hospital development plans.

Advantages of day case surgery and early discharge

Provision of day surgery represents an important element in surgical care. The advance of anaesthetic and surgical techniques means that the opportunity for day surgery is rapidly expanding. Day surgery is now considered the best option for

50% of all patients undergoing elective surgical procedures, though the proportion will vary between specialties. Day surgery has often been regarded by health service planners as providing an opportunity for reducing expenditure during long in-patient hospital stay. In the UK, health service administration and nurse management often regard day surgery as being of low priority, despite the fact that the Department of Health saw day surgery as an expedient for reducing waiting lists.

Day surgery provides a convenient facility which is widely appreciated by many patients. Recruitment and retention of staff, particularly of those with outside commitments, is less of a problem than in other areas of hospital practice. Day surgery can be effective in reducing waiting lists, not simply because in the short run it may allow an increase in the volume of surgery undertaken but because it removes from the list those cases whose admission to the wards is frequently delayed for long periods by the pressure of urgent demand for the treatment of life-threatening disease. Successful day surgery is superior to in-patient care for many conditions. It is welcomed by patients and is satisfying for the surgeons and nursing staff in a well-designed and well-managed day unit.

Care in the selection of patients is crucial, assessment of the general medical status and the home circumstances being as important as the surgical diagnosis. The high standards required demand that both the operator and the anaesthetist must be experienced in the practice of day surgery. Junior trainees should be personally and closely supervised by experienced staff. This may require the transfer of sessions from in-patient to day surgery practice.

When widely adopted, day surgery will alter the balance of the surgical workload and require a higher ratio of consultants and trained surgeons to trainees in many specialties. Day surgery is not likely to be so widely applicable as to exclude from in-patient care sufficient minor surgical cases for the training of registrars and senior house officers. Day patients should also be available for undergraduate teaching. The experience in North America and on the continent of Europe demonstrates the potential for a substantial expansion of day surgical activity in the UK. The trend will be enhanced by the availability of new anaesthetic agents and the development of minimally invasive surgical techniques.

Design of day case surgery

The provision of day surgery is useful for those operations which require a relatively short general anaesthetic and which do not carry the risk of postoperative complications that require management in hospital. The facilities of the day unit will be necessary, although the procedure can be carried out using local anaesthesia or a regional block. Often the decision as to whether a particular condition should be treated on an outpatient basis or by admission to the day surgery unit will depend upon the general condition of patient. The use of the accident and emergency department for elective minor operations is no longer appropriate, although urgent surgery for minor wounds must always continue there. It is recommended that day surgery be provided in the environs of a general hospital. The provision may take three main forms.

1. *Day surgery unit*   The ideal is a self-contained day surgery unit, with its own admission suite, wards, theatre and recovery

area together with administrative facilities. Such a unit should be provided in most district hospitals.

2. *Day case ward*   A less desirable alternative is a day case ward with patients going to the main operating theatre where lists may be made up entirely of day cases.

3. *General ward*   The third possibility, day beds in standard surgical wards, is unsatisfactory both for the patient and the nursing staff and is not recommended. The two main advantages of a day ward, that it can be closed at nights and weekends, and that the beds are booked in advance and never blocked by an emergency admission, are lost by this practice.

In addition to surgical operations and investigations, beds in the day unit may be used for various interventional radiological procedures, for chronic pain relief procedures, for endoscopy, for haematological and oncological treatment, and for other procedures such as liver biopsies. It may sometimes be convenient to reserve certain days in the week for certain categories of patients, e.g. paediatric or gynaecological cases. To foster efficiency each session should be fully utilised by a single surgical team. Not all surgeons are enthusiasts or interested in day surgery. Those who are should be encouraged to devote more sessions to this work and accept referrals from their colleagues. Surgeons often welcome contracts which allow them to concentrate on elective surgery, including day surgery, without a commitment to emergency care. Hospital managers should be prepared to explore innovative contracts to expand day surgery.

Accommodation and facilities

Size

A ward of 20 'bed'- or trolley-spaces is becoming the norm, with a range between 10 and 30. It is sensible for the last cases on an afternoon list not to require a general anaesthetic. Twelve cases per theatre day is a safe calculation. A 20-bed day ward will therefore require two dedicated operating theatres during normal working hours.

A throughput of 1.5 patients per bed per day for 240 days per year is possible in an integrated day surgery unit. With an occupancy of no more than 80%, the annual turnover of a 20-bed unit should therefore be in excess of 5,750 patients. Thus, given the target that 50% of elective surgery may be performed on a day case basis, an integrated unit with 20 beds and dedicated twin theatres should suffice for a hospital with an annual total of operations in all specialties of 12 000. Larger hospitals will be likely to generate a larger workload and the wider adoption of the practice of day surgery will require extra accommodation. Current practice falls far short of the 50% target because few health authorities have been prepared to provide integrated accommodation for day surgery on this scale. The OPCS Monitor showed that 22% of all surgical procedures were treated on a day case basis in 1982 and one regional health authority now estimates 25%–30% of all operations will be undertaken as day cases.

Location

The integrated day surgery unit should have its own ward area in association with the theatres serving it to form a dedicated unit. It enables efficient management, reduces porterage,

encourages a distinct ambience and enhances job satisfaction of the nursing staff who can rotate through the sub-departments of the unit. A ground floor ward with easy external access is desirable to avoid long walks and the use of lifts for postoperative patients. It should be well signposted, and have an adjacent car park; this both assists punctual arrival of patients and saves postoperative patients having to walk in the open. If an integrated unit is not possible, the ward should be as close to the theatre suite as possible. Here a specific theatre should be dedicated to day surgery.

Specifications

The design, specification and equipment of the operating theatre, anaesthetic room and recovery ward are identical to those of the normal inpatient equivalent, with all the associated ancillary areas. The anaesthetic room must be large enough to allow free access around the patient's trolley to permit the use of local or general anaesthesia. Wall-mounted cupboards for drugs must be provided with good lighting, piped gases, gas-scavenging devices, vacuum essential services, basic equipment includes anaesthetic machine, monitoring apparatus.

The operating theatres should be of the same specifications as an inpatient equivalent, able to accommodate surgical equipment: table, diathermy machine, dressing trolleys, anaesthetic machine and monitoring equipment. A good operating light, air conditioning and piped services are required with usual scrub-up and lay-up facilities. Appropriate facilities for each different surgical specialty must be available: blackout for ENT, arthroscopies and ophthalmic surgery; compressed air lines, image intensification and plaster rooms for orthopaedic surgery; irrigation and warm lotion cupboards for urological surgery; high ambient temperatures for paediatric surgery; imaging, laser, laparoscopic equipment, and so forth.

The recovery ward should be equipped and staffed as a high dependency area; the management of the unconscious patient is the same whether recovering from minor or major surgery.

The day surgical ward is most conveniently designed on an open plan; this makes supervision of the patients easier with fewer staff. Male and female changing rooms are needed. A wall-mounted sphygmomanometer is useful. A reception area adjacent to the ward is necessary. This needs to be of sufficient size for patients to wait with their escorts on arrival whilst admission formalities are completed, and to await collection prior to departure. The day unit office should be close to the ward. Here waiting lists are held, the admission letters and instructions are despatched. The secretary and/or receptionist is responsible for: obtaining replacements for patients who cancel their appointments; assembling the case notes and investigation reports preoperatively; preparing patient identity bracelets and completing documentation procedures on arrival; typing and despatching discharge; making outpatient follow-up appointments; contacting general practitioners' surgeries to relay messages regarding postoperative care.

Areas ancillary to the ward will include:
– Staff changing room.
– Staff rest/seminar room.
– Sister's office for administration and interviewing.
– Doctor's room for patient interviews, administration and audit.

– Kitchen, for preparation of sandwiches and beverages for patients postoperatively.
– Lavatories with bidet in the ratio of one for ten patients, fitted with grab rails, safety locks and wash basin. Bathrooms are not required as patients are asked to bath before admission.
– Lavatories for staff.
– Equipment store for video screens, microscope, image intensifier, laser etc.
– Large store for disposable items, linen and furniture used only occasionally.
– Clean utility, for storage of clean dressings, syringes, needles and drugs for premedication and postoperative discharge, intravenous infusion and urinary catheterisation equipment.
– Dirty utility, for disposal of soiled dressings and testing of urine samples brought by patients on admission, bedpan washer and storage for bedpans, urinals etc.

Patient selection

Selection for day surgical treatment requires an assessment of the patient's health and circumstances. The elderly and the infirm will ordinarily be excluded, but the young are often best treated in this way. For surgery under local anaesthesia requirements will be less stringent.

A responsible companion must be available to provide care during the night as well as during the day. In doubtful cases it may be necessary to confirm with the general practitioner, district nurse or health visitor that home circumstances are sufficient to provide for this care. A telephone must be accessible so that in emergencies the hospital can be contacted. All patients must be accompanied home and in no case should the patients be permitted to drive. The patient must clearly understand that he or she may not operate any mechanical device or undertake domestic cooking within 24 hours of the operation. This period may be further prolonged with certain drugs and patients should be advised accordingly. Legal documents should not be signed nor important decisions taken during this period. Alcohol should be forbidden. Rest in bed on arrival home and a light diet initially are advised. Patients must be advised against driving within 48 hours of general anaesthesia. The assistance of a general practitioner or nurse in the immediate postoperative period, with hospital backup, should be available in emergencies.

Suitability of the condition for day surgery will be assessed at the time of outpatient consultation. The length of anaesthetic is a factor: there is a wide individual variation in the speed of recovery after general anaesthesia and operations likely to take up more than 60 minutes or so are generally unsuitable. The nature of the operation and the routine of management are fully explained to the patient after which the consent form is signed. Patients requiring general anaesthesia should normally be of physical status ASA I or II, namely, normal healthy people (I) or those with minor systemic disease not interfering with normal activities (II); ASA III or IV can successfully undergo lower urinary tract instrumentation as a day case under a well-judged general anaesthetic. The upper age limit of 65–70 years should be based on biological rather than chronological age. Patients who are grossly obese should be excluded (body mass index) – unclothed weight (kg) divided by height (m^2) – greater than 30).

The general medical and domestic status should be assessed at the initial outpatient visit. This may be done by the outpatients surgical team, in special anaesthetic screening clinics, or by the nursing staff on the day unit. A pre-admission visit to the day unit has many advantages.

Preoperative routine

On the day of operation the patient should reach the unit in good time. Staggered times of arrival are ideal. The anaesthetist should normally see the patient at this stage.

Anaesthesia and post-anaesthetic recovery

The three stages of recovery from general anaesthesia are:
1. recovery of vital reflexes such that the patient is able to be left unattended;
2. sufficient recovery of physical and mental functions to return home;
3. complete psychomotor recovery needed to drive or to operate other complex machinery safely.

The length of stay in the recovery area is often related to the magnitude of the surgery and the length and nature of anaesthesia. Many of the psychomotor tests used to assess recovery from anaesthesia were established for subjects who had not had a surgical operation. Surgery inevitably interacts with recovery from anaesthesia. There is no single test that will assess the patient's fitness to go home. Postoperative recovery is complex and it is unreasonable to assume that all neurological functions should recover at the same rate. The time taken to recover and safely resume all usual activities will depend on the anaesthetic agents used, the overall dose, their metabolic rate and the individual patient. Moreover, anaesthesia may involve the administration of several different drugs for different effects and the overall combination will have a bearing on the quality of immediate and delayed recovery.

Patients given local or regional anaesthesia should also be cautioned about driving and operating machinery. They should be accompanied home.

Postoperative care

The fundamental difference between day surgery and inpatient care is the discharge of the patient the same day, entailing spending the first postoperative night at home, instead of in hospital with medical and nursing supervision.

Postoperative care encompasses the whole management of the patient from the immediate postoperative period until the patient is seen again in the outpatient department. Control of postoperative pain is an important aspect of day surgery, if a regional/local block with a long-acting local anaesthetic agent has not been inserted in theatre, adequate analgesics must be given on the ward, and a small supply provided for the patient to take home as well. Some doctors may be reluctant to describe sufficiently potent analgesics for domiciliary patients, but such fears are ill-founded, pain must be relieved. The use of sublingual agents and drugs administered in suppository form extend the routes by which effective agents can be administered without requiring injections. Anti-emetics may also be indicated.

Wounds are best closed with an appropriate absorbable subcuticular suture and covered with a transparent dressing. Inspection of the wound should be made on the ward to ensure there is no undue bleeding and dressings are changed if necessary, a small supply being dispensed for patients to take home. All patients should be seen by the medical staff at the end of the operating list and the ultimate responsibility for the patient's discharge must rest with them, though the decision may be delegated to the sister in charge of the ward. If the patient is deemed unfit for discharge either on anaesthetic or surgical grounds, arrangements must be made for inpatient admission; the incidence of this should be less than 2–3%. The 24-hour period of restriction will need to be extended to 48 hours when benzodiazepines, sedatives or opioids have been administered in conjunction with general, regional or local anaesthesia. Patients should be given a contact number to call in the event of any medical problem arising (e.g. persistent vomiting or bleeding).

When local or regional anaesthesia has been given particular warning should be given to patients to avoid injury due to loss of sensation and/or motor function in limbs and eyes. The patient's discharge summary will have been completed, so that the patient may take it home and a copy should be despatched to the general practitioner.

Management, audit and quality control

Effective day surgery depends on all staff being aware of the aims and policies of the unit. A clinician, who enjoys the confidence of his colleagues, should be appointed as director with overall responsibility for coordinating the activities of the unit in addition to controlling the budget.

The day-to-day running is best supervised by the nurse manager who is responsible to the Director. Information regarding the unit's throughout is essential for sound managerial decisions. Computerisation can facilitate this process and enable the attention of nursing and clerical staff to remain patient-centred. A computerised patient information system allows aggregation of data for audit and quality control. Feedback from hospital staff, general practitioners, community services and the patients should be sought. Non-attendance rates, stay-in rates, numbers of patients requiring re-admission and the degree of involvement of community personnel all have a bearing on quality issues and these statistics should be collected, and the reasons behind them, and analysed. The unit should have available for all staff some 'bench books' describing standard clinical practice in each specialty area.

Day surgery for children

The provision of a day surgery service for elective operations on children needs careful planning. Children should be admitted either to a children's day unit or to a general day unit reserved for children on one day (in the week or month, depending on the workload). In some purpose-built units it will be possible to accommodate children in separate rooms, thus segregating them from adult patients. Children require special facilities in recovery rooms, both in terms of accommodation and equipment. Skilled anaesthetists and children's nurses must be available. All children should be offered and encouraged to accept a pre-admission visit to the unit with their parents (and siblings). This allows the child to meet the staff and familiarise themselves with the surroundings.

This is the ideal time for the staff to explain and allay anxieties. Despite this, the duration of anaesthesia for an operative procedure should not exceed 30–40 minutes. In this way it is possible to perform two lists per day, thus increasing patient turnover.

In modern surgical practice probably 50% of all surgical procedures required in infancy and childhood can be performed on a day case basis. These procedures should be performed under general anaesthesia and some 60% of the patients will be under 5 years of age.

Criticism of day case surgery

Many surgeons have been concerned about the management of postoperative pain and about the development of complications where the patient cannot be observed. They have, moreover, often been unconvinced by the economic arguments, because rapid turnover means more operations and more expenditure; the extra costs of district nurses and general practitioners looking after patients following their discharge from hospital (transferred charges) must be remembered. Some surgeons have seen present restrictions upon surgical staffing and availability of operating time as precluding any significant move towards day care. Others have considered the rapid turnover in day surgical units to be risky, likening it to factory production lines.

Short-stay 5-day wards

Some consider short-stay surgery, carried out in 5-day wards, as a safer and less disruptive practice than day surgery. Both systems are useful additions to the surgical services provided but appropriate to different groups of patients.

Medicolegal implications of premature discharge after surgery

A discharge is considered premature if the patient is readmitted with complications after surgery. Surgeons are under increasing pressure to increase the throughput of patients by more efficient use of hospital beds. This has meant an ever-shorter inpatient stay after surgery and increasing numbers of patients are treated as day cases. A common allegation made in negligence claims against surgeons is that the patient was discharged prematurely. This allegation usually follows when urgent readmission has been necessary due to complications. Table 1.15.1 shows an analysis of cases reported to the Medical Defence Union (MDU) over a five-year period in which allegations of premature discharge were made. The 131 cases cover all surgical specialties and illustrate that no specialty is immune from such a claim. Such allegations often prove to be unfounded.

Table 1.15.1   Allegations of premature discharge reported to the MDU over a five-year period

Specialty	No. of cases
General surgery	55
O&G	28
Orthopaedics	26
A&E	7
Cardiac surgery	5
Neurosurgery	3
Thoracic surgery	2
ENT	2
Ophthalmology	1
Dental surgery	1
Plastic surgery	1
Total	131

Premature discharge is never the sole allegation, but is part of a list of factors that have contributed to a patient's readmission with complications of surgery or anaesthesia. Inevitably such an allegation is made with the benefit of hindsight and the clinical scene is viewed through the very familiar retrospectoscope which can impose impossibly high standards. However, it has to be accepted that in some of the cases reviewed it certainly would have been advisable to keep the patient in longer. This may not have prevented the complication which led to the claim, but it would have led to its earlier recognition and prompt treatment. Junior medical staff are under increasing pressure to discharge patients to free beds for new admissions, either elective or emergency and, against their better judgement may send patients home. One can sympathise with them but they should not submit to this pressure. If patients do have to go home earlier than is ideal, arrangements should be made for the district nurse to call and see them. Their GPs should be informed immediately so that if problems arise they know what operation has been done and are aware of any complications that have arisen and any treatment that has been given.

Certain points arise from consideration of the different specialties:

- **General surgery**   The commonest cause for readmission is sepsis, often with severe complications arising from it. There are two contributing factors:

  (1) Many patients rightly receive prophylactic antibiotics when undergoing any surgery on the GIT. Sepsis may be suppressed by prophylactic antibiotics and in any event may not come to light before the patient has been discharged after a short hospital stay.

  (2) Patients are discharged much earlier than they used to be – appendicectomies after 24–48 hours, gallbladders after 48–72 hours (or 24 hours if performed laparoscopically), colonic resections after 4–5 days.

  Naturally patients may be resentful when they have to be readmitted and feel that they have not been treated properly. In a small number of claims the GP or district nurse has told the patient that they should never have been sent home so soon. These cases illustrate the importance of close cooperation between hospital and GP and district nursing services if day case surgery and early discharge is to be safe for the patient. In one hospital the district nurse liaison sister attends ward rounds and knows exactly which patients are going home and when, and can inform the district nurses about them immediately. Thus, wounds are checked and appropriate care is given as soon as needed. If a patient with a wound problem is keen to get home, the nurse informs medical colleagues whether the wound could be coped with at home.

- **A&E**   Patients with head injuries have developed intracranial bleeding at home; road traffic accident patients have been readmitted in extremis with internal bleeding; a patient with missed cervical spine injury was readmitted with quadriplegia. It is likely that employment of more experienced medical staff in A&E departments at unsociable hours would reduce these hazards, but it is hard to imagine that such an ideal will ever be achieved.

- **Anaesthesia**   The five reported cases in which the anaesthetic led to the claim are of interest, and all plaintiffs cited premature discharge on the list of allegations. Two patients claimed for awareness, so the premature discharge allegation had no real substance. Both were day cases and it is likely that junior anaesthetists had kept the anaesthetic as light as possible so that the patient would wake promptly ready to go home. One case of possible halothane jaundice occurred and would have happened even if the patient had been kept in hospital: a child having a day case procedure inhaled and should not have been allowed home. The child was readmitted with a severe chest infection. The remaining case was a patient who was given a spinal persisting paralysis. It would certainly have been advisable to keep this patient in hospital until he had recovered.

Identifiable risk factors

A number of the claims related to elderly patients who died from medical problems unrelated to their recent surgery. Perhaps understandably relatives feel concerned when the patient dies a short time after discharge from hospital, but these deaths could have occurred at any time. These cases require very careful handling by the GP so that relatives understand what has happened and it is explained to them that the condition which caused death could not have been anticipated. Poor selection of elderly patients for day case surgery has led to other claims. It is vital to consider the whole patient, not only the procedure, when listing patients for day case surgery.

Another group of claims occurred in day case patients in whom complications arose which were not recognised at the time. The patients were allowed home and had to be readmitted when their symptoms got worse; for example, visceral injury after laparoscopic sterilisation and endoscopy.

The final group of patients developed complications which perhaps they and their relatives should have been warned about in advance. This raises the vexed question of informed consent. A good example in this group was the clotting of a bypass graft which led to amputation of a leg. The claim was refuted, but the patient had unrealistic expectations from bypass surgery and claimed to be unaware of the possibility of the clot which had resulted in the amputation.

Risk management

How can risks be reduced? Day case patients should be assessed fully – taking into account age, other medical problems, drug therapy and home circumstances. In a busy outpatients department it is very easy to focus on the problems for which patients present and to list them for a day case procedure. There should be facilities to retain day case patients if the anaesthetist or surgeon is unhappy about them returning home.

Patients must be seen before going home to ensure that they are fit and that they understand what has been done and what to expect. Instruction leaflets can be very useful, as it is impossible for patients to recall all that they have been told. The Royal College of Surgeons provides extremely helpful advice in this area. It is essential that clear advice is given to patients on what to do if they are concerned. They should be given a telephone number where they can contact somebody who will either see them or given them advice.

Early discharge of patients after major surgery depends in the UK on the excellent district nursing service now available with the full cooperation and support of GPs. Hospital staff must maintain prompt and accurate communications with the community services so that adequate arrangements can be made to visit discharged patients if necessary and any special arrangements can be made in advance of their discharge. This can put a considerable workload on to junior medical staff, but excellent support can be provided by a district nurse liaison sister as explained above. When problems arise necessitating admission, they must be recognised promptly and treated. It goes without saying that requests for readmission must be dealt with courteously and willingly so that the patient is returned as soon as possible to the care of those who carried out the operation which led to the complication. A number of claims of premature discharge arose when patients were sent back to another hospital when their complications developed and one cannot help feeling that if they had gone back to their own surgeon, these claims may not have arisen.

It should be pointed out that a review of most of these cases shows that a claim of premature discharge could not be substantiated. The problems necessitating readmission were often an accepted hazard of surgery and could not have been predicted. Pulmonary embolism is a good example and there were eight such cases as a result of general surgery, orthopaedics and O&G. In most cases prophylactic measures had been taken and the problem could not have been anticipated. The early discharge now considered proper management inevitably meant that many patients were at home when such an alarming complication arose. In a small number it was fatal, but it is likely that the deaths would still have resulted even if the patient had been on the ward.

Early discharge from hospital after surgery and day case surgery is proving very popular with patients and in the vast majority of cases it is an entirely satisfactory way of handling patients when appropriate selection is made. The claims that have been reviewed should be seen in proportion and they represent only a very small fraction of 1% of the total number of patients undergoing surgical treatment in the United Kingdom.

Evolving practice of day surgery in the light of new NHS reforms

With recent NHS reforms, namely the decentralisation of power through creation of self-governing NHS hospital trusts, separation of health care providers (NHS hospital trusts) and purchasers (district health authorities and GP fundholders) and the use of contracts as links between purchasers and providers, the objective was the introduction of competitive open market principles into the health care system (and hence the streamlining of NHS management executive following the Griffiths Report of 1983; Roy Griffiths was Deputy Chairman and Managing Director of the Sainsbury's supermarket chain) and that the money will follow patients in order to overcome the efficiency trap caused by the use of global budgets for hospitals that provided a fixed income regardless of the number of patients treated (this meant that hospitals were practically penalised for improved productivity because their expenditure increased in line with the number of patients treated but their income remained the same) in order to provide a stronger incentive for hospitals to improve their performance.

The Tomlinson report, 'Making London Better', in 1992 aimed at hospital closures in London by merging six medical school hospitals into three: namely University College Hospital (UCH) and Middlesex on the UCH site, St Bartholomew's and the Royal London hospitals on the Royal London site, Guy's and St Thomas's on one site and at rationalisation of services in west London following opening of Westminster–Chelsea Hospital affecting Charing Cross and Hammersmith hospitals among others, thus reducing the total number of beds in London hospitals by between 2000 and 7000 by the end of the decade. Governmental emphasis on the development of primary health care (provided by general practitioners and community district nurses) and creation of GP fundholders resulted in cost consciousness, with GPs bargaining competitive prices for treatment and short waiting lists for surgery in an open healthcare market. The NHS spending in the UK represents only 6% of gross domestic (national) product GDP while the health service represents 12% of GDP in the USA, and 9% in Germany.

Two contradictory objectives emerge from this competitive market, namely **reduction of costs** and **reduction of waiting lists**; (the latter means more surgery, more staff required to do such surgery and consequently more money! Day case surgery (and minimal access surgery) is seen as the ingenious solution to these two contradictory objectives (reduction in hospital bed cost of patient stay and reduction of waiting lists too). The safety, patient acceptability, high quality and yet cost-effectiveness of day surgery is recognised by purchasers of health care as the best value for money, so that pressure is mounting on competitive providers of surgical services (hospitals) to increase rapidly their volume of day surgery.

General surgical procedures suitable for day surgery

– Excision of skin lesions (benign lesions, basal cell carcinoma, squamous cell carcinoma and melanoma)
– Excision of lipoma
– Muscle biopsy
– Division of tongue tie

- Excision of ranula from the floor of the mouth
- Lymph node biopsy
- Excision of thyroglossal cyst
- Excision of branchial sinus
- Removal of salivary calculus
- Circumcision
- External meatotomy
- Inguinal herniotomy in children
- Orchidopexy for undescended testicles (unilateral and bilateral)
- Bilateral vasectomy
- Reversal of vasectomy
- Repair of hernias (inguinal, femoral, umbilical, para-umbilical, and epigastric)
- Varicose veins surgery (unilateral and bilateral)
- Excision of breast lumps (benign and malignant)
- Microdochectomy
- Segmental resection of breast
- Subcutaneous mastectomy
- Liver biopsy
- Examination under anaesthesia and rigid sigmoidoscopy
- Anal stretch (abandoned now in many centres as it causes uncontrolled multiple sphincteric tears with medicolegally unacceptable rate of permanent incontinence in 38% of cases)
- Haemorrhoidectomy
- Excision of perianal skin tags
- Deroofing of thrombosed external piles
- Excision of perianal warts
- Excision of rectal polyps
- Transrectal resection of villous adenoma
- Diagnostic upper GIT endoscopy
- Therapeutic upper GIT endoscopy
- Diagnostic flexible sigmoidoscopy and colonoscopy
- Therapeutic colonscopic polypectomy

Day procedure but better done as short-stay surgery (2–5 days)

- Laparoscopic cholecystectomy
- Laparoscopic hernia repair
- Laparoscopic varicocele surgery
- Thoracoscopic cervical sympathectomy
- Excision of submandibular gland
- Parotidectomy
- Thyroidectomy

Orthopaedic procedures suitable for day surgery

- Manipulation under anaesthesia
- Excision of ganglion
- Excision of bursa
- Epidermal injection
- Simple nail avulsion
- Radical nail and nailbed removal – chemical ablation with phenol or surgical ablation (wedge excision or total Zadik's operation)
- Amputation of finger or toe
- Release of trigger finger
- Fasciectomy for Dupuytren's contracture
- Joint replacements in fingers
- Operation on De Quervain's syndrome
- Correction of hammer toe
- Operations for hallux valgus
- Ulnar styloidectomy
- Excision of exostoses and echondromata
- Excision of neuromas
- Carpal tunnel decompression
- Nerve repair
- Nerve decompression, e.g. ulnar and lateral cutaneous nerves
- Tendon repair
- Tendon transfers and repairs of rheumatoid hand
- Tenotomy
- Removal of foreign bodies
- Removal of pins and plates
- Removal of external fixator
- Arthroscopy
- Arthroscopic meniscectomy
- Arthroscopic synovectomy

Day surgery is the best option for 50% of all patients undergoing elective surgical procedures, though the proportion will vary between specialties. In the USA, over 50% of elective surgery was day surgery in 1992 and was projected to increase to 60% by 1995 (since the litigation rate in USA is the highest in the world, day surgery must therefore be a safe surgery). In England, by 1989, only 15% of elective surgery was day surgery and by the mid-1990s had risen to just over 20%. Day case activity in the UK varies dramatically from hospital to hospital and between consultants in the same hospital, for instance adult day case inguinal hernia repair rates vary from 0 to 95% (median of 4%), and the mean length of hospital stay is still 5 days (3 days in the 15–65 years of age group). This is despite the fact that in 1985 the Royal College of Surgeons of England considered 30% of elective herniorrhaphy could be performed on a day basis. There are some 80 000 hernias a year in NHS hospitals occupying 5% of all general surgical beds; it can be seen that only by reaching the recommended 30% level of day case hernia repairs across the UK could great savings in hospital beds and expenditure be made. There is overwhelming evidence that day surgery has much lower average costs than equivalent inpatient surgery. There is a unit cost saving of between 19 and 68% depending on the particular procedure being undertaken, as well as home nursing costs, and hospital costs. However, community district nurses are required in 2% of cases. (As day units undertake more complex surgery in future, this percentage may increase.)

Savings, however, do not accrue unless transfer of work from inpatient surgery to day case surgery is accompanied by closure of inpatient beds. Not all of decreased expenditure from this bed loss can be saved, because remaining inpatients are on average more complex cases and require a higher nurse/patient ratio for their care; consequently, unit inpatient costs rise.

Cost however, is not the essential factor in determining the potential application of day surgery. The two critical areas that must be considered are patient acceptability/satisfaction and the safety of day surgery in terms of admission rates, readmission and postoperative complications as important determinants in the applicability of day surgery.

As far as **patient satisfaction** rates for day surgery are concerned, audit revealed over 90% satisfaction in general and orthopaedic surgery; satisfaction increases by 5% over 5 years due to continual audit to improve acceptability. There is an 80% preference rate for day surgery from patients who had undergone a day procedure. Another way (beside audit) of gauging patient acceptability is the number of unsolicited complaints; one hospital study reported the percentage of patients registering a verbal or written complaint was 1.02% for in patients and 0.04% for day cases.

Direct admission rates following day surgery should be less than 2–3% (recommendation of Royal College of Surgeons of England, 1992), yet the Audit Commission in 1992 reported only just under a half of the units it surveyed achieved this or a lower figure (one unit was admitting 18% of its patients). In one study, admission rates were 3% for general surgery, 6% for orthopaedics, 0.8% for other specialties. At least one-fifth of admissions in such studies could have been avoided by *better patient selection*.

Readmission rates after patients have returned home following day surgery were 2% after general surgery, 1% after hernia and varicose veins surgery, 0.07% after orthopaedics, 0.3% after hernia repairs and 0.5% after other specialties. However, there was a significant difference in readmission rates of inpatients (0.3–2.8%) and day case patients (0.2–2.3%) for the same 12 common surgical procedures in five district general hospitals in Oxford; readmission was higher for inpatients.

Overall reported **postoperative complication rates** once the patient has returned home range between 0.9 and 13% (the method of judging is by the number of patients who seek help from the community nurse/GP or hospital). Following day hernia repair, 13% of patients reported postoperative complications; this figure was made up of:

5.8% of patients who treated themselves at home;
4.3% who either with or without a visit were treated at home by their community nurse or GP;
1.7% treated at their GP surgery; and
1.2% sought advice at a hospital casualty department.

It is obvious that postoperative pain and wound infection can be treated by the primary health care team (community district nurses and GPs) and it is unlikely that a patient's prolonged hospital stay will alter the operative outcome. By saving the hospital cost (through reducing hospital bed stay), the cost is shifted to the primary health care sector (transferred costs by increased visit number and work of district nurses and GPs).

However, while 75% of GPs appreciate day surgery, 25% are concerned with increased workload; while 87% of community nurses are in favour, 25% of them think day surgery will increase workload significantly.

It is concluded that day surgery is as safe and uncomplicated as inpatient surgery, but it is also cost-effective; combining this with patient satisfaction, it is surprising that day surgery did not gain momentum in UK until recently because of:

- Intrinsic conservatism and no real pressure for change.
- Fear of losing inpatient beds, which constitute a falsely perceived power base.
- Lack of familiarity with modern surgical, anaesthetic and analgesic techniques.

- Consideration that day surgery requires a low level of surgical skills and should be undertaken by junior staff.
- Lack of adequate facilities and investment in essentials of day surgery prevented surgeons from undertaking this type of surgery.

Day surgery must be a consultant-based unit (run only by an experienced practitioner) for the training of junior staff to embrace day surgery from the beginning in future. There should be information leaflets ready for patients when booked with a 24-hour telephone helpline. It must have a manager and organise regular meetings with nurses to define a policy and shape the audit of practice. Patient selection is the linchpin of successful day surgery.

Poor selection of patients leads to an unacceptable level of admissions after day surgery and of complications at home that may require readmission. Selection is not simply a matter of choosing patients with conditions that may be treated on a day basis, but sifting out those patients who are unsuitable for day surgery due to medical or social reasons. Patient selection involves GPs, consultants, junior medical staff, day unit nurses, and all of these must be familiar with selection criteria (see below). Usually at the request of the GP referral letter, or at the out patients visit, the consultant decision will be made. However, pre-assessment clinics run by junior surgical or anaesthetics staff may be set weekly before proposed operations, and an experienced day unit nurse is equally effective in selection, such as checking haemoglobin in bleeding patients (menorrhagia or haematuria) and ensuring blood will be grouped and serum saved; sickle cell test will be performed in coloured patients.

Contraindications to day surgery (selection criteria)

Medical

- Unfit (not ASAI or II).
- Obese with body mass index > 35.
- Specific problems, e.g. multiple recurrent hernias.
- Size of pathology, e.g. large scrotal hernia.
- Operation over 1 hour, although modern anaesthetic techniques using a short i.v. induction agent such as propofol (Diprivan) for quick induction and recovery of clear-headed patients, allows day procedures to last over 1 hour with comfort.

Patient

- Concept of day surgery unacceptable to patient.
- Psychologically unsuitable.
- Lives more than 1 hour drive from the unit.

Social

- No competent relative or friend to:
    accompany or drive the patient home after operation;
    look after him or her at home for 24–48 h.
- At home no access to:
    telephone;
    indoor toilet and bathroom;
    lift if patient lives in upper floor flat.

These criteria may be liberal, because many patients for social reasons are done as day cases and recuperated in hospital hotel facilities. Hotel care is provided after patients are discharged from the hospital; staff (not nurses) act in place of the patient's relatives, community nurses visit as necessary and the on-call doctor acts as GP. In the UK minimal care wards with low level nursing care act in place of hospital hotel facilities.

Postoperative pain control after day surgery and home analgesia have not been addressed thoroughly. There is a trend towards non-steroidal anti-inflammatory drugs (NSAIDs) administered intermittently by doctors away from opiates and patient-controlled analgesia systems (PCAS) by computerised driven syringe (both of which may cause constipation and bowel smooth paralysis, respiratory depression, nausea and vomiting). An operative site will be infiltrated with local anaesthetic prior to skin closure supplemented with per rectal diclofenac (phenylacetic acid derivative, an NSAID) so that the patient wakes up pain-free; postoperative oral diclofenac or tylex capsules (500 mg paracetamol with 30 mg codiene phosphate) may be sufficient as two capsules 6 hourly. Recently, tramadol (Zydol), a centrally acting opioid non-narcotic analgesic given by mouth or injection, has been introduced in the UK for mild and severe pain control, but with less constipation and respiratory depression than conventional opioids for equivalent pain relief. Tramadol has greatest affinity for μ (mu) receptors; it also inhibits neuronal noradrenaline uptake and 5-HT (serotonin) release (dual action). Studies revealed that it is as effective as pethidine for postoperative and labour pains and as morphine for moderate chronic pain; it is probably not as potent as morphine for severe pain, and the dose frequency is less convenient than modified-release morphine. It is not a controlled drug (which is an advantage). It is, however, more expensive than standard opioids.

Postoperative instructions must be conveyed to the GP (and community nurse if necessary) by a letter dictated immediately on a dictaphone in theatre; this letter can be posted or faxed according to the urgency of the condition. The surgeon is encouraged to close the wounds with subcuticular maxon or vicryl with or without Steristrips to reduce the workload of later stitch removal by GPs and community nurses.

Day surgery, when well managed, is safe and cost-effective and is acceptable to the majority of patients; the high quality of day surgery is dependent on patient selection, good patient information, skilled surgery and anaesthesia, adequate post-operative analgesia, rapid communications and continued audit. By the end of the twentieth century, the majority of elective surgery will be undertaken on a day basis.

Day surgery may be viewed as a surgery of three groups of patients: endoscopy list (upper and lower), minor surgery list under local anaesthesia/regional block, and intermediate surgery under general anaesthesia. Each day surgery case is a contract with health care purchasers and within the NHS is considered a Finished Consultant Episode (FCE) from admission to discharge irrespective of the nature of surgery, so that a costly abdominoperineal resection for rectal cancer under general anaesthesia is one FCE and if admission to ICU is required it is even more costly (2000 sterling per patient bed per day in ICU); an excision of sebaceous cyst under local anaesthesia is also one FCE. Healthcare Related Groups (HRG)

have been introduced as a quality measure (taking into account the nature of the surgery performed) to replace FCE. A hernia repair equivalent operation is considered a measure of quality of operations performed, and a better index than sheer number of minor cases performed, so that for example one may view that:

1 hernia repair   = 4 sebaceous cyst excisions
8 hernia repairs = 1 abdominal aortic aneurysm repair.

However, such quantification of quality is not easy or always practical.

1.16 Surgery of the Elderly

Geriatric patients are arbitrarily defined as those individuals over 65 years of age, though there is no correlation between chronological and biological age. In the USA, individuals 65 years or older comprise 11% of the total population; indeed, 5000 Americans reach age 65 years every day and more than 50% of those reach 75 years of age. It is estimated that 50% of geriatric patients will require surgery before death, and that 30% of total drug prescriptions are written for such patients. The mortality rates for males and females aged over 75 is nearly twice that for over 65, and for those over 85 it is trebled.

The five most frequently performed surgical operations in geriatric patients, with their associated mortality rates, are:
- Cataract extraction (mortality 0.16%).
- Transurethral resection of prostate.
- Hernia repair (mortality 1.6% in males and 0.88% in females).
- Cholecystectomy (mortality 1.8% in males and 3.18% in females).
- Reduction of a fractured femur (mortality 18.9% in males and 13.9% in females). Of those who live to the age of 90, an estimated one-third of women and one-sixth of men will experience a fracture in the neck of femur.
- Aneurysm repair, (mortality 28.3% in males and 40% in females); the high mortality reflects the number of emergency operations performed for ruptured aneurysms.

Although surgery differs very little in elderly patients, its practice in regard to diagnosis, clinical judgement, anaesthesia and postoperative care is more demanding than in younger patients. Morbidity and mortality are increased in geriatric patients undergoing surgery due to coexisting diseases and life-threatening complications (see below), especially if the operation is an emergency. Nevertheless, advanced age alone cannot be considered a contraindication to surgery; avoidance of surgery in high-risk patients (based on age alone) would deny some patients with potentially recoverable conditions the possible benefits of surgical treatment. However, the decision not to operate is as important as the decision to operate, particularly in genuine high-risk patients (based on co-existing diseases). There is some evidence that postoperative morbidity and mortality can be reduced by better medical and anaesthetic management in the pre- and postoperative periods. In Cardiff, for instance, the mortality rates for the general population during two 6-year periods (1958–63) and (1972–7) were 2.9% and 2.2% respectively, reflecting the impact of good medical and anaesthetic care on postoperative mortality.

Elderly patients frequently have multiple-system disease, while the signs and symptoms of the disease may be altered by the ageing process itself. Much of the high postoperative mortality may be due to delayed diagnosis, and therefore more advanced pathology. Furthermore, there may be difficulties in history-taking because of impaired mental acuity or emotional disturbances; many elderly patients accept symptoms as part of the ageing process rather than attribute them to disease.

Improved medical care and advanced anaesthetic techniques have increased the longevity but with minimal contribution to life expectancy; the cure of cardiovascular and renal disease would add only 7.5 years to life expectancy, and cure of cancer only 1.5 years. Thus it is no longer exceptional for octogenerians to undergo major joint replacement, resection of aortic aneurysms and major gastrointestinal resection. The real problem limiting longevity is the ageing process itself, a complex process involving genetics, development and environment.

Objectives of surgery

Objectives of surgical treatment are more limited in elderly patients than in younger age groups. While the prolongation of active, enjoyable and worthwhile life is the principal aim, the successful return to gainful employment or to vigorous leisure pursuits is seldom necessary. Many geriatric patients represent a high-risk group, and the surgeon has to weigh the benefits of operation with its postoperative morbidity/mortality and to time the surgery in the light of improvement by preoperative measures against the progressive nature of the disease for which surgery is indicated. Teamwork is a prerequisite to good management; it must involve the surgeon, anaesthetist, geriatrician, the rehabilitation services, patient's family and general practitioner. Risk factors can only be assessed against the background of knowledge and expertise of the surgical team. Thus, it is the obligation of any clinician active in geriatric surgery to audit the morbidity and mortality rates engendered in the surgical treatment of various disorders in relation to advancing age.

Physiological changes

Care of geriatric patients in the perioperative period must consider altered responses to drugs and changes in major organ function manifested by decreased reserve, i.e. old age is a continuation of life with decreased capacities for adaptation. Such a progressive decline of physiological functions accounts for 1–1.5% annually of major organ systems. However, reduced function can often be demonstrated only by stress testing, e.g. cardiac function sufficient for a sedentary life may become inadequate during the perioperative period should anaemia or infection occur. The ageing process is usually associated with physiological changes in the following systems.

1. **Nervous system**   The progressive decline in CNS activity and the loss of neurons, particularly in the cerebral cortex, as well as gradual slowing of conduction velocity in peripheral nerves can conceivably increase susceptibility of geriatric patients to drugs acting on peripheral and CNS, e.g. require-

ments for local anaesthetics and volatile drugs are known to decrease with ageing.

2. **Cardiovascular system**   Changes often reflect decreased responsiveness to stimulation from the autonomic nervous system, with associated reductions in the ability of the heart to compensate for stress. Cardiac output declines 1% every year after 30 years of age (though cerebral, coronary and skeletal muscle flow are relatively maintained); individuals who maintain physical fitness may sustain relatively unchanged cardiac outputs from age 30 to to age 60, at which point cardiac output may decline rapidly. Also, there are left ventricular hypertrophy, decreased heart rate (due to increased parasympathetic activity), and increased blood pressure (due to thickened elastic fibres in walls of large arteries).

3. **Pulmonary system**   There are poor gas exchange and deteriorated pulmonary function tests. Total lung capacity declines about 10% by 70 years of age, but residual volume and functional residual capacity are increased so that the ratio of residual volume to total lung capacity is increased from a normal of 20% to nearly 40%. There is progressive decline in vital capacity, FEV_1 and forced vital capacity.

4. **Renal system**   There is a progressive decline in the renal blood flow and renal function manifested by decreases in GFR and urine concentration. Creatinine clearance (based on 24 h urine excretion) is more reliable than plasma creatinine concentrations which does not increase despite the low GFR, because of the reduced skeletal muscle mass in the elderly patients. Combinations of decreased renal and cardiac function make geriatric patients more vulnerable to fluid overload with impaired renal elimination of drugs. Impaired distal (but not proximal) tubular function makes geriatric patients less able to concentrate urine after water deprivation with reduced ability to secrete acid load. Mechanisms to maintain volume and composition of extracellular fluid are impaired, thus the reduced ability to conserve sodium would make this age group vulnerable to low total body concentration of sodium, particularly when acute illness leads to diminished oral intake of sodium. Renin activity and aldosterone concentration decrease 30%–50%, leading to hyperkalemia. In addition, associated reductions in GFR make geriatric patients at risk of hyperkalemia during i.v. infusion of solutions containing potassium.

5. **Gastrointestinal and hepatobiliary system**   Gastric changes include reduced perfusion, decreased gastric emptying and decreased gastric cell function, which in turn lead to impaired acid secretion and elevation of gastric fluid pH. Hepatic changes include decreased albumin production, reduced hepatic blood flow and decreased activity of hepatic microsomal enzymes manifested by reduced plasma clearance of drugs known to be metabolised in the liver. Reduction in the rate of clearance of drugs reflects decreased renal elimination or reduced hepatic metabolism.

6. **Endocrine system**   Changes include low basal metabolic rate, a decline in pancreatic function (with high incidence of diabetes mellitus and glucose intolerance), subclinical hypothyroidism and Hashimoto's thyroiditis.

Preoperative assessment

The discovery of a disease that may be amenable to surgery is no more than an indication to instigate full and detailed assessment of the patient. The precise preoperative diagnosis to elucidate the underlying aetiology and the extent of disease is imperative for planning the subsequent management. Therefore, knowing the precise cause of obstructive jaundice will enhance the safety and the speed of management, while discovering hepatic metastases will avoid unnecessary operation, the magnitude of which cannot be withstood by the patient. It is also important to avoid unpleasant, invasive, costly and somewhat hazardous investigations if surgery is not contemplated, i.e. investigations should not be recommended unless they contribute actively to the decision-making and influence the management.

Co-existing concomitant diseases frequently accompanying ageing can influence the management in the perioperative period: they include essential hypertension, coronary artery disease, chronic pulmonary disease, diabetes mellitus, rheumatoid arthritis and osteoarthritis. Therefore, chest X-ray, ECG, full blood count, plasma electrolytes/urea estimations, urine examination especially for glucose, sputum culture and pulmonary function tests including blood gases, and finally assessment of the nutritional status of the patient are essential. Preoperative assessment of the mental state and psychological attitude of the patient is also important in order to correct the underlying causes if possible (underlying metabolic disorder, drug therapy and hypoxia are correctable) and to anticipate postoperative agitation and confusion when the help and advice of the psychiatric department may be sought.

Furthermore, geriatric patients are likely to be taking several different drugs; these should be recorded with dose and duration since they can result in adverse effects or drug interactions with anaesthetic agents during surgery. The drugs commonly prescribed for geriatric patients with their adverse effects and/or drug interactions are:

- Diuretics (hypokalemia and hypovolemia).
- Digitalis (arrhythmias).
- β-adrenergic blockers (bradycardia, heart failure, bronchospasm, and attenuation of autonomic nervous system activity).
- Centrally acting antihypertensives (attenuation of autonomic nervous system activity and decreased anaesthetic requirements).
- Tricyclic antidepressants (anticholinergic effects, increased anaesthetic requirements, and arrhythmias with pancuronium and halothane-reversal with anticholinesterase drugs)
- Lithium (arrhythmias, prolongation of muscle relaxants).
- Antidysrhythmics (prolongation of muscle relaxants).
- Antibiotics (prolongation of muscle relaxants).

Hypovolaemia and anaemia are common preoperative findings. Orthostatic hypotension associated with increased heart rate is suggestive of hypovolaemia. Conversely, orthostatic hypotension not accompanied by increased heart rate is suggestive of a malfunctioning sympathetic nervous system. Deficits of intravascular fluid volume and/or haemoglobin concentration must be corrected slowly prior to surgery. Inadequate preoperative fluid replacement leads to hypotension during induction of anaesthesia.

Preoperative evaluation of the airway should consider the characteristic changes of ageing which may render the intubation risky because:

- Potential vertebrobasilar arterial insufficiency may affect mental status by extension and rotation of the head.

- Some 50% of patients over 65 years of age are edentulous, so poor dentition and dentures must be confirmed because the maintenance of a patent upper airway may be difficult when edentulous patients are unconscious.
- Cervical osteoarthritis or rheumatoid arthritis may interfere with visualisation of the glottic opening by direct laryngoscopy. Preoperative hoarseness can reflect laryngeal involvement by rheumatoid arthritis.
- Weakened posterior membranous portion of the trachea can increase the likelihood of damage during intubation, particularly when a stylet is used to facilitate placement of a tube in the trachea.

Arthritic changes may influence operative procedure, e.g. lithotomy position may be uncomfortable or impossible because of arthritis in hip joints.

Regarding patient consent to operation, the surgeon should allow the patient and the patient's family sufficient time to comprehend the risks of having or not having the operation in order to assimilate the advice of the surgeon. When the offer of surgery is declined, the surgeon should ensure that the possible effects of refusal or delay are fully explained. However, it must be openly acknowledged that refusal to agree to surgery is the patient's privilege, as is the freedom to alter the decision at a later date. Sometimes, it may be appropriate to encourage the patient to take a second opinion, but on no account should patients ever be persuaded or seduced to agree to surgical treatment.

In demented or confused patients, the consent of available relatives is important. In this situation, major surgery will usually be restricted to procedures that will either relieve pain or will make that patient more manageable by those caring for the patient, e.g. excision of an ulcerating tumour, amputation of a gangrenous limb, or relief of intestinal obstruction are operations that will relieve suffering. On the other hand, elective surgery for extensive non-obstructing malignant disease is less easy to recommend in a severely demented patient.

Perioperative measures

There is supportive evidence to justify the routine use of anticoagulant measures during major surgery, particularly in those with increased risk of thromboembolism, such as advanced age, obesity, malignant disease, past or family history of thrombosis, and certain operations, e.g. those on the hip. These measures include low dose heparin or dextran 70, graduated compression stockings, early mobilisation and substitution of regional anaesthesia for general anaesthesia (regional anaesthesia reduces the incidence of deep venous thrombosis and pulmonary embolism). Such prophylactic measures are associated with some bleeding problems, e.g. wound bruising and haematomas, but not with major haemorrhage requiring transfusion.

There is a proven benefit in using prophylactic antibiotics in reducing wound infections following gastrointestinal, biliary and colorectal surgery.

There have been many reports on the beneficial use of enteral and parenteral feeding before and after major surgery in regard to postoperative morbidity and mortality.

Diabetes mellitus is ten times more common in people over 45 years of age; it is associated with increased atherosclerosis (macroangiopathy) of coronary, cerebral and lower limbs arteries, microangiopathy of retinal and renal vessels, infection and obesity. Diabetics therefore, are high-risk patients and require surgery in later life. The mortality rate for diabetics is 3–4% and is mainly due to myocardial infarction and infection; 25% of diabetic patients on surgical wards are newly diagnosed (present *de novo*) and often require emergency treatment. Tight metabolic control requires control of blood sugar in the intraoperative and postoperative period and is associated with a more favourable outcome; this is achieved by the use of controlled insulin and glucose i.v. infusions and best managed in a high-dependency unit.

Postoperative care

Postoperative complications are related to cardiac, pulmonary, renal, or hepatic dysfunction. Monitoring of these four organ systems, therefore, is essential throughout the postoperative period to reduce postoperative morbidity and mortality. The heavy demands on nursing services alone, which on some wards may be difficult to provide continuously, are best satisfied by the provision of high-dependency nursing areas with detailed monitoring of critically ill patients and administration of adequate pain relief. This means acceptance of the concept of progressive patient care so that available resources can be allocated most effectively and efficiently. Specific perioperative measures have already been mentioned. Anticipation, identification and early treatment of complications is also of the greatest importance. Thus a short period of mild postoperative confusion may result in a minor fall which in turn can lead to the most disastrous sequelae in an aged patient recovering from abdominal surgery. This 'cascade effect', whereby minor complications may pave the way for dangerous complications, is a common experience in caring for the elderly.

Due to associated CVS, pulmonary and renal dysfunction, there is a need for intensive support of ventilation of lungs, supplemental oxygen (to offset the ventilation/perfusion mismatch), pulse oximetry (a rapid and reliable non-invasive method of monitoring saturation of haemoglobin with oxygen and thus serves as an early warning of development of arterial hypoxaemia), ECG (to monitor 'potential cardiac ischaemia), i.v. opioids in reduced doses, early ambulation with elastic support stocking (to prevent lung infections and deep venous thrombosis) and, finally, careful fluid and electrolytes balance. The CVP and arterial blood pressure and blood gases may all need to be continuously observed.

Senile atrophy makes the skin more sensitive to injury from adhesive tape and monitoring electrodes used for recording ECG or eliciting response to peripheral nerve stimulating. Geriatric patients are prone to injury from warming blankets, particularly those who have peripheral vascular disease; pressure points must be avoided during positioning for surgery (to prevent decubitus ulcers). Early ambulation should be pursued vigorously by both nurses and physiotherapists.

Progeria

Progeria is a syndrome characterised by premature ageing; it is inherited as an autosomal recessive disorder, with clinical manifestations becoming apparent after 6 months of age. These patients develop all the diseases of old age during the first or second decades of life, e.g. coronary artery disease, hypertension, cerebral vascular disease, osteoarthritis and diabetes mellitus are common.

The cause of progeria is unknown, and there is no effective treatment. Mean survival age is 13 years, with death usually occurring by age 25 from congestive heart failure or myocardial infarction. Surgical procedures must consider changes in major organ system functions that accompany normal ageing; anaesthesia must consider the mandibular hypoplasia and micrognathia that may impose difficulties during intubation. The presence of a narrow glottic opening and need for a small tracheal tube is suggested by the typical high-pitched voice characteristic of these patients. Even minimal laryngeal oedema can compromise the patency of the airway. Careful movement and positioning of patients with progeria are necessary to avoid injury to the thin and fragile extremities.

1.17 Endoscopy and Clinical Surgery

While flexible fibreoptic endoscopy is better tolerated by the patient and provides a diagnostic, therapeutic, research and screening service, there are also some disadvantages:

- Expensive – £7000 per instrument.
- Fragile instruments – a careless bite could cost £2000.
- Cannot readily be sterilised.
- More dangerous than radiology.

However, endoscopy has the advantage of greater accuracy. The conventional barium meal gives about 67% accuracy, while accuracy with endoscopy is about 95%. Endoscopy also has therapeutic uses, e.g. oesophageal dilatation and colonic polypectomy, which are cost-effective.

INDICATIONS FOR OESOPHAGOGASTRODUODENOSCOPY

Diagnostic

The advantages of fibreoptic endoscopy include: direct visualisation of the lesion and organ in question, making possible an assessment of appearance, movement and contents; biopsy specimens for histopathological study and cytological smears can easily be taken, and permanent records of appearance obtained (still photographs, cine-film and video-tape recordings). Thus, endoscopy complements radiology and may be used to confirm or clarify radiological findings, but is also used diagnostically instead of radiology.

Indications in oesophageal disorders include the investigation of dysphagia and the diagnosis and assessment of varices and oesophagitis, as well as the confirmation and clarification of radiological findings. In the stomach, one of the most important indications is the assessment of gastric ulcers, i.e. their possible malignancy. The duodenum is a common seat of disease and radiology often gives equivocal results: endoscopy is extensively used in the diagnosis of duodenal ulcer and of duodenitis. It is also of particular value in assessing the symptomatic patient who has undergone gastric or gastro-duodenal surgery (e.g. recurrent peptic ulcer).

Oesophagogastroduodenoscopy (OGD) is more accurate than radiology in diagnosing the cause of **acute upper gastrointestinal bleeding**, partly as lesions difficult to find radiologically can readily be seen (e.g. Mallory–Weiss tears, acute gastric or duodenal erosions and varices) and partly because the site of recent bleeding can usually be identified when two or more abnormalities are present. Mortality is about 10% and emergency OGD should be done after 4–12 h to allow for gastric emptying and resuscitation of the patient. Up to 48 h, OGD gives a satisfactory diagnostic rate and after 72 h the diagnostic yield falls. The commonest lesion in the UK is duodenal ulcer (up to 35%), followed by gastric ulcer (up to 20%), erosions (up to 15%), and Mallory–Weiss tears (up to 13%). Bleeding varices (3–5%) are uncommon in the UK but carry 50% mortality.

Therapeutic

- Eder–Puestow dilatation of oesophageal strictures (e.g. peptic and corrosive strictures, achalasia).
- Insertion of oesophageal tubes for inoperable carcinoma, injection of sclerosants for varices, removal of ingested foreign bodies, polypectomy, guided small bowel biopsy and laser photocoagulation or electrocoagulation of bleeding or potentially bleeding lesions.
- Local application of drugs (by spraying clotting factors or tissue adhesive; or intralesional injection, e.g. noradrenaline).
- Application of arterial clips.
- Placement of Teflon feeding tubes for enteral nutrition under vision if the pylorus cannot be passed by the usual methods.
- Sphincterotomy for gall stone removal and papillary stenosis as well as palliative intubation.
- Biliary drainage of the bile duct after sphincterotomy and dilatation of the stricture.
- Percutaneous endoscopic gastrostomy (PEG) (Fig. 1.17.1) PEG tube insertion is performed under prophylactic intravenous antibiotics and aseptic conditions when per-oral gastroscopy and percutaneous Seldinger needle insertion into the stomach (via skin incision under local anaesthesia) are performed by an endoscopist and assistant simultaneously; through the biopsy channel of the endoscope a biopsy forceps or polypectomy snare grasps the looped wire threaded via a percutaneous needle cannula and pulled out with the scope. Then the looped wire retrieved orally is interlocked with the loop of PEG tube and the PEG tube is pulled through the abdominal wall (with lubrication and traction) and fixed in place with a fixation ring on the abdominal skin and secured with stitches. A PEG tube may be used as a gastrostomy tube for feeding or other purposes.

Lasers

LASER (light amplification by stimulated emission of radiation) is basically a high-power source of light energy leading

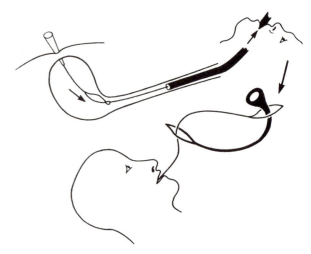

Fig. 1.17.1 PEG procedure of endoscopic retrieval of snare guidewire inserted percutaneously into the stomach under direct vision then passing the guidewire through the loop at the end of the feeding tube which is then pulled percutaneously and the emerging part is fixed to the skin

to coagulation or destruction of tissue protein on striking human tissues.

Endoscopic electrocoagulation requires direct contact between the coagulating probe and the bleeding vessel in the ulcer base; furthermore the depth of thermal injury is difficult to control and coagulum is easily dislodged when the probe is removed. By contrast, endoscopic laser photocoagulation performs its function without touching the lesion. However fresh blood and clot should be cleared from the lesion by using sucking and a high-power water jet so that the bleeding vessel in the ulcer base can be identified and to enable the beam to penetrate to the bleeding vessel. Firing the laser through clots destroys the fibre tip and prevents effective photocoagulation. Coaxial inert gas keeps the tip free from blood and the vessel relatively clean. Photocoagulation should be aimed around the base of the bleeding vessel to produce thrombosis and shrinkage, thus achieving permanent haemostasis. A dual-channel endoscope is especially valuable to allow for continuous lavage during photocoagulation.

There is no irradiation hazard from laser beams but they may cause skin burns if directed at close range. As viewing the laser beams during coagulation is potentially dangerous to the viewer's retina, all laser systems incorporate a fail-safe shutter filter attached to the endoscope eyepiece. Observers should wear protective goggles. A fully installed laser system of any type costs around £30 000.

Laser photocoagulation can be used therapeutically for active peptic ulcer and oesophageal bleeding and prophylactically for those with endoscopic evidence of visible vessels in the ulcer base or stigmata of recent haemorrhage (the two indicators of the risk of recurrent bleeding). Haemostasis is achieved in over 90% of cases and is usually permanent. The risk of perforation is rare.

Laser photocoagulation is also used in the treatment of gastrointestinal vascular malformations, e.g. haemangiomas, colonic angiodysplasia and gastroduodenal telangiectasia as in hereditary haemorrhagic telangiectasia.

Many tumours take up haematoporphyrins preferentially and porphyrins are powerful photosensitising agents which sensitise cells so that exposure to light induces damage. Therefore i.v. injection of tumour sensitiser, e.g. haematoporphyrins, followed by endoscopic photocoagulation can lead to destructive treatment of early tumours in the upper gastrointestinal, bronchial and urinary bladder regions.

There are three types of laser system used currently in medical practice:
1. Neodymium Yttrium Aluminium Garnet (NdYAG) is the most versatile and the one currently used for gastroenterology and experimental surgery.
2. Argon for gastroenterology and ophthalmology.
3. Carbon dioxide for surgery.

Research

No clinical trial of a drug claimed to have ulcer-healing properties would be complete without serial endoscopic control.

Screening

Japanese and European experience has shown that superficial 'early' gastric carcinomas may be diagnosed by endoscopy and that the prognosis of patients who have such lesions operated on is excellent.

Hazards of OGD

Hazards include erroneous diagnosis, complications of medication (e.g. dysrhythmias, apnoea and sudden death), perforation (incidence 0.01–0.1%), pulmonary aspiration, cardiovascular complications induced by medication and instrumentation (e.g. ECG abnormalities during endoscopy), bleeding due to clot dislodgement or biopsying a lesion likely to bleed and rarely the introduction of hepatitis. The overall morbidity is 0.05–0.35% and mortality is 0.01–0.025%. Special risk factors include old age, degree of illness and emergency endoscopy.

ENDOSCOPIC RETROGRADE CHOLANGIOPANCREATOGRAPHY

Endoscopic retrograde cholangiopancreatography (ERCP) is a combined endoscopic (side-viewing duodenoscope) and radiographic technique which can demonstrate the anatomy of the pancreatic and biliary duct systems, obtain pure pancreatic juice for biochemical and cytological examination and permit non-operative removal of gallstones from the common bile duct. It is a difficult and costly procedure which should not be undertaken when simpler methods can provide the same information.

Indications

Diagnostic

● Investigation of pancreatic disease either neoplastic or inflammatory. Grey scale ultrasonography or computerised

tomography are complementary and provide information about pancreatic size.
● Investigation of jaundice, especially when the biliary system is thought to be normal. Percutaneous transhepatic cholangiography (PTC) is simpler when there is dilatation of the biliary system. Preliminary ultrasonography is helpful in deciding which is the more suitable technique. ERCP is safer when percutaneous cholangiography is prevented by a coagulation disorder.
● Suspected biliary disease when cholecystography or i.v. cholangiography is unsatisfactory.
● Postcholecystectomy problems when intravenous cholangiography is unhelpful or when there is an allergy to i.v. contrast materials.
● Preliminary to endoscopic papillotomy for retained common bile duct stones.

Therapeutic

Includes sphincterotomy for papillary stenosis, stone extraction, dilatation of biliary strictures, transnasal biliary drainage and endoprosthesis insertion.

Complications – specific to ERCP

Occur in approximately 2% of examinations; much more common with an inexperienced endoscopist or when contraindications are ignored.
● Acute pancreatitis – very rare unless previous acute pancreatitis existed. More likely after overfilling of pancreatic duct or extravasation. Simple hyperamylasaemia is common but of no consequence.
● Infection of pancreatic pseudocyst – a dreaded complication. Avoid if possible by detecting cysts by ultrasonography. If pseudocyst is opacified urgent surgical drainage should be considered.
● Cholangitis – associated with anatomical abnormalities of biliary system, especially stones. Prevented by giving appropriate antibiotic before or immediately after ERCP.
● Bacteraemia and septicaemia as a consequence of cholangitis – prevented by antibiotics.
● Perforation of passages with cannula or by overdistension with contrast.
● Wrong diagnosis due to inadequate filling of ducts or poor radiology.
● Mucosal dissection of duodenal wall – a nuisance as it may produce swelling and prevent adequate cannulation.

The current place of ERCP in jaundice

First establish:
● Whether the bile ducts are dilated.
● The anatomy of the lesion.

Current methods

Non-invasive
● Grey scale ultrasonography.
● Computerised axial tomography.

Invasive
- Endoscopic retrograde cholangiography (ERC) and endoscopic retrograde pancreatography (ERP).
- Chiba needle PTC.

Efficiency of showing the biliary tree (depends upon experience)

ERC is successful in 70–90% of patients regardless of the size of the ducts. However, PTC is successful in 95% of dilated ducts but in only about 50% of non-dilated ducts.

Special considerations

- ERC may be the procedure of choice for:
  - Pancreatitis causing cholestasis.
  - Tumours of the ampulla, duodenum etc.
  - Endoscopic sphincterotomy.
  - Sclerosing cholangitis.
- ERC and PTC may be complementary in defining the extent of bile duct strictures and tumours.
- Choice is also dependent upon the therapeutic component (drainage, stent prosthesis, sphincterotomy).

NB: In a jaundiced patient, the size of the ducts should first be assessed by a non-invasive method (grey scale ultrasonography). If they are dilated, PTC is the procedure most likely to succeed. If the ducts are not dilated, ERC is most successful. After both procedures, if dilated bile ducts are shown, early surgery or non-operative drainage is advised.

ERCP interpretation

Biliary system (ERC)

ERCP provides information on the *lower duct* but may fail to fill the upper ducts if a block or stenosis is present. Therefore, PTC may provide more useful information on the *upper duct system* where ultrasonography has shown dilated 'intrahepatic' ducts.

The success rate of ERC depends on operator experience but in average hands is about 70%.

Remember the value of *late films* (45 min or later) in demonstrating gallstones not shown on routine cholecystography.

Pancreatic duct (ERP)

ERP is the most accurate technique available for assessing the presence and extent of pancreatic disease. Unfortunately it can be very difficult to distinguish between benign or malignant disease and other methods such as *cytology, ultrasonography* and *CT* may be required to assist in this differentiation.

Radiological signs of value are:
- *Block* or *stricture* of duct system.
- *Leakage* from duct system.
- *Irregularity* and *beading* of side radical.
- *Cysts.*
- *Delayed emptying* of main duct (more than 10 min) in part or all of the duct system.
- *Calcification* in pancreas and relationship to duct.

NB: If a cyst is filled or there is leakage from the duct system at ERP there is a serious risk of secondary complications (e.g. acute pancreatitis or abscess formation) and surgical treatment may be required urgently.

Duodenoscopic sphincterotomy and gallstone extraction

Allowing spontaneous passage   This is the easiest and least traumatic method of eliminating stones; over 70% will pass spontaneously within 4 weeks. However, ascending cholangitis may still occur, and repeat checking by ERCP is necessary. A transnasal biliary catheter facilitates repeat cholangiography and allows flushing of stones.

Extraction of stones   This may be done at the time of sphincterotomy or subsequently using 'baskets' (a strong basket is used for mechanical lithotripsy to crush the stone into fragments) or 'balloon catheters'. Balloon catheters are rather fragile. It is possible for the basket to become impacted if the orifice is inadequate (Figs 1.17.2 and 1.17.3).

Selection of patients

Common bile duct stones
- After previous cholecystectomy when the risk of surgery is high.
- After previous cholecystectomy if the patient does not want a further operation.
- After 'recent' cholecystectomy if other methods have failed.
- Patients with stones in *both* the gallbladder and common bile duct where surgery is contraindicated on medical grounds and common bile duct stone is causing problems.

Papillary stenosis   If this is a cause of the problem.

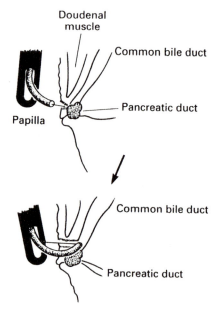

Fig. 1.17.2   Needle-knife sphincterotome followed by traction wire sphincterotome to create choledocho-duodenal fistula (sphincterotomy) is useful in lower impacted ductal stone

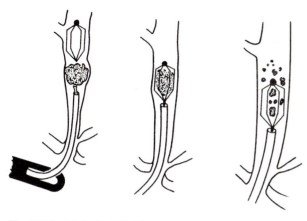

Fig. 1.17.3 Mechanical lithotripsy

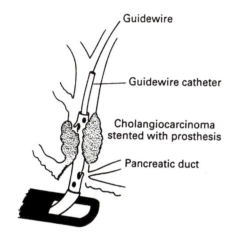

Fig. 1.17.4 Insertion of prosthesis (stent) in malignant stricture by combined technique (radiologist and endoscopist). Note the preliminary sphincterotomy

Papillary tumour For stent palliation (Fig. 1.17.4) or preoperative drainage.

Results

An experienced surgeon should be able successfully to treat over 90% of common bile duct stones with endoscopic sphincterotomy. Complication rates depend on experience and type of patient treated. A mortality of around 1% is anticipated on present evidence.

CHOLEDOCHOSCOPY (RIGID AND FLEXIBLE)

Choledochoscopy is the visual examination of the interior of the bile ducts with a choledochoscope. In **operative choledochoscopy** the instrument is placed directly into the common bile duct during the course of a surgical procedure for gall stones. In **postoperative choledochoscopy** the flexible instrument is passed via a T-tube track into the common bile duct and hepatic ducts during the postoperative period as a means of retrieving retained bile duct stones. This is widely used in Japan, but not in the UK.

Operative choledochoscopy

Postexploratory choledochoscopy

The common bile duct is explored by conventional methods and any stones removed. The choledochoscope is *then* used to provide a postexploratory visual check that the common bile duct and hepatic ducts are clear and no stones or debris have been overlooked. This method of direct visual check is more reliable and quicker than a postexploratory intraoperative cholangiogram which may be difficult to interpret.

Exploratory choledochoscopy

The choledochoscope is placed into the common bile duct as soon as it is opened and used as the exploring instrument. Exploration of the bile ducts for stones is thus carried out by direct vision. This is much less traumatic and more reliable for finding the stones than conventional blind techniques with forceps or bougies.

Stone retrieval

Using exploratory choledochoscopy it is only a short step to stone retrieval under direct vision. Devices which pass along the irrigation channel of the choledochoscope for this purpose include a Fogarty-type balloon catheter, a wire basket, wire stone forceps, a catheter with reversed water jet, and a controllable right-angled curette for dislodging impacted stones and detaching stones from the duct walls. Smaller loose stones are easily flushed out of the ducts by the high-pressure fluid irrigation through the channel of the choledochoscope. These techniques are much less traumatic than blind stone retrieval.

COLONOSCOPY

Indications

Colonoscopy is usually performed after the patient has had a high-quality double-contrast barium enema, although some centres prefer to do colonoscopy or sigmoidoscopy before barium enema. Colonoscopy is indicated for:
- Evaluation of an abnormal barium enema: a suspect area may be inspected and biopsied or cytological brushings taken.
- Persistent symptoms, especially rectal bleeding, with normal barium enema.
- Selected cases of inflammatory bowel disease where it may be helpful in the differential diagnosis to assess the extent of disease or to examine strictures and to search for synchronous or metachronous lesions.
- Assessment of postoperative colonic anastomosis or inspection of bowel segment prior to reconnection.
- Therapeutic polypectomy.

Contraindications

Contraindications to the procedure are those related to the general medical condition of the patient such as recent myocardial infarction, and those directly related to colonic disease such as acute severe colitis of any kind. It is wise to think carefully before performing colonoscopy in those patients who are elderly and frail; those with severe diverticular disease; those who have had extensive previous pelvic or abdominal surgery; and, in particular, after pelvic irradiation and in those with an excessively redundant colon. Newer techniques of intubation and improvements in the instruments, however, make these considerations less important than previously.

Limitations

It may not be possible to pass the instrument and complete the examination because of poor preparation or poor technique, or because of one of the contraindications mentioned above. There may be blind spots at the splenic or hepatic flexure, in the caecum and sigmoid colon, or behind prominent haustral folds. It may not be possible to intubate all strictures or to obtain adequate biopsies at these sites.

Complications

The procedure is an invasive technique. Complications are those associated with medication and those directly due to the procedure.
● Perforation may be due to direct instrumentation, air pressure, biopsy or diathermy.
● Vagal reflex may be caused by traction on the mesentery and result in hypotension which may be associated with myocardial infarction.
● Bacteraemia and retroperitoneal emphysema have also been recorded.
● Polypectomy may be complicated by perforation, haemorrhage or a transmural burn which may lead to the postpolypectomy coagulation syndrome.
Colonoscopy is an accurate diagnostic tool but has not replaced the barium enema. It has, however, replaced diagnostic laparotomy and surgical polypectomy.

1.18 Lasers in Surgery

In 1960, Mainman, working for the Howard Hughes Aircraft Corporation, produced the first working laser, using a ruby as the lasing medium. LASER is an acronym for Light Amplification by Stimulated Emission of Radiation.

Types of laser used in surgery

Lasers are named after the lasing medium that they contain, because it is the medium that gives them their particular characteristics such as the wavelength and power. So far, most of the surgical work with lasers has used just three types, as detailed in Table 1.18.1.

Argon laser

The blue–green light that this laser produces is well absorbed by melanin and also by blood so it is effective at producing

Table 1.18.1 Characteristics & lasers used in surgery

Laser type	Argon	CO_2	Nd-YAG
Wavelength (μm)	0.49 0.51	10.6	1.06
Typical power energy (W)	3–10	3–40	70
Penetration into lightly pigmented tissues: 90% absorbed (mm)	0.5	0.2	2.0

haemostasis. The beam can be passed down quartz fibres and the argon laser is used to stop bleeding in peptic ulcers, in dermatology and in ophthalmology. The results are slightly limited by the power output of present machines being lower than with other surgical lasers.

Carbon dioxide laser

Because its infra-red output is so strongly absorbed by water, this laser is ideal for vaporising tissues and for making incisions with great precision and minimal damage to adjacent tissue. It can seal vessels only up to about 0.5 mm diameter, is less effective than the Nd-YAG or argon lasers. Its effects are not specific to any particular cell types. Flexible fibres to transmit the beam are still in the development stage so it has to be directed at the target by mirrors. The laser beam transport arm can be held or coupled to an operating microscope or colposcope. Because the infra-red beam is invisible, a helium–neon beam is used to aim the laser.

Neodymium-yttrium-aluminium-garnet laser (Nd-YAG)

Not only does the wavelength of this laser give deep penetration into tissue, but the output of the machines presently available can be up to about 70 W, thereby giving very effective haemostatic abilities which allows it to seal vessels up to about 1 mm diameter. The beam will also pass down quartz fibres, allowing it to be used in conjunction with flexible endoscopes.

Other lasers playing a part in surgical practice are the low power helium–neon lasers, which are used to aim CO_2 lasers, krypton ion lasers, which are used to produce fluorescence after administration of haematoporphyrin derivatives, and liquid dye lasers which can produce different wavelengths for greater specificity of effect on certain tissues.

Effects on tissue

The effects of laser light depend on the total energy applied (the product of the power and duration of exposure), the wavelength, the spot size and the optical characteristics of the target tissue, for instance whether it is pigmented or vascular.

The main effect is thermal tissue destruction. As the beam heats the target tissue there is local oedema, denaturation of protein, contraction of tissue due to alteration of fibrous tissue proteins and then boiling of cell water. There are also pressure and elastic recoil effects of the energy and local intracellular thermal effects. These changes can be used to produce a variety of effects on biological tissues. The local swelling, denaturation of protein and contraction of fibrous tissue can block small vessels to produce haemostasis, and the heat may thrombose the blood within vessels, adding to the effect. If the wavelength of the light is such that it is selectively absorbed by blood pigment (e.g. the blue–green light of the argon laser) then vessels can be sclerosed with minimal changes in surrounding tissues. If the wavelength is one which is strongly absorbed by water (e.g. infra-red output of carbon dioxide laser), cells can be vaporised to steam with minimal charring and also minimal damage to surrounding cells, since the latent heat of vaporisation of water absorbs the energy. Studies have shown that the width of the heat-damaged zone, adjacent to the vaporised tissue, is only approximately 100 μm. Small areas of tissue can be removed by this means, and the depth of the effect precisely controlled under vision in contrast to diathermy or cryotherapy. If the beam is drawn across the tissue a linear cut can be produced.

Lasers can also destroy cells by non-thermal effects and this can be used selectively on malignant tissue. Malignant cells have an affinity for porphyrins and ultraviolet light makes the porphyrins fluoresce, providing a method of detecting such cells. Studies have been carried out on a derivative of haematoporphyrin (known as HpD) which is particularly specific for malignant cells and when activated by laser light causes cytotoxic singlet oxygen to be produced in the cell, allowing selective destruction of malignant tumours provided the surrounding normal tissue has a low affinity for HpD.

This photodynamic therapy represents a new form of cancer treatment by systemic injection of photosensitising agent (e.g. HpD or photofrin 1–2 mg/kg) that is selectively retained in tumours and exposure of tumour to visible light (or tunable-dye laser, such as wavelength-specific diode laser) exciting drug molecules and leading to a series of intermolecular energy transfers resulting in liberation of singlet O_2, a highly reactive and cytotoxic agent causing destruction of vascular integrity of the neoplasm through endothelial damage and release of vasoactive substances including thromboxane. Because more sensitiser is present in neoplastic than in most normal tissues, tumours are destroyed with relatively limited damage to surrounding normal structures.

Photodynamic therapy has been used in many malignant tumours, such as transitional-cell carcinoma of the bladder, skin tumours, obstructing pulmonary tumours, brain tumours and GIT tumours. With more refined drug and light delivery systems, this modality will be applied to more tumours with improved results. Cutaneous photosensitivity with photofrin is a bothersome, but not a limiting factor in the treatment.

The localising properties of photosensitising agents have led to the use of these compounds in cancer diagnosis and detection. Exposure of tissues containing tumour to appropriate light wavelengths will cause localised porphyrins to fluoresce and allow visible detection of tumour, such as early stage lung cancer in high-risk patients. Fluorescence devices can be used to detect microscopic metastases in the skin and lymph nodes of patients who have received photofrin for tumour treatment.

Advantages of lasers

Precision   When a laser beam transport system is hand-held, the fine beam can be accurately directed at small targets and drawn across tissue to produce a cut without the distorting drag-effect of a conventional knife. Precision is increased even further when an operating microscope and micromanipulator are used.

Little surrounding damage   This is less than occurs when heating is produced with diathermy. Also diathermy current passes out along blood vessels and can cause thrombosis and therefore further surrounding damage by ischaemia.

Access   The beam will pass down flexible optical fibres and when these are used in combination with flexible endoscopes, access is provided to areas such as the GIT or bronchi. The beam itself does not impede visibility so that when it is passed down a rigid tube such as a bronchoscope or laryngoscope it does not impede visual access to the target. The laser also allows access to areas such as the interior of the eye through the transparent cornea.

No touch   Since the instrument does not touch the target tissue bacterial contamination is avoided. Other methods of haemostasis, such as diathermy, tend to pull off a blood clot when the instrument is taken away and this does not occur with the laser.

Specific for particular cells   The output of the argon laser is selectively absorbed by blood, leaving adjacent non-pigmented cells relatively undamaged. The demonstration or destruction of malignant cells containing haematoporphyrin derivatives is one of the most exciting examples of the specific action of lasers on specific cells (photodynamic therapy).

Other advantages   Other claims have been made for the use of lasers for different surgical procedures, for instance that laser incisions are less painful than conventional incisions and that they heal more quickly. It does appear that healing is more rapid than for incisions made by diathermy, but probably not more rapid than incisions made with a conventional knife, and differences in pain have never been proved. Lasers have been claimed to have special anti-cancer effects by blocking lymphatics and sealing in cancer cells when a tumour is removed but there is no evidence for this; it appears that at least lasers do not increase the risk of spreading cancer cells.

Hazards of lasers

Laser radiation is potentially dangerous to patients, operators or observers and strict safety codes must be followed. Guidelines on these precautions have been published by the Department of Health.

It is the eye which is most at risk from laser radiation. Filters built into the eyepiece of optical instruments and the use of protective goggles for the operator and observers all help to provide protection. Non-reflective instruments reduce stray radiation and signs and locks on doors are essential to prevent people entering the room without realising the laser is being used. The patient's eyes also must be carefully protected.

Fire is another significant hazard and can be avoided by use of non-volatile anaesthetics, using wet swabs, non-reflective instruments and ensuring that all materials that the laser beam might fall on are non-flammable.

PRACTICAL APPLICATIONS

General surgery

Upper gastrointestinal haemorrhage

The significant mortality from upper gastrointestinal bleeding has not decreased in the past 20 years. Rebleeding in hospital is associated with a ten-fold increase in mortality, and if this could be controlled by non-operative means then the high mortality rate for emergency surgery might be avoided.

Endoscopy is now routinely used in the management of such bleeds, and a variety of endoscopic techniques have been tried, such as diathermy, tissue glues and metal clips, but none has proved effective. The 'no-touch' property of the laser is not only more effective but it is also easier to direct accurately on to the site of the bleeding. Argon and Nd-YAG lasers have both been used to stop bleeding from peptic ulcers, with the beam passing along a flexible quartz fibre running before the endoscope is introduced and a clear view of the ulcer must be obtained, if necessary by squirting the area with a jet of water. The quartz fibre is then passed down the endoscope's biopsy channel, and around the fibre is placed a tube through which carbon dioxide gas is blown, both to clear blood off the end of the fibre and off the ulcer. This carbon dioxide is usually vented by a narrow bore nasogastric tube. About six pulses are fired in a tight ring around the bleeding vessel, since direct firing might dislodge the blood clot and increase bleeding. Movement can be controlled with intravenous injections of buscopan or glucagon, and patients can be asked to hold their breath if respiration interferes with the endoscopist's aim.

There is no doubt that active bleeding can be stopped by this technique, but not in every instance because it is sometimes impossible to see the bleeding site clearly and therefore to direct the laser accurately. It is also clear that not all laser-sealed vessels will stay sealed. It is not known whether laser treatment offers a significant benefit, and the reason for this uncertainty is that about 80% of ulcers stop bleeding spontaneously with only a small percentage going on to rebleed, so large, carefully controlled randomised trials may be needed to demonstrate a significant improvement over conventional treatment.

With the argon laser, studies did not reveal any significant overall benefit in treating actively bleeding ulcers, and no evidence that it prevented further bleeds, but other studies found a reduction in rebleeding, that just reached significance, and a lower mortality in the laser group.

With the Nd-YAG laser, controlled studies show a small but significant reduction both in the incidence of rebleeding and in the need for surgery after Nd-YAG laser treatment. The only significant complication is perforation of the duodenum or stomach and this has been reported in approximately 1% of patients treated with the Nd-YAG laser; some of these may heal spontaneously. In general, results of this new treatment technique are encouraging, with the Nd-YAG appearing more effective than the argon laser. It is still not known whether the treatment is cost-effective or indeed whether the difficulties and the time-consuming nature of the technique would ever allow it to find wide acceptance even if the instruments were widely available. At best, it is a short-term measure for avoiding hazardous surgery.

Mucosal vascular malformations of GIT

These lesions are responsible for 35% of acute lower GIT bleeding (mainly colonic caecal angiodysplasia of the elderly) and for 2% of acute upper GIT bleeding. The aetiology of such malformation is unknown, but some lesions are hereditary with positive family history, such as hereditary haemorrhagic telengiectasia (also known as Osler–Weber–Rendu disease) or the blue rubber-bleb naevus syndrome. Laser coagulation via fibreoptic endoscope (colonoscope or gastroscope) can be performed using argon and Nd-YAG lasers.

Early gastric carcinoma

If diagnosed very early without lymph node metastasis (protruded lesions 1 cm or less in diameter or depressed lesions 1 cm or less in diameter without ulceration), in the hands of expert endoscopists early gastric carcinoma can be treated radically without the need for open surgery. This can be achieved with lasers acting as a photothermal source of destruction using high energy (Nd-YAG), and as a photochemical source using the low energy output of the argon laser (photodynamic therapy, using oncotropic porphyrin derivative; the patient should avoid direct sun exposure for 3 months to avoid photosensitivity).

Obstructing or bleeding colorectal carcinoma

Control by use of the Nd-YAG laser can reduce both in-hospital mortality and morbidity by avoiding operative diversion prior to resection/ anastomosis. Obstructing left colonic and high colorectal carcinomas can first be dilated colonoscopically or sigmoidoscopically, using a guidewire and Savory dilators under fluoroscopic control, then the lesion is traversed and photoablated using the Nd-YAG laser endoscopically. Within 24 hours bowel preparation is given, followed by complete colonoscopy and subsequent elective resection/primary anastomosis. Thus, operative procedures currently in use for patients with obstructing colorectal carcinoma include:
1. Classical 3-stage approach (colostomy diversion, resection/ anastomosis, and colostomy closure).
2. The 2-stage approach (colostomy diversion + resection/ anastomosis, and colostomy closure).
3. One-stage primary resection/anastomosis (end-to-end colo-colic) with or without intraoperative lavage.
4. Endoscopic tube decompression followed by elective primary resection/anastomosis.
5. Pre-resectional laser recanalisation followed by elective primary resection/anastomosis.

Liver resection

Many general surgical operations have been carried out using the CO_2 laser as a haemostatic scalpel. Liver resection can be carried out with reduced blood loss, with most vessels being sealed and blood flow temporarily interrupted when the laser is being used. Laser photoablation/resection of liver tumour and selective photovaporisation of deep-seated hepatic metastases can be used. This use has not found favour in clinical practice but the CO_2 laser is being used to excise lesions in the skin, mouth or anus, to remove rectal polyps and also to make incisions where precision and reduced blood loss are important. The sealing of small blood vessels and the absence of surrounding tissue damage allows good takes to be obtained when skin grafts are applied directly to the defects left after laser excisions.

Laparoscopic surgery

Laparoscopic cholecystectomy (photocoagulation of gallbladder fossa), laparoscopic adhesiolysis of intestine and dissection can all be performed using the argon laser with less smoke.

Haemorrhoidectomy

The Nd-YAG laser can be used for excision of first-, second- and early third-degree piles.

Lithotripsy

Laser lithotripsy of residual biliary stones delivered endoscopically is still experimental.

Vascular surgery

The laser has many applications in vascular surgery, such as argon laser endarterectomy; CO_2, argon and Nd-YAG laser angioplasty (whether bare fibre, pulsed laser, hot-tip laser, or smart laser); laser-assisted balloon angioplasty; laser recanalisation of prosthetic graft stenosis; laser-assisted vascular anastomoses (paradoxically welding suture line by coagulum by unknown mechanism); and laser ablation of lower limb telangiectasias.

Thoracic surgery

Early work on the bronchial tract was carried out with the CO_2 laser directed through a rigid bronchoscope. More recently Nd-YAG and argon lasers have been used with flexible fibres to transmit the beam down either the rigid or flexible bronchoscope. The rigid bronchoscope has the advantage that large biopsy forceps can be passed and also that it is easier to control haemorrhage because suction is better, but the flexible bronchoscope can be passed under local anaesthesia and recovery is faster.

The treatment has been used to palliate inoperable bronchial carcinoma but can only destroy those tumours accessible to the bronchoscope. It can palliate without the systemic toxicity of chemotherapy. It is mainly used to reopen the bronchial lumen in patients with breathlessness; it is most effective if it is the trachea that is obstructed and progressively less useful further down the bronchial tree, because a small improvement in the lumen of the trachea may dramatically improve airflow into the lungs. Results show that it can produce clinical improvement in breathlessness in over 50% of such patients. The laser can also be used to control haemoptysis if the bleeding point can be identified.

One of the difficulties that can occur with the technique is the development of hypoxia, particularly if the procedure takes a long time. The smoke is irritant to the lungs and causes troublesome coughing and, together with the heat produced by the laser, causes an exudation of fluid which may temporarily increase the airway obstruction needing repeat bronchoscopy to remove the secretions. It can be reduced by pretreatment with dexamethasone. There is also a risk of pneumonia if a lung is re-expanded after laser therapy, particularly if the collapse has been long-standing. However, a mortality of less than 1% has been reported for the procedure, and is claimed to give a good palliative effect in 60% of patients.

Another exciting use for lasers has been found in the photodynamic diagnosis of bronchial carcinoma. If haematoporphyrin derivative (HpD) is given intravenously it is retained by malignant cells for longer than by normal cells. If bronchoscopy is carried out 48 hours after an intravenous injection of HpD, any that remains in tumour deposits can be made to fluoresce by shining a krypton ion laser (wavelength $450 \, \mu m$ with interference filter). The fluorescence is weak and needs an image intensifier to detect it, and although some encouring results have been obtained there is a significant proportion of both false-positive and false-negative results. Only the part of the bronchial tree that is visible down the bronchoscope can be examined but the procedure may be helpful in directing the bronchoscopist to the best site from which to take biopsies. Future developments of this technique may allow it to be used to treat malignant deposits by using the absorption of a tuneable dye laser by HpD to release singlet oxygen in the malignant cells.

Dermatology

Most work has been carried out on port wine stains (naevus) of the face using the argon laser because of its high absorption by blood. Coagulative necrosis of the vessels can be produced, leaving the other skin structures relatively undamaged. The argon laser is used in short pulses and an anaesthetic is not needed. Results vary, mainly because the lesions alter with the age of the patient, being pink in children because they contain only small vessels, and purple in adults because they develop large blood-filled ectatic spaces. The results are better in adults than in children, because the greater number of red cells in the darker lesions gives better absorption. Test patches are useful in determining the likely outcome, with the results being observed for six months before progressing to treatment of the whole lesion. Skin biopsy has also been used as guide to which lesions will respond well, and if > 5% of the dermis is occupied by vessels, the mean vessel area is over $2500 \, \mu m^2$ and over 15% of vessels contain red cells, there will be a better result.

One complication of treatment is the development of hypertrophic scars, but the results suggest that almost 60% of adults get a satisfactory cosmetic result. It will probably be possible to obtain better results with the tuneable dye laser because its output of $577 \, \mu m$ is absorbed even more selectively by red cells than the argon laser. Histological studies have shown that less energy is required to produce an acute vasculitis and there are minimal changes in other skin structures.

Many other skin lesions have been treated with lasers. The argon laser has been used for other vascular lesions such as haemangiomas and telangiectasias, and the CO_2 laser has been used to vaporise papillomas, viral warts, larger arteriovenous malformations, skin deposits of multiple melanoma and tattoos, using either local or general anaesthesia. With tattoos skin is vaporised down to the cells containing the pigment, so the tattoo is replaced by scar tissue. This can give satisfactory results for line tattoos but hypertrophic scarring is a significant complication.

Ophthalmology

This provides one of the most widely used roles for the laser in medicine. The eye lends itself to laser applications because the internal structures are accessible to laser radiation through the clear cornea and this avoids the damage that other instruments might cause. At the time when lasers were developed, powerful light sources were already being used for photocoagulation in the eye, a technique initially developed in 1949 using the xenon arc light source. It was an obvious application for the laser, which has the advantage that it is brighter and so treatment times can be shorter, the spot size can be as small as 50 μm, and the light is monochromatic.

Diabetic retinopathy

In diabetic retinopathy there are abnormal vessels with micro-aneurysms, dot and spot haemorrhages and obstructed arterioles producing areas of capillary non-perfusion in the retina that can be demonstrated by fluorescein angiography. The retinal ischaemia in turn leads to the formation of new vessels which have increased permeability, leading to lipid and protein exudates, and chronic retinal oedema. Deposition of fibrous tissue along with the new vessels may lead to traction on the retina producing distortion or detachment. These changes can be treated by ablation of the peripheral retina. The aim is to protect foveal vision by destroying the peripheral retina as far out as the equator. The laser is fired at the retina to produce about 3000 spots of 500 μm size, almost touching each other. Some ophthalmologists do this in one session, and some take four sessions over a period of up to 4 weeks. The greatest care has to be taken to avoid burning the fovea, veins, areas of fibrosis and haemorrhage or vessels on the optic disc. The procedure does not usually need even local anaesthetic; it produces a dull pain for several hours, washed out colour vision, poor light and dark adaptation, and contraction of the visual fields. Visual acuity is slightly impaired but does not deteriorate further provided treatment has been adequate, and early treatment can prevent blindness developing in the majority of diabetics. Since diabetes is a major cause of adult blindness in the industrialised countries, and is rapidly increasing in incidence in developing countries, this use of the laser is now providing a very large workload. Other retinopathies have also been treated with laser. Retinal vein occlusion disrupts the fovea with oedema, ischaemia and haemorrhage and many patients develop widespread capillary non-perfusion which may lead to rubeosis iridis with secondary neovascular glaucoma. Treatment by peripheral retinal ablation prevents these changes but cannot restore central vision. Neovascularisation also occurs in Eales' disease, which is a disease of unknown aetiology affecting young adult men in the Middle East and Asia, progressing to blindness, and this has been treated by the laser. The role of the laser is uncertain in sickle cell retinopathy.

Retinal tears and lattice degeneration

Both can be treated with the laser to help prevent retinal detachment occurring, and the laser has also been used as an adjunct to retinal detachment surgery by surrounding the hole or tear with at least three rows of 500 μm spots with their edges touching each other.

Using the ND-YAG laser

This laser has been used in ophthalmic surgery for only a few years. It is possible to use it for a very different set of operations to the argon laser because it can divide non-pigmented tissues within the eye. One such tissue is the posterior capsule of the lens. When an intracapsular excision of the lens is carried out for cataract the posterior capsule is left intact, thereby protecting the vitreous. However, in 30% of patients this posterior capsule eventually becomes cloudy but if this occurs it can be cut open with the Nd-YAG laser. Another use for this laser is to cut through fibrous bands within the vitreous if these are causing retinal detachment or tears. A unique property of the Nd-YAG laser is that very little energy is transmitted beyond the breakdown zone in the fibrous band because a 'plasma' is formed which shields and protects other ocular tissues, such as retina.

Otolaryngology

The CO_2 laser has been used for several years in conjunction with an operating microscope and micromanipulator with the beam being directed down a special laryngoscope. The greatest care is needed to ensure that the endotracheal tube is non-flammable because the risk of fire is increased by the high concentration of oxygen inside it. Polyps, nodules and carcinoma of the larynx can be treated and laryngeal or tracheal stenosis can be incised. The laser has also been used on the tongue to treat areas of leukoplakia, superficial malignant lesions or to carry out hemiglossectomies.

The argon laser has been used in otology. In otosclerosis the stapes may be removed by the non-touch technique and it has been suggested that this gives better inner ear function after operation. In tympanoplasty an ear drum graft of temporalis fascia may be spot-welded onto the ear drum remnant by tiny spots of laser light.

Neurosurgery

Following the removal of a cerebral glioma with the CO_2 laser in 1970, a variety of neurosurgical laser operations have been carried out, including removal of cavitation of acoustic neuromas, intracranial meningiomas, and various other lesions. In Shanghai, a powerful 170 W CO_2 laser has been used in craniotomies. Advantages include ability to operate with a smaller exposure, reduced brain retraction, less mechanical manipulation of the tumour mass, less blood loss, less heat damage to surrounding tissue than with diathermy and decreased operating time. However, agreement is not general about these advantages and there is also disagreement about whether it produces less cerebral oedema. More experience is needed before it can be decided what its place will be in neurosurgery.

Gynaecology

It is the CO_2 laser that has been used principally, the main uses being to treat carcinoma-in-situ of the cervix, vulval lesions and for fallopian tube surgery.

For carcinoma-in-situ of the cervix the laser is coupled to a colposcope and a helium–neon beam is used to aim the invisible CO_2 laser beam. A general anaesthetic is not needed for the procedure. A 3% acetic acid solution is applied to the cervix to clear mucus and to aid assessment of the abnormal tissue. The abnormal epithelium is vaporised by the laser with an adequate border and down to a depth of 7 mm to include the cervical glands. Cone excision can also be carried out with laser. Suction tubes are needed to remove smoke. Healing takes about 3 weeks. Results to date show that the procedure is effective in removing neoplastic tissue with a less than 6% recurrence rate. Since it leaves minimal cervical scarring fertility is likely to be good and the cervix is likely to be competent in future pregnancies and to dilate satisfactorily during delivery.

Vulval lesions have also been treated by the CO_2 laser with areas of carcinoma-in-situ being vaporised under general anaesthetic, localised areas of recurrent vulval cancer being excised and viral warts vaporised.

In fallopian tube surgery, carried out for infertility, the CO_2 laser has been used either free or attached to an operating microscope. Adhesions can be divided with minimal bleeding. However, there is inadequate follow-up data available to know whether this use of the laser produces better long-term results. Experimental studies would suggest that use of the laser to divide fallopian tubes before anastomosis does not give satisfactory patency.

Visible deposits of endometriosis seen at laparoscopy have been destroyed using the argon laser, but this interesting technical achievement would seem to have a minimal part to play in the general management of this disease.

Other uses of the laser

It is still not clear whether the difficulty involved in using the laser makes it worthwhile for the small advantages it offers. For instance, mastectomy can be carried out with the laser producing slightly reduced blood loss, and good healing, but the operation takes significantly longer and the existing instruments are cumbersome to use. In urology, early studies on treating bladder neoplasms with the CO_2 laser after filling the bladder with gas proved that the equipment needed was too cumbersome but Nd-YAG laser has been used by passing a quartz fibre along the cystoscope and filling the bladder with fluid in the conventional way.

1.19 Tropical Surgery

GENERAL CONSIDERATIONS

Surgical procedures carried out in temperate climates can also be performed in tropical areas; however, there are certain diseases which are prevalent mainly in tropical and subtropical areas. These diseases may also be encountered in developed countries due to people movements because of tourism and immigration.

Nutrition plays a major role in the state of health of inhabitants of tropical and subtropical areas. Kwashiorkor and adult hypoproteinaemia are still major problems in many places in Africa. Anaemia, vitamin deficiencies, salt and electrolyte disturbances should be considered in the assessment of patients undergoing surgery, whether urgent or elective.

Acute abdomen

Causes of acute abdomen in tropical areas are different from those in developed countries. The clinician must have a high index of suspicion, take a detailed history, perform thorough physical examination and utilise available investigations before the plan of management is carried out.

Causes of intestinal perforation

- Trauma by:
  - gunshot wounds
  - stab wounds
  - perforation of uterus by cervical dilaters and injury of a loop of small bowel in the pelvis. History is not always obvious and mortality is high.
- Gut perforations due to typhoid fever or ascaris.
- Perforated peptic ulcer.
- Large bowel perforations resulting from:
  - Malignant disease
  - Amoeboma
  - Diverticulitis.
- Rupture of hydatid cysts.
- Acute appendicitis.
- Strangulated hernias of internal and external type.
- Acute intestinal obstruction.
- Pelvic peritonitis secondary to gonococcal infection.
- Pelvic peritonitis due to use of local irritant herbs in enemas for treatment of abdominal pain. These herbs cause sloughing of the mucosa of the rectum and peritonitis.
- Intraperitoneal rupture of liver abscess; amoebic or bacterial.
- Rupture of liver abscess.
- Ruptured ectopic pregnancy.
- Sickle cell crisis.
- Pneumococcal peritonitis.
- Perforated gallbladder in children with typhoid fever.

Pyrexia of unknown origin 'PUO'

When fever persists for many days and weeks and the cause is not clear it is labelled as 'PUO'.

Causes of PUO in tropical areas are:
- Wide varities of infections – see also Malaria, the mimic (below).
- Connective tissue disorders.
- Drug hypersensitivity.
- Tumours, specially lymphomas.

The clinical history, examination and investigations should be repeated, reviewed and analysed; this may clarify the aetiology of fever. Empirical treatment is sometimes required, if the pyrexia persists. An opinion from an unbiased observer is recommended if the patient's condition is deteriorating.

SPECIAL CONSIDERATIONS

Malaria

Malaria is endemic in many places of Africa and may be encountered in patients with surgical problems; it is likely to be confused with some other emergencies too. It is caused by plasmodium species – *P. Malariae, P. vivax, P. ovale* and *P. falciparum*. Conditions simulated by malaria are:

Acute appendicitis

In malaria there is usually a short history of less than 4 hours duration, high temperature (40 °C) and symptoms reminiscent of appendicitis. Blood film is positive in malaria. In such situations it is advisable to give antimalarial drugs and wait for 24 hours before deciding on operation. Drugs used in the treatment are:

- Chloroquine phosphate, 1 g stat and 500 mg after 6 hours and then daily for 2 days.
- Sulfadoxine 500 mg and pyrimethamine 25 mg (Fansidar), this is used as a single dose. It is used when there is resistance to chloroquine.

Backache

Muscular and back pain indicative of disc lesions is observed during malarial attacks in endemic areas. Unnecessary X-rays and traction of the spine should be avoided. A course of antimalarial drugs and analgesics is an effective therapy.

Enlarged malarial spleen

This often causes pain and discomfort in many patients in endemic areas; the spleen is liable to torsion and spontaneous rupture. Splenectomy is indicated to cure these patients and prevent complications.

Postoperative fever

When there is no evidence of wound, urinary tract and respiratory infections, fever could be attributed to malaria.

Malaria, the mimic

Although there were over 2300 imported cases of malaria in the United Kingdom in 1991, most GPs and hospital doctors only come across patients with malaria infrequently. It is therefore all too easy among the many with trivial illnesses to miss the patient with an influenza-like illness who is at serious risk. *Falciparum malaria* is not known as malignant malaria for nothing; each year in Britain there are a few deaths (12 in 1991) from unrecognised or late diagnosed malaria. Many of these deaths are followed by compensation claims which are indefensible. A typical case history is as follows:

A 26-year-old computer programmer travels to Kenya for a fortnight's holiday in a pleasant hotel near Mombasa. He takes chloroquine and proguanil prophylaxis during his stay but is not aware of being bitten by any mosquitoes and stops prophylaxis immediately on leaving Kenya. He has taken no special care to avoid mosquito bites during his stay. Ten days after his return he begins to experience muscle pains, headaches and feels shivery. He takes to his bed and waits for his 'influenza' to improve while treating himself with paracetamol. Two days later his mother, with whom he lives, sends for her GP to attend her young daughter. On his way out of the house the GP is told about the older son who is still in bed with 'flu' and it is casually mentioned that it is unfortunate that he has not been able to show off his sun tan recently acquired in Kenya. The conscientious GP examines him but finds nothing amiss except a pyrexia of 37.6°C. He tells the young man to continue with paracetamol but to call again if he is not better in two days' time. Three days later an urgent visit is requested because the young man is semiconscious. When the GP attends he recognises that his patient is now very ill, with slight jaundice and impaired consciousness. He arranges urgent admission to hospital with a diagnosis of fulminant viral hepatitis.

On arrival at the hospital a full history from the mother reveals that her son has recently been in Kenya and blood films are requested. The laboratory reports that 40% of red cells show rings of *Plasmodium falciparum* and other findings include a very low platelet count, hypoglycaemia and acidosis. The pharmacy has no ampoules of quinine and this results in a 4-hour delay in initiating specific treatment. Later that day the young man dies.

This case brings out the common lack of compliance with antimalarial regimes, the failure of the patient to seek advice early and of the doctor to pick up the clue about travel or to ask specifically 'Where have you been?'. Even if the patient has been conscientious in taking malaria prophylaxis this does not rule out the possibility of severe falciparum malaria. Its clinical course is often that of a non-specific illness in its early stages and the patient is often not obviously ill for the first few days. Non-immune patients may then deteriorate with alarming rapidity over a few hours and die. Children are at special risk of a rapid downhill clinical course.

Common presentations of falciparum malaria

- Influenza-like illness
- Diarrhoea and vomiting
- Jaundice
- Cerebral disturbance or fits
- Progressive anaemia
- Acute renal failure
- Acute respiratory distress syndrome
- Arthralgia
- Severe headache
- Postural hypotension or shock
- Thrombocytopenia, rarely with bleeding

Do not expect to obtain a 'typical' history of rigors on alternate days; though this is more common with vivax malaria. A history of full compliance with prophylactic antimalarials does not rule out a diagnosis of malaria since there is widespread drug resistance. The spleen is not usually palpably enlarged.

In recent years about 2000 cases of imported malaria have been recorded in the United Kingdom each year and the proportion of cases of falciparum malaria has risen to about 50%. About 75% of malaria patients from Africa have falciparum malaria while 90% of imported malaria from Asia is due to *P. vivax*. Groups who are at particular risk include businessmen and overland backpackers. Former immigrants who were brought up in a malarious area may have developed a degree of immunity during childhood but following long years of residence in Europe much of this immunity is lost and when they return on holiday they may experience sharp attacks of malaria. Children of these immigrants who have lived in this country all their lives are just as susceptible as other non-immunes when they visit relatives in malarious areas. Many holiday-makers travelling to tropical Africa are at a much higher risk than they realise when they book a package holiday at the last moment. The risk of malaria during unprotected travel to West Africa is estimated to be about 2% per month spent is an endemic area.

The only way of making a diagnosis of malaria is to ask for a history of travel and to arrange urgent blood films on two or three occasions over the next one to two days. This is particularly important if the patient is taking prophylactic drugs or has had a recent course of treatment since parasitaemia may be below the level of detection for a while. Falciparum malaria in non-immune persons must be treated as a medical emergency; the diagnosis and treatment cannot be left to the next morning.

Other causes of febrile illness

There are many other causes of febrile illness in people returning from the tropics. Some of the commoner ones are:
- Dengue fever
- Typhoid
- Amoebic liver abscess
- Tuberculosis
- Acquired immunodeficiency syndrome (AIDS)
- Acute schistosomiasis
- Visceral leishmaniasis
- Tick typhus

Ubiquitous diseases such as pneumonia and urinary tract infections are also frequent. It is worth remembering that travellers from rural Africa or medical workers might be infected with more dangerous viruses such as Lassa or Ebola. The advice of a specialist in tropical medicine or infectious diseases should be sought if the diagnosis is in doubt.

We all need to appreciate that drug prophylaxis or malaria is often ineffective either because the traveller has not complied fully with the drug regime, most often because he or she has stopped taking the drugs on return, or because of the drug-resistant falciparum parasites in many areas of the world. Emphasis is needed not only in prescribing a correct antimalarial drug regime, but also in advising careful measures to prevent bites from anopheline mosquitoes and in educating travellers about the necessity of telling their doctors where they have been and attending quickly for treatment if they have any illness after return from the tropics. *Inter-*

national Travel and Health, published annually by the World Health Organisation, is a useful source of information about the distribution of malaria in different countries. Current British opinion about prophylactic regimes can be obtained from the British National Formulary or by telephoning the numbers contained therein.

Hydatid disease

Many foci of endemic areas are encountered in Africa and areas of the Middle East, such as Iraq and Iran, and Mediterranean countries. Hydatid disease of the human liver is caused by Echinococcus species in areas in which there is close association between man, dog and sheep. Man is an accidental intermediate host of the larval form of *Echinococcus granulosus* (Fig. 1.19.1). The liver and lung are the most frequent sites affected by the disease. The right lobe of the liver is affected in 75% of patients and the left lobe in 25%. It is important to note that hydatid cysts are breeding places for second, third and further generations of larvae which are derived from the embryo. The condition is diagnosed by a combination of clinical, radiological and serological methods. The liver is usually enlarged and tender. Abdominal X-rays may detect calcification in chronic cases. Ultrasound is valuable in diagnosis and screening in endemic areas. Computerised axial tomography (CT scan) confirms the presence of space-occupying lesions in the liver. Magnetic resonance (MR) is reported to be of great value in detection of intrahepatic rupture of hydatid cysts. The serological tests carried out are: Casoni test which is of historical value as an antigen–antibody reaction with sensitivity of 86%; complement fixation test (CFT) is positive in 60%; enzyme–linked immunosorbent assay (ELISA) is widely utilised in diagnosis and is highly specific. The treatment of hydatid cysts of the liver is primarily surgical. The recommended operations are (Fig. 1.19.2):

Cystectomy or removal of the whole cyst *in toto* without opening it: this is possible for pulmonary or hepatic cysts which are not communicating with the biliary system.

Evacuation of the parasite: meticulous surgical technique is required in order to avoid spillage of cyst material in the peritoneal cavity. Abdominal packs soaked with normal saline or scolicidal solutions are used to isolate the area. A small amount of fluid is aspirated and scolicidal agent such as formalin 10% or hypertonic saline, is injected for 10 minutes. The cyst is carefully opened and the germinal layer

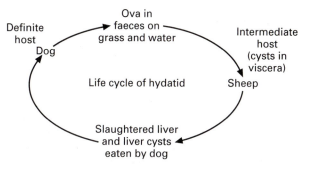

Fig. 1.19.1 Man is only an incidental intermediate host

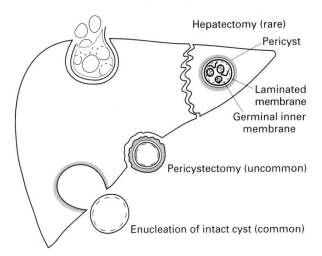

Fig. 1.19.2 Surgical techniques for removal of hydatid cyst

removed in one piece. The residual cavity or dead space can be dealt with in many ways:

1. Left open and drained. This is not recommended, as small bowel may get into the cavity and become obstructed.
2. Cavity is filled with saline and closed.
3. Cavity is packed with omentum. This method is recommended as it gives good results.

Removal of involved organ, i.e splenectomy.

(Rarely) *removal of part of the affected organ*, i.e partial hepatectomy.

Indications for medical treatment:

1. Extensive, widespread disease with many organs involved (hydatidosis).
2. Recurrent cysts.
3. When surgery carries high risk, namely, in elderly, unfit patients with cardiothoracic problems.
4. If the cyst ruptures and the patient presents with acute abdomen albendazole is started in a dose of 10 mg/kg/day for one month with encouraging results. Some reports established that some cysts completely disappeared after one course of medication.

Hydatid disease of the lung

Hydatid cysts of the lung develop from larvae which have passed through the liver sinusoidal system. This means that almost all patients with lung hydatid have liver cysts as well. The lower lobes are predominantly involved, the right more than the left. The percentage of finding multiple cysts is 14–22%. Each lung cyst should be dealt with, independently. An important difference between hydatid cyst of the lung and liver is that daughter cysts are rare to find in the former but they are commonly seen in the latter. Another difference is that adjacent liver cysts may communicate with each other; this does not happen in lung hydatid. The last difference is that calcification is rarely seen in lung hydatid. Hemoptysis, chest pain and dyspnoea are the main presenting features. Chest X-rays are diagnostic and show the size of

the cyst; rate of growth can be assessed by comparing consecutive films.

The treatment of hydatid cysts of the lung is surgical. Operations recommended are:

- Aspiration.
- Cryogenic technique. this is similar to aspiration, but a cone is applied to the opening of the cyst; this method reduces spillage of fluid in the pleural cavity.
- Segmental resection
- Cyst enucleation
- Pericystectomy
- Lobectomy

In the presence of combined hepatic and lung hydatid cysts, the surgeon must operate on the pulmonary cyst first (to improve the respiratory function) and then operate on the liver cyst.

Other worm infestations

Ascaris lumbricoides This is the main offender of the gastrointestinal tract, it may cause:

- Intestinal perforation in children and small bowel obstruction in both children and adults.
- The worm moves down to the appendix and causes obstructive appendicitis; it migrates upwards towards the ampulla of Vater and causes obstructive jaundice. The worm is soft and difficult to feel during common bile duct exploration. The best way of recognising it is to aspirate fluid from the common bile duct and examine it for ova.
- Abscesses: superficial and deep abscesses may be generated by the ascaris worm. Patients in tropical areas with abdominal pain should always be examined for worm infestations (ova in stool) and appropriate treatment administered, otherwise the condition may be misdiagnosed as peptic ulceration, gallbladder or colonic disease. Piperazine as a single dose of 20–30 ml (250 mg per ml), given on an empty stomach and followed by a purgative, cures the condition.

Tape worms *Taenia solium* and *Taenia saginata* are known to cause muscle abscesses. The thigh muscles are the most frequent sites affected. Niclosamide (Taenicide) 500 mg tablets is an effective cure; the adult dose is 4 tablets given once.

- Cysticercosis: Larval forms of a number of tape worms can invade the tissues of man, with serious consequences. Man becomes infected with cysticerci by swallowing eggs on uncooked vegetables, salads and other articles of food and contaminated drink. Embryos liberated from the eggs penetrate the intestinal mucosa and are carried by the blood to the muscles and the brain; however, any tissue can be affected. Dead cysts tend to calcify and may be visualised radiologically. The most characteristic symptoms of cysticercosis are palpable subcutaneous nodules and epileptiform attacks. Fulminating cases may have a picture of acute encephalitis. Excision of cerebral cysticerci for focal epilepsy rarely affects the course of the disease; decompression for hydrocephalus may be worthwhile.

Ancylostomiasis These worms, known as hookworms or *Ancylostoma duodenale* and *Necator americans*, are lodged in the duodenum and upper jejunum. There are some reports which associate duodenal ulceration with them. Ancylostoma are famous for iron deficiency anaemia due to chronic blood loss. Treatment is by:

- Tetrachloroethylene, as a single dose of 0.1 mg per kg body weight, given in the morning on an empty stomach.
- Bepheneum hydroxynaphthoate (Alcopar) in two successive doses of 2 g given on an empty stomach, cures the condition.

Threadworm (oxyuris vermicularis)   The adult worm is an inhabitant of the large bowel. The tiny worms migrate at night to the anus and produce itching (pruritus) due to deposition of ova. They are associated with abdominal pain in the form of appendicular colic in children. There are no reports that associate Oxyuris with the aetiology of acute appendicitis. Piperazine (Antepar), in a dose of 75 mg per kg for a week, gets rid of the condition.

Schistosomiasis

This is a major public health problem in many developing countries like Egypt and Sudan.

Schistosoma haematobium infects the urinary tract and pathological features of pseudotubercles, granulomas, polyps, ulcers, sandy patches and fibrosis are seen in the urinary bladder. Sandy patches are calcification on the subepithelial layer of the bladder around dead ova and they persist throughout life. Metaplasia of transitional epithelium to squamous may occur with bilharziasis. The association of carcinoma of the bladder and bilharzia is not clear and whether bilharzia plays a role in aetiology is controversial.

The main clinical manifestation is terminal hematuria. When the ureters are involved, strictures of the lower third occur, and in long-standing cases, back pressure with hydronephrosis, atrophy of the renal parenchyma and deterioration of renal function is the end-stage of the disease.

Treatment of this complication is aimed at prevention but there is a place for surgical operation in ureteric obstruction. These operations are carried out by urologists and their rationale is combating obstruction by reimplantation of both ureters into a healthier site.

Schistosoma mansoni

Infection begins in the large bowel and ova travel via the radicles of the portal system to the liver where extensive periportal fibrosis develops. This leads to portal hypertension with its sequelae of splenic enlargement, and occurrence of oesophageal varices. Liver functions are maintained within normal limits in most patients with schistosomiasis. Diagnosis is based on clinical grounds and finding stigmata of portal hypertension. *S. mansoni* may be isolated from the stool of patients with portal hypertension. Ultrasound of the liver is useful in estimating the degree of periportal fibrosis and it is considered by some physicians to be as accurate as liver biopsy.

Drugs used in the treatment are:

- Praziquantel, orally in a single dose of 40 mg per kg body weight, is effective in treatment of both types of bilharzia.

- Oxamniquine (Vansil) is used for treatment of *S. mansoni* infections. The recommended dosage is 15 mg per kg given orally once.

The objective of surgical operations is the control of bleeding from oesophageal varices. The types of operation performed are:

- Shunt operations
- Splenectomy and devascularisation of the stomach. This was performed extensively by Egyptian surgeons. Hassab, an Egyptian surgeon from Alexandria, has given his name to the operation. Several surgeons perform the operation with some modifications, i.e. ligation of the left gastric vein and less extensive devascularisation of the stomach and lower oesophagus. It is advisable to attempt sclerotherapy on bleeding patients. The favourable results of sclerotherapy in controlling the bleeding is well documented in many reports. Surgical operations should be reserved for those who experience bleeding despite repeated sclerotherapy (*see* Section 54).

Elephantiasis

This condition is caused by *Microfilaria bancrofti* and *Microfilaria malayi*. Extensive swelling of the lower limbs and scrotum is observed. Tissue swelling associated with elephantiasis is not entirely due to lymphatic obstruction as the swelling tends to disappear with bed rest and elevation of the affected part. There is leakage of lymph from the vascular system into the interstitial tissue. This lymph is rich in protein and exerts a high osmotic pressure which leads to gross lymphoedema. Surgical procedures like anastomosis of superficial lymphatics to the deep system were not successful. Diethylcarbamazine is the only effective drug against microfilaria: 0.25–0.50 mg per kg is started on the first day and doubled each day until 2 mg per kg is reached. This dose is then continued orally for a period of 3 weeks.

Dracunculiasis

This disease is caused by *Dracunculus medinensis* and is known as 'Guinea' worm and 'Medina' worm infection. Larvae thrive in drinking water. The adult worm provokes local inflammation with swelling of the lower limbs near the ankle region. There is severe pain and itching. The mature worm tends to invade the skin and produces ulceration when it is in the process of discharging ova. The old method of tying the worm around a match stick and winding it every day while keeping the skin moist, is still widely practised and effective in removal of the worm. Incisions over the swelling should be avoided.

Typhoid fever

This is a systemic illness caused by *Salmonella typhi* with a mortality of 15% in untreated patients and 1% in those who receive suitable antibiotics. Most deaths in treated patients result from either intestinal perforation or haemorrhage. Perforation has an incidence of 4–7% and lower gastrointestinal bleeding 2% in untreated patients. Diagnosis of perforation is sometimes difficult, but the finding of free gas on abdominal or chest X-rays is a helpful sign. The mortality of perforation is doubled when diagnosis is delayed for more than 24 hours.

Laparotomy, under an umbrella of 1–2 g of chloramphenicol every 4 hours for 14 days, is recommended when perforation is suspected or diagnosed. Peritoneal toilet, simple surgical debridement and meticulous transverse bowel closure to avoid stenosis is an operation with low mortality. Other recommended operations are ileal resection, ileo right colectomy, tube ileostomy and simple drainage of the peritoneal cavity without closure of the perforation. Postoperative sepsis and intraperitoneal abscesses have been reported to be high. Severe bleeding not well controlled conservatively warrants laparotomy and resection of the bleeding site.

Tuberculosis

This is a common chronic inflammatory disease caused by *Mycobacterium tuberculosis* bacillus and is characterised by granuloma. The infection is air-borne, caused by the human bacillus, or by the gastrointestinal tract and this is caused by the bovine type. In the lung, cavitation, pleurisy with effusion, pneumonia and bronchopleural fistula may be detected clinically. Hemoptysis and cough are the usual presenting symptoms. The diagnosis of the disease depends mainly on isolation of the organism from body fluids like sputum, urine and serous effusions. Radiology plays a major role to aid the diagnosis. Tuberculin test does not differentiate between active and dormant infection. Other organs affected are:

- Lymph nodes, especially the hilar and cervical groups. Cold abscesses are the usual presentation. Unlike hot abscesses, the tuberculous type does not heal without anti–tuberculous chemotherapy and evidence of scars may be seen on the neck. Collar stud abscess may present in many sites, especially the neck.
- Genitourinary tuberculosis: the kidney, urinary bladder and epididymis are affected; cystitis, with sterile pus in the urine, should alert the doctor for the diagnosis.
- Pott's disease of the spine: the infection starts in the vertebrae but the first radiological signs occur in the intervertebral disc. A paravertebral abscess may occur and may present itself as a psoas abscess. Pott's paraplegia is a known complication of the disease.
- Tuberculous meningitis: this usually causes irritability and restlessness.

Abdominal tuberculosis

This is the commonest type of the disease in many tropical countries, particularly in India and Africa. The site of predilection of the infection is the terminal ileum. Types of pathology include the following.

Hypertrophic ileocaecal tuberculosis   There is hypertrophy of the submucous and subserous layers and absence of caseation necrosis. Patients present with a painful lump in the right iliac fossa associated with fever and attacks of vomiting in 50% of them.

The differential diagnosis includes:
- Appendicular mass
- Carcinoma of caecum

- Amoebic granuloma
- Lymphogranuloma
- Iliac adenitis
- Paracolic and pericaecal abscess
- Crohn's disease
- Actinomycosis.

Ulcerating type   There are transverse ulcers with cascation which extend from the mucosa to the serosa of the large bowel. Perforations are rare but strictures occur in late cases. The clinical presentation of such patients is ill health and evidence of intestinal obstruction.

Radiological investigations usually show distended loops of bowel and multiple fluid levels. When diagnosis of abdominal tuberculosis is suspected, anti-tuberculous drugs can be started and response is observed in a short time. The drugs used are:
- Rifampicin 450–600 mg daily as a single dose orally.
- Isoniazid 150 mg daily is given with the above drug for a period of 10 months. These drugs are effective but they are expensive and the classical drugs, streptomycin 1 g daily for 3 months combined with para-amino salicylic acid (PAS) in a dose of 200 mg per kg daily and 300 mg isoniazid hydrochloride (INH) daily are used extensively with good results. Pyridoxine in a dose of 30 mg daily is used with the above combination to diminish peripheral neuropathy. This treatment is used for a period of two years.

Amoebiasis

This is a protozoal infection with a worldwide distribution. The amoebae live in the lumen of the large bowel and shed cysts in the stool. Symptoms from intestinal disease may vary from mild intermittent episodes of diarrhoea to a severe form known as:

Fatal necrotising colitis   The clinical findings may be confused with acute ulcerative or granulomatous colitis. Toxic dilatation and perforation of large bowel have been described with this condition.

Management of this complication requires early surgical intervention in addition to amoebicidal agents and intensive supportive treatment. Drugs effective against amoeba are:
- Metronidazole in a dose of 2 g once daily for 3 days or 750 mg 8 hourly for 5–10 days is the treatment of choice in the acute attack.
- Chloroquine phosphate in a dose of 1 g daily for 2 days followed by 500 mg daily for 2–3 weeks is effective.

Amoebic liver abscess   This invasive extraintestinal disease is usually diagnosed and managed medically. Metronidazole or emetine hydrochloride are effective in resolution of the abscess. Aspiration of the characteristic anchovy sauce fluid of the abscess under ultrasound or CT control is essential for diagnostic and therapeutic purposes. Surgical drainage is occasionally required if secondary pyogenic infection complicates the abscess. It should be remembered that amoebic liver abscesses may take up to 6 months for complete resolution to occur. Interestingly, 85% of Indian patients give a history of drinking Toddy (fermented palm juice) which contains large doses of *Entamoeba histolytica* and bacteria. Intraperitoneal rupture represents a secondary complication of liver abscess, the primary complication of intestinal amoebiasis.

Tropical ulcer

This is a superficial skin ulceration of uncertain aetiology and it is commonly associated with presence of *Bacillus fusiformis* and *Borrelia vincenti*. Possible aetiological factors for these ulcers are:

– Filth
– Food (malnutrition and vitamin deficiency)
– Friction (walking bare footed)
– Fusiform bacilli

To those 4 'Fs' local trauma can be added. Debilitating diseases like malaria are frequently existing. The organisms (*F. bacilli* and *B. vincenti*) are isolated from scrapings or slough of active ulcers. The sites commonly affected by tropical ulcer are the exposed parts of the limbs and body; the face is not involved.

Tropical ulcer grows slowly for weeks or months and it is usually very painful, sensitive and itchy. The ulcer has raised edges with a covering of grey, bloody pseudomembrane. Other ulcerative conditions which may be mixed with tropical ulcer are:

● Desert sore.
● Cutaneous diphtheria.
● Leishmaniasis.
● Mycosis.
● Varicose ulcer. In all these conditions evidence of the primary disease can be found.

Treatment of acute ulcer

It is known that removal of the patient from tropical to temperate climate is followed by rapid improvement. Before any local treatment is commenced, the ulcer must be thoroughly cleaned and necrotic material removed; this is done mechanically by use of soap and water. Many types of local antiseptics are effective; local and systemic antibiotics are indicated if there is severe acute inflammation with secondary infection.

Treatment of chronic ulcer

This is indolent to the above measures. Occlusive technique using adhesive tape or plaster for immobilisation gives satisfactory results. In some patients, excision of the ulcer and application of skin graft is required.

Brucellosis

This is an infection of domestic animals; it is caused by *Brucella abortus, B. suis* and *B. melitensis*. The infection yields a granuloma in many organs. The clinical picture is that of fever which is prolonged and tends to relapse. The patients are usually less toxic than individuals with typhoid fever. The spleen and liver are usually enlarged, lymphadenopathy is detected in many sites like the neck, axilla and groin. The surgeon may be consulted about those patients who complain of abdominal pain; this pain is felt in the area of the right hypochondrium as a result of liver involvement. Brucellosis may mimic cholecystitis, Hodgkin's disease and rarely appendicitis. Diagnosis depends on suspicion and isolation of bacteria from blood culture; if this is negative, serological tests

will be of considerable importance. A rising titre of haemagglutinins is diagnostic. Brucellosis should always be considered in postoperative patients with fever and as a possible cause of pyrexia of unknown origin. The condition can be treated by a combination of streptomycin 1 g daily and tetracycline 2 g daily for 3 weeks.

Mycetoma (madura foot)

This disease was discovered first in India. The causative organisms are:

● Maduromycetoma.
● Actinomycetoma.

Mycetoma is a chronic inflammatory lesion which contains granules; these are liable to discharge from multiple sinuses. According to the colour of the granules, madura is classified into white, yellow, red and black. Black madura does not respond to any drugs, unlike the others which respond favorably to many agents. Mode of transmission is direct inoculation of organisms which are commonly present in thorns. All sites of the body can be affected but the feet are involved in 60%. Mycetoma has affinity to fat and bones; muscles are resistant to the infection. Mycetoma is confined by facia and spreads along tissue planes, but later it breaks through them causing widespread infection. It is reported that mycetoma does not spread to lymph nodes. The cardinal features of mycetoma are:

● Swelling
● Multiple sinuses
● Discharge of granules

Mycetoma is usually painless and systemic disturbances are not encountered. Radiological appearances of mycetoma are characteristic and the diagnosis is easy. It is often possible to say with confidence what is the species of the infecting organism by looking at the X-rays.

Treatment

The choice of treatment depends on the type of madura.

● For **actinomycetoma**, chemotherapy and surgery are required.
● For **maduromycetoma**, conservative surgery or amputation are required. Chemotherapeutics agents used are dapsone given in a dose of 100 mg twice daily with 1 g streptomycin daily for a period of 9 months.

   Sulphamethoxazole, trimethoprim – 800 mg of the former and 160 mg of the latter is effective when used with streptomycin.

The principles of surgical management are: wide excision of the affected tissues in a bloodless field; general anaesthesia must be employed; madura operations should never be performed under local anaesthesia; amputation must be conservative as many patients do not accept radical surgery.

Trypanosomiasis

This disease is also known as sleeping sickness. It is prevalent in South America and has the name of 'Chagas' disease appended to it. It is caused by *Trypanosoma cruzi*. In Africa it is caused by *T. gambiense* and *T. rhodesiense*. The central nervous system is the primary site affected but other organs may be affected: lymph nodes, spleen, liver and myocardium are other sites for the infection. The surgeon may see the primary chancre which is the site of tsetse fly bite. Diagnosis of the condition depends on isolation of organisms from the chancre and from puncture of lymph glands. Suramin 1 g i.v in 10% of distilled water is the drug of choice, but care should be taken as it is toxic to the kidneys.

Cancrum oris

This is a severe form of stomatitis caused by *Borrelia vincentii* and *Fusiformis fusiformis*. It occurs in young malnourished children and as a complication of measles. Penicillin and local wound irrigation is the treatment of choice. Healing occurs with gross scarring; the scar tissue needs to be excised and the resulting defect repaired by a pedicle flap.

Ainhum

This is a peculiar disease of unknown aetiology; there is a constricting band in the interphalangeal joint of the fifth toe. There is severe pain and treatment is by Z-plasty or amputation of the affected part.

Leprosy

It is a chronic inflammatory disease caused by *Mycobacterium lepra*. 'Tuberculoid' and 'lepromatous' types are recognised. Skin and the nervous system are the primary sites affected. Diagnosis is by isolation of the organisms from skin smear and identifying them by Ziehl–Neelsen stain. Nerve biopsy is helpful; Lepromin test is a non-specific test. The nerves affected are the ulnar, radial, median, great auricular and common peroneal; most of these nerves can be palpated as thick cords. Dapsone 100 mg daily for 2–4 years is the drug of choice. Treatment is usually prolonged and up to 15 years may be needed for complete cure. Surgical management is sometimes needed for correction of deformities.

Sickle cell disease

Sickle cell disease is a blood abnormality due to persistence of haemoglobin S from fetal life. The pathology of sickle cell disease is due to vascular occlusion caused by the crystallised haemoglobin. The manifestations of the disease depend on the organs affected. Generalised lymphadenopathy, chronic leg ulcers, growth disturbances in children, (avascular necrosis of femoral heads can occur in children). Sudden onset of blindness is the most dramatic presentation of the disease. It is common in west Africa and many children in that area carry the trait. The disease imposes the following clinical problems:
- Difficulties in reaching the correct diagnosis.
- Anaesthetic complications prior to surgery.
- Marked predisposition to sepsis.
- Acute abdomen due to sickle cell crisis: the possibility of sickle cell crisis as a cause of acute abdomen should be considered; it is due to blockage of small vessels by sickle cell deposits resulting in ischaemia and hypoxia of the tissues. Infarcts of internal organs usually occur. Sickle cell

disease occurs in young people and it is rare above the age of 30 years. There may be history of previous attacks of jaundice. Abdominal crisis may be confused with:
- Acute intestinal obstruction.
- Ruptured ectopic pregnancy.
- Perforated peptic ulcer.

Surgery is not indicated when the diagnosis is known or suspected. A sickling test must be carried out before operating on young black patients with acute abdomen.

Burkitt's lymphoma

This is the commonest tumour seen in the paediatric age group. The aetiology of this tumour is obscure and it is linked with the Epstein–Barr virus; it is also more common in areas in which malaria is endemic. The tumour has a swift onset and is rapidly fatal if not treated.

The disease is usually multifocal and sites like abdominal viscera, retroperitoneal tissues and the central nervous system may be affected. It should also be noticed that the lymphoma can occur in any age. The jaw and maxilla are affected and adjacent structures are invaded early in the disease. Abdominal mass is a common presentation of the disease; neurological manifestations occur in 50% of patients with Burkitt's lymphoma. These manifestations vary from cranial nerve paralysis to limb paresis.

The diagnosis of Burkitt's lymphoma depends on the histological appearance of 'starry sky'. Treatment of the condition is by a combination of surgery and chemotherapy.

Keloids and hypertrophic scars

These are benign conditions due to proliferation of connective tissue. The keloids usually grow beyond the skin boundaries, unlike the hypertrophied scars which do not. Certain areas of the body are prone to keloid formation more than others. The type of trauma determines the extent of keloid formation; thermal injuries cause the worst type of keloids. Certain individuals are prone to keloid formation more than others and black people tend to get extra keloids. Many types of treatment have been attempted for keloids with some success. Partial or complete excision was successful in relevant cases; radiotherapy and chemotherapy by oral or local injections has also been attempted. A promising way of treatment is pressure application. All these combinations of treatment are used in different areas and by many surgeons.

Bites and stings

Animal and insect bites

Animal bites

The principles of management are fully discussed below for human bites. With animal bites the only potential danger is rabies. Knowledge of the biting animal's health is extremely important. If this is unknown, the treating doctor is faced with the decision of whether to start anti-rabies vaccine or not.

Snake bites

There are many species of poisonous snakes in different areas. Herpetologists are experienced in identification of poisonous snakes in their localities.

Viper bites result in the typical double puncture wounds made by the snake's fangs. Intense local reaction is shown by victims, and systemic manifestations of shock occur within a short time. First aid measures include killing of the snake without damage to the head; this helps herpetologists to identify the snake's species. The skin of the victim is incised and suction of the area is carried out, this removes a substantial amount of venom. A constricting band is applied above the site of the bite and a check on the distal pulses is done. Anti-venom is given according to the species of the snake.

Insect stings and bites

Stings (body tail ends) from spiders, bees, wasps and bites from ants (mouth piece or jaws) may be severe and produce anaphylactic shock. Death has been reported from some of these bites.

Marine animal bites and stings

Jelly fish and spiny venomous marine species inflict bites which are extremely painful. Heat application destroys the venom. Treatment is aimed at combating venom effect by applying heat, pain by analgesics, and secondary infection by antibiotics.

Human bites

These bites can be penetrating or avulsive in nature; they are commonly seen days after infliction of the injury when home remedies fail and wounds become infected.

Treatment Aggressive cleansing, removal of foreign bodies and debridement should be the aim of the management. Wounds of the face heal well after the above treatment and primary closure. Since human saliva is contaminated with many organisms, prophylactic antibiotics are advisable; they must be effective against streptococci and staphylococci.

Spectrum and presentation While human bites are classified here with other bites and stings, they are by no means tropical conditions. Human bites are an important clinical entity encountered commonly in the trauma surgery at the Accident and Emergency department as well as in general practice.

Human bites represent a spectrum of conditions and therefore merit some detailed discussion. They can take many forms:

- Means of defence, by biting the opponent or inflicted by punching the mouth of attacker (clenched fist injury).
- Means of attack, by lacerating bite injuries during violence.
- Passionate love bites – can be traumatic too, and represent the softest extreme of the human bite spectrum.
- Clinical vampirism and pseudo-vampirism (biting and blood sucking).

- Cannibalism (biting and eating human flesh) represents the violent extreme of the human bite spectrum. This primitive habit is practised on a sacramental basis paying respect to the spirit of the dead by cooking their flesh and distributing soup to all members of the tribe (absorbing and distributing the spirit among them).

The human bite was first described by Hultgen in 1910, who drew attention to human bites in the medical literature. As a pathological entity, however, it was described first in 1930. By 1942, about 790 cases had been reviewed; the violence was considered both as a means of defence and as a method of attack. Curtin and Greeley (1961) illustrated an avulsion in the tip of the tongue and a laceration of the lower lip in two negroes bitten passionately by their girlfriends. The clear description was reported in 1979 by Tomasetti *et al.* in a study of 25 cases of human bites of the face, of which five were due to passion.

Al-Fallouji (1990) described 7 cases of traumatic love bites and highlighted the varieties of the human bites spectrum; he reported one case of epidermoid mass of the neck (with a broken plastic tooth inside after love-making with a woman dressed as a vampire at a Halloween party!), one of abscess of the neck, one breast abscess, one avulsion of nipple and 2 cases of cellulitis of the neck.

The virulent nature of human biting stems from the fact that the oral cavity harbours a wide range of bacterial flora, with α-haemolytic Streptococci and Bacteroides species being the most frequent isolates. Human bites are potentially infective and serious. Indeed, death has been reported due to septicaemia after a pyogenic arthritis caused by a clenched fist injury. Antibiotic cover should be routinely administered in all human bite wounds. Tetanus prophylaxis is important; the assertion that tetanus cannot be transferred by human bites is untenable. A 7-day course of oral metronidazole and flucloxacillin together with tetanus prophylaxis is satisfactory in the majority of cases. Abscesses must be incised and drained (pus usually grow Bacteroides and *Staphylococcus pyogenes* or *epidermidis*). Masses on the neck must be excised, since they may harbour a foreign body inside. Bleeding neck can be cleansed thoroughly and a pressure dressing can be applied. Rarely, surgical reconstruction is needed for deep extensive laceration, or avulsion of nipple, ear, tongue tip, or lower lip.

Clinical vampirism Vampirism has been reported in patients with personality disorders such as schizophrenics and sadists whilst committing a sexual or aggressive act (with or without blood-sucking) on a dead or dying person. This is in contrast to mythical vampirism in which the dead feed on the living. However, in the French literature a strange masochistic phenomenon of auto-vampirism has been reported. Two cases were reported. One patient used to cut his neck veins with a knife whilst in front of a mirror, tilting his head, allowing the blood to trickle on to his cheek and sucking it. Another patient in the hospital used to enjoy pulling out her venous line repeatedly, watching the blood flow freely and sucking it.

In Al-Fallouji's series, the cervical mass and the bleeding neck represent pseudo-vampirism rather than real vampirism, i.e. the bleeding inflicted during biting was accidental and not intentional.

Biting with blood sucking (vampirism) is one of the most gruesome superstitions in the world; it originates from Slavonic

can be displayed on an oscilloscope or photographic paper. The picture obtained cannot be relied on to demonstrate detailed anatomy but since IS is based on count density which can be measured against time it readily lends itself to functional or dynamic studies of the target organ. Using computer analysis, graphs and histograms can present measurements of function in a readily understandable form.

Bone scanning

^{99m}Tc attached to a radionuclide vehicle such as methylene diphosphonate is taken up by bone. In conjunction with normal X-rays it can be used to detect bony metastases from the lung and breast and prostatic primary malignancies. It is also of value in the early detection of osteomyelitis and the diagnosis of Perthes' disease and stress fractures. In these clinical situations detailed anatomical display is unnecessary.

Isotope kidney scanning

Conventional intravenous urography not only gives a suitable anatomical display of the kidney, collecting system and bladder but also provides information about renal function. IS can also give anatomical information but its particular value is in measuring differential renal function. Using technetium-labelled DPTA, perfusion images of the renal arteries can be obtained along with the transit time of the isotope through the renal parenchyma and pelvis separately. Using a computer, differential renal function can be plotted graphically. In a similar manner differential perfusion images of the cerebral hemispheres can be obtained.

Localisation of endocrine tumours

^{75}Se-selenonorcholestrol has been used to differentiate bilateral adrenal hyperplasia from adrenal adenoma. Normal or hyperplastic adrenal glands take up the isotope but with unilateral adenoma the abnormal gland takes up the radionuclide but the normal side is suppressed. Technetium-thallium subtraction imaging is the most sensitive method of localising parathyroid adenomas.

NUCLEAR MAGNETIC RESONANCE (NMR)

NMR imaging device is a large and often a very powerful magnet, capable of accepting the whole body. There are two types of electromagnet depending on the type of core – air or iron. An iron core magnet consists of a large central metal C- or H-shaped block of iron around which the current-carrying coils are wound. Air core magnets are either resistive (copper or aluminium windings) or superconducting (niobium/titanium embedded in copper and submerged in liquid helium). The resultant nuclear magnetism along the direction of the applied field involves nuclei containing an odd number of protons, mainly that of hydrogen (protons).

The main medical indications for the use of NMR imaging are:
- mainly in head scanning in the diagnosis of intracranial meningiomas, particularly when used with CT scan;
- to image the pituitary gland and the ocular orbit;

- site-specific definition of the demyelinating plaques of multiple sclerosis (NMR is the only imaging method capable of this);
- evaluation of ischaemic heart disease, differential diagnosis of cardiomyopathies, evaluation of pericardial disease, neoplastic disease and congenital heart disease.

Biological effects of NMR include:
- static magnetic field inducing significant changes (but no long-lasting hazardous bioeffects) in blood composition, alterations in normal growth, changes in physical activity, alterations in neural function and the augmentation of the amplitude of the T wave of the ECG;
- gradient magnetic fields inducing electric current in a conductor (like a dynamo) which is a potential source of harmful effects, since small currents in nerve fibres may cause muscle contraction, such as ventricular fibrillation;
- pulsed radiofrequency fields, which may induce thermal changes;
- possible hazard to patients with ferromagnetic prostheses undergoing NMR; however, heating of these objects is not believed to be a significant hazard.

INTERVENTIONAL RADIOLOGY

In parallel with non-invasive diagnostic techniques, a variety of invasive percutaneous procedures have been developed. These enable the radiologist to provide the clinician with tissue, cytological and microbiological specimens as well as to carry out a broad spectrum of therapeutic procedures.

The surgeon should familiarise himself with these recent advances and be aware of their availability within the hospital or region. The therapeutic and diagnostic techniques performed by the interventional radiologist encroach on the traditional territory of the surgeon. The most appropriate method of diagnosis and treatment of certain conditions requires close cooperation between surgeon and radiologist since they may benefit the patient by avoiding a traditional surgical procedure. Not only do the patient and surgeon benefit, but in-patient time can be minimised with subsequent benefit to the health-care budget.

Percutaneous biopsy

Percutaneous biopsy using fine-bore needles guided by ultrasound or CT imaging has enabled biopsy specimens to be obtained from areas previously only accessible to the surgeon. Percutaneous needle biopsy of lung lesions, abdominal and retroperitoneal masses and pelvic viscera is now well established. Laparotomy, laparoscopy, thoracotomy, mediastinoscopy and craniotomy may all be obviated. In the presence of coagulation disorders the radiologist can biopsy the liver by the transjugular route.

Drainage and extraction procedures

The obstructed urinary tract

The percutaneous placement of a pigtailed catheter into the obstructed pelvicalyceal system under local anaesthesia may circumvent the need for an open surgical operation in a severely ill patient with electrolyte and acid–base disturbance. Percutaneous nephrostomy is of particular benefit in cases of bilateral obstructive uropathy, the obstructed unilateral kidney or the transplanted kidney. Following percutaneous nephrostomy, microbiological and cytological specimens can be taken and antegrade pyelography carried out. The repertoire of the radiologist can extend to the removal of calculi using a steerable catheter and basket retrieval system, the dilatation of strictures using a balloon catheter and the placement of permanent ureteral stents.

Decompression of the kidney may allow the recovery of renal function and the correction of metabolic disturbances. The cause of the obstruction may have meanwhile resolved spontaneously (the passage of a stone) or may have been improved by non-surgical treatment (radiotherapy, chemotherapy or hormone manipulation) and in these cases operation may be avoided entirely. In other cases the patient may have been rendered fit for anaesthesia and an open operation.

Jaundice and gallstones

Preoperative biliary drainage

In the jaundiced patient who is seriously ill, a period of preoperative biliary drainage to allow the recovery of hepatic function prior to surgery seems theoretically advantageous. Percutaneous drainage is currently being evaluated (probably of no value).

The residual common bile duct stone

The retained common bile duct stone after choledochotomy, which previously could only be tackled by reoperation, can now be treated by endoscopic methods and by the interventional radiologist. Both methods are safer than surgery. If a T-tube is still in situ and a stone is demonstrated in the common bile duct, the tube is left for 6 weeks until a fibrous track to the skin has matured. Using a steerable catheter and basket retrieval system the stone may then be removed. In a patient without a T-tube and in whom endoscopic retrograde cholangiopancreatography is contraindicated, the radiologist can still gain access to the common bile duct by a percutaneous transhepatic approach.

Percutaneous transhepatic prosthetic (stent) insertion (in unfit jaundiced patients)

The removal of foreign bodies

Upper gastrointestinal foreign bodies and those in the intravascular compartment (e.g. catheter tips) have been removed successfully by the interventional radiologist.

Intraperitoneal abscess localisation and drainage

Using abdominal ultrasound guide and needle aspiration under X-ray screening by the radiologist (not surgeon).

Vascular disorders

Percutaneous transluminal balloon angioplasty

Recent advances in balloon catheter technology have allowed the relatively safe dilatation of arterial stenoses and the technique of transluminal balloon angioplasty is now firmly established in the management of peripheral ischaemia, renal artery stenosis and coronary artery disease. The restoration of circulation to ischaemic limbs may be successful in circumventing the need for endarterectomy or bypass surgery under general anaesthesia and may salvage limbs in patients unfit for anaesthesia. Angioplasty of the coronary arteries will prevent the need for thoracotomy or sternotomy.

Percutaneous intraluminal stent insertion Across the stenosis after dilatation is being performed by radiologists or vascular surgeons. Intraluminal stenting of leaking aortic aneurysms or of those unfit for major surgery represents a major development.

Venous thrombosis and pulmonary embolism

In the management of the poor-risk patient with iliofemoral thrombosis and in patients where anticoagulants have failed or are contraindicated, the interruption of the inferior vena cava to prevent pulmonary embolism can be achieved by the placement of an umbrella filter proximal to the thrombus via the transjugular approach.

Massive pulmonary embolus is also amenable to treatment without recourse to surgical embolectomy. Utilising the percutaneous transjugular or femoral approach a catheter can be steered into the pulmonary artery via the right heart. The embolus can either be dislodged into more peripheral segments of the artery or extracted using a suction cup. Following embolectomy an umbrella filter can be placed in the inferior vena cava.

Acute arterial bleeding

Therapeutic embolisation of the arterial tree is a major advance in the management of the poor-risk patient with surgical bleeding. Following the selective catheterisation of the appropriate vessel, absorbable or non-absorbable emboli are injected into the artery. Bleeding from tumours, gastrointestinal and urological lesions, fractures, ruptured viscera, aneurysm and biopsy sites has been controlled successfully in this manner. Provided there is sufficient collateral circulation there is little danger to other viscera.

Bleeding oesophageal varices

In addition to balloon tamponade, injection sclerotherapy, vasopressin infusion and various surgical portasystemic disconnection procedures, the interventional radiologist has added another method of control of variceal bleeding. Via a transhepatic or jugular approach, the portal venous system can be entered and the varices occluded by embolisation.

Arteriovenous malformations

The surgery of arteriovenous malformations may be difficult because of their anatomical position and the difficulty is compounded by their vascularity. Surgery may also be impermanent because of subsequent enlargement of collateral vessels. Embolisation of arteriovenous malformations has been used both as a definitive method of treatment and as a method of reducing vascularity prior to definitive surgery.

In neurosurgical practice a variety of lesions have been treated by this method. Previously, flowguided embolisation of vessels was the only method of therapy but more recent advances have improved the accuracy of the procedure. The introduction of fine flexible catheters now allows the selective catheterisation of cortical vessels and the more accurate placement of emboli. Sophisticated balloon catheters have also been developed which facilitate hyperselective catheterisation of vessels and make flow-guided embolisation less hazardous by preventing aberrant embolisation.

The management of tumours

Preoperative embolisation

Embolisation of certain tumours preoperatively may be of benefit. Not only is the vascularity of the neoplasm reduced, helping to prevent operative blood loss, but the chance of tumour emboli being thrown off by operative handling may be reduced. Some authors maintain there is a theoretical advantage of provoking an immune response against the tumour cells as a result of tumour cell necrosis and the release of their specific antigens.

Palliation of neoplasms

The benefit of pain relief and reduction of haemorrhage from inoperable neoplasms has ensured therapeutic embolisation a place in the palliation of malignant disease. Embolisation of hormone-producing tumours is of value in that the distressing endocrine effects, e.g. sweats, palpitations and diarrhoea in the carcinoid syndrome, can be reduced.

Endocrine ablation

It is now possible to infarct the adrenal gland by the occlusion of adrenal veins using percutaneous embolisation. This has proved to be useful in the management of Cushing's syndrome. It may acquire a place in the management of advanced breast cancer in preference to medical adrenalectomy using aminoglutethimide which is toxic or surgical adrenalectomy which is a major surgical procedure.

Conclusions

Interventional radiological techniques have become firmly established in the management of surgical patients. Their scope will increase as radiologists with the necessary technical expertise are trained. This brief account of just some of the exciting developments in the field will it is hoped spur the Fellowship candidate on to investigate the subject more thoroughly and to become aware of the benefits that are likely for the patient and the surgeon. An account of catheter technology and precise accounts of the procedures can be found in the further reading list.

1.21 Clinical Implications of Contraceptive Pills in Surgery

The contraceptive pill is not free from major side-effects. These include the following.
- Thromboembolism is four times more likely to occur than in non-pill takers. This may be:
  - Venous thrombosis (unrelated to the period of pill use) – in superficial veins (proportional to age and parity), in deep veins and in pulmonary embolism.
  - Arterial thrombosis in both coronary and cerebral arteries. The predisposing factors are: oestrogen dose in the pill; age; cigarette smoking; obesity; other conditions such as diabetes, hypertension and familial hyperlipidaemia.
- Cardiovascular complications such as myocardial infarction – hypertension due to salt and water retention – obesity and cardiac failure.
- Gastrointestinal side-effects: abdominal bloating, persistent nausea, vomiting and weight gain. Breakthrough or withdrawal bleeding may sometimes mimic acute abdomen.
- Cholestatic jaundice with lithogenic bile. Gallbladder disease is common in postpartum primiparas who were pre-pregnancy pill takers.
- The hepatobiliary lesions attributed to anabolic steroids and/ or the contraceptive pill are:
  - Cholestasis – both
  - Gallbladder disease – contraceptive pill
  - Liver tumours and nodules – both
  - Budd–Chiari syndrome – contraceptive pill
  - Peliosis hepatis (blood-filled cysts in the liver parenchyma) – anabolic steroids
  - Sinusoidal dilatation – contraceptive pill
- Breast pains and stimulation of fibroadenosis of the breast. The contraceptive pill may activate breast carcinoma and provokes galactorrhoea in females and gynaecomastia in males.
- Special medical problems, e.g. benign intracranial hypertension and erythema nodosum.
- Special surgical problems:
  - Carpal tunnel syndrome
  - Budd–Chiari syndrome (thrombosis of hepatic veins and portal hypertension)
  - Acute pancreatitis
  - Cholangiocarcinoma (no statistical support)
  - Acceleration of fibroid enlargement
  - Swollen painful legs
- Central nervous system side-effects such as stroke, severe migraine/headache and exacerbation of epilepsy. Anxiety and depression can also occur.
- Increased susceptibility to infections – vaginal candidiasis and even cervical erosions, and various skin conditions, e.g. pigmentation, eczema.
- Interferes with diagnostic tests for hydrocortisone assay, thyroxine level and serum iron because it increases the plasma binding proteins, giving false results.
- Drug interference, e.g. anti-tuberculous drugs, ampicillin and tetracyclines, and hypoglycaemic agents.

1.22 Psychological Implications in Surgical Practice

Psychological factors plays an important role in the pathogenesis of surgical disease, in the surgeon's decision-making choosing one surgical approach rather than another, and in perioperative patient morbidity. Indeed, many diseases can be viewed as psychosomatic with predominant psychological influence. Conversely, many surgical diseases can influence patient's psyche by the shocking diagnosis (e.g. cancer) or by the requirement of an operation (e.g. mastectomy for breast carcinoma in females and orchidectomy for testicular tumour in males). The psychological factor, therefore, can be discussed under the following headings.

Psychological aetiology and pathogenesis in surgical disease

Ulcerative colitis   In highly strung and introspective patients colitis attacks frequently coincide with periods of increased stress. Emotional influences can produce changes in colonic mucosa up to frank ulceration. Clinical improvement is sometimes encountered with psychotherapy. In one study, however, 86% denied any relationship to emotional trauma.

Chronic constipation and faecal impaction   The condition is common among inmates of mental asylums and patients of mental hospitals. This may be partially drug-induced constipation. Acute faecal impaction requires emergency evacuation under general anaesthesia, while chronic constipation may occasionally require resection/anastomosis surgery.

Secondary megacolon   This may result from psychological insult of children and requires early correction of emotional problems during surgical management. Rectal inertia in children may result in bowel overstretching with incomplete evacuation and overflow incontinence of fluid faeces around impacted mass. Late removal of underlying psychological cause at this stage may not result in cure, because secondary changes make the bowel physically unable to empty completely.

Complete rectal prolapse   Prolapse is specially liable to occur in patients suffering from mental disease, and rectal prolapse is found surprisingly amongst inmates of asylums. In a study, 33% of rectal prolapse patients were found to suffer some mental disorder, and 3% were definitely psychotic.

Pruritus ani   Mental strain, anxiety and overwork were incriminated by different patients for precipitating their attacks of pruritus.

Abdominal migraine   This non-specific abdominal pain has no underlying organic aetiology; it affects both adults and children. It constitutes 7% of all recurrent non-specific abdominal pain affecting 10–18% of children (mean age of 7.2 years). The condition is thought to have a psychological aetiology. The pain is in the midline; severe enough to prevent

normal activities (comparable in severity to a migraine headache); usually associated with pallor or flushing (vasomotor), nausea and vomiting; attacks last 2 hours with complete recovery between attacks; and there is a family history of migraine. Simultaneous migraine headache affects 58% of abdominal migraine cases, while abdominal migraine occurs in 25% of children presenting with migraine headache. Treatment is symptomatic by simple analgesia, bed rest in a dark room, reassurance and prevention of triggering stress if possible (excitement, such as a birthday party or trip to the beach may trigger abdominal migraine). Like adults with migraine headache, a prophylactic treatment with 5-hydroxytryptamine antagonist, pizotifin (1.5 mg orally once daily) is useful, but may take 10–20 days to act; it should be given on a regular basis.

Impotence   The cause may be psychogenic, arising from domestic and financial stresses; it must be differentiated from organic impotence (see s. 1.64 Impotence in surgery).

Psychological factors   Peptic ulcer exacerbation, hypertension and ischaemic heart disease can all have an important psychological element.

Psychosomatic disorders   Anorexia nervosa, obesity and pain are examples, of which the last two are implicated in surgical practice.

Psychosis-induced surgical problems

Injuries and violence   Addiction to alcohol or drugs causes psychological (and physical) dependence. The incidence of violence, crime and theft is very high among addicts, because of their demand for money to service their daily habit. Drug doses can cost £200 per day and addicts will sell all their possessions and kill for it. Also, such addicts cannot work when they are low and are more prone to injuries than non-addicts, either during withdrawal or because of drug-induced euphoria (in cocaine, heroin, morphine, and alcohol). Delusion of flying can lead to falls from a height. This is seen particularly in patients addicted to LSD (lysergic acid diethylamide). A psychotic patient may cut the flexor surface of their wrists with a razor or knife. Many self-inflicted wounds and ulcers were reported among patients with unstable psychiatric problems.

During travels, narcotic traffickers hide drugs by packing then in bags or condoms and swallowing them; these bags or condoms may sometimes burst, causing sudden collapse and death, or may cause obstruction. They must be removed endoscopically or extracted via open surgery. Smugglers, particularly poor Columbians and South Americans, may transport bags of narcotics such as crack cocaine (cocaine extracted from leaves planted in South America, processed as paste, dried into white powder, and percolated with sodium bicarbonate to make it into small rocks costing £25 or more each) by incising the skin of the thigh and implanting packets deep under subcutaneous tissue. This needs surgical removal under anaesthesia to be recovered as evidence to trace the origin of the drug once such traffickers are suspected after radiological scanning at the airport.

Heroin and morphine are taken i.v. or by heating the drug on tinfoil and snuffing the smoke with a straw intranasally ('*chasing the dragon*'); heroin and morphine addictions (common among doctors, nurses, pharmacists and dentists) are both treated by substitution with methadone after drug withdrawal to prevent abstinence syndrome. Cocaine (crack) surpassed heroin (also called smack) in 1987 as the biggest drug threat facing Britain; it is taken by snorting intranasally (snuffing via a straw or a tube lines of finely ground powder on a mirror is the most popular way to take cocaine), smoking of crack cocaine, or i.v. injection. Cocaine can cause toxic symptoms of formication (sensation of insects crawling under skin); it requires psychotherapy. LSD may result in suicidal injuries and can be cut short by chlorpromazine. Cannabis (hashish, marihuana, pot) is taken by smoking; it requires psychiatric treatment.

Treatment of alcoholism entails 'drying out', which may require hospitalisation; withdrawal symptoms are controlled by phenothiazines, diazepam, haloperidol or chlormethiazole.

Sexual deviation   Homosexuals, for example, are more vulnerable to transmission of diseases by i.v. injection, particularly AIDS and viral hepatitis. When such patients present with surgical conditions, they impose specific hazards to surgeons and theatre staff, and strict precautions must be adhered to during their surgery.

Surgical diseases resulting in psychiatric problems

Untreated surgical conditions may present to and be treated by psychiatrists. The following diseases are examples.
- Primary hyperparathyroidism: a disease of stones, bones, abdominal groans and psychic moans.
- Acute alcoholic pancreatitis requires life-long psychiatric follow-up.
- Terminal cases of carcinomatosis require TLC (tender loving care) and psychiatric support to endure pain and psychological trauma.
- Severe head injury may result in severe or moderate disability (see Glasgow Outcome Scale) and may need psychiatric assessment and follow-up.
- Organic psychosis may be seen during the course of physical illnesses or postoperative complications which either primarily or secondarily affect the brain. Organic psychosis can either be acute (delerium) or chronic (dementia). Atherosclerotic dementia may be treated surgically by carotid endarterectomy.

Psychological impact of diagnosis and communication with the patient

Clearly, the truth should be told. Any hope for the cure by surgery must be magnified and worked on. However, a diagnosis of cancer for example, may shock the patient psychologically, and should be discussed tactfully and sensibly with the patient, since this may result in depression; indeed, some patients may even commit suicide. A diagnosis of cancer must often be told in the first instance to the relatives and those attending the patient. The diagnosis, however, must be disclosed if the patient is very inquisitive or asks a leading question demanding a specific true answer. Many authorities feel that cancer is the patient's and not the relatives' disease and must be told to the patient always to ensure compliance in treatment later on. Even then, the surgeon should tactfully explain that the cancer may be early and likely to be removed by surgery with good prognosis. Cancer, like all other diseases, is treatable and survival may even be better than many so-called benign diseases. In fact, it may be better to have cancer of skin, bladder, uterus, or thyroid rather than having Crohn's disease of the bowel, chronic pancreatitis or severe low back pain. Death is the natural course of all living creatures, and a treated patient (with cancer) may live long to die from other causes, such as a car accident or heart disease; in such cases, the cancer is considered technically controlled.

However, some surgeons believe that telling the truth from the start may encourage the patient to undergo surgery, take chemotherapy, attend the outpatient clinic regularly and become more involved than the surgeon in fighting the disease.

Careful explanation of the diagnosis and its surgical treatment with postoperative consequences must be conveyed to patient tactfully in a non-committal way, because the patient may develop postoperative anxiety due to a contrast between personal expectations from the operation and what the surgeon has aimed to achieve. A senior member of the team should discuss the diagnosis with the patient in the presence of relatives; privacy should be maximised (if the patient is on the ward then a separate room should be used); interruptions should be minimised (divert the phone and leave your bleep/pager with a colleague); support should be arranged with the ward nurse and/or Macmillan specialist nurse. The patient's GP must be informed as soon as possible regarding what has been said and the patient's reaction to it.

In teaching ward rounds, it is better to avoid bedside discussion in front of the patient on sensitive subjects, such as tumours, amputation and terminal care to avoid psychological trauma and the patient's misunderstanding of medical terminology. Parents may object, for example, to hearing their child called 'Mongol': it is better to refer to Down's syndrome. It was reported that a medical student performed per vaginal examination on a pregnant woman and shouted 'I can't feel the fetal head?', causing the woman to collapse because she thought her baby was congenitally malformed. Furthermore, patients must not be treated as interesting cases for students; the patient's permission must be sought tactfully with prior polite introduction of students or junior doctors before embarking on teaching or clinical examination, which should be gentle (the patient comes first).

Perioperative psychiatric problems

Preoperative apprehension   All patients are anxious before operation (preoperative fear of death under anaesthesia and while undergoing operation); preoperative explanation, premedications prior to surgery and mixing with similar patients (people in the same boat) may relieve psychological trauma immensely. A calm and reassuring approach by ward staff and a truthful explanation of what lies ahead can do much to allay fear. Tranquillisers are necessary. If preoperative anxiety is excessive, operation should be postponed until a full psychiatric assessment has been made. It must be remembered that psychiatric patients develop the same surgical diseases as the general population. On the other hand, some hysterical patients produce a bewildering variety of symptoms in the hope of persuading a surgeon to operate.

Munchausen's syndrome is a condition characterised by habitual presentation for hospital treatment of an apparent acute illness, the patient giving a plausible and dramatic history, all of which is false. Some may undergo many operations, all with normal findings; multiple negative laparotomies may become the source of adhesions and real postoperative abdominal pain which may be difficult to verify whether it is psychological or organic in nature. If careful investigation fails to elicit organic disease, a psychiatric opinion should be sought. Once these patients are diagnosed as 'malingerers', their names must be dispatched to all nearby district hospitals to warn them, so they take precautions before embarking on unnecessary treatment by surgery, wasting their time, money and resources.

Patients with abnormal psychiatric behaviour or a history of psychiatric disorder need careful assessment by a psychiatrist during pre- and postoperative periods. This should be undertaken with the surgeon. Drug therapy should be interrupted as little as possible during operation. Patients with suicidal and aggressive tendencies may require special supervision during their stay in a general hospital.

Metabolic response   The response to surgical trauma may be accentuated by psychological fear of the patient on seeing physical findings of bleeding, burnt tissue and compound fracture in shock states. Pain relief may improve emotions and modify the metabolic response.

Postoperative psychosis   May be due to electrolyte imbalance, or may be drug-induced after anaesthesia. Occasionally, postoperative confusion may result in the patient's fall from bed causing head injury which in turn results in more confusion.

The management of postoperative mental disturbance requires recognition and treatment of precipitating factors, a sympathetic, calm and orderly approach to the patient, and if necessary sedation with diazepam (Valium) 15–30 mg daily in divided doses or 10 mg i.m. repeated in 4 h, or with chlorpromazine (Largactil) starting with 25 mg orally three times daily, or 100 mg by suppository or 25–50 mg i.m. Antidepressant therapy should not be given without psychiatric advice.

When treating mentally disturbed patients the following factors should be kept in mind:
1. Elderly patients in a strange environment often become disorientated, particularly at night. Adequate light and a sympathetic approach may be all that is necessary to settle them.
2. Disorientation may, however, reflect hypoxia and may then be resolved with oxygen and respiratory care.
3. Acute urinary retention in the elderly may cause abnormal behaviour. Catheterisation of the distended bladder will give relief.
4. Mental changes – 'toxic psychosis' – occur in septicaemia and may be the first sign of septicaemic shock. Patients who become confused must be examined for evidence of chest, wound or urinary tract infection. If an intestinal anastomosis has been performed, leakage should be suspected.
5. Postoperative disorientation can occur from withdrawal of alcohol. Excessive alcohol intake may not have been suspected preoperatively or may be denied by the patient. If in doubt, relatives should be consulted and treatment instituted as appropriate.

Postoperative pain   Preoperative explanation and reassurance that such pain is a natural response to surgery and will disappear gradually with recovery can partially reduce the experience of postoperative pain. It has been shown that past experience, good or bad, of postoperative pain relief can affect later experiences. A patient who has had good postoperative pain relief in the past may react very differently to the prospect of surgery from someone who has had poor relief. Attitudes of nursing and medical staff, responses of other patients to pain and the ward environment have been shown to be major factors in the response to pain.

Breast surgery   Breast conservation surgery causes less cosmetic damage than mastectomy. However, psychological effects are not necessarily less than after mastectomy. Psychological problems are common and may occur late. Around a third of women still suffer anxiety and/or depression 2 years after initial treatment, often in relation to deterioration and altered body image, sexual problems and problems with role and resumption of social and work activity. In a study of 101 cases up to 2 years after randomisation to mastectomy or breast-conserving operation women expressed no strong preference for one or other treatment before surgery. Anxiety, depression or both were present in 38% of all women who had undergone lumpectomy compared with 33% of those who had a mastectomy. Those who had a lumpectomy were more fearful of a recurrence, often checking their breasts compulsively for lumps, while those who had had a mastectomy tended to worry about the effect of operation on their relationships and appearance. Over half of women felt that they had been given inadequate information about their illness and its treatment and these women were more prone to anxiety and depression. Women who had been allowed to choose their treatment, or had refused randomisation, might have suffered less, but the study nevertheless questions whether conserving the breast lessens psychological impact of surgery for women with an early cancer.

Psychological support must be offered during and after treatment, but may be difficult to provide in the rushed atmosphere of a busy hospital outpatient clinic. Routine hospital follow-up reassures some patients but for others it may heighten anxiety. Elementary measures to ameliorate the anxiety of follow-up include continuity of care and an appointments system that avoids long delays in crowded waiting rooms. Breast clinics should have a full-time counsellor who is adequately trained. Sympathetic attention should be paid to provision of prosthesls for women who have a mastectomy. Doctors should try to identify patients who may be at risk of serious psychological morbidity, such as those with a history of depression or who lack a network of family support. Liaison with a psychiatrist should be readily available if serious problems are found. A sensitive general practitioner and primary health care team can do much to help the patient and her family. Some surgeries have set up community-based cancer support groups, and all patients should be given information about local and national self-help groups.

Stoma patients   Such patients may suffer from the psychological trauma of the underlying disease (cancer), or from the stoma being an artificially created anus or urinary stoma, making the patient different from other people, or perceiving the stoma as being an interference with the patient's cleanliness, which can cause particular problems for adherents of certain religions. This requires psychological support and the creation of ileostomy support groups, allowing the patient to mix with others who find themselves with similar problems.

Terminal cancer patients

Severe intractable pain, particularly in terminal cancer patients, may be alleviated by various surgical procedures, such as nerve section, sympathectomy (for visceral pain), myelotomy to section spinothalamic fibres in anterior white commissure, posterior rhizotomy, anterolateral cordotomy (knife inserted into lateral aspect of spinal cord and swept anteriorly to cut lateral spinothalamic tract pain fibres while leaving ventral spinothalamic tract touch fibres intact), medullary tractotomy, mesencephalic tractotomy, thalamotomy (thalamic injury may result in thalamic syndrome with peculiar prolonged, severe and very unpleasant pain as an over-reaction to minor painful stimuli or even spontaneously without external stimuli), gyrectomy, or prefrontal lobotomy (postoperatively patients report that they feel pain but it does not bother them, so pain is dissociated from its unpleasant subjective affect).

Psychiatric disorders amenable to surgery

Surgery for mental disorder was discredited by indiscriminate use of frontal leucotomy in the past, but now it is regaining its reputation. Surgery is only recommended after frank discussion with patient and relatives and after full cooperation between the referring psychiatrist and surgeon. Intractable anxiety states which do not respond to medical treatment may be improved by discrete stereotactic leucotomy which interrupts white matter pathways from the limbic system.

Aggressive disorders, particularly when associated with temporal lobe epilepsy, may respond to stereotactic amygdalotomy. Severe hyperactivity is difficult to manage, but stereotactic hypothalotomy is sometimes useful.

Intensive care unit (ICU) syndrome

This encapsulates some physical effects (body fatigue, reluctance to move or feeling unable to move, and pain) and striking behavioural/psychological changes of a distinct pattern manifested by an asymptomatic lucid period of 0–2 days following ICU admission, mild psychosis (confusion/anxiety)

on days 2–4, severe psychosis (hallucination/fear/panic/anger/disorientation to time and place) on day 4–discharge, and finally recovery (usually asymptomatic but occasionally dreams/nightmares) on or after discharge. Contributing factors include certain pathophysiological disorders in critically ill patients such as hypoxia/renal dysfunction. However, the ICU environment is alien to most patients who find themselves, unexpectedly, surrounded by many strange and noisy machines, tubes, and nursing staff. Separation from both partners and family (unable to touch or talk to patient because of muscle relaxation and ventilation) is another factor. Constant interventions through monitoring by staff (particularly medical, nursing and physiotherapy) during the day and night may deprive the patient of mental and physical rest needed for recuperation. Endotracheal intubation may be distressing (when patients are being turned or during endotracheal suction) and may prevent communication with staff. The ICU is a noisy environment, frequently exceeding 50 decibels, a level which would wake a person; noise levels of 70 decibels are as high as the equivalent of a busy street in London. If patients overhear staff conversations which are then misinterpreted, this may increase patients' anxiety about prognosis. Windowless ICUs were found to be less pleasant than ICUs with large windows. Drugs and sedation may further contribute to confusion and hallucinations. The use of paralysing agents in management of ventilated patients is becoming less common; however increased use of invasive measures (e.g. arterial monitoring, venous access) as well as ventilatory tubes, various catheters and ECG leads, may all immobilise ICU patients. Consequently, ICU patients feel helpless and more afraid, being less able to interpret their surroundings.

Prevention of ICU syndrome includes communication using paper and pen, keyword boards, and keyboards that may help alleviate patient frustration at not being understood by clinicians. Clinicians should communicate and give a full explanation before commencing a procedure. Another non-verbal communication is the use of clinical touch which can be defined as either functional (staff touching patients during clinical procedures which can be painful) or therapeutic touch (not related to any procedure) as a strategy to provide gentle touch to socially acceptable areas on a patient's body. This reduces the patient's anxiety. However, there is a danger that ICU staff may go to the extreme by constantly talking to and touching patients; a balance needs to be found between patient survival and recovery.

1.23 Terminal Care in Surgery

The terminal stage of any illness can be defined as beginning at the moment when the clinician says 'There is nothing more to be done' and then begins to withdraw from his patient. At this stage the patient can be managed in hospital, home or hospice. The aims of the palliation are:
- To restore the quality of living (symptom control).
- To take the fear out of dying (spiritual support).

Pain

Terminal cases due to cancer form the majority and about 87% of these patients have pain as the main complaint. Malignancy can produce pain by many mechanisms:

- Nerve compression by tumour or pathological fracture caused by the tumour bony metastases (sharp well-localised pain).
- Infiltration of nerve or blood vessel or their perineural or perivascular lymphatics or lymphoedema (diffuse burning, sympathetic).
- Gastrointestinal or genitourinary tract involvement and obstruction (either dull diffuse colicky or burning, as in cystitis).
- Vascular obstruction by tumour (ischaemic or venous engorgement).
- Tension and distension pain due to tumour infiltration of bones and closely investing fascia, and periosteum (pain-sensitive structures).
- Central necrosis and infection.
- Headache due to raised intracranial pressure.

Pain in advanced cancer is constant, and analgesics should be given at 4 h intervals on a regular basis and not *pro re nate* (PRN). Prescriptions are illogical and lead to inadequate pain control and possible consequent tolerance. Opiate addiction does not occur in chronic severe pain and would be immaterial in dying patients. Dose increase, however, indicates a change in the underlying pathology and not the development of tolerance. The oral route is preferred and injections should only be necessary during the last few days of life.

Analgesics

Peripherally acting non-narcotic analgesics

The effectiveness of aspirin (300–600 mg after food) or paracetamol (500–1000 mg tablets 4-hourly) should not be underestimated. However, osseous deposits (in carcinoma of the breast, bronchus, thyroid and multiple myeloma) produce severe bone pain through release of prostaglandins. Since non-steroidal anti-inflammatory drugs (NSAIDs) are potent prostaglandin synthetase inhibitors, they are effective in bone pain relief, e.g. diflunisal (Dolobid) 250 mg 12-hourly, salsalate (Disalcid) 500 mg 8-hourly or indomethacin sustained release (Indocid) 75 mg 24-hourly. Corticosteroids, although they modulate the inflammatory process by preventing prostaglandin release (stabilise cell membranes), are effective in relieving pain caused by nerve compression but not in relieving bony pain.

Centrally acting drugs

The following drugs, given in 4-hourly oral regular doses, can be extremely effective:

Non-narcotics
- Buprenorphine
- Nefopam

Weak narcotics
- Dihydrocodeine (DF 118) 10 mg
- Dihydrocodeine combined with paracetomol (Paramol 118) – contraindicated in asthma and liver dysfunction

- Dextropropoxyphene (Doloxene) 100 mg – causes drowsiness
- Dextropropoxyphene combined with paracetamol (Distalgesic)
- Aspirin and papaveretum

Strong narcotics may, however, be needed:
- Phenazocine 10 mg sublingually 6-hourly
- Morphine slow-release tablet (MST Continus) 10 mg 12-hourly
- Diamorphine i.m. or orally in chloroform water 4-hourly. Diamorphine (heroin) is the preferred opioid since its high solubility permits a large dose to be given in a small volume. Its euphoric action is necessary for mood elevation in depressed terminal patients. Diamorphine syringe driven pumps are preferable.

When dysphagia, intestinal obstruction and persistent vomiting present, one of three *suppositories* is the choice:
- Morphine hydrochloride 10, 30 or 60 mg
- Oxycodone pectinate 30 mg
- Dextromoramide 10 mg

Morphine and diamorphine are probably the best *injectable analgesics*.

Sublingual analgesics include:
- Dextromoramide 5 or 10 mg
- Phenazocine 5 mg
- Buprenorphine 0.2 mg
- Diamorphine hypodermic tablet 10 mg

Note that a syringe driver can give continuous i.v. infusion in chronic pain. The patient can keep the syringe in a pocket and move around without pain. It is becoming an increasingly popular method since it:
- Maintains plasma level of narcotics, antiemetics and phenothiazine.
- Reduces injections to once daily or on alternate days.
- Reloads 12- or 24-hourly.
- Dosage as for i.m./subcutaneous injection.

Terminal cases in children

Oral weak narcotic analgesics should be administered. Diamorphine can result in excessive sedation and problems in withdrawal should the child go into remission. They should be nursed at home with supportive care from the family and general practitioner. Hospital can provide advice when necessary.

Analgesics to be avoided

Too short effect
- Dextromoramide
- Pethidine (any route)

Too many side-effects
- Pethidine
- Pentazocine (unacceptable dysphoria)
- Levorphanol

Unpredictable analgesics (no place in chronic pain)
- Pethidine
- Pentazocine

Bad mixtures
- Diconal (dipipanone + cyclizine) (profound sedation)
- Nepenthe and aspirin
- Brompton cocktail (contains cocaine and chlorpromazine – a pharmacological nonsense)

Inappropriate use (inadequate dose/ inappropriate drug)
- Partial antagonist used with agonist (partial antagonists are pentazocine, phenazocine and buprenorphine).
- Not given according to duration of action.
- Prostaglandin inhibitors not given for bone metastases.
- Inadequate use of narcotic potentiators.

Non-drug methods

May need sophisticated equipment and technical expertise. Such facilities (discussed in s. 1.2 above, see 'General principles') are available in pain clinics (found in special directory).
- Secondary deposits can be treated with radiation or short or single doses of chemotherapy.
- Pathological fractures are a common source of pain and are best treated by fixation (plaster of Paris or preferably internal).
- Visceral upper abdominal pain (intra-abdominal cancer) can be relieved by coeliac plexus destructive block (alcohol or phenol).
- Unilateral pain below C6 level can be treated by contralateral cordotomy.
- Bilateral or midline pain is relieved by pituitary ablation.

Nausea and vomiting

Nausea and vomiting have different causes and are therefore treated differently (a careful history is essential).

Drug-induced (by narcotics)   Should be treated with prochloperazine mesylate (Stemetil) 12.5 mg i.m. 4-hourly (produces moderate sedation while Largactil 25 mg i.m. 8-hourly is the most sedative but least effective antiemetic of the phenothiazines). The antiemetic of choice is haloperidol (Serenace) 2.5 mg i.m. 8-hourly (minimal sedation).

Hypercalcaemia   Can cause vomiting and anorexia. Occurs in carcinoma with bone secondaries or excess parathormone secretion, e.g. bronchial carcinoma. It is relieved rapidly by prednisolone 5 mg four times a day reducing to 5 mg daily or dexamethasone 4 mg i.m. 6-hourly for 48 h. Calcitonin can also be used.

Primary or secondary cerebral tumour (raised intracranial pressure)   Can cause vomiting, headache, blurred vision and mental confusion. Dexamethasone 4 mg should be given 6-hourly for 48 h by which time there should be a response (in this case a low maintenance dose of 2–4 mg/24 h should continue). If there is no response after 7 days, the patient should be reassessed.

Intestinal obstruction   Treat with i.v. infusion and nasogastric suction if obstruction is complete. If obstruction is incomplete a stool softener should be used, e.g. Dioctyl Forte two tablets twice daily. Analgesics and antiemetics should be given rectally (Stemetil or thiethylperazine malate (Torecan) suppositories). Metoclopramide may be used to increase gastric emptying in gastric stasis (can cause extrapyramidal symptoms as do phenothiazines).

Radiation or cytotoxic-induced vomiting   Is almost impossible to control; however, tetrahydrocannabinol can be effective.

Uraemia   Due to advanced obstructive uropathy.

Constipation

Inactivity, anorexia, low-residue diet and analgesic drugs (occupying opioid gut receptors) can all give rise to constipation. Treated by combined faecal softener and peristalsis-inducing (stimulant) laxative, e.g. Dorbanex 10 ml twice daily. Suppositories, enemas or manual disimpaction may also be required. (Senokot or Dulcolax are also useful stimulant laxatives. Lactulose 15 ml twice daily is an osmotic stimulant – an expensive alternative.)

Diarrhoea

Diarrhoea has many causes. It may be due to constipation with overflow (spurious diarrhoea) and treated as above. In subacute intestinal obstruction antiperistaltics can be used, e.g. loperamide (Imodium) or diphenoxylate with atropine (Lomotil). In malabsorption, usually due to pancreatic insufficiency, two tablets of pancreatin with each meal provide replacement. In rectal carcinoma (with mucus discharge) prednisolone retension enema or suppository is used.

Dyspnoea

Dyspnoea should be treated according to the cause, e.g. diuretics in cardiac failure and bronchodilators (salbutamol and aminophylline) in bronchospasm. In superior vena cava obstruction, dexamethasone 12 mg is given daily prior to radiotherapy. The same is used for lymphangitis carcinomatosa. Treat with antibiotics (in chest infection), drainage and possibly bleomycin instillation (in malignant effusion), opiates to relieve the sensation of dyspnoea (although they cause respiratory centre depression) and hyoscine (Scopolamine) 0.4–0.6 mg to dry up the accumulated secretions (death rattle). Oxygen may also be used. Corticosteroids in patients with short prognosis are the drugs of choice. The patient should be propped up in left ventricular failure, placed semiprone in bronchogenic carcinoma and on one side in pleural effusion.

Depression

Tender loving care is required, along with mood-elevating prednisolone 5 mg twice daily. Amitriptyline 25–75 mg daily is a useful antidepressant. It potentiates the analgesic effects of opiates in addition to its inherent analgesic activity. When giving amitriptyline, oral hygiene is important as it causes a dry mouth. For anxiety diazepam (Valium) 5 mg three times a day is adequate. Largactil 25 mg three times a day can be given in the very last days. Emotional and spiritual support is important.

Muscle spasm

Tumour pressing on or irritating a nerve can produce spasm. It is treated with diazepam or dantrolene (Dantrium) 25 mg daily.

Anorexia

Small amounts of the patient's favourite food attractively presented can work wonders. Periactin (an appetite stimulant) is disappointing. Steroids are the drugs of choice (marked effect).

Pruritus

Pruritus can be produced by bile acid accumulation in the skin as a result of obstructive jaundice. Treated with cholestyramine 4 g three times a day, Betnovate skin ointment or trimeprazine (Vallergan – a phenothiazine with marked antihistamine action).

Fits and convulsions

Primary or secondary brain deposits may produce fits and convulsions. Treat with diazepam 10 mg three times a day, phenytoin 100 mg three times a day or sodium valproate (Epilim) 200 mg three times a day. However, dexamethasone may reduce or eliminate the need for anticonvulsants.

Insomnia

Treat with short-acting benzodiazepines (Temazepam 10 mg at night). Chlormethiazole (Heminevrin) 1 g is a useful hypnotic for the elderly.

Miscellaneous

Urinary frequency and incontinence
- Emepronium bromide (Cetiprin) 200 mg at night
- Condom
- Indwelling catheter

Fungating growths
- Radiotherapy, cytotoxic, hormonal manipulation
- Betadine with liquid paraffin (1/4) cleansing
- Antibiotics
- Desloughing agents (natural yoghurt is good)

Oesophageal carcinoma
- Radiotherapy
- Insertion of oesophageal tubes

Nerve compression
- Strong analgesic
- Steroids, e.g. dexamethasone 4 mg/24 h
- Nerve block (intercostal/intrathecal/epidural 5–7.5% phenol glycerine + lactic acid)
- Tricyclic antidepressant, occasionally

Stretched liver capsule
- Paravertebral nerve block, occasionally
- Strong analgesic
- Methyl prednisolone 125–250 mg/24 h × 7 (i.m.)

Note: The following natural agents could be made use of:
- Yoghurt is a good skin desloughing cleansing agent.
- Honey is an excellent surgical dressing for bed sores and ulcers.
- Pineapple juice is a good solution for oral hygiene.

1.24 Audit and Quality Assurance of Health Care in Surgery

CLINICAL AUDIT

Medical audit is the systematic, critical analysis of the quality of medical care, including the procedures used for diagnosis and treatment, the use of resources, and the resulting outcome and quality of life for the patient. The importance of auditing stems from the patient's expectation of and demand for a high quality of health care during treatment. The way of improving the quality of health care is through audit or surveillance. The term 'clinical audit' has been used to embrace the activities of all health care professionals who work directly with patients, such as nurses, doctors and paramedical staff. Medical audit refers to the assessment by peer review of medical care provided by the medical profession. It should be acknowledged, however, that the quality of medical care is not solely determined by doctors, as other health professionals also have an essential role, and therefore the role of other health professionals will inevitably come under consideration in 'clinical' audit, particularly as the integrated team approach to patient care is so important in modern medicine.

The incidence of potentially avoidable deaths (that is those from conditions amenable to treatment) has been analysed for each health authority and shows large variations between health authorities even after adjustment for social factors. All these may provide some indication of the quality of medical care. The objective of surgical audit is to improve the quality of care doctors provide for their patients. Audit is an essential component of quality assurance of health care. Quality assurance is a system by which provision or performance is measured against expectation with the declared intention of minimising deficiency. Surgical audit provides a systematic approach to peer review of medical care. Its content is primarily clinical and educational as opposed to managerial and its focus is on the process and outcome of medical care. However where deficiencies in care can be attributed to lack of resources it necessarily impinges on resource provision and financial audit. The 'grand round' or 'interesting case' type of clinical meeting does not meet the requirements of audit. Audit is a systematic structured procedure with the express purpose of improving the quality of medical care. Whenever possible it should be quantified.

Audit should lead to changes in the organisation and availability of services, clinical policy and clinical practice with consequent improvement in the quality of medical care as measured by appropriate indicators. It is now increasingly recognised as a component of surgical practice and therefore all doctors should be expected to take part. Audit must be an educational process, and this form of audit should not be used for disciplinary purposes. It should be considered as part of normal clinical practice; therefore all doctors, whether in the NHS or in the private sector, should participate in a properly structured surgical audit programme.

Conduct of medical audit

Auditing is different from performing a review or conducting research; it should lead to changing practice for the better and to an action where practice has not matched the agreed standards so that the quality of medical care is improved. Follow-up action is an absolutely essential feature.

Unlike review, audit is not measuring where you are; it is about measuring how far away you are from where you want to be. One should first identify the problem; unless the activity can be changed in any way, there is no need to audit it. It is also important to stick to common activities that have an effect on patient outcome and those for which it is possible to have agreed standards; it is not worth trying to audit a rare problem with little or no effect on patients and which is an area of disagreement amongst consultants. Objectives and goals must be defined as agreed standards; one can then collect data to check the deviation of current performance from the standard by measuring what is actually achieved and how far one is from the proposed goal.

The use of the autopsy (see below) must be encouraged as it remains a relevant final investigation of considerable value in surgical audit. National widespread audit (CEPOD) can improve the quality of care provided by those whose practice would be considered generally to be less than satisfactory, lead to greater consistency in the quality of care provided overall and encourage those doctors currently regarded as 'good' or 'acceptable' to strive to provide even better care. Ideally the quality of surgical practice should be judged by its outcome. Measurement of outcome is most profitable in studying common conditions and procedures in which special care has been taken to ensure complete and reliable recording of data.

The practical approach to an audit therefore, includes:
1. Identification of subject matter to be assessed.
2. Establishment of suitable criteria agreed locally against which to judge performance. Criteria should be based on the best published figures where available or on criteria provided by the Royal Colleges or agreed by other appropriate group.
3. Identification and analysis of any problems.
4. Refinement of the above criteria in the light of experience.
5. Formulation of recommendations and follow-up action. Follow-up action is an absolutely essential feature of medical audit without which the justification for medical audit is lost. Medical audit should lead to changes in the organisation and availability of services, clinical policy and clinical practice with consequent improvement in the quality of medical care as measured by appropriate indicators.

Audit is not a review or case presentation; it is a cycle of activities.

If audit is 'a systematic quantified comparison against explicit standards of current medical practice in order to improve the quality of care to patients' then audit differs from traditional reviews in several ways:

● Audit uses explicit criteria of good practice: we define openly what we mean, and agree how we should assess the practice.
● Audit involves quantifying current patterns of practice, using representative samples of activity and results.
● Audit compares individual performance in peer groups: this enables individuals to see how their performance varies in terms of process and outcome.
● Audit leads to agreed action for improvement: the jointly owned targets for changing practice are produced and acted on.
● Audit requires documentation: who took part, what was audited, general conclusions reached, what should happen next, who should do it, and when the results should be reviewed.

All this involves much more than counting events or presenting cases; it is a cycle of activities, i.e. the *audit cycle* (Fig. 1.24.1).

Audit is not research. There is much confusion between audit and research. The following points help make the distinction clearer.

● Research is a systematic investigation which aims to increase the sum of knowledge; it usually involves an attempt to test a hypothesis. Audit is a systematic approach to peer review of medical care in order to identify possible improvements and to provide a mechanism for bringing them about.
● Research may involve allocating patients randomly to different treatment groups, while audit never involves allocating patients randomly to different treatment groups.
● Research may involve administration of a placebo, while audit never involves a placebo treatment.
● Research may involve a completely new treatment, while audit never involves a completely new treatment.

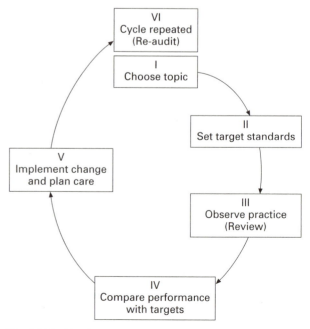

Fig. 1.24.1   The six phases of audit cycle

- Research may involve extra disturbance or work beyond that required for normal clinical management, while audit never involves disturbance to patients beyond that required for normal clinical management.
- Research may involve the application of strict selection criteria to patients with the same problem before they are entered into the research study. Audit may involve patients with the same problem being given different treatments, but only after full discussion of the known advantages and disadvantages of each treatment; the patients are allowed to choose freely which treatment they get.

Audit is not computing. The ability to produce numbers provides only a small part of the audit cycle, and much of this can be done manually.

Audit is not contracts. Purchaser–provider contracts of the NHS may well include paragraphs requiring an effective internal system of medical audit; but the results of audit should not be prematurely used to formulate numerical measures of quality in contracts.

Audit is not resource management. Resource management needs complete and accurate data on the sort of work you do (case mix); so does audit. Audit may take account of resources, but not as a first objective. In reality, good practice is efficient even if it is also expensive.

Administrative organisation of an audit

The essential requirements for audit establishment are appropriate organisational framework, resources, training and trust, including confidentially, to underpin it.

Training   An understanding of the principles of audit must become an established part of undergraduate and postgraduate medical education. Information on audit can be disseminated to all surgeons on a regular basis, perhaps by means of an 'Audit Magazine'. Medical schools should be encouraged in a self-critical approach to surgical methods and practice throughout the curriculum. Clinical firms to which medical students are attached should be expected to demonstrate good clinical practice in all areas, including medical audit. Regional Postgraduate Deans should be expected to recommend disallowance of pre-registration house officer posts in which medical audit is not an integral part of routine practice.

Resources   The effective conduct of audit has important resource implications, particularly in terms of medical and other staff manpower and information technology. The time required depends on length and frequency of regular monthly audit meetings.

Audit co-ordinator   The duties of the audit co-ordinator should be specified. He/she may need to:
- Co-ordinate various specialty groups involved in audit.
- Liaise between consultants and managers in respect of resources required for audit and implementation of recommendations emerging from medical audit and report in a suitable form to the Health Authority on the implementation of medical audit.
- Chair the audit subcommittee.
- Collate information from all sources of audit and make appropriate recommendations.

- Monitor the action recommended.
- Monitor statistics, including performance indicators.
- Arrange interdisciplinary meetings.
- Promote and support education.
- Review the literature on medical audit and disseminate it.
- Give advice when requested on what to audit and how.
- Liaise closely with the department of postgraduate education, district medical education committee and other bodies.

General principles of clinical audit

Criteria of a successful audit

Honesty   The essential nature of audit is a frank discussion between doctors, on a regular basis and without fear of criticism, of the quality of care provided as judged against agreed standards but in a context which allows evolutionary change in such standards. Surgeons who claim no complications in their hands or that their rate of postoperative mortality from cancer is zero, must be assessed objectively to know how many cases that surgeon has performed, and the length of the follow-up. Doctors are prone to self-deceit and self-justification, and lying to a patient is to spare not the patient's anguish, but the doctor's conceit. The habit of being economical with the truth can become ingrained, so that the death certificate of an 80-year-old patient who died after an operation is more likely to be worded 'Bronchopneumonia due to carcinoma of sigmoid colon' than 'Postoperative respiratory failure due to resection for carcinoma of sigmoid colon'. This sort of bias can corrupt clinical audit. It is encouraged by the low autopsy rate in both the UK and USA (about 20–25%, compared with 96% in Sweden), and by the traditional belief, which still lingers, that doctors do not make mistakes. One can only suggest that we should take heart from some of those great surgeons who have not hesitated to report their poor results as well as their good ones.

Audit should lead to action where practice has not matched the agreed standards so that the quality of medical care is improved.

Accurate and standarised forms   These are essential for successful audit. The coding of hospital admissions may need to be improved and streamlined to allow use for audit. Poor coding may be a reflection of the lack of doctors' perception of the importance of accurate and timely coding of patient records. Accurate coding of patient records is a fundamental requirement of audit. Consultants should ensure that summary sheets are completed properly so that records can be quickly and accurately coded by medical records staff. Accuracy in recording data in a computer is a matter for each surgeon to demand. Absolute accuracy is more likely if the information is transferred from case notes to computer forms by a trained clerical assistant who is not medically qualified. Doctors, particularly if they are familiar with the problems of the patient concerned, consciously or unconsciously interpret certain data instead of recording exactly what happened. The forms should, of course, always be checked by the consultant before being entered into the computer.

Consultants both in teaching hospitals and in district hospitals have a duty to train their junior staff. It is up to consultants to make sure that the notes they write to themselves are accurate, and to insist that those of their staff are equally so.

Complete medical records (in so far as is possible)   It should be a rule that everything that happens to a patient in hospital is meticulously recorded in the case notes, and that all reports of special investigations are filed in the case notes; there is no point in asking for a test if the result is not recorded and acted on. It is surprising how often, in completing audit forms, one can find informations in the nursing notes more useful than that in the records of postoperative progress written by house officers and registrars. Surgeons should be meticulous in praising well-kept notes, and in criticising those that are not. Without good case notes, it is impossible to maintain high standards.

Confidentiality   Confidentiality is essential. In audit a patient's clinical records will be open to scrutiny by doctors other than the doctor responsible for the patient's clinical care. This sharing of information is legitimate in that all doctors share the same ethical principles in respect of the confidentiality of patient information. However, those organising medical audit sessions should do their utmost to avoid referring to patients' names or revealing information by which patients may be identified. It is possible to conduct medical audit without using patients' names. Concern has been expressed that any record of the discussions of a audit meeting could be subject to legal problems.

Educational not punishment   The objective of the audit is to improve patients' health care by doctors and staff by learning the lessons from hard experience, the audit meeting should not be a courtyard for exposing surgeons and picking up the mistakes of each other. The environment should provide a sense of educational interaction and should never convey a feeling of inquisition or of witch-hunting for doctors' errors. It is also important that doctors should not feel that they are under a greater threat of litigation because of their involvement in medical audit. Documentation of audit meetings is provided in an appropriately anonymised form so that the general conclusions of the meeting and recommended actions are recorded while the cases used in the discussion are not in any way identifiable.

Relevance to common clinical problems   The audit can thus act as an instrument for change of practice to the better.

Objectivity by peers assessment.

Types of clinical audit

Medical care can be considered in terms of structure, process or outcome. Structure is concerned with the amount and type of resources available, e.g. the condition of buildings, the number of beds available and staffing levels. These are easy to measure but are not necessarily good indicators of the quality of care provided. Process relates to the amount and type of activity expended in the care of a patient (diagnosis, investigations and treatment). Unless resources are severely limited process has more significance than structure, and in many circumstances it is the only measure available. The most relevant indicator of quality of care is outcome. Some outcomes may be difficult to

measure since the final outcome may not be evident until many years later. Examples of outcome measures include post-operative mortality and morbidity, such as perinatal mortality and perioperative deaths, Glasgow outcome scale, APACHE score, POSSUM score, residual disability, relief of symptoms and patient satisfaction.

Audit needs to take into account new knowledge and attitudes, otherwise it is at risk of fossilising the best of today's surgery in its present phase of development.

Ideally medical advances (this would include amongst other things developments in drugs, surgery, advice on behaviour, counselling and in the use and membership of the caring team) should be tested within accepted ethical principles in controlled trials. However, this is not always possible. Some affect diseases that are too rare; others are too operator-dependent for the results of trials to be generally applicable. Controlled trials can only answer one question, or a few questions, at a time and are conducted on clearly defined groups, so that care must be taken in extending their results to unselected patients with the same disease as seen in medical practice. They can be very expensive in time and resources.

Ideally, the quality of medical practice should be judged by its outcome. However, there are several major difficulties in relying entirely on judgement of outcome.

Value of audit

Several studies have demonstrated the value of audit in reducing the number of unnecessary diagnostic tests performed, length of stay and the number of drugs prescribed.

Several studies in general practice have shown that performance in a number of areas can be improved by peer review, including management of common clinical conditions, record-keeping, prescribing and referral practice. The greatest changes occurred in the behaviour of those doctors whose performance was furthest from 'optimal' on the criteria used.

The results of audit involving general surgeons and urologists working in one region showed statistically significant improvements in some clinical practices, including a fall in the number of reoperations and a reduction in deaths associated with a range of surgical operations. Audit data showed the results of arterial surgery were better in units with surgeons who specialised, and it is believed that this was partly responsible for the reduction in deaths and reoperations. Similarly it has been shown that the success rate in a surgical unit for the surgical treatment of biliary atresia is very dependent on the number of operations done. Reductions in wound infection rates have been linked to surgical audit. These improvements were linked to reduction in length of stay and hence released resources for use elsewhere.

Practice of audit

There are two main approaches to the practice of audit. They are (i) retrospective internal audit within a specialty, hospital, general practice or district community in which records are used to review past events, and (ii) concurrent audit which is a continuous assessment of patient management. In both types of audit results are compared with agreed standards, which may be implicit or explicit, protocols or criteria. Retrospective internal audit is likely to be the most appropriate approach for the introduction of audit, but these approaches to audit are not mutually exclusive.

Ideally the basis of audit should be outcome but in practice it is often not. Usually audit of 'process' is carried out on the assumption that good process give rise to good outcome. The subject of audit may include administrative processes (such as medical records, referral and discharge letters), clinical processes (use of drugs, investigations and procedures), clinical condition (classified by diagnostic category) or outcome (return to work, ambulation or unexpected death).

In surgery, however, the most informative audit, whether of process or outcome (or both) is the prospective clinical trial. A well-designed trial sets out with a single question; for example, is it possible to reduce the incidence of burst abdomen to below 1% compared with a previous experience of 4%? Such a trial requires the prospective collection of data about suture materials and methods of suturing, and the results are most persuasive when the controls are not only contemporary but also randomly selected, thus ensuring the minimum of bias and the comparison of like with like. The random controlled clinical trial is an expression of clinical audit at its best. There are, however, some aspects of surgical treatment that are not amenable to the discipline of the random controlled trial.

Complications and deaths occur not only if the process of care was below the best, and not only if the surgery was poorly performed, but if the patients who were operated on were at particularly high risk of complications. It is curious that many reports of the results of operations do not mention the patients who were judged to be so ill that they could not tolerate an operation. This is a serious criticism of the English Confidential Enquiry into Perioperative Deaths (CEPOD); one surgeon's results may be much worse than another's simply because that surgeon operates on patients who are denied by another surgeon the (perhaps slender) chance offered by operation.

Disadvantages of audits

Audits remain controversial issues among sceptics; in a nutshell disadvantages include the following:
1. Time spent on audit would be better spent on clinical work or even research.
2. Audit takes no account of clinicians doing a good job. The definition of audit implicitly assumes that actual clinical practice may not be ideal; audit is about rooting out 'bad' practice and, by implication, bad doctors.
3. If resources are not available for change, what is the point of audit? The long waiting list for hip replacement is a well-known example without the need for audit; without more orthopaedic surgeons and theatre staff, the waiting list will remain long.
4. What evidence is there that adherence to guidelines and protocols results in a better outcome for patients than does reliance on individual clinical judgement?
5. Is there evidence that audit is better than medical education as a method of improving and maintaining standards?

Audit in the hospital

Audit can be practised in various ways. At a local level most specialty groups would favour regular retrospective reviews of clinical practice. Such meetings are able to review workload as well as clinical outcome, including complications and death (morbidity and mortality audit meeting). At such meetings deficiencies in facilities or patient care can be identified and recommendations made to effect improvements.

For such meetings to be successful they have to:
- Take place regularly (at least once a month) at a time set aside from other hospital work. The frequency will depend on the specialty.
- Be attended by all relevant medical staff, especially the consultants.
- Be prepared in advance. Data on clinical activity needs to be compiled and produced for each meeting. Notes of patients to be discussed have to be found.
- Be totally confidential. The identity of patients discussed should never be revealed or be capable of being traced.
- Be able to make recommendations to management or other appropriate bodies where deficiencies in the service have been identified.

Computer facilities will soon be essential within departments for compiling data on which the audit is to be based. The computers needed might range from a small desk top unit to a much larger hospital based system capable of providing patient information to all departments undertaking audit. The selection of the type of computer will depend on the unit and the types of audit undertaken. The need for compatibility has already been noted. Personnel and training to operate such systems will also be required.

Hospital departments will require help in setting up medical audit for the first time and should seek the help of the Medical Audit Co-ordinator.

It will be the responsibility of the Medical Audit Co-ordinator, answerable to the medical advisory committee or its equivalent, for ensuring that medical audit is established in all hospital medical departments.

1. Diagnostic departmental audits

The diagnostic specialties of pathology and radiology have their own particular requirements for audit. These include a review of diagnostic accuracy as well as such matters as timeliness and records.

2. Anaesthetic audit

Anaesthetists, like others, already have morbidity and mortality meetings, the holding of which is one criterion in the College of Anaesthetists' accreditation of training posts. In these meetings individual cases are presented and debated. There is a need for these meetings to be made more comprehensive, involving other relevant disciplines, and also to be directed to the solution of locally perceived problems. The Association of Anaesthetists and the Association of Surgeons together carried out an enquiry into perioperative deaths in three regions (CEPOD); this was extended into a national confidential enquiry at the beginning of 1989. The Health Advisory Service, which was established in 1976, is an example of multi-disciplinary audit; it carries out reviews of hospitals and community health services provided for the elderly and the mentally ill and makes recommendations for the improvement of care.

The collection of reports of critical incidents, as is done by airline pilots, is an important way in which some departments have identified deficiencies in their own structure (such as provision and checks of functional equipment) or process (such as availability of senior support). Many serious problems were revealed in the Survey of Anaesthetic Practice, carried out by the Association of Anaesthetists of Great Britain and Ireland, and these matters must be pursued. This information was acquired by a method which maintained confidentiality.

Other outcomes, such as minor morbidity without prolongation of hospital stay (e.g. nausea, vomiting, headache, minor bruising) and intermediate morbidity with prolongation of hospital stay (e.g. post-dural puncture headache, preparation for operation, postoperative pain relief) are all potential indicators of quality. There are other aspects of the work of anaesthetists which need to be audited, such as obstetric analgesia, intensive therapy and pain therapy services. These three developments have proceeded at very different rates in different parts of the country and audit of these is required nationally, perhaps by the College of Anaesthetists through its regional representatives.

The development of agreed management for a model case by means of discussion by groups of different degrees of experience has started in one region. The protocols which resulted are used as educational tools and are popular. They can also be used in comparison with the management of real cases.

The scrutiny of anaesthetic records is an essential part of audit meetings. This has already resulted in improvements, but considerable financial investment is required in new technology before anaesthetic records can be regarded as satisfactory. It is now possible for routine observations (such as pulse, blood pressure, gas concentrations) to be recorded continuously, automatically and directly on paper. This development is central to any desire for retrospective examination of events during anaesthesia, particularly when rapid physiological changes take place, in order to identify deviations from 'satisfactory' practice.

3. Surgical audit

Surgeons' attitude towards mistakes must change. It is here that ethical reform must begin. It is therefore our task to search for our mistakes and to investigate them fully. We must train ourselves to be self-critical (the so-called self-audit).

Audit of structure

Audit of structure is fairly easy. It involves asking the following questions.
- Are there enough doctors and nurses?
- Are there enough beds?
- Are the beds being used efficiently?
- Are the operating theatres being used efficiently?

Data such as the number of beds occupied, the number of people waiting for admission, and the number of days that patients stay in hospital are easily compiled and are usually complete and accurate. The reports of the British Information Steering Group (the Korner reports) put forward about 450 'performance indicators' that are almost entirely concerned with cost effectiveness. Those that relate to general surgery comprise:
- Actual length of stay
- Expected length of stay
- Standardised length of stay ratio
- Turnover interval
- Actual throughput
- Expected throughput
- Standardised throughput ratio
- Percentage of day cases
- Percentage of cases not operated on
- Preoperative stay
- Postoperative stay
- Theatre sessions/bed
- Waiting list/1000 population
- Notional days to clear waiting list
- Percentage immediate admissions.

The introduction of performance indicators in the UK, which compare local with regional and national average performances presented in graphic rather than tabular form, has gone a long way towards identifying deficiencies in the structure of systems of patient care. These comparisons can bring to light deficiencies and inefficiencies that can be corrected. The purpose of audit of structure is simply the correction of inefficiencies to restore the same standards among various regional health caring areas (consistency); it has nothing to do with the effectiveness of clinical care.

Audit of process

In auditing an industrial process, whether it be in a manufacturing or a service industry, the assumption is made that if the right steps are taken in the right sequence and at the right time, the outcome will be satisfactory. As far as clinical audit is concerned, it has on the one hand the merit of being relatively simple and, on the other, the drawback of not always reflecting the outcome.

Audit of process is carried out by surgeons every day, and it can, and usually does, lead to improvement in clinical practice. A consultant does a ward round with his junior staff. He expects to be told about the history, the physical examination and the special tests done for each patient. If a disaster – such as a burst abdomen – occurs, he will want to be assured that an appropriate suture material was used, that knots were properly tied, and that sufficiently wide bites of aponeurosis were taken (reflected in practice by requiring a record to be kept of the length of each abdominal incision and the length of suture material used, so that the depth of bite could be accurately calculated). The main disadvantage of the audit of process is that it is difficult to quantify. It is, however, difficult to quantify such aspects of care as kindness, courtesy and giving enough time to patients, who are concerned as much with these aspects as with survival without complications.

Audit of outcome

End result analysis is made in terms of postoperative recovery, success rate, morbidity and mortality. The Department of Audit states: 'Comparison is necessary in science. Until we freely make therapeutic comparisons, we cannot claim that a given hospital is efficient, for efficiency implies that the results have been looked into . . . Every hospital should follow every patient it treats long enough to determine whether or not the treatment has been successful, and then to enquire "if not, why not?" with a view to preventing similar failures in the future.' Audit of outcome is the sort of audit surgeons are most suspicious about; many surgeons prefer to place the blame for a failure of treatment on anything rather than their own mistake. The essentials of audit (completeness, accuracy and honesty) apply even more strongly to the audit of outcome than to those of structure and process. We have all met surgeons who tell us that their operation was technically successful, but that the patient died of heart failure on the sixth postoperative day. These are the surgeons who do not ask for autopsies because they do not want to be told the truth – that the 'heart failure' was caused by an anastomotic breakdown.

Ways of auditing oucome in surgery   In order to conduct an audit of outcome in a surgical practice, case notes must be summarised in some way. The easiest way is to enter relevant details about every patient in a log book; these details should include:
- The patient's name and hospital index number (for easy retrieval).
- The diagnosis.
- The treatment.
- The complications.
Keeping a log book is a valuable exercise, but it suffers from the disadvantage that analysis of a whole year's work is difficult to achieve.

The second way in which surgeons can collect data is by entering the names of patients on cards, which are kept in three boxes; this should preferably be done from the log book and at least once a week. One box is for categories of diagnoses, one is for operations and the third is for complications, including deaths. New boxes are started at the beginning of each year. This takes little time and allows an accurate picture of one's practice to be built up over a whole year.

The most advanced way of auditing the outcome of a practice is by using a microcomputer database with specifically created field parameters. Forms are designed that are computer-compatible, and which are completed immediately patients are discharged; if there is any delay, the notes may disappear and the data may never be recorded. These computer forms should not form part of the case notes; on the contrary, the demographic details should be filled in as soon as a patient is admitted and the form sent to the consultant's office. Only in this way can completeness of audit be guaranteed.

Outcome indicators

While structure was defined as the staffing and facilities in which care takes place together with the organisation and financial medical care which had been applied, outcome was the result of medical care assessed in terms of survival, recovery and restoration of function. Process measures are more readily available than those of outcome and this explains why historically process has been used more often than outcome to judge quality of care. This has been justified by the assumption that 'good' medical care of known effectiveness has been applied rather than the determination of whether an intervention is beneficial or not in the long term.

Recently the need to develop outcome indicators has become more pressing, owing to the increasing demand for health care in the face of limited resources and the consequent need to decide priorities in the allocation of resources. Development of outcome indicators has been slow despite considerable research over the past 10 years and the availability of a large amount of data collected routinely on a national basis.

A major difficulty in the development of outcome indicators has been the collection of relevant data on a national basis. Existing indicators of the quality and outcome of health care are few and more work on them is needed. The Korner reports on Health Service Information are now being implemented. Although they are mainly concerned with providing information for NHS management rather than information needed by health professionals to evaluate the results of their care, the Korner data can nevertheless provide a useful basis for the development of some outcome indicators.

Outcome indicators based on routine data include 'avoidable deaths' and some avoidable morbidity indicators such as the rate of admission for diabetic ketoacidosis and coma and readmission rates to hospital following surgery. However, the range of indicators that can be derived from routine data is necessarily restricted, owing to the limited range of data collected. A range of outcome indicators includes preventive services (congenital malformation, infections, cancer, accidents, suicide), treatment services (adverse effects, case fatality, survival data from cancer registries) and overall measures of health (expectation of life, mortality patterns and morbidity patterns from general practice). These data can provide a useful spur for the medical profession to examine current practice. The determination of outcome will often require information about progress of patients whether after discharge from hospital or following treatment in the community. It will be essential to have mechanisms which facilitate follow-up of patients. This could be achieved through the more assiduous use of the NHS number, which is currently used on all general practitioners' records and may feature on many personal health records.

Autopsy in clinical audit

Despite the advent of progressively more sophisticated investigative and imaging techniques, discrepancies between clinical and autopsy diagnosis have remained around the 10% level. For instance, in a study of 100 intensive care unit deaths, 10% of autopsies revealed findings which, if detected before death, would probably have led to a change of management which might have resulted in cure or prolonged survival. Furthermore, 10% of the autopsy findings were of potential therapeutic relevance had they been known before death. In autopsies performed on patients thought to have died of malignant disease there was only 75% agreement that malignancy was the cause of death and in only 56% was the primary site identified correctly. Tumours of the pancreas, liver and biliary tract are the most difficult. In the same way the tendency of doctors to attribute most sudden unexpected deaths to heart disease probably leads to an overestimate of cardiac causes of sudden unexpected death. An audit in a paediatric cardiology unit showed unsuspected abnormalities in 80%, with undiagnosed abnormalities or surgical problems contributing to death in 38%. Such high levels of discordance mean that mortality statistics which are not supported by autopsy examinations must be viewed with caution. It is not possible to predict with any degree of accuracy whch autopsies will yield discrepant diagnoses. Several studies have shown that autopsies are necessary to ensure the accuracy of death certificates.

It is generally assumed that autopsies provide a good index of the quality of patient care, and for this an autopsy rate high enough for analysis is needed. An overall rate of about 35% of hospital deaths has been suggested as adequate. The number of discrepancies between clinical and autopsy diagnoses is an important index of care. However, it has never been shown that there is a correlation between an increase in the autopsy rate and a subsequent decrease in clinicopathologic discrepancies. If this were to be demonstrated then the indispensability of the autopsy in clinical audit would be beyond question.

The decline in autopsies

There has been a progressive decline in autopsy rates throughout the world. This has been not just an absolute decline, but is seen especially in the elderly, where there is a potentially higher discrepancy rate, and a correspondingly higher rate of undiagnosed but potentially treatable conditions.

The reasons for the decline are many and complex. Religious objection is often cited as a cause, but few religions take a stand against autopsies. For instance, the Koran places no restriction on them, but because of Islamic respect for the dead they were not performed in Turkey until 1838, when a medical school was established in Istanbul and an Imperial edict was issued directing that autopsies should be performed as part of the activity of the school. More recently, new legislation in Israel, enacted as a result of religious pressure from Jews, led to a rapid decline.

It is often thought that families may suffer extra distress when an autopsy is requested and reasons for refusal of permission include fear of disfigurement, lack of information about the autopsy, other family member objections and the stress of giving permission for the examination. These considerations may inhibit doctors from requesting permission. However, in a study of the families of patients undergoing an autopsy, 88% considered they had benefited. Their benefits included reassurance that all appropriate medical care had been given, comfort in knowing the cause of death and comfort in advancing medical knowledge. In perinatal pathology, autopsy findings may provide significant evidence for counselling parents about future children.

Medical reasons for the decline include advances in preoperative diagnostic techniques (CT scan and NMR) and increasing faith in their results, failure to obtain consent, fear of litigation and cost. For instance, in the United States, the decline in the autopsy rate in the Mayo Clinic has been associated with the failure of the autopsy service to provide income to the institution, even though it has been shown to play an advantageous role in quality control, cost containment and efficient allocation of resources. It has been suggested that ways should be found to ensure the reimbursement of costs, perhaps by categorising the autopsy as a clinical activity, and by voluntary and government regulation, to assure the role of autopsy in quality assurance programmes.

Obtaining useful information at autopsy

Clinical post-mortems may not be performed without the permission of the deceased's relatives and this is the most important enabling step in the procedure. Permission for post-mortem examination must be obtained positively but sympathetically by the clinicians who appreciate the value of the autopsy in problem-solving and in clinical audit. This appreciation must begin in medical schools where the role of the autopsy is often undervalued in the curriculum. Many schools hold demonstrations of autopsy, and analyse the findings. There should be an increased emphasis on the autopsy in the medical school curriculum where it has a place in developing problem-solving skills.

Great care should be taken in obtaining permission for an autopsy. The responsibility lies with the consultant in charge of the case, but there is frequently uncertainty about who is to undertake this task. Whilst it may be delegated, this should be a positive step and not merely left to the most junior doctor, nurse or manager. Those responsible for approaching the relatives should be trained in a sympathetic and informative approach. Such training should be regarded as a proper duty of consultants for junior staff. Pathologists should also have the right to initiate a request for autopsies on patients when they think that this might be useful.

Histological examination of paraffin sections should be performed in every case. Permanent records of autopsies can be made using a combination of still and video photography. Video recording is of increasing importance in the use of autopsy material for undergraduate and postgraduate teaching as well as part of audit procedures.

In all cases when a death certificate cannot be completed, the death must be referred to the Coroner. As a minimum, clinical autopsies should be requested for all hospital deaths:
1. to verify a cause of death based on a clinical diagnosis and/ or to determine the extent of known or assumed lesions in problematic cases;
2. to investigate cases which are important for training, education and research;
3. to monitor the effects of therapy, especially newly introduced drugs, and the reliability of new diagnostic procedures;
4. to provide a degree of sampling within the patient population. From time to time the sampling may be random or targeted on a particular service. The target figure for sampling general hospital deaths in which there is no perceived prior necessity to perform an autopsy should be at least 10%. Each hospital will need to develop its own system of random sampling, in order to select such cases for autopsy;

5. in the case of perinatal pathology an attempt should be made to obtain permission for autopsy in all cases.

Assessing the results of Autopsy

Regular mortality meetings and clinicopathological conferences should be held to discuss and analyse the autopsy findings in individual patients or groups of cases. The major and primary purpose of these meetings should be educational. There should be frank discussion concerning diagnostic procedures, clinical management and outcome as part of normal hospital procedures.

See Appendix 3: National Confidential Enquiry into Perioperative Death (NCEPOD), the National Audit of UK perioperative mortality.

PERIOPERATIVE MANAGEMENT AND CRITICAL CARE

1.25 High-risk Patients in Surgery

Preoperative assessment

The presence of risk factors increases both morbidity and mortality. Deaths associated with anaesthesia and surgery have been described as 'anaesthetic death' and are usually due to the presence of high risk factors rather than anaesthetic fault. Operative mortality includes all deaths occurring within 30 postoperative days (even if the patient was discharged). These deaths provide useful epidemiological information on risk factors. In 1961, anaesthetic deaths were 21 per 100 000 operations in England and Wales, falling to 4 per 100 000 operations in 1973, despite the rise in inpatient operations from 1.55 million in 1961 to 2.5 million in 1973. In 1990, anaesthetic deaths were around 2.5 per 100 000 operations performed at a rate of 3 million per annum. NCEPOD audit in 1990 revealed an overall death rate of 0.7% in the UK (excluding Scotland); inadequate preparation of the patient may be a major factor to primary anaesthetic causes of perioperative mortality. NCEPOD showed that failures of the delivery of anaesthesia form a small proportion of the total (about 1.5%). The choice of anaesthetic procedure is influenced not only by requirements for surgical access, but also by pre-existing risk factors in the patient.

The influence of risk factors depends whether the planned surgery is of major or minor importance. Therefore, a face-lift surgery in a patient with hypertension, ischaemic heart disease and history of multiple myocardial infarction is deemed unrealistic, but when such a patient is presenting with intestinal obstruction, that person must undergo emergency surgery. Subumbilical or perineal surgery may be performed under epidural or spinal analgesia, e.g. TUR of prostate in cardiovascular or respiratory crippled patients can be carried out under spinal analgesia using bupivacaine. However, nowadays, no high-risk patient need to suffer any more than a temporary postponement of a necessary surgical procedure in order to stabilise and improve their fitness for surgery.

It is essential that the anaesthetist visit every patient in the ward before surgery to assess 'fitness for anaesthesia', as this function cannot always be undertaken by surgical staff. Often, the anaesthetist is frequently under pressure to proceed with planned operating theatre lists, and he or she sees the patients on the ward only 1–2 days prior to the scheduled surgery; cancellation would lead to inefficient use of operating theatre time and inconvenience for patients. Ideally, as a patient leaves the surgical clinic (after being placed on the waiting list), he or she should go to the '*anaesthetic outpatient clinic*', or alternatively, be referred to the anaesthetist for preoperative assessment. The *preoperative visit* aims at establishing a rapport with the patient, obtaining a history and performing quick, selective examination. The anaesthetist assesses the investigations, the risk factors, and, finally, institutes preoperative instructions prior to surgery or decides to postpone the operation.

- All patients have to cease smoking for at least 12 h prior to surgery, because of nicotine action on the sympathetic system, producing tachycardia, hypertension and increased coronary vascular resistance (cessation of smoking improves angina symptoms). Furthermore, heavy smoking reduces available oxygen by up to 23% due to haemoglobin conversion into carboxyhaemoglobin which has a short half-life; abstinence for 12 h, therefore, leads to increased arterial oxygen content. Also, smoking increases postoperative respiratory morbidity by sixfold; abstinence for 6 weeks prior to surgery results in reduced bronchoconstriction and mucus secretion.
- Regular alcohol intake leads to induction of liver enzymes resulting in tolerance to anaesthesia; anaesthetic agents have to be increased during surgery. Postoperatively, delirium tremens may occur. Similarly, regular intake of anticonvulsants (phenytoin), barbiturates, and benzodiazepines may increase requirements of anaesthetic agents and postoperative analgesia.
- Drugs may interfere with anaesthetic agents. In general, most drugs are allowed to continue up to and including the morning of operation, and will be resumed after recovery with the first postoperative oral meal. Antihypertensive agents may interact with anaesthetic agents causing hypotension; reduction of anaesthetics, therefore, is required during surgery.
- Anticoagulant use is of special importance; it may cause bleeding during intubation and during operation. The i.m.

postoperatively. FEV_1 must be 1.21 or more in patients undergoing pneumonectomy for lung cancer. Salbutamol is valuable for bronchospasm; aminophylline suppository is also useful and given with premedication. Ipratropium is an effective bronchodilator in broncho-constriction associated with chronic bronchitis. Broad spectrum antibiotics are dangerous as they may lead to overgrowth of bacteria which are difficult to deal with. Chest X-ray is useful even as negative baseline information. In patients who are deemed fit for surgery, preoperative chest physiotherapy is recommended together with sputum culture for antibiotic sensitivity in the event of postoperative complications. Asthmatics benefit from physiotherapy and salbutamol inhaler.

Postoperatively, there are two problems: hypoventilation (causing rise in Pa_{CO_2}), and inability to cough (causing sputum retention). Sputum retention results in atelectasis and infection; transfusion of non-filtered blood or overinfusion of crystalloids increase lung water, augmenting infection and causing hypoxaemia from shunting. Bronchospasm may be precipitated by laryngeal and tracheal irritation after intubation. Sitting up position, good analgesia, physiotherapy and nebulisation of bronchodilators are the cornerstones of treatment.

When the risk of postoperative respiratory failure is great, thoracic epidural anaesthesia or epidural opiates, or spinal opiate instillation, may be useful. Elective intermittent mandatory ventilation (IMV) is the process of weaning from ventilation and the treatment of choice in early postoperative respiratory failure to encourage spontaneous ventilation after surgery, in preparation for extubation; IMV does not need muscle relaxant, and the patient may or may not be sedated. Late stages of chest infection (particularly atypical pneumonias) are treated by amoxycillin and/or erythromycin.

Patients with diabetes mellitus

Diabetes and its complications predispose to many surgical diseases; patients are usually elderly with peripheral vascular disease, ischaemic heart disease and eventually hypertensive renal diseases. Stress and infection induce insulin resistance, which is also induced by steroids and catecholamines released in metabolic response to surgical trauma, by obesity and by administration of β-blockers (see s. 1.87 Diabetes and surgery).

Management protocols for diabetic patients undergoing surgery, printed on cards and distributed to anaesthetists and junior surgeons, provide a practical, easy and safe guide with instantaneous access (Fig. 1.25.1).

Patients on steroid therapy

Adrenocortical suppression induced by steroid therapy is of major importance as it may lead to postoperative collapse and shock after unrecognised blood loss, myocardial infarction and septicaemia. Patients who stopped steroid therapy, irrespective of duration, regain a normal adrenocortical responsiveness within 2 months and require no cover; others put it at up to 2 years. For minor surgery, 24 hours additional steroid cover will be adequate, while for short procedures such as endoscopy, or D&C, single injection with premedication will suffice. For major surgery, up to 3 days cover is required. Hydrocortisone 100 mg i.m. 6-hourly starting with premedication is the

---

SUGGESTED TREATMENT FOR DIABETICS REQUIRING SURGERY

OP ASSESSMENT

Know the patient is diabetic (screen all urines for glucose)
Assess control in known diabetics
Make a plan for admission if surgery required
        – ? admission early to improve control
                          to start new regime

INPATIENT

Monitor blood glucose by stick QDS

NIDD

Stop chlorpropamide and metformin
Minor operations in patients on sulphonylureas and FBG <8
        – omit drug on day
        – monitor blood glucose
        – avoid i.v. dextrose
        – restart tablets when eating
If having major surgery or poorly controlled, change to insulin

IDD

Obtain good control if possible
? Change long-acting insulin to isophane few days before

WHICH PATIENTS REQUIRE INSULIN

1. All known IDD patients
2. All having major surgery
3. Poorly controlled NIDD
4. Ill patients or emergency surgery

DEXTROSE AND VARIABLE INSULIN REGIME

1. Give normal short acting and 3/4 medium acting dose on evening before with dinner
2. **Day of Surgery**
    i.v. fluid   – 5% dextrose drip 1 litre in 12 hours
    i.v. insulin – Actrapid 50u to 50ml with N saline in syringe

Rate of Infusion

Bl. Glucose (mmol/l)	Regime 1	Regime 2
<4	off	off
4–8	1u/hr	2u/hr
8–11	2u/hr	3u/hr
11–16	3u/hr	4u/hr
16–20	4u/hr	6u/hr
>20	5u/hr	8u/hr

Measure blood glucose hourly perioperatively
Regime 1 suitable for most
Regime 2 if ill, shocked or on steroids
Operations on diabetics best done early on morning list
Continue i.v. regime until 1 hour before 1st postop meal
Restart s.c. insulin with this meal

Fig. 1.25.1 Showing both sides of a quick-reference card displaying the management protocol for diabetic surgical patients

---

recommended regimen. Afterwards, steroid could either be tailed off or even stopped abruptly because negative feedback is a potent stimulus to the pituitary adrenal axis.

Obstructive jaundice

This can lead to hepatorenal syndrome (acute renal shutdown and failure in obstructive jaundiced patients) and bleeding problems. To minimise the risk of renal failure, an i.v. infusion should be started on the night before surgery. Glucose 5%

should be infused at a rate of 100 ml/h. Also mannitol 20 g should be given just before or at induction of anaesthesia. Vitamin K 10 mg i.m. daily preoperatively, and postoperatively for 3 days, may be prescribed.

Hyper- and hypothyroidism

In **hyperthyroidism**, antithyroid drugs take several weeks to render patients euthyroid, may cause agranulocytosis (however rare), may result in intraoperative bleeding due to drug-induced thrombocytopenia or hypoprothrombinaemia, and continued therapy may lead to hypothyroidism; antithyroid drugs are therefore not recommended. Oral iodide, as Lugol's solution, is effective in reducing vascularity of hyperplastic thyroid glands before surgery. Beta-blockers are effective in attenuating manifestations (tachycardia and increased cardiac output) due to excessive sympathetic activity of hyperthyroidism. The combination of oral propranolol (80 mg every 8 h) and potassium iodide (60 mg every 8 h) is effective in attenuating cardiovascular manifestations and reducing T3 and T4.

Thyrotoxic crisis or storm is clinically manifested by hyperthermia, tachycardia, congestive heart failure, dehydration and shock. It is due to severe exacerbation of hyperthyroidism due to sudden excessive release of T3 and T4 into the circulation; it may occur intraoperatively, but is more likely to manifest in the first 6–18 h after surgery, and is nearly always abrupt. Treatment is both supportive and specific. Intravenous infusion of cold glucose crystalloid solution is indicated to replace fluid loss due to hyperthermia. Specific therapy includes sodium iodide 500–1000 mg i.v. every 8 h (effective in acutely reducing the release of T3 and T4), cortisol 100–200 mg i.v. every 8 h (increased metabolism can result in primary adrenal insufficiency, requiring exogenous cortisol), propranolol 1–2 mg i.v. until heart rate declines below 90 beats/min. Propylthiouracil 200–400 mg orally every 8 h can also be recommended to reduce synthesis of new T3 and T4, particularly after administration of potassium iodide. Aspirin may displace thyroxine from carrier proteins and should therefore not be used in lowering body temperature.

In **hypothyroidism**, exogenous replacement of thyroid hormones is essential; restoration of plasma concentration of thyroid hormones must be slow to prevent angina pectoris, cardiac arrhythmias or congestive heart failure. Thyroxine requires up to 10 days to exert action, and therefore is not effective for emergency treatment of hypothyroidism. Conversely, i.v. T3 exerts its effect within 6 h and reaches its peak effect within 48–72 h. Exogenous cortisol is necessary if there is evidence of primary adrenal insufficiency. In heart failure, digitalis is not recommended, since the hypothyroid heart cannot increase myocardial contraction. Hypothyroid cardiomyopathy is reversible with thyroid hormone replacement. Treatment of hypothyroid patients with coronary artery disease poses problems; the attempt to render patients euthyroid with thyroid hormone replacement may produce myocardial ischaemia, for example. In these patients, coronary revascularisation surgery is often attempted first then followed by postoperative thyroid hormone replacement. Elective surgery should not be performed until patients have been rendered euthyroid, confirmed clinically and by normal concentration of TSH.

Immunosuppression (AIDS and transplant patients)

Anaesthesia and surgery can proceed as for immunocompetent patients, but with full precautions to prevent transfer of infection from patient (with AIDS) to hospital staff, and from hospital staff to patients (in transplant patients). (For details see s. 1.13 on AIDS and surgery and s. 1.90 on Transplantation.)

Patients with multi-system organ failure (MOF)

MOF is a complication of polytrauma and intra-abdominal catastrophy associated with gross peritoneal soiling and/or with pelvic or subphrenic sepsis. Septic mediators are implicated; they lead to general breakdown in the integrity of cell membrane function, the so-called 'sick cell syndrome'. Disseminated intravascular coagulation can occur. Increased lung water with protein-rich exudation can cause gross shunting and hyaline membrane formation, the so-called 'adult respiratory distress syndrome' with fatal outcome (see s. 1.34).

POSTOPERATIVE FACILITIES

Risk factors have their maximum impact on the patient in the immediate postoperative period. Fortunately, postoperative facilities are available to monitor high-risk surgical patients; these facilities include the recovery ward, high dependency unit and intensive care unit.

1. Recovery ward

This is an area to which patients are admitted from an operating room, where they remain until consciousness is regained and ventilation and circulation are stable.

2. High dependency unit (HDU)

HDU is an area for patients who require more intensive observation and/or nursing than would be expected on a general ward. Patients who require mechanical ventilation or invasive monitoring *would not* be admitted to this area. Thus, HDU is an intermediate care unit between the general ward and intensive care unit.

3. Intensive care unit (ICU) or intensive therapy unit (ITU) (excluding intensive coronary unit for medical cases)

ICU or ITU is an area to which patients are admitted for treatment of actual or impending organ failure who may require technological support (including mechanical ventilation of lungs and/or invasive cardiopulmonary monitoring).

The role of HDU in postoperative care

HDU was developed (in the UK around 1982) to cater for the early postoperative care of patients undergoing major surgery, and for the seriously ill patients.

Most acute hospitals have ITUs for the care of the critically ill. These allow a concentration of nursing (at a ratio of 1 nurse to 1 patient) and medical skills, as well as specialised equipment in areas where they can be most economically and effectively used. In practice, such units tend to be used mainly for those patients requiring assisted ventilation, and those recovering from major cardiovascular and neurosurgical procedures. However, this often results in a depletion of such skills and equipment in general ward areas, and a net reduction of care for those ill patients who are not considered sufficiently ill to justify transfer to an ITU, for instance elderly patients undergoing major surgery who are in special need of constant observation and detailed care during the early postoperative period. The hospital must be designed with an HDU to reduce the increasing demand on nurses, particularly at night, in maintaining the care of such patients.

In HDU each bed station has piped oxygen and suction, and equipment for continuous monitoring of pulse, ECG and body temperature. Electronically controlled infusion pumps are available for each patient. Postoperative pain relief is provided in over 90% of cases by intermittent i.v. administration of narcotic analgesics, usually morphine. The unit is staffed by fully qualified nurses with a ratio of 1 nurse per 2 patients with all nurses sharing night duties. Financial implications of HDU amount approximately to £30 per patient per day. Clinical care of each admitted patient remains the direct responsibility of the referring consultant clinician and relevant junior staff. Admission to HDU can be elective before major surgery, or on an emergency basis, usually postoperatively. Administration by a panel of four consultants in weekly rotation assists the day-to-day problems which the sister in charge might encounter; the panel is responsible to the Hospital Medical Staff Committee.

In a study conducted in the University Hospital of Wales over a period of 6 months, 320 patients were admitted to HDU, 308 were postoperative admissions from most surgical specialties (general surgery 68%, vascular surgery 12%, ENT/maxillofacial surgery 7%, orthopaedics 7%, and urology and gynaecology 3%), and 12 were acute medical (3%). Average duration of stay of both postoperative and medical patients was similar, namely 38 and 37 hours respectively. About 3% of all patients were later tranferred to ITU because they required assisted ventilation; 3% died in HDU, and 94% were returned to their original wards following clinical improvement and reduced nursing dependency.

HDU, therefore, is a natural evolution of progressive patient care following theatre recovery unit and prior to ITU. The clinical care hiatus between ITU areas and ordinary ward areas in many acute hospitals can be closed by the development of HDU areas for selected high-risk patients. Concentrated staff with careful observation of the patient's cardiopulmonary status allows postoperative pain relief to be managed on an individual basis under close observation. Although HDU introduction results in additional hospital costs, this should be balanced against the need to provide special nurses in ordinary ward areas, or the transfer of patients to very expensive ITU facilities.

PROGNOSTIC SCORING IN HIGH-RISK SURGICAL PATIENTS

There has been great interest recently in quantifying factors preoperatively which correlate with the development of postoperative morbidity and mortality. Some accuracy is possible for this population of patients, but precision does not extend to accurate prediction of risk for an individual patient. Frequently, the decision to proceed can be made only by discussion between surgeon and anaesthetist.

Many surgeons, however, fear that the decision to operate may become a score-driven event rather than a clinical decision based on experience and clinical judgement. However, full POSSUM score (see below) is not available until after operation, and it is impossible to have a mortality/morbidity risk of either 100% or 0%, so that the score can not deprive patients of the possible benefits of an operation. However, the physiological components of the score, when combined with the likely operative severity score, can allow accurate estimate of risk, so that both the patient and relatives can be told.

1. APACHE scoring system (American)

See s. 1.73 Trauma evaluation and prognosis

2. POSSUM scoring system (UK)
(see Tables 1.25.2, 1.25.3)

An acronym for Physiological and Operative Severity Score for the enUmeration of Mortality and morbidity. It has been applied and validated in a wide range of gastroenterological, hepatobiliary, vascular and urological operations. The score is applicable in all circumstances and in all hospitals, and so the variables can be estimated as easily for emergency as for elective cases. POSSUM is accurate and can be useful in surgical audit of morbidity and mortality. British founders of the POSSUM score claim its superiority over the American APACHE score in predicting mortality in general surgical patients (APACHE is not designed to predict operative mortality) and in its general predictive ability in both ICU (ITU) and HDU. POSSUM may be useful for estimation of resources in a high-risk group.

POSSUM is a two-part system that scores both physiological and operative aspects. It is developed of multivariate discriminant and logistic regression analysis of 62 variables reduced subsequently to:
- a 12 factor, 4 grade physiological score; and
- a 6 factor, 4 grade operative severity score.

When these are combined a numerical estimate of both mortality and morbidity is obtained.

The equation for mortality risk is:

$$\log [\text{risk} - (1 - \text{risk})] = -7.04 + (0.13 \times \text{physiological score}) + (0.16 \times \text{operative severity score})$$

The equation for morbidity risk (both minor and major) is:

$$\log [\text{risk} - (1 - \text{risk})] = -5.91 + (0.16 \times \text{physiological score}) + (0.19 \times \text{operative severity score})$$

Example:

A man aged 72 (score 4) presented with a 4 cm diameter aortic aneurysm and requested operation. He was hypertensive (diastolic pressure 105 mmHg) (score 2), and short of breath on exertion (score 2). He took antianginal drugs and a diuretic (score 2), and had had a myocardial infarct a year before (score 4). The other 7 variables scored 1 each: total physiological

Table 1.25.2 Physiological score at time of operation

	1	*2*	*4*	*8*
Age	≥60	61–70	≥71	
Cardiac	No failure	Drug treatment	Oedema/warfarin	Raised JVP
Chest X-ray	Normal	[normal, score 1]	Slight cardiomegaly	Cardiomegaly
Respiratory	Normal	Dyspnoea on exertion	Dyspnoea on stairs	Dyspnoea at rest
Chest X-ray	Normal	Mild COAD	Mod COAD	Fibrosis/consolidation
Systolic blood pressure (mmHg)	110–130	131–170 or 100–109	≥171 or 90–99	≤89
Pulse rate	50–80	81–100 or 40–49	101–120	≥121 or ≤39
Glasgow coma scale	15	12–14	9–11	≤8
Urea (mmol/l)	≤7.5	7.6–10	10.1–15	≥15.1
Haemoglobin (g/l)	130–160	115–129 or 161–170	100–114 or 171–180	≤99 or ≥181
White count (x10^9/l)	4–10	10.1–20 or 3.1–4	≥20.1 or ≤3	
Sodium (mmol/l)	≥136	131–135	126–130	≤125
Potassium (mmol/l)	3.5–5	3.2–3.4 or 5.1–5.3	2.9–3.1 or 5.4–5.9	≤2.8 or ≥6
Electrocardiogram	Normal	[Normal, score 1]	MI >6 mth ago or AF 60–90	MI <6 mth ago or AF ≥91 or ectopics or Q or ST changes

COAD, chronic obstructive airways disease; MI, myocardial infarction; AF, atrial fibrillation.

Table 1.25.3 Operative severity score

Score[a]	*1*	*2*	*4*	*8*
Minor operation	1	[score 1]	[score 1]	[score 1]
Intermediate operation	[score 2]	2	[score 2]	[score 2]
Major operation	[score 4]	[score 4]	4	[score 4]
Major + operation	[score 8]	[score 8]	[score 8]	8
Number of procedures	1		2	>2
Blood loss (ml)	≤100	101–500	501–999	≥1000
Peritoneal soiling	None	Minor (serous or blood)	Local pus	Bowel contents General pus Blood ≥250 ml
Malignancy	None	Primary only	Node metastases	Distant metastases
Timing of operation	Elective	[Elective, score 1]	Urgent, resuscitation	Emergency, within 2 h

[a] Minor: hernia, breast lump, varicose veins.
  Intermediate: cholecystectomy, mastectomy, appendicectomy, transurethral resection.
  Major: other laparotomy, choledochotomy, bowel resection, major amputation.
  Major +: aortic operation, pancreatic, hepatic, oesophageal, abdominoperineal resection.

score *21*. The operative severity score is *16*, made up of major + operation (score 8), blood loss 750 ml (score 4), and 1 each for the other 4 variables.

The equation for risk of mortality is:

$$\log [R - (1-R)] = -7.04 + (0.13 \times 21) + (0.16 \times 16)$$
$$= -7.04 + 2.73 + 2.56$$
$$= -1.75$$

The antilog of −1.75 is 0.1738
If $[R - (1-R)] = X$, then:
$$R \text{ (risk)} = X - XR$$
$$R + XR = X$$
$$R (1 + X) = X$$
$$R = X - (1 + X)$$
$$= 0.1738 - 1.1738$$
$$= 0.148$$

The risk of mortality is therefore 14.8%.

The equation for the risk of morbidity is:

$$\log [R - (1-R)] = -5.91 + (0.16 \times 21) + (0.19 \times 16)$$
$$= -5.91 + 3.36 + 3.04$$
$$= 0.49$$

The antilog of 0.49 is 1.632
If $[R - (1-R)] = X$, then:
$$R \text{ (risk)} = X (1 + X)$$
$$= 1.632 - 2.632$$
$$= 0.62$$

The risk of morbidity is therefore 62%.

1.26 Artificial Ventilation

Anaesthetic sponge steeped in a concoction of aromatics and soporifics was first used by Arab surgeons during the 9th century AD. Artificial ventilation was first used in 1934, using ether. The first British ventilator in commercial use was manufactured by Blease. The patient's breathing can either be spontaneous (without muscle relaxation) or controlled with artificial ventilation (with muscle relaxation).

Methods of artificial ventilation include the following:

Intermittent positive pressure ventilation (IPPV)

IPPV was initially carried out by manual compression of a reservoir bag. IPPV is established after tracheal intubation, administration of muscle relaxant, i.v. agents to produce narcotic-induced apnoea (and thus controlled breathing is necessary), and inhalation agents. In thoracic surgery controlled respiration prevents paradoxical breathing and mediastinal flap. In abdominal operations, controlled respiration by IPPV allows good relaxation with control of patient's oxygenation and carbon dioxide elimination. It allows surgery without deep anaesthesia and many anaesthetists use it during operations when muscle relaxation is not necessary. It may also reduce the amount of thiopentone and relaxant required during operation, thus contributing to speedy recovery of consciousness and muscle tone. IPPV seldom leads to a pressure of $40\,cmH_2O$, but during coughing intrabronchial pressure can reach $100\,cmH_2O$. This may rarely lead (if care is not taken) to rupture of lung and its sequelae, pneumothorax, mediastinal emphysema, pulmonary interstitial emphysema and subcutaneous emphysema.

IPPV results in the following physiological changes:
- Intrapleural pressure during spontaneous respiration is $-5\,cmH_2O$ at the end of expiration, and $-10\,cmH_2O$ during inspiration. In IPPV, pressure rises during inspiration from $-5\,cmH_2O$ to $+3\,cmH_2O$ and falls to $-5\,cmH_2O$ during expiration.
- Damage to lungs. Rupture is unlikely, because during coughing and straining pressure may rise to $100\,cmH_2O$. It is difficult to increase pressure above $50\,cmH_2O$ by bag pressure.
- Compliance. Anaesthesia with or without IPPV, produces 50% reduction in lung compliance.
- Physiological dead space is increased.
- Respiratory alkalosis. This increases affinity of haemoglobin for oxygen, to cause cerebral vasoconstriction and to decrease cardiac output. Blood pressure is likely to fall. Overventilation raises pain threshold.
- Cardiovascular changes. At the end of positive-pressure inspiration, right atrial pressure is raised and hence venous return and cardiac output are decreased. Oxygen consumption is reduced because of abolition of respiratory work.

Continuous positive airway pressure (CPAP)

In CPAP positive pressure is applied to the airway of a patient who is breathing spontaneously. It is advocated in respiratory distress of the newborn, following cardiac surgery, and is valuable during weaning from IPPV. In general, effects of CPAP are similar to those of PEEP.

Positive end-expiratory pressure (PEEP)

In clinical practice this is useful in situations where arterial oxygen tension remains low despite high inspired oxygen concentration. It is useful during conditions such as fat embolism and respiratory distress of the newborn. Despite the importance of PEEP in ITU, there appears to be no place for PEEP during anaesthesia for routine surgical operations.

Indications for PEEP include:
- Respiratory distress syndrome of both the newborn and adults (e.g. fat embolism and multi-system organ failure).
- A trial of PEEP may be considered whenever Pa_{O_2} cannot be elevated to acceptable levels (e.g. 7 kPa or 50 mmHg). PEEP may raise Pa_{O_2} with less danger of oxygen toxicity to lungs than if higher inspired oxygen concentrations are used. Monitoring of blood gases is essential.

Special care is necessary when PEEP is applied in:
- Hypovolaemia, since PEEP may reduce cardiac output and therefore hypovolaemia must be corrected.
- Chronic bronchitis, emphysema and bronchospasm.
- Presence of fractured ribs because of increased danger of pneumothorax. It is safer with a chest tube drain in place.
- Autonomic neuropathy, e.g. in diabetes mellitus.

The possible harmful effects of PEEP include:
- Reduction of cardiac output secondary to decreased venous return to the heart. Any advantage gained by increasing Pa_{O_2} may be offset if reduced cardiac output diminishes the overall oxygen delivery to tissues. A Swan–Ganz catheter will allow measurement of mixed venous oxygen tension, cardiac output, oxygen consumption and delivery.
- Increased airway pressure can result in pneumothorax and even air embolism and pneumoperitoneum. Chest X-ray may be needed.
- Renal function may be impaired. Increased output of ADH may be stimulated with reduced urine output and water retention.
- Rise in cerebral venous and intracranial pressures in parallel with increase in mean intrathoracic pressure.

Intermittent mandatory ventilation (IMV)

IMV has been advocated during weaning from mechanical ventilation. The patient is allowed to breath spontaneously, but ventilation is augmented according to pre-set minute volume. Synchronised IMV allows mandatory ventilation to be synchronised with the patient's own inspiratory effort, and is more effective. Some patients require additional help to inspiration given by a small pressure applied to the airway (pressure support).

High-frequency positive pressure ventilation (HEPPV)

There are three types of high-frequency low tidal volume ventilation: high-frequency jet positive pressure (HEPPV) 1–2 cycle/second; high-frequency jet ventilation (HFJV) up to 7 c/s; and high-frequency ventilation (HFOV) 5–40 c/s.

HFPPV may be delivered using a conventional ventilator circuit, HFJV is given with Venturi equipment, whereas HFOV uses high-frequency solenoid valves.

The technique can be applied using a narrow-bore insufflation tube down the centre of the tracheal tube, in the management of anaesthesia for resection of tracheal stenosis; a tracheal tube is placed proximal to stenosis and insufflation tube advanced distal to it to maintain ventilation while the ends of the trachea are freely mobilised. The method is also used in the care of neonates with respiratory distress syndrome, and also for microlaryngeal laser surgery. The role of HFPPV in acute respiratory failure is controversial. Patients with larger air leaks due to bronchopleural fistula may do well with HFPPV.

Ventilators

The ideal ventilator should be compact, portable, robust, simple to operate and economical to purchase, use and maintain. Ventilators are either automatic or manually operated.

Manually operated ventilators are portable and suitable for emergency or short-term use. Manual ventilators are useful during transfer of ITU patients around hospital. They include:
– reservoir bag with mask or tracheal tube provided there is a source of oxygen or compressed air;
– Ambu bag and Laerdal bag;
– Oxford inflating bellows;
– Cardiff inflating bellows.
– Cardiff infant inflating bag.

Techniques used to reduce bleeding

Such techniques work mainly via induced hypotension or bradycardia. They include:
1. Hyperventilation with halothane.
2. β-blockers.
3. Ganglion blockers.
4. Isoflurane.
5. Epidural or spinal anaesthesia.
6. Tourniquet works via occluding arterial blood flow to the limb under treatment (see Tourniquet under discussion of instruments in s. 4.3 below).

1.27 Incisions, Wounds, Sutures/Implants and Ulcers in Surgery

ABDOMINAL INCISIONS (Fig. 1.27.1)

The abdomen varies in size and shape; it is protuberant and round in the obese patient and scaphoid in the thin patient. Anatomical landmarks can either be constant, such as xiphisternum, anterior superior iliac spine, inguinal ligament and public tubercle, or less constant, such as linea alba, umbilicus (fibrous scar in linea alba containing cords of fibrous remnants of

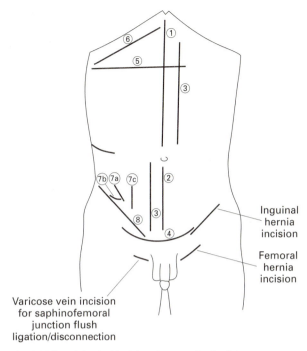

Fig. 1.27.1 Abdominal incisions (see text for details)

umbilical vein, two umbilical arteries, allantois and urachus) and linea semilunaris (extending from pubic tubercle to 9th costal cartilage). Abdominal skin is soft, elstic and mobile; the collagen bundles (Langer's lines) run transversely. Cutaneous arteries accompany cutaneous nerves. There are five pairs of muscles and three aponeuroses in the abdominal wall. Anterior vertical muscles are recuts abdominis and pyramidalis; recti extend from the lower thorax to the pubic bone. Rectus sheath derived from three lateral muscles and rectus muscle is interrupted by tendinous intersections fusing recti to the anterior rectus sheath; the posterior rectus sheath is deficient below the arcuate line. The lateral muscles run in different directions; external oblique muscle fibres run obliquely downwards and forwards; internal oblique muscle fibres run upwards and forwards; and transversus abdominis run horizontally.

Abdominal incisions can be either vertical or transverse.

1. Upper midline incision Ideal for operations on stomach, duodenum, gallbladder, liver (particularly left lobe), spleen and transverse colon. Exploratory laparotomy for undiagnosed disease can be performed by long midline incision skirting umbilicus, or by paramedian incision (equidistant above and below umbilicus); once the peritoneum is opened and diagnosis confirmed, the incision may be elarged upwards or downwards accordingly. Linea alba only can be closed carefully with looped PDS or maxon (absorbed in six months) or using nylon, Prolene, stainless steel, or other non-absorbable sutures taking good bites with equidistance on each side from cut edges of linea alba. Catgut should not be used. Peritoneum is not an essential layer to close, and subcutaneous fat may be closed (though not always) with interrupted catgut after securing haemostasis. Skin is closed with interrupted silk, nylon, or subcuticular Dexon.

2. *Lower midline incision*   Useful for pelvic organ surgery, bladder and prostate. Preoperative urinary catheterisation is imperative. Peritoneum can be closed with catout (though not essential). Linea alba is not well defined as in the upper abdomen and must be closed with non-absorbable suture. There is little point in suturing rectus abdominis muscles to each other.

3. *Paramedian incision*   This incision (1 inch parallel to midline) was popular in the past because it affords strong scar and good exposure of abdominal contents, but it is fading away because of bleeding and time taken to mobilise rectus muscle laterally from its anterior sheath (even when one goes through split muscle fibres along the incision of anterior rectus sheath and skin). Furthermore, the medial half of the rectus muscle will be deprived of its nerve supply and will be followed by atrophy of this part of the muscle. The abdominal wall layers are closed in layers.

In debilitated and septic patients, however, reinforcing deep tension non-absorbable sutures are advocated for deep full-thickness closure for 14 days to avoid wound dehiscence; deep tension sutures are also used in repairing the burst abdomen itself. Tension sutures require careful insertion to avoid penetrating bowel or major vessels, and must be tied over tubing without over-tension to avoid cutting through; they are placed at 2–3 cm intervals throughout wound length.

4. *Pfannestiel suprapubic incision*   This horizontally placed 8–12 cm long incision (curving over pubic bone) is followed by separating rectus muscles vertically. It was designed to prevent incisional hernias following transverse muscle-cutting incisions. It is ideal for bladder and prostate surgery and for gynaecological operations. The incision may result in postoperative inguinal hernias.

5. *Upper abdominal transverse incision*   Extends from costal margin to costal margin and is centred midway between umbilicus and xiphoid process. Muscles are cut transversely and closed in layers. Many surgeons use it for upper abdominal surgery, such as cholecystectomy, since it results in a cosmetically sound scar.

6. *Kocher subcostal or oblique abdominal incision*   Used for surgery on the gallbladder, spleen and colonic flexures with excellent exposure. Again it is a muscle-cutting incision and in patients with narrow costal margin is not recommended. It starts in the midline just below the xiphoid process 1 inch parallel to the costal margin.

7. *Incisions for appendicectomy*   Gridiron incision (advocated by McBurney):
(a) The commonest and safe and sound in healing. The skin is incised obliquely at a point on the medial 2/3 and lateral 1/3 of an imaginary line between umbilicus and the right anterosuperior iliac spine. It is a muscle-splitting incision, separating the external oblique aponeurosis, internal oblique and transversus abdominis.
(b) Lanz incision: similar to gridiron but transverse, providing a cosmetic scar.
(c) Battle (name of a surgeon) pararectal incision: gives better access than gridiron incision. It is vertically placed over the

lateral 1/3 of the rectus muscle, opening the anterior sheath and displacing rectus medially, which may damage the nerve supply of rectus, resulting in lateral partial atrophy.

8. *Oblique muscle-cutting iliac incision* (Rutherford Morison)   Designed for lower ureter (extraperitoneal) and colon (intraperitoneal); it is ideal for right kidney transplantation. It starts 3 cm above the pubic tubercle and passes laterally to 3 cm above the iliac crest, cutting through all muscles along the line of incision.

9. *Incisions for hepatic and complicated hepato-pancreatico-biliary surgery*   Bilateral subcostal incisions meeting with a curved line at the sub-xiphisternum (roof-top incision) or meeting acutely at an angle (chevron incision), or long right subcostal incision with a short left subcostal incision (hockey-stick incision) can all be used for hepatic resection, liver transplantation, high subhepatic bilary reconstructive surgery, Whipple's operation and surgery for portal hypertension. The exposure can be aided by a sandbag below the centre of the back (to bend the backbone and open the upper abdomen), retrosternal retraction with self-retaining abdominal retraction (with blades resting on subcostal margins) or the use of a Omni-tract retractor. Bilateral subcostal incisions can be extended vertically (Mercedes-Benz incision).

Methods of skin closure

Following layered (of all layers) or mass closure (of fasciomuscular component) of the anterior abdominal wall, skin must be closed. There are many methods of skin closure (Fig. 1.27.2):
1. Interrupted suture, which can be either ordinary or eversion (vertical mattress).
2. Horizontal mattress, which can be either fully buried or half-buried.
3. Continuous suture, which can be either over-and-over (overhand) or continuous blanket.
4. Subcuticular continuous suture.
Wound skin can also be closed by means of Steristrips, Michel metallic clips, or by automatic clip applier (stapler).

WOUNDS

A wound is defined as a break in an epithelial surface which may be surgical or accidental (external factors). Burns, ulceration and pressure sores are exluded in this definition, but drain sites should be included. (Ulcer is epithelial discontinuity but due to internal factors.)

Wound strength is dependent on approximation and healing of fascio-muscular layers (sero-submucosa in gut); not skin/subcutaneous fat, peritoneum nor postoperative adhesions can exert equivalent strength.

Phases of wound healing

There are three phases of wound healing:
1. *Lag phase* (postoperative days 1–4): represents the period of inflammatory response with assembly of components for

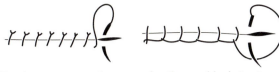

Continuous over and over (overhand) suture

Continuous blanket suture

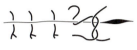

Ordinary simple interrupted

Eversion interrupted/ vertical mattress suture

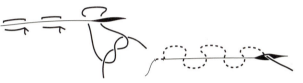

Horizontal mattress suture

Subcuticular continuous suture

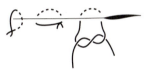

Half-buried horizontal mattress suture

Fig. 1.27.2 Methods of skin closure

collagen synthesis. During this phase wound strength is entirely dependent on external support by sutures.

2. *Proliferative phase* (days 5–20): reflects laying down of collagen lattice and rapid increase of intrinsic wound strength (regaining more than 30% of pre-trauma strength).

3. *Remodelling phase* (day 21 to 1 year): reflects constant collagen replacement and orientation to lines of stress, with wound stability (regaining more than 70% of original strength). The 100% tensile stength can be regained in up to 2 years.

GIT anastomotic healing is similar to wound healing and passes through the above three phases. However, healing in bone fractures differs slightly. Stages for bone regeneration include: haematoma formation, followed by inflammatory response with macrophages demolition and formation of granulation tissue, then soft callus formation (initial scaffolding of woven bone and cartilage), hard callus formation (lamellar bone with Haversian system formation), and finally remodelling.

Factors influencing healing

The oucome of wounding depends on interaction between healing, favourable factors and disrupting, unfavourable factors; the result spells success or failure. These factors may be local or general.

General factors

General, disrupting, unfavourable factors include abdominal distension, coughing (and smoking), obesity, malnutrition, elderly patients, diabetes, steroid therapy, malignancy, chemotherapy, immunosuppression, uraemia, jaundice, anaemia and vitamin C deficiency.

Local factors

Introduction of sutures implies fresh additional trauma to incisional wound trauma. The greater tissue reaction to suture, the more likely are oedema and inflammatory response to weaken the tissue bite; burst abdomen (an acute wound failure) can result from cutting out of an intact suture through the wound edge (like cutting cheese with thread), and also premature absorption of suture material in minority of cases. Suture pressure on tissues is inversely proportional to the diameter of suture material, but large and deep tissue bites must be considered for augmentation of wound strength.

Tissue reaction to suture material is reduced with the introduction of inert synthetic materials, while plain catgut still incites a full reaction; modern processing and chroming can reduce but not abolish tissue reaction to chromic catgut. The naturally occurring non-absorbables, silk, linen and cotton, are grossly reactive, while braided polyglycolic acid absorbable synthetic sutures produce fairly minor tissue response only excelled by monofilaments of nylon, steel, polyethylene and polyproylene (Prolene). Furthermore, tissue reaction is proportional to the quantity of suture material implanted; excessive knotting and long ends may constitute a local foreign body counter-productive to wound security.

Improper haemostasis results in haematoma formation which is an ideal culture for bacteria leading to poor wound healing. Nerve damage inflicted during incision and surgery may cause muscular atrophy weakening abdominal wall closure with possible herniation. Tension, haematoma formation and nerve damage can all be avoidable and must be considered iatrogenic disruption induced by faulty surgical technique.

Infection, too, depends on suture material; silk and naturally occurring non-absorbable materials usually introduce, augment and maintain infection, and resolution may only be achieved by spontaneous ejection by body or by deliberate removal. Multifilament (braided) synthetics may also draw surface infections by capillary action along suture track into the wound. Monofilament synthetics are the best because of inert reaction and relative safety in the presence of infection.

The suture length must be four times the wound length in order to allow for oedema and to avoid tension in an over-taut wound. Sutures must be inserted at right-angles to a line of tissue fibres to avoid the risk of suture cutting out. The loop strength is the sum of linear tensile strength plus knot strength of the material. Tensile strength of suture material is usually measured by Instron Tensiometer. Knot security is important; monofilaments generally have a low coefficient of friction and thus the knot may slip, particularly nylon (Prolene is better). Braiding provides an immediate rise in security. Catgut notoriously 'swells' the knot loose, while polyglycolic acid material produces a secure knot.

Over-tightening of sutures can result in oedema and ischaemic necrosis of devitalised tissues (wound edges must kiss each other without overlapping). However, the choice of a suture material usually depends on the surgeon's preference.

Other local factors include local dead tissues and foreign bodies (e.g. lacerated wound in road traffic accident), which must all be removed and the wound excised with wound toilet; the wound then can rarely be closed with primary suture (if within 6 hours of injury with no wide gap requiring skin graft), or more commonly is left wide open for delayed primary suture (e.g. missile injuries and compound fracture). Blood supply plays a detrimental role in wound healing; excellent blood supply of the face, head and neck is usually associated with good healing despite infection, while poor blood supply of the lower leg particularly in patients with diabetes and atherosclerosis is associated with poor healing of wounds and ulcers despite good infection control.

Types of healing

Healing by first intention

All incised surgical wounds are clean with minimal tissue damage and with edges in opposition (no gaping) due to primary suture; they heal by first intention (i.e. by body first and best inflammatory response). All similar incised wounds within 6 hours of injury can also heal by first intention when wound edges are brought together by sutures, clips or even adhesive material (film or tape). This type of healing is rapid and usually results in an invisible scar (with minimal fibrosis), functionally sound (no contraction) and with a good cosmetic result.

Healing by second intention

All wounds with widely separated edges (gaping) with skin loss and infection heal by second intention (i.e. by body second alternative, excessive granulation and scarring). All lacerated wounds more than 6 hours of injury, missile injuries and compound fracture require wide wound excision with delayed primary suture of skin or delayed skin grafting (if gap is wide); they heal by second intention. Similarly, all ulcers and spontaneously ruptured abscesses heal by second intention. This type of healing is slow and results in heavy scarring with contraction and ugly deformity.

Sterilisation of suture materials

There are three methods employed; each may affect suture material properties to some extent. These methods are:

Gamma radiation   Has the manufacturing advantage of applicability to packed material. However, linen, cotton, PGA and polyprophylene are damaged. It is the best choice for other suture materials.

Ethylene oxide   The poisonous nature of this gas, with requirement for packages to be open prior to sterilisation, makes this choice less attractive. It is method of choice in PGA, polypropylene, linen and cotton: it can also be used for catgut and polyethylene sterilisation.

Autoclave   Readily available but damages catgut, PGA and polyethylene. Silk, linen and cotton can be autoclaved but lose some strength. Polyesters, nylon, polypropylene and metals can tolerate at least three autoclaving procedures. It is the method of choice in metals, such as steel.

Surgical wound infection

A wound is infected if it discharges pus, or if swab from the wound is positive.

A wound developing signs of inflammation or serous discharge is labelled 'possibly infected'; these wounds should be followed daily until they resolve (not infected) or suppurate (infected). Bruising, haematoma formation, serous and lymph collections are complications which may predispose to development of wound infection, and may lead to diagnostic difficulties. Infection should be considered to be present when there is fever, tenderness, oedema and extending margin of erythema. The discharge of clear fluid from a wound does not indicate an infection unless accompanied by cellulitis.

Recently the definition of wound infection has not been dependent on bacteriological result, since false-negative culture can occur and organisms isolated from cultures may occasionally represent either secondary colonisation or mere contamination.

The prospective study by Cruse and Foord (1980) from Alberta (Canada) has improved our knowledge of surgical wound infection; 627 939 wounds were studied over a 10-year period with an overall infection rate of 4.7%. All wounds were allocated to one of the following four categories based on a clinical estimate of wound contamination made by a circulating nurse in the operating theatre.

Clean wound   No infection encountered, no break in aseptic technique, and no hollow muscular organ opened, e.g. inguinal hernia repair, varicose veins operation, mastectomy and thyroidectomy. The infection rate is 1.5%.

Clean contaminated wound   A hollow muscular organ is opened, but with minimal spillage of contents, e.g. cholecystectomy, appendicectomy and hysterectomy. Infection rate is 7.7%.

Contaminated wound   A hollow muscular organ is opened with gross spillage of contents, or alternatively, acute inflammation without pus formation, and operations associated with a major break in aseptic technique (GIT bypass operations and also resection/anastomosis); a traumatic wound within less than 6 hours falls within this group. Infection rate is 15.2%.

Dirty wounds   Pus is encountered at operation or a perforated viscus found, e.g. perforated appendicitis, perforated peptic ulcer, as well as traumatic wounds more than 6 hours old. Infection rate is 40%.

Factors influencing infection rate in surgical practice

Many important recommendations have emerged from this study and contributed to the improvement in surgical practice. These factors include:

1. *Short preoperative stay or hospitalisation.* The longer a patient stays in hospital before an operation, the more susceptible he or she becomes to wound infection. With one-day preoperative stay the infection rate is 1.2%; with one-week preoperative stay it is 2.1%; and for a stay of more than 2 weeks, 3.4%. It is likely the patient's skin becomes colonised with bacteria to which he or she is not resistant. The patient's age is also important, with patients more than 66 years old being 6 times more likely to develop infection than patients 1–14 years old.

2. *Preoperative shower with hexachlorophane.* If the patient did not shower, the infection rate was found to be 2.3%. If the patient showered before operation and used soap, the infection rate was 2.1%, and if hexachlorophane was used in the shower, the infection rate was 1.3%.

3. *Shaving kept to a minimum.* Shaving the operation site increased the infection rate of clean wounds. In patients shaved with a razor, the infection rate was 2.5%; in patients not shaved but having their pubic hair clipped, the infection rate was 1.7%; in patients shaved with an electric razor, the infection rate was 1.4%; and in patients neither shaved nor clipped, the infection rate was 0.9%. Another study used scanning electron microscopy of skin prepared with a safety razor, electric clipper, or depilatory; it showed that the safety razor produced gross cuts, the clipper tended to nip the skin at creases, and the depilatory caused no visible injuries. Another study of clean wounds found an infection rate of 5.6% when the patient was shaved, 0.6% when no shaving was done, and 0.6% if a depilatory was used. Another study stressed the importance of shaving immediately before operation to prevent bacterial growth in razor nicks.

4. *Contamination eschewed.* Contamination can have two sources: endogenous and exogenous.

Endogenous contamination:

- *Skin drapes.* The use of adhesive plastic drapes does not reduce the infection rate of clean wounds. With the usual cotton drapes, the infection rate of clean wounds is 1.5%; with adhesive plastic drapes, the infection rate is 2.3%. This is supported by others who found that the incidence of wound infection was doubled when adherent plastic drapes were used. However, others compared quantitative cultures from herniorrhaphy wounds draped with adherent plastic and those draped with cloth; bacterial density was the same. Furthermore, bacterial density of wounds did not differ from that of adjacent skin. Consequently, adhesive plastic drapes are not used; this also saves money.

- *Skin preparation before operation.* If skin in theatre is vigorously washed for 10 minutes with green soap, then alcohol is applied, the infection rate is 2%. If skin is washed with povidone-iodine scrub sponge on the ward, and in theatre painted with tincture of chlorhexidine (Hibitane) for 3 min, the infection rate of clean wounds is 1.6%.

- *Incidental Appendicectomy.* Infection rate of clean cholecystectomy is 1.4%; when appendicectomy in passing is performed, infection rate is tripled to 4.5% (due to increased endogenous contamination from a break in aseptic technique). Incidental appendicectomy is hazardous and merits scrupulous aseptic technique.

Exogenous contamination:

- *Scrub solutions.* Use of povidone-iodine or hexachlorophene did not affect infection rate of clean wounds. Many surgeons now use chlorhexidine scrub (Hibitane); hexachlorophene became unpopular when a study demonstrated that it was absorbed and detectable in blood.

- *Scrub time.* There is no difference between 5- and 10-minute surgical scrubs after studying bacterial counts on hands of surgeons at the end of 2-hour operations irrespective of the scrub solution used. The economics in terms of scrub time, scrub solution and water conservation are obvious; 10-minute scrub uses 50 gallons of water. The use of a brush scrub with one of the detergent antiseptics for only 3–5 min before the first operation and for 2–3 min with a sponge between operations is a good practice, since it is not associated with an increased infection rate of clean wounds.

- *Gloves.* About 11.6% of gloves are punctured at the end of surgical procedure. Surprisingly, not a single incidence of wound infection has occurred in those patients. Organisms probably escaped from glove punctures in insufficient numbers to be a serious hazard in a clean wound with adequate local resistance. There is probably little risk in operating without gloves, except perhaps to the surgeon in hepatitis and AIDS. Gloves are either starch-powder-containing (Dispo) or starch-free (Biogel). Most surgeons prefer Biogel gloves because starch can cause starch granulomas, adhesions and even starch peritonitis as well as delayed hypersensitivity to both surgeon and patient. Orthopaedic surgeons employ double-gloving to avoid needlestick injuries.

- *Face mask.* Some studies suggested that it is probably unnecessary to wear a face mask in theatre to reduce wound infections. However, there is little evidence to support this belief. Studies showing no difference to contamination of agar dishes 1.2 m above the floor within the theatre suite may be due to a great many people being present which flawed the results; the same argument can be applied to ward work, where many people are moving about and causing considerable contamination from other sources. However, when volunteers were asked to speak at agar plates close to the mouth without and with wearing masks, it was found that surgical face masks were effective in reducing bacterial contamination caused by dispersal from upper airways; findings were of particular interest to anaesthetists peforming spinal block to prevent bacterial meningitis. Type of mask is important; simple paper or cloth masks provide no benefit. The most effective are large soft pleated and pliable masks; the actual material being unimportant. When tested *ex vivo*, good masks remained good bacterial filters for 8 h, though a small increase was seen in agar plate contamination after the mask had been worn for 15 min; although such an increase was statistically insignificant, it may be advisable to wear a fresh face mask for each procedure.

5. *As expeditious an operation as is safe.* There is a direct relation between length of operation and infection rate; the infection rate of clean wounds doubles with every hour. There are four possible explanations:

- dosage of bacterial contamination increases with time;
- wound cells are damaged by drying and exposure to air and retractors;

– increased amount of suture and electrocoagulation may reduce local wound resistance;
– longer procedures are more liable to be associated with blood loss and shock, thereby reducing general patient resistance.

6. *Punctilious surgical technique* with *meticulous haemostasis and coagulation* using an electrosurgical unit. Local wound resistance is more important than patient general resistance. Indeed, the infection rate of clean wounds is usually not influenced by different wards, i.e. ward care does not apparently play a significant role in development of wound infection. Low infection rate can be achieved by gentle and meticulous surgical technique; surgeons with clean wound infection rates less than 1% are those with punctilious and fastidious surgical style. Indeed, the ideal surgeon has been quaintly described as one with a 'harte as the harte of a lyon, his eyes like the eyes of an hawke and his handes, the handes of a woman'. Haematoma formation in operative area (poor haemostasis) is the leading factor in reduction of local resistance. Scrupulous care must, therefore, be performed on elderly, obese, malnourished and diabetic patients.

Infection rate of clean wounds however, is not influenced by performing surgery in one operating theatre than another, or by using one anaesthetic agent than another. In clean operations, in which infection would be disastrous, such as joint replacement, vascular graft, cardiac surgery, and transplantation, the theatre doors are marked 'closed' to restrict traffic; movement and talking in the operating room are kept to a minimum; and anyone with skin infection is excluded. The clean infection rate for total hip replacement is 1.9%.

7. *No drainage* (if feasible). After 24 hours complement level in the wound fluid falls, so opsonisation of bacteria is impaired. Removal of stagnant wound fluid with closed suction drainage allows fresh fluid with opsonins to enter the wound. However, many studies revealed that closed drainage of the gallbladder bed did not reduce infection rate of wounds compared with the infection rate achieved with Penrose drains brought out through a stab wound. The saving was in nursing time: it takes a student nurse 5 min to empty and measure a closed suction drain but 35 min to change the dressing around a Penrose drain. Furthermore, when the Penrose drain was brought out through the main incision, the infection rate rose to 7.8% compared with 4.5% when no drain was used.

8. *Surgical audit.* Data on infection rate of clean wounds must be analysed for each surgeon and compared with the individual's peers.

Commonly used antiseptics in surgical practice

Antiseptics are disinfectant chemical solutions which destroy only the vegetative forms of organisms, leaving intact any spores that may be present; antiseptics can either be bactericidal or bacteriostatic (unlike disinfection, sterilisation is destruction of all living organisms, including spores).

The ideal disinfectant should:
– possess broad spectrum activity against organisms and spores (in practice only a few disinfectants are true sterilisers);
– have a rapid action;
– not be inactivated or vitiated by organic matter like blood, pus and faeces (in practice most disinfectants become impaired by combining to organic matters);

– be non-toxic, irritating or inducing hypersensitivity.
Disinfectants can either be inorganic or organic.

Inorganic disinfectants

These are mainly halogens (Iodine and chlorine) and are true sterilisers (killing vegetative organisms and spores), but their action can easily be annulled by organic matter.

● *Iodine* (Lugol's solution containing 25% iodine and 2.5% potassium iodide in approximately 90% ethanol) is cheap and has a broad spectrum bactericidal activity (best skin disinfectant), but it stains and irritates the skin; hypersensitivity and contact dermatitis are common.
● *Povidone-iodine* (**iodophor**) is iodine solution in non-ionic detergent which has a broad spectrum bactericidal activity with less staining and no stinging; it is moderately expensive with some hypersensitivity and local wound toxicity (though rare), and is rapidly inactivated by blood.
● *Chlorines.* Chlorine is commonly used for sterilisation of water. Chlorinated lime with boric acid has broad spectrum activity, but is moderately expensive, and locally toxic. EUSOL (Edinburgh University Solution Of Lime) dilute hypochlorite solution is cheap and has a broad spectrum activity, but is locally toxic.
● *Oxidising agents*, e.g. hydrogen peroxide and potassium permanganate solutions, are cheap, but with weak and slow bactericidal activity.

Organic disinfectants

● *Alcohols* (e.g. ethanol, isopropyl alcohol) have broad spectrum activity (but not spores), rapid action, but are flammable and moderately expensive; they are most active against bacteria at 70% concentration (pure 100% ethanol is useless as a disinfectant).
● *Phenols.* Phenol is too toxic and expensive to be used as a disinfectant. However, closely related cresol, lysol (cresol in soaps), and Sudol are relatively cheap and less toxic disinfectants and are active in the presence of organic matter, but they have an objectionable odour and can irritate the skin.
● *Dettol* (chloroxylenol) is less irritant and less toxic than others, but with less efficiency; it is inactivated by blood.
● *Chlorhexidine* (Hibitane) possesses a powerful activity against Gram-positive organisms (but not spores) such as staphylococci and streptococci, and moderate activity against Gram-negative bacteria. It has persistent action and is non-toxic, but is moderately expensive with an unpleasant taste.
● *Hexachlorophane* (pHisoHex), unlike Hibitane, is very insoluble in water or even alcohol. Though slow, it possesses cumulative action against staphylococci and streptococci (Gram-positive only); it is moderately expensive and can cause systemic toxicity in neonates with development of Gram-negative infections (in rats it causes cerebral lesions resembling spongy degeneration found in infants). *Triclosan* is less toxic than hexachlorophane but with similar activity.
● *Cetrimide* in benzalkonium chloride or *Cetavlon* (quaternary ammonium compound) is a cheap, odourless, non-irritant,

non-toxic detergent which is readily contaminated with moderate Gram-positive activity, but poor Gram-negative activity.
- *Noxythiolin* is an expensive solution, but has a broad spectrum activity and releases formaldehyde in contact with tissues.
- *Formalin*, 40% solution of formaldehyde gas in water, is a true steriliser; 120 ml of 40% formalin is used for killing hydatid cyst after aspiration of equivalent amount.
- Useful mixtures include:
  – alcohol plus chlorhexidine
  – alcohol plus povidone-iodine
  – chlorhexidine plus cetrimide.

SUTURES AND IMPLANTS IN SURGERY

A suture is a strand of material used to tie (ligate) blood vessels and/or to sew (approximate) tissues together.
- Suture material should have and maintain adequate tensile strength until its purpose is served. It should not shrink in the tissues.
- It should stimulate minimal tissue reaction and should not create a situation favourable to bacterial growth.
- It should be non-electrolytic, non-capillary, non-allergenic, non-carcinogenic (and non-thrombogenic in vascular surgery).
- The material should handle comfortably and naturally by the surgeon and a knot should hold securely without fraying or cutting.
- It should be inexpensive and easily sterilised.

The histological reactions to *all* sutures are essentially the same for the first 7 days as these changes are secondary to trauma of passage of the needle and suture.

Sutures are classified as absorbable and non-absorbable.

Absorbable surgical sutures

A sterile strand prepared from collagen derived from healthy mammals or a synthetic polymer. It is capable of being absorbed by living mammalian tissue but may be treated to modify its resistance to absorption. It may be impregnated or coated with a suitable antimicrobial agent. It may be coloured by a colour additive approved by the Federal Food and Drug Administration (FDA).

Natural collagens (monofilament in behaviour and classification although made originally from two or more ribbons).

Surgical gut Plain or chromic (treated with chromium salt solution before or after spinning into strands in order to resist body enzymes and prolong absorption time); derived from submucosa of sheep intestine or serosa of beef intestine. After 4 weeks, chromic catgut size 0 loses 60% of its initial tensile strength; plain catgut loses strength more rapidly since it is digested relatively quickly by body enzymes. The rate of absorption differs according to the site sutured, e.g. slower in subcutaneous tissues and extremely rapid if exposed to gastric juice.

Collagen sutures Extruded from a homogeneous dispersion of pure collagen fibres from flexor tendons of beef (plain or chromic).

Biological absorbable sutures Of historical interest, e.g. preserved skin, fascia lata strips (also live autogenous), cadaveric dura mater and kangaroo tendon (strong but scarce and expensive).

Synthetic absorbables (multifilament except PDS)

Polyglycolic (Dexon) and polyglactic acid are homopolymers of glycolide and copolymer lactide respectively. Absorption is complete within 4 months.

Polyglactin 910 (Vicryl) B-copolymer of lactide and glycolide absorbed *within* 90 days (it is braided). Dexon loses tensile strength more rapidly and is absorbed significantly more slowly than Vicryl. Their handling property is similar to silk – they knot easily and the knot holds well. Vicryl-rapide is absorbed in 10 days and monocryl (monofilament vicryl) in 20 days, compared to an average of 30 days for vicryl.

Poly Dioxanone Synthetic smooth suture (PDS) is a monofilament synthetic absorbable suture with total absorption at 180 days, thus providing longer wound support. It retains its strength in tissue twice as long as any other synthetic absorbable suture.

Maxon (polyglyconate) artificial monofilament synthetic absorbable suture is prepared from a copolymer of glycolic acid and trimethylene carbonate, available undyed (clear) or coloured green to enhance visibility during surgery. They are available in single and looped sutures. About 70% of suture tensile strength remains 2 weeks after implantation, while 55% remains 3 weeks after implantation. Suture absorption starts at 60 days and completes by 6 months after implantation. Maxon is smooth, with good handling properties and knot security (only one final locking surgeon's knot is required); it elicits only a mild tissue reaction during absorption. It is used for subcuticular skin closure, hernia repair, layered abdominal wall closure, mass abdominal wall closure (using looped Maxon with a non-slip locking knot), vaginal and intestinal anastomosis. It is contraindicated in neural, cardiovascular and ocular tissues.

Non-absorbable sutures

These are strands of material that effectively resist enzymatic digestion in living tissue. A suture may be mono- or multifilament, of metal or organic fibres, rendered into a strand by spinning, twisting or braiding. Each strand is substantially uniform in diameter throughout its length. The material may be uncoloured, naturally coloured or dyed with an FDA approved dyestuff. It may be coated or uncoated, treated or untreated for capillarity (designated as Type B or A respectively). Capillarity refers to the characteristic that allows the passage of tissue fluids along the strand, permitting infection to be drawn into the wound. Type B is resistant to wicking transfer of body fluids.

Natural non-absorbable materials

Surgical silk Derived from raw silk spun by the silkworm larva in construction of its cocoon. Each fibre is processed to remove the natural waxes and gums. Fibres are twisted or braided together to form the suture strand. *In vivo* studies show that it loses all or most of its tensile strength in 1 year and usually cannot be found after 2 years. Thus it behaves as a very slow absorbable suture. Silk is treated to remove its capillary action and to render it serum-proof. It is dyed black for easy visibility in tissues and is used dry because it loses tensile strength when exposed to moisture (the opposite to cotton).

Dermal suture Twisted silk fibres encased in a non-absorbable coating of tanned gelatin or other protein substance.

Virgin silk Consists of several natural silk filaments drawn together and twisted to form a fragile strand of very small diameter.

Surgical cotton Made from individual long staple vegetable cotton fibres combed, aligned and twisted into a strand. It gains tensile strength when wet.

Linen Cellulose material made from twisted long staple flax fibres.

Horsehair and human hair Have been used for plastic and nerve repair.

Surgical stainless steel wire Made of soft annealed iron alloy formula (with nickel, chromium and molybdenum) presenting optimum metal purity, strength, flexibility, uniformity and compatibility with stainless steel implants and prostheses. Both monofilament and twisted multifilament sutures have high tensile strength and low tissue reactivity owing to extreme inertness. Its disadvantages are difficult handling, late fragmentation and the possibility of cutting tissue.

Synthetic non-absorbables

Nylon (Ethilon) Polyamide polymer derived by chemical synthesis. It has high tensile strength and tissue reaction is very moderate. It degrades *in vivo* at a rate of 15% per year (monofilament).

Black braided nylon (Nurolon) Multifilament braided.

Polyester fibre (Mersilene; Ethiflex) Polymer of terephthalic acid and glycolethylene (multifilament braided).

PRESSURE SORE OR DECUBITUS ULCERS
(See also s. 2.2 Leg ulcers)

This is a representative of traumatic ulcer due to direct pressure on bony tissues (while lying supine or sitting down) or shearing forces (while sliding down a bed or a chair).

Normal capillary pressure is about 32 mmHg; external pressure in excess of 32 mmHg over bony prominences can obstruct capillaries in predisposed patients. In the supine position, pressure over the sacrum and heels may reach 40–60 mmHg causing capillary compression and localised tissue ischaemia.

On the other hand, when a patient slides down a bed or a chair, unless repositioned correctly, the skin often remains in contact with the bed or chair whereas the skeleton moves over it causing superficial friction (resulting in skin loss) and deep muscle damage (resulting in a serious penetrating sacral sore).

Immobility, vascular insufficiency, poor diet (hypoproteinaemia, low vitamin C and zinc deficiency), obesity, incontinence, diabetes mellitus, immunosuppression and old age are crucial risk factors predisposing patients to pressure sore.

Pressure sores are attributed to poor nursing care and lack of the surgeon's supervision.

The presence of a pressure sore is now defined (by Department of Health, 1993) as a new or established area of skin and/or tissue discoloration or damage which persists after the removal of pressure and which is likely to be due to the effects of pressure on the tissue. A consensus group has now proposed the **Stirling pressure sore severity scale (Reid J. and Morison M. 1994):**

Stage 0: No clinical evidence of a pressure sore. This includes:
0.0 normal appearance and intact skin
0.1 healed with scarring
0.2 tissues damage, but not assessed as a pressure sore

Table 1.27.1 The Norton 'at risk' scale

Physical condition	Score	Mental condition	Score	Activity	Score	Mobility	Score	Incontinent	Score
Good	4	Alert	4	Ambulant	4	Full	4	Not	4
Fair	3	Apathetic	3	Walk/help	3	Slightly limited	3	Occasionally	3
Poor	2	Confused	2	Chairbound	2	Very limited	2	Usually/urine	2
Very bad	1	Stuporous	1	Bedfast	1	Immobile	1	Doubly	1

Derived from D. Norton et al. (1975) *An Investigation of Geriatric Nursing Problems in Hospital.* Edinburgh: Livingstone

Table 1.27.2 A selection of mechanical methods for relieving pressure

Aid	Use	Advantages	Disadvantages
Sheepskin	Low-risk patients. Norton score 14 or above. Good for under heels	Warm and comfortable. Machine washable. Decreases friction	Does *not* relieve pressure. Hardens and matts with washing. Needs to be changed frequently. *Not recommended* for regularly incontinent patients
Heel and elbow pads: sheepskin, foam, silicone	Norton scale 14 or less or patients on prolonged bed rest	Reduce friction and shearing over the elbow and heel	Often have inadequate methods of keeping them on. Become hardened by washing.
Sorbo ring	Low-risk patients. Norton score 14 or above	At first makes patient feel comfortable	Tends to cause oedema of skin inside the hole of the ring due to pressure of the rim of the ring on surrounding tissues. Can cause venous thrombosis. *Not recommended* for patients with known vascular complications. May be a source of cross-infection
Silicone-filled mattress pad	Norton scale 14 or less or patients on prolonged bed rest, able to move spontaneously	Relieves pressure by distributing it over a greater area. Comfortable. Machine (industrial) washable. Acceptable in community settings as well as in hospital. Can be used for incontinent patients. Relatively cheap purchase price	If the patient is very incontinent of urine, even if the plastic side is uppermost, there is seepage into the core material. Stitching comes undone after several launderings. Reduces self-motivated movements in very debilitated patients
Roho air-filled mattress	Norton scale 10–14, high to medium risk. To wear off pressure-equalising beds	Interlinked air cells transfer air with movement. Patient can be nursed sitting or recumbent. Non-mechanical. Washable	Can be punctured and is expensive to repair. Often incorrectly inflated
Alternating pressure beds (Pegasus, ripple, Alphabed)	Medium risk, 12–14 Norton scale	Mechanical alteration of pressure. Reduce the frequency of (but not need for) repositioning. Available on hire at short notice	Older types prone to breakdown. Must be checked and maintained. May increase pressures in very thin patients. Punctures possible
Mechanaid netbed	Moderate risk patients. Norton score 14 or less	Fits any bed. Easy to assemble and dismantle. Easy to store. No servicing, maintenance or laundry difficulties. Patients can be repositioned by one nurse. Appears to encourage relaxation and sleep. Can be lowered on to the bed surface when a firm base is required	Patients do not always like it. Wedge of pillows needed to sit patient up. Patients may lose heat. Reduces self-motivated movement. Not always easy for patients to communicate with people sitting by bed
Water bed	Moderate risk, Norton score 12–16	Spreads pressure. Is warm and comfortable. Available on hire at short notice	Patient is supported on the skin of the water sac thus reducing the pressure-relieving properties. Difficult to get the patient in and out
Water flotation bed	Moderate to high-risk patients. Norton score 14 or less	Equalises pressure and weight. Heated	Expensive to buy, run and maintain. Makes some patients feel 'sea-sick'. Reduces self-motivated movement. Heavy to move. If not filled correctly can create more pressure than conventional bed. Not to be confused with water trough above
Fluidised air bed	High-risk patients, Norton score 10 or less or indicated because of medical condition	As near to levitation as possible. Warm, sterile air produces a beneficial environment for healing wounds. One nurse can manage even very heavy or debilitated patients on his/her own. Can be used for incontinent patients or those with heavy wound exudate	Expensive to hire, run and in old buildings maintain. Need to reinforce floors before it can be installed. Minimises self-motivation. Can be difficult for the patient to get in and out of bed even with help. Available on hire basis only
Low air loss bed	High-risk patient, Norton score 10 or less. Orientated and immobile patients	Pressure equalising properties equal to the fluidised air bed. Patient can be nursed in any position including prone. (Patient can control position.) Mobilisation easy	Expensive to buy but can be hired. Nurses need education in the use of the equipment

Based on the Manual of Nursing Practice of the Royal Marsden Hospital

Table 1.27.3 Pressure sore grades

Grade	Description
1	(a) Where the skin is likely to break down (red, black and blistered areas)
	(b) Healed areas still covered by a scab
2	Superficial break in the skin
3	Destruction of the skin without cavity (full-skin thickness)
4	Destruction of the skin with cavity (involving underlying tissues)

Based on the Manual of Nursing Practice of the Royal Marsden Hospital, according to David et al., 1983. This is largely superseded by the Stirling Pressure Sore Severity Scale.

Table 1.27.4 A selection of dressings used in the treatment of pressure sores

Dressing	Use	Advantages	Disadvantages
Topical swabs	1 Directly on to clean, dry wounds 2 As a padding over a non-adherent type dressing	Excellent absorbency. Sometimes air permeable. Generally good thermal insulator	Does not provide moist interface. No barrier to infection. Can traumatize wound when removed due to exudate adherence and capillary loop insertion
Dressing pads	As a padding over a non-adherent type dressing	Superior absorbency Partially air permeable. Thermal insulator	No moist interface. No barrier to infection. Exudate often seeps through, providing a fluid pathway for infection
Lyofoam	Non-adherent ulcer dressing	Absorption of excess fluid without dehydration. Conformable. Non-fibrous. Also available with an activated carbon insert (Lyofoam C)	May adhere in presence of dry serum and become hard

Deodorizing dressing for infected/necrotic wounds |
Synthaderm	Non-adherent ulcer dressing	Excellent for varicose ulcers. Air permeable. Impermeable to water. Provides moist interface. Barrier to infection. Thermal insulator. Non-adhesive. Reduces frequency of dressings	Tends to curl away from a wound when first applied. Some adherence occurs when it is dry. Very expensive
Melolin	Non-adherent dressing	Absorbent. Air permeable. Thermal insulator. Minimum trauma when removed	No moist interface. No barrier to infection. Non-adherent part of dressing tends to adhere to wound surface and separate from rest of dressing
Release	Non-adherent dressing	Absorbent. Air permeable. Thermal insulator. Minimum trauma at change. Moist interface	
OpSite/ Tegaderm Bioclusive	Cover for ulcerating wounds	Air permeable. Barrier to infection. Impermeable to water. High elasticity and conformability. Moist interface. Reduces frequency of dressings. Wounds readily visible	Needs considerable skill to apply due to its elasticity. Retention of fluid exudate causes bulging of dressing. Adhesive trauma on removal
Granuflex Duoderm Biofilm	Cover for ulcerating wounds	Air and water impermeable. Provide moist interface. Barrier to infection. Thermal insulator. Reduces frequency of dressings	Adhesive trauma may occur on removal. Disliked by many nurses as they are not able to observe the wound continuously. Tend to crumble after a while
Silastic foam	Non-adherent dressing. Can be tailor-made to wound. Best used on 'clean' wounds	Absorbent. Moist interface. Air permeable. Thermal insulator. Barrier to infection. Minimum trauma at change. Easy to clean. May be used to fill a cavity. Useful for self-caring patients	Needs skill to mix and mould. Need to make two moulds each time (one to wear and one to clean). Not sterile
Scherisorb, Vigilon, Geliperm	Non-adherent ulcer and cavity dressing	Absorbent, non-traumatic debriding of hard eschar by rehydration	May ooze out of wound (Scherbisorb). Cold initially
Sorbsan	Absorbent ulcer and cavity dressing	Highly absorbent, biodegradable, easy to remove by irrigation. Non-irritant	Expensive, may leave material in the wound. Long-term effects not known

Based on the Manual of Nursing Practice of the Royal Massden Hospital.

Table 1.27.5 A selection of agents used in the treatment of pressure sores

Agent	Use	Advantages	Disadvantages
Half-strength Eusol	Infected or necrotic ulcerating wounds	Relatively cheap to purchase. Easy to use. Some antiseptic properties	Short shelf-life (approximately 2 weeks). Relatively long healing times. Caustic to surrounding skin. 'Hospital smell'. Said to be a debriding agent but any debridement that occurs is due to hydration of the eschar or adherence of dried-out dressing to the wound as in wet or dry dressing
Hydrogen peroxide solution	Infected or necrotic ulcerating wounds	Decomposes to liberate oxygen into wound. Antiseptic agent	Caustic to surrounding skin. Considerable skill needed to judge when to discontinue its use. Any debridement which occurs is due to mechanical action of the chemical change (fizzing). Oxygen released insufficiently to have any effect on healing
Varidase topical (streptokinase, streptodornase)	Infected or necrotic ulcerating wounds	Excellent debriding agent. Promotes vascularisation. Rapid healing times. Does not need an aseptic technique for dressings. Reduces odour from wound	Relatively expensive to purchase. Has to be reconstituted using syringe and needle, therefore only available on prescription. Initially increases exudate. *Contraindicated* for use near blood vessels (due to potential effects of streptokinase)
Debrisan/ Iodosorb	Infected or necrotic wounds	Good debriding agents especially on liquid slough. Bacteriostatic	Dry preparation difficult to apply. Pastes or packaged preparations much easier. Must be kept off healthy tissue
Povidone-iodine/ spray	Shallow or superficial clean wounds. Grades 1 and 2	Quick to apply. Good antiseptic	Potential adverse reactions

Based on the Manual of Nursing Practice of the Royal Marsden Hospital

Stage 1: Discoloration of intact skin (light finger pressure applied to the site does not alter the discoloration). This includes:
1.1 non-blanchable erythema with increased local heat
1.2 blue/purple/black discoloration
Stage 2: Partial thickness skin loss or damage involving epidermis and/or dermis. This includes:
2.1 blister
2.2 abrasion
2.3 shallow ulcer without undermining of adjacent tissue
2.4 any of these with underlying blue, purple/black discoloration
Stage 3: Full thickness skin loss involving damage or necrosis of subcutaneous tissue but not extending to underlying bone, tendon, or joint capsule. This includes:
3.1 crater without undermining of adjacent tissue
3.2 crater with undermining of adjacent tissue
3.3 sinus, the full extent of which is not certain
3.4 full thickness skin loss but wound bed covered with necrotic tissue which masks the true extent of tissue damage (until debrided it is not possible to observe whether damage extends into muscle or involves damage to bone or supporting structures)

Stage 4: Full thickness skin loss with extensive destruction and tissue necrosis extending to underlying bone, tendon, or joint capsule. This includes:
4.1 visible exposure of bone, tendon or capsule
4.2 sinus assessed as extending to bone, tendon or capsule

Prevention of pressure sores

Assessment of patients on admission is mandatory so that precautions can be taken for those 'at risk'. Norton *et al.* (1975) developed an 'at risk' scale (Table 1.27.1). Patients with scores of 14 or below run the greatest risk of developing pressure sores, while those with score of 14–18 are not at risk but should be reassessed immediately if any deterioration in their condition is observed. Scores of 18–20 indicate patients at minimal risk.

The most effective way of prevention is by relieving or minimising direct pressure on at-risk areas by correct positioning and regular repositioning 2-hourly. Areas at risk must not be rubbed, since rubbing results in maceration and degeneration of subcutaneous tissues, especially in the elderly. Areas at risk may *only* be washed if the patient is incontinent or sweating profusely; mild soap or liquid detergent may be used

Table 1.27.6 Treatment protocols for superficial and deep sores

---

Superficial sores (Grades 2 and 3)

Action

1. Where possible relieve the pressure on the affected area. Reposition the patient at least 2-hourly and record the position on the relevant chart
2. Clean the wound using an aseptic technique
3. If necessary, cover the wound with the dressing of choice
4. Record any changes in the appropriate documents and amend the care plan accordingly

Rationale

To promote circulation and healing

To prevent infection. The wound should be disturbed as little as possible to allow healing to occur
To prevent leakage of exudate. To provide the optimum microenvironment for wound healing
For accurate evaluation of the progress of wound healing

Deep sores (Grade 4)

Action

1. Where possible relieve the pressure over the area. Reposition the patient at least 2-hourly and record the position on the relevant charts. Use pressure-relieving aids
2. Obtain a specimen of discharge with a wound swab or syringe, as required
3. Clean the wound using an aseptic technique. Use gloved hand in preference to forceps
4. Necrotic wounds should be debrided using suitable tropical agents
5. Cover the wound with an appropriate dressing. Dry topical swabs are not appropriate

6. Cavities should be filled with an appropriate product, e.g. foam, gel or hydrocolloid. Wounds should not be tightly packed with gauze
7. Fix the dressing with hypo-allergenic tape, light bandage or Netelast.
8. Encourage the patient to eat a nutritious diet, rich in vitamin C and trace elements
9. Skin graft may ultimately be required in resistant deep pressure sores

Rationale

To promote circulation and healing
To ensure consistencyin the pattern of positions used

To identify any infecting organisms

To prevent infection
To avoid damage to growing granulation tissue
To allow epithelialisation to take place
To prevent leakage of exudate. To create the optimum microenvironment for healing
Revascularisation and epithelialisation occur into the matrix of the topical swabs. Each time the dressing is removed the new tissue is lifted with it and bleeding occurs. Frequent dressings reduce the wound surface temperature and delay healing
Tight packing increases pressure and leads to further damage

Further damage will occur to broken skin if there is an allergic reaction or if tape cannot be removed easily
If exudate is excessive, substantial protein loss can occur. Vitamin C and trace elements promote healing
Ulcer cannot heal by granulation due to exposed underlying bone without periosteum

---

Modified from the Manual of Nursing Practice of the Royal Marsden Hospital

ensuring that all soap or detergent is rinsed off and the area is patted dry. Excessive use of soap can be harmful to skin. Moisturiser can be used if skin is very dry; thorough gentle drying of the skin promotes comfort and discourages microbial overgrowth; on the other hand, dry skin cracks allow bacterial entry and overgrowth. Barrier creams may *only* be used when indicated to prevent epidermal damage; however, they are occlusive and prevent correct moisture and aeration (oxygenation) of the skin.

Patient education to shift position, to pull or push up regularly and to examine vulnerable areas is important, since self-caring must continue after discharge. Patients must also be encouraged to eat a nutritious diet, rich in protein and vitamin C. A patient mobility programme must also be initiated with the help of physiotherapists or occupational therapists as appropriate. It is also important to keep the patient in a recumbent position whenever possible, supported with bead bags or pillows in bed; bed rests are better avoided since they increase shearing. The period spent sitting in a chair must be reduced if pelvic sores develop.

Mechanical methods using special devices may be employed to relieve direct pressure, particularly if the patient is immobile during surgical intervention or difficult to mobilise because of body deformities or morbid obesity.

These mechanical devices must be chosen to meet the patient's individual needs, according to Norton Scale scoring (see Table 1.27.2).

Treatment of pressure sores

This is the primary responsibility of nursing staff supervised by the surgeon in charge during the day-to-day ward round.

Pressure sores must be graded (according to David *et al.*, 1983) and then treated accordingly (see Table 1.27.3).

Appropriate dressing (see Table 1.27.4) and appropriate cleaning solution (agent) is chosen by the nurse and/or surgeon (see Table 1.27.5). The two commonly used cleaning solutions for infected wounds are normal saline and savlodil, each with advantages and disadvantages. Normal saline is isotonic, non-toxic and non-irritant, but is not an antiseptic. Savlodil is antiseptic but has the disadvantages that it can be irritant and grows bacteria under certain conditions.

Summary of therapeutic actions and rationale

Remember always that unless the source of pressure is removed, the pressure sore will not heal. Progress of wound healing must be documented and recorded daily. Pressure sores are either superficial or deep; they are treated accordingly (Table 1.27.6).

1.28 Perioperative Oliguria

Perioperative oliguria is a urine output of less than 0.5 ml/kg/h or 30 ml/h or 720 ml/24 h (assuming patient's body weight of 60 kg) in the perioperative period (mainly postoperatively). Before labelling the patient oliguric, the fluid balance chart should be checked for errors (unfortunately, all too common) and that all urine passed has been charted. If examination reveals a painfully distended bladder, catheterisation should solve the problem. If a catheter is in situ, it should be checked – the tubing may be kinked or the lumen blocked by clot or even lubricant. If necessary, the catheter should be flushed under sterile conditions with 20–30 ml H_2O. If the patient is catheterised with a patent lumen and no bladder distension, oliguria can be diagnosed. Postoperative oliguria may be considered an undesirable avoidable physiological response to perioperative hypovolaemia (endocrine response to surgical trauma by salt and water retention) rather than an unavoidable pathological response to stress inherent in anaesthesia and surgery which cannot be overcome by simple fluid loading.

- Nearly 50% of the acute haemodialysis instituted in the USA is due to perioperative renal failure. The most common cause of acute renal failure is prolonged renal hypoperfusion, due most often to hypovolaemia. In North America, liberal and sometimes excessive quantities of fluid are given, while in Europe, particularly in the United Kingdom, fluids are restricted severely.
- Oliguria that progresses to acute renal failure in surgical patients produces at least 50% mortality.
- Untreated, this renal hypoperfusion leads to reduced urine output, reflecting reductions in glomerular filtration rate and renal tubule function. The key strategy in reducing the likelihood of oliguria progressing to acute renal failure is limiting the duration and magnitude of renal hypoperfusion. Indeed, renal blood flow, and in particular renal cortical blood flow, is significantly reduced early in acute renal failure regardless of the aetiology. Persistence of renal hypoperfu-

sion for only 30 minutes may be sufficient to lead to acute renal failure. In this regard, undue reliance on laboratory tests (urinary electrolytes, urine osmolarity, derived indices such as renal failure index, or fractional excretion of sodium) to differentiate prerenal causes of oliguria may delay institution of appropriate therapy. None of these tests or derived indices is sufficiently sensitive or specific to predict whether patients have developed or will develop acute renal failure or who will not respond to therapy.

- All these tests and measurements may be misleading in patients who have recently been treated with diuretics.
- Often, the most useful information in the perioperative management of potential acute renal failure is measurement of urine output.

Causes

Causes of perioperative (or postoperative) oliguria can be prerenal, renal or postrenal.

Prerenal causes (decreased renal blood flow)

Low renal perfusion and consequently low urine output is the commonest cause.

- *Hypovolaemia* due to surgical trauma is the commonest cause of oliguria in a surgical patient and must be treated by fluid replacement. The patient is pale, sweaty, tachycardic, cool in the peripheries, hypotensive, with low JVP. Rapid fluid replacement with colloids, such as human plasma protein fraction (HPPF), will increase intravascular volume transiently, leading to increased urine output (positive response to fluid challenge). Surgical patients may suffer fluid losses in various ways.
  - Preoperative losses due to starvation (nil by mouth, or sedated and unable to resume oral fluids), sweating, enemas, diuretics, vomiting (due to premedication), nasogastric aspiration, fever and possibility of salt-losing nephropathy. With increasing age, kidneys become less able to conserve sodium under conditions of deprivation; 50% of elderly patients going to theatre have a salt-losing nephropathy.
  - Operative losses including blood loss and evaporation from skin, exposed viscera, and ventilation.
  - Sequestration of fluid into 3rd spaces. Fluid may be lost from functional extracellular space and be unavailable for normal economy or exchange because of sequestration within the body. Losses may occur in wounds (inflammation and oedema from extensive dissection), damaged muscles, paralytic ileus, ascites (e.g. in pancreatitis, biliary peritonitis, and bacterial peritonitis), pleural effusions, generalised increased capillary permeability (due to lymphokines), and concealed haemorrhage (fractured neck of femur).
- *Cardiogenic shock* with low cardiac output, due to myocardial ischaemia or pulmonary embolism. The patient is pale with tachycardia, hypotension and cool peripheries, but with raised JVP. Treatment should aim at the cause (*see below*).
- Septic shock with initial high cardiac output (hyperdynamic phase) followed by low cardiac output (hypodynamic

phase). Diagnosis of septicaemia may occasionally be difficult; post-genitourinary instrumentation rigors and fever may be replaced in the elderly by subnormal temperature with confusion and restlessness; unexplained tachycardia may be masked by β-blockers or pacemakers; and cold extrimities may be replaced by warm hypotension due to a source of infection or potential infection (e.g. post-GIT resection/anastomosis). Furthermore, septicaemia may be presented with unexplained oliguria, mild jaundice, leucocytosis, and clotting abnormalities. If septicaemia is suspected, blood cultures and cultures of possible sites of infection (e.g. wound, urine, sputum) with full blood count and blood gases must be performed. Arterial, central venous and Swan – Ganz catheters may be necessary to assess fluid replacements. Many litres of crystalloid with additional colloid may be required with appropriate antibiotics.

Renal causes (acute tubular necrosis)

Acute tubular necrosis is uncommon in general surgical practice, but may occur after vascular surgery, hepatobiliary surgery, or in those with pre-existing renal disease undergoing surgery. Diagnosis is by exclusion of prerenal and postrenal causes. Once suspected, urinary and plasma urea, electrolytes and osmolalities should be measured and compared. Urinary Na is inappropriately high and osmolality is low (no tubular absorption of Na or H_2O). Administration of diuretics and dopamine, restriction of fluid and proteins, and control of K and acid–base balance are essential. Renal causes include:

- Renal ischemia and acute renal failure is the principal risk of under-replacement of prerenal hypovolaemia. Those who advocate a liberal approach to fluid claim a drastic reduction in acute renal failure in postoperative and septic patients. In at-risk patients (jaundice, sepsis, the elderly) it is vital to maintain intravascular volume and good tissue perfusion and to preserve adequate urine flow rate, but not at the price of pulmonary oedema. Monitoring CVP (or in the critically ill, pulmonary capillary wedge pressure), core–peripheral temperature difference and body weight, and providing fluids accordingly, will prevent acute renal failure in many surgical patients. Fluid under-replacement may also lead to drowsiness, thirst, headaches, dizziness, malaise and delayed mobilisation.
- Renal nephrotoxic drugs, particularly of the aminoglycoside group of antibiotics (gentamicin, then kanamycin, amikacin, tobramycin, and, least nephrotoxic, netilycin, in this order; gentamicin is three times more nephrotoxic than netilmicin or tobramycin). Neomycin is too toxic for parenteral use; it is given orally since it is non-absorbed from GIT (like other aminoglycosides, a reason why they are given by injections).
- Release of haemoglobin or myoglobin.

Postrenal causes of oliguria are rare. They include:

- Bilateral ureteric obstruction (iatrogenic surgical injury).
- Extravasation due to rupture of bladder.

Postrenal obstruction is rare; it is diagnosed by zero urine output and confirmed by ultrasound. Nephrostomy may be required as a percutaneous upper urinary tract decompression. Thus, the usual differential diagnosis is between prerenal or renal causes.

Differential diagnosis

Oliguria due to prerenal causes is characterised by the kidney's attempt to conserve sodium and to restore intravascular fluid volume. As a result, urinary sodium excretion is often less than 40 mEq/l, and the urine is concentrated to greater than 400 mosmol/l. Excretion of sodium-poor and highly concentrated urine confirms that renal tubular function is intact. Furthermore, the ratio of urine osmolarity to plasma osmolarity is above 1.8.

Oliguria due to renal causes takes a more severe form. It is characterised by reduced blood flow to the renal cortex and a markedly decreased glomerular filtration rate. Indeed, a speculated mechanism for acute tubular necrosis is renal cortical vasoconstriction (acute vasomotor nephropathy), leading to ischaemia of this area of the kidneys. Inability of the renal tubules to reabsorb sodium is evidenced by urinary sodium excretion in excess of 40 mEq/l. Likewise, urine osmolarity is less than 400 mosmol/l (250–300), reflecting washout of osmotically active particles from the renal medulla, due in part to redistribution of renal blood flow from the cortex to the medullary areas of the kidneys. The ratio of urine osmolarity to plasma osmolarity is below 1.1.

Treatment

Aggressive and early treatment of perioperative oliguria is most important for those patients at increased risk for developing acute renal failure. At-risk patients include:

1. Geriatric patients.
2. Patients with sepsis.
3. Those with co-existing renal and/or cardiac dysfunction.
4. Patients with co-existing jaundice.
5. Those undergoing surgical procedures often associated with postoperative renal dysfunction (abdominal aneurysm resection, cardiac surgery, emergency surgery for trauma).

Occurrence of transient oliguria during elective operations in young patients without co-existing renal disease does not require the same aggressive treatment as does oliguria in geriatric patients with co-existing renal disease. However, preoperative fluid deficits should be estimated and corrected as soon as possible before surgery, because anaesthetised patients compensate poorly for even modest deficits. The average 70 kg man undergoing simple surgery without fluid replacement probably loses about 1 litre of fluid; in major surgery, particularly in pyrexial patients, losses and sequestration can be great. Fluid replacement must be provided early to limit activation of neurohumoral response mechanisms responsible for salt and water retention. Fixed fluid regimens are dangerous; perioperative requirement may range between 0.5 and 3 litres, depending on the type and duration of surgery as well as measured losses. Postoperative oliguria may not be completely avoidable, but postoperative acute renal failure certainly should be.

Despite the controversy in the choice of fluids, i.e. colloids versus crystalloids, the fluid replacement must be appropriate to the type of fluid lost (see Table 1.28.1):

Table 1.28.1 Composition of solutions for intravenous use

Colloids	*Na+* *(mmol/l)*	*K+* *(mmol/l)*	*Cl−* *(mmol/l)*	*Ca++* *(mmol/l)*	*Colloid type*
Gelofusine	154	0.4	125	0.4	Succinyl gelatin (MW 30 000, 40 g/l)
Hespan	154	–	154	–	Hetastarch (60 g/l)
Human purified protein fraction (HPPF)	157	2	118	–	Protein (45 g/l) (95% albumin)
Haemaccel	145	5.1	145	6.25	Polygeline (MW 35 000, 35 g/l)
Rheomacrodex (dextran 40)	154	–	154	–	Dextran 40 (MW 40 000, 100 g/l)
Macrodex (dextran 70)	154	–	154	–	Dextran 70 (MW 70 000, 60 g/l)
Dextraven (dextran 110)	154	–	154	–	Dex 110 (MW 110 000, 60 g/l)

Crystalloids	*Na+* *(mmol/l)*	*K+* *(mmol/l)*	*HCO₃* *(mmol/l)*	*Cl−* *(mmol/l)*	*Ca++* *(mmol/l)*	*Monosaccharide* *(mmol/l)*
Normal saline (0.9% saline)	154	–	–	154	–	–
Hartmann's solution	131	5	29	111	2	–
Dextrose saline (0.18% saline in 4% dextrose)	30	–	–	30	–	222
5% Dextrose	–	–	–	–	–	278
Ringer's solution	147	4	–	156	2.2	–

- Losses due to sweating, evaporation, diarrhoea are replaced by 5% glucose or 5% glucose/normal saline (glucose-saline).
- Upper GIT losses and ileus are replaced with normal saline with potassium.
- Burns, peritonitis and crush injury are replaced with albumin. Haemorrhage is replaced with blood.
- However, a balanced salt solution (Hartmann's or Ringer's lactate) may be used to replace losses and sequestration in the perioperative period, but blood losses must be replaced with blood. It is important to note that normal saline supports the intravascular compartment for the short term (several hours) until redistribution occurs. Glucose 5% is essentially water, freely diffusible throughout all compartments and tissues; glucose–saline (20% normal saline) behaves like 5% glucose. Neither glucose (minimal calories) nor saline can expand extracellular volume; given routinely without thought, it is a dangerous drug and is commonly responsible for severe postoperative hyponatraemia. Theoretically, colloids should remain in the intravascular compartment, but in the presence of inflammation or increased capillary permeability may gain access to interstitial space; this leak is particularly worrying in the management of patients likely to develop ARDS, since fluid administration may increase lung water and may result in negative inotropic effect. A mixture of colloid and crystalloid may be indicated in patients with ascites and inflammatory exudate.

A sensible fluid regimen must avoid overhydration during the phase of salt and water retention, as this results in hyponatraemia (the most common risk of fluid over-replacement) and pulmonary oedema. Excessive fluid intake may impair gas exchange, since it increases the distance that oxygen has to diffuse in tissues. In susceptible patients, oedema may increase the risk of ARDS; in critically ill patients, oedema may contribute to multisystem organ failure (MOF). Conversely, under-replacement may result in postoperative acute renal failure. Inappropriate choice of fluid may also result in systemic or pulmonary oedema and hyponatraemia.

Oliguria does not develop in perioperative patients as a result of acute frusemide deficiency; diuretics do not improve GFR. Patients should be euvolaemic, with free drainage of urine ensured before i.v. diuretics are administered to provoke a diuresis. Simply 'pushing fluids' in the hope that the kidney will respond may lead to acute pulmonary oedema; as in all things, not enough is just as bad as too much.

- Oliguria in patients considered at risk for development of acute renal failure is initially treated with rapid infusion of 500 ml of balanced salt solutions (fluid challenge). Administration of diuretics at this point could produce further detrimental effects on renal blood flow if drug-induced diuresis accentuates co-existing hypovolaemia. Brisk diuresis in response to fluid challenge confirms hypovolaemia as the cause of oliguria and will need faster fluid replacement.
- When this challenge does not produce a therapeutic response, additional fluids may be infused with or without monitoring of atrial filling pressures depending on whether patients are at risk for developing cardiac dysfunction.
- When patients are at risk for development of cardiac dysfunction or pulmonary artery occlusion pressures are normal or below normal, treatment with additional i.v. fluids is acceptable. In the presence of elevated pulmonary artery occlusion pressures, the possibility of oliguria and decreased renal blood flow due to low cardiac output should be considered. In this situation, infusion of dopamine, 1 μg/kg/min to 5 μg/kg/min is useful therapy.
- Failure of dopamine to improve urine output may be an indication to administer diuretics such as mannitol

0.5–1 g/kg with or without furosemide 1–3 mg/kg. Combination of low-dose dopamine (1–3 μg/kg/min) and high-dose furosemide (5–15 mg/kg) may facilitate conversion of oliguric to non-oliguric renal failure.

Although easier to treat with respect to fluid and electrolyte replacement, there is no evidence that conversion of oliguric to non-oliguric renal failure reduces mortality.

1.29 Pulmonary Complications after Major Abdominal Operation

More surgical patients probably die of postoperative chest problems than anything else. Such morbidity and mortality can be largely prevented by adequate pre- and postoperative care.

Predisposing factors include the site of operation, sex (males more than females), age (the two extremes of life), chronic bronchitis, smoking, anaesthesia itself (bronchial trauma, prolonged recovery), pain (restricts coughing and deep breathing), patient immobility, dehydration, abdominal distension (leads to paralytic ileus with consequent hypokalaemia which precipitates respiratory failure – vicious circle) and obesity.

After upper abdominal surgery, the vital capacity of the patient's lungs often drops to as low as 25% of its preoperative value. The normal requirement for adequate oxygenation is 10 ml of vital capacity for every kilogram of body weight; if the ratio drops below this, respiratory failure ensues.

This is important in obese patients. For example, if a 120 kg female is undergoing an incisional hernia repair and she is a smoker with a preoperative vital capacity of 4 litres, postoperatively she requires

$$\frac{10}{1000} \times 120 \ = \ 1.2 \, \text{litres}$$

of vital capacity to avoid respiratory failure. However, with the postoperative reduction, she will have a vital capacity of only 1 litre. She will almost certainly be in respiratory failure and will need mechanical ventilation. The situation is also exacerbated by the reduction in intra-abdominal space, causing competition among the contents, which push up the diaphragm and further reduce the vital capacity. The fact that the patient is a smoker means that the lungs will be even less able to cope with the reduction in vital capacity.

Complications

One complication may lead to another.
- Bronchitis: may arise *de novo* or as an exacerbation of pre-existing bronchitis.
- Bronchopneumonia (aspiration pneumonia): commonly by *Haemophilus influenzae* and pneumococci, rarely by drug-resistant staphylococci and *Pseudomonas pyocyanea*. Here the radiological patchy consolidation is associated clinically with systemic manifestations.

- Atelectasis (*see below*).
- Lung abscess.
- Empyema.
- Subphrenic abscess: with the three salient radiological features of basal lung consolidation or collapse, hemidiaphragmatic tenting and subdiaphragmatic pus collection as indicated by fluid level.
- Mendelson's syndrome (*see below*).
- Adult respiratory distress syndrome (*see below*).
  Three of these complications are discussed in detail.

ATELECTASIS

Due to bronchial obstruction by viscid secretions of mucus or pus leading to absorption collapse of the involved lobe. Depression of the cough reflex by pain and/or sedation and/or poor ventilation are predisposing factors. Auscultation for good air entry and chest X-rays are important diagnostic means. It is important to remember that the most likely cause of a high fever within 36 h of surgery is pulmonary atelectasis.

Treatment

The best treatment lies in prophylaxis through endotracheal aspiration at the end of surgery, pain control (not to the extent of respiratory depression, e.g. small repeated doses of pethidine 50 mg), preoperative breathing exercises, no smoking, treatment of pre-existing chest infection prior to surgery and reduction of obesity.

Once diagnosed the treatment must be immediate physiotherapy. Antibiotics do not play any part in the initial management of atelectasis. Bronchoscopic removal of secretions may be required. In extreme cases tracheostomy is needed to reduce the 'dead space'.

MENDELSON'S SYNDROME (USA, 1946) AND VOMITING

Caused by aspiration of vomitus or gastric contents with its irritant hydrochloric acid. Occurs *during induction* of anaesthesia in any patient with a full stomach or intestinal obstruction, or in pregnancy. The condition can occur in *coma*, e.g. after head injury, and *preoperatively* in haematemesis, intestinal obstruction and alcoholic or drug poisoning. *Postoperatively* it may occur after premature removal of the endotracheal tube. The condition can be fatal and is clinically manifested by wheezes, cyanosis, tachycardia, tachypnoea and hypotension. Radiologically widespread lung infiltration occurs more on the right than on the left and more in the lower lobes. Blood gas analysis reveals severe hypoxaemia. Treatment is by prevention, endotracheal aspiration, steroids and bronchodilators.

In 1946 Mendelson published an article about the importance of several hours fluid fast prior to surgery following the risk of gastric acid aspiration pneumonia during obstetric anaesthesia.

However, this prolonged fluid fast is illogical for two reasons:

- –in fasting patients, stomach secretes up to 50 ml of gastric juice an hour; this increase in gastric juice volume is associated with a decrease of gastric juice pH. Both of these factors increase the likelihood and consequences of gastric acid aspiration.
- – ingested clear fluids rapidly leave stomach of healthy people with about half the volume disappearing in 10–20 min.

The Canadian Anaesthetists' Society produced guidelines stating that a fluid fast of more than 3 hr is unnecessary in healthy patients undergoing surgery. Also, gastroscopy can be performed with oesophageal suction even after 2 h fluid fast rather than overnight fast with similar endoscopic mucosal view. Although patients who are ikely to have delayed gastric emptying (through underlying disease or drug treatment) should not drink before anaesthesia or i.v. sedation, there is now overwhelming evidence in favour of allowing patients who fulfill grades I or II of the American Society of Anaesthesiologists classification of physical status to drink fluids up to 2 h before the procedure. This message should now be disseminated to all medical and nursing staff to ensure that patients do not suffer uncomfortable thirst and that their procedure is not cancelled because of an inadvertent drink.

ADULT RESPIRATORY DISTRESS SYNDROME (shock lung)

Leads to pulmonary insufficiency which is a major cause of death in injured patients and patients receiving intensive care.

Clinically shock lung is manifested by tachypnoea and hypoxicaemia in spite of a high inspired oxygen concentration. Radiologically it is seen as diffuse, fluffy infiltrates.

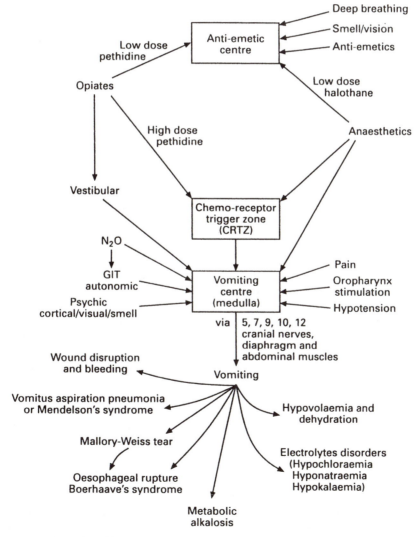

Fig 1.29.1 Stimuli and complications of vomiting

The radiological deterioration usually lags behind the clinical and gas exchange disturbances. This syndrome takes many forms.

- Damage to the pulmonary capillary bed by endotoxin action on vascular epithelium with its swelling, micro-emboli and intravascular coagulation leading to a rise in pulmonary vascular resistance at precapillary and small vein level. Both neurogenic and humoral factors may be involved and the intravascular aggregation of platelets and white blood cells occurs, with local release of vasoactive substances (e.g. prostaglandin $F_{2\alpha}$, 5-hydroxytryptamine, histamine) and lysosomal enzymes.
- Damage to pneumocytes, manifested by interstitial and intra-alveolar oedema (and occasionally haemorrhage) with impairment of gaseous transport.
- Damage to surfactant layer manifested by diffuse patchy atelectasis due to diminished secretion of surfactant (surface-tension reducing substance which normally holds open the smaller air alveoli). The lung compliance is markedly decreased and so it is called stiff lung.
- Pulmonary shunting (bypassing the pulmonary circulation) through dilatation of the arteriovenous communications (which normally exist between the pulmonary and bronchial vasculatures) will further impair gaseous transport. Pulmonary shunting is an excellent guide to the adequacy of pulmonary ventilation and is measured from the oxygen content in arterial and mixed venous blood after the patient breathes 100% O_2 for at least 15 min. The normal physiological shunting should be less than 5%. Acute respiratory failure is defined as an intrapulmonary shunt of 15% or more. A shunt of 40% or more, particularly if it is increasing, is an indication for ventilatory assistance.
- These pulmonary disturbances, although primarily vascular in origin, often tend to be complicated by pneumonitis due to infection by organisms derived from the upper air passages such as those in the klebsiella group and antibiotic-resistant staphylococci (the most lethal).

These are the five elements of shock lung producing a pulmonary vicious circle which can only be broken by achieving improved tissue oxygenation following restoration of blood volume together with intermittent positive pressure ventilation; this is preferably carried out by the technique of positive expiratory end pressure (PEEP) where positive pressure within the lung is maintained throughout the whole respiratory cycle, so that the collapsed alveoli are inflated and the fluid exudation is reversed. Large doses of steroid and antibiotics may also be required. Although the need for oxygen is great and the arteriovenous difference is wide hyperbaric oxygen is useless owing to the failure of oxygen transport in the lungs. Failure of oxygen release from haemoglobin is due to decreased 2,3-DPG concentration, the oxygen dissociation curve swinging to the left.

Shock lung is a dangerous pathological entity because death is likely to result largely from the additional burdens of respiratory failure; it is not only encountered in septicaemia but also follows extensive intravascular coagulation produced by trauma, after massive transfusion and following heart-lung bypass (pump lung), fat embolism, cardiac failure and oxygen toxicity.

1.30 Fat Embolism and Adult Respiratory Distress Syndrome (ARDS)

FAT EMBOLISM

Fat embolism is the main cause of early post-traumatic adult respiratory distress syndrome (ARDS) following fractures of the long bones or pelvis or even after extensive subcutaneous tissue damage. It consists of the blockage of the blood vessels by medullary fragments or fat globules too large (10–40 μm in diameter or even larger) to pass through the capillaries (pulmonary capillaries are 5–7 μm in diameter). Fat emboli can cross the capillary bed or enter the systemic circulation through pulmonary shunts. Furthermore, shock state and lipolytic activity of the lungs increase the quantity of free fatty acids in the circulation thus leading to cerebral, renal and cutaneous damage (petechiae).

Clinical features

Classically, there is a history of femoral fractures, with post-traumatic restlessness, petecheal rash and hypoxia, the diagnosis is fat embolism. Butterfly-like blurred confluent opacities over lung fields are characteristic. a chest X-ray can show bilateral pulmonary infiltrates and haziness only.

Fat embolism can be fatal within days. However, although almost every fracture gives rise to some degree of fat embolism at least 95% of patients remain asymptomatic. Not all of the remaining 5% of cases are fatal, sometimes the clinical picture is incomplete. Late fat embolism is not uncommon particularly after a delayed manipulation of a fracture.

- Fat embolism is clinically manifested by four basic symptoms and signs:
  1. Cerebral: agitation, disorientation, delirium and sometimes coma; funduscopy reveals obstructed retinal vessels with foci of ischaemia.
  2. Respiratory (ARDS): severe hypoxia, dyspnoea, cyanosis, tachycardia, pulmonary oedema, acute respiratory insufficiency and high fever.
  3. Renal: lipuria and often markedly low urine output.
  4. Cutaneous: petechiae of head, neck and upper chest, probably caused by fatty acids released into the blood stream.

  Arterial blood sample for blood gases and acid–base balance must be performed frequently.
- Any clinical evidence of fat embolism requires an immediate treatment with:
  1. Oxygen administration.
  2. Long-term artificial ventilation with physiotherapy and H2-blockers to prevent stress ulcers.
  3. Therapeutic doses of heparin in large i.v. doses or low subcutaneous doses (always given though debatable).
  4. Fluid restriction is imperative in pulmonary oedema (though blood transfusion is occasionally required to restore normal blood pressure).

5. Frusemide administration to stimulate diuresis in order to reduce interstitial pulmonary oedema and haematosis and improve ventilation.

6. High doses of methylprednisolone succinate (1–3 g daily for 3 days) are beneficial in reducing pulmonary oedema by reducing microcirculatory transudation and pulmonary capillary spasm resulting from shock and hypoxia.

Antibiotics, inotropic and vasoactive agents can be used but they are of limited value.

ADULT RESPIRATORY DISTRESS SYNDROME (ARDS)

This syndrome has many synonyms, such as adult hyaline membrane disease, adult respiratory insufficiency syndrome, haemorrhagic lung syndrome, postperfusion lung syndrome, post-transfusion lung, shock lung, solid lung syndrome, stiff lung syndrome, white lung syndrome and respirator lung.

There are about 150 000 cases of ARDS per annum in the USA and 15 000 per annum in the UK. Mortality varies from 50 to 60% and is due to hypoxaemic respiratory failure. ARDS is considered as a pulmonary manifestation of a generalised cellular metabolic disorder with mortality influenced by the failure of multiple organ systems; management must therefore be wide ranging and applied to multiple organ systems. The microscopic damage affecting the alveolar cell and the capillary bed leads to:

1. Hypoxaemia resulting from ventilation–perfusion mismatch and increased shunting due to increased physiological dead space.

2. Pulmonary compliance and functional residual capacity are reduced leading to increase in the work of breathing.

3. Increased pulmonary vascular resistance with increasing pulmonary artery pressures.

ARDS can be complicated by superinfection and barotrauma (due to mechanical ventilation with PEEP) leading to pneumothorax and pneumomediastinum, interstitial and subpleural and subdiaphragmatic air collections.

Common diagnostic criteria of ARDS are:
1. Severe hypoxia
   $Pa_{O_2} < 8$ kPa (60 mmHg) on room air, or
   $Pa_{O_2} < 8$ kPa (60 mmHg) on an F_{IO_2} of > 0.4 (40%) and
   PEEP of 5 cmH₂O or more.
2. New bilateral infiltrates shown on chest X-ray
   plus
   pulmonary capillary wedge pressure < 18 mmHg
   plus
   identification of a predisposing condition

Aetiology of ARDS

Common predisposing conditions to the development of ARDS are:
Respiratory causes:
- Aspiration of gastric contents
- Inhalation of toxic fumes
- Trauma resulting in pulmonary contusion
- Oxygen toxicity
- Bacterial, viral, drug-induced (e.g. bleomycin) or radiation pneumonia
- High-altitude pulmonary oedema.

Non-respiratory causes:
- Major trauma
- Shock (hypovolaemic or endotoxic)
- Massive haemorrhage/multiple transfusions (particularly of mismatched blood)
- Disseminated intravascular coagulopathy
- Massive burns
- Pre-eclampsia
- Fat or amniotic fluid embolism
- Pancreatitis
- Overhydration
- Sepsis from any cause (particularly clostridial and Gram-negative bacteraemia)
- Head trauma/raised intracranial pressure
- Extracorporeal perfusion (cardiopulmonary bypass)
- Heat stroke
- Carcinomatosis
- Bowel infarction

Management

Management is entirely supportive. A patient with ARDS must be transferred to the intensive care unit.

Monitoring Particularly:
- cardiac function parameters;
- arterial pressure;
- CVP and possibly pressure of the pulmonary artery (via Swan–Ganz catheterisation);
- blood gases and acid–base balance;
- urinary output (reflects accurately peripheral blood perfusion and renal function);
- development of bedsores (especially in the occipital, scapular, sacral and trochanteric regions, buttocks, elbows and heels).

Ventilation A prolonged period of spontaneous, assisted or even controlled mechanical ventilation via an endotracheal tube is often necessary. It is best instigated as early as possible. Techniques and devices for artificial ventilation have improved rapidly in recent years. Several alternatives are now available:
- Continuous positive airway pressure (CPAP) when the patient breathes spontaneously through a tightly fitting facemask; CPAP increases functional residual capacity which aids the recruitment of previously collapsed alveoli, improving both gas exchange and compliance. Because peak inspiratory flow rates may easily exceed 70 litres/min, the inspired gas must be in excess of this to maintain a positive airway pressure throughout the respiratory cycle. This is achieved by using a high flow generator. If, despite the use of CPAP, the patient's oxygenation is inadequate (arterial oxygen tension $Pa_{O_2} < 8$ kPa on oxygen concentration of 60% (F_{IO_2} = fractional inspired O_2 concentration = 0.6) or at haemoglobin oxygen saturation $< 90\%$) or there are signs of respiratory failure, mechanical ventilation must be instigated and even high frequency jet ventilation or extracorporeal gas exchange will be required.

● Positive pressure ventilation (to maintain intrathoracic pressure above atmospheric pressure throughout the whole respiratory cycle) either intermittent (IPPV) or continuous (CPPV) and often with positive end-expiratory pressure (PEEP) to counteract the decreased lung compliance and hypoxaemia even before the infiltrates have reached a fluffy, confluent pattern with recognizable air bronchograms. PEEP improves Pa_{O_2}, probably by decreasing shunt and preventing alveolar collapse at the end of expiration, thus facilitating gas exchange and increasing compliance; the increased intrathoracic pressure impedes venous return which may impair cardiac output, and oxygen delivery may, therefore, be reduced. Adequate oxygenation can usually be achieved with 5–15 cmH$_2$O of PEEP; stepwise increments of 5 cmH$_2$O and measuring Pa_{O_2} after 20 min may be required until $Pa_{O_2} > 8$ kPa with $F_{IO_2} < 0.6$.

● Intermittent mandatory ventilation (IMV). The three above techniques are often used in succession; this not only conserves the patient's strength but facilitates the aspiration of endotracheal secretions. The patient's position should be changed periodically during the day to forestall hydrostatic circulatory problems and to ensure a balanced distribution of oxygen. It is vital that the inhaled air should be humidified.

Curarisation may be required for controlled ventilation in order to reduce muscle activity and so decrease tissue oxygen consumption.

Medication

● Intravenous perfusions – consisting of blood transfusions, hyperoncotic solutions (20% albumins or dextran) and normal saline – should be administered with care and precision due to pulmonary damage. Once blood pressure has been restored, fluid restriction is imperative until oxygenation improves. Depletion of circulating volume may result in prerenal failure (though renal impairment may be due to the underlying condition); pulmonary capillary wedge pressure (PCWP), therefore, should be maintained at 8–10 mmHg. Parenteral lipid nutrition may exacerbate lung injury, but lipid metabolism does produce marginally less CO$_2$ than dextrose metabolism, thus favourably affecting lungs; this is important, since in severe ARDS, the removal of CO$_2$ becomes difficult.

● Inotropic and vasoactive drugs should be administered as required (dopamine and dobutamine). In ARDS, a supranormal cardiac output is needed to maintain oxygen delivery in the face of a necessarily low oxygen tension. However, low cardiac filling pressures secondary to a negative fluid balance, high intrathoracic pressures exacerbated by PEEP and elevated pulmonary vascular resistance, all act to impair cardiac performance, and cardiovascular support is nearly always required. Prostacyclin infusion into the pulmonary artery can increase oxygen delivery in patients with sepsis.

● Antibiotics treatment is the subject of much debate. Shock in itself seems to impair immunological defence, and underlying sepsis when present, requires antibiotic treatment. Foley catheters, tracheostomy tubes and endotracheal tubes constitute potential points of entry for pathogenic germs; bronchopneumonia often adds an additional hazard; and the threat of septicaemia from venous catheters is not to be underestimated. Blood cultures, sputum samples and swabs from cannulation sites should be taken at regular intervals. These factors are in favour of prophylactic use of broad spectrum bactericidal antibiotics (penicillin or a third generation cephalosporin). Any occult site of infection, often intra-abdominal, should be identified as it may require surgical drainage.

● Heparin in large i.v. doses or low subcutaneous doses remains controversial. The arguments in favour of systemic heparinisation are that it can sometimes prevent major vessel thrombosis, and that it is an effective means of preventing disseminated intravascular coagulation, particularly in fat embolism. The arguments against are that heparin frequently gives rise to severe (and even fatal) haemorrhage or to embolism – albeit rarely harmful.

● Steroids: early treatment with very large doses of methylprednisolone has been advocated as a means of counteracting the immediate effects of pulmonary contusion. An i.v. dosage of 1–3 g a day for 3 days can reduce the microcirculatory transudation and pulmonary capillary spasms which result from shock and hypoxia.

● Diuretic (frusemide) is now in widespread use. Its effect is to maintain the fluid balance at or below zero and so reduce interstitial pulmonary oedema; both ventilation and haematosis improve quickly, and the prognosis brightens.

● The H$_2$-antihistaminic cimetidine can lower gastric acidity and thereby reduce the risk of stress ulcers.

1.31 Abdominal Wound Dehiscence

Burst abdomen occurs in 1% of all abdominal operations with 10% mortality. The peak incidence is between the 6th and 8th postoperative day.

Predisposing factors

Preoperative Chest infection, systemic sepsis, persistent cough, jaundice, malignancy, anaemia, hypoproteinaemia, diabetes mellitus, steroid therapy, immune deficiency diseases, immune suppression therapy and obesity (general causes – patient's fault).

Operative Septic surgery or operations for peritonitis, poor surgical technique (too tight or too loose suturing, nerve injury and haematoma formation due to vascular injury) (local causes – surgeon's fault).

Postoperative Persistence of the preoperative problem, postoperative distension (gastric or paralytic ileus), premature removal of deep tension sutures, wound infection and haematoma (nurses' and surgeon's fault).

Types and treatment

Revealed (superficial) Gaping of skin and subcutaneous tissues (only) after removal of stitches 2 weeks postoperatively. Due to wound infection or haematoma. The treatment is to evacuate blood clots, treat the wound infection and let the wound heal by secondary intention (granulation).

Concealed (deep) Separation of all layers of the anterior abdominal wall except the skin. Incisional hernia develops eventually. If the condition is recognised in hospital, delay stitch removal, apply abdominal corset and treat incisional hernia on its merit using non-absorbable nylon size 1 or 0 for the repair either in pleating layers pushing the hernial sac into the abdomen without opening (keel operation – Maingot) or opening the sac and repairing the layers from the inside margins of the sac upwards (Cattell's operation). In huge incisional hernia, a preoperative repeated induced pneumoperitoneum may be required to increase the peritoneal reservoir to cope with subsequent reduction of the intestinal contents and to avoid possible respiratory embarrassment.

Complete (burst abdomen) Occurs either gradually with a 'tell-tale' serosanguineous discharge or suddenly with protrusion of a knuckle of bowel or omentum through the wound on the 10th day. Apply *sterile warm* packs (never dry) and do an urgent repair in theatre under general anaesthesia. Resuture with interrupted non-absorbable through-and-through sutures. Do not try to separate the tissues; skin can be included in suturing or left open to heal with secondary intention.

Prophylaxis

In all cases, preoperative predisposing factors should be corrected before any surgery, e.g. reduction of obesity, treatment of chest infection or sepsis, stoppage of smoking and control of diabetes. Attention must be paid to proper aseptic conditions and meticulous surgical technique minimising bowel manipulation to avoid paralytic ileus. Postoperative nasogastric suction (and i.v. drip) to avoid postoperative distension and timely removal of stitches are essential.

1.32 Postoperative Analgesia

Over half of patients have severe pain in the immediate postoperative period. Since pain is a subjective feeling, measurement is difficult. However, thoracotomy and laparotomy associated with painful breathing do permit direct measurement of FEV_1 and PFR and their improvement with analgesia; otherwise, a (rough) linear analogue is used in which the patient makes a mark on a 10 cm line, one end of which is marked as 'no pain' and the other as 'the worst pain you can imagine'. The position of the mark on the line measures how much pain the patient is experiencing. This technique is better than analgesimetry. With the Cardiff Palliator or Newcastle Interactive Demand apparatuses, operated by the patient himself by pressing a button to add a small increment of i.v. narcotic, pain can be analysed quantitatively by the rate of administration of narcotic analgesic.

The incidence of pain was found to be determined by a single factor: the site of operation (which also accounts for its severity), e.g. thoracic (pain incidence is about 70%), upper abdominal (60%) and lower abdominal (50%). Intermittent i.m. injections of narcotics, even when carried out at regular intervals, can produce fluctuating and unpredictable blood levels of the drug. Therefore continuous i.m. (rare) or i.v. (commonly used) infusion of narcotics via mechanically driven syringes is preferable. This means giving more than the conventional i.m. dose, and continuous respiratory monitoring is necessary. However, the respiratory stimulant doxapram can be given continuously for long periods with no effect on the analgesic action of narcotics. It improves pulmonary function and reduces the incidence of postoperative pulmonary complications. It is probably superior to naloxone (a pure narcotic antagonist).

Narcotics

Mild non-narcotic analgesics have no place in the treatment of immediate postoperative pain for four reasons:
1. Rather large doses are needed to produce the maximum effect (equivalent to 6–10 mg morphine).
2. They are given orally at a time when absorption is uncertain after major operation.
3. Immediately after surgery, the inflammatory response, against which aspirin is effective, has not developed so less analgesia will be expected.
4. Increased side-effects such as bleeding may result, e.g. with indomethacin. Postoperative pain should therefore be treated initially with a narcotic (see S.1.2 Pain in surgery) and later with an analgesic and anti-inflammatory agent such as indomethacin.

Inhalational analgesia

Nitrous oxide (e.g. Entonox: $N_2O/O_2 = 50/50$) is a powerful analgesic used with or without mechanical ventilation for not more than 48 h since it depresses the bone marrow and blocks B_{12} activity.

Local analgesic agents

Exert their effect by blocking Na^+ and K^+ channels in nerve membranes. Some have a reliable duration of 3 h, especially if combined with 1:200 000 adrenaline, e.g. 1% lignocaine 3 mg/kg (maximum dose) or preferably long-acting 0.5% bupivacaine 2 mg/kg (maximum dose). Used in, for example, ingrowing toenail operations, circumcision and inguinal hernia. The dose can be doubled if mixed with adrenaline (since their absorption will be slowed down) but adrenaline is contraindicated in digital, penile, nasal and ear infiltration.

Intercostal block

Used in thoractomy, chest trauma with rib fractures, and upper abdominal operations with analgesia duration of 3–18 h. Involves injection of 0.5% bupivacaine and 1:200 000 adrenaline via a needle or indwelling plastic catheter. For upper abdominal incisions seven nerves need to be blocked (T5–T11). Bilateral intercostal block is needed in median and paramedian incisions with the possible risk of bilateral pneumothorax and reduced respiratory function (due to bilateral intercostal muscle paralysis in the presence of impaired diaphragmatic movement). The block is performed posteriorly

7 cm from the midline near rib angles. It is contraindicated in chronic obstructive airway disease. It is superior to the thoracic epidural approach since it is easier to perform and carries no risk of hypotension, leg weakness, urinary retention or early respiratory depression.

Thoracic paravertebral block

Superior to multiple intercostal block. Four nerves can be blocked by one injection. Catheters can be left in for 5 days.

Caudal (sacral epidural) block

Easier in children and used in circumcision, inguinal herniotomy and orchidopexy. Lignocaine + 1:200 000 adrenaline can block up to T12. Lignocaine 1% is used for children under 5 years (0.5 ml/kg) and lignocaine 1.5% for those over 5 years (0.3 ml/kg). Haemorrhage into the sacral canal is a complication.

Continuous caudal block in adults

Continuous brachial plexus block

Carried out by means of catheters inserted via the supraclavicular, axillary and interscalene approaches.

Abdominal wound continous infusion of local analgesic solutions

Fine catheters are used (sited between posterior rectus sheath and rectus muscle) sometimes attached to a bacterial filter. Excellent analgesia is produced but visceral pain remains, and if the patient is unable to sleep, additional sedation may be necessary. Wound healing may be impaired and infection introduced.

Epidural (extradural or peridural) analgesia

For reliable analgesia, the catheter must be placed in the midthoracic region in thoracic and upper abdominal surgery but such positioning involves risks (*see above*, intercostal block). Owing to narcotic absorption the side-effects are similar to those occurring when the parenteral route is used.

Transcutaneous electrical nerve stimulation

Indicated in soft tissue pain (e.g. myalgia), postherpetic neuralgia, cervical and spine metastases, pudendal pain and root pain as an adjunct to steroids and regional blocks.

Cryoanalgesia

Similar to intercostal block but cryoprobe is applied to the nerve. Rapid N_2O expansion causes extreme cold (−60°C) producing local degeneration and interruption of nerve conduction (regeneration of nerves can take place later). This can be done by the surgeon at the conclusion of thoracotomy.

Intrathecal morphine (1–2 mg)

Produces prolonged analgesia of up to 18 h via a needle or catheter. May cause late respiratory depression (after 4 h), itching of unknown mechanism, urinary retention with possible neurotoxicity and arachnoiditis. However, no addiction or classical opiate withdrawal syndrome has been found. Spinal headache is masked by morphine analgesic effect.

PRACTICAL POINTS ON POSTOPERATIVE PAIN

- Intraoperative details must be documented to record:
  - preoperative medications (pre-med);
  - preoperative opioids;
  - NSAIDs or other.
- Type of anaesthesia, whether:
  - spontaneous ventilation, whether under sedation alone or under general anaesthesia;
  - general anaesthesia with IPPV;
  - regional anaesthesia – spinal or
  - epidural
  - caudal
  - local infiltration or anaesthesia
  - nerve block
  - intrapleural
- **Pain score** used postoperatively can either be a linear analogue scale of pain intensity recorded by the patient:

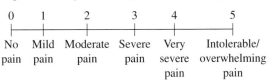

or, more accurately, pain scoring in relation to movement:

Score 0 = Comfortable patient (awake or asleep)
No pain at rest/no pain on movement
For movement ask patient to touch the opposite side of the bed with the hand

Score 1 = Slight pain (only elicited by close questioning)
No pain at rest/slight pain on movement

Score 2 = Moderate pain (bothering the patient but often controllable by lying still; patient will either ask for analgesia or gladly welcome it if offered)
Intermittent pain at rest/moderate pain on movement

Score 3 = Severe pain (dominating consciousness and calling out for urgent relief)
Continuous pain at rest/Severe pain on movement

- **Sedation score** can be used to quantify patient's degree of postoperative sedation following anaesthesia:

Score 0 = None
Patient alert

Score 1 = Mild
Occasionally drowsy, easy to arouse

Score 2 = Moderate
              Frequently drowsy, easy to arouse
Score 3 = Severe
              Somnolent, difficult to arouse
Score S = Sleep
              Normal sleep, easy to arouse

● Nausea can be scored postoperatively as:

Score N = Nausea only
Score V = Vomiting/retching
Score 0 = None

1.33 Nosocomial (Hospital-Acquired) Infection

Nosocomial infection is the result of transmission of pathogenic organisms to a previously uninfected patient from a source in the environment of a hospital. Sources of nosocomial infections are either endogenous, or exogenous, namely:
● Autoinfection: organisms originate from the patient.
● Cross-infection: organisms originate from other patients, from visitors to wards and ITU (community-aquired), and from hospital staff, whether wards, ITU or theatre nurses, surgeons, assistants or spectators.

Microorganisms of concern to surgeons fall into two categories.
1. Those presenting an infection risk to the surgical team and hospital staff, e.g. hepatitis B virus and human immunodeficiency virus (HIV).
2. Those causing postoperative infection with or without added dangers of cross-infection; wounds, presence of surgical prostheses, i.v. lines, and drains are all sites of infection.

Major outbreaks of surgical infection are rare; so too are infections with highly virulent organisms such as group A β-haemolytic streptococci and *Clostridium perfringens* (*welchii*). Most surgical sepsis is caused by staphylococci, Gram-negative aerobic bacilli, and non-spore forming anaerobes (Bacteroides). By and large *E. coli* and *Staphylococcus aureus* are the commonest isolates in these infections.

However, in medical wards, the menace of cross-infection is always present, e.g. patients with open pulmonary tuberculosis, elderly bed-ridden diabetic patients developing resistant decubitus ulcers, bed sores and gangrenous foot, patients with CVA developing staphylococcal pneumonia, and patients with multiple sclerosis or cauda equina lesions with catheterisation developing urinary tract infection due to *Pseudomonas pyocyanea*.

In maternity wards, epidemics of staphylococcal bullous impetigo of the newborn with subsequent maternal breast abscess can occasionally be encountered.

In paediatric wards, explosive epidemics of gastroenteritis (due to enteric bacteria *E. coli*, Salmonella and Shigella organisms) may affect older infants; in children, chickenpox and measles may spread like wildfire.

In mental hospitals, Shigella diarrhoea can be a nuisance. However, in surgical wards, ITU and maternity wards, the incidence of cross-infection reaches its peak, because of wound and/or extensive burns, invasive cardiopulmonary monitoring and maintenance devices, and high delivery rate respectively. However, the most common infecting organisms are *Staphylococcus pyogenes* and Gram-negative intestinal bacilli. Staphylococcal cross-infection manifests itself as skin infections of adults (such as neck boils, gluteal, perianal and/or ischiorectal abscesses, osteomyelitis), particularly in the presence of diabetes mellitus, postoperative wound infections, postoperative atelectasis, ITU pneumonia in ventilated patients, infections of intravascular devices, breast abscesses in lactating women, enterocolitis, as well as newborns' acute conjunctivitis and bullous impetigo.

Gram-negative bacilli are the important cause of autoinfection; they are usually implicated in ITU infections, such as urinary tract infections, respiratory infection in ventilated patients, septicaemia/septic syndrome/septic shock, tracheostomy wounds, extensive burns and occasionally in wound infections, particularly after abdominal surgery. They contaminate theatre humidifiers, infant incubators and, ironically, disinfectant bottles (e.g. cetrimide). By and large, the commonest nosocomial infections are: urinary tract infection followed by operative site infection and then pneumonia (in this order).

Cross-infection plays a major role in maintaining resistant strains of bacteria; antibiotic abuse and cross-infection tend to reinforce each other and set up a vicious circle. The incidence of nosocomial infections varies from 2% to 20% depending on many factors such as patient's age, patient's immune system status, diagnosis of disease, nature of operation, whether contminated or clean, surgical technique, and the hospital in which the patient is treated. Cross-infection is usually transmitted by air-borne spread of staphylococci harboured by man in nose, hair and skin; streptococci harboured in the oropharynx; Gram-negative bacilli harboured in urine and faeces and transmitted by hand contamination (breaking wind into the air may also spread clostridial spores). Hence, the importance of wearing masks, caps and hand gloves (after thorough scrubbing for at least 3 minutes) in theatre, together with ritual application of hygienic habits by hospital staff washing hands with soap and water after examining each patient in the ward.

Despite discovery of potent antimicrobials and sophisticated supportive measures, the infection rate in ITU critically ill patients exceeds that of a general surgical ward by four-fold (20% versus 5%). Intubated patients in ITU are at high risk of developing respiratory infections; indeed pneumonia in intubated ventilated patients is ten-fold more than in patients without a respiratory device. Such nosocomial infections prolong hospitalisation and therefore increase the morbidity and mortality; septicaemia and pneumonia are associated with the highest mortality rate among ITU patients (30%–50%). ITU nosocomial infections, therefore, constitute a major cause of morbidity and mortality; they are very expensive too.

Economic impact of nosocomial infections

According to a SENIC (Study on the Efficiency of Nosocomial Infection Control) audit report from Georgia, USA, on 338 000 patients, published in 1983 and 1986, the commonest site of infection was the urinary tract, but the most expensive in terms of treatment cost and delayed hospital discharge was wound infection; average cost was $1800 per infection (though the hospital was reimbursed only $15) with a maximum of $42 000. The most expensive nosocomial infections were pneumonia (average cost $5000 and maximum $42 000 per infection), followed by septicaemia (average $3000 and maximum $9000), wound infection (average $3000 and maximum $26 000), and urinary tract infection (average $600 and maximum $8000). The SENIC audit also demonstrated that a small reduction in USA infection rates from 5% to 4.7% could cover costs of employing a team consisting of an infection control nurse, a part-time hospital epidemiologist, with clinical assistance and expenses!

The SENIC study concluded that surveillance and reporting of wound infection to surgeons are of great importance in prevention of postoperative wound infection; with better awareness, improved techniques, teaching and good infection control, SENIC audit achieved a remarkable 33% reduction in infection rate (20%–38% lower than in hospitals with less stringent programmes).

In Germany, it was found that in nosocomial pneumonia, average additional hospital stay of 11 days was at a cost of approximately $11 000; in postoperative wound infection additional stay of 14 days was at a cost ranging from $4000 to $7000.

Cost-effectiveness in infection control may be discussed in terms of the most expensive infections, the most costly patients and the most costly patient care and procedures.

The most costly infections
1. Wound infection
2. Pneumonia
3. Septicaemia

The most costly patients
1. Transplant patients
2. Patients in ICU
3. Patients with AIDS
4. Patients with severe underlying diseases (renal failure and chronic obstructive airway disease)
5. Tumour patients
6. Cardiac surgery patients
7. Polytrauma patients

The most costly patient care and procedures
1. Antibiotics
2. Time-consuming nursing procedures
3. Time-consuming disinfection procedures
4. Disposables
5. Buildings and architectural design of barrier zoning, including:
– provision of several ICU rooms
– sluice rooms
– separate septic and aseptic operating theatres

So far as prevention of postoperative wound infections is concerned, *cost containment* can be obtained simply by applying the following recommended highly cost-effective measures (though surgeons may find some measures difficult to practise):
● Reporting surgeon-specific wound infection rates.
● Not talking, less movement, less personnel in the operating theatre.

● No or less disposable material (e.g. forceps, scissors, drapes, gowns, etc).
● No or less dressing after aseptic operations.
● Less disposable wound drainage systems (glass instead of plastic material).
● No protective gown, unless for contact with infected or susceptible patients.
● Preoperative clipping, no shaving of patient's hair with razors (shaving causes folliculitis and often injures skin, thus predisposes patient to wound infection).
● No incision drapes.
● No expensive investments to change architectural design unless proven to reduce wound infection.
● No routine microbiological monitoring (air, surfaces, naso-pharynx of surgeons and other personnel).
● Preoperative hand washing with soap (in minor surgery) for no more than 1 minute.

Perhaps, the cost of managing nosocomial infections is rarely taken into consideration by doctors. It is preferable to provide each department with its own fixed budget from which all consumable and capital items have to be purchased, including everything from light bulbs and typewriter ribbon to antibiotics; any money saved is then re-invested in the department itself.

NOSOCOMIAL INFECTIONS IN SURGICAL ITU

Exogenous and endogenous organisms are responsible for ITU nosocomial infections. Pneumonia and septicaemia with consequent multi-system organ failure account for most of ITU mortality; death rate in either pneumonia or MOF may reach 50% of cases. However, mortality attributed to infection is sometimes difficult to assess in various patient groups; patients with advanced underlying diseases run a high risk of developing life-threatening infection and are likely to die in consequence of infection. Infection *per se* contributes little to the overall mortality in those patients since their risk of dying is high anyway.

Most infections in ventilated patients are caused by bacteria, predominantly. Enterobacteriaceae, Pseudomonadaceae and Staphylococcus *spp.*. Gram-negative aerobic bacilli continue to be the most frequent pathogens of respiratory tract infections and urinary tract infections, whereas Staphylococci predominate infections related to intravascular devices. Most infecting pathogens derive from the microbial flora that colonises the patient's skin and mucosal surfaces of the alimentary canal.

Humans live in peaceful co-existence with their own oropharyngeal and GIT microflora. 'Colonisation resistance' refers to the human's natural ability to resist bacterial colonisation with potentially pathogenic organisms under normal physiological conditions; it includes specific and non-specific skin and mucosal barriers for bacteria, secretory IgA, gastric juice acidity, intestinal peristalsis, gut-associated lymphoid tissue and immune responses to invading bacteria. The stomach therefore, and large portion of small intestine, are almost sterile under physiological conditions. Normally, Staphylococci are restricted to the naso-oropharynx, whereas Gram-negative aerobic bacilli are restricted to the colon and terminal ileum (they constitute a small number of the intestinal flora). In healthy adults, nosocomial infections with Gram-negative aerobic bacilli (with the exception of *E. coli*) are detected irregularly. In contrast, in severely ill patients, the alimentary canal is increasingly colonised by nosocomial pathogens (mainly Gram-negative aerobic bacilli); critically ill patients have therefore been termed 'bacteriologic chameleons' since they easily assume the flora of their medical surroundings owing to their depressed colonisation resistance.

Bacteria may ascend to the stomach and migrate to the oropharynx and tracheobronchial tree; faecal bacteria may also be translocated by contaminated hands of the patient to other body sites, e.g. urinary tract, wounds and upper respiratory tract. The oropharynx becomes an important reservoir of Gram-negative aerobic bacilli in critically ill patients (due to increased adherence to buccal epithelial cells); colonisation is detected in more than 50% of patients within a few days after the beginning of artificial ventilation. Bacterial counts can reach more than 100 000/ml of bronchial secretion. Gastric overgrowth with Gram-negative aerobic bacilli may contribute to oropharyngeal and tracheobronchial colonisation in ventilated patients, and thus predisposing to respiratory infection. Alterations in normal acidity of gastric juice is a contributing factor; high gastric pH in critically ill patients frequently results from alkalising stress ulcer prophylaxis, and also from tube enteral feeding. Since it is impossible to restore normal defences of colonisation resistance in critically ill patients, suppression of gut flora and prevention of nosocomial pathogens by topical non-absorbable antibiotics (called selective decontamination of digestive system, SDD) constitute the strategy for prophylaxis of infection in ITU.

Control of nosocomial infections in surgical ITU

Hygienic measures and special regimens must be vigorously adhered to to decontaminate both the environment (to eliminate cross-infection by exogenous bacteria), and the patient (to reduce autoinfection by endogenous bacteria) respectively.

1. Decontamination of inanimate hospital environment

Includes not only floors, walls, technical equipment and tubing, but also air and fluids coming into contact with patients, nursing and medical staff. Time and energy must be invested in education and training of ITU personnel to decrease transmission of pathogens by hand, instruments, or other material to eliminate cross-infection. Classical hospital hygiene has eliminated cross-infection and epidemics (caused by exogenous bacteria) almost completely, leaving us with the other challenge, endogenous infection.

Measures to prevent cross-infection in ITU

- Staff and visitors change outer clothing on entering the unit.
- Hand washing between cases (handbasin at each bedstation); use of sterile gloves for specific procedures, e.g. tracheal suction.
- Keeping the environment dry.
- Adequate space for each bed (300 sq. ft or 15 × 20 ft).

- Regular cleaning of floor and walls, e.g. with phenol solution.
- Isolation rooms for severely infectious patients.
- No changes of ventilator during a period of IPPV.
- Bacterial filters used on ventilator circuits.
- Use of disposable equipment (tubing and catheters) if possible.
- Proper care of intravascular devices.
- Careful direction of room ventilation air flows.

However, total eradication of nosocomial infection in critically ill patients is difficult, because it is impossible to dispense with life-saving supportive devices (which also increase the risk of infection by endogenous bacteria), such as endotracheal tubes, ventilatory assistance, arterial and venous catheters and parenteral nutrition. The effect of the above measures on the endemic infection rate is minimal, since endemic infections in ITU are frequently caused by pathogens that derive from the patient's own microflora which is difficult to control.

2. Decontamination of the patient

Currently, most nosocomial infections in critically ill patients are due to either primary or secondary endogenous infection. Primary endogenous infections are caused by bacteria normally present at admission, for instance on skin, in oropharynx or in sinuses (e.g. staphylococcal skin infection and streptococcal tonsillitis). Most of these microbes are sensitive to classic non-expensive antibiotics, such as penicillin or ampicillin.

Secondary endogenous infections occur in places not normally their reservoirs; they originate from the oropharynx or digestive flora. After a few days of critical illness with or without antibiotic treatment, predominantly Gram-negative bacteria appear in the stomach, oropharynx and tracheobronchial tree (e.g. pneumonia in ventilated patients is commonly due to Gram-negative bacilli).

Selective decontamination of digestive system (SDD)

Different regimens have been used to prevent secondary endogenous infection:
1. Systemic i.v. antibiotic prophylaxis; the risks and benefits of this approach remain controversial.
2. Topical antibiotic aerosols into the bronchial tree (naso-oropharyngeal decontamination); this led frequently to development or selection of resistant bacteria and an increase of death related to infection. Aerolised polymyxin B administered into pharynx and endotracheal tube represents the commonest practice; polymyxin B was chosen because it is bactericidal against important Gram-negative respiratory pathogens, especially *P. aeruginosa*, *E. coli* and Klebsiella species. Polymyxin B resulted in significant reduction of colonisation and pneumonia-causing organisms (*P. aeruginosa*), but overall rate of pneumonia was not significantly reduced. Infections by organisms resistant to polymyxin B emerged as a new clinical problem. These results indicated the limited spectrum of activity and additional agent was required for broader antimicrobial coverage. Gentamicin addition administered into the trachea of tracheostomised neurosurgical patients reduced colonisation but undesirable new infections remained a problem.

3. Oral administration of non-absorbable antibiotics into the oropharynx and/or the GIT; this regimen is called selective decontamination of the digestive tract (SDD), an expansion of naso-oropharyngeal decontamination. Oral liquid forms of combined polymyxin E 100 mg, tobramycin 80 mg, amphotericin B 500 mg administered via a tube into the stomach 4 times daily with i.v. cefotixin 500 mg 4 times daily represent the commonest regimen. Occasionally, cefotaxime is replaced by daily i.v. trimethoprin 500 mg. A more recent regimen includes polymyxin E 100 mg, neomycin 1 g, and nalidixic acid 1 g given orally 4 times daily, together with topical povidone-iodine solution administered into the oropharynx 3 times daily.

Studies have shown that after 3–5 days, the microflora of the oropharynx and GIT was reduced profoundly (only 10% of patients displayed oropharyngeal Gram-negative bacilli) by SDD as compared with untreated controls. However, up to 14 days are required for colorectal decolonisation, with a 70% decline of respiratory infection (pneumonias). While some studies revealed a significant reduction of overall infection rate, others did not confirm the same benefit. Furthermore, SDD had hardly any effect on infections caused by Gram-positive organisms (which appear to increase in severely ill patients), perhaps because these organisms do not derive from the GIT.

Since naso-oropharyngeal decontamination is essential for prevention of Gram-negative pneumonia, the unchanged overall infection rate by some SDD studies is possibly explained by inadequate effect of intestinal decontamination on naso-orpharyngeal colonisation. Despite the impressive reduced rate of ITU infections by SDD, most studies did not reveal significant reduction of fatal nosocomial infections.

Clinical indications and prophylactic applications of SDD

SDD cannot be recommended in all seriously ill patients. Studies have documented benefits in the following groups of patients:

1. Ventilated patients in ITU to prevent nosocomial Gram-negative pneumonia.
2. Polytrauma patients on artificial ventilation: reduction in mortality following SDD is well established.
3. Patients with longer ITU stay.
4. Elderly surgical patients.
5. Patients with adult respiratory distress syndrome (ARDS).
6. Probably, patients with mid-range APACHE II score.
7. Controversial in multi-system organ failure (MOF), based on the theory of intestinal endotoxin released into the circulation by Gram-negative aerobic bacilli.

None of above-mentioned approaches was able to decrease convincingly the mortality rate from endogenous nosocomial infection. However, SDD appears to be an efficient means of reducing secondary pneumonia in patients requiring prolonged intubation and mechanical ventilation. This may, however, not be true for all types of ITU patients. A French multicentre trial has shown that SDD may not benefit medical ITU patients, whereas it could decrease nosocomial pneumonia and length of hospital stay in high-risk surgical patients. Perhaps, it is imperative to decontaminate environment and patient in severe multiple trauma, in high-risk surgical patients and organ transplantation.

However, measures other than SDD do exist to decrease the load of enteric organisms in the stomach and oropharynx. These measures include:
- Early enteral nutrition.
- Good care of the oropharynx.
- Short-term intubation.
- Means to improve the underlying disease and reduce dysfunction of vital organs.
- Measures to restore body defence mechanisms against infection.

MRSA
(methicillin-resistant *staphylococcus aureus*)

Normally, *Staphylococcus aureus* is present in 20–30% of noses of normal healthy people and is also found commonly on skin; most strains are sensitive to many antibiotics. MRSA bacteria are resistant to all penicillins and cephalosporins, and often to other anti-staphylococcal antibiotics, such as erythromycin and gentamicin. MRSA is transferred between hospitals by a carrier who may be either a patient or member of staff. Some MRSA strains occur in epidemics, e.g. EMRSA-16 and EMRSA-3.

The most common infections associated with MRSA are:
- Bacteraemia from i.v. lines.
- Infection of prosthetic implants and other surgical wounds.
- Pneumonia in long-term ventilated patients.

Once MRSA is established in a hospital, it is difficult and expensive to eradicate, and therefore strenuous efforts should be made by a hospital's Infection Control Team to recognise its introduction and limit its spread. Even in areas of high prevalence of MRSA (large hospitals in the south-east of the UK), it may be possible to concentrate on keeping MRSA out of high-risk units, such as cardiothoracic, orthopaedic and ITU.

1. Once MRSA is isolated from a patient, the individual should be isolated (labelled *Carrier of Methicillin-Resistant S. Aureus*).
2. All patients and staff on the ward must be screened. Recommended screening sites for patients are the nose and the sites of managements (e.g. ulcers, wounds, i.v. sites, catheter urine). For the staff: nose, skin of the hand (web spaces between fingers), hair line, axilla/groin, and skin lesions must be screened.
3. Patient carriers should be isolated, the door closed and management explained to the patient and relatives, who need to be reassured. All equipment used in the room must be decontaminated; the treatment must then be considered. A specially allocated isolation unit (with antiseptic barrier and full precautions by nurses and doctors wearing disposable gloves and aprons when caring for them) is often necessary to achieve a decolonisation process and eradication from a hospital, and temporary restriction of high-risk surgery must be applied. Surgeons who have seen the problems of treating severe MRSA infections are usually happy to comply.
4. The microbiologist should advise on the management of infected or colonised staff. Staff found to be colonised must attend the Occupational Health Department; they will be

screened and then required to be off duty for a minimum of 48 h at the start of the 7 days decolonisation therapy. Rescreening will take place 3 clear days after the end of decontamination. Staff should be advised that if they are admitted to hospital as a patient they must inform the nurse in charge/doctor that they have been caring for patients with MRSA.

- Mupirocin 2% cream should be applied to both nostrils twice daily using a swab rubbing in thoroughly as high as possible into the bulb of the nose.
- Whole body bathing/showering (including the head) with chlorhexidine solution daily.
- Colonised wounds should be treated with povidone-iodine packs for 4–6 h and the application repeated once at an interval of 24 h. The wound should be kept covered. Local Mupirocin 2% should be used if wound colonisation persists.
- All potentially contaminated areas of broken skin should be occluded with sterile dressing (tape should not be used on cannula sites).
- The patient must be re-screened 3 days after completion of the decontamination process; 3 sequential negative swabs are required from previous positive sites before isolation of the patient can cease.
- Systemic antibiotics are only given if the patient has systemic manifestations such as pyrexia. Vancomycin and teicoplanin are classified as glycopeptide antibiotics with bactericidal activity against aerobic and anaerobic Gram-positive bacteria; they are the only fully reliable (and rather expensive) agents. They are indicated in MRSA infections and other serious i.v. line infections and prostheses endocarditis caused by multi-resistant staphylococci. Vancomycin, however, is potentially toxic; it can cause tinnitus (ototoxic), renal impairment (nephrotoxic), agranulocytosis/thrombocytopenia and flushing of the upper body 'red man syndrome' on rapid injection. It must be administered i.v.; recommended dose is 500 mg over at least 60 min of i.v. infusion every 6 h, or 1 g over at least 100 min every 12 h for 7–10 days. Plasma concentration monitoring is needed; *peak* plasma concentration (1 h after i.v. infusion) should not exceed 30 mg/l; pre-dose *trough* concentration should not exceed 10 mg/l. It must also be remembered that vancomycin is also the drug of choice for antibiotic-associated pseudomembranous colitis, for which it is given *by mouth* 125 mg every 6 h for 7–10 days.

Teicoplanin is similar to vancomycin (both are classified as glycopeptide antibiotics with bactericidal activity against aerobic and anaerobic Gram-positive bacteria), but has significantly longer duration of action, allowing once daily administration; unlike vancomycin, teicoplanin can be given by i.m. as well as i.v. injection.

VRSA (vancomycin-resistant *Staphylococcus aureus*)

There has recently been a rise in VRSA due to imprudent use of vancomycin and poor hospital education programmes requiring the active involvement of microbiology laboratories in the detection, reporting and control of VRSA. It is noted that among MRSA strains the are 61 which are resistant to vancomycin too, mainly isolated from ITU. It has been reported that Diprivan (propofol) anaesthetic agent is a lipid-based injection which enhances bacterial outbreak. This is due to easy bacterial contamination of anaesthetic agent propofol. GIT perforations carry a high risk of bacterial contamination with potential resistance to antibiotics. It seems that bacterial resistance is progressively increasing:

- 1950s: resistance to penicillins observed
- 1960s: MRSA observed
- 1980s: MRSA in teaching centres – endemic
- 1990s: Vancymycin Resistant Enterococci, or VRE, encountered as nosocomial pathogen
- 1995: VRSA produced in laboratories
- 1995: Clinical isolation of VRSA

1.34 Sepsis, Septic Syndrome and Multi-System Organ Failure

Sepsis is a spectrum of conditions; it encompasses localised infections, bacteraemia, endotoxaemia, septicaemia (commonly due to endotoxaemia), septic shock and multi-system organ failure (MOF). Approximately 25% of patients entering ITU are already infected, and a further 25% of patients become infected in ITU, due to nosocomial cross-infection with virulent organisms, reduced immunocompetence, or both. Septic shock develops in 40% of cases of sepsis.

Aetiology of sepsis includes:
1. Self-infection with gut organisms in abdominal disease, surgery, and gut ischaemia in trauma and haemorrhage, mediated partly by septic cytokine mediators, and partly by the renin–angiotensin system.
2. Iatrogenic infection via prostheses, indwelling urinary catheters, vascular access catheters, nasogastric tubes and probes.
3. Alteration of lung flora due to mechanical ventilation (IPPV).
4. Alteration of gut organisms due to H_2 antagonists and to enteral nutrition.
5. Primary sepsis due to abscess, burn and cellulitis.

TYPES OF SEPSIS (Fig. 1.34.1)

Localised infections

Minor infections are characterised by moderate alteration of general homeostatic mechanisms, with easy control of microbial invasion by host defences.

Conversely, severe infections, due either to overwhelming bacterial contamination and/or to defective immune defences (defined as septic response), may progress to multi-system organ failure (MOF) and ultimately to death.

Septicaemia

This denotes circulating endotoxins (endotoxaemia), or circulating bacteria (bacteraemia), or both, with or without clinical

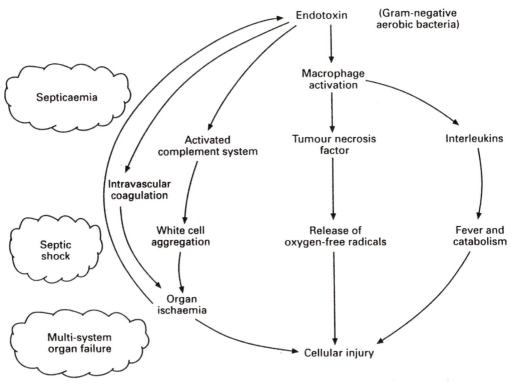

Fig. 1.34.1 Pathogenesis of multi-system organ failure (MOF) revealing cascade of mediators and progress of events from septicaemia and septic shock to MOF

manifestations of septicaemia (clinical syndrome of sepsis or septic syndrome), respectively. Gram-negative bacteraemia is not invariably accompanied by endotoxaemia. Patients who are simultaneously bacteraemic and endotoxaemic, however, have a higher likelihood of hypotension.

Bacteraemia

Refers to circulating bacteria is the bloodstream, being showered from a septic focus (localised infection), or following a surgical procedure. In 0.39%–1.15% of patients admitted to hospitals, Gram-negative bacteraemia is diagnosed. Most bacteraemic patients have clinical manifestations of bacterial infection, most commonly fever, but only a few bacteraemic patients will develop the septic syndrome, which can be complicated by hypotension, coagulation activation, increased vascular permeability and renal failure, and may culminate in a highly lethal syndrome of MOF. Although in the past bacteraemia was considered a gold standard for septicaemia, only 15% of bacteraemic patients develop clinical symptoms of septicaemia (septic syndrome). Moreover, clinical symptoms of septicaemia can develop in patients with negative blood culture.

Transient bacteraemia is a common event in surgical procedures, such as urinary tract catheterisation, sigmoid-oscopy and biopsy, percutaneous liver biopsy, and even barium enema; it invariably has no consequences. It is wise to provide antibiotic prophylactic cover in surgical manipulatory proce-dures, such as T-tube insertion after extraction of common bile

duct stone, percutaneous transhepatic cholangiography, endo-scopic papillotomy, urethral dilatation in presence of stricture, and procedures of similar nature, in order to prevent clinical manifestations of bacteraemia (fever and rigor).

Endotoxaemia due to Gram-negative septicaemia

Refers to circulating endotoxins in the bloodstream. It is well established that clinical symptoms of septicaemia can develop in patients with negative blood culture; this may be partly due to the effect of widespread treatment with antibiotics. The complex lipopolysaccharide (endotoxin) present in the outer membrane of Gram-negative bacteria can induce many biolog-ical phenomena that are observed in septicaemia, so that endotoxaemia may occur in the absence of bacteraemia.

In fact, the outer membrane of Gram-negative bacteria consist mainly of phospholipids, proteins and lipopolysacchar-ides, but it is the bacterial lipopolysaccharides that are responsible for the numerous biological activities including induction of fever, myocardial depression and activation of coagulation, fibrinolytic and complement cascades. It is the lipid moiety in lipopolysaccharide, known as Lipid A, that is responsible for these biological effects. Lipopolysaccharides must be released from bacterial membrane to expose Lipid A in order to exert their biological effects.

Ex vivo, when incubated with human serum, Gram-negative bacteria lose a sizeable fraction of their lipopolysaccharides which form complexes with various serum proteins. One of these proteins, 60 kDa lipoprotein binding protein (LBP) may be important for lipopolysaccharide presentation to macrophages (it binds to CD14 membrane protein); binding of lipopolysaccharide to LBP results in macrophages activation which sparks the release of cytokine mediators, and starts the immunological cascade.

An important factor in assessing endotoxaemia is the timing of the collection of blood samples relative to the development of the septic syndrome. In febrile patients, endotoxaemia proves to be a reliable cause of septicaemia; the average time interval between detection of endotoxaemia and the development of septicaemia is 19.8 h. Endotoxaemia is more likely in bacteraemic and febrile patients; while it is very high in meningococcal septicaemia, endotoxin levels in other septicaemias are too low to be detected. Limulus test and monoclonal antibodies are the only methods for detection (see s.1.11 Monoclonal antibodies in surgical practice).

Septic syndrome

The clinical syndrome of sepsis must be distinguished from microbial infection *per se*. Septic syndrome is the clinical manifestation of underlying septicaemia (usually in the form of endotoxaemia rather than bacteraemia); it can be complicated by hypotension, coagulation activation, increased vascular permeability, and renal failure, and may culminate in a highly lethal syndrome of MOF. It is a complex reaction of various organs and systems to microbial invasion. Septic syndrome is characterised by fever (> 38.5°C) or hypothermia (< 35.5°C), tachycardia (> 90 beat/min), tachypnoea (> 20 respiration/min), and organ failure with oliguria (< 0.5 ml/kg/h), and hypoxia (< 10 kPa). Unfortunately, the clinical criteria for septic syndrome are rather unspecific.

Sepsis, however, is characterised by the following effects:
1. Local effects of sepsis: exudate production and tissue necrosis in the infected site.
2. Systemic effects of acute phase responses to sepsis, which include hormonal, metabolic, haemodynamic and immunological components:
● Hormonal: stress hormones are released; these may include catecholamines, cortisol/ACTH, endogenous opiates, aldosterone and ADH. Insulin level, however, is decreased.
● Metabolic responses mediated by stress hormones include:
 – increased metabolic rate;
 – increased oxygen consumption;
 – increased gluconeogenesis with relative hyperglycaemia;
 – increased glucose oxidation;
 – increased utilisation of endogenous fat;
 – enhanced protein turnover;
 – fluid retention;
 – electrolyte imbalance.
● Haemodynamic responses induced by stress hormones include:
 – tachycardia;
 – decreased vascular resistance (vasodilatation);
 – hypotension.
● Immunological responses include:
 – lymphokine production;
 – leukocytosis;
 – transient decrease in CMI (T-lymphocytes and helper T-cells are decreased);

 – complement system activation;
 – consumption of opsonins;
 – enhanced antibody production;
 – macrophage activation in wounds and infection.

Septic shock

Septic shock can be defined as a generalised failure of tissue perfusion resulting from infection which manifests itself clinically by haemodynamic collapse and by metabolic evidence of impaired blood flow. There are two phases: an early hyperdynamic phase and a late hypodynamic phase (see s. 1.7 Shock).

It should be noted that 'septic shock' can be non-infective, since hypotension induced by severe trauma or bleeding may result in gut ischaemia leading to absorption of endotoxins (derived from the normal gut flora) into the circulation with subsequent septicaemia (endotoxaemia) and septic shock.

Multi-system organ failure (MOF)

The syndrome of MOF was first described by Tilney *et al.* in 1973 following rupture of abdominal aortic aneurysms; it was then given the name of multiple, progressive or sequential systems failure syndrome by Baue in 1975; however in 1981 there were at least seven publications on MOF as a syndrome with clinical and functional alterations and associated with abnormalities of laboratory parameters representative of uncontrolled and disturbed homeostasis.

MOF can be defined as the sequential failure of numerous organ systems, which are commonly lungs (adult respiratory distress syndrome – ARDS), cardiovascular system, kidneys, liver, gut, pancreas, coagulation system following injury such as polytrauma or major surgery (pelvic exenteration or complete GIT cancer extirpation), or following sepsis and septic shock, hypovolaemic shock such as ruptured aneurysms, or following persistent inflammation such as severe acute pancreatitis or transplant sepsis. Thus sepsis is a prototype and the classical example for MOF; MOF pathogenesis, therefore, can be attributed to macrophage activation (angry polymorphonuclear leucocytes) with resultant release of sepsis mediators, such as tumour necrosis factor (TNF), interleukins, activated complement system, prostaglandins, oxygen-free radicals, and disseminated intravascular coagulation. Thus cytokines are involved in the pathogenesis of initial septicaemia which can progress to MOF; endotoxin (produced by Gram-negative aerobic bacteria) is the most potent stimulus for induction of these cytokines.

MOF commonly affects surgical patients staying more than 5 days in the intensive care unit (ITU); it is the major cause of death in surgical ITU patients (MOF accounts for death in 50% of septic cases). Despite significant advances in ITU, MOF remains a major cause of morbidity and mortality.

In a major study of 92 patients (at risk of developing MOF) from University of Minnesota in 1990, many facts have emerged on the MOF patterns and effect of therapy. For practical purposes, criteria for labelling a patient at risk of developing MOF are:
1. Presence of a defined aetiology, e.g. septic shock, haemorrhagic shock, or polytrauma.

2. Surgical intervention within 24 h of the onset of aetiology.

3. Admission to ITU within next 24 h.

4. Development of pulmonary failure (ARDS) requiring mechanical ventilation within 5 days of ITU admission.

5. Patient required ITU more than 5 days.

Thereafter, it is the pulmonary failure that sparks MOF, leading to liver and/or renal failure that may also be accompanied by encephalitis, coagulopathy, GIT bleeding and wound failure. Renal failure may practically be defined as progressively rising serum creatinine and/or the start of dialysis. Liver failure may practically be defined as a progressively rising serum bilirubin with progressively falling serum transferrin despite the presence of nutritional support; it reflects abnormal regulation by the activated Kupffer cells (tissue-specific macrophages of the liver). Sepsis can also be defined as an observed source with a documented bacteriology in the presence of a hyperdynamic, hypermetabolic state.

Patients who expire are older, spend a longer time on a ventilator, and a longer time in the ITU, although not necessarily having a longer hospital stay. Survivors are younger, with less acute lung injury, and without development of renal or hepatic dysfunction. Though their time in ITU was shorter, their hospital stay was long, reflecting the need for rehabilitation and recovery from the catabolic effect of sepsis.

A management team of well-trained and interested personnel is necessary. The management plan should be directed at three levels:

1. Aggressive *source control* through active diagnosis of sepsis, blood culture, searching for pus (usually not apparent in the immunocompromised), and through therapeutic removal of the underlying cause surgically or medically. This includes surgical drainage, 'second look' laparotomy, early stabilisation of fractures, early ambulation of patients, as well as the use of antibacterial drugs (preferably specific to identified organisms) such as vancomycin 2 g/day, flucloxacillin 4 g/day, and third-generation cephalosporin. Also *in vivo* foreign bodies must be removed (if proved to be the cause of resistant sepsis), such as CPV catheters, orthopaedic prostheses and even vascular grafts.

2. *Resuscitation and support* of vital organs with invasive cardiopulmonary monitoring and adjustment of oxygen content and flow to eliminate hypoxaemia and lactic acidosis. Maximising oxygen delivery (> 600 ml/min/m^2) is essential, through using inotropes such as dobutamine 5–10 μg/kg/min, dopexamine 5–10 μ/kg/min, sodium nitroprusside (as a vasodilator), and energy i.v. replacement. IPPV is used to maximise lung function, inotropic agents (dopamine) to maximise cardiac function and renal function (dialysis is often required). Coagulation defects can be reversed by cryoprecipitate. Free oxygen radical scavengers (e.g. 21-amino steroids and chlorpromazine), enzyme inhibitors (indomethacin and OKY-046), IL-1 antagonists (e.g. ibuprofen, *n*-acetyl cysteine), monoclonal antibodies to endotoxin and IL-2, and immunotherapy using antisera can all be tried.

3. *Metabolic support* instituted within 24–48 h after injury and resuscitation by either enteral or parenteral route with the objective of providing:

- 30–35 Kcal/kg/day
- 1.5–2 g/kg/day of modified amino acids
- 3–5 g/kg/day of glucose
- 0.5–1.5 g/kg/day of fatty acids

The regimen may be adjusted every 5–7 days to maintain energy and nitrogen balance.

Apparently, there are three patterns of MOF which differ primarily only in the timing of the development of renal and hepatic malfunction as reflected by increased serum creatinine and serum bilirubin respectively, indicating multiple rather than a single mechanism of pathogenesis. Inadequate micro-circulatory resuscitation is as imporantant as the cell-mediated immunological cascade inducing the endothelial injury during perfusion. Malnutrition is a recognised co-morbidity and co-mortality factor that can be minimised with nutritional support (enteral feeding, however, does not prevent MOF after sepsis). While the association between Gram-negative aerobic bacteria (GNAB) and septicaemia is well recognised, GNAB aetiologies occur at the same rate in both MOF and in survivors; septic episodes characteristic of MOF are due particularly to Gram-positive and fungal infections.

The hypothesis of the gut origin of hypermetabolism and MOF might be questioned as to whether this gut failure is a symptom or a cause of the disease process. Either enteral or parenteral nutrition was used in previous studies. Recent data indicate that after the first few days, there is no route effect of the nutritional support on the outcome from hypermetabolism and MOF. Recent data on gut decontamination is also suggesting that the nosocomial infection rate can be reduced from enteric organisms, but that the incidence and outcome of MOF may not be significantly changed.

PREVENTION OF SEPSIS

'The golden hour'

Trauma is the greatest cause of mortality in the under-40 age group in the Western world. The initial management lies in the hands of the Accident and Emergency Unit physician, surgeon, anaesthetist, and/or intensivist (can be one of the above by professional qualification). The patient's course is largely dictated by events of the first hour, the so-called 'Golden Hour'; the effectiveness of initial resuscitation will determine whether the patient will remain overnight in the ICU, to be discharged to the general ward the following morning, or will suffer a stormy prolonged course involving multi-system organ failure (MOF).

The effective Airway, Breathing and Circulation are well known to us, however the pathophysiology and management during the 'Golden Hour' have an impact on the future outcome.

Hypovolaemia is common after severe trauma. The life-saving response (endogenously released catecholamines by sympathetic system) is to sacrifice blood supply of non-vital organs (skin, muscle and gut) in order to maintain blood flow to vital organs (brain, heart and kidneys). This life-saving response can be life-threatening once deterimental ischaemia affects the blood supply of the mucosal barrier of the GIT (which is a dirty organ), since this may result in translocation of micro-organisms crossing the barrier into the systemic circulation. Overgrowth by intestinal microbes, especially in an alkaline environment is common in seriously ill patients in ITU. However, a disproportionate sensitivity to renin-angiotensin is also important. Bacteraemia, endotoxaemia (septicaemia) and MOF will occur if perfusion to GIT is not rapidly re-established. In fact, bacteraemia is common even after a short period of ischaemia during cardiopulmonary resuscitation. This has instigated the use of non-absorbable antimicrobials in selective decontamination of the digestive system (SDD); indeed, the incidence of septicaemia and nosocomial pneumonia can be reduced by SDD. However, results are not unanimous, and the technique of SDD is expensive, time-consuming and may eventually predispose to the emergence of new resistant organisms.

A more logical solution in polytrauma patients is to increase the integrity of the mucosal barrier to prevent bacterial translocation (early prophylactic approach) rather than to kill micro-organisms within the lumen of the GIT (late therapeutic approach). This is the basis of the importance of the 'Golden Hour'. It is no longer good enough to maintain the function of so-called vital organs (brain, heart and kidneys); the GIT must be considered in these circumstances as a vital organ too. Intestinal ischaemia can be reduced with more aggressive and compulsive fluid transfusion.

'Resuscitation of the GIT'

Ambulance personnel trained in cannulation and rapid fluid infusion, as well as the hospital trauma team, must not only be capable of sustaining life, but of resuscitating GIT mucosa. Practically, skin and GIT mucosa have similar perfusion in shock; if skin is shut down, GIT mucosa is certainly compromised. Skin status, therefore, is an indirect indicator of GIT mucosal status. Fluid must be aggressively transfused until skin of the most distal digit is warm and well perfused. It is almost impossible to over-transfuse an actively bleeding patient with polytrauma, whereas it is very common to under-transfuse them.

Maintaining good blood pressure is not good enough, because blood pressure is maintained at the expense of perfusion to the so-called non-vital organs such as the GIT! By aiming at normal blood pressure together with normal urine output, pulse rate, filling pressures, and skin perfusion, one can guarantee adequate GIT perfusion. However, GIT under-perfusion cannot be recognised immediately; the clinical markers of such GIT underperfusion occur several days later in the ITU as jaundice, renal failure, sepsis and MOF.

It is crucial to give right fluid in the right circumstances; the major problem in polytrauma is hypovolaemia and the most efficient way of restoring intravascular compartment volume is with either blood or colloid transfusion given early and rapidly in actively bleeding patients (retained within intravascular compartment due to oncotic pressure).

Dextrose solutions should not be used for hypovolaemia, since it is hypo-osmolar (once glucose is absorbed), and the water then is distributed to intracellular space. Similarly, because crystalloid solutions are mainly distributed to interstitial space (cannot be retained within the intravascular compartment), they are not efficient for correction of hypovolaemia. Also, salt and water retention is an early metabolic response to trauma; to give extra salt and water encourages pulmonary and peripheral oedema, causing more hypoxia, and decreased oxygen consumption. Salt and water loss is not a

problem in acute management of trauma, it is hypovolaemia from blood loss.

There is no need for monitoring during acute correction of hypovolaemia, but there may be a place for CVP measurements and pulmonary artery wedge pressure in the fine tuning of fluid replacement once the patient is stable.

When the patient requires further investigations (e.g. CT scan, and angiography) or surgery, continued resuscitation during transport and investigations must be provided. The operating room may be an extension of the emergency room, so that early fixation of fractures can be achieved. While early fracture fixation has many advantages in the long-term management, the initial surgery can be prolonged and associated with large blood loss. Furthermore, concurrent pathology must be considered; an urgent laparotomy may be as necessary as a CT scan to exclude intracranial haematoma. Also, thoracic injuries, such as pneumothorax, aortic dissection or lung haemorrhage may become obvious during surgery.

Intra-abdominal bleeding

It is assumed by surgeons that intra-abdominal tamponade is protective in decreasing further bleeding, and that the severity of tamponade can be assessed by abdominal girth measurement. However, it is also important to emphasise that:

- The abdominal girth measurements are of no value in assessing abdominal bleeding.
- While raised intra-abdominal pressure may tamponade bleeding, it may also seriously affect intra-abdominal organ perfusion as well as adversely affecting cardiorespiratory function.

Intra-abdominal pressure can be accurately and easily estimated by measuring intravesical pressure by placing a needle or cannula into a urinary catheter (or by using T-piece attachment); the urinary catheter is clamped distal to this insertion and 50 ml of sterile isotonic saline run into the bladder. A CVP manometer is attached and the readings are taken from symphysis pubis. Less than $20 \, cmH_2O$ is acceptable; $20–25 \, cmH_2O$ causes a reduction in organ flow, particularly to kidneys, and at more than $25 \, cmH_2O$, oliguria occurs, eventually resulting in anuria. Options such as embolisation of venous bleeding or laparotomy may seriously be considered to prevent otherwise certain renal failure and intra-abdominal organ damage. However, the outcome is also influenced by patient's cardiorespiratory status (smoking, chronic lung disease, and ischaemic heart disease), and the patient's drugs (β-blockers, calcium-channel blockers). Aspirin, a very common prophylactic drug in ischaemic heart disease in males over 40 years of age, may be responsible for prolonged and abnormal bleeding after polytrauma.

Cross-infection in ventilated patients in ITU

The best way to treat polytrauma is to prevent it. Prevention of cross-infection is crucial, since the critically ill patient may be immunocompromised, and over half of ventilated patients have GNAB oropharyngeal colonisation due to reduced mucosal fibronectin.

Topical non-absorbable antibiotics (e.g. polymyxin B & E, tobramycin, amphotericin B, povidone-iodine) are used in selective decontamination of the digestive system (SDD), although the influence on infection rates is disappointing.

Maintaining gastric acidity is important in preventing bacterial colonisation of the upper gut, and if anti-peptic ulcer treatment is used, agents that do not severely raise pH are used, e.g. sucralfate. Dopexamine 1–5 µg/kg/min (inotropic sympathomimetic) may be used to maintain gut mucosa oxygenation and integrity.

PROGNOSIS OF SEPSIS

In septic syndrome, septic shock and MOF, mortality is between 50 and 90%. Prognosis depends on:
1. Presence or absence of shock (hypotension/hypoperfusion).
2. Number of vital organs involved (1 organ = 50% mortality; 3 organs = 90%).
3. Disease duration prior to treatment.
4. Adequacy of oxygen supply during crisis.

Clinical bad prognostic indicators include greater tachycardia, cardiac output increases, refractory hypotension, longer disease duration, older age of patient (> 65 years), previous steroid or cytotoxic therapy, previous uraemia, or cardiac failure. APACHE II and III scores of 20 or more reflect these bad prognostic signs.

Biochemical poor prognostic indicators include:
- Sub-therapeutic level of antibiotics (very poor prognosis).
- Admission TSH levels below 0.6 iu/l (90% mortality, while TSH above 3 iu/l is associated with less than 10% mortality).
- Higher lactic acidosis.
- Angiotensin-converting enzyme blood level correlates directly with severity of ARDS.
- Plasma fibronectin level is inversely related to clinical severity of septic shock.
- Circulating levels of antibodies to *E. coli* endotoxin core relate directly to survival in Pseudomonas septicaemia (this has been successfully used to immunise sheep and humans).

SURGICAL ONCOLOGY

1.35 Introduction to Clinical Oncology

Neoplasia (or tumour) is defined as 'an abnormal mass of tissue, the growth of which exceeds and is uncoordinated with that of the normal tissues and persists in the same excessive manner after cessation of the stimuli which evoke the change'. It can be benign (localised, encapsulated, slowly growing by expansion and not fatal unless it causes mechanical obstruction or hormonal imbalance) or malignant (rapidly proliferating and locally invasive with systemic metastatic potential and fatal if not treated early). Histologically a benign tumour is similar to normal tissue while cancer is not. Neoplasia has to be differentiated from:

Hypertrophy – increased organ growth due to an increase in the size of its constituent cells (e.g. prostate).

Hyperplasia – increased organ growth due to an increase in cell number (e.g. thyroid).

Metaplasia – replacement by a cell type not normally present in an organ (e.g. inflammation and squamous cell metaplasia in urinary transitional epithelium).

Wound healing – although the actual mechanism is unknown, the rate of cell and tissue production exceeds that seen in most cancers; however, the presence of chalones, the local inhibitory factors, will prevent further cell division once the wound is healed. Absence of chalones could be a factor in neoplasia.

Development of cancer

Cancer passes through a four-phase evolution (chronic process).

1. Induction phase (15–30 years) with exception of radiation-induced leukaemia (2 years) and genetically determined cancers of infancy (shortly after birth).
2. In situ phase (5–10 years).
3. Phase of invasion – aided by cell multiplication, increased amoeboid cell motility, decreased cell cohesiveness, elaboration of lytic substances and lack of intercellular bridges found in all normal cells (e.g. hyaluronidase).
4. Phase of dissemination – by regional invasion (treated surgically and/or by X-ray therapy) and metastases which initially are micrometastases (treated by chemotherapy).

Types of cancer

The commonest cancers in the UK are, in order of frequency:

Solid tumours (over 90% of all cancers)
Lung
Colon and rectum
Breast
Stomach
Bladder
Prostate
Pancreas
Cervix

Non-solid tumours (haematogenous)
Hodgkin's lymphoma
Non-Hodgkin's lymphoma
Leukaemias

In females, breast and cervix uteri cancers are the leading malignancies.

Incidence

Varies according to the following factors.

Age

Cancers develops at any age but the risk increases with age, with the exception of early childhood cancers (leukaemia and central nervous system tumours) which carry a higher risk in the first 5 years of life than in the following 10 year period.

Sex

Average incidence is similar in both sexes, although the mortality in men is higher. However, under 10 years of age it is higher in males, between 20 and 60 years of age it is higher in females (due to breast and cervix uteri cancers), and over 60 years of age, the incidence tends to be higher in men.

Site of origin

- The rates for cancers of the upper gastrointestinal and of the respiratory tract are strikingly higher in men.
- The rates for gastric, reticuloendothelial and hematopoietic cancers are higher in men but not as markedly so as in the previous group.
- Cancers of the breast, reproductive organs and thyroid are more common in women.
- For all other sites the rates between sexes are similar.

Environmental factors

- Life habits, e.g.
  - Age at marriage, number of pregnancies, breast feeding: breast cancer
- Dietary and smoking habits, e.g.
  - Alcohol consumption: gastric cancer
  - Smoking: lung cancer
  - Reverse smoking (ignited end in mouth): oesophageal cancer in South America
  - Bush tea drinking: hepatic carcinoma in Africa
- Socioeconomic status

Race

Cancers occur more frequently in non-Caucasian than in Caucasian people. Coloured males have more oesophageal, gastric, pancreatic, lung and prostate cancers and myelomas, while white males have more colonic and bladder cancers, melanomas, lymphomas and leukaemias. Coloured females have more oesophageal, gastric and pancreatic cancers and markedly increased rates of cervical cancer while white females have more breast, endometrium and ovary cancers.

Geographical distribution

May be specific to certain cancers although some have world-wide distribution. The following areas of predilection represent the highest incidences:
- Oesophagus (Central Asia)
- Stomach (Eastern Europe, USSR, Japan and Latin America)
- Large bowel (industrialised societies and Hawaiian Chinese)
- Liver (Africa and South East Asia; ? Europe)
- Pancreas (as large bowel)
- Larynx and hypopharynx (Western Europe, Assam, Burma, North Thailand and Egypt)
- Breast (developed communities and Hawaiian whites)
- Cervix uteri (Asia, Latin America and Africa)
- Prostate (Sweden)
- Urinary bladder (Egypt, South Iraq and Sudan)
- Melanoma (Australia)

Prognosis

Not only the length of survival but the quality of life after treatment must be considered. The average cancer mortality rates in developed countries are higher in men than in women. This is due to anatomical differences – in men there is a higher incidence of cancer of low curability (e.g. lung and gastric cancer) whereas in women the most common cancers are reasonably curable (breast and cervix cancers).

The arbitrary '5 year survival rate' is reasonably satisfactory. It includes patients both with and without residual or recurrent cancer; '5 year cure', however, includes only those patients apparently free of disease at the 5 year mark. The 5 year cancer-survival rates (in their localised stage and with regional involvement) are as follows. (These figures should be remembered at least approximately for the final FRCS examination):

Gastric	early 63%; advanced 10%
Bladder	early 72%; advanced 21%
Breast	early 85%; advanced 56%
Colon and rectum	early 71%; advanced 44%
Larynx	early 79%; advanced 37%
Lung	early 33%; advanced 11%
Oral	early 67%; advanced 30%
Prostate	early 70%; advanced 61%
Uterus	early 83%; advanced 46%
Thyroid	early 90%; advanced ?

In fact, only 5% or less of people with cancer of the lung, stomach, oesophagus or pancreas will be alive after 5 years. Factors bearing on prognosis include sex, age, pregnancy, hormone-dependence, histological grade, lymph node metastases, distant metastases and the interval between treatment and local recurrence or metastases.

The nature of the tumour is another factor (spontaneous regression and cure as well as multiple primary cancers). Spontaneous cure is an extremely rare phenomenon seen in neuroblastoma (children), bladder and renal cell carcinoma and malignant melanoma.

Multiple primary cancers may occur at the same time (synchronous) or at different times (metachronous). These are due to pre-existing multiple foci. This phenomenon is extremely common in skin colon and breast cancers, the incidence possibly rising to 20% in patient cured 20 years earlier. In smokers, cancers of the mouth, larynx and lung are frequently multiple and development of cancer at one of these sites indicates an increased risk of cancer at the other site. Papillary thyroid carcinoma is also multifocal. Treatment itself (especially multimodal) may result in a second primary cancer (both radiation and cytotoxic therapy are carcinogenic).

However, certain genetic and immune deficiency states are the predisposing factors.

Tumour spread

Tumour is spread by direct invasion along lines of least resistance in surrounding normal tissues or by infiltration into epithelial structures, e.g. ductal carcinoma infiltrates the overlying epidermis leading to Paget's disease of the nipple. Local invasion without distant metastases occurs in basal cell carcinoma, craniopharyngioma, glioma and well-differentiated fibrosarcoma. Tumour spread occurs via:

- Lymph nodes by embolism or permeation; when lymph nodes are infiltrated and obstructed a retrograde spread occurs. Lymphatic spread becomes haematogenous when cancer cells enter the blood stream through the thoratic duct. Malignant melanoma and tongue cancer invade the lymphatics very early. Squamous cell carcinoma of the skin or lips spreads rather late. Basal cell carcinoma of the skin does not spread to lymph nodes.

- Blood by infiltration through small veins or vascular spaces of the tumour itself or following lymphatic spread. It is the common route in sarcomas. Lung, breast, kidney, prostate and thyroid cancers spread via blood early and lymphatically later. Body tissues have different affinities to metastasis. Liver, lungs, bone, brain and adrenal glands are common sites in that order. By contrast spleen, skeletal muscle and skin are very rarely involved. This selective affinity may be specific, e.g. metastases to spine and pelvis in prostatic carcinoma whilst a solitary lung metastasis would point to a renal carcinoma.

- Implantation, as in serous cavities when cancer cells gravitate to and land in the rectovaginal or rectovesical pouch. Cerebrospinal fluid (CSF) may act as a carrier in brain tumours. Urine may do the same in the spread of renal pelvis carcinoma to the bladder (although the theory of multicentric origin refutes this). Even the surgeon's knife may implant the cells in the operative wound causing recurrence later on.

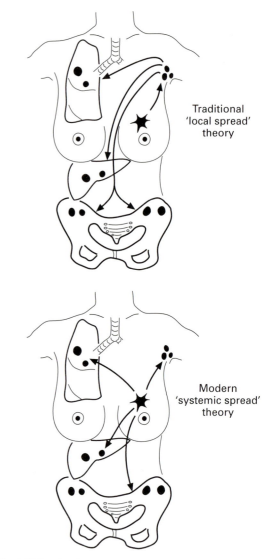

Fig. 1.35.1   Theories of cancer dissemination

THEORIES OF CANCER DISSEMINATION

Traditionally, a malignant tumour was believed to spread initially by local permeation, i.e. by direct centrifugal extension along tissue spaces and by embolisation of lymphatics to the regional lymph nodes. Metastasis to these regional lymph nodes was regarded as the first step in the dissemination of a tumour which thus could be contained as a regional disease. The second step, that of dissemination by the bloodstream, followed later (Fig. 1.35.1). It was this theory which led to the general belief that cancer was 'curable' provided that it had not spread beyond the regional nodes, and to the development of 'curative' radical operations designed to eradicate all malignant cells in the primary tumour and its related lymph nodes. While this theory is still valid in gastrointestinal cancers, it is no longer tenable in cancers of the lungs and breast, and perhaps other cancers.

It is now believed that even at the earliest stage tumour cells invade both the lymphatic and the blood vessels which carry them to regional and distant sites to form widespread micrometastases. Regional lymph node involvement therefore is not regarded as a stage in the progression of the disease but as an indicator that the widespread dissemination has in fact occurred (Fig. 1.35.2). It is this concept which has led to a reappraisal of the role of local treatment, and to recognition of the need for systemic adjuvant (or sole) systemic treatment for long-term control of the disease, i.e. adjuvant chemotherapy and/or radiotherapy following surgery for early cancer.

However, the good documented results following the introduction of total mesorectal excision (TME) as a part of radical resection of rectal cancer (anterior restorative resection or abdominoperineal excision of rectum), together with good results of R2 (D2) radical gastrectomy whether unmodified (conventional Japanese style removing lymph nodes and spleen) or modified (by Professor Johnston and Sue-Ling of Leeds by removing lymph nodes but without splenectomy) can only indicate that the traditional local spread theory is still tenable in gastrointestinal cancers. This means that cancer in

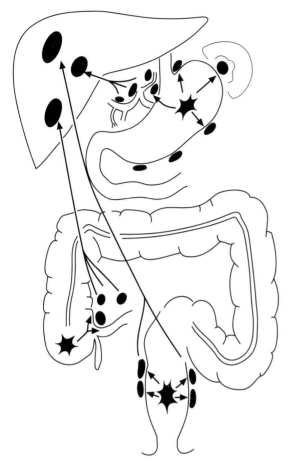

Fig. 1.35.2 Traditional 'local spread' is the valid method of GIT cancer dissemination

different organs behaves differently. Even in early breast cancer, local spread theory is perhaps valid in 25% of patients, while systemic spread theory predominates the 75% of patients.

Tumour structure

Macroscopic (gross) features

Benign tumours may be deep (solid or cystic) or epithelial. The projectile epithelial nodule is morphologically a polyp (pedunculated or sessile); if the epithelium is secretory it is called an adenoma. Cancers may be intraluminal, extraluminal or transmural (according to the direction of growth) and may be fungating (cauliflower), ulcerative (excavating) or annular (stricture) in hollow viscera, e.g. the gastrointestinal tract. In compact organs cancers may be solid (scirrhous) or cystic.

Microscopic (histopathological) features

According to the Broder classification, cancer can be well-differentiated (Grade I), moderately differentiated (Grade II) or undifferentiated (dedifferentiated, anaplastic; Grade III).

Tumour-host relationship

Benign tumours can cause serious mechanical obstruction of natural passages, e.g. trachea, ureter, intestine, intracranial and intraspinal sites. Endocrine tumours (phaeochromocytoma, Zollinger–Ellison syndrome) may also affect the host. Cancers can cause local destruction as well as haemorrhage, ulceration and secondary infection.

Systemically, cancers can cause: anaemia as in gastrointestinal tract cancer (e.g. gastric and caecal) as a result of chronic blood loss, malabsorption and bone marrow replacement; thrombophlebitis migrans in pancreatic cancer; afibrinogenaemia in prostatic cancer (haematological); central nervous system; demyelination, peripheral neuritis, myopathic weakness and dermatomyositis (neuropathic). Non-endocrine cancers, e.g. lung, may produce Cushing's syndrome, hypoglycaemia, hypercalcaemia and hyponatraemia (hormonal). Pulmonary osteoarthropathy could be produced by lung cancer. Immunologically, Hodgkin's lymphoma produces delayed cell-mediated hypersensitivity while lymphosarcoma induces a humoral immunoglobulin-induced hypersensitivity.

Cancer causes death in 50% of patients by virtue of its complications (e.g. ureteric obstruction and anuria in 50% of pelvic cancers, fulminating haemorrhage in cancers of the upper airways and upper gastrointestinal tract, intercurrent infection in cancers of airways, gastrointestinal tract and haematopoietic system). Few patients die from the consequences of the treatment (operative mortality is 25% in oesophageal cancers; operative or radiotherapy mortality is 3–4% in pelvic cancers due to late urinary complications or prolonged radiation of the lumboabdominal region with renal and digestive complications).

Cancer cachexia is the classic cause of death; it is a vague term covering a complex biological course (cancer cells concentrate alanine, methionine, histidine and isoleucine and thus compete with intestinal and hepatic cells leading ultimately to negative N_2 balance ending in death). Other causes of death are cardiac metastases due to direct invasion from primary lung and oesophageal cancers or to secondaries from lymphoma and melanoma. Major endocrine infiltration (e.g. adrenal and hypophyseal) is found in 30–35% of autopsies. Cerebral metastases inducing coma can cause sudden or rapid death.

Diagnosis

Early diagnosis of a cancer is directly related to the educational level of the public. Whether it is done on an individual basis (by history, physical examination and selected investigations, depending on the particular cancer) or on a population basis (mass screening), the aim is to detect early cases for successful treatment. The extent of the disease is evaluated by clinical staging, using either the TNM system or the traditional system (early, Stage 0 in situ; Stages I and II; and advanced, Stages III and IV). A treatment strategy is then planned.

Treatment

The therapeutic armamentarium includes single or multimodal treatment of surgery, radiotherapy and chemotherapy.

Surgical treatment

The major treatment (for most solid tumours). Its main limitation is that it is a localised treatment for a disease which may be systemic at the time of presentation, e.g. carcinoma of bronchus and breast. In early cancer, adequate radical surgery which eradicates the tumour with margins of normal tissue and regional draining lymph nodes is curative (while inadequate initial surgery leads to local recurrences). Surgery may be palliative (prolonging comfortable life), e.g. removal of gastrointestinal tract cancers causing bleeding and obstruction, amputation of limbs with painful bleeding sarcomas, mastectomy of ulcerating bleeding fungating breast, endocrine ablation, arterial infusion of cytotoxics (hepatic and carotid artery), urgent decompression of spinal cord tumours.

Surgery, however has three other therapeutic aspects:
- *Preventive*: by removal of premalignant and in situ lesions, e.g. familial polyposis coli and in situ carcinoma of cervix uteri.
- *Reductive or debulking*: in the hope that chemotherapy and/ or deep X-ray therapy may be able to contain or cure the micrometastases, e.g. childhood tumours.
- *Reconstructive*: for those parts destroyed by initial therapeutic procedures (e.g. plastic procedures to restore the results of aggressive ENT surgery and prosthetic bone replacement for bone tumours).

Diagnostic (e.g. staging laparotomy in Hodgkin's disease, mini laparotomy, exploratory laparotomy and various types of biopsies) should be distinguished from therapeutic surgery.

1.36 Cancer Immunobiology

The cellular immune system normally performs the function of immmune surveillance to eradicate individual tumour cells (recognised as non-self cells) in tissues and circulation; tumour antigenicity may be diverse, though tumours sometimes lack antigenicity, which will hinder the effectiveness of immune response. Failure of the immune system to kill tumour cells may be due in part to immunosuppressive action of tumour cells themselves. Clinically, trauma, surgery, sepsis, nutritional status and chemotherapy can all modify the immune response to tumour cells.

IMMUNOLOGICAL CASCADE

Immune responses are either innate (constantly active), or they are adaptive (learned) responses requiring specific priming stimuli. With introduction of foreign antigens, it is the macrophages (antigen-presenting cells from innate mechanism), which initiate a chain of immunological events or cascade leading to generation of specificity (among T- and B-lymphocytes of adaptive mechanism), thus linking the two immune mechanisms together.

Thus macrophages, when they encounter a cell that is perceived as foreign or abnormal, engulf it and break down the antigens present on the cell surface; these antigen complexes are then presented to T-helper cells and B-cells (lymphocytes) to initiate specific antibody production. Simultaneously, the macrophage (antigen-presenting cell) secretes soluble mediators (cytokines) known as interleukins (IL), locally secreted hormones that regulate cellular activity and act synergistically to augment immune activation. Macrophages secrete IL-1 when presenting antigen to T-helper lymphocyte, and this will stimulate T-helper cells to secrete IL-2 and interferon-gamma (IFN-γ) which enhance T-helper cell activity and boost cytotoxic T-lymphocyte activity and multiplication. Cytotoxic T-cells in turn secrete cytokines, such as tumour necrosis factor (TNF-α) and IFN-γ which further enhance cytotoxic effect.

ONCOLYSIS (TUMOUR CELL KILLING)

Innate responses (Figs 1.36.1, 1.36.2)

Innate responses are capable of lysing non-self cells without the need for specific antigen processing and presentation (unlike adaptive T- and B-lymphocyte responses).

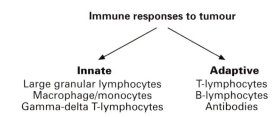

Immune responses to tumour

Innate	**Adaptive**
Large granular lymphocytes	T-lymphocytes
Macrophage/monocytes	B-lymphocytes
Gamma-delta T-lymphocytes	Antibodies

Fig. 1.36.1   Immune responses to tumour

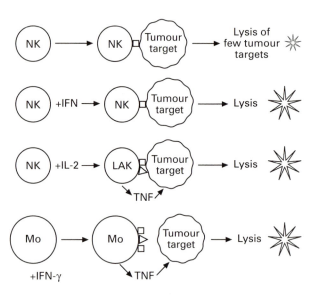

NK = Natural killer cell
LAK = Lymphokine-activated killer cell
Mo = Monocyte/macrophage

Fig. 1.36.2   Innate responses to tumour (oncolysis)

Natural killer cells (NK cells)

Large granular lymphocytes constituting 10% of the total peripheral lymphocyte population. NK cells are effective in lysing virally transformed cells (such as HIV), and cells of some haematological cancers including K562 erythroleukaemia. Lytic activity of NK cells is boosted by interferon-α, β, or γ. This is a normal cellular response to viral infection. Attempts to treat patients with interferon as a single agent anti-tumour agent have so far failed in all but a few uncommon haematological tumours; this is due to resistance of most solid tumours to interferon-enhanced NK activity. Experimentally, NK cells are important in prevention of blood-borne tumour metastases. NK cells are capable of binding to both susceptible and resistant tumour cells, but only when they interact with a susceptible cell are they capable of killing that cell.

Lymphokine activated killer cells (LAK cells)

Whereas NK activity is present naturally in circulating lymphocytes, LAK activity requires a period of lymphocyte activation by high concentration of IL-2. Furthermore, LAK cells lyse *all* tumour cells (killing is not restricted to specific tumour); such fascinating promiscuous killing is attributed to their ability to recognise all types of cancer. LAK cells, however, do not lyse normal cells, unless normal cells are manipulated to alter their surface phenotype.

Macrophages

Monocyte/macrophage (Mo) cells can be activated by bacterial invasion, trauma, interferon, or IL-2. Activated Mo cells are capable of recognising and destroying any abnormal cell they encounter; they may be directly cytotoxic to tumour cells without prior sensitisation to tumour. This is the basis of tumour regression seen in association with sepsis.

Mo cells also process abnormal cell antigen, and display it on their surfaces (in association with major histocompatibility complex class II antigenic molecules) and present this antigen complex to generate adaptive immune responses by T-cells and B-cells. The lytic mechanism employed by Mo cells involves membrane associated molecules such as tumour necrosis factor (TNF), a peptide bound to cell membrane of macrophages and which is cytotoxic by cell-to-cell contact with tumour cells; once released into the environment of a tumour by activated macrophages, soluble TNF itself may also cause tumour cell lysis. Tissue-specific macrophages such as pleural macrophages and hepatic Kupffer cells are more oncolytic than their blood monocyte precursors; this may be due to their enhanced ability to secrete TNF.

Adaptive responses (Figs 1.36.1, 1.36.3)

Generation of adaptive responses involves a period of delay for antigen-processing and presentation to B- and T-cells; it is

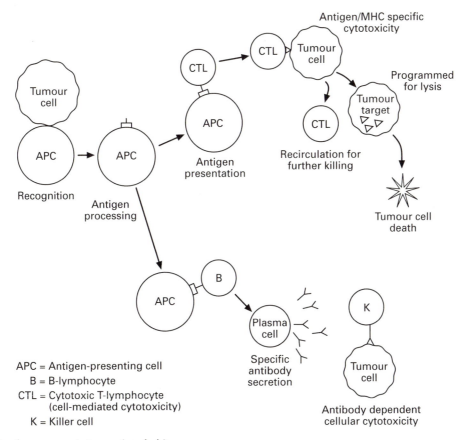

APC = Antigen-presenting cell
B = B-lymphocyte
CTL = Cytotoxic T-lymphocyte
    (cell-mediated cytotoxicity)
K = Killer cell

Fig. 1.36.3 Adapative responses to tumour (oncolysis)

therefore dependent on effectiveness of tissue-specific macrophages (antigen-presenting cells).

T-lymphocytes

Lymphocyte infiltrates within most tumours contain a proportion of T-cells with cytotoxic potential. Most T-cells are of CD8 cytotoxic/suppressor phenotype. If these tumour infiltrating T-lymphocytes are cultured *in vitro* with IL-2, their oncolytic activity will be 50–100 times more than LAK cells.

B-lymphocytes and antibody-dependent cellular cytotoxicity (ADCC)

The role of serum antibodies in a host's response to cancer is uncertain. First, antibodies have to cross from blood into tissues in sufficiently high concentrations to have an effect on tumour cells. However, some tumour cells in the blood are vulnerable to antibodies. Secondly, the heterogenous nature of all tumours may enable part of the tumour to escape specific recognition by the antibody. Once a tumour cell is labelled foreign or abnormal by an antibody, it will be susceptible to lysis by a number of mechanisms, including lytic complement components. ADCC occurs in rejection of transplants.

Certain IgG antibodies can block cytotoxic activity of immune cells (blockers or blocking antibodies).

Mechanisms of oncolysis (Figs 1.36.2, 1.36.3)

Cell-mediated lysis occurs in a number of phases; first, the effector cell recognises and binds to the tumour cell target. If the tumour cell is not susceptible, or the binding is non-specific, the cells separate and each goes its own way unaltered. Binding to a susceptible target, however, initiates an intracellular signal and triggers the second phase: the effector cell induces a metabolic change within the target cell, programming the cell to die by lysis. The effector and target cells then separate; the tumour cell undergoes lysis after a short interval, while the effector cell will be free to kill again. The rate of cell killing is dependent on both the number of effector cells and the time taken to form lytic conjugates with successive target cells. A number of cytotoxic molecules are known to be released from cytotoxic cells. NK cells produce a specific NK cytotoxic factor (NKCF) and a molecule (perforin) that causes the membrane of the target cell to become porous; both molecules disrupt the integrity of the cell membrane and allow influx of other lytic molecules like serine proteases. When NK cells are transformed into LAK cells by IL-2, their molecular secretion changes and the production of TNF and IFN-γ is enhanced; these peptides in combination are markedly cytotoxic to tumour cells.

When molecules such as NKCF, perforin, TNF, IFN-γ and lymphotoxin (derived from T-lymphocytes) are secreted into the microenvironment of the tumour; they act as a lytic cocktail and kill tumour cells independently of cell-to-cell interactions.

Tumours may evade recognition by the immune system in a number of ways:

● Tumour cell either reduces or continually alters its antigenic profile, then it can escape antibodies and T-cell responses directed at specific antigens. This can be observed experimentally, when antibodies raised against primary tumour cannot bind to its metastases.

● Some tumours express a reduced amount of MHC antigens, diminishing their recognition by T-cells.

● Tumour antigens can be shed and this may also block specific immune effector function.

Absence of immune reactions to tumour deposits in lymph nodes remains an unexplained phenomenon, reflecting immune tolerance or an evasive mechanism.

Once an immune response to a tumour is elicited, the tumour is subjected to 'selection pressure' to change in order to survive. Tumour cells capable of inactivating immune responses may grow without interference from the immune system; it is an important mechanism of tumour 'escape' from immune killing.

Patients with large tumour burdens are generally immunocompromised through unknown tumour cell products.

Most epithelia are controlled by many autocrine regulatory peptides, such as transforming growth factor-beta (TGF-β), which is a principal negative regulator of cell growth. It is thought that tumour cells are relatively unresponsive to their own TGF-β, while immune cells infiltrating the tumour are inhibited by this potently immunosuppressive molecule.

IMMUNOLOGICAL RECOGNITION OF TUMOURS

Specific antitumour immune response requires that cells of the immune system recognise the difference between normal and tumour cells. These differences may be tumour-specific or tissue-specific. A number of tumour antigens (oncogens) have been identified in serum and studied with monoclonal antibodies; such antigens include CA19–9 (pancreas), CA50 (colon), CA25 (breast). However, many were proved later not to be entirely tumour-specific, as they were found in some non-malignant tissues. To date, few human tumour-specific antigens exist, against which corresponding monoclonal antibodies have been produced.

Tissue-specific substances are used as diagnostic and prognostic indicators in malignant disease. These include carcinoembryonic antigen (CEA) expressed by gut-derived tissue, alpha-fetoprotein (AFP), acid phosphatase, and human chorionic gonadotrophin (hCG). The clinical applications are well established in monitoring tumour recurrence their concentrations in serum being closely related to tumour bulk.

Clinical applications

There is traffic of lymphocytes within tissues; they travel in repeated cycles between blood, tissues, lymphatics, lymph nodes and back to the blood. The process of recirculation takes a few hours, and is independent of the presence of antigen in tissues. It is uncertain whether these cells have actively infiltrated a tumour that displays 'abnormal' antigens or whether they just represent residual lymphocyte traffic arrested in the tumour environment. In human immunogenic tumours, such as melanoma and hypernephroma, highly active anti-tumour lymphocytes can be isolated from resected surgical specimens. In colorectal carcinoma, however, mild infiltration of immune cells is found, while plasma cell infiltration (non-cytotoxic non-lytic) was found in some breast carcinomas.

Melanoma

In melanoma, spontaneous regression has an immunological basis. Treatment with monoclonal antibodies has been partially successful. Isolation of tumour infiltrating lymphocytes revealed mostly cytotoxic T-cells with 80% specificity for melanoma tumour (from which they were isolated); these cells can be stimulated by non-specific stimulants such as BCG vaccine with clinical tumour response. The use of IFN-α as a stimulant to NK cells results in 30% of patients responding to treatment. The most promising responses were obtained using IL-2 as a direct stimulant to T-cells within the tumour deposits.

Renal adenocarcinoma

In hypernephroma, lymphocyte infiltration contains 50–70% NK cells and 30–50% cytotoxic T cells, reflecting possible diverse immunological responses to the tumour (both innate and adaptive responses). Spontaneous regression in hyper-nephroma is rare (1 in 500 cases) and must follow removal of the primary tumour. The use of IFN-α is partially successful in metastatic disease (15% response); IL-2 use produced 20% response in patients with advanced disease, while the use of adaptive immunotherapy using IL-2 and LAK cells is more effective (30% response).

Breast carcinoma

The relation between improved prognosis and lymphocytic infiltration in breast carcinoma is well established. The infiltrating cell type most strongly correlating with improved diagnosis is the macrophage. Failure of single agent immuno-therapy is perplexing; however, the use of adaptive immuno-therapy has occasionally been encouraging.

Surgical trauma

In trauma increased steroid hormones may suppress immune responses during the period of recovery from trauma. At the start of the anabolic phase of recovery, the concentrations of trophic hormones in the circulation increase. This may aid the growth of tumour cells and encourage seeding to sites that would not otherwise support growth. The suppression of tumour-directed cellular cytotoxicity caused by operations may occasionally be prevented by perioperative modifiers such as IFN-α.

Sepsis

In sepsis, there is an orchestrated endocrine and metabolic response. Coley, in 1893, demonstrated that 35% of patients with untreatable tumours of the head and neck could be induced to respond if severe erysipelas was caused locally by the injection of streptococci. His work led to the treatment of tumours with a partially refined bacterial broth named 'Coley's

toxins'. Coley produced a response rate as good as those obtained by immunotherapeutic regimens used today. The response to sepsis includes the release of many cytokines such as IFN-γ and TNF; these tumoricidal molecules may then kill susceptible tumour cells rendered vulnerable by the prolonged catabolic phase of continuing sepsis.

Chemotherapy

Chemotherapy suppresses bone marrow and lymphocytes. However, during the recovery phase from treatment with cytotoxic drugs, there is a significant augmentation of the ability to generate LAK cells by patients with advanced GIT cancer, perhaps because regenerating bone marrow precursors are more responsive to IL-2.

Nutrition and cancer

Advanced tumours are associated with malnutrition which impairs immune responses. Attempts to correct immune deficiency by i.v. nutrition have led to limited success. While the humoral immune system can benefit, cellular antitumour immune response was significantly impaired by parenteral nutrition. The lipid has immunosuppressive effect.

Immunotherapy (Fig. 1.36.4)

- IFN-α has a place in the management of some haemato-logical malignancies and is the best treatment available in hairy cell leukaemia; 70% of patients with metastatic carcinoid tumours derive symptomatic benefit.
- The use of TNF as a single agent immunotherapy has been unsuccessful and is associated with serious toxicity, because TNF is the initiator of septic shock.
- IL-2 is promising; regimens using IL-2 as a single agent are designed to reduce toxicity and improve response. IL-2 infusion i.v. activates lymphocytes and monocytes and secretes IFN-γ, TNF and yet unknown factors which mediate toxic (and perhaps therapeutic) effects.
- The isolation of cytolytic cells from the blood or tumour of patients with cancer, and their expansion into millions by IL-2, has enabled us to reinfuse them into the same patient to

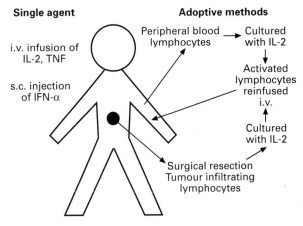

Fig. 1.36.4   Immunotherapy methods

improve the anti-cancer immune response; this approach has been successful mainly in patients with malignant melanoma and hypernephroma after failure of conventional treatment.

1.37 Radiotherapy

Ionised radiations damage both normal and neoplastic tissues (DNA strand breaks). However, normal tissues recover while neoplastic tissues do not, resulting in therapeutic benefit. A radiation dose is defined as the energy absorbed per unit of mass and is expressed in rads or in Grays (1 Gray = 1 joule/kg = 100 rad). Radiotherapy is used mainly for malignant tumours and rarely in benign tumours (e.g. thyrotoxicosis and some skin conditions). It may be palliative or radical.

Cancer response

Varies according to the following.

Type of cell May be very radiosensitive (e.g. reticulosis group, Wilms' tumour and seminoma), moderately sensitive (e.g. rodent ulcer, squamous epithelioma and transitional cell carcinoma) or variable (e.g. melanoma, thyroid carcinoma and osteogenic sarcoma). Sarcomas and recurrent tumours following previous irradiation are generally radioresistant. Note that while seminoma needs 2000 rad, Hodgkin's disease requires 4000 rad and squamous cell carcinoma of the larynx needs 6000 rad.

Differentiation of cells Radiosensitivity is directly proportional to reproductive activity and inversely proportional to the degree of cell differentiation; thus, germinal cells and spermatogonia are very sensitive while neurones are resistant (except medulloblastoma). Anaplastic cancers are generally radiosensitive.

Blood supply Anoxic cells are radioresistant, e.g. in large rapidly growing cancers or in association with syphilis or post-inflammatory scarring. Hyperbaric O_2 increases the radiosensitivity of cancer.

Localisation The more localised the cancers the easier they are to control (e.g. basal cell carcinoma, carcinoma of the cervix) and the better the results (provided they are radiosensitive).

Assessment of tumour

Radiation is administered after the extent of the cancer has been accurately assessed by diagnostic radiography, surface anatomy, examination under anaesthesia and preoperative insertion of radiopaque markers around the target. Radiation dose depends on age, condition of patient, type of cancer and the target volume (the larger the cancer, the greater the number of radiation fractions). Deep-seated cancers are most often treated by multiple convergent beams or by rotational therapy.

Irradiation effects (total body)

Immediate
- Very high dosage (over 5000 rad single exposure) produces cerebral syndrome (nausea, vomiting, tremor, convulsions and death).
- Moderate dosage (800–5000 rad single exposure) produces gastrointestinal syndrome (nausea, vomiting, diarrhoea, dehydration and death).
- Low dosage (under 800 rad single exposure) produces haematological syndrome (mild initial nausea and vomiting but mainly bone marrow aplasia with panocytopenia manifested by infection and bleeding).

Late
- Premature ageing
- Cataract
- Sterility
- Fetal abnormalities
- Malignant disease
- Genetic effect

Local irradiation effect on skin (in chronological order)

1. Erythema followed by pigmentation.
2. Fibrinoid necrosis with vessel thrombosis leading to radionecrotic ulcer (painful, indolent, sloughing base, clean-cut edge).
3. Fibrosis with absent hair follicles and accessory glands (delayed healing in injury). Skin becomes atrophic with telangectasia.

Types of radiotherapy and administration

External beam irradiation

- Conventional X-ray therapy (orthovoltage 10–500 kV) either superficial or deep.
- Megavoltage (1.2–40 MV) from:
  - (a) γ sources ^{60}CO, ^{137}CS teletherapy.
  - (b) X-ray sources from linear accelerator giving sharper, deeper but more expensive radiation.
  - (c) Particle beam (electrons) from linear accelerator.
  - (d) Betatrons (circular electron accelerators).
  - (e) Cyclotrons and synchrotrons producing heavy particles, e.g. neutrons.
  - (a) and (b) are electromagnetic radiations while (c), (d) and (e) are particle radiations.

Brachytherapy

Radioactive sources are inserted within or close to the cancer.

Intracavitory

Used mainly in gynaecology for treatment of carcinoma of cervix and corpus uteri. Radium, ^{137}Cs, ^{90}Y (bladder carcinoma) and ^{198}Au colloid (in malignant effusion – ascites or pleural) are used. One method involves insertion of a special applicator (under anaesthesia) which is left in for 24 h; this procedure should be repeated many times. The cathetron technique involves inserting a shielded ^{60}Co source holder under general anaesthesia after loading it mechanically from another room.

Interstitial

Involves application of moulds under general anaesthesia (e.g. radium and ^{137}Cs needles, ^{192}Ir, ^{192}Ta and ^{90}Y wires; ^{198}Au grains; and radon seeds). Used in tongue and bladder carcinoma. Can be used with surgery (unresectable tumour) in parotid and apical lung cancers.

Systemic radiotherapy

Uses ^{131}I (for thyrotoxicosis and thyroid carcinoma) and ^{32}P (for polycythemia rubra vera). It is given i.v. The materials are taken up preferentially by malignant cells in much higher concentrations than by normal cells.

Clinical uses

Radical radiotherapy (alone), with the aim of cure, e.g. squamous cell carcinoma of skin and oral cavity, vocal cord and laryngeal carcinoma and carcinoma of cervix uteri.

Planned combination of *surgery with radiotherapy*, e.g. seminoma (with improved 5 year survival of from 50% to 80%) and carcinoma of pharynx. Radiotherapy can be preoperative (as in hypernephroma) but is more commonly postoperatively (as in breast carcinoma).

Planned combination of *cytotoxic therapy with radiotherapy*, e.g. late stage malignant lymphoma and head and neck tumours.

Palliative radiotherapy, e.g. in bronchogenic carcinoma to control profuse haemoptysis, bone pain, dysphagia, and obstruction of bronchus (dyspnoea) and superior vena cava; in breast carcinoma to control bone pain (due to metastases) and retrobulbar deposits causing proptosis.

Future advances in radiotherapy

Include administration of chemical and physical radiosensitising procedures such as:
- Hyperbaric oxygen.
- Hyperthermia (lethal to malignant cells).
- Misonidazol (with conventional X-ray).
- Use of particle radiation, e.g. fast neutrons, protons and negative pimesons (O_2 independent).

Special indications for surgery

When complete excision is possible, surgery is preferred to radiotherapy under the following conditions:
- Site is vulnerable to friction (sole of foot), moisture and infection (axillae), which favour radionecrosis.
- Underlying tissue is cartilage or bone, e.g. dorsum of hand, shin and pinna.
- Peritumour area is prone to malignant change so wide excision is indicated, e.g. vulva.
- Peritumour area is already damaged (e.g. by burns, scars, syphilis or previous irradiation) with anoxia prevailing, and radionecrosis of normal tissues is likely.

Radiation hazards

Various diagnostic radiological procedures and therapeutic interventional radiology can cause ionisation leading to chemical changes (free radicals reacting with cell DNA) resulting ultimately in biological changes (somatic and genetic), among which cancer formation is the most serious radiation effect.

Principles of radiation protection include:
- Justification of X-ray exposure.
- ALARA (As Low As Reasonably Achievable) principle.
- Dose limits.

Risk of cancer and genetic defects varies according to different body parts exposed to radiation. Assuming effective whole body dose is 1, then radiation risk is fractionated as follows:

Gonads 0.25
Breast 0.15
Red bone marrow 0.12
Lung 0.12
Thyroid 0.03
Bone surfaces 0.03
Remainder 0.3

The radiation exposure dose varies with radiological procedures as follows (from the smallest dose to the largest dose):

Dental film (the smallest dose)
Chest X-ray
Skull X-ray
Mammography
Thoracic spine
Pelvis
Abdominal (plain X-ray)
Lumbar spine
CT head
Barium meal
IVP
Barium enema (equivalent to 400 chest X-rays)
CT body (equivalent to 800 chest X-rays) (the largest dose)

1.38 Chemotherapy

Drug treatment of cancer is varied. It includes:
- Cytotoxic, antineoplastic, or anticancer drugs
- Endocrine therapy
- Immunotherapy
- Retinoid
- Interferon
- Systemic (metabolic) radiotherapy (i.v. radioisotopes)
- Supportive therapy (e.g. nutrition, antibiotics, analgesics)

CYTOTOXIC THERAPY

Cancer can be completely excised *en masse* (surgery) or it can be covered by a field of radiation (both means are localised and have limited value when the disease has disseminated). Cytotoxics may be used for both local and metastatic cancer. These agents affect both cancer and normal cells and are always cidal drugs unlike antimicrobial agents (affect bacteria only and are either bacteriostatic or bactericidal).

Cytotoxic therapy aims to bring about cure or prolong survival. These aims have been partially achieved in haematological and childhood cancers. Cure by cytotoxics alone has been reported in acute lymphatic leukaemia (children), Hodgkin's disease, Burkitt's lymphoma, Wilms' tumour, Ewing sarcoma and rhabdomyosarcoma. Prolonged survival has been demonstrated in acute leukaemia (adults), lymphocytic lymphomas, multiple myeloma and neuroblastoma. Among adult solid tumours the picture is far less encouraging. Cure has only been seen in relatively uncommon cancer, e.g. chorion carcinoma and seminoma. Prolonged survival has been claimed in ovarian and breast cancers.

Cytotoxics are given either as adjuvant 'prophylactic' chemotherapy over a prolonged period of time for patients presumably cured (by surgery and/or radiotherapy) to counteract subclinical microscopic micrometastases, e.g. early breast carcinoma, or as an aggressive multimodal therapy for certain disseminated cancers (e.g. childhood cancers which are relatively anaplastic and rapidly growing with high growth fraction); hence, a combination of radical chemotherapy, surgery and radiotherapy is used. Such carefully designed multimodal protocols (to treat other solid cancers in adults) are becoming more popular throughout the world.

Tumour growth (Fig. 1.38.1)

Synthesis of DNA occurs in a relatively short interval in the 'cell cycle', the pattern of which was revealed by radioactive-labelled thymidine. Tumour growth in relation to DNA synthesis in the cell cycle is called tumour kinetics. The cycle passes through the following phases:

G_0 Some cells have division capacity but are temporarily removed from the cycle; suitably stimulated they move to G_1
G_1 Apparent metabolic rest
S   Synthetic period (of DNA)
G_2 Premitotic period
M   Mitosis (cell division)

A normal cell divides only to replace a lost cell (total cell number is constant). A cancer cell divides and adds to existing cells (total cell number is continually increasing). Tumour growth is the outcome of three combined parameters and is expressed as tumour doubling time (T_D) (the time it takes a given amount of tumour tissue to double its own volume). T_D

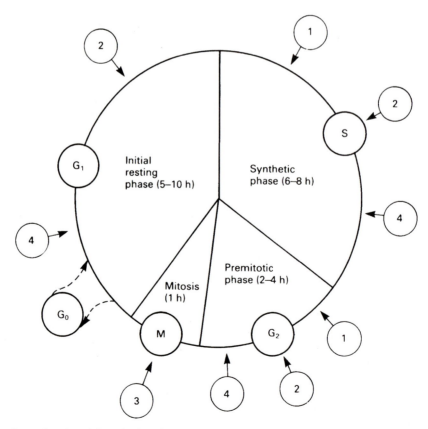

Fig. 1.38.1 Tumour cell growth cycle and sites of action of cytotoxics. 1, polyfunctional alkylating agents; 2, antimetabolities; 3, mitotic spindle inhibitors; 4, antitumour antibiotics

Table 1.38.1 Tumour cells

Dividing	*Non-dividing*
Tumour stem cells $\rightleftharpoons$	Resting tumour cells
Doomed cells (divide 4–5 times and then stop for biological reason)	End cells (though alive never divide)

4. *Antitumour antibiotics* Bind with DNA to block RNA production, e.g. adriamycin, daunorubicin, mithramycin, actinomycin D, mytomycin C and bleomycin.

5. *Miscellaneous*
● Antiproliferative enzymes (L-asparaginase) act on protein synthesis.
● Nitrosoureas affect DNA cross-linkage.
● Inorganic platinum compounds (cis-platinum).
● Others (procarbazine, hydroxyurea).

= 4–500 days. Leukaemia and lymphoma have the shortest T_D followed by sarcoma with carcinoma having the longest T_D.
● Growth fraction (G_f = the ratio of actively dividing cells to resting cells.
● Cell cycle time (T_c) = (for human cells) 40–80 h.
● Cell loss coefficient = the ratio of cells lost to cells produced. It is 100% for normal tissues (zero growth) and 95–99% in cancer. Reduced cell population is due to tumour cell loss caused by exfoliation by friction (skin and gastrointestinal tract), central necrosis, biologically inadequate cells, metastases (washed away) and destruction by host defences, or to the presence of resting cells (Table 1.38.1).

A cancer may therefore be viewed not as a mass of very rapidly dividing cells but as a tissue dividing at an approximately normal rate but failing to lose cells in the normal fashion and therefore gradually increasing in size. T_D is constant for any tumour, i.e. a cancer that can double its size in 2 days will have quadrupled its size in 4 days and be eight times its original volume in 6 days (such proportional increase in size with unit time is termed 'exponential growth'). The human body contains 5×10^{13} cells; a tumour is clinically detectable when it reaches 10^9 cells = 1 g = 1 cm in size and when it reaches 10^{12} = 1 kg the patient is near death. A tumour is therefore clinically detectable and treatable during that last 10–14 of its 35–40 doubling times.

Classification of cytotoxic drugs

This is according to their chemical structure and mechanism of action (Fig. 1.38.1).

1. *Polyfunctional alkylating agents* Interfere with cross-linkage of DNA, e.g. nitrogen mustards (mustine, cyclophosphamide, chlorambucil, melphalan), thiotepa, busulphan and piposulfan.

2. *Antimetabolites* Interfere with nucleic acid synthesis because they are analogues of normal metabolites and act by competition, e.g. folic acid antagonist (methotrexate), purine antagonist (6-mercaptopurine), pyrimidine antagonist (5- fluorouracil) and glutamine antagonist (Azaserine).

3. *Mitotic spindle inhibitors* Cause mitotic arrest and include colchicine and Vinca alkaloids (vinblastine and vincristine).
Plant alkaloids form a broad group (including cocaine, morphine, quinine, atropine and Vinca alkaloids).

Drug resistance and toxicity

Malignant cells may have primary (natural) or secondary (acquired) drug resistance (the latter is due to adaptation and/or mutation).

Toxicity occurs as a result of damage to rapidly dividing normal tissues:
● Bone marrow: anaemia, haemorrhage and infection (most drugs).
● Gastrointestinal tract: stomatitis, vomiting, diarrhoea (most drugs).
● Lymphoreticular: immunosuppression and infection (most drugs).
● Hair follicles: epilation or alopecia (cyclophosphamide, vincristine and adriamycin).
● Lung: damage (chlorambucil and bleomycin) – dose-related
● Urinary bladder: cystitis and sterile haematuria (cyclophosphamide).
● Hepato- and nephrotoxicity (methotrexate).
● Skin: impaired wound healing, vesiculation and oedema.
● Cardiotoxicity (daunorubicin and adriamycin) – dose related.
● Fetus: teratogenesis and abortion.
● Tissue damage if extravasated.

Careful choice of cytotoxic combinations, strict observance of total doses (many effects are dose-related) and serial blood counts with symptomatic control (e.g. antiemetics) will minimise toxicity.

Contraindications

Use of ineffective agent, availability of another superior approach, very advanced disease (fatal toxicity is likely), pre-existing bone marrow depression or active infection and when there are no means of assessing the progress of treatment.

Methods of cytotoxic use (Fig. 1.38.2)

Single-agent continuous therapy

A constant blood level of a single cytotoxic drug is maintained until unacceptable toxicity, drug resistance or cure results.

Combination therapy

Continuous

This uses a number of drugs with various actions continuously; the cancer mass reduces only at the expense of simultaneous

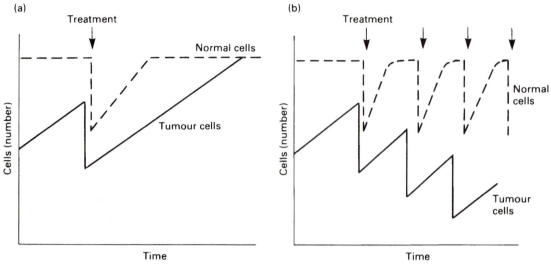

Fig. 1.38.2 Comparison of (a) single and (b) pulsed combined cytotoxic therapies

normal tissue toxicity which necessitates a rest phase for recovery during which time the cancer will repopulate.

Pulsing combination therapy

This is the most widely used treatment. Treatment is split into short intervals each of which is referred to as a pulse. Its advantages are:
- Maximal exploitation of the differential in recovery times between normal and malignant tissues.
- Relative lack of toxicity allows therapy to continue indefinitely so increasing chance of cure.
- Allows higher doses of individual drugs to be given so that a higher proportion of cancer cells are killed.
- Recovery of normal tissues in between treatment pulses includes the restoration of the immune system which has further tumoricidal action against small cancer cell populations.

Sequential therapy

When combination chemotherapy is given in sequence it is called sequential therapy. In Hodgkin's disease stages IIIb and IV there is 70–80% remission following the MOPP schedule:

Mustard (nitrogen mustard)	6mg/m^2	i.v.	Day 1 and 8
Oncovan (vincristine)	1.4 mg/m^2	i.v.	Day 1 and 8
Procarbazine	100 mg/m^2	(0)	Day 1–14 (inclusive)
Prednisolone	40 mg/m^2	(0)	Day 1–14 (inclusive)

Prednisolone is given only during the first and fourth courses. Six courses are given with 2 weeks rest between the end of one course and the beginning of the next.

The early stages of Hodgkin's lymphoma (I, II, IIIa) are treated with radiotherapy (Fig.1.38.3).

Cytotoxic administration

Systemic (oral and i.v.)

More toxic but drug can reach micrometastases.

Local

Similar in effect to the localised methods of treatment (i.e. surgery and radiotherapy). Includes:

Regional cytotoxic therapy

Arterial infusion
- Malignant melanoma recurrence: phenylalanine mustard.
- Head and neck tumours: through the external carotid artery with methotrexate followed by antidote folinic acid for rapid neutralisation.
- Liver secondaries: through the hepatic artery during laparotomy with 5-fluorouracil.

Extracorporeal limb perfusion The main artery and vein to the tumour-bearing area are cannulated to maintain artificial circulation. Limb temperature can be raised (by immersing the limb in a water bath or covering it with hot towels) to cause vasodilation for increased rate of cytotoxic perfusion (also hyperthermia may be lethal to cancer cells). This method is used in malignant melanoma or soft tissue sarcoma of the limb (Fig. 1.38.4).

Intracavitary

For example:
- Pleural effusion due to secondary deposits or complicated malignancy of the breast and bronchus may lead to dyspnoea and may be treated with instillation of cyclophosphamide or thiotepa causing pleurodesis and fibrosis.
- In ascites thiotepa or cyclophosphamide instillation is used with three objectives – control of ascites, control of

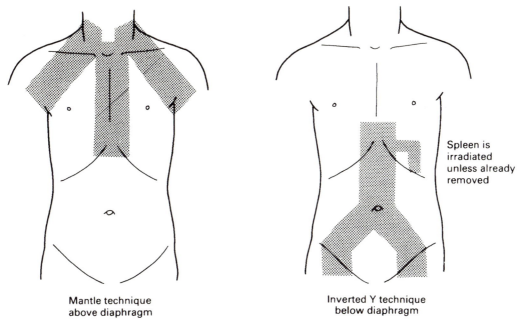

Spleen is
irradiated
unless already
removed

Mantle technique
above diaphragm

Inverted Y technique
below diaphragm

Fig. 1.38.3   Radiotherapy in Hodgkin's disease

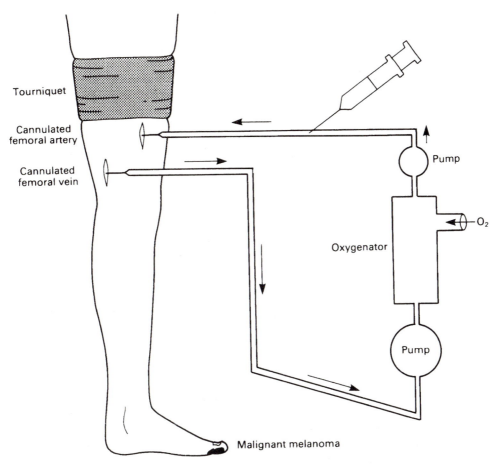

Tourniquet

Cannulated
femoral artery

Cannulated
femoral vein

Pump

O_2

Oxygenator

Pump

Malignant melanoma

Fig. 1.38.4   Extracorporeal isolated lower limb perfusion

advanced primary disease and as adjuvant therapy at the time of resection for primary gastric, rectal and ovarian cancers.

Intrathecal

For example, subarachnoid methotrexate injection in acute lymphatic leukaemia since most cytotoxics cannot cross blood–brain barrier.

Topical

Creams and ointment, e.g. 5% 5-fluorouracil twice daily for 2 weeks in skin carcinoma. It causes intense local reaction and is inferior to other means.

Therapeutic potential of cytotoxic agents

Influenced by drug toxicity, tumour kinetics (the larger the G_f and the higher the cell loss coefficient, the more vulnerable the tumour to cytotoxics and vice versa), drug pharmacokinetics (drug should reach the tumour site and remain there in a sufficient concentration for sufficient time) and the method of cytotoxic use.

The cancer response to cytotoxics is therefore classified as:

Group A   Striking, e.g. Burkitt's lymphoma
Group B   Less effective, e.g. endometrial carcinoma
Group C   Ineffective, e.g. oesophageal carcinoma

ENDOCRINE THERAPY

Therapeutic manipulation of endocrine environment is carried out either by:
- Ablative therapy (surgical removal or radiation destruction of particular endocrine organ); or
- Additive therapy (medical castration) where exogenous natural or synthetic hormones are administered.

Endocrine therapy (unlike cytotoxics) is never curative – eventually all hormone-sensitive tumours will become resistant – and offers only a form of palliation in advanced endocrine-sensitive cancer (in less than 30% of cases) with successful growth control lasting for a maximum of 2 years.

Endocrine pharmacology

Oestrogen

Has many anti-cancer actions: direct action on breast and prostatic tissue; pituitary-mediated effect as anti-prolactin in breast carcinoma and anti-interstitial cell-stimulating hormone in prostatic carcinoma; immune stimulation in both breast and prostatic carcinoma; increases testosterone-binding globulin, thus decreasing free testosterone in prostatic carcinoma. The preparations include (with oral daily doses):

Ethinyloestradiol	0.1–0.5 mg three times daily
Stilboestrol	1–5 mg three times daily
Tripara-anisilchlorethylene (Tace)	12–24 mg

Fosfestrol tetrasodium (Honvan)

Usually inert, but under the action of acid phosphatase of prostatic carcinoma, free stilboestrol will be liberated and leads to sacral and pelvic pain rapidly following injection (daily i.v. dose 250–500 mg) in patients with metastases to these areas (thus it is diagnostic and therapeutic in these cases).

Androgens

Testosterone propionate 100 mg three times weekly (i.m.); may lead to hirsutism, hoarseness, skin changes, increased libido and baldness (in men).

Progestogens

Medroxyprogesterone acetate (Provera).

Antiprolactins

CB_{154}, L-dopa and CG_{603}; used in advanced breast cancer.

Aminoglutethimide (Orimeten)

A steroidogenesis enzyme blocker inhibiting oestrogen synthesis by blocking desmolase, which mediates the first step in the conversion of cholesterol to androgens in the adrenal glands (medical adrenalectomy), and aromase, which mediates the conversion of androgens to oestrogens peripherally. Clinically 250 mg three times daily with hydrocortisone 20 mg twice daily (to prevent a reflex rise in ACTH, which might overcome the adrenal block) is used in postmenopausal or oöphorectomised women with metastatic breast cancers (especially oestrogen positive) producing remission in 30% with results comparable to those of surgical adrenalectomy.

Anti-oestrogens

Inhibit oestrogen by blocking receptor sites in target organs in oestrogen-dependent tumours. They have minimal side-effects, mild oestrogenicity and possible prolactin inhibition. They are (with oral daily doses):

Tamoxifen	10–20 mg twice daily (may cause thrombocytopenia): very popular drug
Nafoxiden	60–90 mg three times daily (causes dry skin, photophobia and cataract)
Clomiphene citrate	50 mg twice daily

Glucocorticoids

Cancer complications such as hypercalcaemia (due to bone metastases, immobilisation with osteoporosis precipitated by oestrogen therapy), cerebral oedema, autoimmune haemolytic anaemia, general depression and anorexia are all treated with prednisolone. However, prolonged glucocorticoid therapy may cause many side-effects – suppression and atrophy of adrenal glands, Na^+ and H_2O retention, K^+ depletion, weight gain and risk of heart failure, hypertension, susceptibility to infection, cushingoid appearance with moon face and buffalo hump, gastrointestinal tract problems (e.g. dyspepsia, peptic ulcer and perforation), osteoporosis, hyperglycaemia and diabetes, psychosis with euphoria, skin changes, cataract and myopathy.

Clinical uses

Breast carcinoma

Only 30% respond to hormonal manipulation. Prediction of the response depends on laboratory tests (positive oestrogen receptors, tumour culture with different hormones and hormonal assay) and clinical factors (older age and long disease-free interval between primary treatment and appearance of first recurrence have a better response; menopausal status also counts).

Early breast carcinoma

Treated by surgery ± radiotherapy. Adjuvant prophylactic chemotherapy is now also given even if axillary lymph nodes are not involved.

Advanced breast carcinoma

Treated by (in order of procedure):
1. Palliative surgery.
2. Radiotherapy: in bone and skin metastases.
3. Premenopausal: ovarian ablation.
4. Perimenopausal (5 years after menopause): antioestrogens or androgens.
5. Postmenopausal: oestrogen but use prednisone in hepatic and lung infiltration. An anti-oestrogen is the drug of choice in soft tissue and pulmonary involvement. Relapses after ovarian ablation need secondary endocrine ablation (adrenalectomy or hypophysectomy). In postmenopausal relapses, stop the treatment and look for a withdrawal response and if none then perform a secondary endocrine ablation.

Cytotoxic therapy is indicated in endocrine failure or is used initially if the tumour is found to be hormone insensitive (e.g. negative oestrogen receptors) and in fairly aggressive diseases like fulminating hepatitis lymphangiosa. Either single or, usually, intermittent combination therapy is used (5-fluorouracil, cyclophosphamide and methotrexate). It is the treatment of choice in rapidly progressing breast carcinoma.

Immunotherapy (by non-specific stimulation of immune defence mechanism) and neutron therapy are still under trial. *N.B.* In male breast carcinoma (1% of total breast carcinoma) bilateral surgical orchidectomy is effective in two-thirds of cases. If relapse occurs, steroid therapy is better than ablative therapy.

Prostatic carcinoma

Ninety per cent are hormone-dependent. Oestrogen (stilboestrol) is the initial treatment. If thromboembolism occurs, whether induced by oestrogens or already present due to malignant infiltration of lymphatics or venous drainage of lower limbs by prostatic carcinoma, then:
- Perform bilateral subcapsular orchidectomy.
- Relapses need steroid or ablative therapy.

- Bone metastases are controlled with megavoltage radiotherapy and obstructive uropathy is controlled with prostatic transurethral resection (TUR).

Cancers of ovary, uterus (endometrial) and kidney (adenocarcinoma)

These organs are the embryological derivatives of the urogenital ridge and their cancers are all treated with progestogens.

Thyroid carcinoma

Thyroxine 0.1 mg three times daily (or alternatively T_3 20 μg three times daily) is given to suppress TSH and to prevent the growth of the primary residual tumour and its metatases (after total thyroidectomy ± block dissection in papillary carcinoma, medullary carcinoma and malignant lymphoma; after hemithyroidectomy in follicular carcinoma). However, T_4 is required as replacement therapy and careful observation for toxicity is needed. Radiotherapy, especially ^{131}I therapy, is indicated in lethal anaplastic carcinoma, for postoperative treatment of residual malignant tissues and in multiple secondaries (especially bone metastases of follicular carcinoma).

IMMUNOTHERAPY

The high incidence of cancers in kidney transplants and immune-deficient states together with the rare phenomenon of spontaneous tumour regression indicate the value of immune defences. Tumours differ antigenically from their host – this antigen difference is evident from host ability for allogenic inhibition (tumour cells lacking antigen will not grow when they are in the company of normal cells) and immunological surveillance to restrain tumour growth. Host immunoglobulins act either as:
- An agent enhancing tumour growth.
- Unblocking antibodies that reverse the enhancement (see above).
- Beneficial cytotoxics that activate the complement system. Cell-mediated immunity against a specific tumour antigen (Type IV) as well as antibody-dependent cell-mediated (killer) cytotoxicity) (Type VI) can be demonstrated in cancer patients.

Clinical uses

Immunotherapy in humans is capable of destroying only very small quantities of malignant cells in subclinical forms, usually after the completion of other therapies. It is either specific or non-specific.

Specific

Stimulation of the host immune exaggerated response can be:
- Active; autologous tumour, e.g. patient's own tumour cells irradiated and reinjected.
- Adoptive: e.g. transfusion of donor-sensitised or immunised cytotoxic cells as well as transfer factor.
- Passive: use of antiserum specific to a particular antigen, e.g. antilymphocyte serum in leukaemia.

Non-specific

To stimulate general immune mechanisms by injecting BCG into melanoma nodules (leads to regression) or intrapleural injection of BCG in pneumonectomy (for lung cancer). *Corynebacterium parvum* and levamisol are other boosting agents.

RETINOIDS

Non-toxic chemical modifications of preformed vitamin A (alcohol retinol). Vitamin A deficiency results in squamous metaplasia which can be converted after vitamin replenishment to actively secreting columnar epithelium; therefore, retinoids prevent squamous metaplasia and their role in differentiation may be used in cancer prevention and preneoplastic conditions. (Vitamin A is inferior to retinoids as it may cause hepatic toxicity.) Clinical regression is noticed in actinic keratosis, basal cell carcinoma and malignant melanoma after topical therapy. Specific retinoid cytoplasmic receptors as well as immunostimulation may explain their mode of action. Further clinical studies are needed.

INTERFERON

Interferon (IF) is a protein which interferes with viral infection. If the inducing agent is a virus or double-stranded inducer it is called Type 1 IF. Type 11 IF is produced if the immunocompetent cells are stimulated by unrelated substances. IF has three actions:
- Binds to a surface receptor in the target cell and sets in motion a series of secondary messengers culminating in a change in the cell's general metabolic state (such changes inhibit virus replication using the genetic machinery of the host cell).
- Complex inhibitory effect on cell growth and division.
- Profound effect on the immune system (acting as a lymphocyte hormone).

According to heterogeneity, there are three families of IF: α (predominantly produced by leucocytes), β (produced by fibroblasts) γ (produced by antigen- or mitogen-stimulated lymphocytes). Including subtypes there is a total of 14 different molecular species of IFs. Clinically the use of IF in myeloma, breast cancer and non-Hodgkin's lymphoma results in objective regression of these tumours. It can cause some side-effects (dose-related) including anorexia, weight loss and central nervous system toxicity (metabolic encephalopathy). Other tumours, such as melanoma, renal cell carcinoma, lung cancer and Kaposi's sarcoma, respond to IF at a low rate (less than 20%). This anticancer potential of IF could possibly be utilised in adjuvant therapy in the early stages of solid tumours as well as in advanced disease.

SUPPORTIVE THERAPY

Consists of non-specific symptomatic measures to control the primary complications of cancer (e.g. cachexia, dysphagia, infection) or to counteract the side-effects of anticancer treatment (e.g. bleeding, infection). Includes nutrition (enteral or parenteral), blood transfusion, antibiotics, analgesics and terminal care measures.

1.39 Tumour Markers and Cancer Screening in Surgery

TUMOUR MARKERS

These are products of the metobolic activity of tumours and are either tumour-derived or tumour-associated, although not necessarily tumour-specific. They may be secreted (into blood, urine or other body fluids) or expressed (at the cell surface) in quantities larger than those in normal tissue. Their concentrations in body fluids are measured by radioimmunoassay or detected on the cell surface (in paraffin sections, smears or fresh biopsy tissue). They include (with their typical tumour):

Hormones with their subunits

ACTH and related MSH	(bronchogenic carcinoma)
ADH	(bronchogenic carcinoma)
Hypothalamic releasing factors	(bronchogenic carcinoma)
PTH	(bronchogenic carcinoma)
Calcitonin	(bronchogenic and breast carcinoma)
Prostaglandins	(colon and breast carcinoma)
HCG	(chorion carcinoma and teratoma)

Notice that these hormones are ectopic (i.e. their production is inappropriate to the tissue of origin of the tumour). Eutopic hormones (i.e. appropriate to the tissue of origin of the tumour) are also markers, e.g. calcitonin in medullary thyroid carcinoma, catecholamines and urinary vanillylmandelic acid in phaeochromocytoma, and urinary homovanillic acid in neuroblastoma.

Oncofetal products and antigens

CEA (carcinoembryonic antigen)	(gastrointestinal tract carcinoma) (Table 1.39.1)
AFP (α-feto protein)	(hepatoma and teratoma) (Table 1.39.1)
Ferritin	(many)
Cancer basic protein	(all)
Pregnancy associated proteins	(breast and teratoma)
Placental type enzymes	(many)

Enzymes and isoenzymes

Prolyl hydroxylase	(hepatoma and breast)
Sialyl transferase	(many)
Prostatic acid phosphatase	

Table 1.39.1 Non-specific rise of AFP and CEA in various conditions in order of frequency

AFP	CEA
Neoplastic	
Liver	Colon and rectum
Biliary tract	Pancreas
Pancreas	Liver
Stomach	Bronchus
Colon and rectum	Breast
Lung	Uterus
Malignant melanoma	Ovary
Non-neoplastic	
Viral hepatitis	Ulcerative colitis
Alcoholic cirrhosis	Alcoholic liver disease
Chronic active hepatitis	Chronic bronchitis and emphysema
Ulcerative colitis	Fibroadenosis
Crohn's disease	

Macromolecules

  Paraproteins (monoclonal immunoglobulins
    with urinary light chain Bence–Jones
    protein)   (myeloma)
  Milk protein   (breast)
  Polyamines   (many)
  Nucleosides   (many)
  Other tumour-associated proteins (acute
    phase reactive proteins and urinary
    hydroxyproline)

Hormone receptors   (breast carcinoma)

? Hormonally induced cancer-associated phenomena (see Table 1.39.2)

Clinically useful markers

Those suitable for routine management and general screening are very limited. They include the following.

HCG

Produced by placenta (reaching maximum concentration in the eighth gestational week) and abnormal trophoblastic tissue. It is composed of α-non-specific and β-specific subunits. It increases in chorion carcinoma and can detect a tumour mass of 1 mg; it is therefore used as a screening test in all cases of hydatidiform mole after uterine evacuation to judge the progress, to monitor chemotherapy and to detect early metastases. β-HCG (above 10 i.u./l) is found in 50% of testicular teratomas and in few pure seminomas. False high levels may occur after orchidectomy and hypogonadism owing to high LH (luteinsing hormone) (identical to α-HCG subunit), and retesting after testosterone administration is therefore needed. HCG also increases in carcinoma of the pancreas, stomach and bronchus.

AFP

Normal range 1–16 μ/l in adults. This is a protein synthesised by yolk sac, liver and gastrointestinal tract and is the major serum protein of the fetus. Levels above 40 μg/l are found in 60% of teratomas and although high levels of AFP are non-specific (see Table 1.39.1), its assay in conjunction with β-HCG gives positive results in 75–95% of testicular teratomas and both levels are crucial in the subsequent management.

Staging   Preorchidectomy high marker levels that fall to normal postoperatively suggest Stage I while persistently high levels after orchidectomy suggest undetected Stage II (retroperitoneal lymph node) or Stage III (supradiaphragmatic node involvement). Slow falls in AFP levels may indicate a residual AFP-producing tumour.

Assessing prognosis   Levels of HCG $< 5 \times 10^4$ i.u./l and AFP < 500 μg/l are associated with 10% mortality whereas levels above 1×10^5 i.u./l and 1 mg/l respectively carry a mortality in excess of 40% (the marker level is proportional to the bulk of metastatic teratoma).

Monitoring therapy   Eighty per cent of metastatic teratomas undergo remission on combined chemotherapy, the duration of which is judged by assay of markers (if they become normal, there is no need for maintenance therapy). If marker levels fall to normal but there is static residual disease (evident on chest X-ray or CAT scan) biopsy of the residual lesions will be consistent with differentiated teratoma or necrotic tissue (further therapy is not indicated). On the other hand advancing disease with static marker levels indicates non-marker-producing tumour cells and change of therapy is indicated.

CEA

A complex glycoprotein synthesised by tumour cells and by normal colonic epithelium. It is carried on the cell surface membrane and normally shed with faeces. In cancer it is shed into surrounding serum and serous fluids. Although raised levels are non-specific (see Table 1.39.1), the serum levels detected in 65% of all colorectal cancers depend on:

- Tumour stage: CEA is raised in 30% of patients with Duke's Stage A tumour and in 90% of those with hepatic metastases.
- Tumour site: CEA levels are low or absent in right colonic and rectal tumours and higher in left colonic, particularly sigmoid cancer.
- Degree of differentiation.
- Functional hepatic status.

CEA therefore has no role in screening among the normal population. However, it is used as a prognostic indicator (very high preoperative levels suggest a poor prognosis) and as an indicator for second-look surgery for cure in early colonic recurrence. In monitoring therapy, falling CEA levels suggest a response to chemotherapy or radiotherapy.

Hormone receptors

Hormones are defined as chemical mediators secreted by cells to affect 'target cells' at a distance, e.g. most hormones (endocrine effect); to stimulate nearby cells to secrete other hormones, e.g. glucagon from α-cells of the pancreas stimulating β-cells to secrete insulin (paracrine effect); or to act as neurotransmitters (neurocrine effect). Each hormone binds a protein situated on the cell membrane or within the cell (receptor) with a high affinity and specificity. There are two types of receptor mechanism.

Hormone-receptor complex

Situated at the cell membrane, this complex activates adenyl cyclase enzyme, leading to the production of adenosine monophosphate (AMP) as a second messenger which in turn stimulates intracellular metabolic events. Such a mechanism can be seen in catecholamines and peptide hormones, i.e. glucagon, LH, FSH, ACTH, while protein hormones, i.e. growth hormone, insulin and prolactin, activate membrane receptors by production of a second messenger other than AMP (probably a peptide).

Steroid hormones

These diffuse through the cell membrane to bind to a specific cytoplasmic receptor protein which then undergoes a change in conformation and translocates to the cell nucleus, acting on the genome to induce transcription (RNA synthesis). Some target cells possess more than one receptor type, e.g. thyroid hormone acts via multiple receptor sites in the cell membrane, on the mitochondria, within the nucleus and in cytoplasm. The receptor assay, e.g. oestrogen receptor, is done by preparation of a particulate fraction from the tissue, incubation with radioactive hormone and separation of the hormone portion bound to the receptor from the free portion; the ratio of these two components is determined by scintillation counting. Receptor assays have considerable clinical impact:

- Development of hormone inhibitors that compete with the natural hormone for binding to receptor sites leading to no response, e.g. anti-androgen (cyproterone) used in prostatic carcinoma as well as in sexual offenders, antioestrogen (tamoxifen) used in breast cancer treatment, histamine H_2 receptor blockers (cimetidine), β-adrenergic receptor blocker (atenolol).
- Testicular feminisation syndrome (male genotypically but female phenotypically) represents end organ insensitivity and/or abnormal androgen receptors.

Oestrogen receptors in breast cancer

A method of predicting hormonal sensitivity of breast cancer

About 32% of breast cancers have no detectable or significant receptor activity and must be spared ineffective endocrine therapy (better treated by cytotoxic therapy). The remaining two-thirds, mainly in postmenopausal patients, must be considered for endocrine therapy with a 50% chance of response. Tumours with high receptor levels are more likely to respond. As samples of metastatic disease for assay may be difficult to obtain, receptor analysis should be an essential investigation in all primary breast cancers (since quantitative differences in the receptor concentration in primary cancers and their later metastases will not disturb the differentiation between receptor-positive and receptor-negative tumours).

Androgen and progesterone receptors have also been discovered. The latter are present in a proportion of oestrogen receptor-positive tumours which respond to hormonal treatment better than those possessing oestrogen receptors alone (70% response versus 25% respectively). Progesterone receptors are only rarely found in tumours without oestrogen receptor activity.

Tamoxifen A potent oestrogen receptor-blocking drug which competes for binding to cytoplasmic receptor sites yielding no response. It is now the initial treatment of choice for advanced breast cancer with oestrogen receptor activity. Tamoxifen has a similar efficacy to high dose oestrogen therapy but *lacks its side-effects*; therefore, it is also the treatment of choice in those with unknown receptor status and is a suitable treatment for asymptomatic early disease (since in the majority of patients, breast cancer is already a systemic disease at the time of presentation, necessitating systemic as well as local therapy). Adjuvant tamoxifen with chemotherapy after mastectomy is therefore more effective in delaying recurrence than chemotherapy alone.

Provide a prognostic guide Recurrence is less and survival rates are better in receptor-positive cancers than in receptor-negative cancers. Oestrogen receptor activity is a sign of a biologically favourable tumour since there is a higher proportion of receptor-positive tumours in patients with well-differentiated (Grade I or II) tumours, those without axillary lymph node involvement and those in whom focal elastosis is prominent.

? Hormonally induced cancer-associated phenomena

Hypercalcaemia

Ectopic parathormone explains a few cases but osteolytic metastases are often associated with biochemical changes not consistent with the hyperparathyroid state. Breast cancers have been found to release prostaglandins E and F which have the ability to mobilise bone calcium, a property that is inhibited by the addition of aspirin or indomethacin. These macromolecular factors (prostaglandins) can explain hypercalcaemia and can have prognostic implications. The cell source is unknown.

Cachexia

The commonest cause of cancer death. The progressive weight loss, anorexia, malabsorption and wasteful pattern of tumour metabolism have a complex underlying cause. Toxohormone and cytotoxic polypeptides have been postulated but remain questionable.

Gastrointestinal changes

The recent recognition of gastrointestinal tract hormones (Table 1.39.2) has helped significantly to explain some of the tumour manifestations. These hormones may be produced ectopically or released by endocrine tumours.

Table 1.39.2 Circulating alimentary hormones

Hormone	Location	Physiological role	Pathology
Gastrin	Antrum	Stimulates acid secretion. Maintains mucosal growth. Causes gastric motor activity	High in atrophic gastritis and achlorhydria. Fasting gastrin level is normal in duodenal ulcer while high in gastrinoma in Zollinger–Ellison syndrome
Secretin	Duodenum	Stimulates pancreatic bicarbonate	Failure of secretion leads to faulty pancreatic bicarbonate mechanism for neutralising acid in duodenal ulcer
Cholecystokinin	Duodenum and jejunum	Stimulates gall bladder contraction Stimulates pancreatic enzyme secretion	High in chronic pancreatitis
Motilin	Jejunum	Causes upper alimentary motor activity	–
Glucose-dependent insulin-releasing hormone (GIP)	Jejunum	Stimulates insulin release	–
Neurotensin	Ileum	Unknown (hypotensive)	High in dumping syndrome (in partial gastrectomy or vagotomy)
Enteroglucagon	Ileum and colon	Maintains mucosal growth. Slows intestinal transit	High after bowel resection but low in massive resection
Pancreatic polypeptide	Pancreas	Anticholecystokinin	High in minor or acute pancreatitis, low in severe pancreatitis and steatorrhoea

VIPomas

Also known as the Verner–Morrison or WDHA syndrome = watery diarrhoea, hypokalaemia and achlorhydria. Occur in non-B-islet cell tumours of the pancreas and 15% of neural childhood tumours (ganglioneuroblastomas). A vasoactive intestinal peptide (VIP) (made up of two amino acids related to the gastrointestinal peptide group) is responsible for this syndrome which may also include diabetes mellitus, hypercalcaemia, tetany and flushing. Death occurs from renal failure. This syndrome should be distinguished from the Zollinger–Ellison syndrome (gastrin-producing islet cell tumour associated with refractory peptic ulceration). Diagnosis may be delayed, leading to metastasis; streptozotocin (cytotoxic) is effective in producing prolonged remission. The diarrhoea may be controlled with high-dose steroids. Early diagnosis is based on suspicion in any case of profuse diarrhoea and hypokalaemia in which case VIP estimation should be done. VIP is usually grossly high and treatment by localised pancreatic resection may be curative. VIP may be normal (pseudo-Verner–Morrison syndrome) and total pancreatectomy may be the only method of treatment to remove the responsible product (other than VIP).

CANCER SCREENING

The aim is to detect and treat the disease in the population at an early curable stage in order to reduce cancer mortality.

Advantages
- Improved prognosis.
- Less radical curative treatment.

- Reassurance for those with negative test results.
- Resource savings from less radical treatment.

Disadvantages
- Longer morbidity for those with unaltered prognosis.
- Overtreatment of borderline abnormalities.
- False reassurance for those with false negative results.
- Anxiety and morbidity for those with false positive results.
- Cooperation from population to accept screening and carry out repeated tests cannot be relied on.
- Hazards of screening test.
- Resource costs from screening, diagnostic investigations and overtreatment.

In the absence of effective methods of primary prevention or effective treatment of symptomatic tumours, screening offers the best hope of controlling the mortality from some cancers. Health education promoting self-examination is also a form of screening, e.g. breast cancer, skin melanoma and testicular cancer. Medical follow-up, e.g. hydatidiform mole by HCG assay for chorion epithelioma is another form of screening.

The *sensitivity* of a test is the number of positive tests per 100 patients with the disease. The *specificity* of the test is the number of negative tests per 100 patients who do not have the disease.

Mass screening tests

Uterine cervix

Cytology with 80% sensitivity and very high specificity. It has the disadvantage of overtreatment of borderline abnormalities. Colposcopic biopsy and laser excision of affected epithelium may reduce this disadvantage. The age and frequency of screening is controversial. Five-yearly repeats may miss up to 40% of invasive cancer.

Stomach

Double-contrast barium meal detects early gastric carcinoma. It carries a radiation hazard and is very non-specific with almost 25% of screened individuals requiring further investigation involving fluoroscopy, cytology and endoscopy. Mortality has been reduced by 20% since the test was introduced but the natural history of this disease is ill understood and it is argued that both incidence and mortality from gastric cancer were falling already.

Breast

This is the only cancer in which screening reduces the mortality rate (proven in randomised controlled trial). Mammography (by a single oblique view) is highly sensitive and specific with low radiation dose and low cost; 20–40% of detected cancers are preinvasive. Breast self-examination needs greater exposure in the general population. Although widely advocated, its sensitivity, specificity and effectiveness in reducing mortality require further research.

CA 15–3 is a mucin marker (that employs two monoclonal antibodies), but lacks specificity and sensitivity for screening. An elevated level is found in 55–100% of advanced breast cancers, in only 10–46% of early breast cancers, and in 2–20% of cases benign breast disease. An elevated pretreatment level is associated with poor prognosis, and a raised post-treatment level may indicate recurrence.

Lung

The multifocal, often bilateral, distribution of lung cancers along with their rapid growth rate make attempts to control mortality by screening disappointing. Chest X-ray and sputum cytology combined and repeated at 4-monthly intervals detect nearly 90% of cases especially in high-risk groups. Neither is sufficiently sensitive on its own: X-rays lack specificity whereas with cytology localisation of lesions is difficult. Health education aimed at primary prevention and measures to curtail cigarette smoking seem much more profitable means of control.

Colorectal cancer

In the United Kingdom there are 31 000 new cases of colorectal cancer each year and nearly 20 000 deaths, the second most common cause of all deaths from cancer in the UK (the four common killing cancers in the UK are bronchogenic carcinoma, colorectal carcinoma, breast carcinoma and gastric carcinoma, in this order). Early diagnosis would significantly improve survival rates as many cases are diagnosed at a late stage when curative treatment is not possible.

Faecal occult blood tests have a low sensitivity and only moderate levels of uptake among screened population. Detecting and removing premalignant adenomas by flexible sigmoidoscopy could be more effective than detecting early localised asymptomatic cancers in reducing deaths from colorectal cancer (see below).

Most (85–90%) colorectal cancers are sporadic (not hereditary). *High-risk groups* include:
- Familial group: the risk of colorectal cancer in a first-degree relative of an affected person is 2–3 times the risk in the general population with an early age of onset.
- Familial adenomatous polyposis (responsible gene on chromosome 5) accounts for 1% of colorectal cancer.
- Hereditary non-polyposis colorectal cancer whether site-specific colon cancer (type a) or colonic and extracolonic endometrial, ovarian, genitourinary cancers (type b) have at least three relatives in two generations with colorectal cancers with one of the relatives having cancer under the age of 50 (gene predisposing to colorectal cancer is hMSH2, one of the DNA repair genes).
- There is an increased risk in longstanding ulcerative colitis and to lesser extent in Crohn's disease. Also patients who have had colon cancer in the past are at higher risk of developing additional colorectal cancers.

Most colorectal cancers, however, arise in people who have no known predisposing risk factors. In future most high-risk groups may be identified by genetic markers, but selective screening of high-risk groups is unlikely to have a major impact on the overall incidence or mortality.

Colorectal cancer screening tests

In the UK screening has not been recommended on a population basis. The American Cancer Society recommends an:
- annual digital rectal examination for people over 40;
- annual faecal occult blood test for people over 50;
- sigmoidoscopy (preferably flexible) every 3–5 years in people over 60.

Digital rectal examination   Easy to perform, but of limited value for screening as only a small proportion of colorectal cancers are within the range of an examining finger.

Faecal occult blood tests   Tests are based on the assumption that cancers bleed and the small amount of blood lost in stool may be detected chemically or immunologically. Haemoccult is the commonest (do-it-yourself) test, in which the person being screened places a small stool sample on a guaiac impregnated filter paper card and sends it off to be tested in the laboratory. The test is quick, cheap and easy with reasonable (but not high) levels of acceptability to the population (distaste for taking faecal sample). Its main disadvantages are:
- Low sensitivity (40% of cancers and 80% of adenomas may be missed by a single screen). It is also a poor marker because most adenomas do not bleed and not all tumours bleed. Because haemoglobin is degraded as it passes via the GIT, these tests are also less sensitive for upper GIT bleeding lesions than for lower lesions. Furthermore, they are less sensitive for rectal lesions than for higher left-sided lesions, possibly because there has been less opportunity for blood to be diffused widely through the whole stool.
- Many tumours bleed only at a late stage in their natural history resulting in a short diagnostic time. Also, blood loss

from colorectal cancers is not constant but intermittent; therefore the test must be performed on 3–6 successive stool specimens.

● Sensitivity is inversely related to the dryness of the stool sample when tested; therefore rehydration (with a drop of water) is recommended. Although this improves sensitivity, it results in a four-fold increase in positive true and false results leading to many unnecessary interventions and colonoscopies; red meat and vegetables containing peroxidase such as tomatoes may all give false positive results and therefore dietary restriction for 3 days before the test is sometimes recommended. In the Minnesota randomised trial of faecal occult blood testing, there was 33% reduction in mortality from colorectal cancer for an annually screened population, but there was no significant reduction in mortality for those screened every 2 years; the rate of false positive results was unduly high (38% of those screened annually and 28% of those screened every 2 years had at least one colonoscopy) with unnecessary invasive intervention and considerable anxiety and greatly increased workload and costs. The large number of colonoscopies carried out in the Minnesota study make it difficult to determine whether the reduction in mortality can be attributed to faecal occult blood testing or to the use of colonoscopy.

Sigmoidoscopy Whereas faecal occult blood tests aim at detecting asymptomatic cancers, most distal colorectal cancers arise as benign adenomas with a slow transition time to malignancy of 10–35 years. Because of this long natural history, prevention of progression to cancer by detection and removal of premalignant adenomas may be a more effective method for reducing deaths from colorectal cancer than detection of early localised asymptomatic cancers. It is a more expensive and invasive initial test than faecal occult blood tests, but it has two distinct advantages:
– it is highly sensitive for lesions as small as 5 mm, so neoplasia is detectable at an early stage;
– lesions can be removed endoscopically at the time of screening in most cases, so the screening procedure can be both diagnostic and therapeutic.

Furthermore, although cancer in the proximal colon cannot be detected directly by sigmoidoscopy, about 30% of those with proximal colon cancers will have an index lesion within the reach of the flexible sigmoidoscope. Features of distal adenomas as markers of *high risk* of developing proximal colon cancer include:
● > 3 adenomas in number
● > 5 hyperplastic adenomas in sigmoid colon
● > 1 cm in size
● villous or tubulovillous (tubular is associated with low risk)
● severe or malignant dysplasia (mild or moderate dysplasia is associated with low risk)

Therefore, not all patients with adenomas are at high risk, but those with high risk distal adenomas are at a four-fold increased risk. About 90% of the colon cancers which developed during follow-up occurred in this high-risk group which comprises 3–5% of the population; selected colonoscopic surveillance of those (3–5%) with high risk distal adenomas detected at screening should thus enable the prevention of at least some proximal colon cancers, with 25% reduction in mortality in those with proximal colon cancer.

The flexible sigmoidoscope (65 cm) is now recommended for screening rather than the rigid sigmoidoscope. It is preferred by patients and may be passed higher into the colon than the rigid sigmoidoscope; it can negotiate the junction of the sigmoid and descending colon (below which over 60% of colorectal cancers are located). Bowel preparation is required, but actual examination takes only 4–8 minutes, depending on the need to undertake biopsy or polypectomy. Screening with flexible sigmoidoscopy could lead to a reduction of at least 30% in mortality from colorectal cancer. If all adenomas detected at sigmoidoscopy are completely removed, the risk of rectal cancer is rendered low for many years (preventing at least 85% of rectal cancers from developing as shown in a retrospective study from St Mark's Hospital).

The Imperial Cancer Research Fund has made a strong case for a randomised controlled trial of flexible sigmoidoscopy; it has been proposed that screening by a single flexible sigmoidoscopy towards the end of the sixth decade, with appropriate colonoscopic surveillance for those found to have high risk adenomas (3–5%), could, if applied nationally, prevent about 5500 cases of colorectal cancer and 3500 deaths in the UK each year.

Bladder

Workers exposed to carcinogenic chemicals in their occupation (e.g. rubber and dye industry) may be screened by urinary cytology at 6-monthly intervals. Its sensitivity, specificity and effectiveness need to be evaluated.

Prostatic cancer

Prostatic specific antigen (PSA) is a widely accepted tumour marker in prostatic cancer. PSA is a glycoprotein secreted exclusively by prostatic epithelial cells and is organ-specific.
● Elevated PSA (> 4 ng/ml) occurs in 65% of localised prostatic cancer and in 30–50% of benign prostatic hypertrophy.
● Serial PSA changes are more useful than a single PSA measurement. Combined PSA, rectal examination and prostatic ultrasound are the best method of detection of early prostatic cancer.
● High pretreatment PSA correlates with prostatic volume and degree of differentiation and is therefore associated with poor prognosis. PSA level falls following surgery, radiotherapy or endocrine therapy.
● Serial rise in PSA indicates prostatic cancer recurrence and can precede the clinical recurrence.

Thyroid

First-degree relatives of patients with medullary thyroid carcinoma can be screened by measuring calcitonin levels (20% of these carcinomas have a familial history with an autosomal dominant inheritance).

QED clinics

QED clinics

Quick Early Diagnosis (QED) aims to detect cancer at an early stage through providing a rapid diagnostic service for suspected patients referred directly through a phone call by the general practitioner or via a computer link with the QED Clinic.

Each day, four mini-clinics are set and each is devoted to one question, e.g. Does this patient have a cancer in the stomach? For 2 hours, four endoscopy rooms (in one mini-clinic) will work simultaneously to investigate up to 30 worried patients. By the end of 2 hours, 29 patients will be reassured and 1 lucky patient with early cancer will have been detected in order to be treated with hope of cure. For the remainder of the day, the unit will concentrate on other sites, e.g. bladder, bowel and breast, in the other three mini-clinics.

About one-third of the population die from cancer, and QED clinics are a quick and efficient way to solve one problem at a time and thus cope with the number of referred patients.

1.40 Skin Markers of Internal Cancers

Skin markers of internal cancer are manifold; they include the following.

Skin metastases

Metastases arise by direct invasion from underlying structures, extension via lymphatics, embolisation through lymphatics and blood vessels, and accidental implantation at surgery.

- Carcinomas most frequently associated with cutaneous metastases originate in breast, stomach, lung, uterus, kidney, ovary, colon and urinary bladder (in this order). Skin metastases carry extremely poor prognosis; the patient often dies within 3–6 months.
- Certain areas of skin are predisposed to metastases. Scalp is a favourite site for metastases from breast, lung and genitourinary system; chest wall from breast carcinoma; abdominal wall, especially around umbilicus, in cancer of the stomach and rest of GIT; and lower abdominal wall and external genitalia from cancers of genitourinary system. Hypernephroma and thyroid carcinoma which metastasise to bone can produce pulsating tumour mass with a bruit detectable through the overlying skin. Implantation of tumour cells in surgical scars is not uncommon.
- Skin metastases may rarely be the first indication of internal malignancy. Histological examination of skin metastasis may indicate the site of the primary tumour; presence of mucin in a glandular tumour suggests GIT origin. Hypernephroma, thyroid carcinoma, hepatoma and seminoma may retain their characteristic appearance in skin metastases.
- In a woman, chest wall metastasis usually indicates breast cancer, while cancer en cuirasse is commonly associated with breast cancer and less commonly from stomach, kidney and lung. Inflammatory carcinoma of skin (usually inguino – thigh flexure) which is sharply marginated and slightly elevated is spectacular; it is commonly associated with breast carcinoma, but may originate from uterus or lung.
- Metastatic carcinoma to liver may produce stigmata associated with cirrhosis: palmar erythema, spider naevi and jaundice. Extensive invasion of mediastinum by tumour produces the superior vena caval syndrome: oedema of the face, conjunctivae and neck associated with a prominently distended venous pattern on the neck, chest and upper extremities.
- Paget's disease of the unilateral nipple and areola is a well-known indicator of underlying breast carcinoma.
- Extramammary (anogenital) Paget's disease is a skin marker of internal malignancy, such as underlying apocrine sweat gland carcinoma and rectal carcinoma; carcinoma of the urethra, prostate, Bartholin's glands and breast have also been reported.

Skin syndromes produced by humoral secretions from non-endocrine tumours

Non-endocrine neoplasms can secrete substances that mimic endocrine disease and produce other distinctive syndromes. The unifying concept to explain various ectopic humoral syndromes has as its cornerstone the APUD cell (high contents of Amino Precursor Uptake Decarboxylases).

The two most commonly recognised disorders are:

- Ectopic ACTH-producing syndrome producing Cushing's syndrome with hyperpigmentation, profound proximal muscle weakness, or myasthenia gravis-like syndrome, and gynaecomastia. The primary is usually a lung cancer. Patients usually die within several weeks after diagnosis of adrenocortical hyperactivity.
- Carcinoid syndrome associated with bronchial adenoma releasing serotonin (5-hydroxytryptamine) and occasionally with ileo-appendicular carcinoid tumours.

Other apudomas include insulinoma, glucagonoma, gastrinoma (Zollinger–Ellison syndrome), calcitoninoma, vipoma (watery diarrhoea, hypokalaemia, and achlorhydria – Verner–Morrison syndrome), secretinoma, phaeochromocytoma, chemodectoma, bronchial adenoma and oat-cell lung carcinoma. Melanoma is a non-humoral-secreting apudoma. Also, familial autosomal dominant syndromes of multiple endocrine neoplasms (MEN), whether MEN type I (tumours of pituitary/pancreas/parathyroid/adrenal cortex); MEN type II, which is also called Sipple syndrome (tumours of thyroid C cell-medullary carcinoma/adrenal medullary phaeochromocytoma/parathyroid adenoma); or MEN type III, which is also called multiple mucosal neuromas (MMN), featuring medullary thyroid carcinoma, phaeochromocytoma in association with a marfanoid habitus and multiple mucosal neuromas with characteristic facies (gross features of thickened everted bumpy lips and thickened slightly everted eyelids and superficial neuromas on tongue). In MEN types I and II, there is development of medullary thyroid carcinoma and calcitonin must be measured in high-risk patients before metastases occur. Total thyroidectomy is indicated because cancers are multifocal in origin; screening of family members for elevated plasma calcitonin is mandatory.

Neurofibromatosis (Von Recklinghausen's disease) is a member of the apudomas too; multiple Schwann cell tumours develop in association with cafe-au-lait spots and sometimes phaeochromocytoma.

Proliferative and inflammatory dermatoses associated with internal cancer

Generalised *pruritus* or *itching* is an uncommon sign of cancer, but frequently accompanies lymphomas, especially Hodgkin's lymphoma, lymphatic leukaemia and mycosis fungoides. Pruritus occurring with cancer is not as severe, generalised or intolerable as it is with lymphoma.

Acanthosis nigricans is probably the most well-known cutaneous marker of internal malignancy. However, it occurs in conditions unrelated to neoplasia, such as congenital or familial lesion, in association with puberty (juvenile, benign and pseudoacanthosis nigricans), endocrine disease and excessive weight gain and with a number of congenital anomalies. Acanthosis nigricans chiefly affects the flexures: neck, axillae, groin, and antecubital fossae; with extensive involvement, lesions can also be found on the areola, around the umbilicus, and in the perineal area. Hyperkeratosis of palms and skin over elbows, knees and interphalangeal joints can occur as well; the skin is thrown into folds. It is associated with adult cancers, mainly abdominal (stomach in 60% of cases, but also uterus, liver, oesophagus, pancreas, prostate, ovary, kidney, colon and rectum). Almost all cancers accompanying this dermatosis have been adenocarcinomas. Tumours associated with acanthosis nigricans are highly malignant, and the average survival after the cancer is discovered or resected is 12 months. In the majority of adults with obesity and acanthosis nigricans (since childhood) there may be an endocrine basis, such as Cushing's disease. Special concern must be given to non-obese adults who develop acanthosis nigricans, for they are the ones in whom a malignancy is almost always present. Differential diagnosis of acanthosis nigricans includes erythrasma (produced by Corynebacteria with hyperpigmentation in axillae and groin), and Addison's disease.

Dermatomyositis may antedate the development of lung, GIT or breast cancer; it is occasionally associated with lymphoma and melanoma. The interval between the onset of dermatomyositis and discovery of cancer may be long as 3–8 years.

Musculoskeletal disorders associated with cancer are: clubbing, hypertrophic osteoarthropathy, pachydermoperiostosis, polyarthritis simulating rheumatoid arthritis, tenosynovitis and fibrositis. Clubbing of fingers and toes is a well-known manifestation of bronchogenic carcinoma, mesothelioma, and metastatic cancer to the thorax.

Migratory superficial *thrombophlebitis* and multiple deep venous *thrombosis* can be associated with carcinoma of the body and tail of the pancreas (observed by Armand Trousseau in 1862), and develop in the neck, chest, abdominal wall and limbs.

Defibrination syndrome, characterised by easy bruising, widespread purpura, and bleeding from multiple sites, may also be a feature of malignancy.

Blistering disease and dermatitis herpetiformis-like disease occurs in chorioncarcinoma, malignant ovarian tumours, uterine, prostate, bladder, rectum and breast cancers. Erythema multiforme, pemphigoid, erythema gyratum repens and urticaria can all occur with internal cancer.

Hyperkeratosis of palms and soles (*tylosis* or *keratoderma*), with wartlike or callous appearance which may be associated with painful fissures and hyperhidrosis, *Tylosis* is a marker of systemic disease, usually oesophageal carcinoma.

Exfoliative dermatitis is a relatively frequent manifestation of lymphoma, leukaemia and mycosis fungoides, but it is extremely uncommon as a marker of solid cancers.

Ichthyosis appearing *de novo* in adults is another relatively specific sign of lymphoma.

Syndromes indicative of systemic or organ-related carcinogenesis

Bowen's disease of the skin (epidermoid carcinoma in situ) is associated with eventual development of internal cancer.

Squamous cell carcinoma can develop in cutaneous scars resulting from third degree burns, lupus vulgaris, lupus erythematosus, dystrophic epidermolysis bullosa, from edges of chronic draining osteomyelitis sinuses and from chronic ulceration, especially on the legs.

Radiodermatitis of the hands, seen commonly in medical personnel and in certain women due to poor X-ray machine calibration and improper shielding, is a premalignant condition and basal cell tumours and squamous cell carcinomas may arise.

Xeroderma pigmentosum is an autosomal recessive disease with rapid development of ageing and neoplastic changes in the skin in response to sunlight, particularly the wavelength of ultraviolet light between 290 and 320 nm. Affected children develop erythema, freckling and increased pigmentation after their initial exposure to sunlight. Dryness, scaling, skin atrophy with fine telangiectasia soon follow. By 2–3 years many youngsters have senile skin and tumours: basal cell tumours, squamous cell carcinomas, haemangiomas, keratoacanthomas and malignant melanomas. Photophobia, keratitis and ectropions are common and responsible for corneal opacities.

Familial adenomatous polyposis (FAP) or colonic polyposis may present with extracolonic manifestations, such as Gardner's syndrome (cutaneous osteomas, fibromas and multiple large disfiguring sebaceous cysts).

Peutz–Jeghers syndrome, with freckle-like pigmentations on lips, nose, buccal mucosa, fingertips, under nails and anus, is associated with hamartomatous polyps of stomach, small intestine and colon.

In *Torre's syndrome* multiple carcinomas, primarily of the GIT, are associated with multiple sebaceous gland neoplasms, mainly on the trunk (not cysts).

Cowden's disease is a multiple hamartomatous syndrome linking musculocutaneous lesions (lichenoid or wart-like papules, keratosis punctata, multiple lipomas and cavernous haemangiomas) with later development of internal cancer.

1.41 Malignant Melanoma

The incidence of cutaneous malignant melanoma in white-skinned people is increasing on a world-wide basis. It is estimated that both the incidence and the mortality are doubling every 10 years. While malignant melanoma is a potentially curable disease in its early stage, it is fatal in the late disseminated stage:

Malignant melanoma arises *de novo* or in a pre-existing benign naevus. The benign melanotic hamartoma (or naevocellular naevus or mole) is derived from a neural crest and may be junctional, compound, intradermal or blue naevus. These naevi may be small or large, pedunculated, sessile or flat, with or without hair. They are benign and usually remain so, or they may undergo spontaneous regression, leaving a halo (or Sutton's naevus) representing an autoimmune phenomenon (which may also occur in malignant melanoma). However, 10–40% of benign naevi undergo malignant change and this should be suspected if there is an increase in size, a change in colour (whether darker, lighter or mottled), bleeding, ulceration, crusting, itching or the formation of satellite spots.

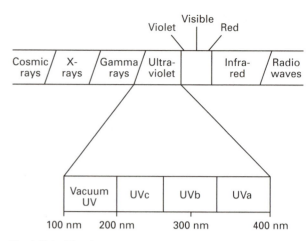

Fig. 1.41.1 The electromagnetic spectrum

Aetiology

- Exposure of fair-skinned people, particularly the Celts, to excessive sunlight. The ultraviolet irradiation causes nuclear damage and collagen disruption. The incidence of malignant melanoma is strongly influenced by the amount of ultraviolet light and duration of exposure.
- Familial or hereditary melanoma with 20% incidence of multiple lesions.
- Precancerous lesions (i.e. the giant bathing-trunk naevus) and in situ melanoma (i.e. conjunctival melanosis and lentigo maligna or Hutchinson's freckle).
- Trauma and hormonal changes (e.g. pregnancy) are doubtful.

Ultraviolet (UV) radiation obviously causes much greater skin injury than the more commonly recognised UV-induced skin cancer. In experimental animals (guinea-pigs), wound tensile strength was found to be significantly lower in irradiated than in control animals. Both UV and UV radiation compromised wound strength. Irradiation produced 'sunburn' cells, swollen vascular endothelial cells and perivascular haemorrhage in papillary dermis. UV radiation led to focal eosinophilic infiltration. Dermal collagen and elastic fibres were unaltered. Thus UV radiation impairs the reparative capacity of the skin through mechanisms that remain to be clarified. Changes caused by environmental levels of UV radiation suggest that tanning sunbeds be avoided and sunscreens and glasses that protect against UV radiation be used.

CLINICAL PATHOLOGICAL ASPECTS

Clinical classification and staging

There are four main clinical types:

Lentigo maligna malignant melanoma develops slowly at the site of a previous Hutchinson's melanotic freckle on the faces of elderly people. It is regarded as a preinvasive in situ melanoma with a relatively good prognosis.

Superficial spreading malignant melanoma represents a flat junctional activity anywhere on the skin with late dermal invasion and nodular transformation (the latter is associated with lymph node metastasis).

Acral lentiginous and mucous melanomas These variants have recently been described as arising on the soles and palms, and on mucosal surfaces respectively. It is characterised by melanocytic abnormalities of the adjacent epidermis or mucosa which is similar to that of lentigo maligna except that actinic damage is not seen. The prognosis is similar to that of superficial spreading melanoma.

Nodular malignant melanoma with early dermal invasion and lymph node metastasis. The prognosis is poor.

There are three clinical stages in the spread of malignant melanoma:

Stage I   No evidence of regional spread.

Stage II   Clinical involvement of lymph nodes by embolism or regional spread by lymphatic permeation producing local satellite nodules and/or 'intransit' deposits between the primary tumour and the regional lymph nodes. However, there is no evidence of distant spread.

Stage III Distant spread: bloodborne metastases are seen in lungs, liver, brain, bones and skin. Secondary black deposits may involve unusual sites, e.g. small intestine, heart and breasts, and may cause melanuria.

Prognostic factors in order of importance are:

1. Tumour thickness.
2. Infiltration level.
3. Presence of ulceration.
4. Mitotic activity.
5. Location.

Factors which on multivariate analysis do not appear to influence prognosis are: sex, age, histogenetic type of tumour, vascular invasion and lymphocytic infiltration.

Histological microtomal prognostic evaluation (or classification)

Tumour thickness (Breslow, 1970) Simple vertical measurement through the tumour centre is a reliable, accurate, reproducible objective and important determinant of the therapy and prognosis, since there is a close correlation between tumour thickness and prognosis. Tumours less than 0.75 mm are very unlikely to metastasise and rarely, if ever, recur if a margin of at least 2 mm clearance is achieved; thus excisional biopsy with 2 mm clearance is recommended generally for diagnosis and may be therapeutic if the tumour thickness is less than 0.75 mm.

Tumour infiltration or penetration level (Clark–McGovern level classification, 1976) Although important, this was proved to be highly subjective with up to 30% variation in the estimate of levels by different pathologists, and the system is replaced by the Breslow tumour thickness measurement. In the Clark–McGovern system (Fig. 1.41.2) the tumour is stated to be:

Level 1 (in situ malignant melanoma). Confined to basal epidermis.

Level 2 Invasion of the papillary dermis (subepidermal connective tissue).

Level 3 Invasion to the junction level between the papillary and reticular dermis.

Level 4 Invasion of the reticular dermis.

Level 5 Invasion of the subcutaneous tissues.

This system is well correlated with patient survival.

MANAGEMENT

Surgery remains the mainstay in Stages I and II. Radiotherapy has no place and chemotherapy is only considered in Stage III. The clinical-histological work-up consists of excision biopsy (with 2 mm clearance margin) to measure the tumour thickness. Incisional, needle and scrape biopsies are contraindicated owing to the risk of tumour spread. Incisional biopsy is now acceptable for very large lesions or where there is little spare skin, e.g. on the face, hands and feet. Shave biopsies should be avoided. For enlarged lymph nodes, fine-needle aspiration cytology is the initial investigation of choice. Surgical treatment follows in the form of adequate excision of the primary tumour, with or without lymph node block dissection. Troublesome metastatic lesions are occasionally removed.

Stage I

Wide excision (3–5 cm clearance) of skin and subcutaneous tissue down to deep fascia (rarely including deep fascia) with split skin graft taken from the unaffected limb is the ideal approach (since the incidence of local recurrence is very low). The exceptions are:

- Lesions less than 0.75 mm thick and invasion level II: treated by local excision and closure without grafting (same as excisional biopsy with 2 mm margin clearance).
- Malignant melanoma of the face: treated by wide excision and rotational flap.
- Subungual malignant melanoma: treated by amputation via the neck of the proximal phalanx (no need for complete disarticulation of the finger).
- Malignant melanoma of the choroid of the eye necessitates eyeball enucleation or removal.

Prophylactic lymph node block dissection is indicated in tumours within the territory of the lymphatic drainage (e.g. groin malignant melanoma) and for tumours of 1–5 mm thickness because of documented increase in 5 year survival. In tumours greater than 5 mm, the survival is so poor that node dissection may be postponed since blood-borne spread will probably appear before lymph nodes reveal evidence of recurrence. For these thick tumours node dissection represents a form of prophylactic palliative surgery for future troublesome locally fungating lesions. With the advent of lymphatic mapping (using blue dye and immunohistochemistry to identify regional nodes most likely to be involved in dissemination) and hand-held isotope neoprobe (to identify involved nodes), prophylactic node clearance cannot be justified because 20% of patients with

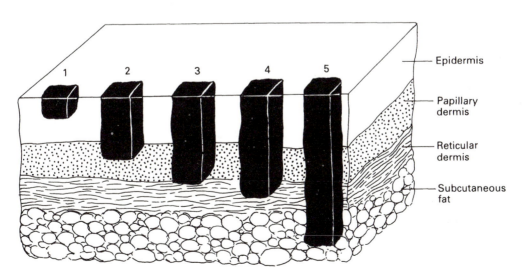

Fig. 1.41.2 Clark–McGovern levle of classification of malignant melanoma

apparent stage I disease have micrometastases in regional lymph nodes proved on lymphatic mapping and isotope neoprobe. Only selective node clearance is advisable now.

Stage II

- For 'in-transit' metastases, it is necessary to perform an in-continuity dissection and remove all potentially contaminated tissue between (and together with) the primary malignant melanoma and the draining lymph nodes, i.e. prophylactic and therapeutic dissection.
- Clinically palpable lymph nodes necessitate careful therapeutic lymph node block dissection (inadequate node-picking operations should be abandoned because of the risk of tumour spillage – local wound recurrence is almost invariably fatal). Such a radical clearance of inguinal lymph nodes (in leg malignant melanoma) or axillary lymph nodes (unilateral in arm malignant melanoma and bilateral in midline back malignant melanoma) is invariably followed by lymphoedema and requires elastic stockings. Axillary dissection must be more radical than that used in breast cancer.
- Theoretically, a central midline back malignant melanoma should be excised with combined bilateral axillary and bilateral inguinal lymph node block dissection. Practically however, in view of the high associated morbidity, some surgeons prefer to excise the melanoma alone and to monitor the patient, performing block dissection only in clinically palpable lymphodenopathy (staged operation).

Stage III

- Palliative surgery is often worthwhile as a debulking procedure and to remove the painful, ulcerated lesions.
- Chemotherapy either i.v. or intralesionally using dimethyl-triazinoimidazole-carboxamide (DTIC) in subcutaneous and pulmonary recurrences. Visceral metastases are difficult to treat.
- Isolated limb perfusion (ILP) with phenylalanine mustard (in limb recurrences), with or without hyperthermia, remains a useful treatment and is occasionally curative for localised metastatic disease (the treatment of Stage II in-transit metastases). While routine use of ILP in primary disease cannot be justified, ILP is very useful for recurrence of limb disease. Patients with recurrent melanoma on a limb should be referred to a centre where treatment options that include ILP and laser therapy are available. Cutaneous recurrence is a poor prognostic sign, but long-term control and survival can be achieved for some patients. While ILP does not change the overall survival, it can prolong the disease-free interval.
- Immunotherapy using BCG intralesionally.
- Heavy neutron radiotherapy is used for recurrences.

INCIDENCE

World-wide incidence of melanoma varies widely; the highest incidence is 35/100 000 in Queensland, Australia (1977). In the UK the incidence has almost doubled over 10 years 1986–1996.

Natural ultraviolet light irradiation in sunlight has three colours:

- wavelength UVa (320–400 nm) is innocuous and responsible for tanning;
- wavelength UVb (280–320 nm) is responsible for sunburn;
- wavelength UVc (200–280 nm) is absorbed by the ozone layer and is highly energetic and dangerous; it is responsible for skin cancer.

Nuclear bombs, or the use of chemical aerosols containing chloro-fluoro-carbon (CFC) refrigerators and air-conditioners, may result in breaks and holes and thus in removal of the protective ozone layer causing more penetration of UVc with more malignant melanoma. Thus the world-wide efforts to replace CFC with more 'ozone-friendly' products.

BIOLOGICAL IMPACT OF COSMIC CHANGES
(ultraviolet radiation, global warming and the ozone layer)

Man's health is greatly influenced by acquired environmental and cosmic changes. Within the cosmos (universe), a delicate balance exists between benefit and danger. The Earth is 4.5 billion years old, positioned within a solar system far from the centre of the Milky Way galaxy, and facing dangers many of which are natural to the cosmos; but others may prove to be of our own doing and avoidable if we can control our destructive proclivities. The Earth, for example, has two protective shields: the magnetic field (which we are presently unable to control), and the ozone layer (which we are in the process of destroying).

The magnetic field

Reversal of the magnetic field can explain one of Earth's great mysteries: the sudden collective death of dinosaurs 65 million years ago after having lived on Earth for 140 million years. Not only dinosaurs were affected; 70% of all animal species vanished and 50% of all the Earth's plants. Ordinarily, the Earth's magnetic field, (generated by the Earth's inner currents and the planet's rotation) coupled with our atmosphere are strong enough to protect the planet from radiation emanating from outer space. Reversal of the magnetic field can weaken this protective shield and can also make Earth more vulnerable to *strikes by meteors and comets* as well as *exposure to strong cosmic radiation*, which can pass through with disastrous effects on living beings. A particular source of radiation would be a nova flare-up (a dying star bursting suddenly into a nova), leaving a black hole and dust cloud behind. A *black hole* may result from a flare up and subsequent implosion and collapse of a dying star, to a state of density from which not even light can escape and which attracts and swallows all other matter within its area of attraction – gases, planetoids, planets, suns and, theoretically whole solar systems.

Furthermore, cosmic dust, dying stars, blasts of meteorites or comets, exploding bombs, seismic and volcanic disturbances may all contribute to *cosmic dust clouds* that cut down the warming effect of the sun, raising the possibility of a *New Ice Age*. Our planet, as part of our whole solar system, makes a round trip within dust-laden areas of the galaxy approximately every 200 million years. New Ice Age theory is posited on an ice increase in Antarctica (5 million square miles and 3 miles thick), the widening of the ice cap in the Arctic, cooling of the North Atlantic, the intensity and lengthening of winters during past decades, and the fact that glaciers in the northern hemisphere – retreating until 1940 – have began once more to advance, all culminating in a gloomy climatic outlook.

However, the theory of a 'new Ice Age' has more recently been superseded by the theory of *Global Warming* or the *Greenhouse Effect*. Currently the amount of radiation we receive from the sun is about one-third more than it was 4000 million years ago due to the entrapped temperature within the atmosphere owing to the carbone dioxide layer (though transparent to short-wave radiation, it absorbs long-wave radiation of more than 1000 nm and becomes warmer) and water evaporation from the oceans, lakes and rivers (absorbing even longer wavelengths) which in turn causes a thicker atmospheric blanket (similar to greenhouse glass) which too is transparent to short-wave radiation but opaque to long-wave radiation, thus trapping heat.

Volcanic eruptions, oil production (burning fossil fuels in the form of coal, oil and gas), industrial pollution, burning of biomass (wood for fuel in Third World countries), and desertation owing to deforestation are the main causes for the increased *carbon dioxide concentration* in the atmosphere. It is estimated that deforestation is responsible for the release of 2 billion tonnes of carbon dioxide into the air each year. Other greenhouse gases include: methane, nitrous oxide and chloro-fluoro-carbons.

Methane – 'swamp gas' – is also released as a natural gas from coal mining and after burning forests. About 120 million tonnes a year are produced from rice paddies (artificial swamps) and 90 million tonnes a year are produced from the eructations of cattle by bacteria living in cows' guts. Each molecule of methane is 20 times more efficient at trapping heat than a single molecule of carbon dioxide. Whereas carbon dioxide in the air has increased by a quarter, methane has doubled over the past 200 years and is increasing at a rate of 1% a year (twice as fast as the build-up of carbon dioxide).

Nitrous oxide is produced from nitrogen fertilisers in arable farming and from burning forests; nitrous oxide may contaminate growing fruits and vegetables and when ingested may become carcinogenic nitrosamines (after reactions with water and gastric juice).

All the greenhouse gases are natural components of atmospheric air; it is simply their quantities that have been increased by human activity. Chloro-fluoro-carbons (CFCs), however, were not present in the atmosphere at all until they were manufactured by industrial chemists in the 1930s. CFCs are the main ozone layer destroyer and are extremely efficient greenhouse gases; molecule for molecule, some CFCs are 10 000 times more effective at trapping heat than carbon dioxide.

Deforestation or mass clearing of tropical rain forests (by cutting for timber or burning to release land for agriculture and cattle farming) can lead to many devastating consequences.

- Forests are delicate and complete ecosystems and represent the lungs of the planet for absorbing accumulated carbon dioxide from atmospheric air by photosynthesis (the process by which green plant carbohydrates and oxygen are produced from carbon dioxide and water through the agency of light) during the daytime and releasing carbon dioxide into the air (in exchange for oxygen intake) during the night, following burn and after plant death or decomposition; thus trees maintain the carbon cycle in nature. Trees are also the biggest sponge for maintaining the water cycle (absorbing water from soil by capillary action and releasing water vapour into the atmospheric air). Trees also maintain the third cycle in nature, i.e. the nitrogen cycle, by absorbing nitrogen from air and soil and fixing it in their roots, and then releasing nitrogen into air and soil on decay and plant death.

- Once a tropical soil is cleared, it no longer has the protection of the forest canopy shading it from direct sunshine and direct scatters of falling rain. Baked by fierce sunshine and beaten by torrential rain, the inherently weak soil is liable to deteriorate rapidly and will be unsuitable for farming or forestry in a distressingly short time.

- Clearance may distort the water cycle; where forests have been cleared high on slopes, the rain has washed away the soil which has then polluted rivers. In the lowlands, exposing the soil to sun and rain may flood the area, turning it into swamp.

- By reducing the amount of water removed from below ground and released as vapour by plants, deforestation may alter the rainfall itself, and thus change the climate. The alteration of land colour from dark green (forest canopy) to a paler colour (farm crops or baked earth) may change the radiation balance of the tropics; more radiation will be reflected into space and less absorbed, leading to a hot climatic change.

- Deforestation will lead to loss of nearly half of all the growing timber in the world, with extinction of rare and unknown species adapted to such particular habitats, together with a scientific loss of genetic information.

- Deforestation deprives mankind of rain forest medicines. About 70% of 3000 plants identified by the USA National Cancer Institute as having anti-cancer properties are found in the rain forest. Alkaloids yielded by the Madagascan forest plant the rosy periwinkle have increased the recovery rate from childhood leukaemia and other blood cancers from 20% to 92%.

Cosmic radiation from a supernova or an abnormally large solar flare coupled with the intermission or magnetic reversal of the planet's poles can cause mass extinction of organisms; such events the may have either killed the dinosaurs outright (extinction) or have caused such genetic mutations that they effectively disappeared as dinosaurs. (One interpretation is that dinosaurs adapted to live in deep water, escaping the total destructive effects of cosmic radiation on Earth's land and shallow water areas. It is conceivable that some of them still exist in the abysses of seas and oceans, giving rise to the legends of the Loch Ness monster in Scotland, the Bahamas plesiosaurus and the sea serpents so often and insistently reported by seafarers and deep sea research vessels).

The Earth has a further protective shield, *the ozone layer*, which exists high in the Earth's stratosphere and to which we owe our continued existence. The atmosphere consists of five layers:

- *Troposphere*, up to 50 km above ground level with a temperature of 15°C (containing the carbon dioxide blanket and part of the ozone layer).
- *Stratosphere*, at 200 km above ground level with a temperature of –65 °C (the ozone layer here contains 95% of all the world's atmospheric ozone).
- *Mesosphere* at 500 km above ground level with a temperature of 1117°C (containing the solar radiation).
- *Ionosphere* at 700 km above ground level with a temperature of 1180°C (containing cosmic rays and Aurora).
- *Exosphere* at 800 km above ground level with a temperature of 1187°C.

This ozone layer is a field of unstable ionisation so that the air contains atomic oxygen (O), ordinary molecular oxygen (O_2), and ozone (O_3) and each time a molecule of oxygen breaks down some ultraviolet radiation (UV) is absorbed; in effect, therefore, the ozone layer maintains a transparent wall between Earth's upper atmosphere and the sun, permitting us to benefit from the life-giving heat and light of the sun and protecting us at the same time from the sun's UV (short-wave) radiation. However, an ozone layer near the ground is highly undesirable, and is building up over northern continents at a rate of 2%. It is another greenhouse gas and contributes to:

- *Photochemical smog* (a poison to humans produced by sunlight action on nitrous oxides, hydrocarbons and carbon monoxide emitted from, for example, vehicle exhausts); its concentration rises with industrial pollution and in Third World countries, where laws and measures to restrict pollution are loose, the results can be seen in such places as the 'Valley of Death' (Cubatao in Brazil), which has one of the highest world rates of infant death, birth defects, lung diseases and skin disorders. The environmental pollution is reported to be second only to what might be expected from a nuclear war.
- *Acid rain*, compounding damage caused by other pollutants, as nitrogen and sulphur oxides emitted from vehicle exhausts and power plants form acid in the air which falls in rain to poison plants, resulting in massive agricultural losses.

However, it is the stratospheric protective ozone shield that really matters most. This is being increasingly damaged by:

- The wide use of extremely stable chemical gaseous compounds, the freons or chloro-fluoro-carbons (CFCs) used in refrigerators, freezers, air conditioners, as propellants in aerosol cans and as bubbles in plastic foam used in making the cushions of modern furniture.
- The worldwide use of spray cans of nitrogen-based pesticides and fertilisers used by farmers may lead to the release of nitrogen oxides in the air, which react with oxygen and ozone to form stable compounds and thus further deplete the stratospheric ozone layer.
- Nitrogen oxides are massively produced by burning fossil fuel in the oil industries and by the engine exhaust of supersonic jets as they pass through the stratospheric ozone layer.
- Thermonuclear testings may add to ozone layer depletion, and nuclear war and its aftermath ('nuclear winter') would be devastating.

SYSTEMIC SURGERY

SURGERY OF THE ALIMENTARY TRACT

1.42 Reflux Oesophagitis

Gastro-oesophageal reflux disease

Gastro-oesophageal reflux disease (GORD) accounts for the greatest number of general practitioner GIT consultations; oesophagitis now surpasses peptic ulceration in upper GIT endoscopic diagnoses. Common presenting symptoms include heartburn, regurgitation, sensation of dysphagia (non-obstructive dysphagia) and odynophagia (pain on swallowing hot liquids); about 30% of patients may present with epigastric pain, cardiac type of chest pain, nocturnal cough or wheeze, hoarseness or an acute upper GIT bleeding (and anaemia).

Perhaps it was the high GORD incidence that led to the new culture of Open Access or Direct Access Endoscopy for GPs (patients are directly referred by GPs from their practices to the Endoscopy Unit without the need for the patient to be seen in the outpatient clinic by a specialist prior to endoscopy in order to diagnose the condition properly and to pick up the disease at an early stage). Direct Access endoscopy can either be true (all referred patients will be endoscoped) or censored (the endoscopist will sift through GP letters to select patients to avoid unnecessary endoscopies). The endoscopist is usually a physician, clinical assistant, or surgeon, but some GPs are directly involved by performing an endoscopy session themselves, sharing the workload and reducing the long waiting lists.

Oesophagitis is usually due to gastro-oesophageal reflux (acid-peptic oesophagitis) and rarely to entero-oesophageal reflux (alkaline oesophagitis). In man, the oesophagogastric junction marks the transition from negative intrathoracic pressure to positive intra-abdominal pressure and is normally 3–5 cm in length. This tonically high pressure zone, called the 'lower oesophageal sphincter' (LOS), maintains a resting pressure of approximately 15–30 mmHg. The LOS relaxes with swallowing, allowing food to pass freely into the stomach. Normally, the diaphragmatic crura, the phreno-oesophageal ligaments, the acute angulation of the oesophageal entry into the stomach, the intra-abdominal segment of the oesophagus and the mucosal rosette all contribute to functioning of the LOS as a mechanical flutter valve (mechanical theory of LOS). However, the LOS is also a specialised tonic muscle which acts as a normal protective barrier to reflux via the excitatory and inhibitory effects of many neurotropic, hormonal and pharmacological agents, e.g. vagotomy leads to reflux while metoclopramide and domperidone antagonise the inhibitory dopaminergic receptors of LOS leading to a pressure rise and prevention of reflux. Gastrointestinal hormones exert excitatory and inhibitory effects (sphincter theory).

Pathogenesis

Gastro-oesophageal reflux has been associated with sliding hiatus hernia and a causal relationship has been established. However, the relationship between hiatus hernia *per se* and reflux is probably of no significance since:

- A substantial number of patients with hiatus hernia fail to demonstrate evidence of reflux.
- 20% of patients with reflux have no demonstrable hiatus hernia.
- Reflux may occur without oesophagitis whether or not a hiatus hernia is present.
- Displacement of the sphincter into the thorax, as seen in hiatus hernia, does not diminish its pressure or competence.

Hiatus hernia, gastro- or entero-oesophageal reflux and oesophagitis are therefore three separate and distinct conditions.

The reflux is due to some abnormality in LOS function which causes the sphincter to become weaker and subsequently incompetent, leading to a retrograde flow across the sphincter into the oesophagus. At least three major abnormalities in LOS function have been described in man:

- Decrease in basal LOS pressure, usually to below 10 mmHg or even as low as 2 mmHg, allowing free reflux of gastric content while the patient is asleep in the recumbent position and in the fasting state.
- Reduction in the adaptive response of the LOS to increase in intra-abdominal pressure. Normally there is an adaptive mechanism that allows the LOS pressure to increase to a greater degree than the intra-abdominal pressure during exercise, Valsalva's manoeuvre or the wearing of tight garments. Patients with reflux disease do not demonstrate this physiological response.
- A defect in the release of the hormone, gastrin, during the ingestion of a meal leading to postprandial complaints. Normally, ingestion of a protein meal leads to the antral and duodenal release of gastrin, which in addition to stimulating acid secretion, is the most potent stimulus for increasing LOS pressure in man. Patients with reflux have less gastrin released during a meal and subsequently show a diminished LOS pressure response to a meal. Other hormones such as glucagon, secretin and cholecystokinin and certain prostaglandins reduce LOS pressure. Foods

rich in fat may greatly reduce sphincter competence by the release of cholecystokinin. The causes of LOS incompetence are:

- Idiopathic (the majority of cases).
- Congenital short oesophagus (brachyoesophagus).
- Chalasia of infancy.
- Pregnancy and obesity.
- Prolonged nasogastric intubation.
- Iatrogenic – after operations that disturb the function of the cardia, including oesophagogastric anastomosis and Heller's oesophagocardiomyotomy (acid and pepsin gastro-oesophageal reflux); or after oesophagoduodenostomy, oesophagojejunostomy, distal gastrectomy with Billroth II (gastrojejunostomy); and occasionally after vagotomy and pyloroplasty (alkaline entero-oesophageal reflux).
- Chronic pyloric or duodenal obstruction, sometimes.

Diagnosis and assessment

It is the reflux disease rather than sliding hiatus hernia that should be called the 'masquerader of the upper abdomen'.

Clinical history

A clinical history is essential. Suggestive symptoms of reflux are burning epigastric or retrosternal pain during or after food ingestion (heartburn), and gastric content regurgitation with effortless vomiting. The aggravation or precipitation of these symptoms by stooping or lying (postural aggravation) is diagnostic for reflux. There is no correlation between the severity and duration of symptoms and the presence or absence of oesophagitis as determined by endoscopy. Some patients complain bitterly of symptoms but with no visible endoscopic evidence of oesophagitis, whereas others present with peptic stricture and dysphagia but with no other symptoms. Inflammation, ulceration and bleeding (melaena or haematemesis) with anaemia occur. Dysphagia is usually a late symptom due to peptic stricture; however, if it occurs earlier it is due to oesophageal spasm triggered by reflux. Other complications of reflux include aspiration pneumonia, abscesses and bronchiectasis. Prolonged reflux can lead to metaplastic mucosal changes with replacement of squamous epithelium by columnar epithelium (Barrett's epithelium); this is rare but considered to be a premalignant condition leading to adenocarcinoma of the oesophagus.

There are no physical signs to be looked for during physical examination.

Investigations

The primary and routine investigations are *radiology (barium swallow, especially in the Trendelenburg position, and fluoroscopic study) and oesophagoscopy with biopsy*. These are the most informative for diagnosing reflux oesophagitis with or without stricture. Histologically reflux oesophagitis is either: acute, when changes are visible microscopically and not macroscopically; chronic, with visible changes and microscopic fibrosis identical to chronic gastric peptic ulcer; or a combination of acute and chronic, i.e. a subacute ulceration of aberrant gastric mucosa. Barrett's (columnan cell lined) oesophagus is acquired (rather than congenital) in elderly patients due to reflux and cephalad migration of gastric mucosa producing patchy distribution of ectopic columnar mucosa amidst squamous epithelium resulting in stricture at the OG junction, large Barrett's ulcers (may lead to massive bleeding) and possible cancer in 10% of cases

Other selective tests are the following.

Intraoesophageal manometry Quantifies the gastro-oesophageal pressure barrier, locates the gastro-oesophageal junction physiologically as a guide to placement of the pH electrode and catheters for other tests, and determines whether other conditions such as scleroderma, spasm or achalasia are present.

pH reflux test (Using a nasogastric pH electrode after introduction of 300 ml of 0.1 N HCl into an empty stomach). The most accurate method for detecting reflux and judging the competence of the cardia.

The acid perfusion test (Bernstein) Perfuse saline at a rate of 6 ml/min for 10 min in a sitting position and switch to 0.1 N HCl (unknown to the patient) at the same rate for 20 min or until the patient spontaneously complains of reflux symptoms or pain. The perfusion is switched back to normal saline. The test is positive when symptoms occur during acid perfusion and not saline perfusion. This test determines whether acid in contact with the oesophagus causes symptoms, and as with the pH reflux test, it may identify the reflux as the cause of the symptoms.

Acid clearing test Measures the motor ability of the oesophagus to empty itself of acid and thus protect itself from damage as a result of prolonged contact with refluxed gastric secretions. It correlates well with the presence of reflux oesophagitis.

Potential difference test Detects whether oesophageal mucosa is squamous or abnormal (non-specific).

The specificity of these tests is shown in Table 1.42.1.

Table 1.42.1 Specificity of tests for reflux

Test	Specificity
LOS pressure (manometry)	+++
Radiology	
Barium swallow	+
Cine barium swallow	++
pH acid reflux	+++
Mucosal integrity	
Endoscopy	++
Biopsy	+++
Acid perfusion	+++
Acid clearing	++

+++ = excellent; ++ = good; + = fair

Treatment

Normal people can have occasional reflux. If gastroduodenal reflux alone without symptoms or complications is demonstrated, no treatment is required. The primary treatment of reflux oesophagitis is medical. The plan of treatment consists of three stages.

Stage I

- Simple therapeutic postural manoeuvres, e.g. patient should sleep with the bed head elevated, avoid reclining immediately after eating and diminish activities that decrease the gravitational advantage of the oesophagus.
- Obesity should be reduced and patients should not wear tight garments or take vigorous exercise after eating. Dietary advice: avoid coffee, smoking, alcohol, chocolate and fatty food (these lower the LOS pressure either through release of cholecystokinin, directly or through an unknown indirect mechanism).
- Gaviscon and antacids neutralise gastric acidity and directly increase LOS pressure and prevent reflux through their alkalinisation effect. Non-calcium-containing antacids are preferred, e.g. Maalox, to avoid hypercalcaemia from prolonged use.
- Stop contraindicated drugs that reduce LOS pressure, e.g. anticholinergic and β-adrenergic drugs.

About 75% of patients with uncomplicated reflux will respond to Stage I medical treatment.

Stage II

Those who have failed to improve with traditional Stage I therapy require specific pharmacotherapy.

- Give drugs that increase LOS pressure and are relatively free of side-effects, e.g. bethanecol chloride and metoclopramide hydrochloride (Maxolon).
- Give drugs that inhibit acid secretion by H_2 receptor antagonism, i.e. cimetidine and ranitidine.

A further 20% of patients respond to this therapy, so that only 5–10% of all patients with reflux disease will require surgical intervention (Stage III).

Stage III

Includes antireflux procedures. In the past, the aim of surgery was to repair the hiatus hernia. This approach, as represented by Allison surgical repair, had limited success and many failures since reflux is unrelated to the presence of a hiatus hernia.

Surgical reconstruction or restoration of the competent LOS mechanism leads to functional improvement and clinical cure and should be the aim of any antireflux operation.

Surgical treatment

Indications

- Failure of medical therapy (Stages I and II) and/or severe initial symptoms interfering with patient's occupation.

Surgical approaches

Either the laparotomy or the thoracotomy approach is used.
The advantages of the laparotomy approach are:

- Less painful (no intercostal neuralgia).
- Safer in middle-aged obese patients.
- Able to provide satisfactory examination and surgical treatment for intra-abdominal associated diseases, e.g. duodenal or pyloric peptic ulcer and gall stones.

Thoracotomy has the advantages of:

- Better access for severe oesophagitis and shortening of oesophagus.
- Being the best approach for para-oesophageal hiatus hernia repair.
- Definite place in peptic stricture treatment, e.g. Thal's patch.

Types of antireflux operation

Mark IV – Belsey repair (Belsey, Bristol, 1966) (Fig. 1.42.1)

A transthoracic approach through the eighth rib bed. After careful and complete mobilisation of the oesophagogastric junction or cardia and intra-abdominal reduction of the peritoneal hernial sac, the repair is performed in three stages:

(a) Reapproximation of the two halves of the right crus of the diaphragm with stout sutures (snug closure of the oesophageal hiatus behind the oesophagus).
(b) Restoration of an acute oesophagogastric angle by plication of the stomach fundus onto the distal oesophagus via the initial row of mattress sutures.
(c) Restoration of an abdominal segment of the oesophagus via the second row of three mattress sutures.

Fundoplication (Nissen II, Switzerland 1964) (Fig. 1.42.2)

A transabdominal approach. The right crus margins are identified and approximated. Mobilisation of stomach fundus by dividing the gastrosplenic omentum is followed by wrapping the mobilised fundus around and suturing in front of the abdominal oesophagus for a 2 cm distance (after incubating oesophagus with a large Maloney bougie) to produce an

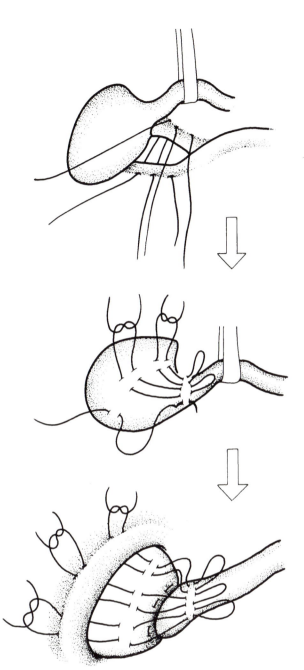

Fig. 1.42.1 Mark IV – Belsey repair of hiatus hernia

- Local complications, e.g. oesophagitis (with ulceration visible on barium swallow), haemorrhage (with anaemia), peptic oesophageal stricture.
- Respiratory complications from reflux, e.g. aspiration pneumonia, abscesses, empyema and bronchiectasis.
- Paraoesophageal (rolling) hiatus hernia (10% of cases; the sliding type represents 85% and the mixed type 5% of cases) with postprandial cardiorespiratory distress and dysphagia.
- Associated lesions, e.g. pyloric or duodenal (peptic) ulcers and gallstones.

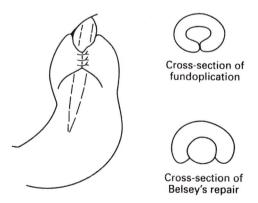

Cross-section of fundoplication

Cross-section of Belsey's repair

Fig. 1.42.2 Nissen Fundoplication. Note the cross-section as compared with Belsey's repair

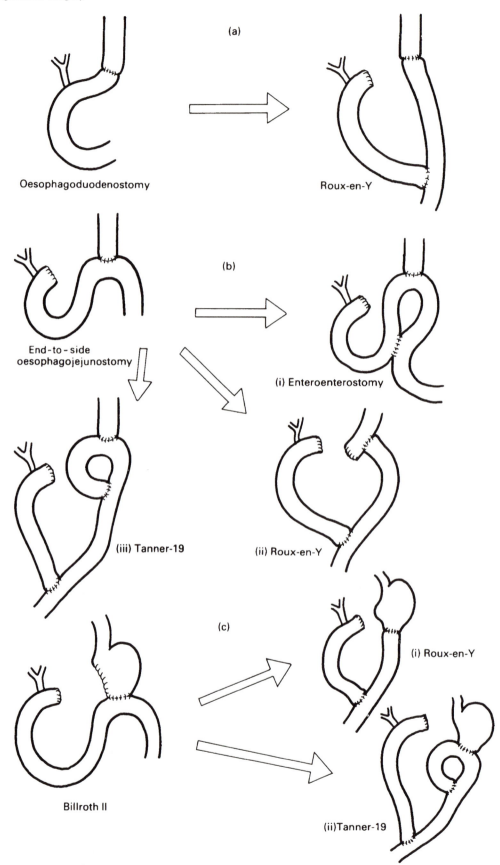

Fig. 1.42.3 Choice of treatments for alkaline reflux oesophagitis

'unspillable inkwell' effect. In the presence of pyloric or duodenal peptic ulcer, vagotomy and pyloroplasty could be added.

Gastropexy

Simple anterior fixation of the anterior surface of the stomach (near the lesser curve) to the linea alba (described separately by Boerema of Amsterdam, 1955 and Nissen (I), 1960).

Posterior fixation by anchoring the gastro-oesophageal junction to the pre-aortic fascia and median arcuate ligament after transabdominal reduction of the hernia and closure of the hiatus posterior to the oesophagus (Hill, 1967).

Others

Collis thoracoabdominal approach with approximation of the right crus in front of the oesophagus and fixation of stomach fundus to the undersurface of the left dome of the diaphragm to maintain an acute angle.

Balanced composite operation (Berman and Berman, 1959): consists of reduction of the hernia, bilateral vagotomy, repair of hiatus, oesophagogastropexy and pyloroplasty.

Silastic ring Angelchick prosthesis placed around oesophagogastric junction – another useful procedure, easy to apply and effective anti-reflux prosthesis that serves to neutralise the elevated intragastric pressure, though it is more expensive. When dislocated, the prosthesis creates problems and necessitates reoperation in just under 1% of cases. Serious complications, such as wall erosion (with opening lumen), downward slippage of prosthesis over the stomach and stricture formation have been observed.

Alkaline reflux oesophagitis (Fig. 1.42.3)

Treated in the following ways:
(a) Oesophagoduodenostomy – convert to Roux-en-Y oesophagojejunostomy.
(b) End-to-side oesophagojejunostomy – (i) add enteroenterostomy; or (ii) convert to Roux-en-Y; or (iii) convert to Tanner-19 modification.
(c) Billroth II – convert to (i) Roux-en-Y or (ii) Tanner-19. Alternatively add an enteroenterostomy.
(d) Billroth I – convert to Roux-en-Y (not illustrated).

1.43 Gastrointestinal Cancer: Precancerous and Predisposing Conditions

Oral cavity

Lips Exposure to sunlight (countryman lips) with actinic cheilitis; skin precancerous conditions (see Section 5: Surgical pathology, Hard skin tumour).

Tongue Leucoplakia due to 7 S's (smoking, syphilis, sepsis, sharp tooth, spirits, spices and susceptibility). Some benign tumours and lingual thyroid can undergo malignant mitotic changes.

Salivary glands Benign tumours such as pleomorphic adenoma may develop malignancy.

Oesophagus

Plummer–Vinson (USA) syndrome (or Paterson–Kelly syndrome – two British ENT surgeons). A premalignant condition which leads to postcricoid and cervical oesophageal carcinomas. It affects middle-aged women and is manifested by dysphagia due to high oesophageal web, iron deficiency anaemia with koilonychia, smooth tongue, stomatitis and achlorhydria.

Achalasia of cardia Auerbach's plexus Absence leads to diverticulA, carcinomA, Aspiration pneumonia, Arthritis (toxic rheumatoid) and Anaemia.

Lower oesophageal carcinoma Develops in 0–20% of achalasia cases after a duration of about 17 years.

Ectopic gastric mucosa Associated with hiatus hernia and reflux oesophagitis may lead to a primary adenocarcinoma.

Leucoplakia In a longstanding area of reflux oesophagitis due to any cause.

Benign strictures From various causes, e.g. lye and peptic strictures. Carcinoma may develop in an oesophageal diverticula (probably insignificant association).

Benign tumours (papillomas and adenomatous polyps) Can undergo malignant changes.

Tylosis (with palmar and solar desquamation).

Reverse smoking (smoking with the ignited end in the mouth – common habit in South America).

Stomach

Diet Carcinoma is uncommon in areas where maize is the staple food. Meat, and green and yellow vegetables also lower the risk. Carcinoma is common in areas where potatoes form a major part of diet. Consumption of pickled vegetables and dried/salted fish, ingestion of secondary amines (fish), less milk, and smoking increase the risk. The preparation of food is also important, e.g. talc-treated rice in Japan was found to have an inverse relationship to gastric carcinoma and atherosclerosis.

N-nitrosamines Produced by bacteria and other nitroso compounds, they are precancerous and seen in chronic gastritis, extensive intestinal metaplasia and following Billroth II gastrectomy and gastroenterostomy.

The risk of developing carcinoma in *partial gastrectomy* stump after 25 years is six times the risk after 15 years (the breaking period is 10–15 years, after which regular gastroscopy check-up is necessary).

Gastric ulcers   Develop malignancy in 3–5% of cases.
Pernicious anaemia   Increases the risk four times and gastric carcinoma develops characteristically in the gastric body and/or fundus.

Familial predisposition   Relatives of gastric carcinoma patients are four times more at risk than those with unaffected relatives.

Gastric cancer and H. pylori   Intestinal metaplasia (precancerous condition) occurs when gastric atrophy is present; gastric atrophy, however, most commonly results from long-standing *Helicobacter pylori* chronic antral gastritis. Furthermore, it is suggested that *H. pylori* may impair gastric antioxidant defences manifested by low gastric juice vitamin C levels in infected subjects. Early acquisition of infection was associated with high gastric cancer rates in a large study from China. Studies that failed to show a relationship between *H. pylori* and cancer were based on inability of identification of *H. pylori* at the time of diagnosis of cancer; such methodology is flawed, because *H. pylori* positivity is often lost in patients who have had longstanding infection with resultant gastric atrophy, as *H. pylori* requires acid secreting mucosa to survive (see also s. 1.45 Critical review of peptic ulcer management).

Polyp   A descriptive term which means a projection into a lumen or cavity. Gastric polyps are classified into:
● Hamartomatous polyps which include:
  – Juvenile polyps.
  – Peutz–Jeghers syndrome (gastrointestinal hamartomatous polyposis with ano-oral melanosis – usually benign).
  – Cronkhite–Canada syndrome (alopecia, nail atrophy and gastric polyposis).
  – Heterotopias: as aberrant pancreatic tissue located submucosally.
● Hyperplastic – regenerative polyps.
● Neoplastic adenomas present in 40% of gastric polyps and are either tubular, villous or tubulovillous.

Giant rugal hypertrophy of the stomach (Ménétrier's disease)   is a benign disease with ancedotal evidence of ?malignant changes.

Others   Gastric carcinoma develops in patients with blood group A (Japanese however claim blood group B). Asbestosis and immunodeficiencies may be associated with gastric carcinoma.

Hepatobiliary system

Gallstones   May be complicated by gallbladder adenocarcinoma.

Clonorchiasis   Has a particular role in the pathogenesis of primary cholangiocarcinoma (intrahepatic bile duct carcinoma) in Hong Kong.

Cirrhosis   A definite precancerous condition, predisposing to primary hepatocellular carcinoma. Cirrhosis is mainly idiopathic or alcohol-induced rather than malnutrition-induced. *Genetic* α_1-antitrypsin deficiency may be an enhancing factor for cirrhosis and even carcinoma.

Natural carcinogens
● Pyrrolizidine alkaloids found in 'bush teas', consumption of which may cause veno-occlusive disease common in the West Indies.
● Cycasin found in camphor oil, cinnamon and bay leaf.
● Ethiopian herbal mixtures and taenicides.
● Nitrosamines found in smoked fish, bacon and mushrooms.

Drugs   Contraceptive pill has been reported to cause liver cell adenomas, hepatoblastomas and hepatocellular carcinoma. This depends on the duration and the dose of both oestrogen and progesterone. However, there is no statistical back-up and it is currently agreed that the contraceptive pill may cause benign hepatic tumours only. Androgen/anabolic steroids can cause benign hepatomas and hyperplasia.

Mycotoxins   Are toxic metabolites of fungi and include sterigmatocystin, luteoskyrin and the best known aflatoxins, a group of compounds produced by *Aspergillus flavus*.

Hepatitis B   There is a significant association between HB_sAg with both cirrhosis and hepatocellular carcinoma and with α-fetoprotein production.

Pancreas

Diet   While fruits and vegetables have a protective value, a high fat diet stimulates bile and increases the availability of bile acids, cholesterol and their metabolites, thus increasing the pancreatic cell multiplication (via cholecystokinin) and causing hyperplasia and possibly carcinoma. While tea consumption was found to be associated with a reduced risk of pancreatic carcinoma, coffee consumption, in contrast, was found to correlate with pancreatic, prostatic carcinomas and leukaemia in males only. Even decaffeinated coffee was found to be associated with pancreatic carcinoma. Later studies were equivocal and the relationship remains to be confirmed (coffee drinkers are usually smokers and the blame probably lies with smoking rather than coffee consumption).

Smoking   Increases the risk of pancreatic carcinoma as documented by the high incidence of pancreatic hyperplasia and atypia in autopsies of smokers. The risk is directly proportional to the amount smoked.

Alcoholism   Predisposes to oral, pharyngeal, oesophageal, laryngeal, hepatic and possibly pancreatic malignancies (weak relationship).

Familial predisposition   Is very rare but definite. It is associated with Gardner's syndrome and hereditary pancreatitis (both autosomal dominant). In multiple endocrine neoplasm (MEN-I), which is also autosomal dominant, the pancreatic neoplasm is usually islet cell functional insulinoma, glucagonoma or gastrinoma and is associated with adenocarcinoma of the pituitary, parathyroid and adrenal cortex. Pancreatic carcinoma is 15 times more common in ataxia telangiectasia than in control relatives. Occult pancreatic adenocarcinoma is also associated with Lindau's disease and with neurofibromatosis.

Diabetes   There is a statistically significant excess of deaths in diabetics due to pancreatic carcinoma in both sexes.

Chronic pancreatitis   Pancreatic carcinoma develops in 30% of families with chronic pancreatitis, but it is probably related to the associated alcoholism or the biliary tract disease (or both).

Small bowel

Coeliac disease   Significantly associated with intestinal lymphoma and lymphosarcoma.

Peutz–Jeghers syndrome   Usually benign but very rarely the polyps undergo malignant changes.

Crohn's disease   Rarely may be complicated by malignancy.

Neural crest remnants   (Apudoma or carcinoid tumours or argentaffinoma.)

Large bowel

Multiple primary cancers occur in 5–20% of cases.

Diet   There is sufficient evidence to indicate that patients with large bowel cancer have a greater consumption of fat or meat than controls. Beer consumption was also associated markedly with colorectal cancer. Vegetables have a protective value.

Burkitt (1971) stressed that the low-fibre content of Western diets may be responsible for the higher incidence of colon cancer and other diseases in the West than in Africa. He rightly suggested that the longer intestinal transit time and the lower stool weight associated with a low residue would tend to increase both the concentration of any faecal carcinogens and their period of contact with colonic mucosa.

Fibre is a group of structural substances present in the plant cells. Crude fibre signifies the heterogeneous residue remaining after plant foods have been treated successively with dilute acid and dilute alkali. Dietary fibre includes all structures of plant foods that are not digested by human digestive enzymes, e.g. cellulose, hemicellulose, lignins and all indigestible plant polysaccharides. There is sufficient epidemiological evidence to indicate that dietary fibre has a protective value in appendicitis, colonic cancer, coronary heart disease, colonic diverticulosis, constipation, haemorrhoids, varicose veins, obesity, gall stones and diabetes which are very common in urban areas and developed countries and by contrast rare in rural areas and developing countries.

There are several *dietary anticarcinogens* active in preventing colorectal cancers (Fig. 1.43.1). All sources of fibre, namely cereal, fruits and vegetables, are protective against development of colorectal cancer. Chemicals in food used to inhibit cancer in laboratory animals include:
1. Plant phenols found in grapes, strawberries, apples.
2. Dithiothiones and flavones found in cabbage, broccoli, brussels sprouts and cauliflower.
3. Thioethers found in garlic, onion and leek. Diallyl sulphide, the flavour and fragrance component of garlic. Organic

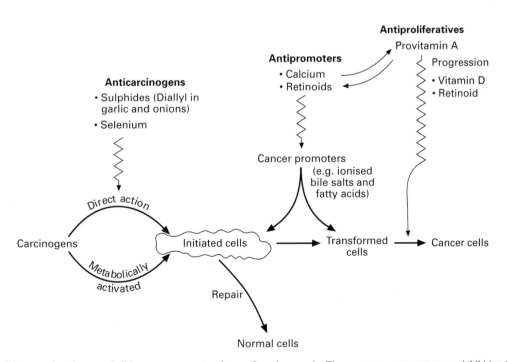

Fig. 1.43.1   Dietary anticarcinogens. Solid arrows represent pathway of carcinogenesis. Zig-zag arrows represent cancer inhibition factors

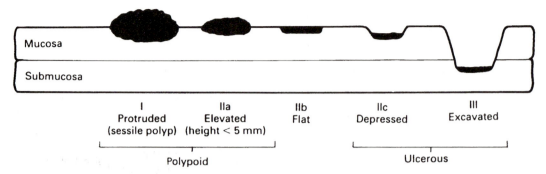

Fig. 1.44.1 Early gastric carcinoma. Classification according to the Japanese Society of Digestive Endoscopy, 1962 (uppermost) and Hermanek and Rosch, 1973 (lowermost)

sulphides found only in garlic and onions are potential antagonists of alkylating carcinogenesis.

4. Terpenes found in citrus fruit.

5. Carotenoids found in carrots, yams and water melon. Carotenoids include also provitamin A and retinoids.

Trace elements, such as selenium and calcium, were found to have anti-carcinogenic effects. Selenium is effective in prevention of carcinogen-induced breast neoplasia in experimental animals. Calcium inhibits the tissue damaging and proliferation-inducing effects of colonic lipids, since combination of lipid and calcium results in inert chemical soaps. Similarly, the proliferation-promoting effect of deoxycholic acid (secondary bile acid) and oleic acid (diet-derived fatty acid) is largely eliminated by adding calcium to the diet (see Fig. 1.43.1).

Aspirin and non-steroidal anti-inflammatory drugs (NSAID) are claimed to have an anti-cancer protection effect. Many Norfolk labourers (England) habitually took aspirin as a painkiller for their rheumatoid arthritis – a reason why they lived so long despite their creaking joints! Aspirin's protective effects against GIT malignancies, mainly colorectal cancer, was evident by the reduction by about one-third in the incidence of cancer when aspirin was taken according to doctor prescription, or about one-half when aspirin was self-prescribed. Aspirin also reduces the likelihood of suffering coronary thrombosis, a transient ischaemic attack, actual strokes and cataracts.

Familial polyposis coli is regarded as a precancerous condition (being an autosomal dominant, the family should be screened with barium enemas). Gardner's syndrome (polyposis coli with osteomas) may be associated with gastroduodenal tumours, e.g. periampullary tumour. Sebaceous cysts in children should always give rise to the suspicion of Gardner's syndrome. (See s. 1.9 Genetic factors in surgery)

Ulcerative colitis Especially in the presence of pseudopolyps which increase the risk of malignancy by 15%. Generally the risk of cancer is in the region of 3.5% which increases to 12% after 20 years.

Crohn's disease Rarely predisposes to colonic cancer.

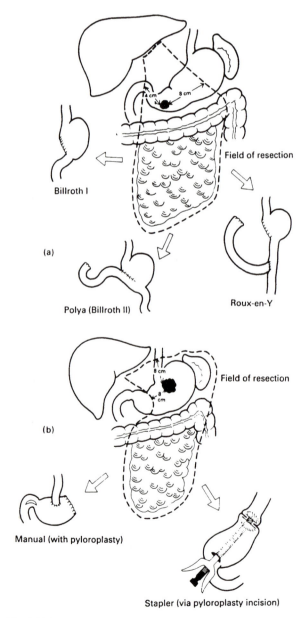

Fig. 1.44.2 (a) Distal gastrectomy (antral tumour) and (b) proximal gastrectomy (fundus tumour), showing alternative methods of repair

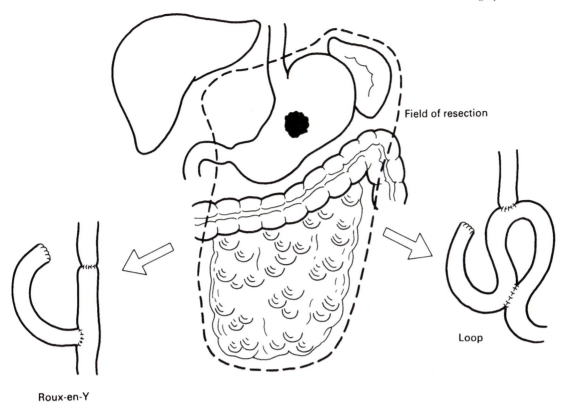

Field of resection

Loop

Roux-en-Y

Fig. 1.44.3 Total gastrectomy and oesophagogastrojejunostomy showing alternative methods of repair (oesophagoduodenostomy should not be done because of risk of alkaline oesophagitis)

Adenoma of rectum (villous, tubular or tubulovillous) A definite premalignant condition, especially if the size is more than 2 cm.

Carcinogenic metabolites of excessive bile salts Hydrolysed by bacterial flora – mainly nuclear dehydrogenating Clostridia – they may lead to cancer. The relationship between cholecystectomy and colonic cancer is debatable.

Bilharzioma (*Schistosoma mansoni*).

Ureterosigmoidostomy May be complicated by colonic cancer.

Anal canal

Radiotherapy (squamous cell carcinoma)

Leucoplakia and squamous cell carcinoma

Usual skin premalignant conditions Note that basal cell carcinoma and melanoma can develop in the anus (very rarely).

Homosexuals are more vulnerable to squamous cell carcinoma.

1.44 Early Gastric Carcinoma

Early gastric carcinoma (EGC) is the term adopted by the Japanese Society of Digestive Endoscopy in 1962 and defined as 'Carcinoma limited to the mucosa and submucosa, with or without lymph node metastases'. Surgical treatment usually leads to cure. The Japanese 5 year survival is 92% and becomes 57% and 29% respectively when muscles and serosa are invaded in contrast to 20% or less in the usual gastric carcinoma which has the distinction of being the commonest fatal cancer in the world. Morphologically EGC is classified into three types (Fig. 1.44.1).

The diagnosis is reached by the use of a double-contrast barium meal (DCBM) as a screening test coupled with endoscopy and biopsy in suspected cases. The DCBM was used widely for stomach examination in Japan in 1966. It is a six-film technique without fluoroscopy using a medium-density, low-viscosity barium suspension with air introduced originally via a nasogastric tube which is then replaced by a 'bubbly barium', effervescent drinks and effervescent tablets. Results are enhanced by using smooth muscle relaxants (glucagon 0.25 mg i.v. or hyoscine butylbromine (Buscopan) 20 mg i.v.) to induce gastric and duodenal hypotonia. The latter drugs are contraindicated in heart failure, angina, prostatism and glaucoma. In this manner it is possible:

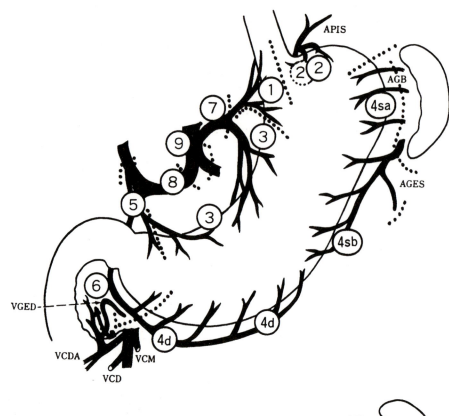

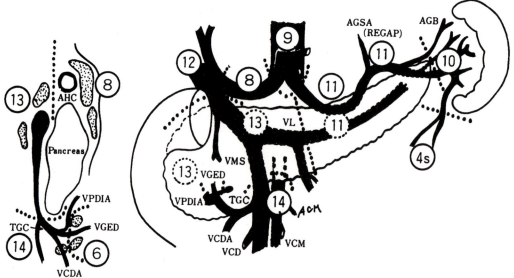

APIs, . . . A. Phrenica inferior sinistra
AGES, . . . A. Gastroepiploica sinistra
AGB, . . . A. Gastrica breves
VGED, . . . A. Gastroepiploica breves
VCDA, . . . V. Colica dextra accessorius
AGSA, . . . A. Gastrica sinistra accessorius
(REGAP), . . . (Ramus esophago-gastricus
                ascednens posterior)

ACM, . . . A. Colica media
VCM, . . . V. Colica media
VCD, . . . V. Colica dextra
VPDIA, . . . V. Pancreaticoduodenalis
                inferior anterior
TGC, . . . Truncus gastrocolica
VMS, . . . V. Mesenterica superior
VL, . . . V. Lienalis
AHC, . . . A. Hepatica communis

Fig. 1.44.4   Grading of radical dissection

Degree of radicality (R) or dissection (D)

$R_0(D_0)$ N_0 LN dissection or incomplete N_1 dissection

$R_1(D_1)$ complete N_1 (LN) dissection

$R_2(D_2)$ complete N_2 dissection ($N_1 + N_2$)

$R_3(D_3)$ complete N_3 dissection ($N_1 + N_2 + N_3$)

$R_4(D_4)$ complete N_4 dissection (impossible)

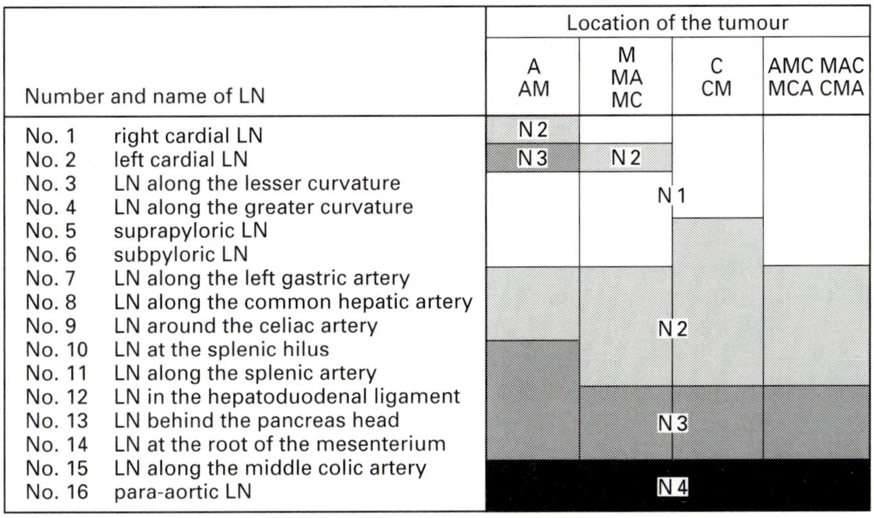

Number and name of LN		Location of the tumour			
		A AM	M MA MC	C CM	AMC MAC MCA CMA
No. 1	right cardial LN	N2			
No. 2	left cardial LN	N3	N2		
No. 3	LN along the lesser curvature			N1	
No. 4	LN along the greater curvature				
No. 5	suprapyloric LN				
No. 6	subpyloric LN				
No. 7	LN along the left gastric artery				
No. 8	LN along the common hepatic artery		N2		
No. 9	LN around the celiac artery				
No. 10	LN at the splenic hilus				
No. 11	LN along the splenic artery				
No. 12	LN in the hepatoduodenal ligament				
No. 13	LN behind the pancreas head		N3		
No. 14	LN at the root of the mesenterium				
No. 15	LN along the middle colic artery				
No. 16	para-aortic LN		N4		

LN, lymph node; A, lower third; M, middle third; C, upper third

Fig. 1.44.5 Regional lymph nodes and N categories depending on the location of the primary tumour

- To detect slight mucosal irregularities, e.g. small cancers, ulcers and ulcer scars.
- To see lesions *en face* and assess the size, shape and margins.

In 1971, a total of 1 886 062 Japanese people were screened (as above) in a mass gastric survey. EGC was detected in 0.15% and the 5-year survival proved to be 63%.

Many British surgeons, however, believe that EGC described in Japan is probably a different disease from gastric carcinoma diagnosed in the UK.

Treatment

Surgery is the only form of curative treatment and is also the main means of palliation in advanced cancer. Preoperative preparation aimed at correction of electrolyte disturbances, dehydration and anaemia is essential. Parenteral nutrition and prophylactic antibiotics may be required.

The choice of operation depends on the site, the extent of the growth and the state of the patient. Curative resection should include the entire tumour and a 7–8 cm margin proximally and distally to ensure adequate macroscopic excision with removal of greater and lesser omentum and lymph nodes *en bloc*. A Polya technique utilising a wide stoma should be used. The transverse colon is usually left in situ, but can be included if necessary. For antral tumours, distal gastrectomy should include 4 cm beyond the pylorus via the abdominal approach (Fig. 1.44.2a). For cardia or fundus tumours, proximal gastrectomy should include the spleen, pancreatic tail and lower part of the oesophagus via a thoracoabdominal approach (Fig. 1.44.2b). For extensive or multiple tumours in the body of the stomach, total gastrectomy should include removal of the whole of the stomach, again via the thoracoabdominal approach (Fig. 1.44.3). If the lower part of the oesophagus is resected, both vagal trunks are divided and pyloromyotomy or pyloroplasty is needed to prevent pyloric obstruction. However, the Japanese believe that a conservative gastrectomy is satisfactory for EGC.

The postoperative prognosis depends on age, length of history, operation type, tumour site and size, depth of invasion, lymph node metastases, tumour-free margin, tumour macroscopy and microscopy and immune response (represented by infiltration of the tumour by lymphocytes and plasma cells and follicular response in adjacent lymph nodes).

Established gastric carcinoma

Japanese surgeons have endeavoured to perform curative radical dissection procedures for patients with an established diagnosis of gastric carcinoma at the time of presentation. Furthermore, they have graded such a formidable undertaking into various degrees of radicality (R) or dissection (D) according to the level of clearance of all lymph nodes (LN) within the area of their potential drainage fields or regions (N group), for instance doing R2 (D2) for N2 (see Figs 1.44.4, 1.44.5). Occasionally, radical dissection is preferably performed to include an N group ahead of its corresponding number, e.g. doing R2 (D2) for N3. Extended total gastrectomy may include (in addition to radical lymph adenectomy) resection of the left lobe of the liver, transverse colon, pancreatic tail and spleen.

However, Professor D. Johnston and Mr H. Sue-Ling at Leeds General Infirmary have modified R2 (D2) by removing all draining LNs but leaving the spleen in situ; they have clearly shown that removal of the spleen can only worsen the morbidity and mortality rates due to post-splenctomy overwhelming infection.

1.45 Critical Review of Peptic Ulcer Management

Aetiology of peptic ulcer

There are three important contributing factors, namely increased gastric acid output, defective mucosal barrier defence system, and infection with *Helicobacter pylori* (previously called *Campylobacter pyloridis* or *Campylobacter pylori*). Such aetiology has a great impact on medical treatment. There are three groups of drugs, i.e. those which reduce gastric acidity, those which enhance mucosal barrier defence system, and those to eradicate infection with *H. pylori*.

Medical treatment of peptic ulcer

Major groups of drugs act via different mechanisms in order to promote healing of peptic ulcers.

1. Drugs which reduce gastric acidity

Gastric and duodenal ulcers respond to one of three groups of drugs:
- Antacids neutralise gastric acid.
- H_2 receptor antagonists.
- Omeprazole.

Omeprazole and H_2 receptor antagonists decrease the volume and the acidity concentration (pH) of gastric secretions. Sudden withdrawal of any of these three drugs (interrupted incomplete course) may be followed by a rebound phenomenon (decreased gastric acid secretion leading to high gastrin hormone due to feedback mechanism).

Antacids are useful in symptomatic treatment of both ulcer and non-ulcer dyspepsia and in reflux oesophagitis. They are best given when symptoms occur or are expected, usually between meals, at bedtime, four or more times daily. They are less effective than anti-secretory agents. They should not be taken at the same time as other drugs as they may impair their absorption. Magnesium-containing antacids tend to be laxative, whereas aluminium-containing antacids may be constipating.

H_2 receptor antagonists include four agents: cimetidine, ranitidine, famotidine and nizatidine; equivalent oral doses are 800 mg, 300 mg and 40 mg for cimetidine, ranitidine and famotidine respectively; ulcer healing rates are 85–90% and prevention of relapse is equivalent for all of them. For i.v. use, both cimetidine and ranitidine are recommended to be given 8- or 12-hourly. The former three compounds are eliminated by the kidneys, therefore dosage reduction is necessary in severe renal impairment. Anti-androgenic effects of cimetidine (gynaecomastia and impotence) especially in high doses are not seen with ranitidine or famotidine. Famotidine has not been shown to increase prolactin levels unlike both cimetidine and ranitidine. Cimetidine is an inhibitor of the cytochrome P-450 and interferes with hepatic blood flow, thus inhibiting the metabolism of drugs such as phenytoin, warfarin and theophylline; ranitidine has only minor effects while famotidine has not been shown to cause any changes.

Famotidine has not been as widely used as cimetidine or ranitidine; furthermore, famotidine is only available as a tablet with no liquid or injectable formulation.

Omeprazole is recently introduced and is a specific inhibitor of the gastric proton pump (H^+– K^+ ATPase) in the gastric parietal cell. It causes a dose-dependent inhibition of acid secretion by binding to the enzyme and effectively reduces gastric acid secretion. It is indicated in benign resistant ulcers unresponsive to conventional therapy, the Zollinger–Ellison syndrome and for healing erosive reflux oesophagitis. There is very little clinical experience of omeprazole and it is 10 times more expensive than the cheapest H_2 antagonist for 1 day's treatment.

2. Drugs which enhance mucosal barrier defence system

These also include three main agents:
- Sucralfate.
- Bismuth chelate (De-Nol).
- Misoprostol.

There are many similarities between sucralfate and bismuth chelate; both have no effect on gastric acid secretion and are without acid neutralizing capacity. Both are complicated molecules; sucralfate being a complex of sulphated sucrose and aluminium hydroxide, and bismuth chelate a complex bismuth salt of citric acid (tripotassium dicitrato-bismuthate). Both form large complexes with proteins (primarily albumin and fibrinogen) in the ulcer bed which adhere to the ulcer to form a relatively persistent barrier against acid, pepsin and bile acid penetration, and thus creating an environment that permits ulcer healing. Furthermore, sucralfate and bismuth chelate possess antipepsin activity and absorb bile salts and pepsin. Their site of action, therefore, is entirely local with only small amounts of the drugs being absorbed. Both seriously impair the absorption of tetracyclines when given concurrently. Antacid may impair their absorption; it should be avoided for 30 min before or after a dose of these drugs. Bismuth chelate possesses equal efficacy with H_2 antagonists in the treatment of peptic ulcer and has a slower ulcer relapse rate. This effect may be partly due to its antibacterial properties against *Campylobacter pylori*, (now known as *Helicobacter pylori*), a bacterium found in the gastrointestinal tract of most patients with peptic ulcers and closely associated with gastritis. However, the exact role of *H. pylori* in the aetiology of peptic disease is unclear.

Most of ingested bismuth is excreted as bismuth sulphide causing blackening of the faeces while the small amount absorbed is excreted in the urine. Bismuth encephalopathy has only been reported in patients receiving high doses over a prolonged period. Similarly, with sucralfate, which is an aluminium salt, and therefore neurotoxic levels of aluminium could theoretically accumulate in patients with renal impairment.

Misoprostol is a synthetic prostaglandin E1 analogue with antisecretory and cytoprotective properties. It is not superior to H_2 antagonists. Furthermore, adverse effects are more common with misoprostol than with H_2 antagonists. However, misoprostol is effective in the prevention of drug-induced gastritis and peptic ulcer, particularly following NSAID therapy. Prostaglandins have uterotropic effects; thus misoprostol can endanger pregnancy.

3. Drug therapy of H. pylori infection

The discovery of an infective basis of duodenal ulcers has been a major breakthrough in our knowledge of pathogenesis of ulcer disease; indeed, the linking of relapse in peptic ulcer with *Helicobacter pylori* infection has been a considerable advance in managing patients with ulcer disease. Infection with *H. pylori* is common in patients with peptic ulceration.

A short course of standard conventional ulcer treatment (i.e. H_2-antagonists or proton pump inhibitor) usually heals ulceration, but about 85% of patients relapse within a year.

However, in patients with duodenal ulceration, if *H. pylori* is eradicated with anti-microbial therapy, the relapse rate falls from 85% to 0–20%, ulcer healing rate increases from 73% to 95%, the time patients have an active ulcer reduces, the need for long-term acid-suppressing maintenance treatment (in most patients) is eliminated once the ulcer has healed and the total cost of treatment is reduced.

H. pylori is Gram-negative, spiral, flagellate bacillus found in the mucus lining human gastric epithelium and in areas of gastric metaplasia in duodenum; the likelihood of infection increases with age. *H. pylori* does not colonise normal intestinal epithelium or areas of intestinal metaplasia in stomach; it is quite distinct from other Campylobacter species that cause enteritis with diarrhoea. Specific serology tests indicate that this infection is common even in healthy people and prevalence increases with age; in the UK it affects at least half of those over the age of 50 (strongly associated with non-NSAID related peptic ulcer).

Only a small proportion of infected people develop peptic ulcer (other factors are needed such as acid hypersecretion, smoking and genetic predisposition). The infection is present in 90% of patients with duodenal ulcer or chronic active antral gastritis, and 70% of those with gastric ulcer; there is some evidence that *H. pylori* may be associated with gastric cancer, but there is no convincing evidence yet (at present) for a relation between *H. pylori* and non-ulcer dyspepsia.

H. pylori infection can now be considered as the world's most common infection. Gastric metaplasia in the duodenal bulb may be induced by increased acid secretion; these foci of gastric metaplasia are colonized by *H. pylori*, the precursors of duodenal ulceration. The effect of *H. pylori* on acid secretion, however, remains less clear.

Diagnosis of H. pylori

Invasive tests (following endoscopy)

- Rapid urease tests (CLO test): The enzyme urease is detected using a commercial assay within the endoscopy suite. The first antral biopsy is taken for CLO test, later biopsies are immersed in formalin for histology and the biopsy forceps tip is then contaminated with formalin which may invalidate CLO test results. The antral biopsy (via endoscopy) is inserted into a plastic slide with agar gel (containing urea, pH indicator, buffers and bacteriostatic agents); if urease enzyme of *H. pylori* is present in biopsy tissue, the resulting degradation of urea causes the pH to rise and the colour of the gel turns from yellow to magenta in minutes, giving an immediate result.
- Histology: *H. pylori* organisms can be identified on stained gastric (usually antral) biopsy samples.
- Culture: Microbiology laboratories routinely culture *H. pylori* from biopsy specimens. Usually, two antral gastric biopsies are sent: one for Gram staining histology (see above), and another to be cultured on Columbia agar supplemented with 5% horse blood and incubated for 5 days under microaerophilic conditions. Culture may be prone to high false-negative rates.

Non-invasive tests

- Serology: IgG antibodies against *H. pylori* can be detected in the serum using laboratory based and near-patient testing serology kits (may be useful in primary health care, although not highly accurate).
- Breath tests: Isotopically labelled carbon dioxide can be detected in the breath of *H. pylori*-positive individuals following ingestion of urea labelled with ^{13}C or ^{14}C.

How to eradicate H. pylori infection

Eradication is defined as the absence of *H. pylori* in the stomach, as judged by a labelled-urea (^{13}C or ^{14}C) breath test, CLO test, histology or culture, but *not by serology*, at least 1 month after completion of treatment. Patients having no infection 1 month after the end of treatment appear to have a low risk of reinfection (less than 1%) for several years. Bismuth salts (colloidal bismuth subcitrate CBS or De-Nol) and several antibiotics, such as metronidazole, tetracycline and amoxycillin, are effective against *H. pylori*. When used singly, these drugs eradicate *H. pylori* in up to 30% of patients; double or triple therapy are commonly used to improve eradication.

Standard triple therapy (usually for 2 weeks)

Bismuth subcitrate	(120 mg qds daily)	plus
Metronidazole	(400 mg tds daily)	plus
Tetracycline	(500 mg qds daily)	

This combination is more effective (93–95% eradication) than combination containing amoxycillin (instead of tetracycline) (73% eradication). Duration of therapy is usually 2 weeks, though recent studies confirm the effectiveness of a one-week short course of triple therapy (as good as a 2-week course), which is safer and tolerated better by patients, leading to better compliance.

Triple therapy requires patients to take a large number of tablets and they are likely to suffer unwanted effects, which occur in up to 50% of patients; these include metallic taste, nausea, vomiting and diarrhoea. Bismuth also causes black discoloration of stools. In countries where metronidazole is widely used for treatment of giardiasis, amoebiasis and non-specific diarrhoea, 80% of *H. pylori* strains are metronidazole-resistant. Clarithromycin, a new macrolide (macrolide is a group of antibiotics comprising erythromycin, the parent compund, and its related derivatives, clarithromycin and azithromycin) is particularly effective against metronidazole-resistant *H. pylori*.

An eradication rate of 95% or over can also be achieved by other triple therapies:

One week of:

Omeprazole	(20 mg bd daily)
Amoxycillin	(1000 mg bd daily)
Clarithromycin	(500 mg bd daily)

Alternatively

One week of:

Omeprazole	(20 mg bd daily)
Metronidazole	(400 mg bd daily)
Clarithromycin	(250 mg bd daily)

Regimen of double therapy Proton pump inhibitor, omeprazole, can temporarily suppress *H. pylori* and is also a potent acid inhibitor that may serve to enhance the effect of acid-labile antibiotics on *H. pylori*. The latest proton pump inhibitor, lansoprazole, does not confer additional benefit over omeprazole, with regard to *H. pylori* eradication but it is much cheaper than omeprazole and can replace it in all regimens employing omeprazole. Double therapy in which omeprazole is given with a single antibiotic is now being assessed. Omeprazole plus amoxycillin (in various doses) eradicates 30–80% of infections and is well tolerated. This cannot be recommended as first-line therapy, although it may be considered in patients in whom triple therapy has failed.

Success of eradication therapy depends on two factors:

● Patient compliance (patients should be counselled concerning the importance of completing the whole course of therapy and warned of side-effects they may experience).

● *H. pylori* sensitivity to antibiotics (metronidazole and tinidazole are less effective in populations with high resistance, including some ethnic minorities).

Vaccination can theoretically be possible by using orally administered mouse/*H. felis* sonicate and cholera toxin as an adjuvant.

When to treat?

Drug therapy to eradicate *H. pylori* is strongly recommended in all patients presenting with *H. pylori*-positive peptic ulcers as well as ulcer patients on maintenance therapy with anti-secretory drugs, envisioning a definite cure of the ulcer diathesis and a significant cost benefit. Future research has to clarify whether or not anti-*H. pylori* treatment should be used more widely in *H. pylori*-positive dyspeptic subjects or even prophylactically in particular circumstances.

However, currently drug therapy should be limited to patients in whom duodenal ulceration is a management problem, such as:

– newly diagnosed non-NSAID related peptic ulcer;

– frequent recurrences requiring maintenance treatment with H_2-antagonist or proton pump inhibitor (in fact all those presently on maintenance therapy should be considered for a course of eradication therapy);

– those who are being considered for elective surgery;

– those who have bled or perforated in the past.

Many of those patients are likely to have had a recent endoscopy and antral biopsy confirmation; it would be reasonable to give patients with active duodenal ulceration a standard anti-secretory therapy *with*, *or followed by*, 1–2 weeks of triple therapy to eradicate *H. pylori*. It is imperative to encourage patients to stop smoking (smoking doubles ulcer recurrence rate), although it may not have this effect once *H. pylori* has been eradicated).

Currently, triple therapy is not indicated in patients with non-ulcer dyspepsia, NSAID ulceration and Zollinger–Ellison syndrome.

Indications for surgery in peptic ulcer

● One of ulcer complications, e.g. perforation, pyloric stenosis and bleeding whether continuous or intermittent; two episodes of bleeding before 45 years, or single episode after 45 (due to atherosclerosis that prevents vascular contraction and spontaneous stoppage of bleeding).

● Failure of medical treatment and/or economic considerations and expediency.

● Combined gastric and duodenal ulcers.

● Serious persistent hourglass deformity due to cicatrized gastric ulcer.

● Suspicion of malignancy, e.g. greater curve ulcer and/or positive cytology, very long ulcer history (size is not criterion for malignancy), ulcer in patient over 60 with short history or ulcer developing in a patient with pernicious anaemia or after 10 years of a partial gastrectomy.

GASTRIC ULCER

Presents in one of two ways.

Combined gastric ulcer + duodenal ulcer (25%)

The duodenal ulcer is the primary and gastric ulcer is secondary. If both are active then gastric ulcer is benign but if duodenal ulcer is scarred then gastric ulcer is probably malignant. Treat medically (while duodenal ulcer is treated as above). If unsuccessful then total vagotomy + hemigastrectomy resecting both ulcers. Alternatively HSV + dilatation with gastric ulcer excisional biopsy.

Gastric ulcer alone (75%)

Ulcer cancer (15% of gastric ulcers) Clinical, radiological, endoscopical (five biopsies) and histological confirmation before operation are needed. Treated by gastrectomy (usually Billroth I–PG).

Prepyloric gastric ulcer (behaves like duodenal ulcer)
● Ulcer cancer: treat as above.
● Benign gastric ulcer with maximum acid output (MAO) more than 40 mEq HCl/h: treat as duodenal ulcer.
● Benign gastric ulcer with normal MAO: treat as gastric ulcer at incisura or lesser curve (Billroth I–PG; see below).

Benign gastric ulcer The acid output level is normal. Serum gastrin level is high. Minority have gastric stasis (with coexisting pyloric channel disease or duodenal ulcer). Pressure within pylorus is abnormally low and reflux of duodenal content into stomach is greater than normal.

The reflux of bile salts and lysolecithin breaks the gastric mucosal barrier, leading to gastritis, and release gastrin, rendering gastric mucosa more vulnerable to the action of irritant drugs, acid and pepsin.

Ulcers occur in the junctional zone between the parietal cell mass and alkaline mucosa of the pyloric gland area. The operative principles therefore should be to:
● Reduce the output of acid and pepsin.
● Reduce reflux of bile into stomach.
● Ensure that gastric stasis does not occur.

Treatment

Conservative

Treat with H_2-antagonist (e.g. ranitidine, cimetidine), carbenoxolone (Biogastrone), antacids, rest, regular meals, no smoking. If these measures do not lead to healing of the ulcer in 6 weeks, surgery is indicated (in duodenal ulcer 6 months' medical treatment is required before operative intervention is deemed necessary after failure).

Operative

● PG (Billroth I). Recurrent ulcer in 2% and operative mortality of 2%.
● Truncal vagotomy and drainage (TV + D) with ulcer excision (indicated in elderly and frail patients and in cases of bleeding gastric ulcer or high gastric ulcer on the lesser curve). Recurrent ulcer on 10% and operative mortality of 1.5%.
● Highly selective vagotomy (HSV) + ulcer excision is a good alternative as it reduces hydrochloric acid and pepsin output and increases intragastric pressure, thus preventing bile reflux.

DUODENAL ULCER

The operative methods of treating duodenal ulcer are compared in Table 1.45.1. These are: partial gastrectomy (PG), vagotomy and antrectomy (V + A), total vagotomy and drainage (TV + D), (whether drainage is in the form of gastrojejunostomy (GJ) or pyloroplasty (P)), and highly selective vagotomy (HSL).

Posterior truncal vagotomy and anterior seromyotomy (Taylor's procedure)

Highly selective or parietal cell vagotomy is associated with high ulcer recurrence (can reach 20% in some studies). Inadequate denervation of parietal cell mass is the comon cause of failed operation. Extensive dissection and division of vagal nerve fibres near antrum and pyloric channel, on the other hand, may lead to gastric stasis. These problems in predicting the extent of vagal denervation led Tylor et al. (1982) to the procedure known as 'posterior truncal vagotomy with anterior seromyotomy'. Effectiveness of anterior seromyotomy was based on anatomic observation that the anterior vagus nerve courses obliquely via seromuscular layers of stomach before innervating the fundic parietal cell mass. Dividing the seromuscular layer along the lesser curvature would thus assure complete fundic denervation. Taylor believed that this technique diminished both the risk of injury to the nerve of Latarget and ischaemic necrosis of the stomach.

The myotomy (dividing longitudinal and circular muscle fibres leaving deeper oblique muscle intact) begins 6 cm proximal to the pylorus, 1.5 cm from the lesser curve and can be extended proximally as far as the gastro-oesophageal junction (may be extended to include the gastric cardia). Anterior seromyotomy does not alter gastric motility or emptying due to vasovagal nerve impulses from the anterior to posterior antrum; pyloroplasty or balloon dilatation therefore are not necessary.

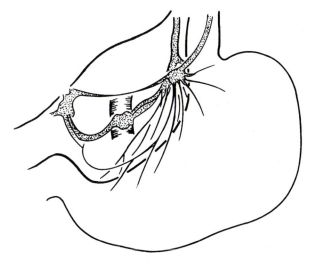

Fig. 1.45.1 Anterior and posterior vagus nerve showing gastric bronchus (of anterior and posterior nerves of Latarget), subhepatic and coeliac plexuses

Table 1.45.1   Assessment of operative treatment for duodenal ulcer

	PG	V + A	TV + D	HSV
Operative mortality	1.5%	1.2%	0.6%	0.3%
Postoperative morbidity	Gastric stasis, loop syndrome, ruptured duodenal stump		Anastomotic leak	Lesser curve necrosis and bleeding 0.1%
Side-effects	Dumping, diarrhoea, dysphagia (heartburn and reflux oesophagitis), bilious vomiting, postprandial distension. Visick clinical grading: Perfect (1), Good (2), Fair (3) and Poor (4). In HSV (1 + 2) represents 96% while in V + A or TV + D (1 + 2) represents 76%.			
Recurrent ulcer after 5–10 years	3%	1%	9% (V + GJ = 7%) (V + P = 11%)	8% Surgeon should clean distal 5 cm of oesophagus downward, leaving only 5–7 cm from pylorus
Long-term metabolic sequelae after 5–30 years (gastric cripple), e.g. weight loss, anaemia (iron and B_{12} deficiency), tuberculosis and bone disease (osteoporosis and osteomalacia)	+++	++	+	None
Carcinoma of gastric remnant after 15–30 years (due to bile reflux and gastritis). Vagotomy also produces chronic gastric mucosal changes of unknown significance	++	++	+	?(unknown)
Relative ease or difficulty of salvage operation if first operation fails	Worst ⟶ Best			

Taylor et al. reported a 6% recurrence rate in patients with duodenal ulcers followed up to 4.5 years after procedure. When compared to truncal vagotomy and pyloroplasty, recurrent ulcers were found more common after Taylor's procedure than TV + P, mean operating time was increased when Taylor's procedure was performed, but dumping and diarrhoea were significantly commoner after TV + P, and better overall Visick grading was achieved with Taylor's procedure. Continued monitoring is required to assess long-term incidence of recurrent ulceration after Taylor's procedure.

Posterior trauncal vagotomy and anterior highly selective vagotomy

Bailey et al. (1991) rekindled interest in this procedure originally described in 1978 by Hill and Barker who reported 73% reduction of basal acid output (BAO) and 65% reduction in stimulated acid secretion in patients undergoing this procedure. Gastric emptying time was found to be identical to the control unoperated patients.

TV + P versus TV + GJ (merits and demerits)

In *total vagotomy and pyloroplasty* the long-term metabolic sequelae are less severe. The operation:
● Is simpler and quicker.
● Maintains the normal pathway.
● Has a definite place in bleeding peptic ulcer.
● Is safer in elderly and high risk patients (with cardiac and/or respiratory and/or renal problems).

● Diarrhoea is a rare problem.
● Higher recurrence rate.
● Difficult to dismantle

Total vagotomy + gastrojejunostomy deals with healthier tissue and, probably, is the best drainage procedure:
● It can be undone easily when a salvage operation is needed.
● Recurrent ulcer rate is less (7% versus 11%).
● Less bile reflux, thus possibly lessens the chance of cancer of the stomach.
● There may be problems with afferent loop and dumping.
● Diarrhoea may occasionally follow.
● Has a definite place in pyloric stenosis

PERFORATED DUODENAL ULCER

Conservative treatment

This consists of continuous suction, i.v. fluids and antibiotics. It is indicated in old patients unfit for operation, in cases of cardiovascular insufficiency or shock and is also used on board a ship or in remote parts of the world. It is not recommended because:
● The underlying cause of the perforation is left undiagnosed and could be gastric ulcer, carcinoma of the stomach or colonic carcinoma.
● No peritoneal toilet means a high risk of abscesses.
● It makes great demands on the time of the nursing and medical staff.

Operative treatment

After preoperative preparation of analgesia, nasogastric suction, i.v. fluids, CVP line and urinary catheter. This is the main method of management and there are two alternatives.

Simple closure and peritoneal toilet

Operative mortality is 7%. Recovered patients require postoperative cimetidine and careful follow-up.

Advantages
- Quick simple procedure.
- Can be done by senior house officers and registrars.
- Healed ulcer already (in minority of patients).

Disadvantages
- Leaves an untreated vicious and dangerous ulcer.
- An overlooked kissing ulcer posteriorly caused by the stress of peritonitis and operation may bleed and lead to death in 2% of cases.
- Reperforation due to friable oedematous tissue.
- Gastric outlet obstruction.
- Long-term complications (30% develop further complications, 40% continue to have symptomatic peptic ulcer and in 30% the peptic ulcer remains silent). Follow-up required.

Definitive treatment at the time of perforation

TV + P converts the actual perforation into a Finney or Mickulicz repair. If perforation is large, PG may be necessary. HSV is hardly ever used as an emergency. Cimetidine 400 mg nightly should be given for 12 months postoperatively.

Disadvantages
- Difficult.
- Higher operative mortality.
- Mobilisation of distal oesophagus in the presence of peritonitis may lead to mediastinitis (theoretical).

PERFORATED GASTRIC ULCER

This is more dangerous than duodenal ulcer because of the advanced age and poor health of the patients, the large perforation, gross peritoneal contamination, haemorrhage from ulcer and ulcer-cancer in 10% of cases. It is treated by:
- Partial gastrectomy (Billroth I) in chronic cases and suspected carcinoma.
- Simple closure with multiple biopsies (if acute).
- Biopsy and closure with TV + D in selected cases.
- Wide ulcer-bearing segment resection, which is both diagnostic and therapeutic.

BLEEDING PEPTIC ULCER

Chronic peptic ulcer represents 60% of bleeding cases, acute gastric erosions represent 10–20% while varices and the Mallory–Weiss syndrome account for the remainder. Unlike perforated ulcer, bleeding ulcer must *always* be treated by a definitive ulcer-curing procedure, however ill the patient may be. Generally the operative mortality is 10% and the surgeon must be an expert. After first aid treatment, a full history is taken, and the patient is managed as follows.

1. Resuscitation by blood transfusion until skin is warm and pink, blood pressure is stable and urinary output is good. Four units of blood are reserved.
2. Cimetidine is given intravenously.
3. The source of bleeding is identified using:
- Emergency oesophagogastroduodenoscopy. This is diagnostic and can be therapeutic (electrocautery, laser photocoagulation, variceal sclerotherapy or polypectomy according to the nature of the bleeding lesion).
- Radiography (double contrast).
- Angiography. This is sometimes done and is diagnostic of the site and therapeutic (selective injection of vasopressin and therapeutic embolisation).
4. Central venous pressure (CVP) line, two i.v. cannulae, nasogastric suction, urinary catheter, ampicillin or cephalosporin with good anaesthesia are required (since hypotension and arrhythmias during induction are common).
5. The operation is via a midline incision (palpate the stomach and duodenum). Adhesions indicate the ulcer site and duodenotomy is performed and the bleeding ulcer is underrun by X-stitches of 00 Dexon or vicryl absorbable suture. TV + P is carried out by suturing the gastroduodenotomy transversely, producing a Mickulicz repair. The recurrent ulcer rate is 13% and mortality is 8% (about half that of the alternative Polya PG, which is 15%). In the absence of adhesions, separate duodenotomy and/or gastrostomy (without damaging the pyloric sphincter) and underrunning of the bleeding points with HSV are performed.

In bleeding gastric ulcer, a PG (Billroth I) is done with operative mortality of 20%; however, if the patient is unfit, the ulcer should be underrun, biopsied or excised with vagotomy. The ulcer base could be excluded by leaving it attached to the pancreas. Acute gastric erosions are better treated conservatively. However, if bleeding continues, then operation can be done – either TV + P or HSV. Subtotal Billroth I is another option.

In stress ulcer, operation should be avoided in often septic, seriously ill patients. However, if required, TV + P with underrunning of bleeding points can be performed, but this carries high mortality in a sick patient.

Mallory–Weiss syndrome rarely requires a relatively simple underrunning of the tear via gastrostomy.

PYLORIC STENOSIS

This may be due to fibrosis and/or oedema and/or spasm. Clinically there is copious vomiting, succussion splash and stomach compensation by hyperperistalsis.

Gastric outlet obstruction secondary to peptic ulcer is differentiated from carcinoma by barium meal, gastroscopy and biopsy, BAO and MAO (the latter is normal or high in peptic ulcer and low in carcinoma). Treatment is by repeated gastric lavage, correction of anaemia, dehydration and electrolyte imbalance, with chest physiotherapy, vitamin C supplement and treatment of dental caries; followed by total vagotomy + Finney's pyloroplasty or highly selective vagotomy + digital or Hegar (size 16) dilatation via a gastrostomy or highly selective vagotomy + duodenoplasty.

POST-GASTRECTOMY SYNDROMES AND COMPLICATIONS

Severe intractable side-effects occur in 5–20% of patients undergoing ulcer surgery. They can follow gastric resection for carcinoma. The term 'postgastrectomy' is a misnomer, because symptoms may occur prior to ulcer operations or develop after non-resective gastric surgery. The pathogenesis is mostly attributed to ablation or bypass of pyloric sphincter, rather than gastric resection *per se*. Mixed presentation is common. Careful history, physical examination and endoscopy are essential. Following gastric surgery, complications occur in the early postoperative period, while syndromes occur in the remote postoperative period. Early postoperative complications can either be non-specific (pulmonary atelectasis; deep venous thrombosis; cardiac arrhythmias, infarction and hypotension), or specific complications of gastric operations. The latter group include anastomotic haemorrhage (treated with blood transfusion and gastric lavage; if severe, relaparotomy to oversew anastomosis with continuous through-and-through suture); paralytic ileus (treated with drip and suction); stomal obstruction (due to stomal oedema treated with drip and suction, or due to retrograde jejunogastric intussusception, see below); acute postoperative pancreatitis; and, more importantly, duodenal stump blow-out (fistula), a rare but serious complication of Polya PG. The latter occurs on the fourth postoperative day and is due to avascular necrosis following difficult duodenal closure or increased tension within afferent jejunal loop. This can be prevented by careful duodenal stump closure with inverted suture (crushing clamp should not be used), avoiding operation on hot duodenum (by choosing another alternative such as TV and GJ); the leak must be safeguarded and led out by a multi-lumen tube drain. Should the leak occur, it must be treated urgently since it accounts for 60% of deaths after gastrectomy. Operation consists of providing free duodenal drainage with peritoneal suction only. The external fistula usually closes spontaneously.

Post-gastrectomy syndromes are usually delayed for many months if not years after gastric surgery. They include the following complications (of surgical interest).

Dumping syndromes

Early (vasomotor) dumping syndrome   The most common side-effect of gastric surgery. Symptoms include weakness, dizziness, headache, fainting, feeling warmth, palpitations, sweating and dyspnoea as well as fullness, distension, epigastric discomfort, nausea, vomiting, excessive borborygmi and diarrhoea. Symptoms occur during or immediately after eating and are precipitated by high carbohydrate meals. Only severe persistent dumping is associated with weight loss and malnutrition.

The pathogenesis is due to rapid emptying of hyperosmolar chyme from residual stomach into small intestine

leading to osmotic diarrhoea with hypovolaemia (due to fluid shift from vascular compartment into bowel lumen), resulting in the vasomotor manifestations. The syndrome is diagnosed clinically, or by dumping provocation test by administering hyperosmolar liquid (50% carbohydrate); if radiolabelled, the rapid emptying can be observed with an external camera.

Treatment is conservative by dietary adjustment, by having frequent small meals rich in protein and fat, and low in carbohydrate, avoiding taking fluids during meals. Agents to delay gastric dumping include:

– Pectin (non-absorbable vegetable carbohydrate).
– Granulated guar gum (soluble fibre).
– Somatostatin or its long-acting synthetic analogue, octreotide (they inhibit secretion of gut regulatory peptides and decrease intestinal motility and secretion). Their side-effects include diarrhoea and paradoxical hypoglycaemia.

Surgery is indicated only in 5% of patients with severe intractable symptoms. Surgical options include:

● Dismantling of gastrojejunostomy, or pyloric reconstruction (indicated in those having truncal vagotomy and drainage).
● Isoperistaltic jejunal interposition, using a jejunal segment 10–15 cm long, interposed between gastric remnant and duodenum (indicated in dumping following partial gastrectomy).
● Roux-en-Y diversion is sometimes considered the best option in dumping following partial gastrectomy. However, Roux-en-Y anastomosis itself acts as a functional obstruction and can lead to Roux-en-Y syndrome, namely chronic abdominal pain, persistent nausea and vomiting, gastric retention, stomal ulceration (in absence of complete vagotomy), stasis, bacterial overgrowth, kinking or strangulation of Roux-en-Y, and afferent loop syndrome. All patients treated with isoperistaltic jejunal interposition or Roux-en-Y diversion must be maintained on H_2-receptor blockers to prevent marginal or stomal ulceration, obviating the need for vagotomy.

Late dumping   Late dumping due to reactive hypoglycaemia is less common, occurs 1–3 h after a meal and is characteristically relieved by ingestion of carbohydrate. It is due to rapid emptying of carbohydrate into intestine, rapid glucose absorption, hyperglycaemia leading to excessive insulin release (reactive hypoglycaemia). Diagnosis is confirmed by an extended oral glucose tolerance test, which should demonstrate late hypoglycaemia. Treatment is usually conservative, by small frequent meals rich in protein and low in carbohydrate. Somatostatin and glucomannan (gel-forming dietary fibre) are useful too.

Enterogastric reflux

Also called reflux alkaline gastritis, bile gastritis, duodenal reflux syndrome, and postoperative gastritis. It is seen after pyloroplasty, gastrectomy, gastroenterostomy and rarely after highly selective vagotomy. There is reflux of upper intestinal secretion (bile, pancreatic juice and succus entericus) into the stomach and lower oesophagus resulting in erosive gastritis/oesophagitis. Causes of bile vomiting after gastric surgery include recurrent ulceration, enterogastric reflux, reflux oesophagitis and afferent or efferent loop obstruction. Clinically, enterogastric reflux leads to epigastric pain (constantly aggravated by eating and not relieved by antacids or vomiting), vomiting (bilious or food mixed with bile), and weight loss (decreased oral intake due to pain and vomiting). Patients occasionally present with iron-deficiency anaemia, melaena and rarely haematemesis. Intestinal metaplasia may be seen in long-standing cases. Diagnosis is established on clinical ground (particularly history), endoscopy with multiple gastric biopsies (histology). There is no correlation between symptoms and histology or endoscopic findings. Treatment is conservative and includes cholestyramine (binds bile salts), mucosal protective agents (e.g. sucralfate), prokinetic agents (e.g. metoclopramide and cisapride which promote gastric emptying), and H_2-blockers (beneficial but not known why).

Surgical options are similar to those used in dumping but with different objectives, diverting pancreatico-biliary and duodenal secretions from the stomach.

Recurrent peptic ulcer

Peptic ulcer is a disease with recurring symptomatic periods. Postoperative symptomatic recurrence can take one of three forms.
- Ulcer dyspepsia with endoscopically proven ulcer.
- Ulcer dyspepsia without endoscopic evidence of peptic ulcer.
- Endoscopic silent recurrence.

There is no relationship between preoperative gastric acid output and subsequent recurrence.

Causes of recurrence (in order of frequency)

1. Technical errors: incomplete vagotomy; insufficient gastric resection; poor antral drainage.
2. Failure in the choice of operation.
3. Ulcerogenic drugs, e.g. aspirin, steroids, phenylbutazone (Butazolidin) NSAIDs and alcohol or smoking.
4. Others: Zollinger–Ellison syndrome (ZES), G-cell hyperplasia, parathyroid adenoma, hypercalcaemia, multiple adenoma syndrome, long afferent loop, rarely polycythaemia and liver cirrhosis.

Diagnosis (history of symptoms after operation)

- Endoscopy (to confirm peptic ulcer and to see whether gastric or duodenal).
- Barium meal to evaluate gastric emptying rate only; it cannot confirm peptic ulcer in an operated case because of deformity and scarring.
- Serum gastrin is measured to exclude pancreatic gastrinoma, retained gastric antrum and antral G-cell hyperplasia.
- Insulin test.
- If the ratio of basic acid output (BAO) to maximal acid output (MAO) is more than 1:3 then ZES is not present.
- If BAO/MAO is 1:1 then do: basal and food-stimulated gastrin level (possibility of ZES), serum calcium and phosphate (parathyroid adenoma) and blood glucose (hypoglycaemia) with skull X-ray showing ballooned sella turcica in multiple adenoma syndrome.

Treatment

Conservative　Give cimetidine and antacids and withdraw alcohol, smoking and ulcerogenic drugs.

Operative
- Revagotomy with or without antrectomy (Billroth I) after TV + D or HSV. Sometimes, Polya PG may be needed.
- Exclude ZES if there is recurrence after PG. Stomal ulcer after PG is treated with vagotomy.
- If gastric ulcer recurs after an operation for duodenal ulcer, it is due to gastric stasis. However, ischaemic gastric ulcer may follow HSV. Do antrectomy including the gastric ulcer.
- ZES ulceration is treated with total gastrectomy if medical treatment with omeprazole (proton pump inhibitor) fails.

Prevention

Avoid Albatross syndrome (failures in gastric surgery due to wrongly selected patient developing side-effects; called albatross syndrome due to patient 'hanging about the surgeon's neck'). Such cases include patients with atypical pain and young patients with short peptic ulcer history who smoke and drink, are absent from work and on anti-depressant drugs.

Remember that recurrence after complete vagotomy is usually gastric while after incomplete vagotomy it is usually duodenal.

How to test for complete vagotomy

Intraoperative tests (Fig. 1.45.2)

Burge test (UK, 1964)　A manometer is applied via an oesophagogastric balloon, the pylorus is occluded with a clamp, and then the vagotomised area is stimulated. Any detected increase in pressure indicates incomplete vagotomy.

Grassi test (Rome, 1971)　A glass electrode inserted through a small gastrostomy is used to measure pH after vagotomy and MAO stimulation. A pH of 1.2–2 surrounded by a pH of 5.5–7 indicates the presence and actual location of incomplete vagotomy.

Postoperative tests

Peak acid output after pentagastrin　A 50% or more reduction compared to the preoperative value indicates complete vagotomy.

Insulin (Hollander's) test　Performed 1 week after vagotomy; an insulin test has a prognostic value. If it is positive within such a short time, the chance of recurrence is high; if it is negative, the chance of recurrence is low. The insulin test is contraindicated in epileptics, patients over 65 years of age, those with a history of ischaemic heart disease and diabetics.

Post-vagotomy diarrhoea

This is a misnomer, since diarrhoea is mainly due to the drainage procedure rather than due to vagotomy. The incidence

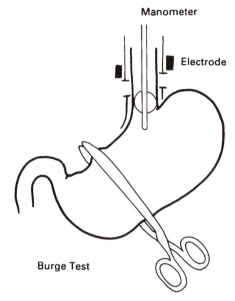

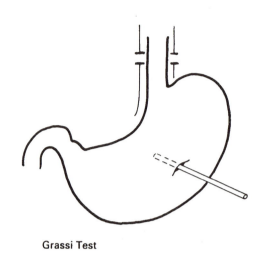

Fig. 1.45.2   Intraoperative tests for incomplete vagotomy

of diarrhoea is highest after truncal vagotomy and drainage (2–40%). It is uncommon after gastric resection and highly selective vagotomy. There are three forms of diarrhoea seen after gastric surgery: frequent loose motions, intermittent short-lived episodes and severe explosive diarrhoea. Severe intractable diarrhoea occur in 1–2% of patients undergoing truncal vagotomy and drainage, and is characterised by urgency, and occasionally faecal incontinence. The causes for this infrequent (though troublesome) postoperative diarrhoea are multifactorial; it may be attributed to the following factors:

1. Rapid gastric mechanical emptying following drainage procedure (gastrojejunostomy usually and pyloroplasty occasionally) due to bypass or damaged sphincter (removal of halting valve mechanism).
2. Dumping of hyperosmolar chyme from stomach into the intestine can result in osmotic diarrhoea, by shifting fluids from intestinal mucosal vessels into the lumen.
3. Post-vagotomy spasm of sphincter of Oddi will lead to gallbaldder overflow incontinence of bile. This continuous uncontrollable flow of unnecessary bile with bile salt malabsorption can irritate the large bowel, resulting in cathartic action.
4. Intestinal motility is functionally decreased following vagotomy; slowed peristalsis can lead to bacterial colonisation and overgrowth resulting in infective diarrhoea due to disturbed delicate balance of intestinal bacterial flora (with each other).
5. Vagotomy can induce (by a yet unknown mechanism) gastric and perhaps intestinal mucosal changes directly, similar to subtotal villous atrophy of coeliac disease (as confirmed by jejunal biopsies using special peroral capsule). This can result in a mini malabsorption state with associated diarrhoea.

Diagnosis is based on history and clinical manifestation. It must be differentiated from any correctable pathology, such as coeliac disease or blind loops.

Treatment is conservative by dietary adjustment (diet low in animal fat) and drugs, such as intestinal sedatives (e.g. lomotil

and codeine phosphate) and bile acid binding agents (e.g. cholestyramine). Surgery is indicated for severe intractable diarrhoea; surgical options include (Fig. 1.45.3):

- distal onlay reversed ileal graft, designed to create a passive, non-propulsive, 10–20 cm segment situated about 30 cm proximal to the caecum;
- Reversed jejunal segment: consists of the reversal of a 10–20 cm segment of jejunum about 100 cm distal to the ligament of Treitz. This may result in bacterial overgrowth, enterogastric reflux, postprandial colic and episodes of intestinal obstruction.

Other syndromes

Cancer after gastric surgery   Gastric stump carcinoma (after PG) varies from 0.4 to 8.9% with latency of 10–30 years. Aetiological factors include hypochondria and enterogastric reflux. Hypochlorhydria encourages bacterial overgrowth, including anaerobes converting ingested nitrates in food and drinking water into nitrites, which combine with ingested nitrosamines to form N-nitroso compounds. Enterogastric reflux can lead to formation of endogenous carcinogens by bacterial action on refluxed bile acids; it also promotes atrophic gastritis, intestinal metaplasia and dysplasia, which are all associated with gastric carcinoma. Gastric stump carcinoma is suspected in patients with recurrent ulcer or postgastrectomy syndromes 10 years after operation.

Diagnosis is established by endoscopy with multiple biopsy and brush cytology. *Treatment* is either radical excision of gastric remnant with extended lymphadenectomy, or palliative excision of tumour, depending on stage and time of diagnosis. The disease has a bleak outlook due to the aggressive nature of the lesion and late presentation. The need for endoscopic surveillance to screen for gastric stump cancer is probably justified, though controversial.

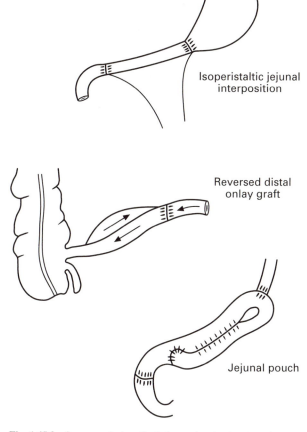

Isoperistaltic jejunal interposition

Reversed distal onlay graft

Jejunal pouch

Fig. 1.45.3 Some surgical methods for postgastrectomy syndromes

osis and jejuno-gastric intussusception. The risk factors include long, redundant afferent loop and inappropriate positioning of stoma. It may be acute, but more commonly chronic and intermittent.

Acute afferent loop obstruction presents with severe abdominal pain, vomiting, abdominal tenderness and occasionally upper abdominal mass. Plain abdominal X-ray, barium studies and abdominal ultrasound are needed before emergency laparotomy is carried out to relieve the obstruction.

Chronic afferent loop obstruction presents with intermittent episodes of epigastric fullness, abdominal pain (related to meals), and vomiting (bilious, projectile, and usually relieves the symptoms). It may also present as blind loop syndrome due to bacterial overgrowth.

Acute jejunogastric intussusception refers to herniation of jejunal loop into the stomach. Efferent loop is more frequently involved than afferent limb. It presents with severe epigastric pain, vomiting, haematemesis and palpable epigastric mass. Abdominal X-ray reveals soft tissue mass surrounded by gastric air. Emergency barium meal displays a coiled spring appearance in the gastric remnant. Endoscopy can confirm the diagnosis. Urgent surgery is required to avoid strangulation and gangrene, which are associated with high mortality.

Small stomach syndrome   This is encountered after extensive PG (> 75%). It may present with epigastric fullness, early satiety, abdominal pain, vomiting and weight loss. Food aggravates symptoms resulting in limited oral intake.

Treatment is conservative by increasing calorie intake, small frequent meals and elemental nutrition by tube feeding (Silk feeding tube). Surgery is indicated after failure of medical treatment; it involves reconstruction of the jejunal pouch and restoration of duodenal continuity.

Postsurgical gastroparesis   Though rare, the condition is disabling. It is gastric atony without mechanical obstruction, with prolonged gastric emptying. It is usually seen after TV without drainage or TV with PG. Patients may present with nausea, vomiting, postprandial pain and weight loss. Diagnosis is difficult and is made by exclusion.

Treatment is with drugs, such as bethanicol, metoclopramide and cisapride may help in gastric stasis. Surgery is indicated for those not responding to medical treatment. Options may include adding the drainage procedure in patients with TV, or performing a combined gastrectomy with reconstruction of jejunal pouch, or 50 cm Roux-en-Y jejunal loop.

Reflux oesophagitis   This may result from enterogastric reflux. Other common causes are gastric stasis and gastro-oesophageal incompetence (caused by excessive oesophageal mobilisation with damage to phreno-oesophageal membrane during gastric resection or vagotomy). For diagnosis and treatment, see s. 1.42 Reflux oesophagitis.

Extrinsic loop obstruction   This is rare and usually involves afferent loop; it is seen after truncal vagotomy and gastroenterostomy or Billroth II resection. Causes include internal herniation, kinking of anastomosis, adhesions, volvulus, sten-

Bezoars   Most bezoars are composed of undigested vegetables, fruit matter, or hair. They develop in the stomach or small intestine. Patients may have psychiatric problems. Presentation is non-specific, such as nausea, vomiting, epigastric fullness, pain, halitosis (foul breath) or early satiety. Complications include ulceration, bleeding, perforation, malnutrition and small bowel obstruction.

Treatment consists of oral enzymatic agents, e.g. cellulase to digest component fibres. Endoscopic crushing may be tried. Surgical extraction is reserved for failed medical therapy and complications; patients are advised to remain on a low fibre diet to avoid recurrence.

Cholelithiasis   Increased incidence of gallstones is reported after TV. It is debatable whether highly selective vagotomy or gastric resection alone predispose to gallstones. It is believed that truncal vagotomy causes increased resistance to flow of bile via the sphincter of Oddi, gallbladder dilatation and bile stasis.

Pulmonary tuberculosis   The acid defence barrier to combat infection is lost in gastrectomised patients who may have reactivation of latent focus due to diminished nutrition; they show slight but definite increased susceptibility to pulmonary tuberculosis.

Nutritional deficiency syndromes

Weight loss

Seen particularly after total and Polya gastrectomy, main causes of weight loss are inadequate calorie intake due to postprandial symptoms, poor appetite and early satiety (due to reduced gastric capacity). Other less important causes are bacterial overgrowth, fat malabsorption and increased small bowel transit. Weight loss can be prevented by adequate calorie intake with nutritional follow-up, and dietary education.

Anaemias

Anaemia is seen after PG as well as TV + D. Anaemia is commonly due to iron-deficiency and less commonly due to vitamin B_{12} and folate deficiency.

Iron-deficiency microcytic hypochromic anaemia occurs 10–20 years after gastric resection, affecting women more than men. Aetiology is multifactorial:
- impaired conversion of ferric iron in ingested food into ferrous (absorbable) state due to increased gastric pH;
- loss of gastric factor (gastroferrin) which facilitates iron absorption
- bypass of duodenum by gastric resection or gastrojejunostomy;
- diminished splitting of iron-protein binding complexes (iron carrier).

Iron-deficiency anaemia may not be nutritional, but caused by underlying reflux oesophagitis, recurrent ulcer and gastric carcinoma; these must be excluded therefore before starting the treatment. Prophylactic treatment with oral iron, 300 mg qds, is recommended in all patients after gastric resection or TV + GJ. Megaloblastic anaemia (due to lack of vitamin B_{12} and rarely to folate deficiency) may take many years to develop, because of large body stores of vitamin B_{12}. After total gastrectomy, vitamin B_{12} malabsorption is due to loss of intrinsic factor (abnormal Schilling test). Patients require vitamin B_{12} injections every 3 months. Following PG + TV, vitamin B_{12} deficiency is due to lack of acid that facilitates release of vitamin B_{12} bound to ingested food (normal Schilling test); treatment with oral crystalline vitamin B_{12} is adequate.

Folate deficiency is rare, but is seen occasionally after extensive surgery or inadequate dietary intake; it is treated by oral supplements.

Bone disease

Osteoporosis and osteomalacia are seen after total and Polya gastrectomy. These long-term sequelae are mainly due to diminished dietary intake or malabsorption of vitamin D and calcium. Hypocalcaemia, raised alkaline phosphatase, and radiological rarefaction usually predate clinical symptoms. Presentations include generalised bone pain, weakness from associated myopathy and stress fractures. Treatment is conservative, by improving nutrition and vitamin D supplements.

1.46 Stress Ulcer Prophylaxis

Stress-associated gut mucosal erosions (SAGME) are usually asymptomatic superficial multiple lesions in acid-producing mucosa (gastric body and fundus) in patients with no recent gut pathology who are subjected to physical stress, such as multiple trauma, head injury, major surgery, sepsis, severe burns, respiratory failure (defined as > 48 hours on a ventilator), failure of liver, or kidneys (risk factors for stress ulcer bleeding for patients in ICU); presence of coagulopathy remained significant on multivariate analysis. These lesions may be present on admission to ICU and can form within hours after stress. SAGME usually cause upper GIT bleeding which can be significant in 39.6% of cases at or after admission to ICU; in 37% of cases the bleeding is from more than one site. Average bleeding duration is 6 days.

SAGME are assessed directly by endoscopy. Traditionally, they also include:
- Curling ulcers (1842): classically are deep gastric or duodenal ulcers or both that bleed extensively and may perforate. Today, Curling ulcers describe multiple superficial erosions in the stomach of patients with 1/3 or more burn of the body surface.
- Cushing ulcers, in association with primary CNS trauma and surgery, are deep ulcers of the oesophagus, stomach, or duodenum associated with hypersecretion of gastric acid, pepsin and gastrin.
- Drug-induced ulcers are associated with ingestion of ethanol and administration of aspirin, other inhibitors of prostaglandin synthetase and glucocorticoids.
- Exacerbation of chronic acid-peptic disease may occur in a critical care setting with shallow or deep ulceration, and scarring, in the non-acid producing areas of the stomach (antrum) and duodenum (bulb).

Pathophysiology

The pathogenesis of stress ulceration is multifactorial; most mechanisms are speculative and include:
- Part of the endocrine/metabolic response to stress with stress triad: GIT erosions/ulcers, adrenal enlargement and atrophy of thymus, spleen and lymphoid follicles.
- Excess protons and pepsin in gut lumen.
- Bile reflux.
- Mucosal permeability.
- Mucosal ischaemia.
- Intramucosal alkalinisation.
- Broken mucus proton barrier.
- Prostaglandins (PGE_2 and PGI_2).
- Epithelial renewal defect.

Prevention of SAGME

Identification of patients at greater risk

This is essential, though some ICUs provide routine protection against SAGME to all patients admitted to ICU. Prevention currently is by antacids, H_2-antagonists or both (see below).

Drug prophylaxis

Antacids can prevent SAGME in most studies. Continuous intragastric infusions are more effective than hourly injections in maintaining consistently high intraluminal pH (by infusing 20–160 ml/h).

Antacids may be said to have a cytoprotective effect against NSAID (e.g. aspirin) damage. In routine SAGME prophylaxis, aluminium hydroxide gel or magnesium antacids, adjusted according to colonic output, may be given continuously with intermittent measurement of pH of aspirated luminal fluids.

Histamine H_2-receptor antagonists are also protective. Those now marketed include cimetidine, ranitidine, famotidine and nizatidine (others in clinical trials include ebrotidine, mifentidine, roxatidine, sufotidine, and zaltidine). In a meta-analysis of 16 trials in 2133 patients, the incidence of overt bleeding was 15% in those treated with placebo (702 patients), 3.3% in those given antacids (458 patients), and 2.7% in those given H_2-antagonists (402 patients). Infusion of H_2-antagonists are more effective with mechanical infusion devices. Cimetidine, up to 50 mg/h was more effective in maintaining gastric intraluminal pH > 4 than equivalent doses given as bolus injections.

Anacidity from antacids and H_2-antagonists compromises the antimicrobial activity of gastric acid. Enteric pathogens spread rapidly from stomach to trachea. Patients with consistent alkalinisation may be at greater risk of pneumonitis with these organisms. This risk of SAGME prophylaxis, resulting in tracheopulmonary colonisation with enteric bacteria, must be considered in prevention of nosocomial infection (pneumonia) in ICU seriously ill patients. Careful monitoring, intermittent gastric acidification by interrupting H_2-antagonist i.v. infusion occasionally (to permit transient acidity to sterilise the stomach), or prophylactic use of poorly absorbable antimicrobials (to minimise the risk of nosocomial pneumonia) may be considered.

Sucralfate is the basic aluminium salt of sucrose octasulphate; it does not raise intragastric pH (lesser suppression of gastric intraluminal acid). Its use is associated with a lower incidence of nosocomial pneumonia than therapy with antacids and H_2 antagonists. Nosocomial pneumonia was observed three times more often in patients on mechanical ventilation treated with antacids than in those receiving sucralfate. It is considered by many as the first choice of prophylaxis, since it is effective, cheap and has few side-effects; for high risk patients, a combination of sucralfate and cimetidine may be given (but unproven by studies).

Proton pump inhibitor, e.g. omeprazole, may produce long-lasting suppresion of gastric acidity; its role in SAGME is not yet identified.

Prostaglandin analogues, e.g. enprostil, misprost and enisoprost, are effective in preventing NSAID and aspirin gut damage.

Other agents of some useful value in SAGME prophylaxis include pirenzepine, allopurinol with dimethylsulfoxide (DMSO), cytoprotective drugs, epidermal growth factors, antimuscarinic agents, somatostatin, tranexamic acid and glucagon.

Enteral nutrition and resuscitation

The risk of stress ulcer bleeding is low in patients who are receiving enteral nutrition. This is not the result of a rise in intragastric pH, but due to improved mucosal gut barrier. There is increased awareness of the dangers of non-functioning gut and limitations of total parenteral nutrition encouraging clinicians to commence enteral nutrition (feeding) early, and this is very likely to further reduce the incidence of stress ulcer bleeding.

Furthermore, improvements in general management of critically ill patients have contributed to the reduced incidence of stress ulceration, particularly if shock and sepsis (major risk factors) are prevented. In one study, where intraluminal gastric mucosa pH (pHi) was measured, no bleeding occurred if pHi was maintained at > 7.24 (prophylaxis); patients with lower pHi were at risk of bleeding despite antacids therapy and successful alkalinisation of gastric contents (therapy).

1.47 Surgery for Chronic Inflammatory Bowel Disease

Colon concern and rectal bleeding clinics

In September 1992, Colon Concern, the campaign to promote greater awareness of colorectal disease and patient care, convened a round-table meeting of general practitioners, specialist physicians and surgeons to agree a set of objectives for management of bowel disease. Health care providers and purchasers need a blueprint for consultation; providers want to ensure the best treatment available for their patients; purchasers want to know the extent of the services required and the necessary budget allocation.

The objectives of Colon Concern were two-fold:
1. To enhance awareness of the need for early diagnosis of rectal bleeding.
2. To draw guidelines on diagnostic and clinical management so that high standards of care could be encountered throughout the United Kingdom.

Colon Concern recommendations

1. A campaign to educate the general public on the potentially serious nature of rectal bleeding and need for immediate investigation should be vigorously pursued.
2. It was agreed that an educational campaign for GPs would stress the importance of conducting a digital rectal examination on every patient presenting with rectal bleeding.
3. It was agreed that GPs should be encouraged to acquire rigid sigmoidoscopes and use them wherever the cause of rectal bleeding was not determined by digital examination; some GPs may wish to become trained to perform flexible sigmoidoscopy as well for their own and neighbouring GP practice clinics.
4. Referral for specialist opinion or further examination should be accomplished within 2 weeks. Hospital gastroenterology units should make provision for all patients with rectal bleeding

to be seen within 2 weeks. Fast-track clinics issuing appointments within 2 weeks are already available in some hospitals.

5. A system of shared care between GPs, specialists and patients should be encouraged in the management of bowel disease. Another concept is the 'Open Access Clinic or Direct Access Endoscopy' where patients need only obtain a letter of referral from their GPs, and then walk in for on-the-spot flexible sigmoidoscopy.

6. Patient-held cooperation cards are proposed as a means of keeping specialists, GPs and patients themselves informed as to what treatment and advice has been prescribed. The cards might detail investigations, results, current treatment (drug and dosage). Cards would possibly also include a diagrammatic representation showing the extent of the patient's disease to enable a check to be kept on its progression.

7. Local diagnosis and managment protocols were called for to ensure optimal 'shared care'.

Rectal bleeding clinics

Rectal bleeding is a common problem, with a prevalence of between 10 and 20% of the population in any 6-month period. It may be the only sign of serious large bowel disease, and hence the importance of rectal bleeding clinics.

Patient may either present with rectal bleeding or bloody diarrhoea. In rectal bleeding, PR examination, proctoscopy, rigid or flexible sigmoidoscopy with biopsy are the main outpatient diagnostic tools to diagnose rectal carcinoma, polyps and inflammatory bowel diseases (haemorrhoids are diagnosed on proctoscopy, while most cases of diverticular disease are diagnosed by flexible sigmoidoscopy/colonoscopy and/or barium enema). The patient is then referred to a colorectal surgeon for treatment. If no diagnosis is established and the patient is more than 45 years of age, then double contrast barium enema and/or colonoscopy is performed; if the patient is less than 45 years of age, he or she can be observed and once the rectal bleeding recurs, then barium enema and/or colonoscopy is performed.

In rectal diarrhoea, stool microscopy and cultures must initially be performed; if positive, then antimicrobial chemotherapy is instituted accordingly (e.g. in amoebic dysentry, metronidazole is the drug of choice). If the stool microscopy and cultures are negative and the diarrhoea resolves, then only observation is required; however, persistence or recurrence of bloody diarrhoea will be investigated as in rectal bleeding (see above).

MANAGEMENT PRINCIPLES

Ulcerative colitis

In ulcerative colitis, both the extent (total colitis, rectosigmoid colitis, or proctitis) and severity of colitis (mild/moderate or severe) must be determined before treatment. Acute severe colitis is defined as passage of more than six stools per day with blood and evidence of a systemic disturbance such as:
- fever (more than 38°C);
- tachycardia;
- anaemia;
- tender colon;
- hypoalbuminaemia (less than 30 g/l).

Total colitis patients have 19 times the risk of the general population of developing colorectal cancer; after having the disease for 20 years the highest incidence is around 10%. It is recommended that every patient with total colitis for 8 years or over should receive annual surveillance by colonoscopy and those with left-sided colitis should probably commence surveillance after 15 years of disease.

In mild/moderate colitis in acute episodes and for maintenance during remission one of the oral 5-amino salicylic acid (5-ASA) drugs or rectally administered steroids (prednisolone suppositories) or 5-ASA preparations is required. The 5-ASA drugs include the following:
- sulphasalazine is a combination of 5-ASA and sulphapyridine; the latter constituent is responsible for adverse effects in 5–50% of users such as rash, aplastic anaemia (and other blood disorders), azospermia (male infertility), and lupoid syndromes, in which case other 5-ASA drugs without a sulphapyridine constituent are preferred;
- balsalazide (Colazide);
- mesalazine is the 5-ASA itself (Asacol if coated, or Pentasa if slow release);
- olsalazine is composed of 2 molecules of 5-ASA bonded together which will separate in the large bowel (hence the name Dipentum); thus it is well tolerated by patients. However, it may cause diarrhoea in 10–20% of users.

One of the last-named drugs must be tried if the patient develops side-effects to sulphasalazine; however, all drugs retain side-effects profiles associated with the 5-ASA moiety, such as diarrhoea, nausea, headache, salicylate hypersensitivity, and interstitial nephritis and reversible pancreatitis.

High doses of 5-ASA drugs, high-dose corticosteroids and bland diet (non-fibre diet such as varieties of meat, dairy products, eggs, tea, coffee, clear soups, soft drinks) are the mainstay of treatment in acute colitis. Preventing toxic dilatation is a more urgent consideration that a clinician's worry about the side-effects of steroids (steroids, however, are to be avoided where possible in the maintenance of remission, because of side-effects).

In severe colitis, hydrocortisone or prednisolone enema or suppositories (Predenema and Predsol) for localised rectal disease will induce remission; foam preparations (hydrocortisone Colifoam and Predfoam) are useful in patients with difficulty retaining liquid enemas. More extensive disease requires oral corticosteroids and severe extensive or fulminant disease needs hospital admission and i.v. prednisolone 40–60 mg in the morning daily (reduced over 4 weeks). In resistant cases, cyclosporin A 4 mg/kg may be tried but with no proven benefit (it represents a minor addition to therapy acting through interference with immune response by stopping proliferation of colitis antigen-primed T cells which normally produces interleukin-2 which, via positive feedback, causes T-cell proliferation to produce more antigen-primed T-cells).

However, in chronic active ulcerative colitis unresponsive to 5-ASA in patients reluctant to lose their colons, azathioprine 2 mg/kg/day can be given together with systemic steroids to maintain the disease in remission. Azathioprine may cause nausea in high doses (requires gradual dose increase) and rarely may lead to a toxic shock syndrome-like condition with hypotension and diarrhoea.

Antimotility drugs such as codeine and loperamide should not be used in severe colitis as they can precipitate paralytic ileus and megacolon; they have limited value in mild disease too. For similar reasons, antispasmodics should not be used in ulcerative colitis. Paradoxically, in proctitis some surgeons advocate high-fibre diet and bulk-forming laxatives (e.g. methylcellulose) to facilitate bowel movement through inflamed rectum.

If the patient shows no signs of improvement, surgery should be considered early, before the patient becomes severely malnourished or toxic. If they are treated with high-dose steroids and 5-ASA drugs, they should show improvement within 48 hours; if there is no improvement at this time then surgery should be performed. Similarly, if they have not gone into remission after a week (judging by above criteria of severe acute colitis), surgery should be considered.

About 20–25% of patients with acute severe colitis will not go into remission (no response is demonstrated with no medical control of disease activity); they will need surgery (total colectomy with ileostomy and rectal mucous fistula, total proctocolectomy and ileostomy, or restorative proctocolectomy with ileoanal pouch, or total colectomy with ileorectal anastomosis).

Crohn's disease

In Crohn's disease, roughly 50% of patients have both terminal ileal and colonic or anal disease; 25% have small bowel disease; and 25% have colonic disease only; and a small number of patients have perianal disease, perhaps with fistulation into the vagina or around the sphincter. While Crohn's disease can be viewed as an immunological disorder of intestinal mucosa, recent research suggested that many cases of Crohn's disease may be due to atypical mycobacterial infection (there is a striking similarity with ileocaecal tuberculosis, but as yet anti-tuberculous treatment remains experimental).

The treatment particularly of colonic disease is similar to that for ulcerative colitis (toxic dilatation, though rare, may occur in colonic Crohn's disease). In small bowel disease, 5-ASA drugs are of doubtful value. Oral prednisolone suppresses the inflammation, and metronidazole may be beneficial, possibly through antibacterial activity for overgrowth. Cholestyramine and aluminium hydroxide mixture bind unabsorbed bile salts (which themselves have cathartic action) and provide symptomatic relief of diarrhoea following ileal disease or resection and bacterial colonisation of the small bowel. In both colitis and Crohn's disease general nutritional care and appropriate supplements are essential. Maintenance therapy in chronically active disease should include mesalazine and immunosuppressives (azathioprine and 6-mercaptopurine). Steroids have no role in maintenance therapy.

Thrombotic complications after surgery are much more frequent in patients with Crohn's disease and anticoagulant prophylaxis is essential. Anastomotic breakdown, disease recurrence and malnutrition following bowel resection are all potential problems.

There is no evidence that performing an anastomosis through affected tissue is dangerous; the biggest danger is to operate on a patient who is malnourished and it is important to get the patient in the best nutritional state prior to surgery. Similarly, there is no evidence that steroids affect breakdown of the anastomosis. In order to protect against 'short-bowel' syndrome, if resection is necessary (e.g. for fistula or perforation) only the affected area should be resected. Provided there is no distal obstruction then any breakdown with fistula formation will eventually close. Stricturoplasty is the accepted treatment for strictures, even those of up to 15–20 cm in length, and is better than resection. Results are good, even long stricturoplasty will show normal appearance on barium study in 1–2 years. Even short strictures close together are better converted into one long stricturoplasty.

As a general principle in Crohn's disease, the surgeon must only deal with the area giving problems, even if other areas have disease. Patients with Crohn's disease will often have 3–5 operations in their lifetime. Recurrences will occur whether all macroscopic disease is removed or not and these recurrences will often respond to medical therapy. The surgeon should never leave stenosed bowel and one should always do a stricturoplasty; a Foley's catheter passed along the bowel lumen will detect strictures which are not obvious to external examination. Above all, the general principle for all inflammatory bowel diseases is to 'do a safe operation'. If in doubt, bring the ends of the bowel out to the surface. Once the patient's nutrition is improved and everything is under control, definitive surgery can be planned. Most of the complications of surgery in Crohn's disease occur through surgeons trying to do that little bit more rather than doing the minimum necessary to treat the complications. Finally, dietician plays an essential role in postoperative management, the role is similar to that of the physiotherapist and stoma nurse in abdominal surgery.

SURGICAL MANAGEMENT

Ulcerative colitis

Indications for surgery

- Chronic: stricture and carcinoma.
- Acute: bleeding, perforation, toxic megacolon and obstruction.
- Extraintestinal manifestations, e.g. eye, joints and skin: ameliorated by surgery.
- Intractability: in spite of medical treatment in chronic recurrent cases (salazopyrine, bland diet, diarrhoea control and steroid retention enema) and in acute cases (i.v. fluid replacement, parenteral feeding, i.v. prednisolone 60 mg/24 h, blood transfusion and twice daily steroid retention enema).

Surgical options (Fig. 1.47.1)

Proctocolectomy and ileostomy
- Most widely used.
- Complete excision of entire colonic mucosa.
- No risk of recurrence or stump carcinoma.
- Impaired sexual function in some patients.
- Ileostomy for life but it is well managed by young patients and the adherent stoma bag is followed up by a stoma therapist.

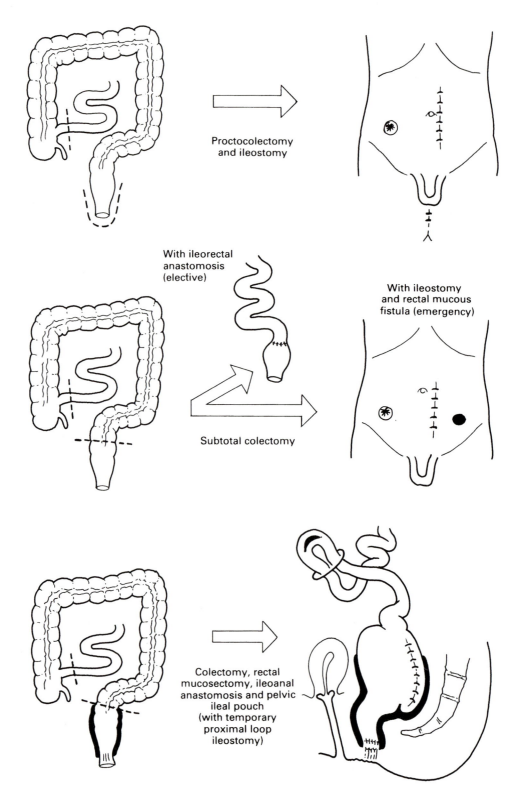

Fig. 1.47.1   Surgical options in ulcerative colitis

Subtotal colectomy and ileorectal anastomosis
- Increasingly used operation particularly in the UK.
- Incomplete excision of colonic mucosa.
- Risk of recurrence and carcinoma in rectal mucosa.
- Life-long sigmoidoscopic and rectal biopsy follow-up.
- No ileostomy and no sexual function impairment.
- Loose stools in some patients (mean frequency of 3.5/24 h, range of 1–6/24 h).

Colectomy, ileostomy and rectal mucous fistula
- Performed in emergency situations.
- Incomplete excision of colonic mucosa.
- Safe emergency operation as it is less extensive and can achieve remission via diversion of faecal stream.
- Retains the option of a subsequent restorative procedure such as subtotal colectomy and ileorectal anastomosis.

Proctocolectomy and Kock's continent ileostomy
- Similar to proctocolectomy and ileostomy with complete excision of entire colonic mucosa.
- 'Mini' stoma requiring regular catheterisation.
- Such a reservoir stoma with an intussuscepted nippled valve could become dilated with contents, or could malfunction and produce incontinence (leakage).

Colectomy, rectal mucosectomy, ileoanal anastomosis and pelvic ileal pouch
- Complete excision of entire colonic mucosa.
- No risk of recurrence or cancer.
- Temporary loop ileostomy for 6–8 weeks (to protect the ileoanal anastomosis), but no permanent stoma and no psychological trauma (in young man concerned about sex and marriage).
- Continence is maintained by anal sphincters.
- Sexual function is intact.
- Probably the most promising operation of the future.

The pelvic ileal pouch is constructed either by a J-shaped anastomosis using a stapler or by a triple S-shaped sutured anastomosis. Removal of the rectal mucosal cuff down to the dentate line followed by anastomosis may lead to infection and anastomotic dehiscence – therefore routine ileostomy protection is needed. Postoperative diarrhoea may be troublesome and anastomotic stricture may be marked requiring dilatation.

Crohn's disease

Indications for surgery

- Anal manifestations, i.e. abscesses, fistulae and strictures.
- Intestinal obstruction, haemorrhage and perforation (perforation is rare because of transmural thickening).
- Extraintestinal manifestations, i.e. uveitis, recurrent polyarthritis and pyoderma gangrenosa.
- Failure of medical measures to suppress the active disease or to aid healing of anal lesions (i.e. salazopyrine, steroids, azothioprine, correction of anaemia and hypoproteinaemia; control of diarrhoea by low-fibre bland diet and administration of codeine, lomotil and cholestyramine to overcome the cathartic action of non-absorbed bile salts on the colon).

Surgical options

Gastroduodenal disease
Gastroenterostomy or duodenoenterostomy with vagotomy are indicated only in severe stenosis (never resect).

Small bowel disease
Crohn's disease is precancerous and has a tendency to recur. Therefore, resection is generally better than exclusion surgery. Resection also avoids the risk of the blind loop syndrome. However, resection should be restricted to the diseased segment in order to leave the small bowel for normal absorption and secretion:
- Resection (including lymph nodes) is performed in complicated Crohn's disease, i.e. obstruction, abscess, fistula, perforation, bleeding and carcinoma.
- Resection should always be avoided in diffuse small bowel disease and in acute florid non-obstructive ileal disease. Acute ileitis may be due to *Yersinia enterocolitis* and even if not recurrence is rare if acute ileitis is treated medically.
- Emergency appendicectomy can be performed if the caecum is intact, since postoperative fistulae are rare.
- If both the terminal ileum and caecum ± appendix are involved by the chronic process then ileocaecal resection (limited right hemicolectomy) is done.
- In multiple skip lesions if intervening segments of macroscopically healthy bowel are less than 10 cm apart they can be sacrificed and if the segment is less than 20 cm from the ileocaecal valve then resection should include the caecum.
- If longer segments of intervening bowel are present, multiple small resections or frequent stricturoplasty may be indicated.

Large bowel disease
The indications are less precise here:
- Defunctioning loop ileostomy: in the hope that colonic disease will be improved by faecal diversion in acute active colonic disease not responding to medical treatment.
- Defunctioning split ileostomy: Faecal diversion is better than the above.
- Colectomy and ileorectal anastomosis: there is a risk of recurrence in rectal mucosa and life-long sigmoidoscopic and barium follow-up is required.
- Proctocolectomy.
- Abdominoperineal excision of rectum.

Perineal disease
- Drainage of abscesses.
- Strictures dilated.
- Fistulae are left alone (spontaneous healing occurs in 50% of cases).
- However, low fistulae could be laid open safely.

1.48 Restorative Proctocolectomy or Ileoanal Reservoir Anastomosis

Ileoanal reservoir anastomosis, preferably called restorative proctocolectomy (RP), is now the operation of choice for ulcerative colitis and familial adenomatous polyposis.

Stages of restorative proctocolectomy

RP is usually performed in two stages.

1. *Colectomy*, with upper rectal excision, mucosal proctectomy of most distal rectal segment (preferably carried out via abdomen than per anum), creation of ileal reservoir, and pouch–anal anastomosis protected by proximal loop ileostomy.

Mucosectomy is now being replaced by extending the rectal excision down to the transitional zone 1.5 cm above dentate line and stapling it via the abdomen with linear stapler 30 or 52, using PI (3 M) or GIA reusable staplers, then using anvil and circular stapler to staple ileal reservoir to anal stump per anum. Alternatively, the anal stump can be manually sutured (with or without inversion) to the ileal reservoir.

2. *Loop ileostomy is closed*. In toxic megacolon, however, or indeterminate colitis (doubt exists whether colitis is due to ulcerative colitis or Crohn's disease), a preliminary colectomy with terminal end ileostomy and rectal stump preservation as either mucous fistula, or as a Hartmann's type procedure (rectum closed and left inside pelvis), converts the procedure into *three-stage-operation*, allowing for more definitive histological examination. Furthermore, in severe ulcerative colitis and patients on systemic steroids a three-stage procedure is in the patient's best interest. Neither low albumin levels nor steroid intake were in isolation predictors of increased complication rates (pelvic abscess and intestinal obstruction); however, in conjunction they were powerful predictors of a poor outcome.

The *single-stage operation*, without loop ileostomy cover, has been used in polyposis coli and colitis patients who have already undergone colectomy or are not receiving oral steroid therapy (interferes with wound healing), particularly if patients are young (though not widely recommended).

Absolute indications

1. Ulcerative colitis.
2. Familial adenomatous polyposis (FAP).

Relative indications sometimes include:
3. Indeterminate colitis.
4. Multiple colon cancer.

Very controversial is the role of RP in:
5. Certain types of severe, disabling constipation.
6. Megarectum/megacolon.

Prerequisites for RP with ileal pouch–anal anastomosis

1. Good sphincter tone.
2. No toxic colitis.
3. No Crohn's disease.
4. No cancer in the lower third of rectum.
5. No desmoid tumour in the mesentery of the small bowel.
6. The patient is fully informed about the operation.

Contraindications

Absolute

1. Poor sphincter tone. Incontinence as reported by the patient is usually due to urgency and significant rectal inflammation and diarrhoea. Therefore, this is not per se a contraindication to pouch surgery. However, one will take a careful history relating to trauma (obstetric, sphincterotomy), evacuation disorder, spinal injury or surgery, diabetes and assessment of sphincteric tone clinically (per rectal examination) and manometrically (more reliable).

2. Toxic state/megacolon. In toxic megacolon, subtotal colectomy with ileostomy and rectal fistula (rectum is preserved) is the safest option, allowing for pathological evaluation of resected colon and it can later be converted into an ileoanal reservoir anastomosis when the disease is controlled, toxicity settles down and the patient is well and off steroid therapy. In some cases of toxic megacolon, loop ileostomy and blow hole colostomy technique is particularly helpful in being simple, quick in a very toxic patient, and allows control of the disease very well, following which elective ileoanal reservoir anastomosis can be made. Emergency proctocolectomy and ileostomy is never indicated as it is associated with high mortality.

However, when megacolon toxicity, such as tachycardia, active colonic bleeding, mild leucocytosis, requirement of large doses of steroids, albumin level < 30 gm/l, low-grade fever, is mild or these signs are present singly, the experienced pouch surgeon may choose to proceed with RP (with covering loop ileostomy), and usually this can be done safely.

3. Cancer in the lower third of rectum. The procedure of choice here is proctocolectomy and ileostomy (whether usual spouting incontinent ileostomy or Cock's continent pouch ileostomy) (*see below*).

4. Crohn's disease and diagnostic dilemma. Crohn's disease is a contraindication to RP. Yet the diagnosis is not always easy to make. Ileal disease, granulomas demonstrated on biopsy, patchy distribution of colitis, aphthous or deeply penetrating linear ulcers, cobblestoning, indurated skin tags and anal fistulas are major 'red flags' (contraindications to proceed). In the absence of the above features, while typical ulcerative colitis appearance is lacking, one may still proceed with RP, but long-term outcome for such '*indeterminate colitis*' is still to be determined.

Alternatively, and for patients keen on RP, a staged operation of subtotal colectomy allows for pathological evaluation of the resected specimen and future conversion to RP.

5. Mesenteric desmoid (found in FAP). This will usually prevent adequate reach of a pouch to anus. Ileorectal anastomosis is then preferred. For patients with extensive polyposis in upper rectum with few polyps in the lower third colectomy, partial proctectomy and ileal J-pouch–low rectal anastomosis can be made.

6. The patient with few or no concerns about a permanent ileostomy – this is likely in patients over 50 years of age – can be strongly recommended total proctocolectomy and ileostomy (the gold standard).

Relative

7. Previous small bowel surgery. Adhesions and bowel shortening may make construction of a pouch and its low anastomosis diametrically difficult if not impossible.
8. Aged patient. While IPAA is inferior in those over 50 compared to those under 50 years, surgeons have performed the procedure in patients over 60 with apparently good results. Physiological age is more important than chronological age, but still manometric studies must confirm the clinical impression of good sphincter before embarking on IPAA.
9. Metastatic cancer. Ileorectal anastomosis is the preferred option.
10. Obesity and a narrow pelvis. The experienced surgeon can still perform RP and IPAA. Alternatively, colectomy and ileostomy (to allow steroid withdrawal and weight reduction before later performance of IPAA), or proctocolectomy and ileostomy, or even colectomy and ileorectal anastomosis, can all be technically easier to perform.
11. Anal fistula. In most cases, perianal or anovaginal fistula are features of Crohn's disease. Yet, provided histological, endoscopic and clinical work-up strongly favour the diagnosis of ulcerative colitis, one is prepared to do IPAA in rare circumstances, such as low fistula, and only after prior warning to the patient of the possible sequelae.
12. Co-existing severe illness.
13. FAP with few (< 20) rectal polyps.
14. Colonic haemorrhage.

Additionally, for the stapled IPAA, in which the anal transitional zone is preserved, the following should also be considered contraindications:

Absolute

– rectal dysplasia;
– colorectal cancer;
– likely poor follow-up compliance.

Relative

– extraintestinal manifestations of ulcerative colitis. These commonly respond to proctocolectomy.

Despite the above contraindications, the majority of patients with ulcerative colitis are suitable for surgery in the form of RP or IPAA. Indeed, 80–90% of all surgically treated causes of ulcerative colitis have undergone RP in recent years.

Surgical techniques

Pouch shapes and construction (Figs. 1.48.1, 1.48.2)

The S-shaped triplicated pouch was originally introduced with great optimism. However, the inability to evacuate the S-pouch spontaneously has always been the Achilles heel of the triplicated reservoir. Realisation that long efferent limbs were the major reason for poor evacuation has instigated modifications with shorter pouch outlets, but even then, there is still a small though significant incidence of catheterisation. Thereafter, the introduction of a duplicated J-pouch (constructed as

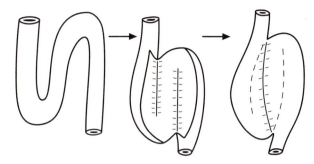

Fig. 1.48.1 Construction of triplicated ileal reservoir

isoperistaltic double-barrelled reservoir with equal limbs 2 × 15 cm) resulted in functional stability attained in the shortest time (as compared to other designs), soiling was not problematic and evacuation was always spontaneous.

The quadruple W-pouch (4 × 12 cm) was introduced later, but like the S-pouch (3 × 7.5 cm), the obstruction of the efferent limb of the pouch remained a problem as only 41% of W-pouches could evacuate spontaneously; it may also be technically difficult to place it within the pelvis and anastomose it to the anus. Interestingly, intraoperative volumes of reservoirs were 325 ml (W), 177 ml (S), and 172 ml (J) as compared with 322 ml (W), 416 ml (S) and 197 ml (J) respectively when measured after ileostomy closure; increasing the volume of the ileoanal reservoir results in improved functional performance, particularly to frequency and nocturnal evacuation. Functional outcome, however, is dependent on the lack of damage to the anal sphincter mechanism (while creating ileal pouch–anal anastomosis, as proven manometrically by postoperative pressure studies of anal sphincter) rather than the size or the shape of the pouch (J, or S, or W-pouches, though J-pouch is widely recommended). With attention to internal anal sphincter, the surgeon may guarantee good faecal control and a comparative lack of any incontinence or seepage in the majority of patients even if they are over 60 years of age.

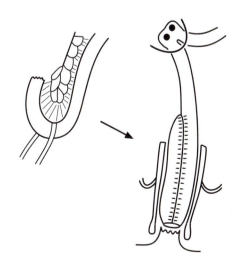

Fig. 1.48.2 Construction of J-pouch

Pouches can either be hand-sewn or stapled using a linear stapler via apical enterome and purse-string prior to circular stapler application; after firing the pouch is telescoped over the gun which then can be fired once more up to 4 times (a stapled pouch can also be performed using multiple enterotomies). The same apical site is also used for ileoanal anastomosis. As there are no hand-sewn enterotomies, stapled pouch incidence of leak is less, there is no septum within the pouch and, like stapled anastomoses, it is faster to construct.

Rectal cuffs and mucousal proctectomy

Long rectal cuffs were thought important initially to improve continence by preserving receptors in perirectal tissues, but very acceptable functional results can be achieved with short rectal cuffs. Furthermore, a long rectal cuff may require abdominal mucosectomy. Mucosal proctectomy (stripping of rectal mucosa preferably with prior injection of 1/200 000 diluted adrenaline solution) can be performed abdominally (from above) or endoanally (from below), or after rectal stump eversion from below.

Haemostasis of bleeding points must be secured meticulously with diathermy, since any haematoma between rectal cuff and pouch may be a cause of prolonged postoperative sepsis resulting in poor functional outcome. Currently, rectal excision down to transitional anal canal with double stapled technique is proving effective and becoming increasingly popular.

Ileoanal anastomosis

This is usually performed by endoanal hand-sewn full-thickness anastomosis using 10–15 interrupted 2/0 vicryl sutures; the pouch apex (preferably with the catheter inside) is grasped with tissue forceps or pulled through to the perineum (with 4 stay sutures inserted into the pouch) without twisting of, or tension on, the pouch. If there is no apical enterotomy, this can be created by a simple slit, cruciate incision or excision of a small elipse. In current practice peranal anastomosis can be stapled with a circular stapler applied and fired at the anorectal ring after conventional mucosal proctectomy; a purse-string suture may be inserted into the denuded rectal stump, performed from above, or from below (endoanally or after rectal eversion). Alternatively, the rectum can be transversely stapled and transected with a linear stapler (e.g. TA55 or ILA52) to avoid the need for a purse-string, then a new Premium EEA circular stapler or Roticulator is used through the suture line of the rectal stump closing the pouch to the rectal stump before firing to complete ileoanal anastomosis. This double-stapled technique may leave an area of rectal mucosa above the dentate line. The hand-sewn method may damage the anal sphincter by manual dilatation, eversion and hand manipulation resulting in poor functional outcome (faecal incontinence). The stapled technique (particularly, double-stapling) produces better functional results, since the stapler is used without the need for anal dilatation, with less incidence of pelvic abscess and stricture formation when compared with the hand-sewn method; the good functional outcome in elderly patients outweighs any potential long-term disadvantages of leaving a residual rectal mucosa.

Surgical procedure with emphasis on double-stapled technique

In performing colectomy on the right side, it is important to maintain the ileal branch of the ileocolic artery. Terminal ileum is transected flush with the ileocaecal junction. Previously, concern as to inability to bring the pouch down to the anus led to division of mesenteric vessels, which may be unnecessary. Individual colonic vessels are ligated and divided in midsection without the need of dissecting them out to their origin. Higher up in the pelvis, a total mesorectal excision (TME) is recommended to remove the shelter mesorectum of a potentially premalignant disease with better haemostasis, clearance and technical access to the lower rectum after removing its mesorectal tissues (it should look like a buttock or baby's bottom); one should be well forward of the sacral promontory to avoid damage to sympathetic nerves (presacral nerves). Within the pelvis the dissection will then be kept very close to the rectum on both sides to avoid damage to the parasympathetic nerves in lateral ligaments and to keep well behind the seminal vesicles to avoid damage to final common pathway of these nerves for bladder and sexual function.

It is important to dissect all of the rectum down to the levators circumferentially to the point where retrorectal mesentery disappears as the rectum passes through the levator mechanism. At this point the rectum is closed shut with a PI 30 mm stapler or 52 stapler-3 M as low as possible and with the aid of a perineal operator with a finger in the rectum making sure that that stapled closure is literally 1 cm from the dentate line. The specimen can then be removed and haemostasis can be secured totally in the pelvis.

The ileum should be mobilised right up to the pancreas to gain as much length into the pelvis as possible. A loop of ileum which will adequately reach to the pelvis is then selected for the apex of the J-pouch. There is no set size or distance, but most commonly it is 15 cm in length (occasionally 18 cm). Using a double-stapled technique, the pouch does not have to go down as far as it does by performing transanal ileoanal anastomosis. Tension is not a problem with double-stapling, and the pouch should reach in every patient without major difficulty.

The pouch is constructed by creating an enterostomy at the apex of the selected ileal limb; two linear firings of a ILA 100 stapler are adequate to make the pouch (haemostasis is usually good). The pouch is tested by distending it with an injection of Betadine solution. A purse-string suture is then placed in the apex of the pouch and the detachable head of a CEEA 28 mm stapler is placed in the pouch and the purse-string tied. With the aid of the perineal operator, the CEEA stapler is inserted into the anal canal with the spike withdrawn. The spike is then advanced through the central point of the stapled rectal stump to reach the pelvis; the spike is withdrawn and the pouch is clicked into place with the detachable head into stapler shaft. The stapler is then closed, fired and removed without difficulty. The pouch is tested with intrarectal Betadine and/or air proctoscopically following digital examination to confirm the adequacy of the anastomosis.

Faecal diversion by proximal spouting temporary loop ileostomy is preferably created as close to the pouch as possible without tension through a preoperatively marked site in the right rectus muscle. Following full haemostasis, the abdomen is closed with or without pelvic suction drainage, and the loop ileostomy is constructed over a rod. The anstomotic leak is low, with minimal pelvic sepsis or stricture formation, and the patient is continent.

The average distance of anastomosis from the dentate line is 1 cm in females and 1.5 cm in males; this does mean leaving some cells of ulcerative colitis or FAP rectal mucosa, and biopsy is required for subsequent elective cauterisation of residual mucosa, which may be needed one year or more postoperatively should the biopsy reveal a positive result. Postoperatively, the patient is better decompressed with an intra-pouch Foley's catheter, urinary catheter and antibiotics.

Malignancy and pouch surgery

Colorectal adenocarcinoma has been discovered in resected specimens from patients undergoing ileoanal reservoir surgery; Kaposi's sarcoma has also been reported in a resected specimen for a HIV-negative ulcerative colitis patient undergoing pouch surgery. In the Mayo clinic study (1985), 518 ileoanal reservoir operations were performed over 5 years and 17 of these patients (3.3%) had a co-existing carcinoma. Of those 17 patients, 13 were colitis patients with an average history of 16 years while 4 had polyposis coli. Hospital stay was slightly prolonged compared with non-malignant cases, and postoperative morbidity, especially due to intestinal obstruction, was increased. In another series of 177 patients undergoing ileoanal anastomosis with endorectal pull-through, 7% had colorectal cancers at the time of operation.

These reports conclude that if the principles of radical surgery can be adhered to with complete excision of rectal mucosa, then RP is not contraindicated should a carcinoma be found; and hence the emphasis on total mesorectal excision during RP. However, the necessity for conventional mucous proctectomy over retaining the whole anal canal and transition zone has been questioned and the standard stapled pouch–anal anastomosis with retention of the whole anal canal transitional zone mucosa intact can result in improved continence with better sampling (discrimination between fluid and flatus) over mucosal proctectomy.

On the other side, colo-anal sleeve anastomosis for both benign and malignant lesions was performed by the late Sir Alan Parks, but as with straight ileo-anal anastomosis, and low anterior resection (sphincter-saving), faecal urgency was severe, frequency excessive and the patient was rendered semi-incontinent despite the sphincter preservation (**anterior resection syndrome**). It has been considered that the lack of any pelvic capacitance organ may be responsible for the poor results.

A pelvic pouch constructed from colon has therefore been proposed and reported in many recent studies. This endoanal J-shaped (2 × 10 cm) colonic pouch–anal anastomosis can be protected by a temporary transverse colostomy. The functional results of colonic pouch–anal anastomosis are better and more predictable than straight coloanal anastomosis.

Complications

The complexities of the technique, the nature and severity of underlying disease and therapeutic modalities employed prior to surgery have all contributed to a significant number of complications. These are either non-pouch-specific, or pouch-specific complications; the latter affect 10% of patients and can even endanger the viability of the reservoir, leading ultimately to pouch removal in 6% of cases. Thus the operation is successful in 94% of patients (irrespective of complications) with a failure rate of 6% only requiring excision of pouch and/ or establishment of a permanent ileostomy. In Mayo Clinic experience with more than 1300 operations, the operation is safe, with a low 0.2% mortality; in contrast, the morbidity is significant, ranging between 15 and 55% (average 30%).

The most frequent causes of failure have been pelvic sepsis, poor functional results (gross incontinence at night and/or frequent stools), later appearance of granulomatous disease, and, very rarely, recurrent recalcitrant pouchitis (2% of all failures). All failures have occurred in ulcerative colitis patients, suggesting that earlier referral of less ill patients and careful selection of patients are paramount to ultimate successful outcome. Salvage operations for pouch-specific complications are safe; none of the reoperated patients has died. However, the risk of further complications and reoperations including pouch excision is high, and should not be undertaken unless the surgeon has already gained considerable experience in primary construction of ileal pouch–anal anastomosis. Meticulous technique and timely intervention and reoperation of pouch-specific complications should minimise the risk of operative failure.

Non-pouch-specific complications

Small bowel obstruction is the most common complication seen in 15% of patients. In half the patients, the obstruction will resolve spontaneously, but other patients will require surgical intervention. Other non-pouch-specific complications include wound infection in 3%, transient urinary retention in 5%, sexual impotence in men in 1.5% and dyspareunia in women in 7%.

Pouch-specific complications and management

These may be categorized as strictures, perianal sinus–fistula–abscess formation (due to anastomotic leak), pelvic fistula–abscess formation (due to anastomotic leak, but also disease-related), unsatisfactory function, pouchitis and other complications.

Strictures Stenosed ileoanal anastomosis can be observed either before or after closure of temporary ileostomy. When the patient returns for closure of ileostomy, a per rectal examining finger may feel a short, soft web of tissue at the anastomosis; this is an asymptomatic benign stricture that can be treated with digital dilatation at the time of ileostomy closure. True anastomotic stricture is observed after ileostomy closure, and is often long, dense, non-pliable and more difficult to treat even by reoperation. The association of perianastomotic sepsis may also result in fibrosis and loss of compliance of pelvic floor structures. Though simple dilatation can prevent progress in some, the majority (60%) are recurrent and will need repeated dilatation or even operation. The surgeon may elect to excise the strictured segment peranally, advancing and sewing the pouch mucosa distally to the dentate line, or totally mobilise the pelvic reservoir, via an abdominal approach, excising the strictured segment and reanastomosing the repaired pouch to anal canal mucosa. In either method, great care must be taken to avoid damaging the internal sphincter. Satisfactory functional results can be achieved in 69% of patients; in 14%, however, pouch excision is required.

Perianal sinus/fistula/abscess formation   Pouchography may reveal asymptomatic radiological sinus prior to ileostomy closure. Such sinuses represent incomplete anastomotic healing and are simply managed by deferring ileostomy closure.

True pouch–perianal and pouch–vaginal fistulas have been reported in 5% of patients, and only in ulcerative colitis patients. Pouch–perianal fistula is usually associated with low-grade fever, perineal or low back pain, and intermittent purulent drainage. Surgical management includes fistulotomy, dilatation of anastomotic stricture, re-establishment of a diverting ileostomy and, commonly, good local drainage with antibiotics. Some low, readily accessible abscesses may also be amenable to CT-guided drainage. Satisfactory functional results were achieved in 70% of such complications. Postoperative complications, however, occurred in over two-thirds of these patients, and ultimately 17% of them have to have their reservoir removed.

Pelvic abscess/fistula formation and anastomotic leak   This is a feared complication of pouch–anal anastomosis and is the most significant prognostic factor influencing ultimate functional outcome after RP. Anastomotic dehiscence varies from 1% to 8%. The complication rate increases with the frequency of emergency procedures or performance of more complicated designs. Pelvic sepsis is more common in patients who are underweight, or suffering with malignancy or systemic toxicity preoperatively; it is more serious in female patients. It is also a disease-related complication, as it is observed after ileoanal anastomosis for ulcerative colitis and not for FAP. Major symptoms include fever, peritonitis and pelvic or low back pain; leucocytosis is often present. Pouchography may demonstrate a fistula behind the reservoir; CT scan may help define the nature of the infectious process and whether it is amenable to CT-guided drainage.

Treatment usually requires abscess drainage via the abdominal route. Care must be taken not to disrupt pouch integrity, and if ileostomy has been previously taken down (closed), it should be re-established. If loop ileostomy is in place but with incomplete faecal diversion, the loop ileostomy should be converted into an end ileostomy. Complications after surgical treatment of pelvic abscess are frequent and may include recurrent intra-abdominal abscesses, intra-abdominal fistulas, and stricture. About 59% of these patients will require further operation, and eventually 34% of pouches need to be excised.

Unsatisfactory function   These patients include those with:
- Faecal incontinence or seepage, most likely due to damage to the internal anal sphincter during the construction of the ileoanal anastomosis. Overflow incontinence may also be

related to too small or too large a reservoir. Partial or total reservoir reconstruction may be necessary. Recurrent pouchitis can also be associated with poor neorectal emptying.
- Poor neorectal emptying due to long afferent limb after construction of S-shaped, or W-shaped (H-shaped) pouch. Some of these patients may require shortening or total amputation of the afferent limb, or even reservoir excision with construction of a new reservoir (if technically feasible) via an abdominal approach.
- Obstruction secondary to J-pouch septum. Transanal transection of septum can usually be performed easily with a GIA stapler.
- Outlet obstruction due to mucosal prolapse.

Salvage operations for pouch-specific complications are safe, but the risk of further complications is high and 20% of reservoirs will need to be excised. Satisfactory functional results can be achieved in 60% of these patients; of these 70% can be expected to have a stool frequency and continence similar to those without complications after pouch construction.

Pouchitis (15%)   This is clinically characterised by sudden onset of watery and sometimes bloody diarrhoea, low abdominal cramps, urgency, malaise, anorexia, fever and rarely uveitis, arthralgia and erythema nodosum, reminiscent of the ulcerative colitis the patient experienced preoperatively. As such, pouchitis is considered a temporary dysfunctional failure of the operation. Patients with ulcerative colitis, especially those with extracolonic manifestations, are at great risk, while those with ulcerative colitis alone are at lesser risk. Pouchitis is very rare in FAP patients, and therefore must be considered as ulcerative colitis recurrence. Mucosal pouch ischaemia can also cause pouchitis occurring very soon after construction; it usually requires pouch excision.

Endoscopy and biopsy (congestion, mucosal petechiae, excessive mucous secretion and frank ulceration), microscopy and culture of pouch effluent, use of ^{111}In-labelled granulocyte scanning and faecal granulocyte excretion may be required in investigations.

The majority of patients with pouchitis can be treated successfully with antibiotics, especially metronidazole, even if pouchitis recurs. This suggests bacterial aetiology, particularly anaerobes, Campylobacter, or Salmonella. Pouchitis alone has very rarely been a cause of failure in operation. Moreover, in these rare cases, it has not always been possible to rule out the possibility of Crohn's disease. Poor emptying was also implicated in aetiology; if more than 10% of isotope emptying counts (using labelled stool) remain in the pouch following evacuation, the patient may benefit from catheterising the pouch at regular intervals (every 1–2 h). Pouchitis not responding to antibiotics (such as metronidazole, ciprofloxacin, or augmentin) requires topical corticosteroids or mesalazine with regular catheterisation.

Other complications   These are rare or uncommon; they include carcinoma of the rectal cuff, anastomotic haemorrhage, pouch leak (less than 5%), pouch haemorrhage, pouch necrosis and superior mesenteric artery syndrome.

1.49 Restorative Resection of Carcinoma of the Rectum

PERSPECTIVES IN COLORECTAL ANASTOMOTIC LEAK

Anastomotic leak or dehiscence remains the most challenging mortality and morbidity problem in restorative rectal resection. Although minimal leaks, especially after high anterior resection, often pursue an innocuous, subclinical course, major leaks are life-threatening and prolong convalescence. Anastomoses between the colon and extraperitoneal rectum, classified as 'low', leak more readily than intraperitoneal 'high' ones when the rectum has a serous peritoneal coat. The lower the anastomosis, therefore, the greater the likelihood of leakage. The mortality is 20–22% in leaking cases compared with 7% when the anastomosis is intact. The anastomotic leak is a spectrum and diagnosed clinically (postoperative faecal fistula, local or general peritonism), radiologically (suture line barium enema – diluted barium under low pressure performed towards the end of the second postoperative week can diagnose silent subclinical leaks), rectally (the examining finger reveals pus or feels the anastomotic gap) or sigmoidoscopically. Radiological evidence varies from 6 to 35% and is higher than the clinical evidence (2–18%).

Anastomotic healing

Intestinal anastomotic healing passes through the same phases of wound healing as occur elsewhere in the body. In general, first-intention wound healing consists of three distinct phases:
1. The lag or substrate phase (occurs within the first 4–6 postoperative days), when fluid containing plasma, blood cells and fibrin exudes from tissue into the wound.
2. The healing or proliferation phase (6th–14th postoperative days), when fibroblasts multiply rapidly, bridging wound edges and restoring continuity. Collagen is secreted from cells and formed into fibres. Healing begins rapidly and terminates about the 14th day.
3. The maturation phase (14th–21st postoperative day), when there is sound scar formation.

The collagen concentration in the large bowel is low in the immediate postoperative period and does not increase subsequently (in contrast to that of the small bowel). Mucosal collagenase activity increases after surgery and in the colon there is a predominance of collagen breakdown during the first 4 postoperative days, whereas synthesis predominates in the second week. Factors influencing collagenase activity are: infection, a collagenase inhibitor in plasma and intestinal obstruction.

Decisive factors in anastomotic leak

These can be divided into general and local factors.

General factors

Age (over 60 years), malnutrition and vitamin C deficiency, severe protein malnutrition, zinc depletion, jaundice, uraemia, diabetes, immunosuppression and large doses of steroids all have adverse effects, enhancing anastomotic dehiscence. These factors are patient-related and of no great interest surgically.

Local factors

These are more important.

1. Colonic contents and infection

About 40% of the dry weight of faeces consists of bacteria and 97% of this is obligatory anaerobes. Without antimicrobial prophylaxis a 50% abdominal wound infection rate can be expected. Combined metronidazole–cefuroxime prophylaxis (i.v. 500 mg and 750 mg respectively three times a day starting with premedication and continued for 24–48 h postoperatively) is effective enough to abolish abdominal wound sepsis. It can improve anastomotic healing although not eliminate complications completely. Attempts to sterilise the faeces are impossible and dangerous. However, mechanical colonic emptying before surgery is essential. Whole gut irrigation was found popular neither with patients nor nurses but 500 ml of 20% mannitol given orally as an osmotic laxative may be used (can lead to explosion if diathermy is used). However, Picolax (two sachets) given orally 1 day before surgery was found to be very successful. (Laxatives are principally of four types: stimulant, e.g. Picolax, cascara, senna; osmotic, e.g. oral mannitol, lactulose, magnesium sulphate; faecal softners, e.g. liquid paraffin, acting by lubrication; and finally bulk-forming drugs, e.g. bran, spaghula husk, methylcellulose.) Rectal enema (phosphate retention or soap water), suppository (Dulcolax) or washout (using a lavage tube with syphon principle) should be done routinely. In the event of occasional failure, peroperative on-table irrigation is done.

2. Shape of the pelvis

The low anastomosis lies in the presacral space which is deep (especially in males) and has a rigid curved posterior wall. Blood and exudate accumulate here easily and become infected resulting in an abscess bursting through the suture line. Drainage of the presacral space is therefore important (for 5 days using a sump drain or Redivac). In high anastomoses the dead space should be filled with living tissues, e.g. small intestine or omental wrap, to seal any possible leak.

3. Suturing techniques

Staplers undoubtedly make the operation quicker and easier and are very practical in low anastomoses. However, the overall results are only slightly better than those of hand suturing and the radiological leak rate is not altered.

There was no difference clinically between single-and two-layer hand suturing in high intraperitoneal anastomoses.

Single-layer anastomoses, however, were superior when constructed below the peritoneal reflection. The inverted interrupted serosubmucosal (partial-thickness) single-layer hand technique was found to be simple and effective for difficult anastomoses low in the pelvis (circular staplers can give a comparable result in such cases and may be even simpler in difficult access). Experimentally, the single-layer technique provides a larger lumen (no stenosis), minimal tissue strangulation (mucosal sloughing occurs with two-layer technique) and better anastomotic strength. The inverted technique was superior to everted techniques when performed expertly in a clinical situation.

Whichever technique is used, the anastomosis should be gas-tight, not strangulating and there should be no mesocolic vascular tension.

Thus suturing techniques include the comparison between:

- hand-sewn *versus* stapler,
- single-layer *versus* two-layer,
- interrupted *versus* continuous,
- open *versus* closed,
- inverted *versus* everted.

4. Suture materials

The ideal suture does not exist. In colonic anastomoses, however, a suture should not potentiate infection, be non-braided, dissolve slowly and exhibit low irritancy and knot easily and securely. The normal colon takes approximately 30 days to regain full breaking strength after injury. This healing period can be lengthened by local infection. Absorbable sutures, with the exception of polydioxanone (PDS) lose strength too rapidly. Braided materials, notably silk, produce a prolonged tissue response and harbour bacteria. Monofilaments, either absorbable (PDS) or non-absorbable (polypropylene or nylon) are possibly the sutures of choice since they are unreactive and appear least likely to delay healing; therefore, they should be incorporated into one layer of any sutured colonic anastomosis. For surgeons, however, it is the handling properties rather than any other factor that determines a surgeon's choice of a particular material.

5. Blood supply

There should be pulsatile extramural blood flow. The documented extramural avascular critical points of Sudeck (1907), Toupet (1951) and Griffiths (1956) at the rectosigmoid junction (between the last sigmoidal and superior rectal arteries), the sigmoid colon (between the sigmoidal arteries) and the splenic flexure respectively (see Al-Fallouji, 1988), are macroscopic points in an extramural pattern without intramural counterparts but act as physiological points for blood flow gradient and as a buffer zone between the high and low regional blood flow patterns of various segments in the left colon and rectum.

The terminal colorectal vessels constitute minicollateral vessels easily compromised by intramural haematoma or complete transmural suturing. Therefore intramural haematoma necessitates re-resection and re-anastomosis. There are two primary transmural plexuses – at the subserosal and submucosal (the most important and extensive) sites – with two subsidiary plexuses at the intermuscular (fed by subserosal) and mucosal (fed by submucosal) sites. Single-layer (hand) suturing, therefore, should be partial (seromuscular) and from the outside-in, using submucosal grooves as landmarks for entry or exit bites. The mucosal layer is optional; although it reinforces the gas-tight barrier, careless deep strangulating suturing predisposes to leakage and also leads to late stenosis. As the cut ends of the intramural transverse vascular circles have variable shapes, there is an unavoidable percentage of leakage, theoretically caused by microvascular mismatch between the uncompensated vascular circles in the free cut ends of the anastomosed segments.

The physiological properties of the colonic microcirculation are important – shock, haemorrhage and hypotension during anaesthetic induction may predispose to leakage. Lowering of the systolic blood pressure by more than 50 mmHg below the base line for 15 min or longer during the operation results in a 150% increase in the rate of leakage. Homeostatic visceral vasoconstriction usually occurs to preserve cerebral and coronary blood flow at the expense of intestinal blood flow. A loss in blood volume of 10%, while producing only small changes in blood pressure and cardiac output, can reduce colonic blood flow and oxygen availability by 28%, as shown in dogs. The worst possible clinical combination is inadequate volume replacement using only blood (dextran or Hartmann's solution should be used instead, see below). Measured haemodilution, done by withdrawing blood and replacing with Hartmann's solution until haemoglobin is around 11 g/100 ml, was found to decrease viscosity and improve oxygen transport at the microcirculation level. Anastomotic leak was found to be associated with a mean haemoglobin level of 14.6 g/100 ml as compared to 12.5 g/100 ml when leak was not present. Furthermore, perioperative blood transfusion is associated with significant colorectal recurrences and bad long-term prognosis.

6. Intra-abdominal sepsis

In the absence of infection leak occurred in about 7.9% of cases while it occurred in 20.5% when infection was encountered during the operation. This represents a 150% increase in the incidence of postoperative leak. Primary colostomy, therefore, is required in the presence of local, general or spreading peritonitis.

7. Emergency operation

The leak rate increases by 150% when compared with elective operation due to poor bowel preparation. Local blood supply especially may be jeopardized by the intraluminal distension that occurs following intestinal obstruction, and a delay in new blood vessel formation has been demonstrated in experimental anastomoses constructed in distended bowel. Primary anastomosis in acutely obstructed colon was considered to be contraindicated because of risk of delayed healing. Later experimental studies, however, suggested that primary anastomosis of the obstructed left colon is not contraindicated by haemodynamic considerations, namely: increased left colonic and ileal blood flow; decreased caecal blood flow; and blood shunting from the mucosa to muscular layers. Immediate primary anastomosis without colostomy is currently the accepted procedure, even in acute large bowel obstruction.

8. Anastomotic rest

Intracolonic pressure is generated by colonic segmentation and peristalsis. The latter are activated by neostigmine used to reverse effects of relaxants in the recovery from anaesthesia and some advocate the use of pyridostigmine instead. Parasympathomimetics (bethanicol, distigmine, neostigmine and pyridostigmine) and laxatives particularly the stimulant group (Bisacodyl, senna, danthron, figs and Picolax) must therefore, be avoided. Peristalsis is also activated by morphine (peripheral direct action), metoclopramide, food ingestion and emotion and these should be avoided. Colonic segmentation, however, is paralysed by propantheline bromide and reduced by pethidine. Postoperative antiemetics such as metoclopramide or Maxolon should be avoided due to their effect on gastrointestinal motility. Suction drainage may adhere to the anastomosis and damages it. Immediate postoperative anal digital stretch or rectal tube insertion may be practised (though without controlled studies) to overcome any anal sphincteric spasm that might strain the anastomosis through high intracolonic pressure. Fizzy drinks must be avoided, since they strain the anastomosis by distension with gas bubbles.

9. Preoperative radiotherapy

Irradiation may be administered as an adjunct to surgery for colorectal carcinomas. The induced microangiopathy mitigates against primary healing. Radiation causes intestinal microcirculatory changes which are dose-dependent. Clinically, there is a three-fold increase in anastomotic dehiscence following radiotherapy. Experimentally colonic healing is significantly delayed following irradiation, particularly when treatment immediately precedes surgery. Further experiments on dogs indicate that low anterior resection with either an EEA stapled or handsewn anastomosis cannot be done safely after 6000 rad (chy) preoperative irradiation.

10. Colostomy

Usually one out of 10 postoperative patients will leak clinically (10% of cases).

Indications for prophylactic primary protective colostomy are:

- Presence of local, general or spreading peritonitis.
- Opening of the bladder or vagina in order to remove the lesion adequately.
- A very low anastomosis particularly if the anastomosis has to be made by hand per anus.
- Doubt about the blood supply to the colonic cut end or about the degree of tension at the suture line. As experience increases, this indication should become rare.
- Previous high-dose pelvic irradiation, usually for uterine carcinoma.

Indications for emergency secondary colostomy (performed usually between the 5th and 10th postoperative days) are one or more of the following:

- Unsettled fever.
- Signs of spreading pelvic peritonitis.
- Surgical emphysema around pelvic drain site.
- A large and persistent faecal fistula.
- A large palpable gap in the suture line on rectal examination.
- Persistent and troublesome diarrhoea caused by a presacral abscess cavity following a low anastomotic dehiscence.

SPHINCTER-SAVING RESECTION

The majority of large bowel growths are found in the lower sigmoid colon and upper rectum. Sphincter-saving resection has stood the test of time and is comparable in results to abdominoperineal excision of the rectum with permanent colostomy. For Duke's B and C tumours of average malignancy, there was no difference between sphincter-saving resection and abdominoperineal excision of the rectum in terms of 5 year survival. If the rectal stump was well irrigated at operation (sphincter-saving resection), malignant implantation in the suture line was very rare. It was thought that the possibility of recurrence was higher in sphincter-saving resection because it is less extensive than abdominoperineal excision of the rectum.

While both operations deal with upward spread it was the distal and lateral spread of tumour cells which led to the debatable 5 cm distal clearance rule in sphincter-saving resection. However, distal intramural spread is rare and usually extends for less than 1 cm. Spread greater than this indicates advanced C or D with poor prognosis and patients usually die of distant metastases before they develop local recurrence. Distal extramural lymphatic spread was found less than 2 cm from the distal margin of the tumour. The amount of tissue that can be removed laterally is just as extensive in radical sphincter-saving resection as in abdominoperineal excision of the rectum. The minimal 2 cm distal clearance from the tumour is therefore adequate.

For anorectal function 6–8 cm anorectal preservation was thought necessary but studies showed that very low colorectal or even coloanal anastomoses will achieve continence and sensation after a period of 18 months' adaptation. The quality of life is certainly better in sphincter-saving resection because the social and/or psychological trauma of permanent colostomy is avoided.

In terms of operative mortality and morbidity sphincter-saving resection is probably safer. The morbidity of permanent colostomy in abdominoperineal excision of the rectum is comparable to that of anastomotic leak in sphincter-saving resection.

SOME PRINCIPLES IN COLONIC SURGERY

- Sigmoidoscopy and biopsy are the keystone investigations in both emergency and elective cases. Emergency barium enema is indicated in acute cases (to identify the level of colonic obstruction) when emergency operation is contemplated on the day of admission.
- Bowel preparation should be perfect in the partially obstructed bowel: use laxatives (Picolax), enema, suppositories or rectal washout preoperatively; and if the bowel is still not clean, use operative on-table antegrade colonic irrigation.

- Do not operate without antibiotic cover or prophylaxis (start i.v. or i.m. with premedication and continue for 24 h, e.g. metronidazole, cefuroxime).
- Full mobilisation is essential, especially of the splenic flexure, to cut the congenital bands so that anastomosed segments are floppy and tension-free; otherwise ischaemia and/or leak may occur.
- Early vascular interruption to prevent intravascular dislodgement of tumour cells.
- Always identify the ureter in left colonic surgery (no need for preoperative IVU). In right colonic surgery identify the ureter operatively as well as preoperatively (IVU).
- Recurrence in anterior restorative rectal resection or sphincter-saving resection is higher than in abdominoperineal excision of the rectum owing to intraluminal exfoliation of malignant cells; therefore, always irrigate the rectal stump operatively (prior to anastomosis) with 1% noxythiolin (Noxyflex) solution. This minimises suture line recurrence.
- The anastomosis should be made gas-tight, not strangulating and with no tension using a single-or double-layer (hand) technique in high anastomosis and a single-layer (hand) or stapler technique in low anastomosis. It should be covered by living tissue such as the small intestine or omentum.
- In low colorectal anastomosis drainage of the presacral space is important to prevent haematoma bursting through the suture line (drain is removed on the fifth day). Mobilised splenic flexure area may necessitate another drain because of excessive exudation (such a drain does not influence the anastomotic integrity).
- Colostomy does not influence the anastomotic leak but is certainly a life-saving procedure when the leak occurs. Therefore a primary anastomosis can be constructed without protective primary colostomy, but in this case the surgeon should be prepared to perform secondary colostomy when the leak occurs (roughly in 1 out of 10 cases post-operatively). A primary colostomy is indicated, however, in the presence of intraperitoneal sepsis or when a low anastomosis is insecure because of difficult suturing or unavoidable tension.
- Postoperative and digital dilatation is recommended (though not proven) to decompress the intracolonic pressure. Similarly drugs increasing intracolonic pressure or enhancing peristalsis should be avoided, e.g. neostigmine, narcotic analgesia (morphine) and Maxolon.

BOWEL PREPARATIONS

Chemical sterilisation and mechanical emptying before surgery are essential. However, attempts to sterilise the faeces are both impossible and dangerous.

1. *Two days before surgery* (or colonoscopy or barium enema), the patient is allowed a light diet with no fibre, such as cheese, eggs, fish, clear soup, white bread, tea, coffee; *but* no fruit, vegetables, meat, brown bread, cereals, or other high roughage diet are allowed.

2. *On the day before surgery* or examination, the patient is asked not to eat any more until after surgery or examination.

However, plenty of fluids such as tea, coffee, clear soup and water are encouraged. One of the two following preparations is widely and commonly used in surgical practice with the following instructions.

- Picolax:

  Two sachets of a strong stimulant laxative, Picolax, are required to cleanse the bowel prior to surgery or examination.

  Each Picolax sachet contains 10 mg sodium picosulphate, 3.5 g magnesium oxide, 12 g citric acid with excipients and flavour given orally 1 day before surgery was found to be very successful.

  The first sachet is taken before breakfast, the second is taken 2 h after lunch. At 8 am. the powder contained in one sachet or envelope is dissolved in a little water (3–4 tablespoons) in a glass. The solution will become hot. The patient should wait for about 5 min, then half fill the glass with cold water and drink the solution. About 2 h after lunch the powder contained in the second envelope should be taken in exactly the same way. The patient should be prepared for their bowels to open 1 h after the first dose and several other times during the day. By 8 pm it is preferable that the patient abstain from taking any food or fluid. A rectal wash-out is done at 10 pm. Alternatively, Klean-Prep is used (see below).

- Klean-Prep (polyethylene glycol and electrolytes or PEG + E). This is an iso-osmotic bowel cleansing solution, thus avoiding net water absorption and the risk of dehydration; it is neither osmotic nor a stimulant laxative (no abdominal cramps). The patient should be instructed to eat no solid food 3–4 h before starting to take Klean-Prep until after the medical procedure. Clear fluids may be drunk during this time. Iron tablets should be discontinued 4 days beforehand and no constipating agents (e.g. codeine) taken on the day of examination. Metoclopramide or domperidone may be given to accelerate gastric emptying. The solution may be started at 2 pm and finished after 6 h; by 8 pm the patient must abstain from taking food or fluids. A rectal wash-out is done at 10 pm.

  For adults, including the elderly and patients with cardiac or renal insufficiency, four sachets are required. The contents of each sachet must be reconstituted with 1 litre of water. One glassful (250 ml or ½ pint) must be drunk rapidly every 10–15 min until all solution has been consumed. The solution has a pleasant vanilla flavour for enhanced patient acceptance; it may be more palatable if chilled. The procedure's to be repeated with all four sachets until the rectal effluent is clear and free of solid matter; the first bowel movement occurs after approximately 1–2 h. The solution from all four sachets should be drunk within 4–6 h. It can be administered by nasogastric tube at 20–30 ml/min.

  The reconstituted 4 litre solution provides 235 g of polyethylene glycol 3350 (Macrogol 3350), 22.74 g of sodium sulphate, 6.74 g of sodium bicarbonate, 5.86 g of sodium chloride, 2.9 g of potassium chloride, and 0.2 g of aspartame. The sodium content is present mainly as the sulphate to minimise absorption; the small amount of sodium absorbed is balanced by comparable secretion into the gut; furthermore, PEG-3350 is not absorbable nor does it undergo fermentation (like mannitol). The solution should be kept in a refrigerator after reconstitution, and must be discarded if unused after 48 h.

It is contraindicated in GI tract obstruction or perforation, gastric retention, ileus, toxic colitis or megacolon, and body weight less than 20 kg.

Precautions must be taken in patients with impaired gag reflex, unconscious patients (possibility of regurgitation or aspiration), pregnancy, ulcerative colitis and reflux oesophagitis.

Side-effects include nausea, bloating, abdominal cramps (usually transient – reduced by taking more slowly), rarely vomiting, anal irritation, urticaria, rhinorrhoea and dermatitis.

3. *On the day of surgery* or examination:

● At 8 am rectal wash-out (rectal tube siphoning normal saline into the patient from a bottle and then letting it out into a bucket washing faecal debris out) immediately before surgery or examination is performed.

● A combined metronidazole/cefuroxime prophylaxis (i.v. 500 mg and 750 mg respectively three times a day starting with premedication and continued for 24 h postoperatively) is effective enough to abolish abdominal wound sepsis. It can, therefore, improve anastomotic healing though not completely.

The rectal stump must be washed out prior to anastomosis for two reasons: first, to reduce bacterial content of the stump and second, to minimise the risk of local recurrence. Sodium hypochlorite was found better than povidone-iodine or saline as a rectal wash-out for colorectal anastomosis both as an antiseptic and as a cytocidal agent (it kills free floating viable tumour cells on contact, does not delay anastomotic healing in dogs and is not toxic).

The combination of oral neomycin and metronidazole has been the preferred oral antimicrobial regimen with an infection rate varying between 2 and 10%. Nevertheless, without excellent mechanical cleansing of the colon, oral antimicrobial agents have had little impact on the incidence of postoperative wound-related sepsis. The use of parenteral antibiotics prophylactically appeared to be of little value until recent studies revealed their benefit. There is absolutely no additional benefit that can be demonstrated for receiving antibiotics beyond the immediate perioperative phase, i.e. first 24 h. Another study compared oral kanamycin plus metronidazole with the same agents given parenterally at the appropriate time intervals. All patients had been prepared by an excellent mechanical cleansing regimen. Postoperative sepsis occurred in only 7% of patients assigned to receive parenteral antibiotic prophylaxis while infection developed in 36% of those managed by the oral antimicrobial preparation. Bacteria causing postoperative wound-related sepsis are almost always resistant to the antibiotics used and appeared to have been selected out by just a few hours of oral therapy. Thus, the expeditious parenteral administration of antibiotic such that protected tissue concentrations can be achieved before bacterial challenge is apparently the most important step of all. Should resistant strains evolve, the parenteral route of administration will be the only reliable method.

Other types of large bowel preparations include:

● Whole gut irrigation or Hercules wash-out (Hercules, son of Zeus diverted the river to cleanse the stables of Aegeus) was not popular with patients or nurses. Furthermore, saline absorption can lead to water and salt overload in patients with incipient heart failure, cirrhosis and renal disease; it may cause acute intestinal obstruction and perforation in patients with completely obstructive colonic lesions. A careful selection of patients, therefore, is absolutely imperative.

● Alternatively, 500 ml of 20% mannitol given orally as an osmotic laxative may be used. Unfortunately, it can dehydrate patients and increase the risk of sepsis, because mannitol is an excellent substrate for various anaerobic

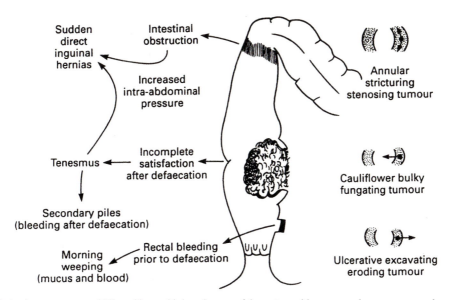

Fig. 1.49.1 Correlation between upper, middle and lower third carcinomas of the rectum with macroscopic appearances and corresponding clinical presentations.

3. Local tumour invasion (Dukes staging)

Extensive local invasion is a critical factor in determining survival; it is as important as lymphatic metastases, histological grading or extramural venous invasion, and was closely related to all these factors. Dukes' Stage B (American Astler–Coller B2) and C, particularly for tumours below 12 cm from the anal verge, are classified 'high-risk' cancers by the North Central Cancer Treatment Group (NCCTG). Dukes' A (Astler–Coller A + B1) lesions and tumours more than 12 cm from the anal verge are classified as 'low-risk' cancers and usually have better prognosis. It is the lateral and posterior tumour spread (circumferential invasion) which accounts for poor prognosis; if following restorative resection, positive infiltration of the cut lateral edge or mesorectum were found, the outlook is bleak, and may indicate the need for adjuvant radiotherapy or combination chemotherapy. In doing restorative resection of rectal carcinoma therefore, it is absolutely mandatory to be aggressive in local resection by cutting all of the lateral edge of the tumour and by removing all mesorectal fat generously and meticulously, and this perhaps is associated with low morbidity. Multiple organ resection, however, may be accompanied by higher operative mortality.

Total mesorectal excision (TME), pioneered by Heald from Basingstoke, has immensely improved the local recurrence rate. TME was developed from anatomical understanding based on what is surgically feasible. Precise sharp dissection is undertaken around the integral mesentry of the hind gut, which envelopes the entire mid-rectum. Meticulous TME encompasses the whole field of tumour spread and can improve the cure rates and reduce the variability of outcome between surgeons. TME has claimed to eliminate virtually all locally recurrent disease after 'curative' surgery. For high-risk cancers (Dukes B and C and tumour below 12 cm from the anal verge), results by surgery with TME alone performed on 135 patients over a 13-year period from 1978–1991 (5% local recurrence at 5 years and 22% overall recurrence) were superior to the best reported (NCCTG) results using conventional surgery plus radiotherapy (25% and 62.7% respectively), or surgery plus combination chemotherapy (13.5% and 41.5% respectively), implying viable local tumour residues remaining in the two latter modalities. The excellent results of TME were objectively scrutinised to dismiss statistical aberration (the result of case mix and analytical techniques).

The operation is defined as *curative* when, at the end of the procedure, the surgeon believes that all grossly detectable cancer has been removed. Local and overall *recurrence* are defined as disease detected or suspected within the pelvis (local) and anywhere (local or systemic) during life or necropsy, respectively. *Non-curative* procedures include mainly tumours with distant metastases and a small group with locally non-invasive but residual disease believed to remain on the side wall of the pelvis.

The findings are at variance with the notion that cancer is a systemic disease, and clearly rectal cancer is not, since spread of rectal cancer is confined within the mesorectal envelope, and rectal carcinoma is far more curable by surgery alone than has generally been believed or is currently accepted. In poorer countries, health care providers wrestle with the cost of chemo radiotherapy, and TME does not require adjuvant therapies and reduces the number of patients requiring combination therapy.

The technique of TME involves an anterior restorative resection with meticulous precise and sharp dissection of the avascular plane between mesorectum and parietes completed under direct vision; the excised specimen, therefore, includes the entire posterior, distal and lateral mesorectum out to the plane of the inferior hypogastric plexus, which is carefully preserved in order to preserve the principal parasympathetic erigenti nerve root on each side of the pelvic wall. Anteriorly, dissection proceeds with seminal vesicles in front and Denonvillier's fascia behind; the specimen must include intact Denonvillier's fascia and the peritoneal reflection. Posteriorly, the specimen shows the characteristic smooth bi-lobed lipoma encapsulated appearance and distally reflects the contours of the pelvic floor and the midline anococcygeal raphe. Implantation is prevented by aqueous washout below the clamp before the anorectum is divided, and in the pelvis itself.

Dissection, therefore, avoids autonomic nerves by defining the place within them (holy plane) which is subjected to sharp dissection under direct vision throughout. Complete excision of enveloping mesorectal tissues in a covering of thin but recognisable fascia protects the pelvic walls, genito-urinary structures, presacral nerves, parasympathetic roots and neurovascular bundles, and creates a specimen with a thin mobile covering of areolar tissue; this requires specific surgical skills and strengthens the case for specialised referral patterns. Efforts and resources into surgical training in the technique would pay great dividends in the management of this common visceral malignancy. The improved local excision reduces metastatic disease developing subsequent to local failure.

The cost of TME success, however, is not inconsequential; it is more difficult, time-consuming (but not more radical), and can be associated with relatively high anastomtic leak. Meticulous dissection requires additional operating time (operation lasts up to 2.5 h) and blood transfusion requirements increase. Anastomoses at 3–6 cm from the anal verge have led to 17.4% anastomotic leak rate for TME, and may need temporary protective colostomy. Long-term anastomotic failure, significant morbidity, and permanent stoma have marred the recovery of 5% of patients, but these drawbacks seem justified in terms of local recurrence improvement.

4. Lymphatic metastases (particularly the number of palpable lymph nodes and fixity)

Increasing numbers of positive lymph nodes are associated with a progressive decline in survival; for rectal carcinoma with one lymph node involved the corrected 5-year survival was 63.6% falling to 36.1% when 2–5 lymph nodes were involved. If more than 10 nodes were replaced by tumour, survival was only 2.1%. If lymph nodes are fixed by malignancy, they carry a poorer prognosis compared to inflamed and/or mobile lymph nodes. Rectal cancer is spread by lateral, circumferential and posterior invasion via mesorectum; the staging, therefore, is closely related to patient prognosis. Staging, however, is difficult to assess preoperatively. The finger (per rectal examination) cannot tell about tumour and lymph node fixity. CT scan is increasingly used in rectal carcinoma. Endoluminal ultrasound is useful, particularly in tumour invasion of mesorectal fat (with accuracy of 85–93%). Recently, laparoscopy is being used to assess tumour spread to lymph nodes.

5. Extramural venous invasion

There is considerable evidence to suggest that venous invasion by tumour is associated with a high incidence of distant metastases and significant reduction of survival. This is a matter of some importance since patients with colorectal carcinoma are said to die from vascular spread (metastasis) more commonly than from lymph node metastases or local spread. Venous spread is one of several important indices of tumour invasiveness; it may indicate a patient at high risk of developing distant metastases, particularly to the liver, and who may benefit from adjuvant chemotherapy. It is doubtful whether any specific surgical manoeuvre will have any influence on the process once established, although Turnbull's 'no-touch' technique, if it can reduce i.v. tumour embolism, may have a place. However, many patients were found to have vein invasion in the absence of distant spread.

6. Histological grading of tumour differentiation

Grading of tumour differentiation on biopsy is important; patients with poorly differentiated tumours had a decreased survival compared to those with well-differentiated tumours. However, venous invasion, perineural invasion, number of mitoses, tumour infiltration of tumour margin and lymphatic infiltration may all carry a poor prognosis.

7. Distant metastases

Metastases to the liver particularly (occurs in 15–25% of patients) usually indicates a dismal prognosis. Of all factors known to influence survival in colorectal cancer, none carries more ill-foreboding than the presence of liver metastases; most patients with untreated liver metastases are dead within 2 years of diagnosis. Patients with solitary liver metastases fare better than those with multiple deposits; they are also candidates for liver resection with the possibility of cure. However, despite contraindications to hepatic resection (proposed in the past), 5-year survival has been obtained in patients with extrahepatic disease resected simultaneously (with colorectal resection), patients with bilobar liver metastases, patients with multiple metastases and patients with positive margins. A computerised assessment of the percentage of hepatic replacement by cancer may relate directly to patient survival rate. Unfortunately, only 10% of patients with liver metastases have solitary lesions. Primary tumour resection, however, has an important bearing on the outcome for patients with hepatic metastases; it affords considerable palliation with relief of symptoms and improvement in survival. Resection of multiple liver deposits, systemic cytotoxic therapy, cytotoxic agents via portal vein infusion and hepatic artery ligation with (5-Fu) or without infusion chemotherapy, were all advocated with inconclusive results. The poor overall survival for patients with liver metastases is influenced therefore by two factors; the extent of secondary spread in the liver and the treatment of primary tumour.

8. Large intestinal obstruction

Whether intestinal obstruction has any influence on survival is arguable. Obstruction resulting in diverting colostomy as first operation is found to be of no significance. Certainly there is a high operative mortality after resection for an obstructing carcinoma compared with a non-obstructing tumour. However, studies confirmed that intestinal obstruction may indicate a transmural advanced local spread; thus obstructing tumours are associated with poorer prognosis than non-obstructing tumours. Caecum and rectum have a larger lumen than other parts of the bowel; tumour at these sites needs to be of greater size to produce intestinal obstruction. Resection of tumour, whether staged (wiser) or otherwise, is always recommended. It is dubious whether decompression by transverse colostomy without resection of offending tumour can be recommended even in high-risk patients because, first, emergency colostomy is not without mortality and can be associated with serious complications; secondly, there is undue delay between decompression and subsequent tumour resection with a risk of dissemination; and lastly, since most tumours are situated in the sigmoid or rectosigmoid region of the left colon, a left iliac colostomy is often preferable to transverse colostomy allowing better clearance and possible excision of colostomy along with primary tumour if so required.

9. Perforation or tumour spill during operation

Whether spontaneous or by the surgeon from extraluminal or intraluminal sites, spill or perforation, particularly at a tumour site, carries a bad prognosis independent of stage of fixity, with 5-year survival of 12–25%. This is due to increased intraluminal pressure and particularly exfoliation of tumour cells.

10. Anastomotic leak

Anastomotic leak following restorative resection is associated with high future local recurrence, and therefore is considered as poor prognostic factor. It is debatable whether stapled anastomoses are associated with more local recurrence than handsewn ones. Postoperative infection, and in particular postoperative fever, is a most unfavourable prognostic clinical factor.

11. Perioperative blood transfusion

Transfusion in colorectal surgery is associated with a high rate of local recurrence (long-term harmful effects), perhaps because it lowers the patient's immunity as well as enhancing anastomotic leak (which itself can lead to high local recurrence).

12. CEA level

This tumour marker correlates well with extent of tumour spread and is important in postoperative monitoring for tumour recurrence; CEA may also help in locating tumour recurrence and selecting patients likely to benefit from 'second-look' surgery.

13. Other indicators

Mucin production, tumour DNA status, tumour-associated antigens and oncoproteins, particularly mutated P53, may all indicate poor prognosis. Mutated P53 is present in 40% of lung carcinoma, 70% of hepatocellular carcinoma, 50% of ovarian malignancies, and 49% of colorectal cancers; the more advanced the tumour, the more mutated P53 and vice versa.

1.52 Common Anorectal Conditions

RECTAL PROLAPSE

Complete full-thickness rectal prolapse is a relatively uncommon but distressing condition for the patient. Some patients are elderly and infirm, others are otherwise fit. The two main objectives of treatment are: first, to carry out a procedure that safely corrects the prolapse with minimal morbidity and no mortality; and secondly, to improve associated incontinence and underlying defaecatory disorder.

Aetiology and pathogenesis

- Thought to represent a sliding hernia.
- Mobile mesorectum allowing the rectum to straighten with loss of normal rectal curvature.
- Radio-opaque markers confirmed the theory that rectal prolapse represents a rectal intussusception (widely accepted). Perhaps, rectal prolapse is a spectrum of progressing conditions of mucosal prolapse, solitary ulcer syndrome, to rectorectal and rectoanal intussusception, and thence to full-thickness rectal prolapse.
- Associated with pelvic floor denervation, since majority are females after childbirth (rare in nulliparous). Chronic neurophysiological damage may result in chronic straining at defaecation. A significant association with spinal cord injury was also found.
- Failure of rectal support by levators and pelvic floor fascia due to defective collagen maturation in pelvic floor following stretching in childbirth.
- Prolapse initiates a persistent recto-anal inhibitory reflex so that internal anal sphincter remains chronically relaxed with poor contraction in response to raised intra-abdominal pressure. Indeed, following repair, pressures improve.

Investigation

1. Clinical assessment: up to 58% of patients have incontinence and reduced anal sphincter tone on rectal examination. Incontinence is probably due to combination of pudendal neuropathy associated with straining and perineal descent.
2. Anorectal physiology tests reveal shorter sphincter, low resting anal pressure, low squeeze (voluntary external anal contraction) pressure, poor anorectal sensation to electric stimulation and requirement for higher balloon size to appreciate its volume. Prolapse is usually associated with anorectal incontinence.

3. Defaecation proctography can confirm the diagnosis and can confirm the presence of intussusception in incontinent patients without overt prolapse. Parks flap valve theory of continence based on anorectal obliquity is not supported by evacuation proctography. Continence depends on sphincter ability to respond to raised intra-abdominal rectal pressures. Perineal descent at rest and straining is present.

Management

Correction of associated constipation is very important, since some prolapse patients have impaired colonic transit. However, conservative management has nothing to offer in full-thickness rectal prolapse; it is justified in high-risk patients only.

Injection of sclerosant may fix mucosa to underlying muscle in mucosal prolapse.

Perineal local operations

1. *Thiersch encirclage*, using silver wire (Porter, 1962), pursestring nylon (Baker, 1970), or silicone rubber or silastic thread (Jackman, 1980) to tighten the anus and retain the prolapse without treating the underlying pathophysiology. Anal relaxation during defaecation is restricted resulting in constipation and faecal impaction.
2. *Delorme procedure* is non-invasive, in which prolapse is fully everted then rectum is denuded of its mucosa for the length of prolapse, and underlying rectal musculature is then plicated, and mucosal defect is subsequently repaired by suturing proximal and distal resection margins over plicated rectal wall. The results are good but inferior to abdominal operations since no attempt is made to repair main anatomical or physiological defects. There is a significant long-term relapse rate. It is reserved for elderly or infirm patients.
3. *Altmeir procedure* is more common in the USA than the UK. Instead of a mucosal excision, full rectum thickness is resected starting at the upper end of the anal canal. This allows prolapsing rectum and sigmoid colon to be dissected in stages via the anus. After redundant bowel has been resected, the colon is anastomosed to the top of the anal canal at the dentate line. Levator ani and puborectalis can be plicated to improve continence. Rectal removal in this method will be replaced by sigmoid colon which is often diverticular and non-distensible resulting in faecal urgency which may exacerbate incontinence. There is no recurrence and this procedure may be recommended to elderly and infirm patients, because of their anxiety about recurrence. Resting pressure may improve, but such low anastomosis may damage the anal sphincter. It is superior to Delorme procedure and inferior to abdominal operations.

Abdominal operations (Figs. 1.52.1, 1.52.2)

Despite sling operation, colopexy, colonic plication and reversed intussusception, the current modern management is abdominal rectopexy, with or without resection of redundant bowel.

Mobilisation of bowel for rectopexy Via transverse lower muscle-cutting incision, upper rectum and distal sigmoid colon are mobilised, lateral peritoneal reflection is incised and

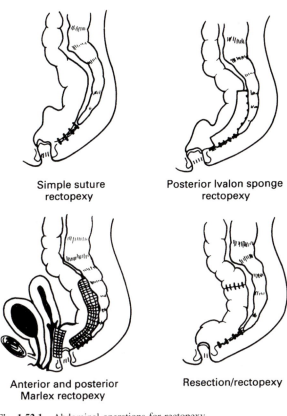

Simple suture
rectopexy

Posterior Ivalon sponge
rectopexy

Anterior and posterior
Marlex rectopexy

Resection/rectopexy

Fig. 1.52.1   Abdominal operations for rectopexy

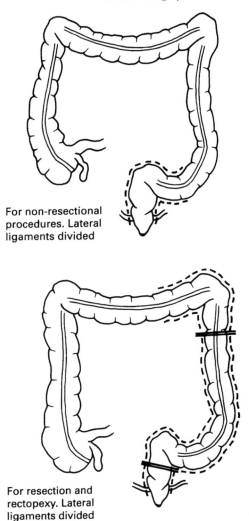

For non-resectional
procedures. Lateral
ligaments divided

For resection and
rectopexy. Lateral
ligaments divided

Fig. 1.52.2   Colorectal mobilisation for rectopexy

dissection is carried distally to levators safeguarding autonomic nerves (otherwise, there will be unacceptabl urinary, faecal and sexual morbidity). The lateral ligaments of the rectum are divided. For resection and rectopexy, splenic flexure is mobilised to provide a healthy descending colon for anastomosis without tension. Low anastomoses are more liable to leak and remove most of the rectal reservoir; it is not justified.

1. Ripstein rectopexy (Ripstein 1972)

This procedure is common in the USA. After full mobilisation, the rectum is fixed to the sacral promontory with an encircling sling of Teflon mesh. The recurrence rate is 1.5% and constipation may result from a combination of the sling and redundant sigmoid colon. If the sling is too tight it obstructs proximal bowel; the sigmoid is commonly partially obstructed in the angulation at the mesh attachment point. Redundant sigmoid bowel prolapses into the pouch of Douglas.

The four commonly used rectopexy procedures in the UK are: simple suture rectopexy, posterior Ivalon sponge rectopexy, anterior and posterior Marlex rectopexy, and resection rectopexy.

2. Simple suture rectopexy

This procedure is the easiest and is reserved for elderly patients; the rectum is fixed to the pelvic floor and presacral fascia by four prolene sutures (two distal and two proximal) to

prevent rectal intussusception leading to incontinence and recurrence, but not so high to cause the rectosigmoid angulation seen in Ripstein rectopexy.

3. Posterior Ivalon (polyvinyl alcohol) sponge rectopexy (Wells, 1959)

Ivalon sponge is secured by non-absorbable sutures to presacral fascia posteriorly and to the back of the rectum. Prosthetic material enhances dense fibrous reaction that fixes rectum into sacral curvature preventing recurrence. Unlike other materials, Ivalon is thought to be absorbed and so associated with less septic complications seen with non-absorbable materials. Recurrence rate is 2.7%.

4. Anterior and posterior Marlex rectopexy

The anterior rectum is well supported, particularly in women (in addition to posterior rectum) to prevent prolapse by anterior rectal wall descent, since a deep pouch of Douglas in females and rectovesical pouch in males is considered to be an important component of prolapse. Many elderly women have rectoceles which are the end result of pelvic floor weakness and obstetric trauma.

A sheet of Marlex is sutured posteriorly (as in Ivalon sponge fixation). Then the anterior rectal wall is separated from the vagina in females; in males Denonvillier's fascia is incised above seminal vesicles and dissection continued distally on rectal muscle tube to avoid injury to nervae errigentes. Following this mobilisation, a strip of Marlex is fixed in place on the distal anterior rectal wall in the rectovaginal septum to provide additional anterior support.

5. Resection rectopexy (sigmoidectomy-rectopexy by Frykman and Goldberg 1969)

After mobilisation, anastomosis is constructed without tension 12 cm from the anal verge. Redundant sigmoid and distal descending colon is resected. Splenic flexure mobilisation allows healthy well-vascularised descending colon to be used for anastomosis rather than sigmoid which may have a compromised blood supply, especially in elderly. In addition to resection, the distal rectal remnant is fixed to the pelvic floor and presacral fascia in a similar manner to simple suture rectopexy. The recurrence rate is 1.9%.

6. Anterior resection alone

There may be a 9% recurrence rate, some morbidity associated with risks of anastomotic complications, and 1% mortality. It is rarely performed.

Overview analysis

Abdominal operations are safe with no operative mortality (except in anterior resection) and no serious morbidity. Postoperatively, they do not cause significant alteration in bowel function. Most options achieve their primary objective (control of rectal prolapse); it is perhaps in the secondary objective (restoration of continence) that comparison between functional results is important.

Simple suture rectopexy and resection rectopexy are the most successful at restoring continence in incontinent patients; they result in a significant rise in resting anal pressure. Such internal anal sphincter improvement is probably due to removal of sphincter inhibition caused by presence of prolapsed rectum. In implant rectopexy, the presence of prosthetic material may interfere with sphincter recovery due to the inflammatory response that ensues; the implant makes the rectum less compliant and this may contribute to lack of improved sphincter function (no sphincteric recovery confirmed by persistent postoperative low resting anal pressure). Implant rectopexy is claimed to have a low recurrence due to fixation of rectum, but suture rectopexy and resection rectopexy have shown similar results.

Disadvantages of prosthetic implant rectopexy are probably balanced by the risk of anastomotic complications in resection rectopexy. There is no significant improvement in somatic muscle function following any procedure, probably due to partial denervation of external anal sphincter and puborectalis

documented on pre- and postoperative electromyography and histology; clearly rectopexy cannot improve this damage. There is improved postoperative sensory awareness (rectum and upper anal canal) in all rectopexy patients, with reduction in volume of first rectal sensation in the postoperative period. Radiologically, the anorectal angle and degree of perineal descent may not show any significant alterations; the lack of correlation between operative success and radiological changes is well documented.

If the patient is frail and unfit for major surgery, one of the perineal procedures should be chosen under regional anaesthesia. However, with modern safe anaesthesia, many patients can withstand abdominal operation with advantages of rendering the patient continent and reducing recurrence rate to minimum.

Recurrence following surgery is a major problem, and although surgery may be successful, the probability of restoring continence following secondary procedure is much lower; sphincter-tightening procedures can be tried as back-up, but overall success rates are low. Resection rectopexy may be the operation of choice for some surgeons, because continence rates are high and there is no recurrence; colonic resection may also cure the associated constipation due to slow colonic transit, but radical resection with ileorectal anastomosis is contraindicated in prolapse patients with weak sphincter, since severe incontinence can result. It is unusual for incontinence to become worse although this has been reported in a few patients after Frykman resection rectopexy, anterior resection and Wells Ivalon rectopexy (ranging between 5% up to 32%).

Postoperative constipation may be due to obstruction by sling compression, kinking of rectum over the sling, fibrosis and rigidity of the rectal wall, and aggravation of slow transit constipation; it varies from 8% to 44% and is more seen after Ripstein rectopexy, followed by Wells Ivalon rectopexy, and less frequent after Frykman resection rectopexy.

Results are worse in elderly females who are parous and in those patients with marked incontinence preoperatively. Finally, the management of prolapse remains a challenging problem; there is a great deal to learn.

PROLAPSE-RELATED SYNDROMES

Internal intussusception of rectum in the pre-prolapse evolution may lead to two syndromes: descending perineum syndrome and solitary ulcer syndrome.

Descending perineum syndrome

This refers to patients with anal symptoms who, when asked to strain during examination, showed marked descent of the perineum and loss of angulation between rectum and anal canal. Symptoms include anorectal bleeding, mucous discharge, sensation of incomplete emptying of rectum, and obstruction within the anal canal, and 'bearing down' discomfort with a long history of difficulty with defaecation and of excessive straining. Physical examination reveals perineal descent and weakness of anal sphincter and prolapse of anterior rectal mucosa into the upper anal canal which results in sensation of incomplete rectal emptying leading to straining which further aggravates anterior mucosal prolapse (vicious circle). If untreated, it results in pelvic floor weakness and incontinence. Re-education of bowel habits and prevention of anterior mucosal prolapse is achieved via injection sclerotherapy, elastic band ligation, or operative excision. If incontinence has already developed, then post-anal repair of pelvic floor muscle is the treatment of choice.

Solitary ulcer syndrome

This is related to complete rectal prolapse and descending perineum syndrome of unknown aetiology and pathogenesis; it is characterised by ulcerated anterior lower rectum presenting as tenesmus, anorectal bleeding, mucus discharge and feeling of anal obstruction with occasional history of straining. Perrectal examination reveals induration on palpation, while sigmoidoscopy reveals a well-demarcated, shallow ulcer, covered with a slough; biopsy is taken to exclude other conditions. Treatment is unsatisfactory, but the patient's instruction of avoidance of straining and better regulation of defaecation are essential. Co-existing complete rectal prolapse is treated on its own merit and can be of value in treatment of the ulcer.

HAEMORRHOIDS

It has been suggested that the progressive decline in the occurrence of haemorrhoids both in the USA and in England/ Wales over the past 30 years may be attributed to high-fibre diet, but such a decline remains speculative, since many patients are keen on high-fibre medications (non-surgical treatment) and are treated in Accident and Emergency departments or by primary care general practitioners on an outpatient basis without consulting surgeons, and therefore are not surgically registered.

Nature and aetiology

The aetiology of haemorrhoids remains controversial; varicosities of the internal haemorrhoidal plexus with dilatation of the terminal superior haemorroidal venous plexus (vascular piles), or sliding downwards of thickened mucous membrane concealing the underlying veins (mucosal piles or partial prolapse) were proposed due to either straining during defaecation when intra-abdominal pressure increases and anal sphincteric pressure decreases (forming a high pressure gradient), or an improperly functioning anal sphincter to cope with increased intra-abdominal pressure causing compression of low pressure superior haemorroidal veins in an effort to expel constipated stool in the lower part of rectal ampulla, respectively. Lord expounded his theory of constricting pectin bands encircling the lower part of the anal canal situated between mucous membrane and external sphincter.

Haemorrhoids are rare among Africans on high-fibre diet. However, not all patients with piles are constipated, and raised intra-abdominal portal vein pressure does not always result in piles (rectal varicose veins rather than haemorrhoids), and veins of the superior haemorrhoidal plexus contain no valves and cannot therefore become varicose. Urethral strictures,

Table 1.52.1 Degrees of haemorrhoids and associated complications

Degree	Bleeding	Prolapse
First	+++	None
Second	++	↓↑ Spontaneous or reduced by hand
Third	+	↓↓ Hanging out permanently with improper cleaning after defaecation, mucus dischange, and pruritus ani
Complicated piles	Strangulation Thrombosis Gangrene	

enlarged prostate, or benign pelvic tumour may result in increased straining to void, but not necessarily in haemorrhoids.

There is no evidence that patients with chronic respiratory disease with increased intra-abdominal pressure due to coughing have increased incidence of haemorrhoids. In pregnancy, haemorrhoids often develop before the fetus is large enough to mechanically obstruct venous outflow. Furthermore, aspiration of piles does not yield blood (vascular plexus rather than dilated veins) and bleeding of piles is usually bright red arterial blood, not dark blood of congested veins. The venous plexus of the upper anal canal is considered by others as physiological (not pathological) corpus cavernosum recti with direct arteriovenous communications, hyperplasia of which results from failure of mechanisms controlling arteriovenous shunts; others consider it normal vascular cushions playing a part in continence. Haemorrhoids may therefore be considered displaced and prolapsed cushions resulting from disruption of supporting tissues and mucosal suspensory ligament.

Diagnosis (Table 1.52.1)

High rectal or colonic disease must be excluded before treating haemorroids, particularly co-existing inflammatory bowel disease through history, physical examination and rectal biopsies.

Development of piles may be arrested by high-fibre diet, avoiding constipation and straining at stool with bulk laxative. Treatment depends on the degree of haemorrhoids: first and second degree piles can be treated conservatively. In patients with chronic fissure and piles, treatment should be directed at the fissure (as it is the cause of most severe symptoms).

Treatment

Open surgical haemorroidectomy Entails V-shaped incision, transfixing ligation and excision of the three piles leaving an intervening mucocutaneous bridge for epithelialisation to avoid stenosis formation. The bridges have to be undermined in order to remove secondary and large external piles and can be sutured (interrupted 3/0 chromic catgut) to the level of the dentate line (converting the operation into closed haemorrhoidectomy). A proctoscope must be inserted at the conclusion of operation to make sure there is no bleeding and no stenosis of the upper anal canal. Surgical haemorrhoidectomy remains the operation of choice for most cases of third-degree large prolapsing piles associated with skin tags and complicated haemorrhoids whose symptoms will not be controlled by any form of conservative treatment; there is postoperative pain, although operation can be done as day case surgery. Patients are put on preoperative bulk laxation in order to have easy postoperative bowel movement to enable a short hospital stay without the need for catheterisation and with an early discharge after 24 h% or less, using pain management on an outpatient basis.

Non-surgical methods of treatment
- Sclerosant injection of 5 ml of 5% phenol in almond or arachis oil (up to 20 ml can safely injected at a time) into the submucosa around the pedicle of the first-degree and small second degree pile aiming to produce a chemical thrombosis in internal haemorrhoidal plexus, and to produce fibrous reaction in submucosa fixing the loose redundant mucous membrane to inner muscle and pulling the pile up. The patient can be examined 6 weeks later for further injection if deemed necessary (persistent symptoms). Sclerotherapy is painless, quick and complication-free. Recurrence may occur within 5 years.
- Barron rubber band ligation, ideal for large first- and second-degree piles (with long pedicles to grasp) in the absence of associated skin tags. The band must be applied to the correct site, which is the false pedicle drawn out at the base of the pile at the top of the anal canal at least 1 cm above the dentate line (not the prolapsing part of the pile). Should the dentate line or anal papilla be included in the band, considerable pain will result. The ligated pile will necrose after 48 h (with dull aching pain) and slough off after 7 days. Most patients find the discomfort greater with rubber band ligation than with sclerotherapy.
- Cryosurgery employing cryosurgical probe using liquid nitrogen at a temperature of −160 °C for first- and second-degree piles; the iceball forms a white area delineating tissue to be sloughed. The procedure takes 15 min and the patient is observed for 30 min before going home. The procedure is performed without bleeding and is moderately painful (most pain is associated with postoperative oedema). The main disadvantage is profuse watery discharge (with potassium) starting within 3 h and lasting for up to 4 weeks, with several days off work. It is not practised widely.
- Lord's procedure of manual dilatation of anus (uncontrollable sphincteric stretch of anal canal including area above dentate line using 4 fingers for 4 minutes) under general anaesthesia to break the constricting pectin bands followed by insertion of a large lubricated polyvinyl sponge inserted with forceps to produce pressure and prevent bleeding and haematoma formation (removed after 24 h); this can be followed by a regimen of anal dilators over a period of 6 months. However, complete and permanent incontinence do occur with ruptured anal sphincters, particularly in the elderly and those with poor sphincteric tone. The procedure is not practised nowadays because of litigation problems associated with iatrogenic faecal incontinence.

- Laser haemorrhoidectomy is painless and gives good results. It is becoming a popular method of treatment.
- Infra-red coagulation.

Prolapsed thrombosed or strangulated haemorrhoids   A common and painful surgical emergency. There are three methods of treatment:
- Conservative method, commonly recommended, with elevation of bed foot, lubricated warm gauze after reduction, injectable analgesia, antibiotics and stool softner with bed rest. Piles gradually subside after a few days and can then be treated as indicated according to the degree of piles.
- Severe pain can be controlled quickly by carrying out manual dilatation of the anus (Lord's procedure), and the patient may need definitive treatment later.
- In the presence of history of severe attack of prolapsing piles or thrombosed prolapsed piles which have become gangrenous, emergency haemorrhoidectomy should be undertaken safely (postoperative pain is less than preoperatively).

Thrombosed external piles (wrongly called thrombosed perianal haematoma)   May arise spontaneously or may follow strenuous exercise or lifting, sexual intercourse, or excess alcohol. There is a painful lump lasting for 3 days and disappearing in weeks. Treatment is by incision under local anaesthesia and expression of the clot.

ANORECTAL FISTULAE (Figs 1.52.3, 1.52.4)

The majority of fistulae arise from previous non-specific cryptoglandular infections, or improperly drained or ruptured abscesses (whether perianal, ischiorectal, intersphincteric, supralevator, or deep postanal space abscess). The commonly employed system is the Parks' classification system categorising fistulae into:
- *Inter-sphincteric* between internal sphincter (caudal continuation of circular smooth muscle of the rectum) and the encircling external sphincter (cylinder of skeletal muscle composed of three components; subcutaneous, superficial, and deep portions).
- *Trans-sphincteric* fistula may have a circumferential component in addition to axial component so that the tract will lie around the anal canal on one side, or both, resulting in infra- or supralevator horse-shoe fistula; they always originate in the midline posteriorly
- *Extra- or supra-sphincteric or high* fistulae due to injudicious probing by a surgeon trying to determine the extent of trans sphincteric fistula with a supralevator extension (a supralevator extension is rare with inter-sphincteric fistula). High fistulae may not be associated with anorectal disease at all, but rather a downward extension of intraabdominal or pelvic disease or a tract resulted from perforation of rectum by a foreign body, such as wood or a fish bone

Diagnosis

Physical examination of the external opening can give a clue to fistula track; Goodsall's rule states that if the external opening is located posterior to the transverse anal line, the fistula tract

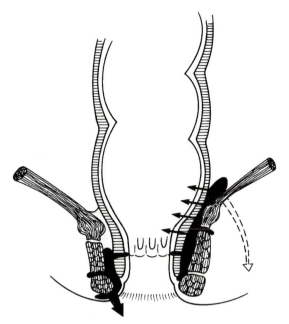

Fig. 1.52.3 A perianal abscess (low intermuscular wrongly called submucous), with a low intersphincteric fistula (*left*) revealing primary radial track-gland abscess-extension commonly into intersphincteric radial track (solid arrow for rupture or drainage) or occasionally into trans-sphincteric track. The deep intermuscular abscess (*right*) shows primary radial track–gland abscess–upward extension in the intersphincteric plane before bulging radially into the trans-sphincteric plane below puborectalis or above levator ani. It is treated by long open internal sphincterotomy (*solid arrows*); it must never be opened via perineum (*dotted arrow*) or a suprasphincteric fistula will result

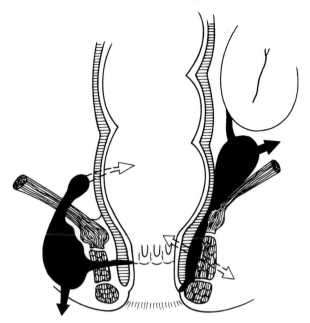

Fig. 1.52.4 High fistulas. Ischiorectal abscess (*left*) with a supralevator extension with primary track at the dentate line. Prompt primary drainage via skin prevents uncommon upward extension (*solid arrow*); it must never be opened into rectum (*dotted arrow*) or an extrasphincteric fistula will result necessitating colostomy and the use of a seton. The supralevator abscess (*right*) follows the bowel (diverticulitis or Crohn's) or pelvic disease. It must be drained suprapubically and managed from above (via abdomen); there is no need to cut external sphincter unless the track passes through the muscles trans-spincteric extension (*dotted arrows*)

will curve posteriorly to the posterior midline crypt. Fistulography can be helpful. Careful history to exclude inflammatory bowel disease, immunodeficiency, and suppurative disease, e.g. hydradenitis suppurativa and pilonidal disease. Manometric studies are needed to document status of anal sphincters.

Treatment

Conservative treatment through expectant therapy with antibiotics and sclerosing injection of fistulae can occasionally work. The surgical principles include the identification of anal opening (with proctoscopy), assessment of course of fistula tract, assessment of involved sphincter muscle encompassed within fistula tract, and choosing an appropriate technique that maximises the healing and minimises sphincteric injury, thereby preserving continence.

Surgical options include:

1. Laying open the fistula or fistulotomy is suitable for intersphincteric or low trans-sphincteric fistulae, where the tract is layed open between internal and external openings, cutting through the skin, internal sphincter and, in case of trans-sphincteric fistula, portions of external sphincter muscle; granulation tissue is curetted and may be sent for pathology. Marsupialisation of cut skin edges helps haemostasis. Fistulotomy is preferred over fistulectomy (in which the entire fistula tract is excised via a larger wound with prolonged

healing time and potential injury to sphincter resulting in compromising continence). Re-routing technique can be used to re-route the fistula tract by cutting sphincteric muscle with immediate reconstruction of external sphincter behind the tract, thereby converting a high trans-sphincteric fistula into an intersphincteric one which can be dealt with by conventional method once healing of the external sphincter has occurred.

2. Placement of a seton as a cutting or marking (non-cutting) device is indicated in trans-sphincteric with supralevator extension (wrongly termed high fistulae) wherever the surgeon thinks excessive muscle is involved within the fistula tract so that cutting through muscle may result in incontinence, e.g. if greater than one-third of the external sphincter is involved or if the fistula is anterior in a woman. The primary complex is laid open and the upward supralevator cavities are carefully curetted and drained. The opening through the levator muscles must be enlarged so that a finger can be inserted. When cutting out these cavities, care must be taken not to produce a secondary high opening into the rectum (it is not uncommon to have the primary opening at the dentate line and to pass intersphincterically below or through the lower portion of puborectalis to enter the ischiorectal fossa).

The rationale of seton use includes:

– it provides on-going drainage;

– it stimulates fibrosis of spincteric muscle so that subsequent cutting will not result in retraction of cut ends;

- it provides a means of the assessing the depth and extent of sphincteric muscle involvement while the patient is not under anaesthesia.

There are various ways of using a seton, such as two-stage fistulotomy using silk as the seton (second stage performed 4–8 weeks after seton placement), cutting technique where the seton was tightened gradually to cut through and divide the anal sphincter (Barron band ligature instrument can be used for tightening seton), or the use of a seton as a short-term drainage device with subsequent removal and healing of the fistula tract with fibrosis.

3. Temporary defunctioning colostomy in high anorectal fistulae together with the lower tract laid open and supralevator extension opened widely (so that the rectal wall can be seen above puborectalis). The defect is then closed with interrupted wire sutures and the wound allowed to granulate. The colostomy can be closed after 3 months, when the wound has completely healed.

Closure of internal opening with anorectal mucosal advancement flap technique   Endorectal advancement flap was used originally for rectovaginal fistulae and extended in the management of complicated anal fistulae, with the surgical principles of closing the internal opening, curettage and drainage of the external opening, without disturbing the sphincteric mechanism. A well-vascularised rectal flap is assured by broad base at the apex, and adrenaline infiltration and tension-free suturing are mandatory.

Primary fistulotomy with drainage of perianal abscess   Patients with perianal abscess with intersphincteric extension present with pain on defaecation and throbbing in the anal canal; treatment is by simply laying open (deroofing and drainage). If a fistula is apparent, this is *laid open at the same time (primary fistulotomy)*. Large ischiorectal abscesses, on the other hand, should be drained and any fistula must be treated later when the acute condition has resolved. It is interesting to know that when no fistula is present, the pus from the abscess grows *Staphylococcus pyogenes* on culture, whereas if a fistula is present (but not apparent at operation), the swab grows intestinal flora (Bacteroides). Primary fistulotomy offers the advantage of a lower recurrence rate but the disadvantage of potential creation of a false tract or injury to the sphincter muscles in the face of active acute inflammation. Adequate drainage of abscess via good deroofing is essential (cruciate incision can be converted into a diamond by trimming the triangular edges), because the skin may heal while the abscess has not been drained adequately.

FISSURE-IN-ANO

This is a common and painful condition. Fissures most commonly present in the midline posteriorly following the traumatic passage of a large constipated stool causing acute tear leading to spasm and pain after defaecation and passage of a bright red streak of blood. If acute fissure is not healed, it becomes hypertrophied with skin papilla and tag and termed as sentinel tag. The incidence is the same in men and women and peak incidence is in the third decade. A fissure is frequently found with haemorrhoids.

Fissure pain is severe and the patient is apprehensive and must be examined gently. Inspection and digital examination is with liberal 2% lignocaine gel; inability to pass the finger confirms the provisional diagnosis and requires the patient's examination under anaesthesia.

Conservative outpatient treatment of acute fissure-in-ano is effective and consists of St Mark's anal dilator size 2 lubricated with 2% lignocaine gel and performed by the patient him- or herself (auto-dilatation) before leaving outpatients. This may continue twice daily at home for 3 weeks and can result in healing of the fissure.

Chronic fissure, however, does not heal by conservative means; it requires operative treatment in one of three forms.

- Open or closed (subcutaneous) lateral internal sphincterotomy (unilateral on one side is as good as bilateral on both sides) is commonly used, cutting and dividing full thickness of internal sphincter from its margin to at least 0.5 cm above the dentate line; postoperative recurrence rate is low (1–2%). The procedure can be done under local anaesthesia in jack-knife position.
- posterior sphincterotomy is carried out if there is intersphincteric abscess deep to chronic fissure, or fistula with a fissure.
- Lord's manual dilatation of the anus under general anaesthesia is effective and simple, but its simplicity is marred by iatrogenic uncontrollable incontinence, ecchymoses and resultant fibrosis with 16% recurrence (it is not widely performed).
- Excision of fissure (fissurectomy) was found to be an unnecessary operation.
- Landscaping: excision of proximal papilla and distal anal tag without excising the fissure can also be performed but results are less satisfactory than unilateral lateral internal sphincterotomy.

PILONIDAL DISEASE (PND)

Pilonidal – *Pilo* (hair), *nidus* (nest) – disease may either be congenital or acquired. The association of eyebrows crossing the midline and familial incidence favours the congenital aetiology. The acquired aetiology is suggested by low incidence among those using bidet or water ablution after defaecation as compared to those using paper ablution. Differential diagnosis includes hidradenitis suppurativa, fistula-in-ano, and actinomycosis.

Usually PND presents as painful abscess (draining sinuses are usually painless). Incision and drainage with removal of hairs, bathing or waterpic irrigation are mandatory. Antibiotics are not necessary.

Various methods of treatment of pilonidal sinus may include:
- Wide local excision with (closed method) or without (open method) primary closure after methylene blue injection to identify sinus ramification for thorough excision.
- Incision and marsupialisation with or without suturing can be done in outpatients. The cavity is opened, epithelium is curetted, lateral one-third of cyst wall is removed and the edge of the cyst base is either affixed to skin with non-absorbable suture or left open. Dressing and waterpic irrigation twice daily speeds healing, which occurs in 2–6 weeks.

- Phenol injection to destroy epithelium and dissolve the hair (1–2 ml of 80% phenol solution); repeat injections are occasionally necessary.
- Local conservative excision of skin ellipse containing sinuses, probing and brushing of the sinus track, with circle excision of external opening, and daily postoperative shaving of perineal region (Lord's conservative procedure).
- Excision and Z-plasty, lateral flap, or gluteus maximus myocutaneous flap are too extensive procedures for a simple PND.

PAINFUL ANORECTAL LESIONS

Common lesions

Include:

- *Anorectal abscess*

  Perianal — commonest type; adequate drainage through cruciate incision with trimming of skin edges.

  Ischiorectal — adequate drainage as above; immediate or subsequent exploration to exclude fistula-in-ano; if present lay open track (some units practise incision, curettage and primary suture under antibiotic cover).

  Submucous — open into rectum as visualised via proctoscopy.

  Pelvirectal is a pelvic abscess with no pain in anal region usually.

- *Anal fissure*

  Severe pain during defaecation with slight bleeding, some discharge. Sentinel skin tag often seen.

  Acute — conservative treatment (analgesic ointment, bulk-forming agent and avoid costipation and patient's own finger auto-dilatation under analgesic ointment). If unsuccessful then surgical digital dilatation of anus (condemned, as it may cause permanent incontinence in 36%).

  Chronic — sphincterotomy and excision of skin tag.

- *Strangulated/thrombosed piles*

  Complication of second- or third-degree haemorrhoids; treatment may either be conservative (analgesia, bed rest, ice pack, compresses, aperients) or operative (immediate emergency haemorrhoidectomy)

- *Perianal haematoma*

  Thrombosed external haemorrhoid; treatment within 48 h (incision/deroofing with evacuation of haematoma followed by analgesics, hot baths, aperients).

Less common lesions

Include:

- *Sexually transmitted diseases*

  Gonorrhoeal proctitis

  Genital herpes and *Condylomata acuminata* (viral infection)

  AIDS

  Primary chancre and *Condylomata lata* (syphilis)

  Non-specific proctitis

- Anal carcinoma
- Acute exacerbation of pilonidal sinus/abscess
- Proctalgia fugax
- Crohn's disease

FAECAL INCONTINENCE

The involuntary loss of faeces is a distressing social disability. Normally the anorectal mechanism is made up of two tubular-shaped parts, one ensheathing the other. The innermost structure is the termination of the gut (*visceral* part); this is surrounded by pelvic floor *skeletal* muscles, the lower part of which form the *external anal sphincters*. The lower rectum and anal canal are innervated by the autonomic nerves and are therefore not subject to voluntary control. It is the surrounding skeletal muscle sphincter that is essential for establishing normal continence. The upper part of the visceral component is lined by unstratified, mucus-secreting columnar epithelium which is almost devoid of sensory receptors. Fortunately, the terminal 2 cm is atypical in that the visceral mucosa has been replaced by squamous epithelium which does not secrete mucus; the perineum is therefore not continuously soiled by mucous discharge.

This lower 2 cm is supplied with somatic sensory nerves which supply information to the spinal centres and is a valuable part of the mechanism of continence. The terminal part of the circular muscle is greatly enlarged to form the *internal sphincter muscle*. Its visceral tone is the most important factor in maintaining a closed anal canal, but it is autonomically supplied and there is no control over it. Outside this there is a relatively thin layer of longitudinal muscle that has no significant function in this area.

The external sphincter muscles maintain control over the outlet. In addition they have an antigravity function in maintaining a closed pelvic outlet against the forces of abdominal pressure. However, surgical division of the internal sphincter rarely results in any serious disability. Similarly extensive division of the external sphincter (in anal fistulae) leads to only a slight disability. The forward pull of the fibres of the puborectalis muscle creates an *anorectal angle* (normally 60–105°) which is maintained involuntarily by a spinal reflex; once this angle is exceeded, faecal incontinence occurs. *Faecal continence therefore appears to be related principally to the preservation of a normal anorectal angle which in turn is dependent on a normally functioning puborectalis muscle with a flap-valve mechanism accentuated by the intra-abdominal pressure.*

The sensation of continence is conducted through receptors lying within the rectum and the nearby pelvic floor muscles which cradle it (and therefore coloanal anastomosis does not interfere with this sensation).

Diagnosis

A careful history (current complaint and duration, gastro-intestinal symptoms, neurological symptoms, past history of congenital defect, operative trauma or neurological disease), rectal examination (to exclude rectal neoplasm, assess sphincteric function and test anal skin sensation) and sigmoidoscopy. Intra-anal pressure recording and preoperative electromyographic exploration of the perineum may be helpful in mapping out the deficient skeletal muscles.

Classification of causes with treatment

True incontinence

Partial incontinence

This occurs in the presence of partial or complete rectal prolapse or commonly as a complication of minor surgery, e.g. sphincterotomy, fistula surgery, haemorrhoidectomy or manual dilatation of the anus. There is normal function within the pelvic floor muscles and external anal sphincter.

This group may need no treatment or simple conservative treatment (constipating agents). Complete rectal prolapse, however, may need a purse-string procedure or even rectopexy.

Complete incontinence

Usually there is a normally functioning internal anal sphincter and a markedly deficient or dysfunctioned skeletal muscle component.

Idiopathic   No apparent underlying neurological or anatomical causes. However denervation of pelvic floor muscles and the external sphincter with anal reflex delay is thought to be the cause as proved by microscopic and special histochemical examination of muscle biopsies (*localised neuronal damage*). Spontaneous occurrence of incontinence in women is due to a prolonged second stage of labour with possible perineal tears. Prolonged straining at defaecation may lead to the *descending perineum syndrome* due to pudendal nerve stretch injury. There may be pudendal nerve entrapment within Alcock's canal (comparable to carpal tunnel syndrome).

Postanal repair (muscle-tightening procedure) may be indicated in which the levator ani, puborectalis and external sphincter muscles are apposed behind the anorectal ring. The gracilis sling procedure or free autotransplantation of the palmaris longus or sartorius muscle placed as a U-shaped sling around the rectum may also be used.

Traumatic   Due to anal injury, fistula surgery damaging the integrity of the puborectalis sling and abolishing the anorectal angle; treatment is by sphincteroplasty (see comment below) which necessitates a temporary defunctioning colostomy.

Neurological   As in tabes dorsalis or multiple sclerosis, paraplegia and cauda equina. Conservative measures may be used (not very effective) and include pelvic floor faradism, external sphincter stimulation by direct electrode implantation and external anal plug stimulation.

Congenital   As in anorectal agenesis and anal ectopia. This needs accurate siting of the *neoanus* and rectum in relation to the pelvic floor and necessitates preoperative electromyography.

False incontinence

Incontinence may be secondary to organic colorectoanal disease or occur in severe diarrhoea. The commonest cause in the elderly is dyschesia; this is a spurious diarrhoea due to liquefaction of impacted faeces. Treatment is that of the primary cause.

Sphincteroplasty

Surgical repair of the injured sphincter basically includes apposition, overlapping and reefing. In principle the surgeon usually attempts to repair the external sphincter muscle or puborectalis sling or both. Gracilis muscle transposition or a Dacron-impregnated Silastic sheet sling can be used to supplement the sphincter mechanism.

Construction of a neoanal sphincter by transposition of gracilis muscle and prolonged neuromuscular stimulation via implanted electrical stimulator has been pioneered by N. Williams (1990) and indicated in selected patients with faecal incontinence.

OUTLINE OF ANORECTAL PHYSIOLOGY STUDIES

There are many gastrointestinal motility centres in the world. Among all tests performed on GIT motility, the anorectal studies are considered to be the most useful and relevant to the clinical practice of colorectal surgery.

Even when the results of various anorectal studies are negative (in 30% of cases), the centre provides a psychological reassurance to both the referred patients and the referring doctor.

In America, anorectal tests are performed, occasionally for medicolegal reasons, before and after anorectal operations (such as fistulectomies) to confirm or refute the presence of faecal incontinence prior to surgery in order to safeguard surgeons from patients claiming incontinence caused by operation.

Anorectal physiology centres can provide diagnostic services as well as academic research activities in the three major fields of colorectal surgery, namely faecal incontinence, pelvic floor disorders and obstructed defaecation.

Faecal incontinence

To confirm the clinical diagnosis, identify the underlying aetiology and thus influence the therapeutic modality used to treat patients with 'Faecal incontinence'. It also promotes the academic research in various conditions leading to faecal incontinence.

Faecal incontinence can be due to damage to the internal anal sphincter (IAS) and/or the external anal sphincter (EAS)/ puborectalis complex; it may be due to disruption of any component of the nervous reflexes that control these muscles. The disturbances in sphincter function responsible for faecal incontinence can be grouped into several clinical entities, that can be characterized and discriminated by manometric and electrophysiological studies.

Table 1.52.2 Causes of faecal incontinence that can be identified by physiological testing

Causes	Features	Possible treatment
Pudendal neuropathy (neurogenic)	Perineal descent. Weak conscious and reflex EAS contractions. Normal electrical responses	Post-anal repair
Obstetric trauma (myogenic)	Weak sphincter. Circumferential electrical gap	Sphincter repair
Impaired rectal sensation	1. IAS relaxes at volumes that fail to induce sensation and EAS response 2. Delayed EAS response	Retraining
Low spinal lesion	Impaired rectal sensation. Reduced rectal tone. Absent EAS responses to rectal distension and increases in intra-abdominal pressure	Training
High spinal lesion	Absent rectal sensation. Little or no conscious control of EAS. Enhanced reflex control	Training
Irritable bowel syndrome	Enhanced rectal sensitivity. Reduced rectal compliance. Increased rectal contractility, and anal relaxation in responce to rectal distension	Drugs Diet Psychotherapy
Transient IAS relaxation	Inappropriate IAS relaxations under resting conditions and after squeeze and strain	?Drugs
Impaired IAS function	Very low pressures. No IAS relaxation on rectal distension	?Sympathomimetic drugs

The commonest causes of faecal incontinence in surgical practice are in this following order:
- Myogenic injury of the anal sphincter as a postoperative complication following haemorrhoidectomy, fistulectomy and episiotomy.
- Occasionally, neurogenic injury after delivery due to the pressure effect of the fetal head crushing the pudendal nerve(s).
- Rarely, peripheral neuropathy in diabetics, alcoholics and in AIDS patients may all produce incontinence.
- Idiopathic anorectal incontinence leads to a short weak sphincter, reduced rectal compliance, abnormal sampling (sampling is the rectal sensation to discriminate between flatus and faeces), and diminished anorectal sensation. EMG reveals denervation and subsequent reinnervation of striated muscle of EAS and pelvic floor.

The identification of the mechanism underlying faecal incontinence provides a useful basis for selection of an appropriate treatment option (see Table 1.52.2).

Pelvic floor disorder

Pelvic floor disorders are common and cause much disability. They form a group of functional disorders of the pelvic floor musculature that cause anorectal, urinary and gynaecological problems. The pelvic floor disorders have inter-related underlying causative mechanisms. The underlying functional disturbance can be assessed clinically, pathologically and electrophysiologically (Table 1.52.3).

Identification of causes of obstructed defaecation

Defaecation is a stereotyped sequence of actions, usually initiated by a conscious mechanism and involving a number of

Table 1.52.3 Pelvic floor disorders

Anorectal incontinence
Urinary incontinence (genuine stress incontinence)
Double incontinence
Anorectal prolapse
Genital prolapse
Pelvic pain syndrome
Intractable constipation
Solitary rectal ulcer syndrome
Complications of childbirth
    Sphincter injuries
    Vaginal and uterine prolapse
    Incontinence
    Delayed complications, e.g. altered bowel habit, incontinence of
      urine or faeces

pelvic reflexes that are controlled and coordinated by a centre in the brain stem.

Faeces are propelled into the rectum by propagated colonic contractions. If the stool is large enough, the rectal distension (and proably also the weight of the stool on the pelvic floor) induces a desire to defaecate. This sensation is usually associated with a rectal contraction and a relaxation of the IAS which serves to tamp the stool down into the proximal anal canal, increasing the defaecatory urge. If conditions are appropriate, the subject sits or squats, contracts the diaphragm, the abdominal muscles and the levators, while relaxing the external sphincter and possibly also the puborectalis (to open up the anorectal angle), and faeces are extruded. Once it has commenced, defaecation can continue with no conscious effort; presumably, as a result of strong propagated colonic contraction.

Table 1.52.4   Causes of obstructed defaecation that can be identified by physiological testing

Causes	Features	Possible treatment
Anismus	Paradoxical puborectalis/EAS contraction during defaecation	?Retraining
Short segment Hirschsprung's (or myenteric aganglionosis in adult constipation)	High anal pressure. Failure of IAS to relax on rectal distension (absent recto-sphincteric reflex) Requires full-thickness rectal biopsy for histological confirmation	Sphincterotomy
Megarectum	Increased rectal compliance and capacity. Reduced rectal sensation	Defaecation training
Low spinal lesion	Impaired rectal sensation. Weak or absent conscious EAS contraction Absent EAS response to rectal distension and increased abdominal pressure. CT scan and MR imaging can confirm cauda equina compression caused by intervertebral disc prolapse	Training
Irritable bowel syndrome	Enhanced rectal sensitivity. Reduced rectal compliance. Increased rectal contractility, and anal relaxation in response to rectal distension	Drugs Diet Psychotherapy
Non-prolapsing haemorrhoids	Ultraslow waves. High resting pressures. Failure of outermost anal canal to relax during rectal distension	Banding Electrocoagulation Haemorrhoidectomy
Partial rectal prolapse	Very low resting pressures. Failure of anal pressure to increase above rectal pressure during increases in intra-abdominal pressure	Banding ?Post-anal repair

Defaecation may be impaired by failure of the internal anal sphincter to relax, inappropriate contraction of the external anal sphincter and puborectalis, failure of the levators to lift the pelvic floor and open the anorectal angle and luminal obstruction by haemorrhoids and partial prolapse of the rectum into the anal canal. Many of these conditions can be identified and discriminated by combined anorectal manometry, electro-myography and test of the rectal sensation (see Table 1.52.4).

In contrast to obstructed defaecation, chronic constipation is either due to prolonged transit time or due to a hypertensive anal canal (anismus or paradoxical puborectalis contraction). The operation of choice in chronic constipation due to slow transit time is total colectomy with ileorectal anastomosis; sigmoid colectomy is followed by a high incidence of recurrence and, therefore, is not recommended.

In hypertensive anal canal, a skeletal muscle relaxant anti-spasmodic may be tried (e.g. Baclofen) initially. However, various operations may also be performed, such as Lord's procedure, lateral sphincterotomy, myectomy and division of puborectalis on both sides.

Diagnostic procedures performed in the centre

Primary major studies

There is no need for bowel preparation prior to investigations. There are three sets of basic investigations performed in the left lateral position:

1. Manometric studies using a Multichannel Pressure Recorder to measure the pressure and record the findings on paper as graphic material evidence for permanent documentation of the physiological status of the anorectal sphincter.

The pressure transducer is connected to a water-filled microballoon mounted on a 5 FG ureteric catheter which is prefilled with water (no air) via a 3-way tap and a syringe. The catheter is lubricated and the pressure is recorded at the level of the anal cleft before insertion (baseline pressure recording) and after insertion inside the anorectum (resting pressure recording of IAS) which is roughly around $20\,cmH_2O$.

When the patient is asked to squeeze or contract the anus, the pressure shoots up to around $60\,cmH_2O$ or more. False pressure rise may be due to buttocks contraction or thigh adductors contraction and, therefore, EMG is better and more informative than manometry.

2. Single Fibre EMG is used to record muscle action potential obtained via the single muscle fibre electrode needle inserted through the post-anal puborectalis portion of levator ani; the other electrode plate is wrapped around the patient's thigh.

Uni- or monophasic action potential is normal; biphasic or polyphasic action potential is indicative of muscle partial denervation (and nerve regeneration). Complete denervation or surgical muscle excision will give rise to a flat tracing.

Concentric fibre EMG is used for recording muscle potentials in multiple sphincteric muscle defects or tears (this can be confirmed with transanal ultrasound to localise sphincteric tears). It is also used in obstructed defaecation cases, where any muscular spontaneous activity can be recorded (via the needle myography).

3. Bilateral pudendal nerve stimulation: using the St. Mark's pudendal electrode for investigating patients with pelvic floor neuromuscular disorders.

The electrode is wrapped around the gloved index finger and the wrist; the finger is lubricated and introduced into the anus to stimulate each side of the pelvis separately by redirecting the finger laterally to the right and left. Nerve stimulation (indicated by a flashing green light) and consecutive electrode recording can easily determine the pudendal nerve latency or the conduction period between the electrical stimulus and the anal sphincteric response.

Muscle contraction will be absent only if the pudendal nerve is absent (surgical excision) or totally damaged (late stages of damage).

As a rule of thumb, if the pudendal nerve is absent, EMG is abnormal. However, pudendal nerve normally supplies EAS, so if the pelvic floor and/or IAS contracts (with absent pudendal nerve), one can still get some action potential on EMG, (a very rare situation).

Secondary minor studies

4. Anal canal functional length is recorded when the pressure transducer is pulled out gently until no IAS pressure wave is seen; the length of transducer from the anal verge is then measured (using a ruler) to represent the functional length of the anal canal.
5. Rectal sensation is assessed on balloon distension using a syringe, and a rectal tube with a big balloon filled by air or by cold water. Water volumes causing the patient to sense the first feeling, urge for defaecation and pain are termed 'threshold volume', 'urge volume', and 'maximal tolerance volume' respectively.

If the tube and the balloon are inside, one can inject 50 ml of air and quickly withdraw it to check for the so-called 'recto-sphincteric reflex' producing a gradual rise in IAS pressure with its immediate relaxation (the reflex is absent in Hirsch-sprung's disease).
6. Rectal sensation on electrical testing using a special electrode mounted on a catheter and connected to the EMG machine.
7. Perineal descent (using a perineometry) during rest and strain can be classified as mild, moderate and marked.
8. Rectal compliance.

Supportive and complementary tests

- Anal ultrasound with a rotating probe introduced via a water filled sigmoidoscope (water is needed for accoustic contact). Anal ultrasound can clearly demonstrate any defect in IAS and/or EAS.
- Defaecating proctogram using 120 ml of Microtrast enema followed by asking the patient to defaecate under screening, while sitting on a commode. Internal rectal intussusception can be symptomatic in rectal prolapse, solitary rectal ulcer syndrome and incontinence, but can also be asymptomatic; it can be detected on rectal examination and sigmoidoscopy by an experienced surgeon, but is usually confirmed on evacuation proctography.
- Shapes test: the patient must abstain from taking laxatives for one week and then takes 20 pieces of radio-opaque marker with breakfast. After 3–5 days, the plain X-ray film normally should not reveal more than four unexcreted pieces. Presence of more than four pieces indicates a slow transit time.
- Pelvic CT scan.

1.53 Critical Review of Abdominal Stoma

Abdominal stoma includes:
- Surgically designed gastrointestinal stoma constructed percutaneously, i.e. gastrostomy, jejunostomy (for feeding in e.g. proximal advanced malignancies), ileostomy and colostomy (intestinal content diversion) whether temporary or permanent, terminal end or looped fashion.
- External stoma. Include fistulae due to a variety of causes (diseased bowel such as Crohn's or diverticular disease, following penetrating abdominal trauma, postoperatively after resection and primary intestinal anastomoses, following radiotherapy and rarely congenital umbilical fistula).
- Urostomy in urinary diversion, i.e. ileal conduit. We will deal here only with ileostomy and colostomy problems, abdominal fistulae and urostomy.

ILEOSTOMY AND COLOSTOMY

Stoma site

Preoperatively the intended site of the stoma should be marked on the skin of the abdominal wall while the patient is standing. The selected site should be visible to the patient and should take account of the proposed site of the laparotomy incision. To ensure that the appliance sits squarely on the skin the opening should be sited away from the umbilicus and bony points, and as far as practically possible should avoid previous abdominal incisions. The patient should try out an appliance before the operation and should meet the stoma therapist who will help with after-care.

Construction of stoma

In the construction of an ileostomy it is necessary to evert 6 cm of ileum to produce a 3 cm spout. The deeper layer of the ileum needs to be anchored to the abdominal wall either from within or at the level of the external oblique aponeurosis. Whichever technique is chosen care should be exercised in the placement of the sutures. The bite into the bowel should go only through serosa.

The formation of a pericolostomy fistula or a pericolostomy abscess which bursts onto the skin with the subsequent formation of a fistulous track requires surgery. The track should be laid open and left to granulate. In the case of an ileostomy the whole stoma may have to be revised.

Stoma appliances

There are two basic designs of stoma appliance. The one-piece unit consists of a bag which is attached to the skin directly either by adhesive, Stomahesive or karaya gum. The bag itself may be drainable or closed. The two-piece unit consists of a plastic flange which is either attached directly to the skin or bonded to a karaya gum or Stomahesive square. The collecting bag can be detached from the plastic flange and disposed of separately. The two-piece system makes stoma management easier and minimises skin irritation due to constant removal and reapplication of the bag, but it is bulkier than a one-piece bag.

Skin problems

Skin problems associated with an ileostomy are more common since its efflux is liquid and contains proteolytic enzymes. The contact of the efflux with skin rapidly causes irritation, maceration, excoriation and digestion. For this reason an ileostomy is constructed as a spout protruding 2–4 cm beyond the skin of the abdominal wall so that the motions pass directly into the collecting appliance.

Leakage of the stoma efflux may be due to faulty site selection, failure of adherence of the appliance or to complications in the stoma itself which allow escape of the efflux directly onto the skin. Adhesive sensitivity is another cause of skin problems.

Skin problems in relation to a colostomy are seldom so severe since the motions are semisolid and are non-irritant. Leakage of the faeces from a colostomy may be due to faulty site selection; problems of the stoma itself (rendering adherence of the bag difficult) or a loose colostomy appliance which causes skin maceration.

Too frequent change of the one-piece appliance

The use of a one-piece system may result in skin soreness due to the constant minor trauma of removing the bag. If this is the cause of the skin irritation, then the patient should be advised to use a two-piece system. A Stomahesive or karaya square is cut to cover the injured skin and a hole made in it to accommodate the stoma. The square should be left on the skin for as long as possible. A plastic flange is mounted onto the square or may be integral with it. The bag is merely unclipped from the flange at the appropriate time and replaced with a new one. Once the skin has had time to heal the patient can go back to the old appliance or may continue with the new method.

Problems with the two-piece appliance

In applying the plastic flange of a two-piece ileostomy set, care should be taken to ensure that it does not chafe the spout; otherwise it may cause bleeding or pressure necrosis of the stoma and a fistula may develop at skin level. Should this occur the efflux will discharge directly onto the skin, causing excoriation, and the stoma will have to be revised.

Sensitivity to adhesive

Sensitivity to the adhesive can be tested by placing a similar appliance on another part of the patient's body. If a skin reaction occurs, the patient should avoid appliances using adhesive and be advised to use those utilising either a Stomahesive or karaya washer since sensitivity to these materials is virtually unknown.

Established skin excoriation

Established ulceration or weeping macerated skin can be dressed with Stomahesive squares upon which a flange and clip-on bag can be mounted. Healing of the skin below the Stomahesive takes place.

Control of the stoma efflux

Most ileostomies settle to a discharge of 500 ml/24 h and the stool becomes sloppy rather than liquid in its consistency. For those patients with a persistently loose ileostomy which drains large volumes (up to 1500 ml/24 h), leakage and the development of skin irritation can be a major problem. Attempts to improve the consistency of the efflux should be made by the administration of hydrophilic agents such as ispaghula, sterculia or methylcellulose. Kaolin may sometimes help and certain drugs such as codeine phosphate, loperamide and diphenoxylate which reduce intestinal motility can be tried. Should these manipulations prove unsuccessful and the patient cannot manage, then, as a last resort the revision of the ileostomy is contemplated. A reversed interposed loop of ileum proximal to the stoma has been tried and the conversion of the ileostomy into a continent reservoir has also been advocated.

Control of the colostomy is usually much more straightforward. It responds well to dietary and pharmacological agents. A loop colostomy fashioned in the right upper quadrant can be loose and fixture of the bag a problem, but by the measures outlined above the stool can be rendered firmer and the colostomy controlled better.

Stoma complications

Necrosis

Following the fashioning of an end colostomy, necrosis of the bowel adjacent to the mucocutaneous suture line may occur as a result of inadequate intraoperative assessment of the viability of the blood supply of the terminal portion of the bowel, or as a result of thrombosis in the vessels constricted by a tight external oblique aponeurosis.

This complication can be avoided by paying attention to the placement of ligatures on the mesentery when mobilising the sigmoid colon, ensuring that the opening in the abdominal wall is adequate and that there is no tension on the suture line.

Slight separation of the mucosa from the skin merely requires observation since the mucosa will rapidly re-epithelialise the defect. If the colostomy necroses for more than 1.5 cm, the stoma should be revised since the granulating area will fibrose and a stenosis of the stoma will result.

Stenosis (more dangerous than prolapse)

When stomas were not immediately completed by direct mucocutaneous suture stenosis was commonplace. Direct mucocutaneous suture has made this complication rare. It may occur if the distal bowel becomes gangrenous and circumferential granulations undergo fibrosis. It can be remedied by excising the stenotic rim, mobilising the stoma so that viable bowel can be brought to the skin surface without tension and performing direct mucocutaneous suture.

Obstruction

Faecal impaction

Large bowel obstruction may be due to faecal impaction with or without spurious diarrhoea. A glycerine suppository, a colostomy washout or digital evacuation may remedy the situation.

A search should be made for an underlying stenosis of the stoma. This may be at skin level or at the level of the external oblique aponeurosis as revealed by digital examination.

If the stoma is of normal calibre the patient is advised to keep the stool soft by taking a high fibre diet or a faecal softener can be prescribed. If a stenosis is the underlying cause of the faecal impaction then the stoma may have to be revised.

Prolapse of the small bowel through pelvic peritoneum

Following the excision of the rectum and repair of the pelvic floor, if the suture line in the pelvic peritoneum gives way a knuckle of small bowel may herniate into the pelvic space. This may give rise to an obstruction. If at laparotomy the defect cannot be resutured easily, the pelvic peritoneum is opened in its entirety so that the complication cannot recur.

Lateral space obstruction

This complication has been eliminated by the extraperitoneal technique of stoma fashioning. If a direct colostomy or ileostomy is fashioned care should be taken to close the lateral space by suturing the mesentery of the bowel to the lateral wall of the abdominal cavity or, alternatively, a flap of mobilised peritoneum is sutured to the bowel in order to prevent the prolapse of small bowel around the lateral side of the emergent limb of the stoma.

Fistula

The placement of sutures through the serosa of the colon to anchor it to the deeper layers of the abdominal wall should be avoided. It is unnecessary and a misplaced suture which passes through the whole thickness of the bowel is an invitation to a fistula.

Prolapse

Colostomy

Prolapse is a much commoner complication of loop colostomies than of end colostomies. Once a colostomy prolapses it becomes oedematous and the mucosa splits. It may also become abraded by the stoma appliance and bleed. Most prolapses cause little discomfort but may make changing the bag difficult or cause the bag to be pushed off the abdominal wall. The bulk of a prolapsed colostomy may be a social embarrassment.

With a right transverse loop colostomy prolapse of the distal loop is usually more troublesome than prolapse of the the proximal loop. Prolapse of the proximal loop can be avoided by making the colostomy as far to the right of the middle colic vessels and as near to the hepatic flexure as possible. For the same reasons, when fashioning a defunctioning loop left iliac colostomy, the stoma should be placed as near to the descending colon as possible.

An oedematous prolapsed colostomy can be left alone if it is small and not troublesome. A large problematical prolapse can usually be reduced on the ward by patient gentle digital manipulation. Closure of a loop colostomy is the best method of cure but if restoration of the continuity of the bowel is not contemplated, it may be necessary to convert the loop into a single barrel provided there is no distal obstruction. If there is distal obstruction a divided colostomy or double-barrelled colostomy can be fashioned. If it is not possible to close a right transverse loop colostomy on its own, it can be closed if a defunctioning loop ileostomy is constructed proximally at the same time. The prolapsed problematical end colostomy may need to be revised. This is usually a simple matter of amputating the redundant bowel.

Ileostomy prolapse and recession

When the ileostomy is being fashioned, approximately 8 cm of terminal ileum is brought through the abdominal wall uneverted at the site of election. The inner tube of bowel is fixed either by suturing the mesentery of the bowel to the abdominal wall from within the abdominal cavity or by suturing it to the anterior rectus sheath from without. Alternatively, very superficial sutures are passed directly between the ileal serosa and the rectus sheath. The ileum is then everted and the distal mucosa sutured directly to skin. The final ileostomy bud should project between 2.5 and 4 cm.

A fixed excessive projection of the bud may force the appliance off the abdominal wall, while fixed inadequate projection predisposes to seepage of efflux onto the skin, leakage and skin problem.

Failure to secure the inner tube of ileum to the abdominal wall or subsequent collapse of the fixation may result in a sliding prolapse of the ileostomy or a sliding recession. Leakage of the appliance becomes a problem.

Fixed excessive projection can be treated by straightforward amputation of the stoma bud to the desired length. Alternatively, all of these stoma problems can be dealt with by revising the stoma completely. The mucocutaneous junction is circumcised and adhesions between the two limbs of the bud broken down. The outer tube is uneverted, the bowel is amputated to the desired level, the inner tube of ileum is fixed to the rectus sheath, the spout is everted and the mucosa sutured to skin. The presence of a large defect at the level of the posterior rectus sheath which predisposes to prolapse may have to be closed at laparotomy and the ileostomy resited – possibly even in the left iliac fossa.

Parastomal hernia

Para-ileostomy and paracolostomy hernia result from making too large a hole in the abdominal wall. The extent of the hernial bulge is variable but large bulges result in problems with the appliance. In a large number of instances the herniation can be controlled by the fitting of a surgical corset with an aperture for

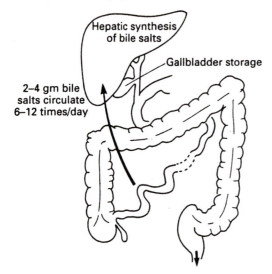

Fig. 1.53.1 Enterohepatic circulation of bile salts. About 95% is absorbed from the terminal ileum resulting in faecal excretion of 0.2–0.6 gm/day only

the stoma. Should this be insufficient, then a repair of the hernia may have to be carried out. This may be difficult. The operation may entail merely the tightening of the abdominal wall around the stoma or it may necessitate a major repair using non-absorbable mesh and the resiting of the opening.

Recurrent Crohn's disease

The recurrence of Crohn's disease in the spout of an ileostomy may be associated with the formation of fistulae. The extent of the diseased segment will have to be gauged and the offending segment resected with the fashioning of a new stoma.

Stone formation (Fig 1.53.1)

Ileostomy diarrhoea (due to resection of halting ileocaecal valve, or to diseased or resected terminal ileum with consequent cathartic action of unabsorbed bile salts) and loss of bile salts interfere with enterohepatic circulation of bile salts. This disturbs the cholesterol/bile salts ratio, ultimately leading to gall stone formation. Dehydration and selective uric acid and oxalate absorption are also claimed to cause renal stones.

The quest for continence

The search for reliable methods to establish continent stomas has had more success in relation to the small bowel than the large. A number of mechanical devices have been invented to achieve a continent colostomy but they are not particularly successful. These include the implantable Erlangen magnetic closing device, hinged clips and the implanted Silastic cuff. A method of constructing a new sphincter for the emergent colostomy limb from transplanted colonic muscle has also been described.

Some patients prefer the method of colostomy irrigation to control the efflux from the bowel. Each morning the patient irrigates the colostomy with 1.5 litres of warm water, and the colostomy is drained into a collecting bag. For the rest of the day the patient wears a vented cap over the stoma and can dispense with the use of a cumbersome appliance. The problem with this method is that it is time-consuming.

Reservoir ileostomy

A reservoir is constructed within the abdomen from loops of terminal ileum. A small bowel loop from the reservoir to the abdominal skin is intussuscepted to produce a nipple. This projects into the reservoir and acts as a valve. The emergent limb from the valve is fashioned flush with the abdominal wall. The initial reservoir is constructed with a capacity of approximately 200 ml but with the passage of time its capacity increases to 1 litre. The reservoir can be emptied via a catheter introduced through the valve and into the liquid stool. The construction of such a device is not without its problems: extrusion of the valve results in incontinence; necrosis of the reservoir can result in the loss of a large absorptive surface area of small bowel; and perforation of the reservoir is possible by the passage of the catheter.

INTESTINAL FISTULAE

We deal here briefly with the principles of management of intestinal fistulae. Broadly speaking fistulae can be divided into two large groups. In those that arise due to an *underlying intestinal disease* with the diseased segment of bowel remaining *in situ*, treatment should be aimed at the underlying pathological lesion – the bowel needs to be removed before the fistula will heal. Fistulae that arise as a result of the *dehiscence of an intestinal anastomosis* following the removal of a diseased segment of bowel can be expected to close spontaneously provided there is no distal obstruction and the fistula has not become epithelialised.

Small bowel fistulae

Small bowel fistulae present a greater challenge in management than do those arising from the large bowel. The efflux of a small bowel fistula contains proteolytic enzymes which can cause severe skin problems, and the daily losses from the fistula cause metabolic and nutritional disturbances. The higher the fistula the greater are the associated metabolic problems. Fluid and electrolyte and acid–base disturbances rapidly follow gastric, duodenal and jejunal fistulae. Ileal fistulae do not as a rule cause marked metabolic upset.

Initially, the daily losses from the fistula need to be calculated accurately. The volume of the efflux and its electrolyte content are estimated and the acid-base status and nitrogen balance of the patient monitored. Appropriate replacement of the losses is required with maintenance of the nutritional status of the patient being of paramount importance. A regimen of total parenteral nutrition is instituted with the patient kept in positive nitrogen balance. Provided there is no distal obstruction, spontaneous closure of the fistula is expected.

Operative intervention to close a persistent fistula is done when the patient is fit.

Small bowel fistulae discharge their liquid efflux containing proteolytic enzymes directly onto the skin. In the problem patient there may be multiple openings onto the abdominal wall at points where it is difficult to fit collecting appliances. Stomahesive is now available in large sheets and its use in such a form has considerably aided in the management of these stomas. Irregularities in the abdominal skin can be filled with Stomahesive or karaya gum before placement of the Stomahesive square into which apertures have been cut to conform exactly to the site and shape of the fistulous openings. Collecting bags can be attached to the square and changed without disturbing the skin. Transparent tubed covers can allow irrigation of large defects without disturbance.

Large bowel fistulae

These fistulae are not as problematical as small bowel fistulae. However, they may discharge at 'inconvenient' points on the abdominal wall – through through an abdominal incision or near to bony points. Since the stools are not corrosive to the skin, excoriation is not a problem. Ingenuity is required to keep a suitable collecting appliance on the skin according to the above principles, in the expectation of final healing.

PROBLEMS ASSOCIATED WITH AN ILEAL CONDUIT

The ileal conduit is a more complicated construction than an ileostomy or a colostomy and the complications that may arise are more numerous.

The surgical construction of an ileal conduit consists of three stages, if a total cystectomy is omitted. (1) A 15 cm piece of ileum is isolated on a vascular pedicle and the continuity of the intestine re-established. (2) The two ureters must be anastomosed to the proximal end of the ileal segment. (3) The urostomy must be constructed as a 2 cm spout through the abdominal wall.

Dehiscence of the intestinal anastomosis

This may present as peritonitis or as a small bowel fistula. This must be treated on its own merits.

Postoperative urinary fistula

Leakage of urine from the site of anastomosis of the ureters to the ileum usually presents as a urine leak from the drain site. Contrast medium can be introduced into the spout of the urostomy to confirm the site of leakage. If the ureters can be visualised and are in continuity with the ileal segment then the fistula can be expected to close spontaneously. If the ureters are not visualised an intravenous urogram is indicated. Complete lack of continuity with the ileal segment will demand reconstruction.

Vascular problems of the ileal segment

The stoma may appear dark red immediately after operation but as oedema of the operation subsides it should regain a healthy pink colour. A persistent dusky stoma or one that turns black indicates that the blood supply to the ileal loop is imperilled and this demands reconstruction.

Control of the urostomy efflux

Unlike for an ileostomy or a colostomy a large volume output from the urostomy is desirable. No efforts should be made to diminish output since large volume flows of urine discourage ascending infections.

Ascending infection and renal failure

Ascending infections are common, and can lead to calculus formation and destruction of renal parenchyma.

1.54 Portal Hypertension

Normal portal venous pressure is 80–120 mmH$_2$O and depends on splanchnic blood flow, resistance to outflow from the liver and pressure in the inferior vena cava. In portal hypertension it reaches 400 mmH$_2$O or more. Bleeding from oesophageal varices starts when portal pressure exceeds 250–300 mmH$_2$O. The portal vein is formed of two main vessels – the superior mesenteric and splenic veins (Fig. 1.54.1). It has no valves. As a result of portal hypertension, extrahepatic portasystemic anastomotic channels become engorged and dilated (i.e. oesophageal varices with profuse painless haematemesis, caput medusae around umbilicus and haemorrhoids). Hypersplenism with pancytopaenia, stasis in the portal circulation with portal vein thrombosis and infarction of the intestine, as well as ascites, also result.

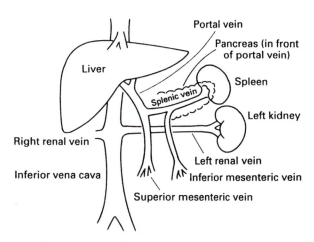

Fig. 1.54.1 Anatomy of the portal vein

Causes of portal hypertension

- Prehepatic presinusoidal (liver is normal) include umbilical sepsis (neonatal), clotting diathesis (polycythaemia), malignant portal vein obstruction and idiopathic causes.
- Intrahepatic presinusoidal (liver is diseased) include schistosomiasis, congenital hepatic fibrosis, sarcoidosis and liver intoxication.
- Intrahepatic postsinusoidal group includes cirrhosis and veno-occlusive disease (Jamaican bush tea).
- Posthepatic postsinusoidal include hepatic vein obstruction (Budd–Chiari syndrome) and constrictive pericarditis.

Schistosomiasis and cirrhosis are the commonest causes of portal hypertension world-wide.

Indications for elective surgery in portal hypertension

Bleeding oesophageal varices (once they have bled they will bleed again) is an absolute indication. Hypersplenism and ascites are relative indications.

Diagnosis and assessment of portal hypertension

Liver function tests; chest X-ray; barium swallow (soap-bubble appearance of varices); barium meal; i.v. urography to evaluate left renal function (for lienorenal shunt); splenoportography and ultrasound (may show patent or obstructed portal vein); transhepatic venography and endoscopy especially in emergency bleeding to confirm the site of bleeding from chronic peptic ulcer or erosive gastritis which may account for 40% of misdiagnosed bleeding varices. Peptic ulcer is more common in cirrhotics and the presence of varices does not necessarily mean that they are the source of upper gastrointestinal tract bleeding. The severity of liver disease is graded according to Child's classification into A, B and C and modified into a flexible system using points.

Serum bilirubin			
(mg/100 ml)	< 2 (1),	2–3 (2),	> 3 (3)
(μmol/1)	< 34 (1),	34–51 (2),	> 51 (3)
Serum albumin			
(g/100 ml)	> 3.5 (1),	3–3.5 (2),	< 3 (3)
Prothrombin time			
(seconds prolonged)	< 2 (1),	3–5 (2),	> 5 (3)
Ascites	None (1), Mild/moderate (2), Gross (3)		
Encephalopathy	None (1), Minimal (2), Moderate/severe (3)		

The added points are classified as follows:

A =   5–7   points
B =   8–9   points
C = 10–15 points

A liver biopsy is essential and liver scan may be required to exclude hepatomas. The ideal patient for a shunt operation should be under 45 years of age, category A or B, with inactive liver disease and should look and feel well.

Elective treatment of portal hypertension
Surgical (shunts) (Fig. 1.54.2)

The most effective method of permanent control. Includes portacaval, lienorenal, mesocaval (jump graft or graft interposition) shunts and selective decompression (Warren's operation – distal lienorenal shunt and gastrosplenic isolation with spleen left in situ.

Non-surgical approach

- Injection sclerotherapy of oesophageal varices, via rigid and flexible endoscope.
- Percutaneous transhepatic embolisation of varices.
- Propranolol for prevention of recurrent haemorrhage (not fully established).

Emergency treatment of bleeding varices
Conservative approach

Blood replacement, i.v. vasopressin 20 units in 200 ml of 5% dextrose (or somatostatin given as i.v. bolus injection of 250 μg to be followed by continuous i.v. infusion of 7.5 μg/min or preferably Terlipressin given in initial 2 mg i.v. bolus dose and repeated 4–6 hourly up to a maximum of 24 h) and Sengstaken–Blakemore balloon tamponade for 24–48 h with vitamin K and prehepatic coma prevention (oral non-absorbable antibiotic, colonic washout, lactulose and restriction of proteins) remain the mainstay of the medical therapy.

Bleeding varices can be injected with 5 ml of 5% ethanolamine oleate using a rigid oesophagoscope and a long Macbeth needle followed by tamponade.

Direct surgery to varices

- Transthoracic, transoesophageal ligation of varices (Boerema–Crile operation).
- Transthoracic, oesophageal transection (mucosal or complete) (Milnes–Walker operation) with variceal ligation or reanastomosis by hand or stapler.
- Subcardiac porta-azygous disconnection (Tanner operation) – gastric transection.

Emergency or urgent shunt surgery

- Emergency portacaval shunt has an overall operative mortality of 57%, which is directly related to the degree of hepatic dysfunction.
- Mesocaval shunt (jump graft) side-to-side Dacron graft between the superior mesenteric vein and inferior vena cava – claimed to have acceptable mortality.

Encephalopathy is caused by:

- Diversion of portal blood from the liver.
- Deteriorating liver cell function.
- Haemodynamic changes precipitated by shunt operation.

The encephalopathy ranges between 12% and 45% but it is around 10% if intestinal antibiotic, lactulose and protein restriction are used for control. Surgical procedures such as subtotal colectomy or colonic exclusion are also claimed to be helpful in reducing this risk.

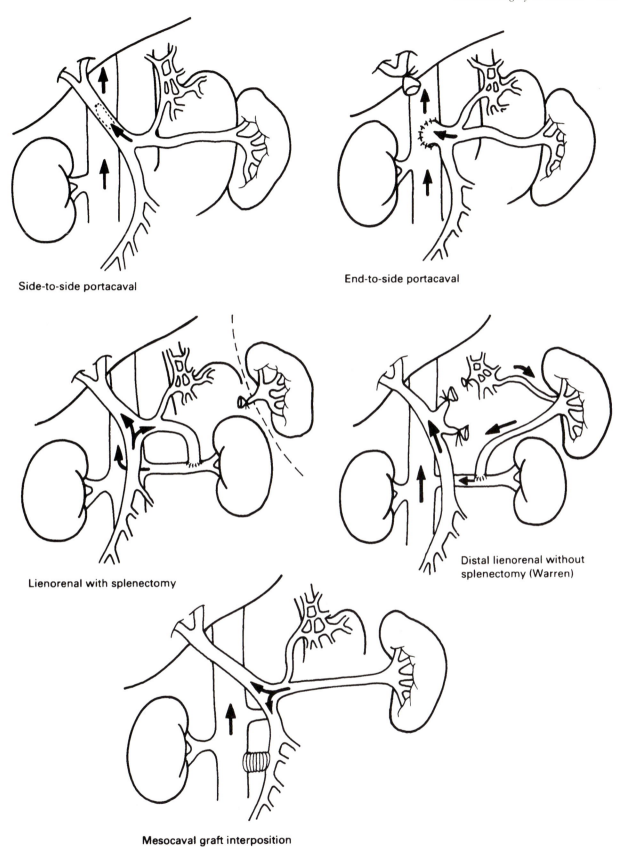

Side-to-side portacaval

End-to-side portacaval

Lienorenal with splenectomy

Distal lienorenal without splenectomy (Warren)

Mesocaval graft interposition

Fig. 1.54.2   Shunting procedures in portal hypertension

gests biliary disease; a normal scan does *not* exclude gall-stones). CT scan may localise pancreatic slough and necrotic tissues accurately.

Elucidation of aetiology and treatment according to severity

Mild cases

All mild cases irrespective of aetiology need peripheral i.v. infusion, nasogastric suction (to prevent the release of pancreozymine and cholecystokinin which stimulate the diseased pancreas), nil by mouth, urinary catheter and subclavian catheter *if necessary* (i.e. in the presence of myocardial insufficiency), regular analgesia (if narcotic drug is used it should be administered with an anticholinergic drug, e.g. atropine or hyoscine butylbromide (Buscopan) to counteract the spasm of sphincter of Oddi) H_2-antagonists. Once the patient has recovered, operation for gallstones should be carried out within 1 week.

Severe cases

Should be admitted to the intensive therapy unit and given peripheral i.v. infusion, with nasogastric suction, urinary catheter, ECG monitoring, subclavian CVP line and peritoneal dialysis (claimed to be of therapeutic value). Good analgesia (pethidine and Buscopan) and total parenteral nutrition are required. The current trend is to investigate such cases extensively and if they are proved to be acute pancreatitis with gallstones endoscopic papillotomy is recommended within the first 48 h for stone retrieval if facilities are available in hospital, or alternatively operative removal with cholecystectomy and T-tube insertions (Carter, 1984). Surgery in severe alcoholic pancreatitis is highly debatable.

Indications for laparotomy

- Diagnostic uncertainty: if the pancreas is normal treat other causes as appropriate. Where acute pancreatitis is diagnosed feel for gallstones and if found proceed to cholecystectomy and exploration of the common bile duct. If acute pancreatitis is not due to gallstones, close the abdomen, leaving a catheter inserted through the foramen of Winslow into the lesser sac for peritoneal lavage.
- Patients with acute pancreatitis and multi-system organ failure who do not respond to intensive treatment within 48 h (especially alcoholic patients), or those with extensive retroperitoneal slough who decline over a period of 5–7 days despite intensive treatment.
- Increasing jaundice and biliary sepsis.
- Late complications of pseudocysts or abscesses.

Follow-up

Since the operative treatment of severe alcoholic acute pancreatitis is debatable, follow-up should be regular and might include social and psychiatric follow-up. All patients with acute pancreatitis should be followed for life.

Questionable therapeutic manoeuvres

- Do not give aprotinin or glucagon (they are expensive and of no proven value).
- Antibiotics are of no proven value in routine management. They are indicated in:
  - Patients with suspected cholangitis.
  - Patients undergoing surgery – give routine prophylactic preoperative cover.
- Nasogastric aspiration is under review and may be unnecessary in mild cases with normal bowel sounds on admission.

SEVERE ACUTE PANCREATITIS

Natural history of severe acute pancreatitis (SAP)

SAP is associated with extensive and prolonged pancreatic and retroperitoneal inflammation with patchy or generalised areas of tissue necrosis and haemorrhage in and around the pancreas. The course can arbitrarily be divided into two successive phases (early toxaemic and late necrotic). Massive pancreatic inflammation with regional necrosis and haemorrhage characterises the early toxaemic phase with the life-threatening complication of multi-system organ failure (MOF). Pancreatic enzymes (trypsin and phospholipase A2) released into the circulation play the key role in this auto-intoxication, since they result in activation of the kallikrein–kinin, complement, coagulation and fibrinolytic systems; pancreatic inflammation activates macrophages sparking the release of septic mediators, such as tumour necrosis factor and interleukins (play a pivotal role in MOF pathogenesis). The main route of this auto-intoxication is direct transfer into pancreatic and retroperitoneal lymphatics draining into cisterna chyli which then becomes thoracic duct which in turn drains its contents into the origin of the left innominate vein.

After 2–3 weeks regional pancreatic inflammation subsides, and the late necrotic phase of ASP starts. Up to 70% of patients undergo uneventful resolution of necrotic areas. About 10% develop pseudocysts. About 20% develop septic complications due to bacterial gut contamination; they range from early infected pancreatic necrosis (liquefactive necrosis confirmed by needle aspiration within 14 days of onset) with poor prognosis due to mixture of proteolytic enzymes and bacteria (MOF), to late pancreatic abscess, a well-encapsulated collection of pus with better prognosis.

Understanding the pathophysiology of ASP has led to development of new management strategies resulting in a precipitous fall of mortality to below 25%.

There are two extremes of therapies ranging from surgical removal of necrotic material (to minimise devitalised tissues and to reduce MOF), to an intensive conservative approach leaving surgery to deal with late complications only.

Therapeutic modalities of SAP

Peritoneal lavage

Though its therapeutic value is controversial, alcoholic SAP with 'prune juice' ascitic fluid does benefit from lavage due to limiting systemic absorption of vasoactive substances released into the peritoneal cavity.

Thoracic duct drainage (of debatable value)

Owing to the crucial role of lymphatic pathways in the transfer of toxic substances released by the pancreas, thoracic duct drainage is advocated by some intensivists to prevent and treat life-threatening remote complications of SAP. The thoracic duct is surgically exposed via a left supraclavicular incision, and, 7 F Swan–Ganz catheter can be passed after distal ligation of the thoracic duct; substantial amounts of enzymatically active trypsin and leucocyte myeloperoxidase can be isolated from thoracic lymph. As a result of drainage, cardiorespiratory dysfunction can rapidly be corrected and patients can survive the early shock (toxaemic) phase. Like peritoneal lavage, thoracic duct drainage did not reduce the incidence of late complications (infection and pseudocysts). Both peritoneal lavage and thoracic duct drainage can remove the potential mediators of MOF; with endoscopic papillotomy they form the pillars of intensive conservative therapy to keep SAP patients alive through the toxaemic phase (see below).

Endoscopic papillotomy

ERCP and emergency endoscopic papillotomy for impacted ampullary stones undertaken within 48–72 h of admission is the best therapeutic approach for SAP with reduction in mortality and morbidity (no exacerbation, haemorrhage and pseudocyst formation). Cholecystectomy may be delayed safely during the same hospital admission until SAP subsides since early surgery may carry higher mortality in those severely ill patients.

Surgical approaches

While surgery in SAP is indicated in diagnostic uncertainty, cholecystectomy/common bile duct exploration (severe gall-stone pancreatitis with or without jaundice), and complications, it is still practised by surgeons in the following circumstances.

During toxaemic phase
- Early subtotal or total pancreatectomy failed to stop systemic effects of inflammation and necrosis; overall mortality raised by 30% with additional morbidity of postoperative diabetes.
- Massive haemorrhage is fatal under conservative treatment. Embolisation and subsequent surgical ligation and thorough debridement to stop bleeding and prevent sepsis are required.
- Persistence of overwhelming MOF with regional sepsis is the most frequent indication for surgery in the early phase of SAP. Necrosectomy and drainage with or without local lavage of the lesser sac resulted in removal of infected necrotic tissues and elimination of activated enzymes with reduction of mortality to 10–20%.

During necrotic phase
- Acute pseudocyst should be drained internally as soon as haemorrhage, infection or organ compression occur (exter-

nal drainage may be complicated by fistula and abscess formation).
- Undrained pancreatic abscess is always fatal. It must be drained either transperitoneally, via the flank, or retroperitoneally. Drainage with or without lavage resulted in good survival rates (75–95%). Early aggressive and thorough debridement of necrotic areas with opening of infected spaces are essential. A preoperative CT scan is helpful in localisation; multiple reoperations may be needed due to fistula, haemorrhage and ongoing sepsis.

CHRONIC PANCREATITIS

Chronic pancreatitis can be defined as a continuing inflammatory disease of the pancreas, characterised by irreversible morphological change, and typically causing pain and/or permanent loss of function.

Calcified acinar tissue (chronic calcific pancreatitis) is common in alcoholism. While several factors are implicated in the aetiology of chronic pancreatitis, alcohol consumption appears to be the dominant factor. Gallstones are present in

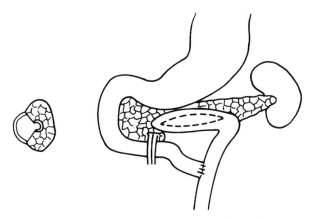

Fig. 1.55.1 Longitudinal pancreaticojejunostomy (Puestow)

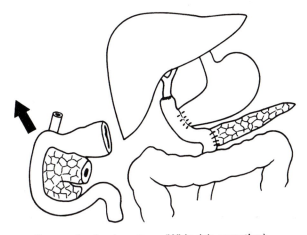

Pancreaticoduodenectomy (Whipple's operation)

Fig. 1.55.2 Surgical treatment of chronic pancreatitis

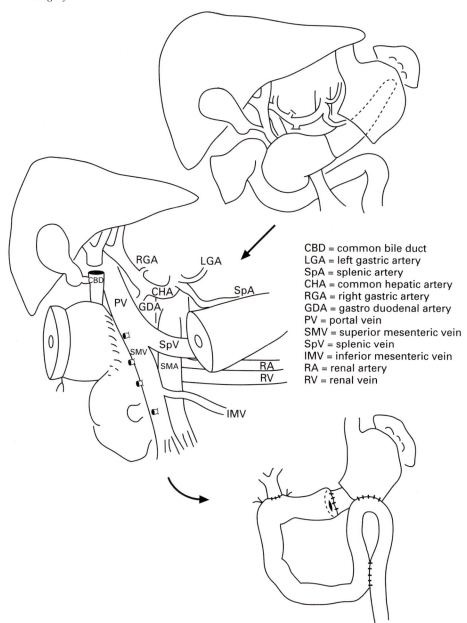

CBD = common bile duct
LGA = left gastric artery
SpA = splenic artery
CHA = common hepatic artery
RGA = right gastric artery
GDA = gastro duodenal artery
PV = portal vein
SMV = superior mesenteric vein
SpV = splenic vein
IMV = inferior mesenteric vein
RA = renal artery
RV = renal vein

Fig. 1.55.3 Whipple's operation (a common reconstruction method), done occasionally in chronic pancreatitis but commonly done for carcinoma of the head of the pancreas, low cholangiocarcinoma and ampullary carcinoma. IMV may also drain into the splenic vein.

15% of patients (most likely incidental finding, but may be a contributing aetiological factor). Hypercalcaemia is a less common cause, and so is protein malnutrition, obstructive chronic pancreatitis (due to pancreatic carcinoma, ampullary carcinoma, or duodenal polyp), and failure of secretory control (due to diabetes, coeliac disease, gastric resection and vagotomy). Isolated lipase deficiency, though anecdotally reported, is exceedingly rare. Familial chronic pancreatitis is rare (probably inherited as autosomal dominant) and present during adolescence with recurrent pain and exocrine insufficiency; in childhood cystic fibrosis and Shwachmann–Diamond syndrome (pancreatic atrophy with fatty infiltration, without

inflammation with cyclical neutropenia, skeletal abnormalities, and dysgammaglobulinaemia) are more common. In the last two similar conditions, recurrent chest infection is also prevalent, but hip dysplasia usually settles the diagnosis in favour of Shwachmann–Diamond syndrome. Rare congenital ductal malformation can also be implicated in the aetiology of chronic pancreatitis.

Clinically, abdominal pain is the principal presenting symptom in 70–90% of patients with chronic pancreatitis. The severity varies from mild epigastric discomfort to severe upper abdominal pain radiating to the mid-thoracic back region and requiring opiate analgesia. Delay in diagnosis may lead to addiction. The pain may be relieved by leaning forward with the patient adopting a stooping position. Alcohol consumption may exacerbate the pain after 24–48 h. Weight loss is attributable to steatorrhoea and to anorexia (in severe pain). Steatorrhoea and associated diarrhoea has sudden onset after many attacks of pain, and leads to malabsorption (painless pancreatic insufficiency is rare). Intermittent jaundice (due to biliary decompression by inflamed swollen pancreas) occurs in 15–30% of patients.

Strictures of the common bile duct can be demonstrated by cholangiography in over 80% of patients, and cause persistent jaundice. Endocrine pancreatic function is also abnormal; diabetes can occasionally be a presenting feature in up to one-third of patients. Carcinoma of the pancreas appears to be slightly more common in chronic pancreatitis; it may be difficult to distinguish between the two. Patients may attempt suicide (may be due to opiate addiction) or die as a result of diabetes, cyst/abscess formation, or pancreatic surgery. In alcohol-induced chronic pancreatitis, 50% survive 20–24 years after onset. Survival in non-alcoholic pancreatitis is 20% greater than alcoholics. The major non-pancreatic causes of death are malignancy (particularly tumours related to smoking), and cardiovascular diseases.

Diagnosis is based on clinical grounds with faecal excretion of more than 5 g/day (steatorrhoea due to exocrine dysfunction), glucose tolerance test (for endocrine dysfunction), as well as radiological and imaging investigations (plain X-ray of abdomen reveals calcifications, ultrasound, CT scan and ERCP reveal pancreatic cysts).

Treatment should include abstinence from alcohol. Pain is better controlled by simple analgesics and non-steroidal anti-inflammatory drugs; opiate analgesia must be avoided if possible to prevent addiction. Coeliac plexus block may relieve the pain temporarily, but is not successful in long-term management; it is more successful in the pain relief of pancreatic carcinoma than in chronic pancreatitis.

Exocrine functional deficiency is replaced with enzyme preparations (Cotazym B, Nutrizym), though these may be degraded by gastric acid so addition of an H_2 antagonist may be helpful. Diabetes, if present, must be controlled, though this is difficult due to variable needs to insulin; patients must have an adequate supply of glucose.

Surgery is mainly indicated in intractable pain. However, 75% of patients with chronic pancreatitis can become pain-free within 8 years, as pancreatic function declines and calcification increases, so that pain relief after operation may be due to continuing disease rather than a result of surgery. The objective of surgery is to preserve functional pancreatic tissue by providing adequate drainage, or to resect the diseased portion of the gland. Pain associated with pancreatic cyst may respond to drainage, but definitive surgery for underlying pancreatitis is recommended. Sphincteroplasty drainage is rarely successful, since multiple strictures throughout the length of the duct may fare better by slitting open – 'filleting' – the gland and anastomosing a Roux loop of jejunum to the whole length of pancreatic duct (pancreatic duct decompression) to construct a pancreaticojejunostomy (particularly if the pancreatic duct is dilated) with better results (Fig 1.55.1). If drainage is not feasible, part or all of the pancreas may have to be resected, since localised chronic

pancreatitis can respond to local resection of either the head or the tail. However, partial pancreatectomy for diffuse disease gives disappointing results. The disease is usually most severe in the head, so that pancreaticoduodenectomy (Whipple's operation) (Figs 1.55.2, 1.55.3) gives immediate pain relief in almost all patients with lasting benefit in 73% of cases; operative mortality can be high together with morbidity (anastomotic ulcers and cholangitis). Occasionally, the disease is limited to the tail so that distal pancreatectomy may be needed. However, the disease may be diffuse and total pancreatectomy may be performed with permanent diabetes and exocrine deficiency. Surgical outcome is more favourable in patients abstaining from alcohol.

1.56 Non-Surgical Treatment of Gallstones

The non-surgical methods employed in the treatment of gallstones leave the gallbladder intact and the patients at risk of recurrent stone formation. Cholecystectomy remains the effective operation and the cornerstone treatment with low rates of morbidity and mortality; it must remain the treatment of choice for most patients with symptomatic gallstones. It is the 'gold standard' by which any other treatment should be measured. Cholecystectomy also removes the risk of carcinoma developing in a diseased gallbladder. It nevertheless involves considerable discomfort to the patient, 1 week of hospitalisation, and 1 month off work with all the attendant financial implications. Furthermore, in patients in whom the risks of operation are greater than normal and in those not wanting a surgical operation for other reasons, the non-surgical procedures provide viable alternatives. The non-surgical methods include the following:

1. Percutaneous extraction of retained residual common bile duct stones, provided that the T-tube placed in the common bile duct at the time of surgery is not removed (T-tube should be of 14 FG size or more with the shortest and straightest course to skin). At least 4 weeks should elapse (with the T-tube clamped) after surgery to allow some fibrosis of the T-tube track.

Analgesia and prophylactic antibiotics are required with premedication 1 h prior to the procedure.

Under X-ray screening control, preferably with T-tube cholangiogram, the T-tube is then removed and a 13 FG steerable catheter is passed down the T-tube track with a Dormia basket to slowly extract small residual stones within the common bile duct or intrahepatic radicals (cystic duct stones are inaccessible). Stones larger than 10 mm will require fragmentation (with the wire basket prior to extraction) or endoscopic sphincterotomy/surgery. At the end of the procedure a suction catheter is manipulated into the duct system and sutured to the skin. Multiple stones may require repeated procedures. The success rate is about 95% with negligible morbidity or mortality.

2. Peroral extraction, i.e. endoscopic removal of stones (ERCP), provides a viable alternative treatment for retained

stones in the cystic ducts and occasionally for unoperated cases of biliary stones in elderly patients (high-risk patients unfit for surgery). It requires a generous sphincterotomy (with diathermy at 35 grade). In ERCP, the standard ordinary (blunt end) cannula is preferred to the traumatic sharp end cannula (even in a tight sphincter) injecting a small dose of Urografin 15% solution on every attempt to enter into the sphincter. The ordinary Dormia basket is used to entangle the stone and pull it out, while the big strong Dormia basket provides a mechanical lithotrite to fragment and crush big stones. Failure to fragment large biliary stones may require ESWL (extracorporeal shockwave lithotripsy) which may necessitate insertion of a nasobiliary tube to provide a radiological measure of the progress of the stone (see below). A nasobiliary tube is a soft fine 300 cm long catheter (with multiside holes and self-retaining pigtail coiled end) introduced over a guide wire via the biopsy channel of a side-viewing duodenoscope; the guide wire is removed and the contrast is injected to confirm its intrabiliary location. Thereafter, the tube is pushed down while the scope is being pulled out gently from the mouth. A nasopharyngeal tube is then inserted via the nose, delivering its pharyngeal end through the mouth in order to thread the oral biliary tube through it. Finally, the nasopharyngeal tube is removed through the nose leaving the nasobiliary tube in situ.

Therefore, a nasobiliary stent can be used for various purposes; it can be placed in the biliary tree with the pigtail end left above a stricture for drainage. An alternative use would be for perfusion of stone-solubilising solutions in the case of retained stones following endoscopic sphincterotomy. Following unsuccessful sphincterotomy, a nasobiliary stent provides drainage and protects the patient against stone impaction. If a cholangiogram performed via the stent, several days later demonstrates that the stone is still present, the sphincterotomy may be extended if feasible, or various agents can be infused in the common bile duct in an attempt to dissolve the stone. Alternatively, ESWL may be employed with the aid of cholangiographic localisation using the nasobiliary stent.

3. Gallstone dissolution therapy is effective in small or medium sized radiolucent cholesterol gallstones with mild symptoms. The gallbladder must be functioning on oral cholecystography, and the stones should be non-pigmented, non-calcified (non-radio-opaque stones), less than 1 cm in diameter and few in number. Patients should preferably be supervised in hospital because radiological monitoring is required. Fewer than 10% of patients coming to cholecystectomy fulfil these criteria. Chemical cholelithotomy can be achieved via:

● Oral route using bile acids (chenodeoxycholic acid and ursodeoxycholic acid). The procedure takes many months to be effective and is associated with side-effects and with a stone recurrence rate of more than 50% at 5 years. Long-term prophylaxis, therefore, may be needed after complete dissolution of gallstones has been confirmed (preferably with cholecystograms and ultrasound on two separate occasions). Side-effects include diarrhoea, pruritus, minor hepatic abnormalities and transient rise in serum transaminases; drugs are therefore contraindicated in pregnancy, chronic liver disease and inflammatory diseases of the small intestine and colon.

Other drugs acting on the gallbladder include dehydrocholic acid and terpene; the former improves biliary drainage by stimulating the secretion of thin watery bile, and is given after biliary tract surgery to flush the common duct and drainage T-tube and wash away small calculi obstructing flow through the common bile duct. Terpene raises biliary cholesterol solubility; it is less effective than the bile acids but may be a useful adjunct.

● Direct catheter infusion through percutaneous cholecystostomy (see below). The most suitable solvent is methyl tertiary butyl ether (MTBE) which can dissolve non-calcified, cholesterol gallstones in a few hours. An oral cholecystogram is performed before the procedure to ensure patency of the cystic duct. A CT scan is also performed to ensure that the stones are not calcified. A small catheter is positioned percutaneously in the gallbladder and small amounts of MTBE are injected and aspirated repeatedly (by hand or using an automatic pump) until dissolution of the stone(s) is achieved. Total or subtotal (more than 95%) dissolution of gallstones can be achieved in more than 90% of patients. Average time for stone dissolution is approximately 12 h. Complications include catheter dislodgement, cystic duct obstruction by stone fragments, haemorrhage into the gallbladder, bile leakage and sedation (caused by spillover of MTBE into the cystic duct).

4. Percutaneous cholecystostomy is used to drain the gallbladder in patients with cholecystitis, but who are too ill for surgery. Under ultrasonic and/or X-ray control, the gallbladder is punctured transhepatically via an anterolateral approach, aiming for the upper third of the gallbladder (where it is attached to the liver) to reduce the possibility of bile leakage. A one-step procedure, using a small catheter (5 FG) on a hollow needle guide, is often possible.

Clinical improvement normally occurs within 24–48 h. Complications are generally minor, but gallbladder puncture can, rarely, provoke an acute vagal reaction requiring immediate resuscitation. Most patients will require cholecystectomy at a later date, although the presence of a catheter within the gallbladder enables percutaneous gallstone dissolution therapy.

5. Extracorporeal shock-wave lithotripsy (ESWL). Gallstones are localized by ultrasound or X-ray image intensifier, and are subjected to repeated pulses of focused shock-waves from the lithotriptor. ESWL was developed in Germany in 1980 for the treatment of renal calculi. The original apparatus, manufactured by Dornier, required the patient to be anaesthetised and submerged in water. With the advent of the second and third generation lithotriptor, the X-ray targeting of shock waves or the use of ultrasound facility as a primary system for the anatomical location of the stones improved and neither water sink nor anaesthesia are required anymore. A generously applied gel is needed, while the sparks are synchronised with heart beats to deliver about 2000 shocks adjusted automatically by ECG monitor. A new spark plug is needed for each patient. The procedure is almost painless, and analgesia is not normally required, with the potential of using gallstone lithotripsy as an outpatient technique.

The selection criteria are those for dissolution therapy (only one-quarter of patients with gallstones are suitable for ESWL). Currently, only those patients with a maximum of 3 uncalcified or faintly calcified stones are selected for ESWL. The cystic duct must be patent to allow subsequent oral bile acid therapy (chenodeoxycholic acid and ursodeoxycholic acid) to dissolve the resulting stone fragments. In a series of 175 patients with gallbladder stones treated with ESWL followed by oral bile acid therapy, there was clearing of stone fragments from the gallbladder in 30% of cases at 2 months and 91% at 12–18 months and with very few or negligible complications. Fragmented particles might migrate and obstruct the biliary or pancreatic ducts giving biliary colic, jaundice or acute pancreatitis (may require sphincterotomy). Other side-effects are due to soft tissue damage inflicted by ESWL; they include cutaneous petechiae in 14% of patients, transient haematuria in 3% and mild pancreatitis in two patients.

The risk of recurrence is, presumably, the same as for that for dissolution therapy alone (40–50% at 4 years). There is as yet no contraindication to treatment. The high capital cost of lithotriptors, the necessary staff and the expense of dissolution therapy must be weighed against the costs of surgery to the hospital service. This is balanced by the economic benefits reaped by the patients, who do not need a long period of convalescence.

ESWL has also been used successfully to fragment stones in the common bile duct that cannot be removed by other methods (such as ERCP). A nasobiliary tube may be required to provide cholangiographic confirmation of fragmentation of large stones during and after ESWL and dissolution therapy.

6. Percutaneous cholecystolithotomy is used to remove stone fragments from a functioning gallbladder in patients in whom ESWL is not possible and to relieve obstructive symptoms caused by stone fragments after ESWL. A rigid nephroscope is passed into the gallbladder via a percutaneous track and the stones are removed with forceps under direct vision. A subcostal, transperitoneal approach to the gallbladder is used to avoid trauma to the liver. The gallbladder is localised with ultrasound and punctured with a fine needle by the radiologist. A track is dilated to approximately 20 FG using a combination of serial dilators and a balloon catheter. A hollow sheath is then placed along the track to facilitate insertion of the nephroscope.

A Foley's catheter is left in place in the gallbladder for 10 days after the procedure. Patients are normally able to leave hospital after the fourth day. This technique, however, requires general anaesthesia. A study of CT scans from 100 consecutive patients showed that gallbladders were accessible to transperitoneal puncture in only 17% of patients.

7. Non-surgical cholecystectomy has passed its experimental phase. Methods to ablate the gallbladder lumen by the injection of sclerosants are being developed, but unless the cystic duct is occluded, the ablated gallbladder may reform. Animal experiments have shown that the cystic duct can be permanently occluded with electrocautery.

Laparoscopic cholecystectomy (performed via infraumbilical hole with three more holes) is performed widely with promising results (see s. 1.14 Minimal access therapy).

1.57 Clinical Aspects of Obstructive Jaundice

Jaundice is clinically detected when serum bilirubin is greater than 40 mmol/l with yellowish discoloration evident mainly in the skin and the sclera. Normal serum bilirubin is 3–17 mmol/l. Extrahepatic jaundice is due to mechanical obstruction of the common bile duct (CBD) which can be corrected surgically. Obstructive or surgical jaundice, as it is termed, may be a life-threatening condition because of the interplay of various factors, e.g. ascending cholangitis, acute renal failure, hampered defence mechanisms with poor antibiotic penetration, high serum fibrinogen/fibrin degradation products, peripheral and portal endotoxaemia. Biliary operative decompression is, therefore, important and also relieves the attendant unpleasant symptoms. Recently, non-operative decompression has been performed with prostheses via percutaneous transhepatic or endoscopic retrograde routes.

Common causes

The pathological distribution of obstructive jaundice in a district general hospital represents a more natural cross-section (among the population) than that seen in specialised centres in which the pathological distribution is skewed as a result of selective referral patterns. Thus in a district general hospital the common causes are:

Benign	CBD Stone	(38%)
	Chronic pancreatitis	(8%)
Malignant		
Primary	Carcinoma of head of pancreas	(30%)
	Extrahepatic CBD carcinoma	(8%)
	Carcinoma ampulla of Vater	(6%)
	Primary duodenal carcinoma	(2%)
Secondary	Portahepatis obstruction	(8%)

Other miscellaneous causes such as traumatic CBD stricture, hydatid disease, chronic duodenal ulcer and sclerosing cholangitis are rarely seen in UK surgical practice.

Diagnosis

Clinical assessment

1. *History* Age, occupation (hydatid disease in farmers), surgery (stricture), alcohol intake (cirrhosis), drugs and contraceptive pill, biliary colic with fever and jaundice (Charcot triad), injections or transfusions (hepatitis B). Family history of anaemia, splenectomy and gallstones (hereditary spherocytosis). History of present illness, e.g. fluctuating obstructive jaundice (CBD stone and ampullary carcinoma) or progressive obstructive jaundice (other malignant causes), the sudden onset (gallstones) or gradual onset (cirrhosis or malignancy), painful (CBD stone) or painless obstructive jaundice (malignancy or viral hepatitis), fever and rigor (cholangitis in CBD stone and rarely in ampullary carcinoma), dark-coloured urine and clay-coloured stool, pruritus due to irritation of cutaneous nerves by raised bile salts, weight loss (suggests malignancy) or weight gain (suggests gallstones).

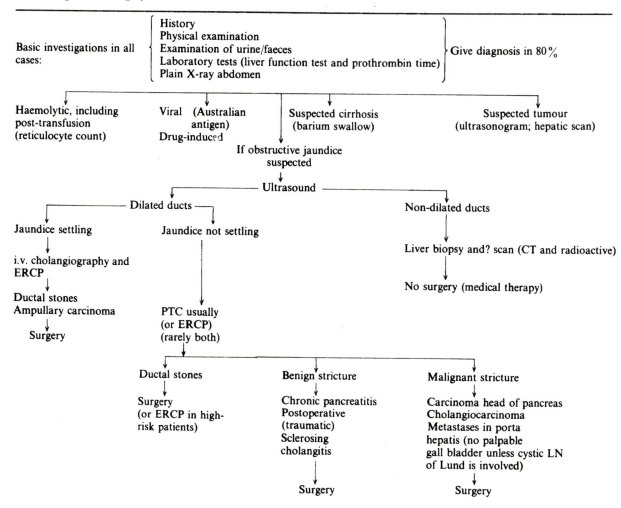

Fig. 1.57.1   Investigation plan of jaundiced patient

2. *Physical examination*   The depth of jaundice, signs of liver failure (spider naevi, ascites, fetor hepaticus, gynaecomastia, testicular atrophy, flapping tremor, clubbing, ankle oedema, palmar erythema and ecchymoses), scratches (due to pruritus), xanthomas (primary biliary cirrhosis), supraclavicular lymph nodes (metastatic carcinoma) and fever (due to cholangitis or viral hepatitis). Notice also abdominal scars from previous operations, palpable gallbladder (carcinoma pancreas), hepatomegaly (slight in obstructive jaundice, hard nodular in secondaries and fine nodular in cirrhosis), splenomegaly (in portal hypertension or haemolytic anaemia), caput medusa (portal hypertension), abdominal mass (malignancy), ascites and rectal examination (remember LUMPS; see section 2.1, Abdominal masses).

Investigations (Fig. 1.57.1 and Tables 1.57.1 and 1.57.2)

Start with the cheapest, simplest relevant non-invasive tests:
1. Urine. Absent urobilinogen in obstructive jaundice and absent bilirubin in haemolytic jaundice.
2. Stool. Colour, absent bile pigment in obstructive jaundice, occult blood in ampullary carcinoma.

3. Blood.
(a) High serum bilirubin confirms jaundice and its level gives an idea of severity.
(b) Alkaline phosphatase can differentiate obstructive jaundice (greater than 100 i.u./l) from hepatocellular and haemolytic jaundice (raised but less than 100 i.u./ l). Alkaline phosphatase has four sources – liver, bone, intestine and placenta. It is therefore high in liver diseases (including jaundice), bone diseases (and growing children), intestinal lymphoma and pregnancy.
(c) Prothrombin time – prolonged but correctable (with vitamin K) in obstructive jaundice; prolonged uncorrectable in hepatocellular jaundice; and normal in haemolytic anaemia.
(d) Australian antigen (HB_s Ag) indicates viral hepatitis. Spherocytosis (full blood count), red cell fragility, reticulocytosis, positive Coomb's test and absent haptoglobins indicate haemolysis. Reversed albumin/globulin ratio (normally 2:1) in chronic hepatocellular jaundice. Autoantibodies (especially antimitochondrial) indicate primary biliary cirrhosis.

Table 1.57.1 Investigations results in jaundice

	Prehepatic (haemolytic)	*Hepatic*	*Extra- or posthepatic obstructive surgical*
Bilirubin	Unconjugated (indirect) ↑	Direct and indirect ↑	Conjugated (direct) ↑
Albumin	Normal	↓	Normal
Globulin	Normal	↑	↑
Transaminases (GOT and GPT)	Normal	↑	Normal or mild ↑
Prothrombin time	Normal	Prolonged uncorrectable with vitamin K injection	Prolonged correctable with vitamin K injection
Alkaline phosphatase	Normal	↑	↑↑↑
γGGT	Normal	↑	↑↑
HBs Ag	Normal	↑	Normal
Antibodies	Normal	Mitochondrial M antibodies in primary biliary cirrhosis	Normal
α Fetoprotein	Normal	↑ in primary hepatoma	Normal
CEA	Normal	Normal	↑ in cholangiocancer
Cholesterol	Normal	Normal	↑
Urine	Urobilinogen ↑↑ No bilirubin (normal colour)	Normal colour	No urobilinogen Bilirubin ↑↑ (dark colour urine)
Faeces	Bilirubin ↑↑ (dark stool)	Normal colour	No bilirubin (pale stool)

A provisional diagnosis should be made now. If the above clinical and laboratory assessment points to a hepatocellular jaundice then radioactive (e.g. gallium) liver scan and liver biopsy are indicated. If the provisional diagnosis is obstructive jaundice (surgical jaundice) then proceed as follows:

4. Ultrasound scan to illustrate intrahepatic bile ducts, biliary stones and the state of the liver and pancreas. If there is any suspicion of pancreatic disease or if the ultrasound scan is inconclusive, as in obese patients or because of excess overlapping bowel gas, then CT scan is used, as its resolution is better.

5. The next step is percutaneous transhepatic cholangiography (PTC) if the intrahepatic ducts were dilated, or endoscopic retrograde cholangiopancreatography (ERCP) if the intrahepatic ducts were not dilated. Both PTC and ERCP are invasive techniques and need expertise. PTC necessitates a normal clotting screen, prophylactic antibiotics and a Ciba fine pliable needle inserted under local anaesthesia with injection of

Table 1.57.2 Differences between benign and malignant obstructive jaundice

	Benign	*Malignant*
History		
Age/sex	Middle-aged/young female	Old male or female
Build	Fatty	Cachectic/weight loss
Appetite	Good	Poor (anorexia)
Pain	Colicky	Painless
Jaundice	Fluctuating	Progressive (fluctuating in ampullary carcinoma)
Fever/rigor	+++	– (occasional fever in ampullary carcinoma)
Diarrhoea	–	+++ (steatorrhoea and pale stool)
On examination		
Jaundice	Lemon	Green (deeper)
Hepatomegaly	–	+++ (due to biliary obstruction rather than liver metastases)
Palpable gallbladder	–	+++ (Courvoisier's law)
Investigations		
ESR	Normal or mild ↑	↑
Faecal occult blood (FOB)	–	+ (silvery stool due to presence of small amount of blood)
Barium meal	–	Wide C-loop of duodenum (pad sign) with rose thorning in pancreatic head cancer or reversed 3 sign in ampullary cancer
ERCP	Ductal stone	Malignant pancreatic stricture or ampullary cancer

contrast medium for diagnosis. Therapeutically PTC external biliary drainage is used in the elderly or as preoperative biliary decompression.

Surgical treatment of obstructive jaundice

Preoperative preparations are essential and include vitamin K injection, correction of prolonged prothrombin time (subsequent bleeding is rare), and infusion of 500 ml of 10% mannitol pre- and peroperatively (with urinary catheterisation). Perioperatively the fluid balance is controlled to maintain a high urine flow (and prevent hepatorenal shut down), and external intermittent pneumatic calf compression (rather than Minihep injection) is used to prevent deep venous thrombosis. Prophylactic antibiotics are also required, and a blood sample is grouped, crossmatched and saved.

The treatment protocol depends on the cause of the obstructive jaundice and is summarised as follows.

CBD stone Cholecystectomy and stone extraction via exploration of the CBD supraduodenally, transduodenally or both. In cases with multiple stones packed in the CBD and in primary biliary stone (i.e. CBD stone developing after 2 symptom-free years following cholecystectomy with no evidence of cystic duct stump or distal CBD stenosis and the stone morphologically is soft, crushable and brown), a choledochoduodenostomy is the prophylactic permanent drainage procedure of choice. CBD stones with carcinoma of head of pancreas may be treated by cholecystectomy and choledochoduodenostomy or choledochojejunostomy (if the CBD is dilated) or extraction of the stone with cholecystojejunostomy without gallbladder removal (if the CBD is not dilated).

Chronic pancreatitis Supraduodenal exploration and dilatation or preferably transduodenal sphincterotomy to treat CBD stenosis. Cholecystectomy is performed routinely.

Early traumatic CBD damage End-to-end reconstruction over a T-tube is recommended. Late strictures are managed with reconstruction and Roux-en-Y hepaticojejunostomy, splinting the anastomosis with a latex tube brought out via the anterior abdominal wall through jejunum or liver.

Pancreatic carcinoma Whipple's operation (radical pancreatoduodenectomy) is performed in early cases less than 3 cm in size with no local invasion or distant disease (with operative mortality approaching 34% in good centres) although palliation by bypass is preferable, i.e. cholecystojejunostomy + gastrojejunostomy + jejunojejunostomy (triple, double or single bypass does not make much difference and the rationale for constructing an enteroenterostomy to prevent food entry via the cholecystojejunostomy with subsequent ascending cholangitis is theoretical).

Carcinoma of ampulla of Vater and primary duodenal carcinoma Whipple's operation.

Extrahepatic CBD carcinoma and porta hepatis obstruction Hepaticodochojejunostomy (± prosthetic tube insertion). In advanced cases, laparotomy and biopsy are the only practical procedures.

Advanced cases or in ill patients Non-operative biliary decompression via endoprosthesis insertion or external biliary drainage are now used more frequently.

Comments

The overall postoperative mortality (16%) of operated obstructive jaundice cases is directly related to preoperative serum bilirubin (especially greater than 250 μmol/l). Age, co-existent cardiac or respiratory disease and the magnitude of operation performed are important contributory factors. However, most if not all operative deaths usually occur in the malignant group.

The bile culture state (e.g. infection) is intimately related to the morbidity, i.e. postoperative complications, rather than to the operative mortality.

Recently eight useful parameters were viewed collectively in the prediction of risk in biliary surgery and correlate well with mortality, i.e. serum creatinine (more than 130 μmol/l), serum albumin (less than 30 g/l), serum bilirubin (more than 100 μmol/l), WBC (more than 10 000 cells/mm^3), haematocrit (less than 30%), malignancy, serum alkaline phosphatase (more than 600 units/l), and age (more than 60 years).

BREAST SURGERY

1.58 Early Breast Carcinoma

TYPES OF BREAST CANCER

Breast cancer is an adenocarcinoma arising from epithelium lining ducts and acini. Cancers arise in the terminal duct-lobular unit and are divided into ductal and lobular types. Both ductal and lobular cancers may be invasive (infiltrating) or non-

invasive (non-infiltrating) or in situ. Only invasive cancers metastasise.

Types of invasive cancers

Duct cancers

Duct cancers represent 80% of all invasive cancers; the common scirrhous carcinoma and the rare Paget's disease of the nipple are basically a duct cancer which has broken through the basement membrane. Duct cancer is usually of nondescript histological pattern; however, specific histological features may occur, such as medullary cancer (5%), tubular cancer (10%), and the rare mucoid colloid cancer (2%).

Lobular cancer

Six per cent of all invasive cancers are of lobular type; invasive lobular cancer accounts for 5–10% of breast cancers. It is typified by the bland homogenous nature of its small cells distributed in linear or concentric fashion; as with duct carcinoma, various histopathological types are described, including cribriform, solid and tubular types. The differentiation between lobular and ductal cancers is not easy and there is no single criterion by which they can be identified.

Carcinoma in situ

This is a microscopic lesion, often visible on mammography by fine speckled calcification. It is a non-invasive cancer of the breast confined to ducts and acini which have not penetrated the basement membrane of the epithelial cell layer. Lobules are enlarged and ducts dilated. There are few mitoses and the condition affects the opposite breast in more than half of the patients. Furthermore, it is multifocal within the breast in 75% of those in whom it occurs. Lobular carcinoma in situ is usually an incidental finding in biopsy specimens of postmenopausal women. Areas of non-invasive lobular carcinoma in situ often appear with invasive lobular carcinoma, since the two tumours are related.

AETIOLOGY AND PROGNOSTIC FACTORS IN BREAST CANCER

In the UK, at least 7% of women develop the disease. In Japan, Africa and South America its incidence is 1/6 of that in Europe and North America. The geographical variation may reflect differences in diet (particularly high fat diet which promotes cancer formation in animals) and early menarche, marriage, pregnancy and menopause. Factors increasing the risk of developing breast cancer include:
1. Early age at menarche.
2. Late age at first pregnancy. Pregnancy and lactation (breast feeding) have protective effects.
3. Nulliparity.
4. Late age at menopause.
5. Upper social class (related to diet).
6. Previous history of certain types of benign breast disease, such as intraduct papilloma. Frank in situ cancer and atypical hyperplasia (evolving from ductal epithelium in fibroadenosis) of the breast associated with a family history of the disease are proven antecedents of invasive cancer.
7. Family history of breast cancer.
8. Genetic factors. Those with Klinefelter's syndrome with gynaecomastia are said to be 66 times more liable for breast cancer than normal men. Wet wax in Western women is also blamed, because both the breast and the wax gland of the ears are modified sebaceous glands. Japanese women have dry wax and a low incidence of breast cancer.

9. The risk in mastectomised patients of developing new primary breast tumour in the contralateral breast is about 1% per year of survival.
10. The state of axillary lymph node (tumour-positive or tumour-negative) at mastectomy influences the rate of future local recurrence and survival.
11. Biological aggressive behaviour of the tumour, such as histological differentiation, tumours expressing differentiation antigens, rich in oestrogen-receptor activity, or with DNA diploid cells, have a more favourable prognosis than undifferentiated, oestrogen-negative and aneuploid tumours.
12. Other factors include radiation (two-fold risk), patients with uterine body cancer have a two-fold risk of developing breast cancer (conversely, breast cancer patients have a two-fold risk of developing endometrial carcinoma), patients on thyroid medications, and Bittner milk factor (mouse mammary tumour virus) in animals.
13. Cancer predisposition gene – BRCA1 gene (BReast CAncer) – is known to cause the rarer familial cancer syndromes (with autosomal dominant mode of inheritance of specific cancer, usually at an early age) and a proportion of the common cancers. Currently, family history is the only practical way in which inherited predisposition for breast and ovarian cancer can be recognised. Identification of predisposing gene carriers in the near future will have a considerable impact on the ability to recognise those at risk by using genetic testing as a screening for breast and/or ovarian cancers and planning prophylactic surgery. About 40% of families with several cases of breast cancer, and more than 80% of families with breast and ovarian cancer, are due to predisposition by the BRCA1 gene, which have been mapped to a small region of chromosome 17. BRCA1 may possibly also confer risks of colon and prostatic cancer. Strongly disposing BRCA1 mutations may account for 2–4% of all breast cancer (with higher proportion at younger ages) the greater part of the risk falling at ages 30–50 and carriers who have developed one cancer will have a high risk of developing a second breast or ovarian cancer. Prophylactic surgery is a consideration for those women at very high risk.

PRESENTATION

At presentation, 20% of breast cancer cases represent advanced disease (M_1) and 80% are potentially curable (by surgery) = early breast carcinoma (Stage I and II or T_1, T_2, N_0, N_1, M_0). At least 40% of the latter become advanced after 10 years.

Early breast carcinoma (T_1, T_2)	Advanced breast carcinoma ($T_3N_2M_1$)	
80% at presentation	20% at presentation	
40% (N_0) → 20%	=	8% after 10 years
40% (N_1) → 80%	=	32% after 10 years

Thus, about 60% end finally with an advanced disease, and so early diagnosis and treatment are essential.

Breast cancer is the commonest cause of death in females between 35 and 55 years of age, and over 10 000 females per year die from breast carcinoma in the UK. Below 35 years the breast is dense in young females and is difficult to assess by mammography.

Diagnosis

The usual work-up includes:

- Clinical examination and staging.
- Good mammography (for patients over 35 years of age, should include two views oblique and craniocaudal showing all the beast tissue). Signs of malignancy include micro-calcification, increased density and architectural disturbance.
- Aspiration to differentiate between solid or cystic lesions (outpatient).
- Fine needle aspiration biopsy-cytology (FNABC), or Tru-cut needle biopsy under local anaesthesia (if FNABC not available), is a desirable outpatient procedure for pre-operative diagnosis of solid tumours. This approach is much better than the policy of 'excisional biopsy – frozen-section –? proceed with mastectomy' because one can tell the patient in advance whether she is going to have a mastectomy or not.

The above four methods are done routinely. However, one can also search for distant metastases: up to 25% of early breast carcinomas diagnosed clinically show skeletal metastases on bone isotope scanning, leading to the belief that the breast cancer is a systemic disease from the start. The search includes:

Physical means

- Conventional chest X-ray.
- Skeletal survey.
- Skeletal isotope scan. Metastases show as 'hot spots' and so does a healed fracture, Paget's disease of bone and degenerative osteoarthritis; X-ray of doubtful areas may resolve this ambiguity.
- Isotope-labelled colloid scanning for liver secondaries – if hepatomegaly present.
- Grey scale ultrasonography.
- CT scan for mediastinal and retroperitoneal masses, if suspected.

Biochemical markers

- Alkaline phosphatase and glutamyl transaminase – raised in liver metastases.
- Urinary calcium and hydroxyproline – raised in bone metastases.
- Calcitonin, carcinoembryonic antigen (CEA), specific milk protein – may indicate residual tumour after mastectomy.

Comment

- FNABC is becoming a very popular means of diagnosis of almost all solid tumours (e.g. thyroid, breast, lymphadenopathy, salivary tumours, prostate, testis) with no documented risk of tumour spread into blood vessels. The procedure is very simple. A 20 ml plastic disposable syringe with a No. 1 or 21 gauge needle is inserted into the tumour after skin cleansing with an injection swab. Then suction is applied while the syringe is passed into the mass of the tumour in three or four directions to disturb and dislodge tumour cells. The syringe is withdrawn and the contents are blown onto a clean slide which is dried in air, labelled and fixed in ethanol and stained by Papanicolaou or haematoxylin and eosin for direct microscopic examination. The remaining tumour fragments and tissue juice in the syringe can be mixed with saline and injected into a test tube for cytological examination of the floating cells. Remember that in splenic, hepatic and abdominal puncture, clotting factors should be normal and local anaesthesia is required. There is no need for prophylactic antibiotics.
- Any discrete breast mass or mammographic abnormality is best removed so that the surgeon is certain that it has been removed and it can be examined histologically. Also psychologically, the patient is happier without it.
- Breast lipoma should not be trusted – perform mammography since it may be a pseudolipoma with underlying breast carcinoma (producing a fibrofatty mass due to infiltration along Cooper's ligaments).

TREATMENT POLICY

Current concepts of surgical treatment

- Breast carcinoma gains direct access to blood and to vital organs early in the course of its development (systemic disease).
- Tumour cells reaching a lymph node (LN) are not necessarily trapped there but can either traverse the LN intact or bypass the LN via lymphovenous communications.
- Internal mammary LNs are involved in 28% of all breast cancers, 25% of laterally placed cancers and 50% of medially placed cancers; in 5–10% of cases they are involved before axillary LNs.
- If axillary LNs are involved, 40% of internal mammary glands are involved already.
- Lymph nodes themselves are regarded as actively hostile to the proliferation of tumour cells owing to the inherent tumoricidal capacity of immunologically competent host cells in these lymph nodes. Therefore if lymph nodes are not involved, this represents a favourable tumour–host relation which may be unbalanced by removal or radiation of such immunologically competent lymph nodes. If lymph nodes are involved, this indicates that the disease is already widely disseminated owing to exhaustion of host-restraining factors and in this case the treatment of lymph nodes is important for symptomatic relief, but it does not increase the cure rate. Lymph nodes are not a nidus for secondary spread and their involvement is merely a sign of poor prognosis. The outcome of treatment is predetermined by the extent of micrometastasis at the time of diagnosis and not influenced by the extent of local therapy.
- The breast should be removed for the following reasons:
  - To prevent local recurrence.
  - To control the disease locally so that at the very least if the patient dies of her metastases, she is not also troubled by an ulcerating, painful, offensive lesion on her chest which may be further complicated by lymphoedema of the arm due to malignant infiltration of axilla. Lymphoedema is non-pitting unlike pitting oedema due to venous obstruction.
  - In order not to leave the patient in doubt.

– Removing the bulk of the tumour and involved regional lymph nodes leaves a sufficiently small tumour burden for which host defence factors may be adequate, and gives radiotherapy a better chance of achieving palliation. Recently wide excision of a tumour followed by radiation of the breast and draining lymph node areas has given promising results with minimal disfiguration (see Table 1.58.1).

Current concepts of radiotherapy

- Normal tissues should never be irradiated prophylactically because of X-ray complications:
  - Skin reaction.
  - Lung fibrosis.
  - Painful bone atrophy, joint destruction and stiffness.
  - Lymphoedema.
  - Decreased immunity, which may accelerate the appearance of metastasis and reduce survival.

As a primary modality in early breast cancer, radiotherapy alone has been used with cure in some cases but the uncertainty about the long-term outcome compared with surgery (no controlled trials) and the danger of radiation-induced neoplasia make such an approach unwise.

- Aims of radiotherapy are:
  - To control possible residual disease at the margins of a surgical resection.
  - To destroy cells implanted or seeded in the operative field.
  - To sterilise lymph nodes not removed at operation.
- Postoperative radiotherapy does protect against local and skin recurrence but treatment of recurrence by radiotherapy when it appears is equally effective. The number of patients with local recurrence persisting until death is the same in the two groups.
- Ten-year survival is identical in extended radical mastectomy and simple mastectomy; thus the extension of treatment by surgery or radiotherapy beyond the breast and axillary lymph nodes does not improve survival.
- Recurrence-free survival rate is identical in simple mastectomy and radical mastectomy when both are followed by radiotherapy, indicating that surgery and radiotherapy are equally effective in treating axillary lymph nodes when these are involved by metastatic disease.
- It is important not to irradiate the axilla after radical or modified radical mastectomy because the combined treatment is a major cause of clinically significant arm lymphoedema.

Table 1.58.1   Treatment policies for early breast carcinoma

Surgery/treatment	Radiotherapy	Reference and remark
Supraradical mastectomy (clavicle and supraclavicular LN removal + as below)	– –	Wangensteen, 1950 Andreassin and Dahl-Iversen, 1949 (abandoned)
Extended radical mastectomy (internal mammary LN removal + as below)	–	Urban and Baker, 1952 (abandoned)
Radical mastectomy (breast + axillary LNs + pectoral muscles)	Variable	Halsted, 1894 (uncommon)
Extended simple mastectomy = modified radical mastectomy (as above leaving pectoralis major)	Variable	Patey and Dyson, 1948 (common)
Simple mastectomy (breast only)	– Postop. X-ray	Crile, 1961 McWhirter, 1955
Subcutaneous mastectomy + breast reconstruction	–	Watts, 1976 (limited use)
Simple mastectomy with pectoral or lower axillary LN sampling	Variable, depending on LN involvement	Forrest and Kunkler, 1968 (very common) particularly in a large tumour in a large breast
QUART = QUadrantectomy + Axillary dissection and Radio Therapy	Postop. X-ray	
Extended tylectomy	Postop. X-ray	Atkins, 1972 (common)
Lumpectomy or tumorectomy	Radium implant Postop. X-ray	Keynes, 1930 Porritt, 1964 (common)
–	Radiotherapy alone	(uncommon)
Surgery + adjuvant chemotherapy CMF (cyclophosphamide, methotrexate and 5-fluorouracil) or tamoxifen	–	Milan Study, 1981 (Rossi *et al.*, 1981)
Tamoxifen alone		Preece *et al.*, 1982 (common in women over 70 years of age)

Modified from A.P.M. Forrest, Cancer of the breast. In: *Recent Advances in Surgery*, No. 7 (ed. S. Taylor), London, J. & A. Churchill, 1969

Treatment rationale (Table 1.58.1)

The aim is to achieve local control of the disease with minimal morbidity. The principles are:

- Surgery or radiotherapy should be given only to sites of proven involvement.
- Excessive removal or radiotherapy of normal tissues which are not involved by tumour increases morbidity but not cure.
- The presence of substantial axillary lymph node involvement indicates that the disease is incurable.
- Involved lymph nodes are equally well treated by radiotherapy as by surgical clearance of axilla.

The most commonly used policy is simple (total) mastectomy with axillary sampling (followed by radiotherapy if nodes are involved). This prevents intraclavicular hollowing and lymphoedema. The disadvantages are false negative axillary sampling (inadequate staging) and a high local recurrence rate; postoperative radiotherapy may therefore be required.

Patey's modified radical mastectomy is also employed and has the advantage of no infraclavicular hollowing. Intramuscular recurrence is rare, and leaving the pectoralis major gives a better cosmetic result with no bridle-like tight scar. With an axillary clearance as good as in radical mastectomy this procedure represents a good compromise and avoids the need for postoperative radiotherapy. Local excisions of macroscopic tumour (lumpectomy, tylectomy), formal quadrantectomy, or partial mastectomy with or without axillary sampling can all have a beneficial cosmetic and psychological result. Since breast cancer is multifocal in 30% of cases the recurrence rate is high and unacceptable without routine postoperative radiotherapy in local approaches. Adjuvant early radiotherapy or chemotherapy (CMF or perioperative cyclophosphamide) or hormonal therapy (tamoxifen) could be used in addition to the surgical treatment.

Breast conservation versus mastectomy – conclusions

Breast cancer is increasingly regarded as a systemic disease from the outset, in which control of micrometastases is the key component determining long-term survival. Primary surgery aims to conserve the breast where this is possible, but at the same time must be effective in preventing local recurrence.

Either quadrantectomy or lumpectomy (with margins histologically free from tumour) performed for tumours less than 4 cm diameter, and followed by radiotherapy to the breast (with an additional booster dose to the tumour bed at the site of resected tumour) can achieve as good local control and survival as mastectomy. Axillary dissection further reduces the risk of local recurrence and gives important information for prognosis (tumour-positive or negative is one of the most important prognostic factors in early breast cancer), allows accurate staging of disease (essential for detailed assessment of treatment and clinical trial outcome), and determines rational use of adjuvant systemic therapy, which can improve survival. The effectiveness of disease control in the axilla and the quality of the histological data depend on the extent of surgery (axillary clearance or limited sampling) and the skill of the surgeon, but in experienced hands precise techniques of sampling provide reliable data with low morbidity, reserving

full axillary clearance for those who prove to have positive nodes.

Factors that predispose to local recurrence in patients treated conservatively include incomplete excision of tumour and presence of extensive intraduct carcinoma in and around the primary tumour. Such intraduct tumours are particularly common in young women. A minimum of 1 cm of macroscopically normal tissue should be removed around the primary tumour. Even then, one report estimated that foci of tumour would remain in 59% of patients. For these women, prevention of local recurrence depends heavily on efficacy of postoperative radiotherapy (or other adjuvant therapy). With the excision of a 3 cm tumour-free margin, the possibility of persisting tumour fell to 17%.

Mastectomy + axillary node dissection, however, is more appropriate in women with extensive intraduct permeation or clinical or mammographic evidence of multicentric disease. Furthermore, tumours greater than 4 cm diameter, particularly in small breasts, and tumours beneath the nipple, where good cosmetic results are difficult to achieve, are best treated by mastectomy. Some women may request a mastectomy because they fear recurrence in the remaining breast tissue. Irradiation of the chest after mastectomy should be reserved for patients with high risk of local recurrence, e.g. patients with tumour at the resection margin and those with large or poorly differentiated tumours. Radiation to the axilla should not be used in addition to full axillary dissection because of the high risk of lymphoedema.

Psychological sequelae following breast conservation and mastectomy are discussed in s. 1.22 Psychological implications in surgical practice.

Planning and timing surgery   Surgery should be planned after outpatient FNACB and mammography (rather than frozen section during operation). It has been suggested that, in premenopausal women, surgery during the phase of unopposed oestrogen (day 3–12) increases the risk of relapse and shortens survival; though this is debatable, surgery should preferably be timed to avoid operating before the 12th day of the menstrual cycle.

ADJUVANT SYSTEMIC THERAPY

An overview analysis of 133 randomised trials of systemic therapy (hormonal, cytotoxic, or immune) conducted worldwide in women with early breast cancer, beginning in 1985–1992 and involving 75 000 women, has shown clearly that adjuvant therapy can reduce the risk of recurrence and improve 10-year survival when cancer is detected early.

Tamoxifen reduced the annual death rate by 17% and the recurrence rate by 25%. Improvements in survival were greater in women over 50 and in those with oestrogen receptor-positive tumours, although patients with oestrogen receptor-negative tumours also benefited significantly. Prolonged treatment (2–5 years) was more effective than shorter courses. Tamoxifen also reduced the risk of developing cancer in the opposite breast by 39%. Tamoxifen should be offered to all patients past the menopause.

Ovarian ablation by surgery, radiotherapy or drugs in women under 50 reduced the annual rate of death by 25% and of recurrence by 26%. Ovarian ablation or combination chemotherapy should be offered to all patients before the menopause, particularly those at high risk of relapse (see below).

Combination chemotherapy reduced the annual rate of death by 16% and of recurrence by 28%. Benefit was greatest in women under 50 and 6 months' treatment was as effective as treatment for 12 months. In patients aged 50–69, chemotherapy + tamoxifen appeared better than tamoxifen alone, whilst for women under 50 chemotherapy + ovarian ablation seemed better than chemotherapy alone.

In postmenopausal women, tamoxifen is generally well tolerated (though it can cause hot flushes, vaginal bleeding and GIT symptoms) and should be offered to all patients past the menopause irrespective of prognosis. Before the menopause ovarian ablation or combination chemotherapy (6 cycles) should be offered to women at high risk of relapse because of positive axillary lymph nodes or other adverse prognostic factors. The unwanted effects of treatment are harder to justify in women with a good prognosis; identifying such patients in future may mean looking at a range of cellular factors, not just lymph node status.

Whenever there is a choice between mastectomy and more localised surgery, every woman should be given enough information to make the decision for herself if she wishes. To take full advantage of this improved outlook every effort should be made to detect breast cancer as early as possible.

SCREENING

The forrest report

The potential benefit of breast screening was evaluated in 1985 by a committee chaired by Professor Sir Patrick Forrest of Edinburgh Royal Infirmary; the evaluation was based on data from randomised controlled studies undertaken in New York and Sweden, and two case control studies from Netherlands.

The **USA Health Insurance Plan (HIP)** study was undertaken in New York in 1963, randomising 80–300 women aged 40–64 years between screened and control groups with 67% uptake. Screening was by two-view mammography with clinical examination. Those who attended initial screen were invited to attend on three further occasions at 12-monthly intervals. All women involved were followed for subsequent development of cancer. As would be expected, there was initially an excessive number of cancers detected in the screened group compared with controls, but by 5 years this was almost equal (304 screened: 295 controls) and by 10 years it was identical. Tumours detected in the screened population were, however, smaller than those of the control group, with reduced lymph node involvement and a greater incidence of in situ disease. Annual mortality after 18 years of follow-up indicated that at 10 years there were 30% fewer deaths from breast cancer in the screened group than in the control population; this difference was 23% after 18 years.

In the **Swedish Two-Counties Trial** in 1977 162 891 women aged over 40 years of age were randomised into 2:1 in Kopparberg and 1:1 in Östergotland between screened and control. Primary screening was by a single mediolateral oblique mammogram but, if an abnormality was found, this was followed by full three-view mammography. If these pictures were suspicious, a clinical examination and full assessment were undertaken. Second screen was requested at 24 or 33 months for women aged 40–49 or more than 50, respectively. Subsequent screen was performed at 24 months. There was 89% compliance for the prevalent round and 83% for the second round screen with a detection rate of 5.56/1000 women screened in the prevalent round. As in the HIP study, there was an excessive number of cancers detected in the first few years of the study; the 'catch-up point' has not yet been reached. A reduction in mortality from breast cancer in the screened group had become apparent by 1981 (4 years after screening), and persisted at 30% by 1986 after 8-year follow-up.

In the **Netherlands Case Control Studies** women in Nijmegen aged 35–64 years were screened by single-view mammography every 24 months, and compared with age-matched controls; a 52% reduction in mortality from breast cancer was demonstrated in screened women. In Utrecht, women aged 40–64 years were screened on five occasions at intervals of 12, 18, 24 and 48 months. When the screened population was matched with controls, a 70% reduction in mortality was shown, but this difference was only achieved for women over 50 years of age.

Conclusions

The Forrest Committee concluded that high-quality mammographic screening had the potential to reduce the mortality in women over 50 years of age by up to 30%, but that there was no substantiated evidence for the effectiveness of clinical examination or breast self-examination alone. The report was subsequently published in 1986, with proposals on how a breast cancer screening programme could be introduced in the UK.

Since publication of the Forrest Report, further justification for breast cancer screening has been published, based on the following trials and studies.

- UK Trial of Early Detection of Breast Cancer (TEDBC): a comparative study of mortality from breast cancer in health districts in the UK, started in 1979. The first group was offered screening by annual clinical examination and biannual mammography (over 7 years in Guilford and Edinburgh); the second population group received instruction in self-examination of their breasts; and the third group served as controls. In the screened population, all women aged 45–64 years (45 841) were invited with uptake of 66%, resulting in cancer detection rate of 5.2/1000 women screened in the prevalent round. No significant reduction in mortality emerged between the study and control populations. Breast cancer mortality in screened districts was reduced by only 14%, but if the figures are adjusted using the standarised mortality ratio for each district, mortality was reduced by 20% in 1984 (not statistically significant).
- *Malmo* randomised trial and Edinburgh randomised trial: neither trial of mammographic screening has shown a significant reduction in mortality from breast cancer.
- Breast Cancer Detection Demonstration Project (BCDDP)
- Florence case control study
- Further results from HIP and Swedish ongoing studies.

The randomised control trials and UK trial indicate an approximately 25% reduction in mortality, even though not everyone accepts the invitation for screening.

Information now available indicates that:
– a reduction in breast cancer mortality of at least 25% is obtainable in the over-50-year group by mammographic screening;
– any value of self-examination of the breasts in reducing mortality remains unproven.

Adverse effects of mammographic breast screening

No medical intervention is without possible adverse effects, and with screening studies and trials of large women populations, some facts emerged.

1. Radiation risk: with current screen-film mammography using grids, in women over 50 years of age, it is estimated that one extra breast cancer might develop each year after a latent interval of 10 years for every million women screened each year; this is less than 0.05 of the natural incidence in this age group
2. Psychological and physical morbidity: the discomfort during screening can be minimised by selection and training of radiographers; potential morbidity is associated with recall for further assessment and particularly with biopsies which have a benign outcome (i.e. false-positive screens). However, 5% of cancers, in over-50-year-olds will always be mammographically invisible, even with modern techniques. Long-term psychological morbidity is eliminated by a sensitive approach with these women by specially trained, multidisciplinary teams.
3. Unnecessary procedures: in the early phases of screening programmes cancer detection at the preclinical stage may be overdiagnosed. However, overdiagnosis was excluded by various trial results.
4. Resource costs: sceening programmes are expensive, even if the test itself is of low cost.

UK National health service breast screening programme

NHSBSP was launched in 1987 with the aim of screening all women in the 50–64 years age-group every three years, based on the following recommendations of the Forrest Committee:

● All women in the 50–64 years age-group should be invited to basic screening by single-oblique-view mammography in static or mobile units at 3-year intervals with the option of self-referral for older women.
● Women with a mammographically detected abnormality should be recalled to specialist assessment units staffed by teams including a clinician, radiologist and a pathologist, all trained in the diagnosis of screen-detected lesions and supported by radiographers and breast counsellors. Full facilities should be available for investigation of mammographic lesions by clinical examination, ultrasonography, special view mammography and fine-needle aspiration cytology (FNAC). Surgeons trained in the management of screen-detected lesions should be associated with each unit, and be responsible for carrying out marker biopsies and subsequent management of diagnosed cancers, particularly when impalpable. The aim of this specialist assessment

approach was to allow rapid and accurate diagnosis of women with cancers, while causing minimum psychological and physical harm to those without cancer.
● Quality assurance must be based on national quality guidelines.

AXILLARY DISSECTION

There are three levels of axillary node dissection.

Level I   extends from the axillary tail of the breast up to the lateral border of pectoralis minor.

Level II   extends up to the medial border of pectoralis minor (located behind pectoralis minor and thus necessitating transection of pectoralis minor; interpectoral nodes between pectoralis minor and major must also be removed).

Level III   extends up to the apex of the axilla.

It is reasonable (in the light of available information) to perform an axillary node sampling in patients with impalpable breast cancers where the rate of axillary node positivity is less than 20% and to perform a level III axillary node clearance in patients with palpable disease (postmenopausal node-positive women do gain significant survival advantage from adjuvant chemotherapy). To avoid axillary dissection and to give axillary radiotherapy instead to all postmenopausal women simply violates the principles of safety of breast management because this ignores the prognostic information which axillary dissection provides and ignores the morbidity of radiotherapy.

SILICONE BREAST IMPLANTS

Between 1962 and 1994, about 1–2.2 million women may have received silicone breast implants in the USA and Canada alone (no figures are available for other countries). In 1964, hypergammaglobulinaemia was reported in two patients who had received silicone and paraffin injections; 18 years later, the first three patients with silicone breast implants and connective tissue diseases were reported on. Since then, 293 patients with connective tissue diseases or complaints have been described in the English language medical literature.

In 1992, the US Food and Drug Administration banned silicone implants for cosmetic reasons, although they may still be used for reconstruction as part of clinical trials and research. In Britain, the Department of Health maintains that there is no scientific evidence to justify a ban. A judge in Birmingham, Alabama (USA), in September 1994, approved $4.25 billion compensation deal for more than 90 500 women worldwide with silicone breast implants with legal suits, the biggest product liability settlement in legal history in the USA; the deal was struck after thousands of women sued manufacturers (including Dow Corning, Bristol–Myers, and Union Carbide) for damages for alleged complications following silicone leak into their body tissues. American women who can show that they suffered from one of a range of illnesses will receive payments ranging between $105 000 and $1.14 million, depending on severity and age at onset.

Diseases and complications must fall into one of three categories:

- Serious systemic diseases and immune disorders, such as scleroderma and scleroderma-like disorders (linked most convincingly to environmental causes, e.g. exposure to silica, polyvinyl chloride, toxic oil and tryptophan), systemic lupus erythematosus, rheumatoid arthritis, inflammatory myopathies, Sjögren's syndrome, and an ill-defined syndrome inappropriately termed 'human adjuvant disease' characterised by malaise, low grade fever, aches and pains. However, most reported cases were anecdotal patients; there was no controlled study to detect any association.
- Neurological syndromes, such as memory loss.
- Silicone disease in the form of rashes, chronic fatigue, muscle weakness, memory loss, breast pain and tension.

What should doctors advise women who have silicone breast implants? If they are well and have not had local problems such as hardening or rupture of the implant, it is recommended to do nothing; they should be reassured by epidemiological studies (all of which show no association). Patients with connective tissue diseases or rheumatic complaints and silicone breast implants need to be treated on a case basis. Whether removing the silicone breast implants alters the course of a connective tissue disease is unknown; among 12 reported cases, some improvement was described in 7; 4 of 9 patients with scleroderma had cutaneous improvement (one of them also had visceral improvement). In 2 cases of systemic lupus erythematosus, both clinical and serological manifestations improved; in one case of 'human adjuvant disease' some improvement was noted. (No firm conclusion can be drawn from these reports.) Whether silicone breast implants are associated with connective tissue diseases remains controversial. Despite the increased number of cases reported in the literature, no association has been convincingly established.

ONE-STOP FAST-TRACK BREAST CLINIC

Such a clinic provides a one-stop diagnostic service for symptomatic breast disease. The team is consultant-led (surgeon, radiologist, pathologist) and the clinic's objectives are:

- Channelling patients from general practitioner (GP) practices to a consultant-led properly specialised outpatient clinic to optimise patient management, sorting malignant from benign in one session, thus avoiding the long wating time between two or three outpatient appointments. Patients with benign disease can be discharged immediately; those with breast cancer can be treated according to the stage of cancer.
- Diagnosing the disease at its early (treatable and cheaper) stage with quick management decisions made in 96% of patients at the first outpatient visit and thus maximising utilisation of hospital outpatient resources. In the St Bartholomew's study (1995), the main wait from appointment until surgical consultation was 37.7 min and that for investigation to clinical review was 56.9 min; 72% patients had a total wait of less than 2 hours and 95% were seen in under 3 hours. Patients seen in the latter half of the clinic were limited by time for investigation, reporting and recall at the same visit. Whenever possible, such patients were recalled with results of their tests within 1 week.
- Alleviating the anxiety associated with symptomatic breast disease (after confirming the benign nature of the disease). Women are investigated with mammography, ultrasonography and fine needle aspiration biopsy cytology (FNABC) (in this order if these three investigations are combined) with immediate reporting. Mammography and ultrasonography must be done first to locate the breast abnormality before FNABC; they must be performed prior to FNABC because the latter may distort breast architecture resulting in a false reporting. Furthermore, FNABC may be performed under ultrasonic guidance.

A one-stop diagnostic clinic provides high-quality health care delivery, better consultant input and patient satisfaction in terms of early diagnosis, management plan and anxiety relief by the appropriate skilled counselling.

The one-stop clinic approach has so far been successful in symptomatic breast disease; it can also be applied in rectal bleeding (perhaps requiring two-stops due to the prolonged barium enema procedure, better termed fast-track rectal bleeding clinic), and leg ulcers (one-stop ulcer diagnostic clinic).

UROLOGY

1.59 Urinary Stone

Stones are formed as Carr concretions or Randall's plaques. They are either primary (metabolic in origin in a normal urinary system and normal acidic urine pH) or secondary (non-metabolic in origin; due to infection, dehydration and alkaline urine pH).

There are four types of urinary (or renal) stones according to composition:
- Calcium oxalate – mulberry calculi (80–85%).
- Triple phosphate, i.e. calcium, magnesium and ammonium phosphate – staghorn calculi (10%).
- Uric acid stones (10%).
- Cystine calculi and xanthine stones (1%).

Urinary stones are classically radio-opaque in 90% of cases. Uric acid and xanthine stones are radiolucent (10%).

Aetiology

Metabolic causes

- Hypercalcaemia in primary hyperparathyroidism, sarcoidosis, vitamin D intoxication, milk-alkali syndrome and ectopic parathormone secretion, e.g. hypernephroma and bronchogenic carcinoma.
- Primary hyperoxaluria.
- Hyperuricaemia in gout, protein catabolism, e.g. leukaemia, and in cytotoxic drug therapy.

Non-metabolic causes

- Dehydration in tropical areas (e.g. Burma) and chronic diarrhoea cases (e.g. Crohn's disease and ileostomy).
- Infection with urea-splitting organisms, e.g. *Escherichia coli, Bacillus proteus*, streptococcus and staphylococcus, leads to alkaline urine and stone formation which leads to obstruction, stasis and perpetuation of infection (vicious circle).
- Residual stagnant urine (stasis) due to immobilisation or distal obstruction leads to infection and stone formation, e.g. a stone-causing pelviureteric junction obstruction and hydronephrosis can lead to a secondary stone in the proximal urine (different in composition from the primary one).
- Congenital, e.g. medullary sponge kidney with congenital calyceal cystic calcification (a similar condition is papillary necrosis which occurs in drug abuse and other, rare, conditions).
- Diet (e.g. excess milk or oxalate-containing food) or deficiency of urinary inhibitors of crystallisation (decreased acid mucopolysaccharides or increased uric acid) together with less fluid intake may lead to supersaturation of urine with crystalloids (increased calcium, oxalate, pH or decreased volume).

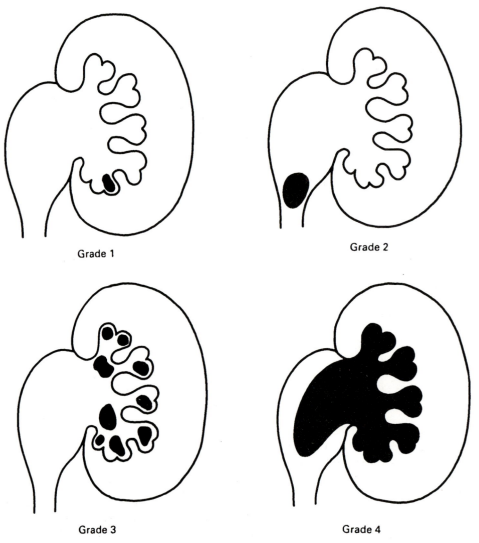

Grade 1

Grade 2

Grade 3

Grade 4

Fig. 1.59.1   Clinicoradiological grading of renal stones

Clinicoradiological types (Fig. 1.59.1)

Grade 1 A small stone usually metabolic (Mulberry spiky stones) subdivided into: (A) immobile, e.g. asymptomatic stone in lower calyx (no need for surgery); or (B) mobile (surgery indicated if over 0.5 cm in diameter or symptomatic, i.e. causes haematuria or is intrapelvic with ball-valve obstruction).

Grade 2 Usually metabolic in origin causing pelviureteric junction obstruction possibly with haematuria, backache and urinary tract infection (minimal symptoms). Pyelolithotomy is required.

Grade 3 Usually infective in origin; occasionally metabolic with multiple calculi in pelvicalyceal system of the kidney (soon forms staghorn calculus). Nephrolithotomy is required.

Grade 4 Infective in origin. The staghorn calculus moulded to the shape of the pelvicalyceal system with kidney calcification as an end-result of Grade 3. Nephrectomy is required if nephrolithotomy is impossible.

Investigations

- Abdominal plain X-ray, intravenous urethrography to see function and whether one or two kidneys are present (urgent IVU in renal colic), MSU (look for red blood cells – microscopic haematuria) with culture and sensitivity.
- If there is fever, but the loin pain is decreasing, do urgent IVU to see if there is obstruction to relieve it with nephrostomy.
- Blood urea, creatinine and serum electrolytes, calcium and phosphorus with blood protein (low proteins lead to false low calcium level).
- Alkaline phosphatase and acid phosphatase (in case of skeletal metastases from prostatic carcinoma with hypercalcaemia), uric acid and 24 h urinary calcium (normally 2.5–7.5 mmol/24 h urine collection) phosphate, urate and oxalate.
- Parathormone (PH) assay is required in suspected primary hyperparathyroidism (increased PH and increased Ca^{2+}).
- Radioactive isotope scan (renogram) to assess bilateral renal function is important. Nephrectomy can only be indicated if scan reveals 10% or less functioning kidney tissues.

Types of treatment

Prophylactic conservative

Used in small (less than 0.5 cm in diameter) asymptomatic stones. Includes:
- High fluid intake achieving high daily urine output.
- Dietary advice (avoid excess milk and oxalate-containing food). In areas with hard water supplies, ask patients to use water softener before drinking. (Hard water is bad for the kidneys but claimed to be good for the heart and cancer, i.e. the incidence of coronary heart disease and cancers is low in hard water areas.)
- Treatment of urinary tract infection (combined high fluid intake, urinary antiseptic and urinary alkalinisation).

- Thiazide diuretics – useful hypocalcaemic agents in recurrent calcium-containing stones. Allopurinol is used in hyperuricaemia and uric acid stone prophylaxis.

Surgical treatment

Prophylactic

- Correction of hyperparathyroidism by removal of parathyroid adenoma because in these cases the nephrocalcinosis is irreversible. The patient feels better and further stones are prevented (hyperparathyroidism is a disease of stones, bones, abdominal groans – peptic ulcer and pancreatitis and psychic moans).
- Correction of any distal urinary obstruction responsible for proximal stone formation. Similarly, prostatic obstructive uropathy should receive treatment priority over associated renal stones.

Therapeutic

Surgery is indicated:
- For obstruction. Manifested clinically by pain, chemically by high urea and creatinine, and radiologically by impaired renal function both on IVU and renogram.
- For infection. Especially in obstructed cases since the change of hydronephrosis into pyonephrosis has a grave outcome.
- For stones over 0.5–1 cm in diameter, whether symptomatic or not, and below that if symptomatic, causing severe pain and/or haematuria. All staghorn calculi should be operated on once diagnosed.

Principles of surgery

To preserve as much as possible of the functioning renal tissue and to prevent complications (e.g. obstruction, infection and severe pain, malignancy and rarely stricture formation).

Anaesthesia (by induction, halothane) may lead to decreased urine output after renal surgery in an already dehydrated patient. Thus, there is no place for hypotensive anaesthesia in renal surgery.

Special considerations

- In bilateral kidney stones, operate on the most painful side first then on the other side.
- In bilateral kidney stones with one non-functioning (bad) kidney, operate on the healthy side first then perform nephrectomy on the bad kidney.

Available approaches (Fig. 1.59.2)

A lateral approach through a subperiosteal 12th rib excision or lumbotomy (lumbar sympathectomy-like incision) provides direct posterior intrarenal access for stone removal (impossible anteriorly owing to the renal vessel). One of three methods can

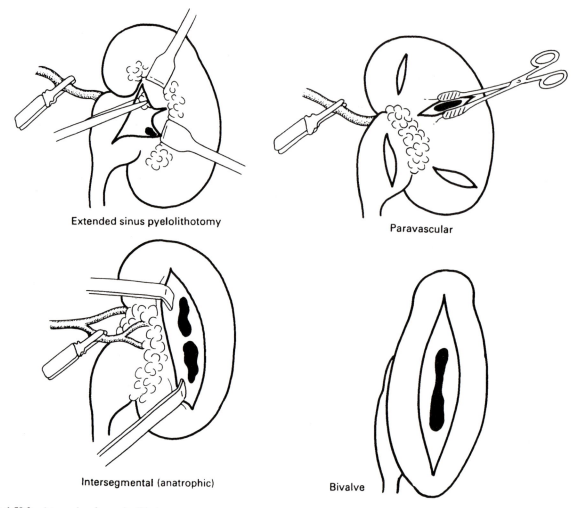

Extended sinus pyelolithotomy

Paravascular

Intersegmental (anatrophic)

Bivalve

Fig. 1.59.2   Approaches for nephrolithotomy

be used (the functional renal reduction is expressed in percentage terms).

- Simple or extended sinus pyelolithotomy of Gil-Vernet, 1965 (0%). Extended pyelolithotomy is done by dissecting through the renal sinus and lifting the kidney substance from the renal pelvis.
- Paravascular radial approach of Wickham *et al.*, 1974 (20%).
- Intersegmental anatrophic approach of Boyce and Elkins, 1974 (30%).

The bivalve approach (50%) is very traumatic and should not be used. While the operation is in progress, vascular arrest may be necessary and hypothermic preservation is achieved with slush ice, external coils or by the intra-arterial method. Sometimes systemic i.v. inosine is used. Arterial clamping is used frequently while cooling the kidney and the clamp should be released every 10 min (a 1 h operation therefore requires six clamping releases and applications). An ischaemic time of 60 min leads to 70% intrarenal depression which will return to normal in 14 days; 120 min ischaemia leads to 100% depression with only partial recovery; 180 min ischaemia leads to 100% depression and no recovery.

After stone extraction (in order that all residual stone fragments are discovered and extracted):

- Carry out a contact nephrogram on the table checking the preoperative IVU on the viewing box from time to time.
- Use syringe and good irrigation with saline.
- Use finger manipulation.
- Carry out pyeloscopy on table (like choledochoscopy).
- Rarely coagulum pyelolithotomy is used. A material is injected that sets and moulds with the stone pieces and can then be extracted in one large piece (the pelviureteric junction should be secured beforehand).

Recurrent renal stone

Usually due to a missed metabolic cause (hyperparathyroidism) or persistent urinary tract obstruction or infection. The patient should be investigated thoroughly, e.g. stone screen including serum, calcium, phosphorus urate, oxalate and alkaline phosphatase as well as 24 h urine collection for calcium, phosphate and urate. Prophylactic conservative and surgical treatment should be stressed. Percutaneous nephroscopy has a place in the treatment.

Ureteric stones

- Upper ureteric and pelviureteric junction: approached like kidney stones.
- Mid-ureter. iliac lumbotomy (like lumbar sympathectomy).
- Lower ureter. approached either cystoscopically (using Collin's knife meatotomy and manipulation with ureteric catheter or Dormia basket extraction) or through a suprapubic open approach.

Recently, flexible fibreoptic ureteroscopy has been introduced for intraureteral litholapaxy, biopsy and fulguration of ureteric transitional cell carcinomas.

1.60 Minimally Invasive and Non-Invasive Nephrolithotomy

Percutaneous nephroscopy/nephrolithotomy (PCNL) and extracorporeal shock-wave lithotripsy (ESWL) are the two available alternatives to open nephrolithotomy and/or pyelolithotomy.

Percutaneous nephroscopy or nephrolithotomy

PNCL is used in intrapelvic renal stones or residual recurrent ones. A good interventional radiologist is needed to create the track into the renal pelvis using IVU and ultrasound guidance. A fascial dilator is used followed by an angioplasty balloon catheter and then rigid concentric rods to prepare for the nephroscopic stone retrieval. Direct stone extraction is done by:

- Ultrasonic disintegration 27 000/s (lithotripsy denotes crushing stone in situ while litholapaxy denotes crushing the stone, and washing it out).
- Extracorporeal electrohydraulic spark shock wave destruction with the patient lying in a water bath under general anaesthetic.

Some ureteric stones, occasionally, can also be extracted endoscopically with a ureteroscope.

Percutaneous nephrolithotomy demands two precautions:

- A prior cystoscopic insertion of a special occluding ureteric catheter, which is self-retained after inflating its balloon at the distal end, in order to occlude the ureter and prevent any stone fragment from blocking the ureteric lumen.
- A Malecot catheter is left in situ (percutaneously) as a nephrostomy tube (like a T-tube left after biliary stone extraction), and a nephrostogram is performed 24 h later so that any remaining fragment can be seen and removed.

PCNL, however, may lead to the following complications:

- Residual renal stones.
- Ureteric obstruction by fragmented stone.
- Retroperitoneal extravasation.
- Bleeding from the renal artery, which requires renal arterial embolization and even nephrectomy which will be an extremely hard decision to take in such a patient.

PCNL is contraindicated in

- Staghorn calculus.
- Higher stones under 12th rib.
- Embedded peripheral calyceal stones.
- Stones in solitary or horseshoe kidney.
- Stones in malrotated kidney in a fatty patient.

Extracorporeal shock wave lithotripsy

ESWL is the non-invasive method of disintegrating kidney stones, developed by the Dornier Company of Germany. It was first introduced into clinical practice by Chaussy *et al.* (1980). The technique revolutionised the treatment of upper urinary tract stone disease. It rapidly gained acceptance and is now the treatment of choice for more than 80% of upper tract stones, particularly renal calculi measuring up to 2–3 cm in diameter (results are better in small stones). ESWL has also been used to treat ureteric stones either in situ or following manipulation of the stone into the kidney: the 'push and bang' technique. Recently, the indications for ESWL have been extended to include the treatment of staghorn calculi either as monotherapy (usually needs many sessions) or in combination with percutaneous nephrolithotomy. The mean number of shock waves/treatment is 1724 for all stones and 2325 for staghorn calculi (the larger the size of the urinary stone, the more shock waves required to achieve fragmentation).

The original lithtriptors (Dornier HM1, HM2, and HM3) are replaced by a new Multi-Purpose Lithotriptor (Dornier Lithotriptor MPL 9000) generation, making the procedure painless, the X-ray or ultrasound anatomical location of the stones and targeting of shock waves better, and obviating the need for immersing the patient in a water sink under general anaesthesia.

The stones are localised by an integrated, dual ultrasonic locating system with the X-ray complementary locating system (image intensifier); the patient is subjected to repeated pulses of focused shock-waves from the lithotriptor.

A generously applied gel is needed, while the sparks are synchronized with heart rate beats to deliver about 2000 shocks adjusted automatically by ECG monitor. A new spark plug is needed for each patient. The procedure is painless, and analgesia is not normally required, with the potential of using lithotripsy as an outpatient technique and for day cases.

The immediate stone fragmentation rate is 90% and the 3-month clearance rate 88%. Secondary treatments are required in 19% of patients and additional procedures in 17%.

However, the complications following ESWL include:

- Postoperative ureteric colics in 25% of cases due to small fragments of the stone passing through the ureter. This is initially treated with analgesia. Obstructing ureteric fragments, however, may require one of the following procedures:

  repeated ESWL alone,
  retrograde push and ESWL,
  ureteroscopic extraction,
  percutaneous extraction,
  cystoscopic Dormia basket extraction,
  percutaneous nephrostomy.

Ureteric stricture may follow in 1% of cases; it requires ureteroscopic dilatation.

- Fever of more than 38.5 °C with mild dilatation of the urinary collecting system in 8% of cases. This requires antibiotic therapy and possibly one of the above procedures. Perinephric abscess may occur in 1.5% of cases, while pyonephrosis in 1% and may require nephrectomy.
- Septicaemia can follow severe dilatation of the urinary collecting system in 0.6% of cases. This requires an urgent decompression by placing a percutaneous nephrostomy catheter.
- Rarely, perirenal haematoma and pancreatitis may follow ESWL.

1.61 Urinary Diversion

Indications

- To maintain renal function by relieving the obstructive uropathy and clearing the infection.
- To improve urinary continence, e.g. in cystectomy, ectopia vesicae, neurological bladder and an incurable vesicovaginal fistula.
- When sphincteric mechanism is diseased or removed.

Types

Temporary diversion

- *Nephrostomy*   Indicated in:
  - Uraemia or acute obstruction in a solitary kidney.
  - Pelvic or gynaecological operation with ureteric damage – percutaneous nephrostomy.
  - Congenital urethral valves in male children (Foley's or Malecot's catheter could be inserted through the thin cortex of the kidney).

  Percutaneous nephrostomy can: serve as a temporary or permanent urinary diversion; provide diversion to allow distal fistula to heal; provide a route for splinting the ureter as well as extracting renal stones. In adults, kidney mobilisation and opening through the kidney pelvis (not cortex) are important. There are two types of nephrostomy in adults – percutaneous and ring nephrostomy. The catheter in the latter can be changed and irrigated easily and works very well.
- *Pyelostomy*
- *Ureterostomy (not very satisfactory)*   Constructed as loop or Y-shaped in children. In adults a ureterostomy in situ is used (via an appendicectomy-like muscle-cutting incision and ureteric catheterisation).
- *Suprapubic bladder drainage*
- *Urethral drainage*

Permanent diversion

- *Reservoir*   Includes ureterosigmoidostomy with various modifications, trigonosigmoidostomy and rectal bladder. Ureterosigmoidostomy could be done with a colonic conduit or rectal bladder (and permanent colostomy). It is contra-indicated in the presence of:
  - Upper urinary tract dilatation.
  - Urinary incontinence (neurological problem) since this leads to faecal incontinence. Complications include:
  - Infection. If there is increased pelvic colonic pressure, longitudinal colonic myotomy is indicated together with the treatment of infection with antibiotics.
  - Ureteric obstruction with recurrent pyelonephritis.
  - Troublesome diarrhoea with hyperchloraemic hypokalaemic metabolic acidosis (with vomiting, thirst, acidotic breathing and coma). Hypokalaemia damages the kidney further.
  - Development of malignant disease is not uncommon in diversion. In rectal bleeding therefore one should not do a barium enema (causes ascending infection) but colonoscopy to see and biopsy the possible bleeding rectal polyp.
- *External stoma*   Includes cutaneous ureterostomy in children, vesicostomy (difficult to attach bag to) and anterior transposition of urethra in females (rarely done).
- *Intestinal conduit*   Using ileal, colonic or ileocaecal segment. Most common is the ileal conduit formed by anastomosing the two ureters to one end of the segment and bringing the other end to the surface as a spouting ileostomy (or urostomy). Complications are:
  - Stomal stenosis, needing revision (since increased intra-ureteric pressure eventually leads to kidney infection).
  - Pyelonephritis (in 18% of cases).
  - Renal stone formation (in 10% of cases), due to urine stagnation and kidney infection.
  - Intestinal obstruction – early postoperative complication in up to 15% of cases.
  - Pyocystis is a problem in neurological bladder cases, if the bladder is not removed.
  - Hyperchloraemic acidosis in ileal conduit – may occur but rarely.

Criteria for successful ideal diversion

- Continence with voluntary control of urine and faeces.
- Complete separation of urinary and faecal streams.
- Functioning urinary reservoir without absorptive problems.
- Absence of unnatural or artificial orifices.
- Accessible to endoscopic assessment.

1.62 Urothelial Tumours, Kidney Tumours and Testicular Tumours

UROTHELIAL TUMOURS

Include tumours arising from the transitional cell epithelium of the urinary tract, i.e. transitional cell carcinoma of the urinary bladder, renal pelvis and ureter. Rarely urothelial metaplasia

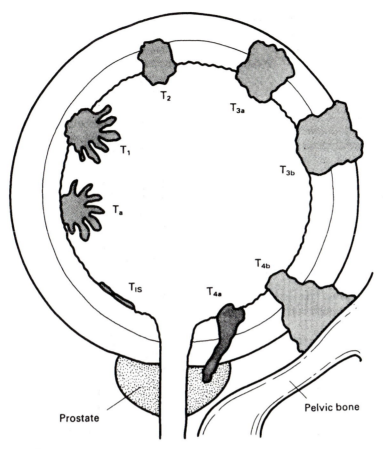

Fig. 1.62.1 Bladder cancer – staging

with subsequent squamous cell carcinoma occurs in the urinary bladder (due to bilharziasis) and in the renal pelvis (due to chronic irritation of a renal stone). They generally present with haematuria and are diagnosed by midstream urine examination (MSU), urine cytology, intravenous urography (IVU) and cystourethroscopy.

Aetiology

- *Occupational*, e.g. aniline dye workers exposed to α-or β-naphthylamine, benzidine, auramine or magenta dyes (carcinogenic).
- *Inflammatory*, e.g. bilharziasis (*Schistosoma haematobium* infestation) or chronic inflammation due to bladder stone.
- *Congenital*, e.g. urinary diverticulum or adenocarcinoma developing in the urachus (remnant attaching bladder fundus to umbilicus).
- *Miscellaneous*, e.g. smoking and abnormal tryptophane metabolism (leading to a carcinogenic metabolite). Benign bladder papillomas are rare and may transform into the usual malignant tumours by the time of presentation.

Histological grading

G1 Well differentiated.
G2 Moderately undifferentiated.

G3 Highly undifferentiated (or dedifferentiated or anaplastic).

Staging

Determined by a combined clinical (bimanual examination under anaesthesia), cystoscopic evaluation and histology (Fig. 1.62.1).

T_{IS} Flat carcinoma in situ confined to the epithelium.
T_a Papillary carcinoma confined to the epithelium.
T_1 Papillary carcinoma involving the epithelium and invading lamina propria.
T_2 Tumour has invaded detrusor muscle layer.
T_3 Tumour has extended into the perivesical fat but is still mobile.
T_4 Tumour has infiltrated into the contiguous structures and is fixed.

Lymph node spread is only assessed during operations on bladder tumours (N_1: regional lymph nodes involved; N_2: juxtaregional or bilateral lymph nodes involved; N_3: fixed). Metastasis in bladder tumours is uncommon. The prognosis depends on *staging* and *histological grading*.

Salient features of bladder tumours and management

T_{IS}

There is no exophytic tumour, but abnormal mucosa with positive cytology. Occurs mostly in males and presents mainly with unusual symptoms (e.g. frequency, dysuria, urethral and/or perineal pain). Haematuria is not a predominant presentation. If T_{IS} is localised diathermy is required but if widespread then cystourethrectomy is necessary. There is a role for intravesical adriamycin or i.v. cyclophosphamide (but not for radiotherapy).

Superficial tumours (T_a, T_1)

- Are the commonest and respond best to treatment.
- Usually well differentiated and do not invade beyond the lamina propria.
- Sometimes invasion is limited to the core of the papilla but may be deeper.
- Have a tendency to recur rather than to invade.
- Overall 5 year survival is 80%.
- Treatment is by any of the following approaches:
  - Endoscopic diathermy (destruction) or resection (TUR) are the commonest treatments.
  - Open excision.
  - Partial cystectomy.
  - Cystourethrectomy.
  - External radiotherapy.
  - Intracavitary radiotherapy.
  - Intracavitary chemotherapy, e.g. thiotepa, ethoglucid (Epodyl), can give 60% of patients a disease-free period of 1 year.
  - Helmstein balloon therapy (cystodistension under epidural anaesthesia for half an hour) is rarely successful.
  - Hyperthermia.
  - Mucosal stripping.

Invasive tumours T_2, T_3 and T_4

T_2

- Difficult to diagnose (since the invasion may be superficial and just beyond lamina propria).
- Tumour less than 2 cm and G1 or G2 is treated endoscopically (TUR).
- Tumour greater than 2 cm or G3 is treated with radiotherapy.
- There is a role for partial cystectomy.
- 5-year survival is 50%.

T_3

- Incidence of positive lymph node at operation.
- Cystourethrectomy alone (5-year survival is 25%).
- Radical deep X-ray therapy (6000 rad) + salvage cystourethrectomy (5-year survival is 40%).
- Preoperative deep X-ray therapy (4000 rad) + radical cystourethrectomy (5-year survival is 38%).
- Flash deep X-ray therapy (2000 rad) + radical cystourethrectomy (5-year survival is 40%).
- Urethra must be removed because:
  - It is involved in 18% of bladder tumours (urothelial tumour is multiple).

- Risk of carcinoma in situ.
- Poor prognosis in urethral recurrence.

T_4

Inoperable, poor prognosis. Treated with:
- Palliative radiotherapy or
- Chemotherapy (methotrexate or cis-platinum).

Renal pelvis tumour

When the *pelvicalyceal system* is involved the tumour tends to be more invasive and highly malignant. Treatment is by partial nephrectomy or even more radical excision, i.e. nephroureterectomy with sleeve resection of the bladder.

When the *pelviureteric junction* is involved, treatment is by radical excision, i.e. nephroureterectomy with partial cystectomy.

Ureteric tumours

- Midureter: treatment is local resection with end-to-end anastomosis or cross-ureteroureterostomy.
- Lower end of ureter: the treatment is by local excision, opening the bladder and making a Boari flap or transureteroureterostomy, especially if a long segment is involved.
- Upper end of ureter: nephroureterectomy and partial cystectomy.

KIDNEY TUMOURS

Wilms' tumour of children (10% of renal tumours)

A connective tissue tumour accounting for 20% of all malignancies in children, usually within the first 7 years of life (adult Wilms' tumours are very rarely reported); presents mainly as a loin mass and less frequently as haematuria. Should be differentiated from hydronephrosis, multicystic kidney and neuroblastoma.

Investigations

- IVU shows grossly distorted kidney. Bilateral kidney involvement occurs in 10% of cases.
- Abdominal ultrasound is helpful in children.
- Chest X-ray (and no further investigation).

Management (depends on age of child)

Below 2 years of age Adjuvant chemotherapy within 24 h before surgery. The tumour should be removed via the anterior abdominal approach to allow for extension (into a long subcostal or thoracoabdominal incision in case the intestine is stuck to the tumour when performing nephrectomy) and also for examination of the other kidney which if involved requires partial nephrectomy. Postoperative adjuvant radiotherapy is also used.

Over 2 years of age   Combined chemotherapy using two agents, actinomycin D and vincristin, is curative in 80% of cases.

Clear cell carcinoma or adenocarcinoma (75% of renal tumours)

A common tumour that originates from cortical proximal tubular cells (adenocarcinoma) and affects males over 40 years of age. Usually mixed and its presentation is disguised in a number of ways.

Loin pain, lump and haematuria   Occur in a third of cases and should be differentiated from splenomegaly or hepatomegaly and, if the pain is diffused, from renal stones.

Systemic manifestations   Due to immunological reaction pro-voked by kidney tumour, e.g. profound anaemia (6–9 g/dl), increased ESR (greater than 100), pyrexia of unknown origin, abnormalities in liver function tests such as high alkaline phosphatase or high calcium. The patient may be intolerably ill and miserable (carry out IVU to reveal renal cancer).

Endocrinal manifestations   Due to hormonal secretion (nor-mal or ectopic), i.e. renin (secreted by ischaemic part of the kidney distal to the tumour) leads to hypertension, abnormal ectopic parathormone secretion leads to hypercalcaemia and erythropoetin secretion leads to polycythaemia (though gen-erally anaemia is commoner).

Metastatic manifestations for the first time   e.g. backache, collapsed vertebra, fractures (skeletal); or lung (solitary usually) or brain deposits.

Rare presentations   e.g. Budd–Chiari syndrome and left testicular varicocele.

Investigations

- IVU especially its nephrogram phase in 1 min film. If inconclusive then 1–2 ml/kg contrast medium is needed with tomography to see the outline of the kidney showing a lump at one pole.
- Abdominal ultrasound can confirm whether the lump is solid or cystic with 95% accuracy; if cystic can be aspirated for cytology followed by injection for cystogram to see its outline (ultrasonic guided aspiration leads to 99.9% cure of simple benign cysts).
- If the lump is solid, or the cystic aspirate is bloody, the surgeon can proceed with operation without the need for arteriography (and its complications). However CT scan is now regarded as the third step to produce the final diagnosis (CT scan has replaced arteriography).
- Venogram (rather than arteriography) is sometimes needed to see if the vena cava is involved, especially in right renal tumours.
- Chest X-ray to discover any solitary metastasis (relevant to the management since lobectomy could be performed).

Treatment

Mainly surgical. Nephrectomy via the anterior abdominal approach is preferred. However, subperiosteal lateral extraper-itoneal approach is recommended if it is certain that the inferior vena cava is clear of tumour lumps. Pulmonary lobectomy is practised in solitary metastasis.

Radiotherapy and chemotherapy are useless but hormonal therapy is worth trying by giving Provera 100 mg three times daily – response is good in 30% of males and 5% of females. If there is no response testosterone 100 mg three times weekly can be given.

The prognosis is directly related to the stage of spread (Stage 1: kidney; Stage 2: perinephric fat; Stage 3: vascular/lymphatic involvement; Stage 4: distant spread). In Stage 1, 5-year survival is 65%.

Renal pelvis tumours (10% of renal tumours)

See Urothelial tumours.

TESTICULAR TUMOURS

Usually occur in men under the age of 40 years. They are fortunately rare as there are no benign testicular tumours (all are malignant). The types are closely related to age: in babies – orcheoblastoma; in young men (20–30 years) – teratoma; in middle-aged men (30–40 years) – seminoma; and in the elderly – lymphoma. The germinal group represents 96% of all testicular tumours (seminoma and teratoma) while the non-germinal group (Sertoli cell, Leydig cell tumours) and paratesticular tumours (lipo-, lienomyo-, fibro-, neuro- and rhabdomyo-sarcomas) together constitute less than 4%.

There are various types of teratoma, named differently according to the British and American classification:

Teratomas (British)	Non-seminomas (American)
Malignant teratoma differentiated (MTD)	Teratoma
Malignant teratoma intermedia (MTI)	Teratocarcinoma
Malignant teratoma undifferentiated (MTU)	Embryonal carcinoma
Malignant teratoma trophoblastica (MTT)	Choriocarcinoma

Chemotherapy is effective and can change MTT into MTI and MTI into MTU.

Local spread of testicular tumour is exceptionally rare because of encapsulation within tunica albuginea. However, it spreads to iliac, para-aortic, mediastinal and supraclavicular lymph nodes and sometimes to lung (extralymphatic).

Testicular tumours are staged accordingly into:

Stage I   Tumour is confined to testis.
Stage II   Para-aortic abdominal lymph node involvement.
Stage III   Supraclavicular (thoracic supradiaphragmatic) lymph node involvement.
Stage IV   Lung involvement (extralymphatic).

Carcinoma in situ has recently been recognised in infertile males (found in testicular biopsy), in males with undescended testicles, in contralateral testis of patients with testicular tumours and in intersex patients.

Diagnosis

- Painless rapid testicular enlargement (heavy with increased size and same shape).
- Painful testis in 15% of cases after minor trauma.
- Secondary hydrocele in 5% of cases.
- Advanced spread, e.g. para-aortic abdominal masses, supraclavicular lymph nodes, haemoptysis (lung metastasis).
- Gynaecomastia.

Clinical examination with fingers is the most reliable method of detection.

Investigations

- Blood for β-human chorionic gonadotrophin and α-fetoprotein (tumour markers).
- Chest X-ray.
- IVU to exclude ureteric displacement by para-aortic lymph node enlargement.
- Urine examination and full blood count are sent routinely to differentiate testicular tumour from epididymo-orchitis. Post-traumatic haematocele is difficult to differentiate since testicular tumour may also start after trauma; exploration will therefore be the final answer.
- Early exploration via inguinal incision (never scrotal since this leads to local spread). A soft clamp is applied to the cord at the internal inguinal ring, the testis delivered and examined (any procedure can be freely carried out after clamping with no risk of blood-borne metastases). If it is obviously cancer then carry out orchidectomy; if in doubt, slice open and send for a frozen section taken from the cut surface (if proved to be cancer carry out orchidectomy but if a benign lesion is discovered then tunica albuginea incision can be sutured with no risk of atrophy). The scrotum remains untouched.
- Once the histological confirmation is obtained, a meticulous search for metastases is to be followed by lymphangiography and CT scanning of retroperitoneal tissues and mediastinum as well as whole lung tomography (staging for proper treatment).

Treatment

In seminomas (always treat one stage ahead, i.e., therapeutic treatment of the clinical stage plus prophylactic treatment for possible subclinical microscopic spread):

Stage I   Orchidectomy and prophylactic retroperitoneal radiotherapy.

Stage II   Orchidectomy and prophylactic retroperitoneal and mediastinal radiotherapy.

Stage III Orchidectomy with combined (retroperitoneal and mediastinal) radiotherapy and chemotherapy.

Stage IV   Orchidectomy and chemotherapy.

The common agents are cis-platinum, vinblastine and bleomycin. The 5-year survival in Stage I has dramatically improved by cis-platinum to 90%.

In *teratomas* the treatment is similar but prophylactic chemotherapy is given first and if it fails then radiotherapy. (If radiotherapy is given first, it may damage the bone marrow and restrict the dosage of chemotherapy that can be given subsequently.) Surgery (thoracotomy or laparotomy) is needed for removal of bulky masses and for radical retroperitoneal lymph node dissection (marginally better than retroperitoneal radiotherapy). It is acceptable now that the cure rate is 90% in stage I and 80% in the presence of metastases.

1.63 Prostatic Carcinoma

There are three main groups seen in prostatic carcinoma.

Clinical carcinoma is diagnosed clinically on the basis of combined obstructive uropathy and findings (on rectal examination) of hard, irregular prostate with obliteration of sulcus or with a nodule. The clinical diagnosis is confirmed histologically.

Latent carcinoma is found incidentally with no clinical evidence of the disease.

In occult carcinoma the primary tumour manifests itself by secondaries in its first presentation.

The incidence of prostatic carcinoma is low in populations with short life expectancy (it is rare before the age of 40 years). It is claimed to be greater in married men and urban people, less in Jews. There is evidence for a hormonal association, based on:

- Regression following castration or oestrogen therapy.
- Multiple endocrine changes in postmortem specimens.
- Correlation with male breast carcinoma.
- Biochemical studies.
- Incidence of prostatic carcinoma in cirrhotics.

The carcinoma usually arises from the peripheral prostatic zone; thus, open prostatectomy (for benign glandulocystic fibromuscular prostatic hyperplasia which arises from the central zone) does not guarantee against future development of carcinoma.

Staging is based on T (primary tumour) progress:

T_0 No palpable tumour. Includes cases with incidental finding of carcinoma in an operative or biopsy specimen (also called Stage A).

T_1 Intracapsular tumour nodule surrounded by palpably normal tissue.

T_2 Tumour is still confined to prostate with smooth nodule deforming the contour of prostatic lobe or lobes but lateral sulci and seminal vesicles are not involved.

T_1 and T_2 are termed Stage B. Early cancer includes Stages A and B only.

T_3 Extraprostatic spread ± involvement of lateral sulci ± involvement of seminal vesicles.

T_4 Tumour is fixed and invading nearby tissues.

T_3 and T_4 are Stage C in the absence of metastasis and Stage D in the presence of distant metastasis. C and D are advanced cancer stages.

Such minimum requirements for assessment expressed by T_x cannot always be met and further investigations are required:

- Rectal ultrasound probe can assess the size, site and nature of the tumour. Ultrasound scanning can be done per urethram or transabdominally.
- Plasma biochemistry, i.e. urea, electrolytes, creatinine, acid and alkaline phosphatases.
- Radiology, i.e. chest X-ray, intravenous urogram, and skeletal survey.
- $^{99}Tc^m$-polyphosphate bone scan.
- Cystourethroscopy and examination under anaesthesia.
- Biopsy (fine needle or Tru-cut punch needle via perineal (better) or transrectal routes) or transuretheral resection (TUR) biopsy (of prostatic chippings). Needle biopsy may lead to infection, bleeding, bacteraemia and septic shock. A prophylactic antibiotic is therefore recommended especially for the transrectal route.

Treatment options

Radical prostatectomy + radical inguinal lymphadenectomy Popular in the USA (not UK); used for Stages A and B and claimed to have very good long-term results but with permanent impotence and urinary incontinence.

Radiotherapy Popular in the UK and used alternatively for Stages A, B and C. The current trend is to use interstitial radioactive isotope therapy via needles inserted under ultrasound guide into the tumour area (after first being diagnosed with rectal ultrasound and then confirmed by biopsy). The prostatic carcinoma is a slow radiosensitive tumour, necessitating prolonged local radiotherapy applied to the disease area.

Hormonal therapy For advanced Stage D. This is the treatment of choice since skeletal metastases melt away and prostatic obstructive uropathy improves. Anti-androgen therapy is either medical or surgical. Medically, stilboestrol is commonly used initially in a low dose (e.g. 2–3 mg daily for 1 week) followed by a maintenance dose of 1 mg/24 h indefinitely. Alternatively, TACE (Tripara-Alnisil-ChlorEthylene) fosfestrol sodium (Honvan), or cyproterone acetate (testosterone antagonist) could be used in the presence of some stilboestrol side-effects (see S. 1.21). However, in patients with thromboembolic complications of stilboestrol or with a history of myocardial infarction, stroke or deep venous thrombosis (due to lymphatic or venous obstruction of the lower limbs or as a thrombotic complication of prostatic cancer *per se*) a surgical approach is preferred in the form of bilateral subcapsular orchidectomy. LHRH agonist Zoladex is commonly used as a form of hormonal orchidectomy.

Others TUR may be diagnostic, therapeutic (if 25% of the resected prostatic chippings prove to be cancer) or palliative in prostatic obstructive uropathy. On occasions no treatment is required apart from indefinite indwelling urinary catheterisation.

Currently there is emphasis on early diagnosis using ultrasound rectal probe and prostatic biopsy followed by curative treatment with radiotherapy or radical prostatectomy. Hormonal therapy is used less frequently.

Prostatic TUR versus open prostatectomy

TUR is indicated commonly in benign prostatic hyperplasia and in carcinoma when there is:

- Acute urinary retention. ⎫
- Chronic retention with overflow. ⎬ Obstructive indications
- Prostatic bleeding.

Poor selections for TUR:

- Recent cardiovascular accident, Parkinsonism and neurological deficiency.
- Abdominoperineal resection of rectum (rectal examination is impossible for assessment of size or lifting the prostate during TUR).
- History of urinary frequency (nocturia, urgency and enuresis) due to detrusor instability which may become worse after TUR.
- Patients under age 55.

Open prostatectomy is indicated in:

- Very large prostate. May be best treated by an open operation, although an experienced surgeon (who can resect more than 1 g/min) can treat almost any size by TUR.
- Bilateral hip osteoarthritis or arthroplasty making lithotomy position of the patient impossible.
- Large bladder stones, which are impossible to crush and wash out endoscopically (litholapaxy).
- History of urethral stricture (relative).
- Bladder diverticula which require excision during operation (relative).
- Very long penile urethra (relative).

Complications of TUR

Bleeding May be primary (due to large gland or bleeding disorder). This should be treated by:

- Gauze tamponade on catheter pulled snugly on bladder neck.
- Local hypothermia.
- EACA (aminocaproic acid) intravesically to prevent further bleeding or intravenously.
- Hydrostatic pressure using continuous irrigation to wash out bladder clots (which encourage further bleeding).
- Evacuation of clots and blood transfusion.
- Bimanual pressure, e.g. one hand suprapubically and another rectally pressing against each other.
- Traction on the catheter to pull the balloon against resected prostatic bed (pressure haemostatic effect).
- Occasionally exploration ± direct intravesical pressure packing (removed after 48 h). Antibiotic prophylaxis is required.

Bleeding may be secondary due to: increased venous pressure on the 10th to 21st day postoperatively; bleeding prostatic bed granulations; or infection. This requires catheterisation with irrigation (see above) and antibiotics. Sometimes, endoscopy may be needed to diathermise the bleeding vessels.

Infection (± septicaemia)   Originates from either the surgeon or the patient himself (either from pre-existing intravesical bacteria, bladder tumour or stone).

Epididymitis   May occur. Prophylactic vasectomy is recommended for repeated TURs.

Incontinence   Caused by sphincteric damage. Rare when special attention is given to the verumontanum. More common after TUR than open prostatectomy.

TUR syndrome   Dilutional hyponatraemia due to water intoxication secondary to excessive fluid absorption leading to decreased level of consciousness, fits and cardiac arrhythmias. Treated by decreasing the irrigation rate (with limited resection time and positioning the irrigating reservoir from less than 60 cm above the symphysis pubis), thiazide diuretic and Digoxin. TUR syndrome occurs even though the irrigating fluid is 1.5% glycine solution – a natural isotonic amino acid which does not conduct electrical current and does not affect the patient when absorbed (NaCl conducts and dissipates the electrical current, making electrical resection impossible). Absorption of distilled water causes haemolysis; cutting is difficult with distilled water (does not conduct electricity well and will bubble after two to three attempts). The 5% glucose behaves just like distilled water once the glucose is absorbed (poor solution).

Bladder wall perforation with extravasation of urine   Requires urethral catheterisation for at least 7 days, decrease or stoppage of continuous irrigation and prophylactic antibiotics. Also nasogastric suction and i.v. fluids in intraperitoneal bladder perforation (with signs of peritonism).

Urethral stricture and bladder neck stenosis (rare)   Anterior urethra is left unresected to encourage epitheliisation as a mucosal bridge, just like haemorrhoidectomy.

Prophylactic antibiotics in urology are indicated in:

● Urological conditions, i.e. bladder stone, large bladder tumour and preoperative urinary tract infection.
● Non-urological conditions, i.e. heart valve diseases, prostheses (including pacemakers) and immune suppression cases.

1.64 Surgery for Impotence

Impotence is the inability to have an erection sufficient for sexual intercourse (applied to men only). Sterility is the inability to reproduce; it affects both sexes.

Impotence is a baffling disorder of great medical antiquity; it has frustrated physicians to both Babylonians and Pharaohs in ancient times and to Presidents in more recent times. Patients are socially and psychologically disturbed; they feel helpless and hopeless, spreading despair (to partners) through the home and workplace. Physicians' failure is reflected by the availability of a plethora of materials claimed to enhance potency (dubious effects), such as ginseng, herbs containing vitamin E, bees' honey, royal jelly and propolis, rhinoceros horn, caviar, snake's blood and bile.

Penile erection is a complex act involving coordinated interaction of neuroendocrine and arterial/venous sinusoidal systems. Discovery of testosterone in the late 1930s and its use to relieve impotence of hypogonadal men was a major step in andrology.

CLINICAL ASSESSMENT

History of intermittent failure can be revealed, followed by inability to sustain erection for more than 2–3 min, followed by inability to penetrate while having firm early morning erections, and finally by penis failure to react to reflex or psychogenic stimuli. Impotence is either organic or psychogenic. Organic erectile dysfunction (at least 50% of impotent men, usually neurogenic and/or vascular) can be caused by failure to initiate (neurogenic, e.g. diabetes mellitus), failure to fill (arteriogenic, e.g. myocardial ischaemia/atherosclerosis and Leriche syndrome), failure to store (venogenic, e.g. venous leak), and end organ diseases with inability to erect properly (e.g. priapism, penile fracture, perineal hypospadias with severe chordee, Peyronie's disease); it tends to correlate with age and is slow to develop. However, spinal or intrapelvic nerve damage is followed by immediate loss of penile erection. Testicular failure and oestrogenic therapy of prostatic cancer results in impotence too (hormonal inhibition of testosterone). Psychogenic impotence occurs during stress which may be marital, economic or occupational with history of depression, use of psychogenic drugs, situations fostering low self-esteem or chronic domestic tension. Alcohol excess is associated with progressive decline in early morning erection. The relative contribution of organic and psychogenic factors needs to be assessed in all patients. Physical examination must be thorough, paying particular attention to vascular and neurological status of the lower limbs (deep tendon and cremasteric reflexes, pinprick and vibration sensation). The genitalia must be examined; size and consistency of the testicles, softening or atrophy would suggest a primary testicular disorder while an indurated penile shaft with distinct plaques suggests Peyronie's disease (erected penis deviates from the midline but not tender or severe enough to prevent intromission).

INVESTIGATIONS

Hormonal levels must be estimated (see below). A history of alcohol excess warrants tests of liver function, gamma glutamyl transferase (gGT) being the most sensitive; if gGT is normal, liver disease is unlikely. Cardiovascular risk factors (cholesterol, triglycerides, and high density lipoprotein cholesterol) are not measured in the absence of specific indications. Investigations include evaluation of various systems.

1. Evaluation of penile arterial system
- Penile blood pressure measurement.
- Doppler pulse-wave analysis.
- Penile blood flow studies.
- Radioisotope penogram.
- Arteriography – a specific, mandatory study to be considered if rearterialisation is contemplated.

2. Evaluation of penile venous system
- Induced erection (ICI) cavernosography.
- Infusion cavernosography.

The diagnosis of venous leakage with cavernosography can best be made after induced erection because injected drugs may be washed out more quickly.

3. Endocrine evaluation Includes testosterone, LH, FSH, prolactin and thyroxine. Low serum testosterone indicates hypogonadism (primary or secondary testicular failure due to hypothalamic or pituitary diseases). LH, FSH concentrations are significantly lower in hypogonadotrophic patients (secondary testicular failure) than in normal individuals. High LH, FSH concentrations are found in primary testicular failure. Hyperprolactinaemia is occasionally associated with impotence; prolactin measurement is therefore required in patients with low serum testosterone but with normal serum LH level.

4. Neurological evaluation Patients suspected to have organic impotence should have a thorough physical examination, as well as nocturnal penile tumescence (NPT), and penile biothesiometry (sensory testing). NPT is an electronic computerised test to detect and measure penile erections that occur during rapid eye movement (REM) sleep; penile circumference is monitored by a fine strain gauge (elastic band) fitted on the penile shaft. The electroencephalogram and electro-oculogram are recorded from 9 pm to 6 am, on two successive nights (after the patient has watched 'blue' movies and read 'soft porn' magazines). Should the patient have normal increases in penile circumference, this would indicate that the impotence is of psychogenic origin; however, if there are no erections or only brief episodes of small amplitude or duration, impotence is organic.

While NPT has been an important objective differentiator of psychogenic from organic impotence, it is not sufficiently sensitive or specific and is being replaced by dynamic studies, such as intracorporeal injection and/or cavernosogram.

More neurological tests should be reserved for impotent patients with metabolic diseases or those with abnormalities on neurological, physical or biothesiometric examination.

5. Rigiscan This is an ambulatory monitor that measures concurrent penile tumescence and rigidity. Parameters in normal erection include:
- Changes in circumference of 3 cm or more at the base of the penis and 2 cm or more at the tip of the penis.
- A rigidity of 70% or more represents a non-buckled fully erected penis, whereas rigidity of 40% or below is considered a flaccid penis.

- Rigidity duration of less than 3 minutes may be proved to have corporeal venous leak. The success rate following revascularisation and venous ligation procedures may be determined by rigiscan.

6. Intracorporeal injection Both diagnostic and therapeutic (see below).

TREATMENT

Medical treatment

Local glyceryl trinitrate paste has been moderately successful, but a condom is recommended to prevent partner-headaches. Potential oral treatments include α_2-adrenergic antagonists (idazoxam, yohimbine), opiate antagonists, and bromocriptine. Testosterone is the mainstay of treatment in androgen deficiency whether from primary testicular disease (Klinefelter's syndrome) or from gonadotrophin deficiency. Testosterone undecanoate (Andriol) at a replacement dose of 160–240 mg/day is recommended (methyl testosterone is no longer used because of potential hepatotoxicity); oral androgen therapy is useful in patients on anticoagulants or those who cannot tolerate injections. A response to 3 month trial necessitates a change to testosterone enanthate (Primoteston Depot, 250 mg) or testosterone esters (Sustanon, 250 mg) by i.m. injection every 4 weeks. Once again, a response to 3 month injections necessitates the need for testosterone pellets for long-term therapy (subcutaneous implantation by trocar and cannula under local anaesthesia via a small incision of lower anterior abdominal wall of 3×200 mg pellet lasting for 6 months).

Hypothyroidism requires slow introduction of thyroxine 25 µg/day for 1 month doubled to 50 µg/day for 2 months, and so on up to 200 µg/day (patients are around 60 years of age). However, adequate treatment of hypothyroidism does not guarantee return to normal sexual function.

Hyperprolactinaemia (rare) causes loss of libido and impotence; it is treated by 2.5 mg/day of bromocriptine (Parlodel) to reduce secretion and reduce the size of both micro- and macroadenomas (the latter requires 20–30 mg/day). Surgical intervention may be required to treat local compression.

Intrapenile or intracorporeal or intra-cavernosal injection (ICI)

The introduction of ICI for diagnosis and treatment of impotence has been a most exciting advance, with immediate results providing instant relief from the anxiety that inevitably accompanies sexual frustration and restoring the patient's self-esteem; it can be undertaken in outpatients or self-injection by the patient at home prior to sexual intercourse. Virag (1982), Brindley (1983) and Adaikan *et al.* (1984), in their innovative work, demonstrated that a smooth muscle relaxant, papaverine hydrochloride (derived from opium poppy), α-adrenergic blockers, such as phenoxybenzamine (Dibenylamine) and phentolamine, and prostaglandin E_1 (alprostadil or PGE_1) can induce penile erection when injected locally into the corpus cavernosum. The most commonly used agents for vasoactive intracavernous pharmacotherapy are papaverine hydrochloride alone or in combination with phentolamine mesylate. Papaver-

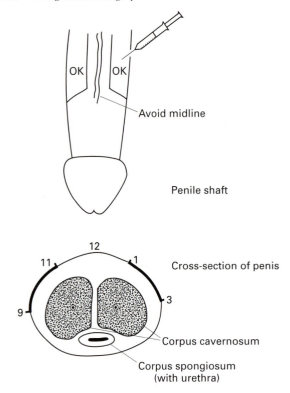

OK   OK

Avoid midline

Penile shaft

12

11   1

9   3

Cross-section of penis

Corpus cavernosum

Corpus spongiosum
(with urethra)

Fig. 1.64.1   Correct intracavernosal injection

ine hydrochloride is a potent, non-specific direct smooth-muscle relaxant. Anxiety and lack of privacy may inhibit the effect of these drugs presumably, because such environment results in the release of adrenergic substances. Other pharmacological agents that may induce penile erection on ICI include theophylline, vasoactive intestinal polypeptide and nitroglycerin.

The response rate is usually related to the aetiology of the impotence (100% in psychogenic and hormonal impotence, 98% in neurogenic; and 82% in vasculogenic impotence); careful determination and regulation of dosage is mandatory to reduce the complication rate. In general, the response rate is higher and the quality of erection is far better in patients with psychogenic, neurogenic, or hormonal impotence; a 5 μg dose of PGE_1 (supplied as 500 μg/ml ampoules diluted into 20 μg/ml) or doses containing 10 mg papaverine and 0.1 mg phentolamine (from a mixture of papaverine hydrochloride 30 mg/ml and phentolamine mesylate 0.5 mg/ml) using an insulin syringe with an ultra-fine needle (26 G, 0.5 in long) injected into the lateral aspect of the penile shaft 4 cm from the tip to avoid the urethra and dorsal neurovascular bundle. Pressure with gentle massage is applied at the site of injection for 3 minutes to avoid fibrosis. Future repeated doses are adjusted according to the initial observations of:
1. The time to complete erection.
2. The quality of erection.
3. The duration of erection.
4. Development of any side-effects.
A good response to 5 μg PGE_1 suggests that the patient has psychogenic or neurogenic impotence (e.g. due to division of

pelvic nerves during colonic resection). Responses at higher doses (usual increment is 5 mg papaverine and 0.05 mg phentolamine) suggest incomplete organic disorder, such as partial arterial occlusion, early diabetic neuropathy and vascular disease, or a venous leak. Complete failure indicates arterial occlusion or idiopathic disorder of corpora cavernosa.

Complications of ICI are either local or systemic. **Local complications** include: priapism (less than 5%), haematoma (due to careless puncture of subcutaneous veins or tunica albuginea with needle), cavernositis, papaverine-induced cavernosal fibrosis (not reported with PGE_1 and therefore may replace papverine as the ICI agent of choice), swelling and penile angulation. These complications may be avoided with careful patient selection and correct application of the procedure. Early intervention to reverse prolonged erection (more than 6 h) is imperative, since ischaemic tissue damage may occur. The patient is advised to take a warm shower, simple analgesia and then sleep (if necessary temazepam 10 mg may be given). Failure demands an antidote with 2 ml infiltration of 2% ligocaine laterally into the penile shaft, with a 21 G needle inserted 3 min later into the centre of corpus cavernosum for immediate partial detumescence (blood flow) followed by injection of 1 mg of metaraminol (diluted in 2 ml of normal saline). Another α-adrenergic drug used to relieve sustained erection, is phenylephrine hydrochloride (Neo-Synephrine), 10 mg diluted in 500 ml of normal saline, and 10–15 ml of this solution is used to irrigate the corpus cavernous bodies after aspiration of the same amount of blood. This procedure can be repeated several times until complete detumescence is achieved. Owing to the risk of sustained erection (priapism), patients must sign a 'Request for Treatment of Impotence' consent form with full explanation of the procedure and its potential complications.

Systemic complications include: orthostatic hypotension, elevation of liver enzymes and metallic taste.

Arterial bypass (venous arterialisation) and venous ligation

Vascular surgery and penile implants are only indicated when ICI has failed or is found unattractive by patients.

Vascular surgery is mainly indicated in young patients suffering from vascular impotence (arteriogenic and/or venogenic) who are unfit or have refused other modalities.

Virag (1982) has described six types of corporeal revascularisation utilising venous arterialisation depending on the availability of inferior epigastric artery and flow requirements to maintain rigidity:

Virag I   Inferior epigastric artery to deep dorsal vein end-to-side; proximal vein left open.

   II   Inferior epigastric artery to deep dorsal vein end-to-side; proximal vein tied.

   III   Saphenous vein graft to deep dorsal vein end-to-side; proximal vein tied.

   IV   Virag I operation plus a shunt between dorsal vein and cavernous body.

   V   Virag II operation plus a shunt between dorsal vein and the cavernous body.

VI Virag III operation plus a shunt between dorsal vein and the cavernous body.

The procedure providing the greatest success of corporeal revascularisation with least complications (thrombosis of vascular anastomosis and priapism) is the Virag V procedure (end-to-side anastomosis of the inferior epigastric artery to deep dorsal vein with simultaneous proximal vein ligation and shunt construction between dorsal vein and the cavernous body).

Technique of Virag V procedure An incision is made along the lateral aspect of the rectus muscle beginning just above the umbilicus and carried along the base of the penis; the lateral border of the rectus muscle is mobilised, and the inferior pedicle is carefully dissected. Perforating vessels are secured. About 20 cm of the vessels are mobilised, the distance to reach the deep dorsal vein is measured and the dorsal vein is dissected. Superficial penile veins are ligated, through an infrapubic incision, Buck's fascia incised in the midline, and the large deep dorsal penile vein is seen. Care must be taken to protect both penile nerve and artery. A long length of the dorsal penile vein is dissected, and the perforating veins are tied; about 6–7 cm of vein are freed. The penis is clamped with a suitable clamp at the proximal end. Then an opening of 1.5–2 cm is made in the dorsal vein, after valvulotomy of the dorsal vein up to the glans penis, then an incision of 1.5–2 cm long is done in the tunica albuginea beneath the vein, after an anastomosis between the dorsal vein and the corpus cavernosum is made. A small tunnel is done in the inguinal area to bring the inferior epigastric artery to the incision at the base of the penis, and (under microscopic magnification) an end-to-side anastomosis to dorsal vein of the penis is consructed proximal to the anastomosis of dorsal vein to corpus cavernosum.

In venogenic impotence, erection is transient, soft and with inadequate rigidity, which may be sufficient for vaginal penetration but with unsatisfactory results; impotence develops gradually (several months prior to presentation). Dissection and ligation of penile venous channels can restore or improve erection in selected patients. The drainage of corpora cavernosa normally occurs through crural veins, cavernous veins and the deep dorsal penile vein. Venous ligation is indicated in patients with venous drainage into a superficial system only, as confirmed by persistent filling after ICI and cavernosography; they are likely to have good results if drainage is eliminated.

Complications of revascularisation and venous ligation Complications include: oedema (mild to moderate), haematoma, and infection, penile shortening (fibrosis in infrapubic incision), priapism (venous arterialisation), hypervascularisation (venous arterialisation).

Penile implant prosthesis

Penile bone implants were used but found to be ineffective due to bone resorption. Scott, Bradley and Timm (1973) as well as Small and Carrion (1975) pioneered the implantation of a functional device intracorporeally (in organic impotence) with gratifying results. Impotence, therefore, must be determined whether it is psychogenic or organic in aetiology. Surgical implants can offer a more impressive 'angle of dangle', but at a price (over £500); they provide the stiffness, but not the size of normal erection. They usually come in three forms: malleable (but permanently erect), self-contained inflatable and multipart inflatable. Penile prostheses, therefore, are structurally divided into two main groups: semi-rigid malleable rods or inflatable prostheses. Both types have undergone subsequent improvements and modifications.

Semi-rigid malleable implant, e.g. AMS Malleable 600 (American Medical Systems) Consists of two silicone malleable rods with a tightly wrapped stainless steel core to help it bend to the erect position for intercourse, or down for concealment at will.

Inflatable penile prosthesis A hydraulic system that allows the transfer of fluid from one space to another and permits the penis to be rigid or flaccid at will. These sophisticated mechanical devices may eventually fail and require replacement; it is imperative therefore that each patient is informed about the need for an additional surgery.

The AMS 700CX is a self-contained implant consisting of two individual cylinders planted into both corpora, with a pump bulb in the scrotum, and reservoir planted suprapublically. Inflation is produced by squeezing the pump bulb in the scrotum as many times as necessary to make the penis firm and erect. Compressing the release valve on the side of the pump returns the penis to a relaxed detumescent position. Located within the fluid passage is a one-way check valve between the reservoir and the pump. This valve prevents fluid from returning to the reservoir inadvertently and thereby causing spontaneous deflation.

This prosthesis is available in 11 and 13 mm diameters and 13, 16, 19 and 22 cm lengths to which one or two rear tip extenders can be placed for a correct anatomical fit. A pulling suture is provided at the distal tip of each cylinder for ease in implantation.

Implantation is carried out commonly through a penoscrotal incision at the penoscrotal junction. After thorough skin preparation with povidone-iodine (Betadine), a 5 cm longitudinal incision is made. This is deepened by sharp dissection until Buck's fascia covering the bluish corpus spongiosum surrounding the urethra is reached and safeguarded. The subcutaneous tissues are then dissected off the lateral aspect of each corpus. A site is selected at 4 or 8 o'clock, avoiding as many encircling veins as possible, and two stay sutures are placed. A 3 cm longitudinal incision through the tunica albuginea exposes the erectile tissue. There is an immediate gush of blood, but dilatation controls this. The corpus is first dilated both distally and proximally with a 9 or 10 mm Hegar dilator and then with a dilator having the same diameter as the prosthesis. After proximal and distal dilatation of the corpus, a suitably sized device is first placed distally with the aid of a Furlow passer and the distal pulling suture then the proximal tip is placed. Tunica incision is closed with a continuous 3/0 Dexon or Vicryl suture. The same procedure is then performed on the contralateral side. Haemostasis should be achieved carefully to prevent a haematoma, with possible subsequent infection. Subcutaneous tissues are approximated with a continuous 4/0 polyglycolic acid suture, and the skin with a subcuticular closure using the same material.

This closure is preferred to other techniques, since there is no external suture to allow the entrance of infection. Betadine ointment is applied liberally to the incision, and the penis is covered with a gauze dressing. Often a 14 F catheter is inserted and removed the next day. Broad-spectrum antibiotics are initiated preoperatively and are continued for several days after surgery. All patients have some postoperative pain; they should be warned preoperatively. Coitus is allowed after 4 weeks.

The device is prefilled with saline. Prosthesis failure is either due to fluid leak or hydraulic mechanical failure.

Complications of penile implant prosthesis:

● Intraoperative perforation of tunica albuginea is likely whether distal or proximal while dilating corpora cavernosa. In such case it is better to back off from placing the prosthesis. Alternatively a sleeve of GoreTex is fashioned for the proximal end of the prosthesis to a length that will allow it to be sutured to the tunica albuginea in the corporotomy area. Care should be taken to avoid undue pressure on the prosthesis for 6–8 weeks.

● Postoperative infection and extrusion of the implant is a serious complication and may necessitate removal of the prosthesis. Some surgeons believe that an infected prosthesis can be removed and a sump drain placed into corporeal wound at the same time. After several days of continuous antibiotic irrigation of the corpus cavernosum a new prosthesis is placed. Alternatively, an infected prosthesis is removed, instituting copious antibiotic irrigation of the corpora and reimplanting another penile device simultaneously. The success rate is reported to reach 84%.

External suction devices

An external vacuum device is an ideal alternative for patients with partial or temporary impotence. The invention of suction devices to produce penile tumescence at will that was then maintained by constriction bands placed at the penile base goes back to the second decade of this century. These devices are expensive (often over £200). The induced erection is hanging rather than standing (see below).

ErecAid System   This system was originally called the Youth Equivalent Device and later the Vita-Life System. The inventor of this system (Osbon) became partially impotent at about the age of 60 years. To remedy his problem, he devised the system, which he personally used for more than 20 years, reportedly without failure.

Mouth suction was used to achieve the vacuum. The device consists of a vacuum pump connected to a transparent plastic penile cylinder, connecting tube and constriction bands. The cylinder is open at one end and closed at the other (except for a small opening to which the vacuum tube is attached). Before using the device, a suitable constriction band is placed around the base of the cylinder. Water-soluble jelly is applied to the open end of the cylinder, then the cylinder is placed over the flaccid penis – an air-tight seal should be obtained. A vacuum within the cylinder is obtained (using a suction pump); the negative pressure created in the cylinder will draw blood into the penis, which consequently becomes erect. When adequate tumescence has been achieved, the constriction band is slipped from the cylinder around the base of the penis in order to trap venous drainage of the penis maintaining sufficient erection for vaginal penetration and intromission.

The cylinder is removed by interrupting the vacuum seal and allowing air into the cylinder. The constriction band is not recommended to be left around the penis for more than 30 min. If a longer erection is required, the band should be removed for a short time and tumescence is repeated.

The erection-like state obtained by the use of such a device differs from a normal erection in following ways:
1. Distension of superficial veins due to congestion of extra corporeal tissues.
2. Blood flow into the penis decreases, causing a drop in penile skin temperature (approximately 1°C degree).
3. The penis is rigid only distal to the constriction bands. Tissue proximal to the constriction band is not engorged so that the patient has a 'hanging' rather than a 'standing' erection.
4. The ejaculate is trapped in the posterior urethra.

Synergist Erection System (Super Condom)   This is shaped like a large condom made of soft transparent silicone rubber with walls thick enough to support the penis. The area on the undersurface near the tip is thin in order to increase sensitivity during intercourse. The device is rigid enough to permit vaginal penetration, and has a small tube connection to allow air evacuation from its interior. There is a thin collar at the proximal open end that acts as a valve to form a seal around the penis following air evacuation. The penis and the inside of the device are thoroughly lubricated with a water-soluble jelly. The penis is brought up to the open end of the device and vacuum created by mouth suction on the attached tubing. The vacuum pulls the flaccid penis into the device while simultaneously producing tumescence. After proper positioning, the tubing is occluded with the attached vacuum-lock valve. When properly positioned, the penis should feel stretched and be slightly tight, a state that resembles a normal erection. Water-soluble lubricant should then be applied to the exterior of the device and intercourse accomplished. Tumescence is retained as long as the device is worn. After inercourse, the vacuum lock valve is opened. The device can then be removed cleaned, and stored.

Possible adverse reactions to this device include:
1. Penile irritation (redness, swelling, and small blisters).
2. Penile enlargement.
3. Vaginal discomfort (can be avoided by lubrication of device outer surface prior to intercourse).
Advantages of the device, however, include:
1. Sexually transmitted disease is less likely to be passed to the partner.
2. Impregnation of the partner is less likely, which may often be desirable.

Comment on premature ejaculation   This must not be confused with psychogenic impotence. Premature ejaculation is the man's inability to delay ejaculation long enough to allow the woman to reach orgasm in at least 50% of couple's sexual encounters. This is possibly due to early masturbation or sexual

activity having established a low excitability threshold for the ejaculatory reflex. The treatment of choice is to reverse this low excitability threshold by:
1. Employing a 'start/stop' intervention, by penile stimulation (e.g. foreplay or masturbation) until the man feels sensations of 'ejaculatory inevitability'. Stimulation is then discontinued until sensations subside. This process should be repeated until penile stimulation can be tolerated for longer periods of time without ejaculation.
2. Intravaginal containment and slow gradual thrusting is then added, first with the woman superior, then with the man in the superior position, until a satisfactory intercourse is obtained. Success rate is around 90–95%.

1.65 Surgery for Urinary Incontinence

The involuntary loss of urine is the most distressing disability in urological practice. Successful storage of urine demands that the bladder does not contract inappropriately (remains stable) and that the sphincter mechanism be competent. These two criteria differentiate non-surgical from surgical urinary incontinence. In the former, which affects up to 10% of the population, there is *idiopathic instability* or *urgency incontinence* (though uninhibited detrusor hyperreflexia also occurs in neurological bladder). The latter is genuine *stress incontinence* – the involuntary loss of urine due to a sudden rise in intra-abdominal pressure. It is an exceedingly common condition affecting up to 50% of young healthy nulliparous women. However 80% of incontinence

case are in the perimenopausal age group, especially multiparous women.

Under normal conditions urine is retained in the bladder because the intravesical pressure is very much less than the intraurethral pressure. This is achieved by suppression of the sacral reflex arc by the higher centres which prevents detrusor contractions occurring during filling of the bladder.

The urethral lumen is kept occluded at a higher pressure than the bladder by a combination of the actions of the smooth- and striated-muscle components and the engorgement of the venous plexuses and elastic tissue around the bladder neck. The urethra is also held forwards and upwards by the pubourethral ligaments so that rises in intra-abdominal pressure are equally transmitted to the bladder and upper third of the urethra, which lie above the pelvic floor, thus maintaining the pressure gradient between the two. In addition a reflex contraction of the levator ani compresses the mid-urethra.

Diagnosis

A careful history (current complaint with urological symptoms, duration and severity, neurological symptoms, gynaecological symptoms integrated with urological complaint, medical disorders, psychiatric disorders and drug therapy; also past history of urinary operations, drugs, obstetric history (in females), enuresis, retention and urinary tract infections), examination (general, neurological, vaginal examination in females and rectal examination in males) and investigations (intravenous urography, voiding cystourethrogram, rarely ascending urethrogram which may demonstrate urethral stricture, cystourethroscopy and particularly urodynamic studies in the form of cystometry, voiding cystometrogram or urethrocystometry) are important.

Table 1.65.1 Types of urinary incontinence

Incontinence	Likely symptoms	On examination	Therapy
True stress	No urgency/no frequency Reproducible, small leaks on abdominal straining (e.g. cough or sneeze)	Cystocele, urethrocele Atrophic vagina Post TUR (bladder neck) (bladder neck weak or open)	Gynecological repair Oestrogens Urologist
False overflow obstruction	Poor flow (stream)/hesitancy (interrupted stream)	May be prostatic enlargement Meatal stenosis	Urologist
Urge detrusor instability (overactivity), especially in children	Urgency/urge incontinence of large leaks/frequency (even if bladder is not full)	NAD May have CNS signs (bladder neck is normal)	Reduce detrusor activity
Atony or hypotonic bladder disorder	Frequency/interrupted stream on abdominal straining	Large bladder (which may or may not be palpable) ? Diabetes ? CNS signs	Increase detrusor activity Neurologist
Reflex	Frequency/no sensation of bladder filling with involuntary control of micturition	Spinal cord lesion /trauma	Neurologist

TYPES OF URINARY INCONTINENCE

Table 1.65.1 summarises the types of urinary incontinence and their diagnosis and treatment. They are discussed further below.

Male urinary incontinence

Causes and treatment

Congenital

● Ectopia vesicae: treated by re-forming the bladder and the abdominal wall and constructing a *neourethra*; however urinary diversion may be required.
● Ectopic ureter: inserted into the urethra below the sphincter. Can be divided and reimplanted into the bladder; in the presence of ascending kidney infection a nephroureterectomy is preferable.

Postprostatectomy urinary incontinence

This occurs in up to 1% in prostatectomy and 20% in radical prostatectomy. The risk is minimised by removal of adenomatous tissue leaving no residual tags behind. In open prostatectomy the urethral mucosa at the apex should be severed sharply and well above the urogenital diaphragm.

During transurethral resection (TUR) it is important to avoid resecting or coagulating extensively at or below the verumontanum. With established mild postprostatectomy urinary incontinence, expectant therapy (time will cure or ameliorate a percentage of all types of urinary incontinence) and possibly pharmacological manipulation (Table 1.65.2) are of value.

In severe cases, urodynamic studies are needed to ascertain whether the patient has an unstable detrusor. A stable detrusor can be treated by passive urethral compression (detachment and crossing of penis crura to compress bulbous urethra – *Kaufman* I; approximation of crura together in the midline with the aid of Teflon mesh tape placed around them to compress bulbous urethra – *Kaufman* II; or placement of silicone-gel prosthesis to compress bulbous urethra with the aid of Dacron straps passed around crura – *Kaufman III*). An unstable detrusor can be managed by use of an implantable inflatable *Rosen compression prosthesis* or an implantable inflatable *Brantley–Scott hydraulic cuff prosthesis*. Electric and electronic stimulation of the pelvic floor (similar to that used for faecal incontinence) may also be used. Other surgical methods include urethral reconstruction, urethral angulation, suspension and sling procedure (not as successful as in females).

The prostheses and devices generally give a success rate of at least 60%, although morbidity may occur in the form of infection, fistula or device failure, and reoperation may be required. Nevertheless they have superseded urethral reconstruction operations.

Neuropathic bladder (with urge or overflow urinary incontinence)

● Spina bifida, myelomeningocele.
● Spinal trauma causing paraplegia or tetraplegia.

Table 1.65.2   Pharmacological manipulation of postprostatectomy urinary incontinence

Action	Drug
Acting on the bladder	
Stimulation (used in retention)	Bethanechol (Myotonine Chloride) Distigmine (Ubretid) Phenoxybenzamine (Dibenyline)
Inhibition (used in frequency, enuresis and incontinence)	Atropine Propantheline (Pro-Banthine) Methantheline (Banthine) Oxybutynine (Ditropan) Dicyclomine (Bentylol) Flavoxate (Urispas) Imipramine (Tofranil) Emepronium (Cetiprin)
Acting on the bladder and proximal urethra	
Stimulation	Ephedrine Pseudoephedrine (Sudafed) Imipramine (Tofranil) Phenylpropanolamine (Eskornade)
Inhibition	Phenoxybenzamine (Dibenzyline) Guanethidine (Ismelin) Methyldopa (Aldomet)

The bladder is either spastic (upper motor neuron lesion with involuntary detrusor contractions, high pressure and hypertrophy, and reduced capacity) or flaccid (lower motor neuron lesion with infrequent detrusor contraction, low pressure and large capacity). Spastic bladder is managed satisfactorily by regular manual squeezing of the abdomen, genitalia or thighs. A large capacity bladder (whether flaccid or spastic) requires intermittent self-catheterisation (with Texas condom catheter) or regular intermittent catheterisation (with silicone Foley catheter). Pharmacological manipulation can be tried. TUR sphincterotomy (of bladder neck, or internal or external sphincter) is used to overcome the spastic obstructing outlet. Ileal conduit diversion is the final answer.

Established urinary incontinence

Can be treated by:

● Texas condom catheter with collecting bag tied to the thigh or calf.
● Drainage with indwelling Foley catheter with small balloon or fine 8 Fr Gibbon catheter.
● Cunningham or Baumrucker penile clamps.
● Absorbent pads.

Remember that overflow urinary incontinence is a false incontinence since it is due to urinary retention, the underlying causes of which should be treated on their merit.

Female urinary incontinence

Causes

Urethral

- *Stress urinary incontinence* (surgical) due to urethral sphincter incompetence following childbirth trauma, cystocoele, TUR of bladder neck, denervation in hysterectomy or sphincter atrophy.
- *Overflow urinary incontinence* due to outflow obstruction (surgical fibrosis or elevation of bladder neck and urethral stricture) or neurological lesions (spinal shock, cauda equina, tabes dorsalis, poliomyelitis and diabetes).
- *Urge urinary incontinence* (non-surgical) due to detrusor instability because of impaired corticospinal inhibition of the sacral reflex (normally a result of stress, but can also result from psychosis, nocturnal enuresis, congenital defects such as spina bifida, trauma, multiple sclerosis, stroke, or intracranial or spinal malignancy).
- *Reflex urinary incontinence* occurs in spinal cord lesions and trauma and prevents sensation of the bladder filling and involuntary control of micturition.

Extraurethral urinary incontinence (surgical)

- *Ureterovaginal fistula* due either to congenital ectopic ureter (draining upper kidney moiety and inserted into vaginal vault or close to external urethral meatus) or traumatic pelvic surgery, e.g. hysterectomy in which case the ureter is injured by direct trauma and/or pressure necrosis from a ligature and/or avascular necrosis particularly after pelvic irradiation.
- *Vesicovaginal fistula* due to obstetric cause in developing countries (obstructed labour, associated with infection and pressure necrosis of bladder base) or to gynaecological surgery in developed countries (during abdominal or vaginal procedures especially where there has been distortion of the anatomy by either infection or irradiation).

Treatment

Stress urinary incontinence

- *Pelvic floor strengthening* Physiotherapy and electrical stimulation can be tried first.
- *Urethral suspension*
  - Fascial sling using pyramidalis, rectus muscle, Mersilene mesh, Teflon strips.
  - Marshall–Marchetti–Krantz cystourethropexy.
  - Burch retropubic bilateral colposuspension.
  - Anterior colporrhaphy.
  - Modified Peyrera needle suspension procedure with cystoscopic Stamey modification.
- *Urethral lengthening* Urethroplasty, urethral narrowing and plication of bladder neck have all been tried.
- *Periurethral Teflon paste injection*
- *Prosthesis surgery* The Brantley–Scott sphincter hydraulic inflatable cuff, with many modifications, has been used for female urinary incontinence.

Overflow urinary incontinence

The aim is to reduce the urethral obstruction and enhance detrusor activity. Urethral dilatation or Otis urethrotomy to a depth of 2 mm at 3 and 9 o'clock is recommended. To promote bladder-emptying, detrusor activity can be stimulated electrically or by a parasympathomimetic drug such as Ubretid. Intermittent self-catheterisation is also recommended.

Urge urinary incontinence

With unstable bladder is treated by one of the following:
- Drugs, e.g. anticholinergic or sympathomimetics (orciprenaline and propantheline) or prostaglandin inhibitors (indomethacin, aspirin and flurbiprofen) are used to subdue detrusor instability with symptomatic amelioration in 50% of cases.
- Cystodistension under epidural anaesthesia.
- Bladder training – intensive bladder drill.
  Bladder denervation.

Ureterovaginal fistula

May close spontaneously; however treatment should be monitored by IVU. Surgical treatment should aim at reimplantation of the ureter with possible Boari flap or psoas hitch or even by an intervening ileal conduit between the ureter and the bladder.

Vesicovaginal fistula

Preoperatively, urinary infection treatment with antibiotics, indwelling urethral catheterisation and treatment of vaginal mucosal ulceration with stilboestrol are recommended. The aim of surgery is to excise the fistula tract completely and to close the bladder and the vaginal defect in layers without tension preferably with an intervening mobilised omentum pedicle graft (or labium majus mobilised subcutaneous fat or mobilised gracilis muscle) to promote healing in such extensive tissue devitalisation. Gynaecologists use the vaginal approach while urologists prefer the retropubic extraperitoneal intravesical approach.

Comment on vesicointestinal fistulae These are due to diverticulitis, colorectal carcinoma, bladder carcinoma, Crohn's disease and trauma in this order of frequency. Common findings are faecaluria, recurrent urinary tract infections and pneumaturia. Cystography or barium enema and cystoscopy may reveal the fistula. In other cases the diagnosis is very difficult to prove. The fistulae rarely close spontaneously, though they may be symptom-free. Preoperative sterilisation of urine and bowel contents with antibiotic and bowel preparation are needed.

The decision whether to perform a single-stage or a multistage operation can only be made during operation. If there is a walled-off abscess associated with the fistula or a very large inflammatory mass, then preliminary faecal diversion by transverse colostomy may be wise (with excision of the fistula-bearing segment of the bowel and bladder, intestinal anastomosis and closure of the bladder). This can be followed later by colostomy closure and restoration of bowel continuity (two-stage procedure, used especially in colonic malignancy which is treated occasionally by faecal diversion alone if inoperable). If the surgical situation looks relatively simple, bowel excision, intestinal anastomosis, closure of fistula, closure of the bladder and diversion of the urine by suprapubic cystostomy and urethral catheterisation may be performed (one-stage). Use of pedicled omental flap is often desirable. The decision whether to perform a protecting colostomy after bowel excision and fistula closure should be made by the surgeon in the course of the operation.

SURGERY OF TRAUMA

1.66 Multiple Injuries

ADVANCED TRAUMA LIFE SUPPORT (ATLS) COURSES

The 'developed' world is at war – a trauma war. In the UK alone, the annual number of deaths from trauma is 14 500–18 000; in the USA the figure is approximately 10 times greater. A third of the victims are killed on the road, and just under a third in incidents at home. As in all wars, it is the youth of the country which takes the heaviest losses. Trauma remains the most common cause of death in industrialised nations in people under 35. In the USA, there are 70 million non-fatal injuries per annum. These patients occupy 12% of all hospital beds in the USA. In the UK annually, 60 000 are admitted to hospital following road traffic accidents, and 26 000 from industrial incidents.

Overall casualties from this 'trauma war' occupy more hospital beds, and cause the loss of more working days, than cancer and cardiac patients combined. For the British taxpayer the cost is high: £2.22 billion per annum, that is around 1% of the gross national product. In USA, the figure is put at $75–100 billion, approximately equal to 1.5 times the total military expenditure on the Gulf war. The final cost is even higher, because there is also a loss of national talent and tax revenue, in addition to emotional and material consequences suffered by affected families. The cumulative effect of trauma patients who survive, but crippled, adds to this financial nightmare.

In 1988, the Royal College of Surgeons of England published its report on the Management of Patients with Major Injuries. The report concluded after a survey of 1000 trauma deaths that at least 1 in 5 patients presenting to hospitals in the UK alive subsequently died unnecessarily. These avoidable deaths were due to medical mismanagement at every level and throughout the specialties. The report proposed many initiatives designed to reduce this appalling toll, often of the youngest and most productive members of our society; improvement in medical and paramedical education were amongst other suggestions. The Advanced Trauma Support (ATLS) course for doctors was introduced late in 1988, followed by the Advanced Trauma Nursing Course (ATNC). More recently (1993), the Pre Hospital Trauma Life Support (PHTLS) programme was initiated for paramedics. The educational packages have truly changed behaviour in ambulances and resuscitation rooms nationally and have resulted in better early care. Also a pilot Trauma Centre has been established in Stoke and nationwide Accident and Emergency Consultants have established Trauma Teams to initiate rapid assessment and resuscitation of trauma victims, particularly in the first 'Golden Hour'.

ATLS courses provide intensive theoretical and practical instruction in the management of the multiply-injured patient during the 'golden hour'. The course is designed to enable doctors (of all grades) to demonstrate concepts and principles of primary and secondary patient assessment and establish management priorities in a trauma situation. Topics covered include initial assessment management; airway management; spinal cord trauma; thoracic trauma; abdominal trauma and practical skill stations in surgery; head trauma; shock; extremity trauma; injuries due to burns and cold; paediatric trauma; trauma in pregnancy; stabilisation and transport of the trauma patient. The course style includes multiple choice questions, simulated teaching, lectures, practical skill stations, and discussion groups. Each ATLS course is limited to 16 participants per course and lasts for 2.5 days; each participant is given a card on completion with 4-year validity and which will have to be updated thereafter by another course. The Pre-Hospital Trauma Life Support (PHTLS) courses are designed for doctors, nurses and qualified ambulance technicians and paramedical staff.

GENERAL PRINCIPLES

The management in the first few minutes is crucial for the final outcome. The luxury of obtaining a clinical history may not be possible because of clinical urgency or the absence of witnesses at the time of the accident. The surgeon, therefore, should assume the worst and proceed as if the airway is compromised, the neck fractured, the intravascular space contracted and the stomach full. The 3 R general management plan is useful: resuscitate, review, then repair.

Management plan

Resuscitation

First aid measures on the spot or on arrival in the Accident and Emergency Department, done within the first minute, are:
- Ensure patent airway (intubation or tracheostomy may be needed).

- Breathing (occlude sucking chest wounds quickly or assisted ventilation may be required).
- Circulation (check blood pressure and pulse and establish an i.v. life-line for fluid replacement, crossmatch blood and save).
- Stop severe external bleeding.

Review

Includes assessment and monitoring, history, physical examination, special tests.

A detailed relevant history is essential, paying special attention to the exact time and mechanism of accident and the presence of concomitant diseases for which the patient may be receiving treatment. Physical examination (include vital signs, general and special examinations) should be quick, thorough and methodical, e.g. in systems or anatomical order (no orifice should be left unchecked). Special tests include:

- Full blood count grouping and crossmatch, urea and electrolytes.
- X-ray of suspected fractures, chest and deep lacerations with foreign bodies.
- Specific tests according to injury.

Tests must not interfere with life-saving treatment. The aim of such assessment is to identify the injuries as precisely as possible and to determine which systems need to be monitored later on. Arrangement of injuries in order of priority in management is essential.

Highest priority
- Cervical spine injuries (immobilisation).
- Respiratory impairment (thoracic injuries).
- Cardiovascular insufficiency (tamponade decompression and bleeding arrest).
- Severe external bleeding.

High priority
- Intraperitoneal and retroperitoneal (abdominal) injuries.
- Brain and spinal cord injuries.
- Severe burns or extensive soft tissue injuries.

Low priority
- Lower genitourinary tract injuries.
- Peripheral vascular, nerve and tendon injuries.
- Fractures, dislocations.
- Facial and soft tissue injuries.
- Tetanus prophylaxis.

Shocked patient
The following procedures are required for differential diagnosis of shock and monitoring:
- Wide-bore i.v. cannulae.
- CVP line.
- ECG monitoring.
- Bladder catheterisation.
- Core/peripheral temperature.
Further monitoring in an intensive therapy unit (ITU) should continue when necessary.

Repair (definitive treatment)

The aims are to:
- Restore intravascular volume.
- Restore cardiac output and ensure its distribution.
- Ensure adequate gas exchange and protect lungs from excessive fluid loading, aspiration and infection.
- Ensure renal perfusion and output.

General measures

- Fluid replacement and blood transfusion.
- Immobilise fractures with splints until specific treatment is performed by orthopaedic team.
- Analgesia should not be withheld from injured patients. In the absence of head injury, judiciously administered narcotic analgesics do not mask the signs or symptoms of skeletal or visceral trauma and where pain is the limiting factor pulmonary ventilation may be improved. Pethidine, buprenorphine and morphine could be given i.v. to provide a steady level. Nerve or plexus block is recommended in rib fractures, and upper and lower limb injuries.
- Assisted ventilation is required when there is excessive respiratory work or ventilatory inadequacy with hypercapnoea. Hypoxia (Pao_2 less than $65\,mmHg$) demands positive end-expiratory pressure (PEEP) ventilation. In coincidental head injury, ventilation should be considered in certain situations.
- Continuous monitoring recording in ITU:
  - Conscious level.
  - Heart rate and rhythm and blood pressure.
  - Respiratory rate and rhythm and blood gas analysis.
  - Core/peripheral temperature difference (non-invasive indication of peripheral perfusion adequacy and reflects changes in cardiac output).
  - Urine output through urinary catheter (indicative of total renal blood flow).
  - Abdominal girth.
  - Haemoglobin/haematocrit (PCV).
  - Electrolytes/acid-base balance.
  - Chest X-ray.
- Antitetanus prophylaxis.
- Antibiotics (prophylactically).
- Care of comatose patient (patent airway, position, feeding, bed sores, urination, defaecation and temperature control).

Special measures

The specific injuries – head, cervical, thoracic, abdominal and hand injuries – should be treated on their merits.

PULMONARY CONSIDERATIONS IN TRAUMA

All severely injured patients suffer from hypoxia to varying degrees and immediate oxygen administration is indicated. Hypoxia may be central (in head injury and injudicious morphine overdose) or peripheral (airway obstruction, pneumo- or haemothorax), anaemic (from blood loss) or stagnant (due to associated shock). The precise causes of hypoxia in multiple trauma are:

Respiratory system:

- Head injury (central respiratory depression).
- Maxillofacial trauma (asphyxia, aspiration of blood, teeth, bone, debris and vomitus).
- Rib cage trauma (pneumothorax, haemothorax, subcutaneous/mediastinal emphysema).
- Ruptured diaphragm (abdominal contents herniation and compression collapse of lung).
- Ruptured oesophagus (mediastinitis, pleural effusion and sepsis).
- Tracheobronchial trauma (ruptured bronchus, trachea with massive air leak – subcutaneous/ mediastinal emphysema, pneumothorax).
- Pulmonary trauma (contusion, haematoma, laceration).
- Increased capillary permeability (non-cardiogenic pulmonary oedema, injury oedema, chemical pneumonitis, acid aspiration, smoke injury, disseminated intravascular coagulation, fat embolism).
- Left ventricular failure (cardiogenic pulmonary oedema).
- Adult respiratory distress syndrome.

Cardiovascular system

- Hypovolaemic hypotension, e.g. bleeding, burns (decreased preload, increased afterload, decreased cardiac output).
- Tension pneumothorax, mediastinal emphysema, pericardial bleeding (cardiac tamponade).
- Myocardial injury, contusion ischaemia, acidosis, valve injury (pump failure, conduction defects).

Respiratory management

The first priority is to ensure that the patient's airway is free and his or her ventilation is unimpaired.

1. Obstructing elements should be removed under direct vision using a laryngoscope and low-vacuum sucker, e.g. dentures, broken teeth, debris, foreign bodies, blood or vomitus.
2. If laryngeal and pharyngeal reflexes are present, forward tongue retraction by insertion of an oral mouthpiece or nasopharyngeal tube may suffice.
3. If reflexes are absent then low-pressure cuffed endotracheal intubation is needed.
4. Tracheostomy is rarely needed as an emergency procedure unless intubation is impossible because of pharyngolaryngeal obstructing injury.
5. Laryngotomy is an alternative to tracheostomy.
6. Thorough tracheal and bronchial toilet should be performed. An asphyxiating plug may require emergency bronchoscopy.
7. Large-bore nasogastric tube aspiration of gastric contents may be needed but should be performed cautiously (or even abandoned) in CSF rhinorrhoea to avoid infection. Extreme care must be taken in intubation of patients with unstable cervical fractures.
8. In pneumothorax, an apical chest drain should be inserted through the second anterior intercostal space (*above* the third rib border to avoid injury of subcostal neurovascular structures) in the midclavicular line. An additional large drain is inserted

through the fifth, sixth or seventh intercostal space (depending on the position of the spleen) in the midaxillary line in haemothorax.
9. In rib fractures with or without pneumothoraces, chest drainage on the fracture side is mandatory prior to artificial ventilation and advisable prior to general anaesthesia. In bilateral fractures with haemothoraces, bilateral apical and basal drains must be inserted.
10. In tension pneumothorax the use of intermittent positive pressure ventilation can kill a patient in seconds. This should be relieved temporarily by a wide-bore i.v. cannula (inserted through the second anterior intercostal space in the midclavicular line) until a chest drain is available. Respiratory distress and cyanosis should always raise suspicion and on examination shifted positions of trachea and apex beat are confirmatory.

The choice between crystalloids (water and electrolyte solutions) and colloids (plasma, albumin, gelatins, dextrans) and their effect on pulmonary gas exchange is controversial. Those who favour colloids claim that colloid osmotic pressure (COP) is maintained and any extravasated albumin is cleared quickly by pulmonary lymphatics while crystalloids reduce COP and increase pulmonary extravascular water and pulmonary oedema. Those favouring crystalloids maintain that with colloids pulmonary lymphatic drainage is rapidly overwhelmed and extravasated albumin increases extravascular COP and oedema (wet lungs are infected lungs since macrophages lose their antibacterial effect).

CRYSTALLOIDS AND COLLOIDS

In a recent randomised controlled trial of postoperative patients with hypovolaemia and/or severe pulmonary failure, there was no significant advantage for colloid over crystalloid in fluid resuscitation. Because colloid is so much more expensive than crystalloid, the conclusion is that crystalloid therapy is preferable. However, in bleeding many intensivists still prefer blood to normal saline, and normal saline to 5% dextrose, and 5% dextrose to giving nothing.

1.67 Abdominal Trauma

GENERAL CONSIDERATIONS

Often combined with multiple injuries which tend to be more obvious than abdominal ones. They are either penetrating (open – after gunshot or knife stabbing) or blunt (closed – usually after road traffic accidents). The management starts with first aid resuscitation (for shock or associated injuries, see s. 1.66), followed by clinical assessment, then definitive treatment (whether conservative or operative intervention).

Clinical assessment

History

In penetrating injuries ascertain the nature and direction of penetration (e.g. knife or bullet) as well as patient position at the time of injury. Pathological visceromegaly should be asked about (e.g. in tropical areas – malaria, hepatitis or kalaazar) as well as drug treatment (e.g. steroids). Shoulder pain is deliberately asked about in splenic injuries.

Examination

For vital signs of revealed or concealed haemorrhage and shock (hypotension, tachycardia and decreased CVP). Obvious cutaneous bruising from a seat belt or underwear may indicate deep injury. Other signs are abdominal distension, tenderness guarding, rigidity, flank fullness and dullness on percussion, hyperaesthesia over the shoulder (referred pain due to subdiaphragmatic irritation by blood – Kehr's sign). The abdominal girth is measured and the abdomen marked with indelible pen for repeated measurements. The pelvis is sprung to detect fracture. Rectal examination to detect the prostate position (normal or floating) and abnormal swellings; note whether there is any blood on the finger. Failure to pass urine may indicate urethral injury. Physical examination may be difficult in comatose patients.

Ancillary procedures and investigations

- Erect chest X-ray to show:
  - Diaphragmatic injury.
  - Rib fractures close to liver or spleen.
  - Subphrenic gas due to ruptured abdominal viscus.
- Supine abdominal X-ray to show:
  - Splenic, hepatic, renal shadows.
  - Outline of psoas muscle (masked in retroperitoneal haematoma and splenic injury).
  - Gastric bubble shape and situation (deviated medially in splenic injury).
  - Ground-glass appearance of intra-abdominal bleeding.
  - Pelvic fractures.
- Four-quadrant tap (needle paracentesis) is a quick test for intra-abdominal bleeding and is done with a wide-bore needle and syringe.
- Peritoneal lavage: more sensitive but time-consuming; carried out if the tap is negative in suspected intra-abdominal bleeding. The bladder should be empty (e.g. via a catheter), then a peritoneal dialysis catheter is inserted subumbilically via a trocar stab or a small incision under direct vision with local anaesthesia. One litre of normal saline is passed intraperitoneally and siphoned out into a plastic bag (with gentle abdominal palpation). A false-positive may be due to traumatic instrumentation.
- Urgent intravenous urography (IVU) may show:
  - Presence or absence of functioning kidney on each side.
  - Hitherto unexpected pathology, e.g. horseshoe kidney or tumour.

When IVU reveals a non-functioning kidney, renal arteriography should be carried out immediately to detect the remediable damage to the renal vasculature in time to save the kidney; otherwise renal transplantation should be considered.

Continuous monitoring

Two days of continuous monitoring in hospital followed by re-examination at intervals is an absolute necessity in abdominal trauma. Nasogastric aspiration is done to prevent acute gastric dilatation (may occur in trauma even without viscus rupture). Blood pressure, pulse rate, abdominal girth, CVP, and i.v. fluid balance are monitored. A decision on whether to pass a urinary catheter is made carefully, in the presence of urethral injury; however, a urethral catheter is needed in all cases of severe urethral injuries and shock to monitor urinary output.

Definitive treatment

Conservative treatment

This is all that is required for the majority of cases after careful monitoring.

Laparotomy

Indicated in:
- All eviscerations (even with a small tag of protruding omentum). The wound itself should be enlarged via laparotomy and protruding viscus (covered with sterile wet dressing preoperatively) replaced, followed by methodical exploration for visceral injuries.
- All gunshot wounds.
- Some stab wounds selectively. A separate laparotomy incision is indicated when there is significant blood loss and peritonitis (otherwise treatment is conservative). If the patient is presented with a knife in situ, do not remove unless in theatre after laparotomy.
- Some closed abdominal injuries when:
  - Frank blood detected by four-quadrant tap and/or peritoneal lavage.
  - Persistent signs of peritonitis, e.g. tenderness, guarding and loss of bowel sounds or signs of spreading peritonitis.
  - Signs of internal bleeding.
  - Urinary damage as revealed on urgent IVU.
  - Blood in stomach, bladder or rectum.

Operative intervention should only be considered after adequate haemodynamic resuscitation and stabilisation except in:
- Horrendous bleeding outstripping all attempts at fluid and blood replacement.
- Evisceration with obvious strangulation of the protruding viscus.

The abdominal incision may be a quick midline or paramedian. Can be extended into a thoracoabdominal or into the flank by a T-shaped lateral extension. Generous access with good exposure is essential. A transverse supraumbilical incision is useful only in children under the age of 5 years. Exploration should proceed methodically with examination of spleen, liver, diaphragm (in that order) then stomach (anterior and posterior wall through a window in the lesser omentum or gastrocolic ligament), duodenum, pancreas, small and large bowel, rectum and bladder (and uterine tubes and ovaries in female) and kidneys, recording the findings of each organ. Quick mass closure, leaving a drain behind, is best.

SPECIAL CONSIDERATIONS

Liver

The largest organ in the abdomen (1.5 kg), the liver, with the spleen, is the most frequently injured abdominal organ. Many studies point out that the incidence of liver injuries is almost the same as that of splenic injuries. The overall mortality rate for hepatic trauma is 15% (20% from blunt trauma and 2% from penetrating injuries). A combination of injuries involving the gut often results in death from sepsis and/or multiple organ failure. Conservative management is the rule.

- Liver injuries that are not bleeding at the time of laparotomy are best left alone, clots should be evacuated and the perihepatic area drained.
- Large bleeding lacerations: suturing of bleeding points and/or ligation of isolated bleeding points. Deep sutures should not be tried first since they cause local ischaemia, necrosis and infection. For temporary haemostasis Pringle's manoeuvre (compressing the lesser omental free edge between finger and thumb) should be maintained for 15 min only. For longer periods gauge packing may be required for 48 h with generous drainage. Ligation of the main hepatic artery (healthy liver can survive on portal blood alone) or one of its branches is the last resort in controlling active bleeding.
- Absorbable vicryl mesh can be used to wrap the liver, both the right and left hepatic lobes, and the mesh can be sutured to encapsulate the liver. Total hepatic mesh wrap technique is effective in securing haemostasis in patients with severe diffuse parenchymal bleeding in severe exsanguinating liver injuries.
- Debridement of devitalised liver is necessary in 10% of cases.
- Lobar or sublobar hepatic resection may be required in 5% of cases and reserved for bursting injuries and those with hepatic venous and intrahepatic vena caval injuries. Hepatic lobectomy has a 50% mortality rate. Adequate blood and platelet transfusion, monitoring of coagulation parameter, parenteral nutrition and prophylactic antibiotics are needed. Hepatic lobectomy is a formidable operation and is not advised for hepatic injury unless there is no alternative. The bile duct should not be drained unless it is injured (T-tubes cause stenosis in normal-calibre common bile duct).

Spleen

Injuries are dealt with routinely by splenectomy. Lethal postsplenectomy sepsis and pneumococcal infection in children have lead to more conservative approaches in such injuries of children and adults below 40 years of age. Blunt abdominal trauma often results in a subcapsular haematoma, cracks in the parenchyma and fragmentation of the pulp.

- Attempts should be made to preserve the splenic tissue by suturing lacerations with mattress sutures supported by pledgets of Teflon felt or omental tissue (splenorrhaphy).
- In fragmentation, partial splenectomy is carried out by ligating the artery that supplies the damaged sector and removing the part of the spleen that subsequently becomes devascularised.

- If splenectomy must be done, spleniculi should be sought and carefully preserved because they may undergo hyperplasia with eventual preservation of splenic function. Pneumococcal vaccine and long-term oral prophylactic penicillin may be administered postoperatively.
- Autotransplantation of splenic tissue into muscle, omentum or retroperitoneal tissues is technically feasible (but still experimental).

Colon

Mortality is high and is related to associated organ injuries, to faecal peritonitis, and postoperative incisional and intraabdominal complications due to faecal contamination. Preoperative preparation consists of i.v. fluid, nasogastric suction and various monitoring procedures with prophylactic metronidazole and cefuroxime antibiotics. Treatment is as follows.

- Caecal injuries: caecostomy.
- Right colon injuries: right hemicolectomy with primary ileocolic anastomosis.
- Perforated transverse splenic flexure and descending colon: primary closure with proximal protective colostomy, which is later closed.
- Large sigmoid lacerations: Hartmann's operation, bringing up the damaged colon as a terminal left iliac endcolostomy and closing the rectal end. They are reanastomosed together later as a cold operation.
- Rectal wounds: proximal colostomy, perirectal drainage and irrigation of faeces from rectum. The rectal perforation should be closed if accessible.

No wound of the colon should ever be closed if there is:

- Profound hypovolaemic shock (blood pressure of less than 60/40 mmHg).
- Blood loss of more than 25% of anticipated blood volume.
- Massive faecal contamination.
- Eight hour delay after injury.
- Destructive bowel wound demanding bowel resection.

Instead, the primarily repaired colon is temporarily exteriorised as a potential colostomy. It should be kept moist with frequent dressing changes. The exteriorised segment is resected after 48 h and closed after 6 weeks.

Small bowel

Double-layer inverting sutures are used.

- Perforation: closed transversely to avoid stricture.
- Mesentery damage: bowel resected with end-to-end anastomosis.
- Difficult duodenal injuries: Kocherisation and closure of small rent transversely.
- Larger duodenal tears: a Roux loop is brought up to anastomose the defect, and feeding jejunostomy or even gastrojejunostomy bypass of the pancreatic duct is performed.
- Pancreatoduodenectomy: rarely used as it carries a high mortality.

Kidneys

Exploration is indicated in bleeding open wounds involving the kidney, expanding perirenal extravasation (with progressive swelling) or massive haematuria. Treatment is according to the urgent IVU results and operative wound findings. Polar or partial nephrectomy is always preferred. A tense retroperitoneal haematoma may be ignored lest the incision and drainage lead to uncontrollable bleeding. Such a conservative approach produces good results with further follow-up.

Bladder

Injury is diagnosed later but fortunately mortality is low. Urethral catheterisation with closure of the vent via laparotomy is indicated.

Urethra

Treatment is debatable (see s. 1.66 Multiple injuries).

Diaphragm

Injury occurs in 4–5% of patients with blunt or penetrating trauma and mainly on the left side as the liver protects the right hemidiaphragm. The mechanism in blunt injury is sudden intrathoracic or intra-abdominal force applied against the fixed diaphragm. The injury is often masked by associated injury of the stomach, spleen and/or splenic flexure and sometimes overlooked during exploration. Blunt chest injuries with an elevated or obscured hemidiaphragm or penetrating wounds below the nipple should raise suspicion. The patient may experience shortness of breath and chest pain, or there may be no signs or symptoms at all. As the injury may be difficult to repair from the abdomen the abdominal incision is converted into a thoracoabdominal one. It is not advisable to repair purely through the chest unless the surgeon is experienced because of the possibility of contaminant intraabdominal injury. Once the abdominal exploration is finished interrupted figure-of-8 non-absorbable sutures are applied through the chest followed by chest tube drainage with underwater seal. Chronic diaphragmatic injury with diaphragmatic herniation is approached through the chest because the herniated viscera are adherent to the lung in most cases.

Pancreas

The main operative principles are:
- Complete haemostasis.
- Removal of devitalised tissue.
- Drainage of pancreatic juice.
  Pancreatic trauma is classified into four types:
1. Superficial non-ductal.
2. Deep lacerations (involving duct).
3. Severe transection of the head.
4. Combined pancreaticoduodenal injury.

If the tail is injured simple closure or resection is done. A Roux loop of jejunum may be used to anastomose the cut end. Partial pancreatectomy and very rarely total pancreatectomy are required.

1.68 Thoracic Trauma

GENERAL PRINCIPLES

Approximately 25% of trauma deaths are due solely to thoracic injuries and 50% of patients who die from multiple injuries have significant thoracic injury. They are either penetrating (open – by gunshot, knives or other weapons) or blunt (closed) injuries. The mortality rate from penetrating chest wounds was 56% in World War I, decreasing to 8% during World War II and to 3% in the Vietnam War as a result of improved transport systems which enabled critically injured patients to reach medical care alive. Generally, mortality ranges between 4% and 12% and increases to 12–15% if extrathoracic regions are involved.

Initial steps in the treatment of penetrating chest injury are:
- Securing an airway and ventilation (occlude sucking chest wound and establish artificial endotracheal ventilation if necessary).
- Restoring circulation and stopping obvious bleeding.
- Tube thoracostomy (chest tube) if necessary – see below

The above measures are all that are required in 70–85% of patients with open chest trauma.

A brief history is taken from the patient or witnesses about the time of injury, weapon type and its direction, the patient's position at the time of injury and the patient's progress during transport. On examination the medicolegal aspects of trauma should be considered. All physical evidence of the weapon should be preserved and neither fingerprints nor adherent tissue, hair or clothing should be removed from the weapon. A quick thorough examination of the anterior and posterior aspects of the chest for associated injuries is carried out, and vital signs and breathing sounds on the side of injury are looked for.

The amount of initial chest tube drainage is recorded and the decision for thoractomy is based on subsequent drainage rather than the initial amount. *Thoracotomy* is indicated in:
- Persistent bleeding (more than 100 ml/h).
- Exsanguinating bleeding.

If the patient is *haemodynamically unstable* (tachycardia, hypotension and there are no breathing sounds on side of injury) then:
- Insert large-bore chest tube (underwater drainage) immediately on the side of injury without prior chest X-ray (under local anaesthesia in the 7th intercostal space immediately above the 8th rib – to avoid injury of the 7th subcostal neurovascular structures) at the midclavicular line and push the tube upward (apical – in pneumothorax), or keep it low (basal – in haemothorax), or both (in pneumohaemothorax).
- Insert at least two large-calibre i.v. cannulae for rapid fluid replacement. Simultaneously blood is aspirated for a baseline PCV, grouping and crossmatching.
- Arterial blood gases if ventilation is compromised.
- Obtain upright posteroanterior chest X-ray during inspiration (only when the patient is haemodynamically stable).

- In addition to chest X-ray, an aortogram should be obtained if:
  - The missile traversed or passed close to the mediastinum.
  - Absent or decreased pulse or bruit.
  - Wide mediastinum on chest X-ray.
- Thin barium swallow should be obtained if:
  - Missile traversed mediastinum.
  - Mediastinal emphysema.

Abdominal injuries are investigated on their merit (see s. 1.66 Multiple injuries).

SPECIAL CONSIDERATIONS

Penetrating heart wounds

Only 20% of such patients reach hospital alive and gunshot wounds are responsible for 80% of deaths due to intracardiac injuries, e.g. valve disruption, septal defects and major coronary transections. Patients present with either haemorrhagic shock (hypotension, tachycardia, low CVP and brisk bleeding through the wound or via tube thoracostomy, which demand immediate thoracotomy on the wound side) and/or cardiac tamponade (triad of paradoxical pulse, high CVP and muffled heart sounds).

CVP is the most reliable test for determining whether the shock is due to blood loss, cardiac tamponade or both. It is essential that the zero level of the manometer be at the midaxillary line in the 4th intercostal space: the saline column in a manometer fluctuates freely during respiration and blood flows back if the bottle is positioned below the heart level. Measurement is obtained while the patient is quiet and if the pressure is above 12 cm of saline a diagnosis of tamponade is fairly certain. However false high CVP is frequently present as a result of:

- Shivering.
- Straining from pleural or peritoneal irritation.
- Malpositioning of CVP catheter.

On balance, patients with any mediastinal wound, high CVP and hypotension should be assumed to have cardiac tamponade until proven otherwise.

Pericardiocentesis with a large-gauge needle may be used diagnostically and therapeutically initially. However, as clotted blood often leads to a false-negative result the best way of accomplishing decompression is subxiphoid pericardial exploration (diagnostic and therapeutic) under local anaesthesia – while the patient is breathing spontaneously to avoid profound hypotension and a drop in cardiac output which accompany general anaesthesia and endotracheal intubation. If blood is found in the pericardium the tamponade is relieved, the patient is given a general anaesthetic and intubated with controlled ventilation. The incision is extended into a standard median sternotomy and the heart wound is repaired with simple techniques (ventricular wounds are controlled with large mattress sutures reinforced with Teflon felt atrial or great vessel wounds can be controlled with a partially occluding clamp and then sutured at leisure with a running vascular suture). The venae cavae may need to be compressed digitally to decompress the heart and control bleeding. Cardiopulmonary bypass may be used selectively but is never necessary routinely as it necessitates prolonged hospital stay and undesirable heparinisation.

Blunt cardiac injury occurs in 20% of cases and produces either cardiac rupture and tamponade or myocardial contusion (ECG reveals ST elevation and sometimes Q wave with arrythmia and the patient has chest pain). They are rarely fatal and treated like myocardial infarction.

Penetrating transmediastinal injuries

A rapid systemic approach is adopted to detect structural damage by:

- Bilateral tube thoracostomy.
- Oesophagoscopy or contrast study of oesophagus.
- Bronchoscopy.
- Aortography.

Intrathoracic aorta injury (in penetrating or blunt chest injuries)

Occurs mainly in high-speed road traffic accidents and usually results in immediate death. In 50% of cases there is no external sign of injury and therefore traumatic aortic rupture should be highly suspected when any of the following is present:

- Pulse amplitude difference between the upper and lower extremities (as in coarctation of aorta).
- Upper hypertension.
- Widening of superior mediastinal shadow seen in chest X-ray. Other radiological signs are obstructed aortic knob, deviation of oesophagus or trachea to the right, downward displacement of left main stem bronchus, hemithorax and fractured ribs.

Rupture at the isthmus (ligamentum arteriosum) is responsible for 90% of aortic injuries and is possibly caused by horizontal deceleration of the aorta with its fixation at the ligamentum arteriosum. Vertical deceleration (e.g. falls) cause rupture of the ascending aorta as a result of aortic lengthening. Thoracic aortography by the femoral or brachial route is essential. In the treatment, associated abdominal injury may take precedence because of continuous bleeding from visceral tears. Aortic rupture is treated by direct repair or restoration of continuity by a tube graft without or with (rarely) cardiopulmonary bypass (or femoral artery-to-vein cardiopulmonary bypass).

Subclavian and innominate artery injuries

Injuries can be penetrating or blunt (blunt rupture with dissecting haematoma or false aneurysm is rare). In penetrating injuries, audible bruit, absent pulse, widening of the superior mediastinum, expanding haematoma, brachial plexus injury or haemodynamic instability are confirmatory signs. Aortography is essential in the presence of these signs.

Proximal vascular control (via median sternotomy for subclavian, innominate and left common carotid injuries) and distal control (incision in the deltopectoral groove for subclavian vessels and extension of the sternotomy incision in a 'hockey stick' fashion along the anterior border of the sternomastoid muscle for innominate arterial branches) are essential. Excision of part of the clavicle may be required for repair of the subclavians. Direct repair or use of a tube graft is recommended.

Oesophageal injury

Although rare, this is a rapidly progressive and fatal injury because of mediastinal contamination by saliva and gastro-intestinal contents. There is a high incidence of associated injuries, e.g. trachea and vessels. The *causes* generally are:
- Iatrogenic perforation during endoscopy or dilatation.
- Spontaneous rupture during emesis (called Boerhaave's syndrome – a longitudinal mucosal tear of the gastro-oesophageal junction during emesis is called the Mallory–Weiss syndrome).
- Ingestion of a foreign body with immediate perforation or erosion.
- Blunt or penetrating external trauma (discussed here). Oesophageal injury results in either:
- Fulminating mediastinitis (if mediastinal pleura is intact); or
- Fulminant pleuritis with massive pleural effusion and hypovolaemia (if mediastinal pleura has ruptured). The effusion results in hypovolaemia, sepsis and cardio-respiratory embarassment due to mediastinal shift.

Cervical oesophageal perforation is confined by the deep cervical fascia. The upper two-thirds of the intrathoracic oesophagus perforates and drains into the right pleural space. The distal one-third perforates and drains into the left pleural space only if the mediastinal pleura is not intact. Rarely the last 4 cm of the intra-abdominal oesophagus perforates and drains into the peritoneal cavity. The most common site of injury is at the tracheal bifurcation – rarely traumatic tracheoesophageal fistula results. Clinical features are fever, tachycardia, hypotension, leucocytosis and pain, deep subcutaneous emphysema confined to deep cervical fascia from the mandible to the clavicle. Mediastinal emphysema on chest X-ray is highly suggestive. Diagnosis is confirmed with a thin barium swallow with immediate and delayed films in the posteroanterior and lateral views. Early recognition with urgent operative intervention is mandatory. Secured two-layer closure (continuous non-absorbable mucosal suture followed by continuous non-absorbable muscular suture) with drainage is essential. Late perforations of the intrathoracic oesophagus may best be treated by oesophageal exclusion rather than by primary intrathoracic repair.

Tracheobronchial injuries

Classified into three groups:
- 'Straddle' injury in which the main-stem bronchus (usually the right) is avulsed at the carina, caused by anteroposterior compression of the chest.
- Tracheal blow-out fractures, caused by a sudden increase in endotracheal pressure against the closed glottis.
- Transverse lacerations, caused by rapid deceleration.

These are rapidly fatal and only a few patients reach hospital alive. Mainly caused by road traffic accidents. Signs and symptoms of tracheobronchial injuries are similar to those of oesophageal perforation depending on the site and nature of the injury and the degree of obstruction of the airways. However, dysphagia and hoarseness as well as cervical emphysema from the mandible to the clavicle (confined to the distribution of the deep cervical fascia) also occur in tracheal injury. Distal blow-out fractures cause massive mediastinal emphysema (if the mediastinal pleura is intact) or right pneumothorax (if the mediastinal pleura is ruptured). In straddle injury of the main-stem bronchus at the carina there is minor haemoptysis, but massive air leak through the chest tube drain with lobar atelectasis is common. Bronchoscopy is both diagnostic and therapeutic to retain control of the airway. Primary repair is achieved with interrupted non-absorbable sutures (e.g. 3/0 Prolene). It is important to debride all fractured tracheal cartilages and suture the intact cartilaginous ring. Pneumonectomy may be required for straddle injury of the main bronchus. Minor lacerations may require only a tracheostomy (through the penetration itself or distal to it) for decompression of the tracheobronchial tree.

Chest wall trauma

Either crushed (closed) or penetrating (open). In both cases the outcome depends on the severity and extent of the underlying structural damage.

Respiratory insufficiency

Caused by:
- Pain interfering with coughing.
- Instability or chest wall deformity.
- Presence of blood or secretions in the bronchial tree.
- Underlying pulmonary contusion.
- Associated haemo- or pneumothorax.
- Associated head injury and depressed respiration. Chest X-ray in two views is essential in all cases and blood gas analysis (and sometimes bronchoscopy) is required in complicated cases.

Rib fractures

Simple isolated

Commonly affect the fourth to the ninth and more often occur on the left than on the right side. Usually result from road traffic accidents, falls or beatings.
- First rib fracture is a hallmark of severe thoracic trauma and multiple system injuries in road traffic accidents. Locally it can produce injury to the brachial plexus or subclavian artery, Horner's syndrome, or thoracic outlet syndrome. The aorta is injured in 7.8% of first rib fractures and arteriography is indicated.
- Sternum fracture, usually caused by steering wheel trauma. Cardiac contusion or rupture is the most life-threatening associated injury. A displaced sternum should be stabilised by suturing. Careful observation, chest X-ray (especially lateral view) and ECG are important.
- Scapula fracture: indicates severe thoracic trauma (like first rib) with significant associated injuries (e.g. rib, clavicular, pulmonary, brachial plexus, vertebral), and even abdominal injuries. Local pain and tenderness and chest X-ray confirm the diagnosis. Immobilisation of the arm in a sling is

important for a few weeks until the fracture is stable and the pain resolves. Treatment of associated injuries may take priority.

Complicated fractures

- Multiple fractured ribs in a row on one hemithorax.
- Stove-in-chest multiple rib fractures with permanent indentation and depression of the chest wall.
- Flail chest with a flaccid unstable anterior chest wall (sternum) caused by bilateral multiple fractures or two rows of fractured ribs on one hemithorax with unstable segment, accompanied by paradoxical breathing.
- Traumatic pneumothorax with a sucking chest wound and late tension pneumothorax (total lung collapse and mediastinal shift towards the opposite side detected by tracheal and apex beat shift and manifested by acute cardiorespiratory failure. It is fatal if not relieved by immediate occlusion of the sucking wound and urgently by chest tube underwater drainage.)
- Traumatic haemothorax or haemopneumothorax.
- Pulmonary contusion and laceration.

Complicated fracture is managed in the following way.

1. Stabilisation of chest wall (strapping or internal fixation with wires or better still tracheostomy).
2. Artificial ventilation via tracheostomy or endotracheal tube.
3. Pain relief, using injectable analgesics (e.g. small doses of morphine) or intercostal nerve block.
4. Pleural decompression of blood and air via chest tube underwater drainage.
5. Tracheobronchial secretions are aspirated bronchoscopically or via tracheostomy.
6. Exploratory thoracotomy following primary chest drainage is indicated in:

- Blood loss sufficient to cause shock (more than 200 ml/h over 4 consecutive hours) or if haemothorax is clotted.
- Massive air leak (tracheobronchial injury).
- Tamponade in most cardiac wounds.
- Oesophageal injury indicated by surgical emphysema or thin barium swallow.
- Open sucking wounds, if skin loss has occurred, as they lead to tension pneumothorax.

7. Treatment of shock lung by colloid replacement for blood, restricting crystalloid solutions, and giving i.v. diuretic (e.g. frusemide 20 mg twice daily for 3 days, and methylprednisolone 30 mg/kg).

1.69 Craniospinal Trauma

HEAD INJURY

Head injury is the cause of 9 deaths/100 000 of the population each year in the UK and 22 deaths/ 100 000 in the USA. About half the deaths occur before arrival at hospital. Most of these have overwhelming multiple injuries or irreparable brain damage. Over half the head injuries are in those less than 30 years of age (head injury is the commonest cause of death in the 15–24 year-old population). Much of the mortality and morbidity (potentially preventable) is attributable to secondary brain damage after the patient reaches hospital.

Causes

The major ones are:
1. Road traffic accidents – the commonest.
2. Assaults – in Scottish men aged 15–25 years assault is as common as road traffic accidents as a cause of head injury.
3. Falls.
The minor ones are:
4. Sporting injuries.
5. Birth trauma.
6. Industrial accidents.

Compulsory use of seat belts (started in Australia and then in the UK) has resulted in 50% less brain damage and 40% fewer fatalities in car occupants involved in road traffic accidents. Very occasionally a disease may precipitate head injury, e.g. myocardial infarction, collapse or epileptic fit. Ingestion of alcohol is a common associated factor and 50% of head injuries were found (in some studies) in drunk pedestrians and those involved in assault.

Pattern of injury

1. Adult pedestrians tend to suffer from more limb, pelvic and femoral injuries, while small children are more likely to be run over and suffer injury to the trunk.
2. The highest incidence of head injury, whiplash neck injury and chest trauma occurs in car drivers and front seat passengers. Twenty per cent of in-car deaths include fatal cervical spine injuries.
3. Domestic trauma (falls in the home): high incidence of limb fractures with 40% sustaining head injuries.
4. Industrial trauma: the head is involved in less than 2% of cases.

Classification

Minor

No or a very brief loss of consciousness and no fracture (clinically or radiologically). Presence of fracture however, is no measure or indication of severity; a linear fracture may be present and the case is still minor.

Severe

Prolonged or profound loss of consciousness or post-traumatic amnesia or lucid period of consciousness (as in intracranial haematoma). Fracture may or may not be present.

Closed   Intact scalp with no communication between intracranial contents and the exterior but often associated with fairly diffuse brain damage. Fracture may or may not be present.

Open   Communication between intracranial contents and the exterior and often associated with focal brain damage. It is caused by a small sharp object, e.g. a stone, bottle or missile. Fracture is always present and is usually of the depressed compound type.

The Glasgow Coma Scale is the proper charting for quantifying the severity of injury (see p. 342). A patient who is alert and fully orientated as regards place, person and time scores 15 while one with severe head injury scores 7 or less.

Pathology

A combined pathology is commonest (e.g. contusion and laceration or contusion and intracranial haemorrhage or subdural haematoma and contusion with laceration).

Immediate impact injury (at the moment of injury)

Scalp Bruises and laceration.

Skull Fractures in vault or base, fissure or depressed, closed or open (compound). The fracture itself is of no consequence unless it is compound.

Brain
- *Concussion* (transient loss of consciousness with diffuse neuronal damage with quick recovery – this is a clinical rather than a pathological term).
- *Contusion* (bruised brain with oedema later on).
- Lacerations (cerebral tear).
- Diffuse white matter damage.

Cranial nerves Any may be involved but I olfactory is the commonest and XII hypoglossal is the rarest. Paralysis is due to laceration by fractured ends (immediate and permanent) to blood clot compression (after a few days with recovery), or to scar or callus (after weeks and permanent).

Blood vessels Vessels torn at the time of injury give rise to bleeding with later formation of pressing expanding haematoma.

Extracranial injuries
- Very common (neck, chest, abdomen and limb fractures).
- Metabolic (fat embolism).

Primary complications

Although initiated by head injury they develop some time after the injury and are distinguished by their amenability to treatment.
- Intracranial haemorrhage (intracerebral, subdural and extra-dural haematoma) with brain shift and herniation due to a space-occupying lesion.
- Brain swelling (brain swells first because of increased blood volume due to cerebral autoregulation in traumatic shock and second because of cerebral waterlogging with oedema fluid due to contusion).
- *Cushing* stress peptic ulcer (extracranial).

Intracranial haematoma accounts for one-third of the deaths of patients who have talked at some stage after head injury. These deaths are due to delayed evacuation of an intracranial

haematoma as a result of late diagnosis. Haematoma is also a common source of disability in survivors. Occurrence of intracranial infection after head injury (see below) is also often a consequence of delayed or inadequate initial care. Such mortality and morbidity are preventable with better management.

Secondary complications

- Brain damage secondary to raised intracranial pressure.
- Hypoxic brain damage (less obvious but disastrous – it is found in 90% of patients who die in hospital after head injury. It is due to inadequate cerebral perfusion secondary to systemic hypotension and/or raised intracranial pressure).
- Infection (meningitis and cerebral abscesses).

Other complications

- Late bleeding (chronic subdural haematoma due to osmotic expansion of a trivial surface clot).
- Permanent cerebral damage (local signs of hemiparesis, hemiplegia, dysphasia, and blindness). In mid-brain (signs of ataxia, tremor, rigidity, dysarthria). Measured sometimes by post-traumatic amnesia:
  0–1 h (slight)
  1–24 h (moderate)
  1–7 days (severe)
  over 7 days (very severe).
  About 70% of patients with less than 24 h post-traumatic amnesia return to work in 8 weeks.
- Retrograde traumatic amnesia.
- Epilepsy (early 5% and late 5%). Presents as a fit within the first 24 h (due to brain oedema), as true post-traumatic epilepsy occurring between 6 months and 21 years after injury (due to contracted scar) or idiopathic epilepsy which becomes evident within days or weeks of head injury. Diagnosed clinically and by EEG and encephalography. If the scar is focal it should be excised, and the dura grafted with fascia or sutured with nylon membrane to prevent more fibrosis. Anti-epileptic drugs are needed.
- Coma causes many problems but the Mendelson (1946) syndrome is fatal. This is fulminating aspiration pneumonia caused by inhalation of irritant vomit (containing hydrochloric acid) during coma or induction of anaesthetic. Dyspnoea, cyanosis and tachycardia with adventitious lung sounds and bronchospasm are followed by gross pulmonary oedema and death. X-ray shows irregular mottling scattered through lung fields but no lung collapse. Small quantities of free hydrochloric acid may be responsible for death.
- Psychiatric disturbance (post-concussion syndrome – lack of concentration, and defective memory and emotional control).
- Post-traumatic hydrocephalus.
- Diabetes insipidus.
- Inappropriate ADH secretion.
- Pneumatocele, meningocele, CSF leaks and carotid–cavernous fistula.

MANAGEMENT

First aid measures

Airway, breathing, circulation and stoppage of external bleeding.

Assessment and monitoring

History

Precise mechanism of injury, patient status after injury, duration and presence of any previous diseases, and whether patient is an alcoholic.

Examination

General examination

For lacerations, CSF or blood leak from the nose or ear – periorbital haematoma, retromastoid bruising. Associated injuries should be looked for, particularly of the cervical spine. Neck stiffness (meningism) indicates subarachnoid bleeding caused by trauma, ruptured Berry's aneurysm or spontaneous intracerebral haematoma. Signs of malignancy may indicate intracranial metastases.

Neurological examination

Consciousness Degree and duration is the best index of the amount of diffuse damage caused by acceleration–deceleration forces. Changes in consciousness level in the first few hours provide the most reliable guide to whether recovery will occur or whether intracranial complications will develop.

The Glasgow Coma Scale (GCS) is the best means of assessing, recording and displaying the level of consciousness. The score ranges between 3 and 15 when the full scale is used. A score of 7 or less indicates severe head injury, while a score of 15 indicates minor head injury. The parameters with response and score are as follows:

Eye opening

Spontaneous	(4)
To speech	(3)
To pain	(2)
None	(1)

Best verbal response

Orientated	(5)
Confused conversation	(4)
Inappropriate words	(3)
Incomprehensible sounds	(2)
None	(1)

Best motor response

Obeys commands		(6)
Localises		(5)
Flexes:	Normal	(4)
	Abnormal	(3)
Extends		(2)
None		(1)

The scale is charted so that medical and nursing staff can readily see the changes (this is particularly important since personnel change many times a day).

Pupil size and reaction Light reflex tests optic (II) and oculomotor (III) nerves. Failure of pupil to react to both direct and consensual light implies a III lesion. Reaction to consensual light only implies II or retinal lesion. III lesion is the most useful indicator of an expanding intracranial lesion. Increased intracranial pressure leads to bilateral fixed dilated pupils. An ipsilateral dilating pupil is a sign of extradural haemorrhage. However, a fixed dilated pupil in coma is not pathognomonic of an intracranial lesion (and mid-brain compression due to uncal herniation from a tentorial hiatus). Since direct eye injury leads to traumatic mydriasis, associated hyphaemia (blood effusion in the anterior eye chamber) should be looked for. An epileptic fit can also produce transient fixed dilated pupils. Bilateral pinpoint pupils are due either to drug overdose or pontine haemorrhage.

Eye movements Abnormal eye movements indicate structural damage.
- Conjugate deviation to the right indicates damage to the right frontal visual field (Brodmann's area 8) or left pontine gaze centre and vice versa.
- Oculocephalic (doll's eye) reflex: head movement in a comatose patient produces transient reflex eye movements in the opposite direction. Normally visual fixation prevents this reflex. Failure to elicit this reflex in coma carries a grave prognosis and implies severe brain stem damage.
- Oculovestibular reflex (caloric test): in coma with intact brain stem the eyes drift slowly towards the side of injection of ice water in the external auditory meatus when the head is elevated 30°. Persistent absence of this reflex in coma implies brain stem damage with poor prognosis. The normal response is nystagmus with fast eye movement away from the injected area.
- Dysconjugate eye movement (eyes do not move in parallel): especially in upward gaze may indicate compressing intracranial lesion.

Limb deficit (assessed as part of GCS). Asymmetrical weakness, hemiparesis or hemiplegia occurs in limbs contralateral to lesion side. However, ipsilateral weakness may be due to uncal herniation pushing contralateral cerebral peduncle onto opposite edge of tentorium cerebelli (termed a false localising sign).

More neurological signs
- Systemic hypertension, reflex bradycardia (dissociated signs), papilloedema are indicative of raised intracranial pressure.
- Localising signs apart from pupil and fracture/ bruise site include:
  - Jacksonian epilepsy.
  - Hemiparesis/hemiplegia.
  - Dysphasia or aphasia (clot pressing over left dominant hemisphere in right-handed patient).

– Homonymous hemianopia of half visual field opposite to the visual cortex or optic radiation compressed by expanding haematoma.

- Low temperature may be due to shock (rarely due to intracranial bleeding but usually due to associated injuries, e.g. thoraco-abdominal or fractures) but a high or progressively rising temperature (in the absence of infection) indicates damage to the thermostatic centre of the hypothalamus and should be kept below 38.5°C (by fan, ice bag and chlorpromazine).
- Impaired facial movements on one side in response to a bilateral supraorbital pain stimulus indicates VII facial nerve weakness.
- Corneal reflex (tests V and VII nerves): loss of blink response in both eyes indicates V lesion on the stimulated side, while loss of blink in one eye irrespective of the side stimulated indicates VII lesion.
- Cerebral lesion may produce slow respiration or Cheyne–Stokes periodic respiration. Drug overdose, respiratory failure and CO_2 narcosis may also be responsible and blood gas analysis is indicated.

Investigations

Skull X-ray A well-penetrated AP skull, true lateral skull and cervical spine and AP chest X-rays are essential in all coma cases. The presence of one or more of the following clinical criteria indicates a need for skull X-ray in patients with a history of recent head injury.

- Loss of consciousness or amnesia at any time.
- Neurological symptoms or signs.
- Cerebrospinal fluid or blood from the nose or ear.
- Suspected penetrating injury or scalp bruising or swelling. Simple scalp laceration is not a criterion for skull X-ray.
- Alcohol intoxication.
- Difficulty in assessing the patient (e.g. the young, epilepsy).

However, many advocate routine skull X-ray in all cases of head injury for medicolegal reasons.

CT scanning A non-invasive facility which should not be used as a substitute for clinical assessment. It is done after resuscitation is complete, in selected cases:

- Deteriorating, fluctuating or prolonged unconsciousness.
- Localising signs (including focal epilepsy).
- Severe head injury (GCS 7 or less) in the absence of localising signs.
- Penetrating head injury.
- Differential diagnosis of coma.
- Head injury with known intracranial pathology
- Late indications (CSF fistula, infection, hydrocephalus, chronic subdural haematoma).

Intracranial pressure (ICP) monitoring Used by some neurosurgeons (see s. 3.7) Head injury and burr hole procedure). The difference between ICP and systemic arterial pressure (the cerebral perfusion pressure) has an important influence upon the maintenance of cerebral blood flow. An extremely high ICP can shut off cerebral blood flow. ICP is a good indicator of a space-occupying lesion, e.g. intracranial haematoma.

Echo encephalography Simple, non-invasive method of detecting a shift in the cerebral midline.

Multimodality evoked electrical potential (by computer) To record visual, somatosensory and auditory near-field and brain stem reflexes. It provides a prognostic index (limited use).

The last three investigations have practical limitations and are used only when clinical assessment is impossible as in comatose patients under controlled ventilation.

Continuous monitoring of the clinical state

- GCS.
- Pupil size and reaction.
- Limb movements.
- Vital signs (blood pressure, pulse rate, temperature, respiratory rate).

Definitive treatment

Minor head injury

Patients with no fracture, who are walking and talking (orientated) can be allowed home provided the relatives are warned to return the patient to hospital if headache, vomiting, drowsiness, visual disturbance or coma occurs.

Hospital admission after recent head injury is indicated in the presence of one or more of the following:

- Confusion or any other depression of the level of consciousness at the time of examination.
- Skull fracture.
- Neurological signs or headache or vomiting.
- Difficulty in assessing the patient, e.g. alcoholics and epileptics.
- Other medical conditions, e.g. haemophilia.
- Unsuitability of the patient's social conditions or lack of responsible adult/relative.

Note
- Post-traumatic amnesia with full recovery is not an indication for admission.
- Patients sent home should be given written instructions about possible complications and appropriate action.

Head injury with expected risk of complications

Patient should be hospitalised for observation as described (admission is indicated for all vault and basal fractures, all closed head injuries with altered consciousness or localising signs, multiple injuries with coexisting medical diseases (e.g. diabetes), known intracranial pathology (e.g. tumour, alcohol or drug ingestion), absence of responsible adult relatives or friends and if clinician is in doubt). If a patient deteriorates and an obvious extracranial cause such as hypoxia, hypotension or dehydration cannot be found, intracranial bleeding should be suspected and transfer arranged to a neurosurgical unit.

Consultation with and referral to a neurosurgical unit is indicated in the presence of one or more of the following:
- Skull fracture in combination with:
  – Confusion or other depression of the level of consciousness;

– Focal neurological signs; or
– Fits (including epilepsy).
- Confusion or other neurological disturbance persisting for more than 12 h even if there is no skull fracture.
- Coma continuing after resuscitation.
- Suspected open injury of the vault or the base of the skull (risk of CSF leak, meningitis).
- Depressed fracture of the skull.
- Deterioration.

In these cases decompression is required in the form of burr hole(s) or craniotomy (osteoplastic flap is preferred since it provides wider exposure and better decompression).

Head injury with coma (but without intracranial haematoma)

- Patient needs special care (to keep the airway open with tracheostomy care if applicable, positioning, nutrition, urination and defecation). Medical management of severe head injury is the only treatment for those in whom there is no intracranial lesion.
- Respiratory function is of the utmost importance. Controlled ventilation is indicated in the following groups:
  - Missile head injury.
  - Head injury associated with severe respiratory trauma.
  - Head injury with pulmonary pathology, e.g. pneumonitis.
  - Head injury with severe generalised brain swelling especially in children.
  - Status epilepticus.
  - Acute reduction of intracranial pressure during coning or brain shift.
  - As part of anaesthesia for all urgent surgery in injured patients.
  - For all investigations requiring immobilisation, e.g. CT scanning.
- Steroids (dexamethasone) have been used in closed head injury but there is no substantial clinical or experimental evidence as to their efficacy.
- Mannitol and other osmotic diuretics could be given as a bolus 1.5–2 g/kg body weight in the early post-injury period. *N.B.* Many centres prohibit the use of steroids and mannitol for reduction of cerebral oedema since possible associated subclinical intracranial haemorrhage may expand when the brain shrinks (they also lead to false interpretation of CT scans by masking the magnitude of brain swelling). They should therefore be used only after strong confirmation of absence of intracranial bleeding and when there is no indication for CT scanning. Giving mannitol in head injury is just like giving narcotics (morphine) in acute abdomen, since it masks physical signs. It is given after CT scan to confirm no double pathology is present.
- Cimetidine 200 mg three times a day with 400 mg at night is effective in controlling gastric acid output and possibly preventing stress ulcer.
- Broad-spectrum antibiotics are given only in pulmonary complications, compound fracture or CSF leak.
- Anticonvulsants are given for fits and prophylactically for extensive open head injury (risk of future epilepsy is more than 50%): phenytoin 300 mg or phenobarbitone 60 mg three times a day orally or i.v. is recommended. Acute epilepsy requires i.v. diazepam. Status epilepticus needs controlled ventilation.

Prognosis

The majority of head injuries are trivial. Of patients with severe head injuries 50% die, 10–12% are severely disabled or vegetative and 40% make a good recovery or have only a moderate disability.

The Glasgow Outcome Scale provides a practical means of classifying the outcome in terms of overall social disability:
- *Death*.
- *Vegetative*: sleep/wake cycles with eyes open but no sentient activity.
- *Severely disabled*: dependent, physically or intellectually, on another person at some point in every day.
- *Moderate disability*: independent but unable to resume fully their previous activities.
- *Good recovery*: may have residual neurological signs.

There is correlation between such outcome with the initial scoring of head injury by the GCS: a score of more than 11 is associated with 87% moderate disability or good recovery and 12% dead or vegetative while a score of 3–4 is associated with 87% dead or vegetative and 7% moderate disability or good recovery.

CERVICAL SPINE INJURY

The commonest vertebral column injury and the most dangerous when associated with spinal cord damage. Such injury is often missed or misdiagnosed because of:
- Pre-existing medical problem, e.g. rheumatoid arthritis.
- Multiple injuries (diverting attention from the neck).
- Head injury with unconsciousness making the clinical assessment difficult (in which case cervical X-ray is the only means of assessment and should be done routinely).
- Alcohol/drug abuse.
- Mild weakness and lack of physical signs (painful movement limitation, tenderness, retropharyngeal haematoma seen through the open mouth in Cl or C2 injuries and head rotation to one side in unilateral dislocation, all rarely present).
- Lateral cervical X-ray visualisation is often incomplete in the upper or lower parts of neck.

Therefore a *lateral complete cervical X-ray* (while the arms or shoulders are pulled down and the head is steadied with a halter) is the keystone of diagnosis and should be practised routinely (in addition to X-ray of the odontoid process taken through the open mouth). Myelogram is indicated in neurological deterioration and in stable but incomplete deficit due to cord compression.

Classification

Either dislocation or fracture (complete or incomplete with or without interruption to cord continuity respectively and stable or unstable).

Stable injuries

When bones will not displace further in the course of ordinary nursing care. They require neither reduction nor immobilisation (for bone healing) but may require a collar or skull traction to control pain.

- Whiplash injury in acceleration–deceleration head injury (extensor–flexor strain) leading to soft tissue injury, rarely with fracture or dislocation manifested by severe pain and stiffness. Treatment is by collar and gentle massage.
- Central cord syndrome due to forward fall with extension strain in elderly patients leading to paralysis of all four limbs (tetraplegia). Paralysis is greatest in the arms and least in the legs with flaccid hand paralysis and spastic leg paralysis. The bladder is paralysed. The syndrome is due to haemorrhage and oedema in the central area of the cervical spine over several segments (involving the anterior horn cells). Treatment is the same as for body paralysis. The neck requires no treatment. The condition is not painful.
- Simple extension lesion with a flake fracture of the inferior edge of the body.
- Fractures of atlas (spinal cord injury uncommon).

Unstable injuries

Require reduction of any displacement, and immobilisation which should continue until spontaneous healing of fractures and torn ligaments occurs.

- *Dislocation* following hanging: occurs between the atlas and axis with forward displacement of the atlas after transverse ligament rupture.
- *Hangman's fracture* at C2–C3 by direct extension: caused by hanging or lifting the head with the hands encircling the neck from behind.

In both the above cases death is immediate as a result of brainstem injury and paralysis of the respiratory muscles.

- Axis fractures (X-ray through open mouth) with the odontoid process displaced forward or backward. Forward displacement of the odontoid may press on the brain stem and kill the patient immediately. Endotracheal intubation (for respiratory paralysis) may accentuate the cord compression and should be done with great care by an expert anaesthetist.
- Burst fractures (C3–C7): caused by vertical compression (due to diving into shallow water and striking the head on the bottom).
- Fracture – dislocations.

Cord injury

Produced by three factors:

- Long axis stretch causing concussion or rupture of nerve fibres and vessels within the cord.
- Nipping of the cord between the fractured bony edge and vertebral lamina.
- Disc protrusion leading to compression.

$$
\text{Mechanical forces} \rightarrow
\begin{cases}
\text{axon injury} \longrightarrow \text{spinal cord necrosis} \\
\text{vascular injury} \rightarrow \text{spinal cord necrosis} \\
\text{(ischaemia and} \\
\text{infarction)} \\
\qquad \downarrow\uparrow \\
\text{biochemical injury}
\end{cases}
$$

The cord traumatic haemorrhage may be:

- Intramedullary (haematomyelia).
- Extramedullary into CSF (haematorrachis), either:
  - Extradural: with progressive cord compression and paraplegia (Thorburn's gravitation paraplegia); or
  - Intradural: with root irritation (blood detected in lumbar puncture).

Segmental injury

Upper cervical injury C1–C4 $\rightarrow$	Respiratory paralysis (since phrenic nerve is derived mainly from C4) with tetraplegia.
C5 $\longrightarrow$	Tetraplegia only (breathing OK).
C6 $\longrightarrow$	Tetraplegia but patient can abduct shoulder by deltoid muscles.
C7 $\longrightarrow$	Paraplegia with triceps paralysis in upper limbs.
T1 $\longrightarrow$	Paralysis of small hand muscles and Horner's syndrome.

All cord injuries result in spinal shock (complete flaccid paralysis below the level of the lesion with urinary retention). In cord contusion this lasts for 48 h followed by return of reflexes (recovery), followed by a third stage of septic complication. If no recovery is seen after 48 h, the injury may be either partial cord lesion (spastic paralysis in extension appears and urinary retention continues) or complete cord lesion (spastic paralysis in flexion appears with mass reflex).

Treatment

Management includes four phases:
1. Injury – first aid means.
2. Transport – immobilisation of neck.
3. Diagnosis (usually radiological though suspected clinically).
4. Treatment. The treatment aims are:
- To avoid incidents that could cause fresh damage to the spinal cord.
- To promote recovery from the damage already sustained.

Accurate clinical assessment of the severity of the damage may be impossible in the first few hours because of spinal shock. Radiological assessment (lateral and transoral X-ray and sometimes myelogram) is therefore essential. Reduction of unstable fractures is done by simple traction with skull calipers and graded increments in weight (also constitutes immobilisation if maintained until bony union occurs). The patient should be confined to bed. A minerva jacket (or halo vest) may be required for ambulant immobilisation. Reduction may be done quickly by closed manipulation under anaesthesia. Once reduction has been achieved spontaneous stabilisation by bony fusion is anticipated in 90% of cases over 9–10 weeks. If by that time X-rays do not show stability on flexion or extension, the patient should undergo an internal fixation with bone grafting. Laminectomy or decompression is not beneficial as cord compression occurs at the time of injury.

Early management of paraplegia and rehabilitation

● High-protein diet (to compensate serum exudation from bed-sores).
● Positioning to prevent bed sores.
● Intermittent urinary catheterisation – to prevent urinary infection (retention is present only initially).
● Active and passive movements and splints (quadriplegia).
● Treatment of respiratory failure.

1.70 Hand Injury, Infection and Surgery of the Rheumatoid Hand

HAND INJURY

Main causes are:
● Industrial accidents (machinery in 40% of cases).
● Home accidents.
● Transport accidents.

Contributory factors include age (usually young in work-related accidents) and experience. The effects of severe hand injury are:
● Economical.
● Personal.
● Psychological.

Types of hand injury

● Incised wound (treated with primary suture).
● Crush injury with oedema, either open (treated with secondary suture) or closed (necessitates decompression incision).

The aim of treatment is to achieve the best possible result in the shortest possible time.

Assessment

1. The injury sustained (see below).
2. The functional loss.
3. The functional requirement of the patient.

Assessment of the injury sustained

● Is there any tissue loss? (e.g. bone, tendon, muscle).
● What structures are exposed?
● Viability of the skin.
● What structures are damaged?
  – Tendon injury is assessed by finger movements.
  – Nerve injury is assessed by sensation (not the motor power which is impaired already).
  – Bone injury by X-ray.
  – Joint stability only under general anaesthesia.

Treatment priorities

1. Skin cover.
2. Tendon repair.
3. Nerve repair.
4. Bone and joint injury treatment.

Principles of skin loss repair

1. Free partial-thickness skin graft.
2. Free full-thickness skin graft.
3. Local skin flaps
   – Rotation flap
   – Cross-finger flap
   – Advancement flap
   – Neurovascular island flap.
4. Pedicle grafts.
5. Vascularised free grafts.

Principles of tendon repair

Tendons heal rapidly when held in apposition and strong union occurs at 4 weeks. Tendons easily become adherent to surrounding tissues, limiting their gliding movement. Such adhesions can be reduced by using *Klinert's traction*. The fingertip, e.g. nail, is attached by a rubber band to the plaster splint of the forearm. Because of rubber band recoil, the patient can actively extend his finger with a passive flexion. A reflex antagonistic relaxation of the flexor hand muscles prevents any mounting tension on the repaired tendon.

The results of immediate repair of extensor tendons are better than those of flexor tendons (due to flexor sheath in the latter).

Flexor tendons are sutured with primary repair or secondary late repair using tendon graft from palmaris longus or plantaris.

Extensor tendons are sutured with primary repair (in open wounds) or treated conservatively by immobilisation (in closed wounds).

Nerve injury

Should be treated by primary immediate repair and tested by nerve conduction study.

Hand bones fractures

K-wire internal fixation is indicated in:
● Fractures involving a joint surface.
● Metacarpal and proximal phalangeal fractures causing shortening, rotation or malalignment.
● Multiple fractures.

Principles of hand surgical technique

1. Tourniquet is essential to provide an adequate bloodless field; good light is important.
2. Anaesthesia – general is better than regional and local. If the latter is used, adrenaline is contraindicated.

3. Careful wound toilet and cleansing.

4. Excision of devitalised tissue and haemostasis of bleeding vessels after release of the tourniquet.

5. Antibiotic and antitetanus toxoid should be administered routinely.

6. After treatment:

● Position of function (not ease) (i.e. flexion of metacarpophalangeal joints, extension of interphalangeal joints, abduction of thumb and dorsiflexion of wrist).

● Elevation of the hand.

● Proper Cramer wire splintage.

● Early physiotherapy.

Cut flexor aspect of the wrist

● Quick assessment with fluid replacement if still bleeding from cut arteries.

● Immediate repair of at least one artery (radial and/or ulnar artery) with 7/0 Prolene.

● Venous injury, however, can be ignored and the vein ligated.

● Immediate primary nerve repair (nearly always median nerve) should always be attempted (see s. 1.71 Nerve injury. Secondary nerve repair is rarely done (because of poor results).

● Immediate primary tendon repair should always be performed as there is abundant areolar tissue which prevents adhesions (providing the conditions permit). End-to-end repair should be carried out using Bunnell (criss-cross) stitch or Kessler (grasping) stitch (Fig. 1.70.1). All tendons should be sutured with the exception of palmaris longus which can be resected to reduce bulky scarring and prevent gross adhesions.

● Skin closure is essential as raw areas (uncovered by skin) predispose to infection and fibrosis.

● Antibiotics and antitetanus toxoid should be administered routinely.

Tendon injuries on the hand palmar aspect

Zone 1 (from the wrist to the distal palmar crease). Both flexor digitorum profundus and superficialis are repaired primarily (if conditions permit).

Zone 2 (from the distal palmar crease to the proximal interphalangeal joint) is called 'no man's land' or 'the danger area'. Traditionally if both flexor tendons are divided, close the skin alone. At the second operation resect flexor digitorum superficialis and repair flexor digitorum profundus by tendon graft. If only flexor digitorum profundus is divided, disregard lest repair endanger flexor digitorum superficialis. However, in expert hands, good results have been achieved after primary repair of both flexor tendons when combined with Klinert's postoperative rubber band traction.

Zone 3 (distal to proximal interphalangeal joint). Divided flexor digitorum profundus is repaired primarily (if conditions permit); otherwise flexor tendon graft via terminal phalanx with a pull-out wire is performed.

If flexor tendon injuries in the wrist and palm, Zones 1 and 3, cannot be repaired primarily, then secondary repair, tendon grafting or arthrodesis of the distal interphalangeal joint is performed later.

HAND INFECTIONS AND TREATMENT

Hand infections are either superficial, deep or unclassified.

Superficial (Fig. 1.70.1)

Nail fold infection (paronychia)

Can be complicated by chronic paronychia or pulp space infection.

Pulp space infection (whitlow, felon)

Due to fibrous bands intersecting the space between the phalanx, tendon sheath and the skin; pus collection is rapid and painful leading to necrosis of the pulp tissue and the skin. Untreated it leads to osteomyelitis, pyogenic arthritis and even flexor tenosynovitis.

Subcutaneous infections

Apical subungual abscess and volar space infections.

Web space infections

Occur between the dorsal and volar skin. Spaces are filled with loose fat bulging between divisions of palmar fascia and

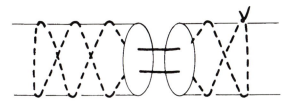

Bunnell

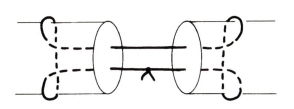

Kessler

Fig. 1.70.1 Tendon repair

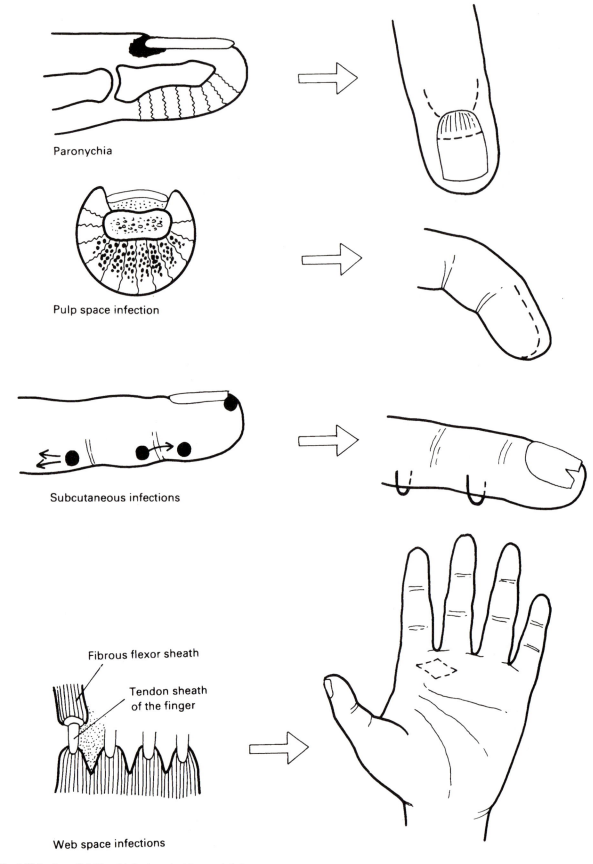

Paronychia

Pulp space infection

Subcutaneous infections

Fibrous flexor sheath

Tendon sheath
of the finger

Web space infections

Fig. 1.70.2   Superficial hand infections: incisions and drainage

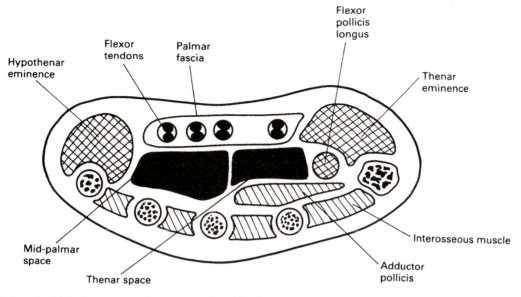

Fig. 1.70.3 Deep hand infections: anatomy (transverse section of hand)

straddling the deep transverse ligament. Treated by a diamond-shaped incision over the affected web space.

Deep (Figs 1.70.3–1.70.5)

Thenar space infection

The thenar space lies deep between adductor pollicis behind and flexor tendon of the index finger in front. It is separated

from the mid-palmar space medially by the intermediate palmar septum (extending from palmar fascia) and laterally by the thenar eminence muscles. True infection of this space is rare and is usually an extension of a web space infection.

Mid-palmar space infection

The mid-palmar space lies between the interossei and meta-carpal bones behind and the flexor tendons of the middle, ring

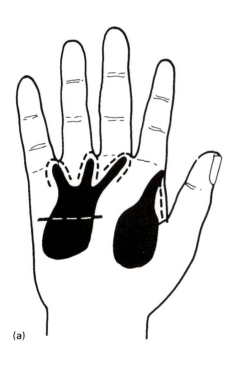
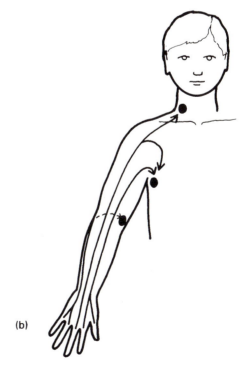

Fig. 1.70.4 Deep hand infections (a) drainage sites; (b) lymphangitis

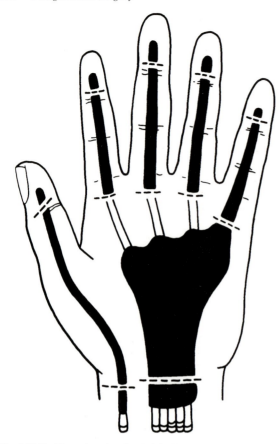

Fig. 1.70.5 Sites of tendon sheath infections

and little fingers in front. This infection is usually an extension of subcutaneous palm abscesses. In deep palmar spaces lymphangitis occurs.

Tendon sheath infections (tenosynovitis) (see Fig. 1.70.5)

There are three classical signs:
- Symmetrical swelling of the entire finger.
- Flexion of the finger (Hook sign) with exquisite pain on extension.
- Tenderness over the infected sheath.

Each tendon infection is treated with two incisions. It is a very serious condition and is complicated by:
- Forearm infection after ulnar or radial bursa rupture into the space of Parona between pronator quadratus and interosseous membrane dorsally and flexor digitorum profundus ventrally.
- Chronic tenosynovitis.
- Pyogenic arthritis.

A stiff digit is treated by amputation. Paralysis of the median nerve requires urgent decompression (similar to carpal tunnel syndrome).

Unclassified infections

Include human bite, orf (contagious pustular dermatitis of sheep) and Barber's pilonidal sinus.

General principles of hand infection treatment

1. Antibiotics, e.g. flucloxacillin.
2. Rest and elevation.
3. Diagnosis and localisation of pus.
4. Evacuation of pus and/or debridement of abscess cavity wall.
5. Adequate after-treatment (position of function, dry dressing and change of wet dressings, physiotherapy and rehabilitation).

SURGERY OF THE RHEUMATOID HAND

Careful selection and patient motivation to undergo prolonged postoperative splinting and therapy are absolutely imperative for successful outcome. Surgical correction of diseased carpo-metacarpophalangeal (CMP) joints of the thumb or of fingers have their own advantages and disadvantages.

Thumb

Arthrodesis (such as using Micks external compression device) produces good pain relief and stability at the expense of the following disadvantages:
- decreased dexterity with age as MCP joint motion decreases;
- inability to flutter hand to pick up objects;
- thumb protrudes when placed in a confined space;
- with trapezium arthritis, other sides of articulation might cause pain;
- difficulties in fusion with prolonged immobilisation.

Resectional arthroplasty produces pain relief, good mobility and is a relatively simple procedure. However, it lacks stability for busy tasks, is associated with decreased strength and it shortens the thumb.

Implant arthroplasty (best with silicone implant) produces pain relief, maintains mobility, is not associated with thumb shortening, allows normal positioning of the thumb and increases strength. Disadvantages include dislocation, fracture of the implant and reaction to the implant.

In flexor tenosynovitis, treatment by release of the proximal pulley *per se* is not satisfactory, but pulleys should be preserved and the contents of the tendon sheath must be reduced. Synovectomy is useful in balancing arthroplasty.

Fingers

MCP joint replacement can be achieved with cemented metallic Schultz finger joint prosthesis or Swanson silicon prosthesis with *collateral ligament release and reattachment*, with daytime dynamic splint and nightime splint.

Diseased interphalangeal joints may develop extension or flexion deformities, swan-neck or boutonniere deformities. Treatment of diseased interphalangeal joints without bone destruction may include *simple manipulation* (to adequately correct the deformity) and *pinning of distal joints in extension* (to cause fibrosis in corrected position), or *joint arthroplasty with soft tissue reconstruction of extensor mechanism of the finger*. If there is bone destruction, *arthrodesis* then is indicated (possibly with proximal joint arthroplasty).

1.71 Nerve Injury and Entrapment

Types of injury

Neurapraxia Physical paralysis of conduction due to stretching or distortion without any organic rupture. Recovery is complete.

Axonotmesis Intrathecal rupture of nerve fibres within an intact sheath. Wallerian degeneration and slow but good recovery by proliferating axons and intraneural fibrosis with fusiform neuroma formation.

Neurotmesis Partial or complete division of the nerve sheath and fibres due to penetrating wounds; central and/or lateral neuroma with retrograde Wallerian degeneration and Schwann cell proliferation. Recovery is poor without nerve repair. Even accurate nerve suture may lead to an imperfect result owing to wastage of axons in scar tissue at the suture line and maldistribution of those fibres reaching the distal segment (maldistribution is greatest in mixed nerves and motor nerves supplying a large number of small muscles). The density of scar tissue at the suture line is increased by local sepsis and inflammation and by tension at the suture line.

NERVE REPAIR

Immediate primary suture is the ideal treatment for a divided nerve in tidy clean incised wounds (no sepsis and no tension). In untidy contaminated wounds, early secondary suture 3–4 weeks after injury is recommended for the following reasons.

- Primary suture requires enlargement of the wound to mobilise the nerve ends without tension. Since the wound is potentially infected, exposure of previously uncontaminated tissues should be avoided.
- Normally the nerve sheath is a delicate structure which is easily torn by the slightest tension. The sheath is also weakened by longitudinal tears but 3 weeks after the injury, epineural fibrosis occurs resulting in a thicker and tougher sheath and accurate coaptation of nerve ends by that time is greatly facilitated.

If a divided nerve is encountered accidentally in an open untidy wound it should be marked with fine silk for future identification but on no account should an attempt be made to identify or scrutinise a nerve.

Technique

After adequate exposure, the two ends of the nerve are identified, freed and freshened with a scalpel until projecting fibres are seen and blood oozes freely from the cut surface. Apposition of the two ends is accomplished by:

- Mobilisation.
- Relaxed position of the limb.
- Transposition, e.g. of ulnar nerve in front of the medial epicondyle and the radial nerve in front of the humerus.
- Nerve anchoring with tension stitches.

(Resection of bone is rarely required.) The sheath is sutured with non-irritant material, e.g. 7/0 Prolene mounted on an atraumatic needle or tantalum wire. Catgut should never be used. Tension or torsion should be avoided.

Principles of neurorrhaphy

- Elimination of tension.
- Use of atraumatic technique.
- No tourniquet.
- Proper mapping and aligning of fascicles.
- Prevention of fascicular gaps.
- Avoidance of lengthy mobilisation which has a devascularising effect.
- Use of meticulous intraneural haemostasis.
- Minimisation of foreign body reactions.

Aids in the repair

- Microsurgery of at least × 4 magnification with straight microsurgical forceps held in the left hand and curved microsurgical forceps (also acting as a needle-holder) or microscissors in the right hand. Interfascicular nerve repair is now the treatment of choice in cleanly incised fresh nerve injuries in which correct fascicular matching is feasible (90% of cases); by checking the rotational orientation of the alignment of the longitudinally running blood vessels in the epineurium, the corresponding fascicular groups can be readily identified.
- Nerve electrostimulation.
- Nerve glues (thromboplastin).
- Nerve wrapping, e.g. tantalum foil, Silastic or Millipore to prevent epineural fibrosis and the spurting of axons from the suture line which may produce a painful local lesion.
- Embedding – sutured nerve may be embedded among muscle fibres through an opening in the muscle sheath.
- Plaster cast – advisable after placing the limb in a suitable position to prevent any nerve strain.

Results

Depend on:
- Preoperative factors
  - The nerve affected: maldistribution is great in mixed nerve repair.
  - Infection.
  - Time.
  - Preoperative management of injured muscles and tendons.
- Operative technique
- Postoperative factors
  - Absence of infection.
  - After treatment, maintenance of relaxation of paralysed muscles, massage, electrical treatment and muscular effort.
  - Patient cooperation.
  - Vicarious movements of other muscle groups.

IRREMEDIABLE INJURY

When primary neurorrhaphy is impossible, owing to actual loss of the nerve substance, one of the following procedures is advisable.

- Nerve grafting from autogenous sural or lateral cutaneous nerve of the thigh to bridge the gap created by the injured nerve.
- Nerve anastomosis, e.g. part of the hypoglossal nerve to the distal end of the facial nerve.
- Tendon transplantation, e.g. in radial paralysis.
- Arthrodesis.
- Amputation.

Compression–entrapment nerve injury

May include:

- Root lesion, e.g. cervical spondylosis and intervertebral disc protrusion.
- Plexus lesion, e.g. thoracic outlet syndrome.
- Cranial nerves (rarely), e.g. conductive deafness in Paget's disease due to bony entrapment of facial nerve.
- Peripheral nerves (commonly).

The compression is either external (e.g. cast, plaster and bandage) or internal (e.g. haematoma due to anticoagulant therapy). The entrapment is the compression in the natural pathways in fascial planes or fibro-osseous tunnels especially during movement. Examples of nerve entrapment are:

Median nerve

- Pronator syndrome (between pronator teres heads): causes signs of median nerve palsy confined to the hand.
- Anterior interosseous syndrome (via interosseous membrane): affects pinch grip with severe pain.
- Carpal tunnel syndrome: acroparaesthesia, tingling and burning pain worse at night and wasting of thenar muscles. The pain is relieved by hanging the hand from the bed. Commonly affects females, usually in the dominant hand. Predisposing factors act either via carpal tunnel narrowing (e.g. rheumatoid arthritis, wrist fracture, tenosynovitis, gout and ganglion rarely) or via enlargement of tunnel contents (e.g. venous engorgement due to dialysis and shunt, contraceptive pill, pregnancy, myxoedema, acromegaly). However, commonly carpal tunnel syndrome is idiopathic. Treatment is by deroofing of the median nerve (decompression via longitudinal incision of flexure retinaculum).

Ulnar nerve

- Old supracondylar fracture of humerus with cubitus valgus leads to tardy ulnar nerve palsy. Fixation of the nerve (due to adhesions following osteoarthritis) or injury can occur in the cubital tunnel (i.e. elbow tunnel syndrome) after it passes behind the medial humeral epicondyle under the arcuate ligament into the forearm between flexor carpi ulnaris and flexor digitorum profundus. There is sensory loss of the medial one and a half fingers and wasting of the hypothenar, interossei and medial two lumbrical muscles (claw hand). Treatment is by anterior transposition of the nerve to the front of the medial epicondyle.
- Entrapment at wrist, palm or in Guyton's canal towards the little finger (no sensory loss). The small intrinsic muscles of the medial aspect of the hand are affected.

Radial nerve

- In the spiral groove of the humerus due to heavy sleep with the arm over the sharp back of a kitchen chair (Saturday night paralysis).
- Posterior interosseous nerve (entrapped between two heads of the supinator muscle). The extensors of the wrist and fingers are affected.

Thoracic outlet syndrome

Due to cervical rib in 0.5–1% of the population. Fibromuscular band may cause the same syndrome. C8/T1 (lower trunk of brachial plexus) is affected with selective wasting of hand muscles (neurological). The vascular component is due to thromboembolism of the poststenotic dilated segment. The pain does not wake the patient at night. Electromyography (EMG) can determine whether the pain is due to cervical rib or to carpal tunnel syndrome.

Meralgia paraesthetica

Entrapment of lateral cutaneous nerve of the thigh as it passes through the inguinal ligament leading to hyperaesthesia and tingling in the lateral aspect of the thigh.

Anterior tibial compartment syndrome

Due to common or lateral peroneal nerve entrapment as the nerve winds around the fibular neck deep to the tendinous arch of the origin of peroneus longus. The condition occurs after unusual exercise, trauma (fracture, soft tissue injury or bandage) and arterial thromboembolism of the iliac, femoral or anterior tibial artery. Treatment is by fasciotomy through a 5 cm longitudinal incision of the lateral aspect of the leg.

Tarsal tunnel syndrome

The tibial nerve is entrapped in a fibro-osseous tunnel deep to flexor retinaculum behind and below the medial malleolus. Clinically, the condition is equivalent to carpal tunnel syndrome. A sphygmomanometer cuff inflated up to systolic blood pressure, applied around the calf for 1 min may reproduce the symptoms. Treatment is by decompression.

Morton's metatarsalgia

Due to neuroma (intermetatarsal bursitis) on the interdigital nerve between the metatarsal heads. Treatment is by excision of bursa.

1.72 Burns Management and Principles of Skin Grafting

BURNS MANAGEMENT

Burns present clinically in four stages:
1. Shock.
2. Infection.
3. Healing.
4. Contracture and scarring.

Generally burns are classified according to their depth into partial thickness (pin-prick pain sensation is present) or full thickness (pain sensation is lost) irrespective of the cause (whether thermal, electrical, chemical or radiation burns). Mortality depends on the percentage of burned surface area (Rule of Nine), patient age and the efficiency of the treatment. Generally, if the age + the percentage area affected is over 100, the chances of survival are very poor.

Treatment

General

- Ensure non-obstructed airways and remove clothes.
- Estimate the percentage of surface burns (Rule of Nine) and the body weight (in kg).
- Via an i.v. or venous cut-down a transfusion of Dextran 110 or plasma solution is given to all adults with 15% burn and all children with 10% or more burn. Deep burns require blood transfusion in addition. In 10–25% burn, the second ration is replaced by blood transfusion, while in 25–50% burn the second and sixth rations are replaced by blood transfusions (see below).
- The volume of colloid to be transfused is six equal rations over six consecutive periods of 4, 4, 4, 6, 6 and 12 h.

$$1 \text{ ration (ml)} = \frac{\% \text{ surface burn} \times \text{weight (kg)}}{2}$$

- If colloid is unavailable, then crystalloid (normal saline and dextrose) can be used.

$$1 \text{ ration (ml)} = \% \text{ surface burn} \times \text{weight (kg)}$$

- The need and rate of infusion subsequently depend on clinical and laboratory observations, e.g. blood pressure, pulse rate, CVP (should be 10–15 cmH$_2$O), urine output (via a catheter), vomiting and packed cell volume (PCV).
- Analgesic morphine 10–20 mg i.v. (as required).
- Oral fluids are given as 60 ml/h increased to 100 ml/h (if there is no nausea). Burn of 35% or over needs nasogastric suction hourly.
- Curling peptic ulcer and the possible need for cimetidine therapy should be remembered.
- Antibiotics are required, particularly against Pseudomonas, the main intensive therapy unit microorganism (e.g. gentamicin and carbenicillin).

Local

The aims are to achieve skin cover and prevent infection and further skin loss.
- Exposure treatment (after skin cleansing with cetrimide–chlorhexidine solution) is practised in head and neck burns and those on a single surface of the trunk or limbs.
- Antiseptic dressing (after skin cleansing) is used in other burn sites. It is done in three layers, i.e. silver sulphadiazine (Flamazine) ointment with Soframycin is placed immediately next to the skin, followed by cotton gauze then absorbent wool held in place with crêpe.
- In full-thickness burns the black slough is separated in 3 weeks through frequent baths and hypochlorite solution (Eusol). Recently there is a tendency to use early excision and skin grafting to speed up the healing and to reduce the risk of infection. Then a split skin graft (autograft) is used for cover; alternatively lyophilised skin (xenograft) or amnion dressing is used.
- Deep localised burns, e.g. electrical, need early local excision and grafting.

Complications

1. Respiratory damage due to smoke inhalation (requires oxygen therapy and/or tracheostomy).
2. Infection, especially Pseudomonas.
3. Anaemia due to deep burns (destroying red cells) and/or gastrointestinal tract bleeding due to curling ulcer.
4. Acute renal failure due to hypovolaemic shock.
5. Metabolic complications, e.g. hypokalaemia, hyponatraemia (sick cell syndrome) – treated with dextrose solution, insulin and potassium chloride. Also hypoxia and acidosis (due to tissue underperfusion, lung atelectasis – smoke inhalation and immobility – and increased oxygen needs). Glycosuria and hyperglycaemia can also occur.
6. Burn encephalopathy due to water intoxication, hypertension (caused by stress) and pyrexia.
7. Late burn contractures and deformities.
8. Eschar: escharotomy to divide eschar in the chest (to relieve breathing) and in the limbs (to maintain blood supply in deep burn.

PRINCIPLES OF SKIN GRAFTING

Indicated in:
- Trauma (fingers and skin).
- Burns.
- Certain diseases (e.g. varicose ulcer).
- Surgical excision of a neoplasm (e.g. malignant melanoma).

The aim is to cover the raw area and obtain healing in order to limit deformity and/or disability.

Free skin grafts

Are used when the raw surface is healthy vascularised tissue (e.g. subcutaneous tissue, deep fascia, paratenon) or clean granulations.

Split-thickness graft (Thiersch)   Consists of one-third to two-thirds of skin thickness. The skin is usually taken from the thigh by a Watson's knife or dermatome. The graft is taken easily and can be fixed by sutures, but it has a tendency to shrink. After being taken, the graft is placed on a wood board and covered with tulle gras. It is then applied to the area with a pressure dressing to secure cohesion between the two surfaces and prevent oedema, haematoma or seroma formation. A split graft can be punctured to spread it over a wide area (*mesh graft*), e.g. in extensive burns. When cut into postage stamp size pieces it is called a 'patch graft' and this is done to ensure escape of exudate without hindrance and facilitate the take.

Full-thickness graft (Wolfe)   Consists of full skin thickness, which is defatted (no subcutaneous fat). It is not easy to take but has no tendency to shrink and is of a better colour and texture than a split-skin graft. May be taken from the postauricular area to cover excised rodent ulcer of the face; from the supraclavicular area again for use on the face; or from the groin to use on the hand. Cone-shaped pieces (*pinch grafts*) indicated mainly in infection (diabetes) and in venous ulcers can be taken, providing a hardy graft with better survival in sepsis but with slow healing, scarring and poor cosmetic results.

Pedicle flaps (Fig. 1.72.1)

Indicated to cover areas with exposed cartilage, open joints, bare cortical bone or bare tendon, and if the vitality of the recipient area has been depressed by scarring or radiotherapy. Also in defects involving a cavity, e.g. full thickness excision of the lip or cheek. The flap is skin with subcutaneous tissue which remains attached to the body by one end to maintain its blood supply.

Types include:

- *Local flaps* to repair skin defects by *local V-Y or Z-plasty adjustment,* by *skin transposition* or by *rotational flaps.*
- *Direct flaps,* e.g. *cross-finger flap, cross-leg flap* and *abdomen-to-hand flap.*
- *Indirect flap via an intermediate carrier site,* e.g. from the abdomen to the face or to the lower limb using the wrist as a carrier.
- *Pedicle vascular flap* (retaining its vascular or neurovascular axial pedicle) e.g. *island flaps* of amputated finger tip.
- *Myocutaneous flap* is another modification, e.g. *latissimus dorsi flap* for postmastectomy reconstruction, *tensor fasciae latae flap* used for closure of defects overlying the greater trochanter.

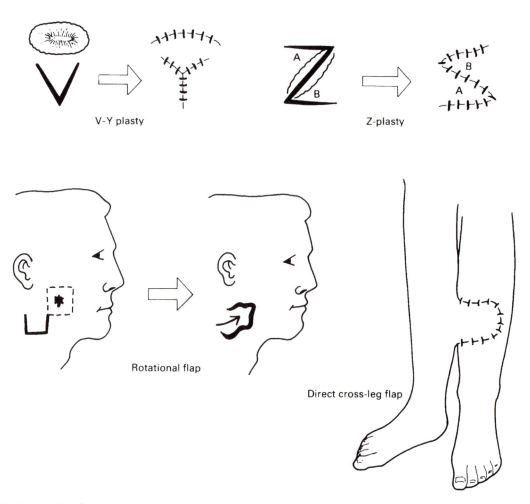

Fig. 1.72.1   Some pedicle flaps

Free vascular transplant

Necessitates microvascular reanastomosis of the skin flap artery to the recipient artery.

Tissue expanders

Recently developed tissue expanders are being increasingly used to repair local defects. These are prostheses implanted adjacent to the defect and inflated gradually over a 2–3 week period to expand the overlying tissue which can subsequently be used to close the defect.

Factors affecting take

- Recipient site nature (e.g. cartilage, bone or bare tendon), vitality (e.g. depressed by radiotherapy) and type of defect (e.g. involving a cavity).

- Technique (proper graft for proper area).
- Ischaemia.
- Infection.
- Haematoma or seroma formation.
- Mobility damages graft take.

1.73 Trauma Evaluation and Prognosis

TRIAGE AND TRAUMA SCORE

At the accident site, first aid treatment must be provided to establish a clear airway and adequate oxygenation as the

Table 1.73.1 Trauma score (trauma index) assessment of general physiological stability

		Value	*Code*	*Score*
A. Respiratory rate		10–24	4	
		25–35	3	
		>36	2	
		1–9	1	
		0	0	A = ...
B. Respiratory effort		normal/retractive	1	
		none	0	B = ...
C. Systolic pressure		>90	4	
		70–89	3	
		50–69	2	
		0–49	1	
		0	0	C = ...
D. Capillary refill		normal	2	
		delayed	1	
		none	0	D = ...
E. Glasgow Coma Score				
Eye opening				
spontaneous	4			
to voice	3	TOTAL GCS SCORE 14–15	5	
to pain	2	11–13	4	
none	1	8–10	3	
		5–7	2	
		3–4	1	
Verbal response				
orientated	5			
confused	4			E = ...
inappropriate words	3			
incomprehensible	2			
none	1			
Motor response				
obeys commands	6			
localises pain	5			
withdrawal on pain	4			
flexion on pain	3			
extension on pain	2			
none	1			

TRAUMA SCORE = A + B + C + D + E

Survival is about 99% for a score of 16 – walking wounded: priority 4
90% for a score of 12 – treat and transport: priority 2
50% for a score of 8 – treat and transport: priority 1
10% for a score of 4 – treat and transport: immediate priority 1

INTENSIVE THERAPY UNIT		APACHE SCORING SHEET				NAME:				
POINTS >	4		3		2		1		0	SUM
TEMP °C	>41	<29.9	39–40.9	30–31.9		32–33.9	38.5–38.9	34–35.9	36–38.4	
MEAN S.B.P.	>160	<49	130–159		110–129	50–69			70–109	
HEART RATE	>180	<39	140–179	40–54	110–139	55–69			70–109	
RESP. RATE	>50	<5	35–49			6–9	25–34	10–11	12–24	
FiO$_2$ > 0.5 A–aDO$_2$	>68.8		46.7–68.7		26.7–46.6					
FiO$_2$ > 0.5 PaO$_2$		<7.3		7.3–8.0			8.1–8.3			
ART. pH	>7.7	<7.15	7.6–7.69	7.15–7.24		7.25–7.32	7.5–7.59		7.33–7.49	
SERUM Na$^+$	>180	<110	160–179	111–119	155–159	120–129	150–154		130–149	
SERUM K$^+$	>7.0	<2.5	6–6.9			2.5–2.9	5.5–5.9	3.0–3.4	3.5–5.4	
SERUM CREATININE	>301		169–300		125–168	<53			54–124	
PCV	>60	<20			50–59.9	20–29.9	46–49.9		30–45.9	
WBC	>40	<1			20–39.9	1–2.9	15–19.9		3–14.9	
AGE RANGE	>75		65–74		55–64		45–54		<45	
AGE POINTS	6		5		3		2		0	

GLASGOW COMA SCALE	BEST EYE RESPONSE ------> 1–4 POINTS	TOTAL	15 MINUS TOTAL
	BEST MOTOR RESPONSE ------> 1–5 POINTS		
	BEST VERBAL RESPONSE ------> 1–6 POINTS		

CHRONIC HEALTH SCORE
Cirrhosis or portal hypertension
Cardiovascular status NYHA class IV
Severe chronic respiratory disease
Renal dialysis patients
Immunosuppression due to disease/drugs/therapy

NO --------> SCORE 0
YES – ELECTIVE POST-OP?
    ├── YES ──> SCORE 2
    └── NO ──> SCORE 5

SCORING DOCTOR	SIGNATURE	DATE	TOTAL APACHE SCORE	PTS.

Fig. 1.73.1 A typical APACHE scoring sheet

first priority in an unconscious patient (**ABC**, **A**irway, **B**reathing and **C**irculation). This also includes occluding any sucking chest wound (to stop the progress of open pneumothorax), applying pressure to external bleeding and placing patients on their side in anticipation of first vomit (handled with care until spinal injury can be proved later). Urgent tracheal intubation and pain relief may be practised too.

Then comes disaster categorisation in a scale to conform with severity and action required (**Triage**). Triage includes primary survey to categorise victims for priority and type of evacuation. The 6-category triage includes:

Priority 1   life-threatening but savable.
Priority 2   serious injury but stable and can wait a little.
Priority 3   non-walking wounded.
Priority 4   walking wounded.
Priority 5   life-threatening but unsavable (e.g. high velocity head injury).
Priority 6   dead.

Trauma can then be scored (**trauma score** or **trauma index**), after assessing general physiological stability of the individual triage categories, according to a trauma scoring system (see Table 1.73.1).

PROGNOSIS SCORING OF CRITICALLY ILL PATIENTS

Apache II and III (USA)

An acronym for Acute Physiology And Chronic Health Evaluation (APACHE). The tests used for the scoring system show correct prediction of mortality, and can be useful for inter-unit comparisons and multicentre trials. The APACHE prognosis score is used in early assessment of recently admitted patients to the Accident and Emergency Unit, or to the Intensive Care/Therapy Unit (ICU or ITU). APACHE II and III are developments of APACHE, based on general health, severe organ insufficiency or immunocompromised state, giving:

5 points for non-operative or emergency postoperative cases; and
2 points for elective postoperative cases.
Organ failure is defined as:
– Proven cirrhosis, portal hypertension or hepatic failure.
– Cardiovascular – NYHA class IV.
– Respiratory – severe exercise restriction, unable to climb stairs, respirator dependency, pulmonary hypertension > 40 mmHg.
– Chronic renal dialysis.
– Immunocompromised by drugs, radiotherapy or advanced disease, e.g. leukaemia, lymphoma, AIDS.

Age points: < 44 years   = 0
                       45–54   = 2
                       55–64   = 3
                       65–74   = 5
                       > 75 = 6

Worst values = are scored for 12 physiological measurements during the first 24 h after admission to the Accident and Emergency Department or ITU, as follows. Each parameter is scored from 0 (normal) to $+4$ (abnormally high or low).

1. Rectal temperature points, °C: $> 41 = 4$; $> 39 = 3$; $> 38.5 = 1$; $36–38.4 = 0$; $34–35.9 = 1$; $32–33.9 = 2$; $30–31.9 = 3$; and $< 29.9 = 4$.
2. Mean arterial pressure, mmHg: $> 160 = 4$; $130–159 = 3$; $110–129 = 2$; $70–109 = 0$; $50–69 = 2$; $40–54 = 3$; and $< 49 = 4$.
3. Heart rate, bpm: $> 180 = 4$; $140–179 = 3$; $110–139 = 2$; $70–109 = 0$; $55–69 = 2$; $40–54 = 3$; and $< 39 = 4$.
4. Respiratory rate, bpm: $> 50 = 4$; $35–49 = 3$; $25–34 = 1$; $12–24 = 0$; $10–11 = 1$; $6–9 = 2$; and $< 5 = 4$.
5. Oxygenation points. $AaDO_2$ on $Fio_2 > 0.5$, KPa: $> 66.8 = 4$; $46.7–66.7 = 3$; and $26.7–46.5 = 2$; Pao_2 on $Fio_2 < 0.5$, KPa: $8.1–8.3 = 1$; $7.3–8 = 3$; and $< 7.3 = 4$.
6. Arterial pH points: $> 7.7 = 4$; $7.6–7.69 = 3$; $7.5–7.59 = 1$; $7.33–7.49 = 0$; $7 25–7.32 = 2$; $7.15–7.24 = 3$; and $< 7.15 = 4$.
7. Serum Na^+ (mmol/l), points: $> 180 = 4$; $160–179 = 3$; $155–159 = 2$; $150–154 = 1$; $130–149 = 0$; $120–129 = 2$; $111–119 = 3$; and $< 110 = 4$.
8. Serum K^+ (mmol/l) points: $> 7 = 4$; $6–6.9 = 3$; $5.5–5.9 = 1$; $3.5–5.4 = 0$; $3–3.4 = 1$; $2.5–2.9 = 2$; and $< 2.5 = 4$.
9. Serum creatinine (mmol/l) (points are doubled for *acute renal failure*): $> 300 = 4$.
10. Haematocrit.
11. White cell count.
12. Glasgow Coma Score (rating = 15 – actual GCS).

A total score of 10 relates to a mortality of about 10%.
A total score of 20 relates to a mortality of about 20%.
A total score of 30 relates to a mortality of about 40%.
A total score of 35 relates to a mortality of about 75%.
A total score of 40 relates to a mortality of about 90%.
A total score of 55 relates to a mortality of about 100%.

APACHE III allows for developments of the patient's condition while in the ITU, and decision-making about stopping active treatment. Figure 1.73.1 shows a typical APACHE scoring sheet.

ORTHOPAEDIC SURGERY

1.74 Common Surgical Conditions Affecting the Hip Joint

CONGENITAL DISLOCATION OF THE HIP

True dislocation of the hip at birth is rare. The condition referred to as congenital dislocation of the hip (CDH) is a dysplastic condition of the joint which predisposes to dislocation.

Incidence

Examination of the newborn in the UK reveals unstable or subluxating hips in 1.7%. However, 68% of these will stabilise within a week and 88% by the end of 2 months. After this time 1.5 per 1000 will have a true dislocation.

The incidence is affected by a number of factors.

Sex   Higher incidence in girls (7:1).

Epidemiology   The variable incidence in different population groups may have a genetic basis:

UK	1.5/1000
Sweden	1/100
Lapps/North American Indians	5/100
Chinese	Very low incidence

This may be explained by nurture. The higher incidence groups tend to swaddle babies with their hips extended and adducted, while the Chinese carry their children with hips spreadeagled in flexion-abduction.

Familial   Ten times higher incidence than general population in siblings of affected children. Incidence of 40% in second monozygous twin if first affected. There may be familial joint laxity.

Joint laxity   In boys there may be a genetic basis. In girls there may be a hormonal basis. Circulating maternal relaxins may be responsible.

Fetal position   In one series 16% of CDH were breech born. In another study 50% of breeches had CDH. Extended breech births have a still higher incidence.

Aetiology and pathogenesis

The two constant features of CDH are acetabular dysplasia and ligamentous laxity, but the relationship between the two in the initiation of the process which leads to dislocation and how much instability itself contributes remain unknown.

Anteversion of the femoral head accompanies dysplasia of the acetabulum and the two worsen the longer the joint is unstable or dislocated. It is thought that anteversion and acetabular dysplasia contribute in a complementary fashion to the pathogenesis of the condition.

Primary acetabular dysplasia in a typical case may be evidenced at birth. There is osseous hypoplasia of the roof of the acetabulum but the cartilagenous contribution is intact. Provided concentric pressure from the femoral head can be applied to the cartilage, it responds by ossification and spontaneous correction. In the majority this does not occur and the acetabulum remains hypoplastic. The femoral head migrates upwards and outwards and the femoral neck becomes anteverted. An anteverted head applies pressure to the anterior part of the acetabulum and flattens and everts the fibrocartilagenous limbus. The acetabular cartilage deforms. As the socket flattens its ossification becomes delayed. Actual dislocation of the hip occurs when the femoral head passes over the fibrocartilagenous rim and the head loses contact with the acetabular floor. The limbus inverts as a result of its inherent elastic recoil. Reduction of the femoral head is prevented by the secondary soft tissue changes which occur.

Pathology

The head of the femur is in a 'false acetabulum' on the outer surface of the ilium with capsule interposed between it and periosteum. The cartilagenous head is large in comparison with the empty acetabulum, and flattened medially and posteriorly. Its ossification is delayed. The femoral neck may be anteverted up to 90°.

The acetabular floor and outer surface of the ilium lie in a straight line. The floor of the acetabulum becomes overgrown with fibrocartilage to which capsule often adheres. The ligamentum teres is either attenuated or hypertrophied. At the point where the psoas tendon crosses the capsule, it becomes constricted and resembles an hour glass; the head of the femur is in the upper chamber and the lower one contains the acetabular contents. The muscles attached to the femur either lengthen, resulting in their mechanical disadvantage, or shorten, so that they act as blocks to reduction of the head.

Clinical presentation and radiological features

Neonatal period

All neonates should be examined for abnormalities of the hip joint. The examiner should note assymetry of the skin folds of the thigh, eccentricity of the labia and widening of the perineum (bilateral CDH). An abduction contracture may or may not be present. Shortening of the femur may be apparent (Galeazzi's sign) and the trochanter of the affected side will be above Nélaton's line. On testing movements abduction is limited while internal rotation is often increased. Ortolani's manoeuvre may reveal subluxation of the hip as a 'click' or jerk as the femoral head rides over the acetabular margin and goes back into the socket. On the basis of Barlow's test the severity

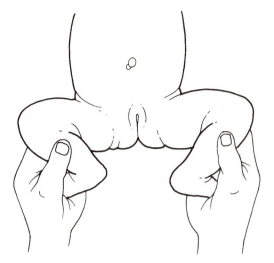

Fig. 1.74.1   Ortolani–Barlow test (abduction of flexed hip and knee joints)

of the instability of an abnormal hip can be graded (Fig. 1.74.1). Hips will generally be normal, minimally unstable, severely unstable or truly discolated.

In the neonatal period radiological screening for CDH is generally of no value. However, signs that may be of value include increase in the acetabular angle and lack of definition of the lateral lip of the acetabulum. A line drawn along the shaft of the femur should pass through the triradiate cartilage (Von Rosen's line) but in CDH it does not. X-rays of the femur in different positions should show the depth from the ossified femur to the acetabular floor to be the same; if not, subluxation can be inferred.

Infants

A dislocated hip may be suspected in the presence of assymetry, clicking of the hip or difficulty in putting the child in nappies because of limitation of abduction on the affected side. When the child starts to walk, assymetry may become more obvious and the child may limp (Trendelenburg gait). In bilateral CDH a 'rolling sailor's gait' is observed and lumbar lordosis is exaggerated. Normally, the secondary ossification centre for the femoral head appears between age 4 and 6 months, but in CDH its appearance is delayed, sometimes up to the age of 12 months. Drawing vertical lines from the lateral edge of the acetabulum and horizontal lines through the triradiate cartilages (Perkin's lines), the secondary ossification centre of the femoral head should be located inferomedially. In CDH the ossification centre lies superolaterally. The acetabulum is obviously shallow and anteversion of the femoral neck may be obvious. A false acetabulum, seen as a shallow depression in the ilium, is sometimes visible. The labrum is folded in the acetabular shallow cavity, the ligaments are lax, muscles are shortened and the capsule is elongated.

Management

The majority (90%) of clicking hips at birth stabilise within 2 months. For minor instability double nappies worn for 2 weeks

will normally suffice. More severe instability at birth or persistent minor instability beyond 2 weeks warrants application of an abduction splint. If at the end of a 3 month period the hip is stable and developing normally, as judged by X-rays, the splint can be restricted to use at night only. Follow-up is for 18 months and frequent out-patient checks are made in this period.

Residual instability at 3 months or the discovery of an unstable hip beyond the neonatal period requires concentric reduction of the femoral head. This can usually be achieved by gentle traction and closed reduction. The child's hip is held in a 'frog plaster' in abduction until stability is achieved.

Secondary changes in the soft tissues as described above may prevent concentric reduction, in which case operative treatment is indicated. Soft tissue release and derotation osteotomy will usually suffice in children up to the age of 3 years, but beyond this age an additional innominate osteotomy is usually required.

Operative treatment

Soft tissue procedures

Release of the psoas tendon may be sufficient to allow concentric reduction of the femoral head. However, excision of the joint capsule, removal of the acetabular contents, including the ligamentum teres, or an inverted limbus may be required.

Derotation osteotomy

Approximately 80% of cases of CDH diagnosed late have significant anteversion of the femoral neck. Concentric reduction of the femoral head and abduction in a frog plaster will result in spontaneous correction of anteversion in some cases. Persistent anteversion exceeding 60% requires subtrochanteric derotation osteotomy. This may also be required if the femoral head displaces after closed reduction.

Innominate osteotomy

CDH presenting between the ages of 18 months and 6 years is associated with the complete gamut of soft tissue and bony problems and requires operative intervention. In addition to soft tissue release and removal of interposed soft tissues plus derotation osteotomy, innominate osteotomy is required to ensure concentric reduction of the femoral head. The Salter osteotomy swivels the acetabulum to cover the anterolateral defect. The Pemberton osteotomy or acetabuloplasty rotates the anterosuperior acetabulum laterally and downwards and has the advantage over the Salter osteotomy of not creating a defect posteriorly. The Chiari osteotomy displaces the acetabulum medially and creates an extension to its root laterally.

PERTHES' DISEASE

Aetiology

This condition of the hip joint affecting children between the ages of 3 and 10 years is not an inflammatory condition but is considered to have an ischaemic aetiology resulting in the upper capital epiphysis becoming wholly or partially avascular.

Depending upon the extent of the avascular necrosis the capital epiphysis becomes deformed and the hip dysplastic. The average duration of the disease is between $2\frac{1}{2}$ and 4 years.

The aetiology of the condition is unknown but genetic, anatomical and environmental factors have been implicated; 80% of those affected are boys. The sharply defined age range correlates well with a period when the capital epiphysis is nourished principally by a precarious blood supply from vessels crossing the lateral epiphyseal line. Four percent have associated major genitourinary abnormalities (the hip and genitourinary system are derived embryologically from the mesonephric ridge). The skeletal maturity of children with Perthes' disease is delayed.

Clinical presentation and radiological features

Clinically the child presents with pain in the hip and a limp. There may be limitations of hip movements, muscular wasting of the buttock and thigh, and shortening of the limb if the femoral head collapses.

Radiological studies indicate that changes occur in the femoral epiphysis and metaphysis, the acetabulum and joint cavity. The earliest feature is flattening and sclerosis of the lateral anterosuperior quadrant of the epiphysis associated with translucency of the adjoining metaphysis. As the head undergoes avascular necrosis it becomes dense, flattened and broader, and a linear translucency can be seen within it. As revascularisation takes place the epiphysis assumes a fragmented appearance with translucent areas. The metaphyseal area of the femur is also affected: it becomes broader and rounded off and the neck of the femur shortens relatively. Cysts often appear on the metaphysis. Within the acetabular cavity the distance between the medial side of the capital epiphysis and the acetabulum appears increased, owing to an increase in thickness of the articular cartilage. The acetabulum becomes dysplastic, adapting itself to the changes in the head of the femur.

Radiological classification and prognosis

Perthes' disease is a self-limiting condition with an overall fair prognosis which is better in boys and the younger child. The problem has been to identify those children with the disease likely to have a poor outcome if untreated.

A radiological classification based upon the extent of involvement of the femoral head and identifying the 'head at risk' has been made by Catterall. Using this classification treatment is reserved for those children with 'head at risk'.

Group I	Only anterior epiphysis involved.
	No collapse of the femoral head occurs.
Group II	More of anterior epiphysis involved with appearance of a dense oval collapsed sequestrum.
	As this sequestrum is absorbed collapse of the head occurs.
	Metaphyseal cysts may be seen.
Group III	Only a small part of epiphysis not sequestrated.
	As collapse occurs lateral segment displaces and metaphysis broadens.
Group IV	Whole epiphysis sequestrated.
	Mushrooming of femoral head.
	Extensive metaphyseal changes.

'Head at risk'	Small V-shaped osteoporotic defect of lateral epiphysis accompanied by similar defect in metaphysis – Gage's sign.
	Lateral calcification.
	Lateral displacement of the femoral head.
	Diffuse or extensive metaphyseal changes.
	Horizontally disposed growth plate.

Management

- Rest for the irritable hip.
- Careful supervision and radiological follow-up until revascularisation complete.
- Treatment for 'head at risk' aimed at containment of the femoral head concentrically within the acetabulum.

OSTEOARTHROSIS OF THE HIP

The nomenclature of this condition is disputed. It is primarily a degenerative disease of the joint and therefore some clinicians use only the term osteoarthrosis. Others prefer the term osteoarthritis since they argue that it only becomes symptomatic when secondary inflammatory changes take place in the soft tissues.

Secondary osteoarthrosis can follow trauma, inflammatory and pyogenic arthritis, haemophilia, gout and avascular necrosis.

Primary osteoarthrosis is used to describe the degenerative joint disease where none of the above factors apply. In this condition, a myriad of clinical syndromes have been described but its aetiology is ill-understood. Occupation and obesity are implicated and there are poorly defined genetic factors. There is a rising non-linear relationship with age. Fifty per cent of all adults have at least one joint affected and 7% are disabled by osteoarthrosis. Between the ages of 55 and 65, 80% have radiological evidence of the condition and this rises to 98% between the ages of 65 and 74 years.

Pathology

Osteoarthrosis is not primarily an inflammatory condition but a degenerative one. The primary lesion is the articular cartilage with secondary inflammation in the soft tissues.

In the hip joint it has been demonstrated that in 71% of joints the primary degeneration of the articular cartilage occurs in the non-weight-bearing areas, in 3% it starts in the pressure areas and in 26% in a combination of both. The cartilage receives its nourishment by intermittent compression causing imbibition of synovial fluid. The absence of this pumping mechanism in the non-weight-bearing areas would support the theory that the lack of nutrition begins the degenerative process.

The non-weight-bearing cartilage becomes soft, heaps up and undergoes fibrillation. In response the subchondral blood vessels hypertrophy and invade the cartilage which then undergoes calcification with osteophyte formation. The loss of cartilage results in fissuring and cleft formation, and also exposes the underlying bone which becomes dense and eburnated. Cysts form beneath the pressure areas; their enlargement is probably caused by synovial fluid being forced into them through cracks in the cartilage as a result of pressure from joint movement. Trabecular fatigue fractures result in decrease in bone height and irregularities of the articular surface. Areas of hyperaemia with venous stasis develop in the bone ends and venous engorgement is said to contribute to night pain which is a feature of the disease.

Biochemical changes in the cartilage precede the visible changes. There is a loss of matrix proteoglycans and collagen. Death of chondrocytes occurs in the degenerating areas. Increased cell division in the cartilage that is left and increased glycoaminoglycan synthesis cannot maintain cartilage repair. Release of enzymes from the chondrocytes into the synovial fluid aggravates the process and, together with the detritus of cartilage flakes, causes synovitis. The synovium undergoes hyperplasia with villous formation. The cartilage flakes and small pieces of bone enter the synovium and the underlying joint capsule becomes involved in the inflammatory process. The capsule and synovium thicken and become fibrosed with consequent shortening and reduction in the range of movement of the joint.

Loose body formation occurs as a result of detachment of osteophytes and pieces of bone and cartilage from the joint surface and shedding of cartilagenous synovial polyps into the joint space. These further damage the joint and give rise to locking.

Clinical features

Aching is usually the first sign of the disease and is probably due to synovitis. It gradually becomes severe and constant. Night pain prevents the patient from sleeping. Pain may be referred to the knee.

Stiffness is a prominent symptom and is worse after resting. It is due to fibrosis and oedema in the capsule. Deformity arises from muscular spasm and capsular fibrosis. The patient limps as a result of a fixed flexion deformity associated with adduction and external rotation of the femur.

The patient walks with an antalgic or a Trendelenburg gait and the affected limb may be obviously adducted and externally rotated with a fixed flexion deformity. Quadriceps wasting may be noted.

The examiner should note old scars and sinuses around the hip joint. Apparent shortening of the limb is greater than true shortening. Thomas' test may uncover a fixed flexion deformity.

The classic X-ray features of osteoarthrosis are joint space narrowing, osteophyte formation, subchondral sclerosis and subchondral cyst formation.

Management

Conservative measures result in improvement in approximately one-third of sufferers. Weight loss is to be encouraged. A walking stick held in the opposite hand should be used. A heel raise may prevent pain and limping. Short-wave diathermy is often helpful and non-steroidal anti-inflammatory drugs are indicated.

Surgery is principally reserved for pain relief but other indications include stiffness and deformity. Age is an important consideration in patient selection. The older patient with a more sedate life-style will do well. However, total hip replacements are carried out in younger age groups.

Total hip replacement

Total hip replacement (THR) has revolutionised the treatment of arthritis of the hip, superseding arthrodesis, femoral osteotomy and excision arthroplasty. THRs have given some patients 15 years of service and those being inserted now are expected to last over 20 years.

The THR prosthesis consists of:
- A femoral component – made of stainless steel, titanium or cobalt-chrome. The head size varies between 22 mm and the natural size. The smaller the head the lower the friction, but the larger ones have a greater range of movement.
- An acetabular cup – utilises high-density polyethylene or ultra-high molecular weight polypropylene which minimises friction at the joint surface.
- The components are fixed into place using methylmethacrylate. This is prepared just before insertion as a putty which hardens into a cement by an exothermic reaction once inside the body. Certain cements are antibiotic-loaded.

Operative technique

To minimise complications of THR – infection, dislocation, loosening of the components and fracture of the stem of the femoral component or fracture of the shaft of the femur – scrupulous attention to insertion technique is mandatory.

The patient should have no focus of infection. Preoperatively a prophylactic antibiotic is administered. The operation should be conducted in an ultra-clean laminar flow enclosure. The surgeon and all assistants wear Ventile gowns with an exhaust system.

In the preparation of the bone surfaces, the acetabulum is reamed so that it will accommodate the largest available cup and it is cleared entirely of all soft tissue, cartilage, fibro-cartilage and osteophytes. Keying holes for the cement are drilled into the ilium, pubis and ischium. The acetabular component is cemented into position 40° to the horizontal and in a neutral position.

The femoral head is removed with a Gigli saw. If an oscillating power saw is used the blade should be cooled with saline to prevent heating with consequent thermal destruction of osteocytes. The femoral shaft is reamed and cleared of all cancellous bone. A trial femoral component is inserted and reduction attempted. The prosthesis must not sit in a varus position. The trial prosthesis is removed, a cement restrictor placed in the femoral shaft and cement introduced into the reamed femur. The definitive prosthesis is inserted and held until the cement has cured, after which reduction is effected.

Revision arthroplasty

Revision of hip prostheses with complications are being carried out in increasing numbers. Loosening of the prosthesis and infection are the two major indications for revision surgery.

Revision arthroplasty should be regarded as a salvage operation.

TRAUMATIC DISLOCATION OF THE HIP

Posterior dislocation of the hip

The majority of posterior dislocations of the hip result from the 'dashboard' injury – force along the long axis of the femur while the thigh is adducted and flexed. Some arise as a result of blows to the back with the person stooping or kneeling, e.g. mining accidents.

Clinically the limb is adducted, medially rotated and shortened. It is important to exclude an injury to the sciatic nerve.

Radiographs may show a concomitant fracture of the posterior lip of the acetabulum.

The majority of these dislocations can be managed by closed reduction. Under a general anaesthetic using muscle relaxants, one of two manoeuvres can be used to reduce the dislocation:

● The hip is flexed, abducted, laterally rotated and then brought into extension in a neutral position (Bigelow's manoeuvre); or
● The hip is flexed, brought into a neutral position and the head of the femur lifted gently into the acetabulum.

Then, Hamilton–Russell traction is applied for 3 weeks, after which the patient is allowed up on crutches. Full weight-bearing is allowed at 6 weeks.

Anterior dislocation of the hip

Posterior dislocation of the hip is 20 times more common than anterior dislocation.

High type

As a result of forced external rotation and abduction of the extended hip, the head of the femur comes to lie on the pubic ramus opposite the iliopectineal eminence.

Clinically the hip is held in full extension, slightly flexed with up to 60° of abduction.

Low type

An external rotation and abduction force on the flexed hip results in the head of the femur coming to lie near the obturator foramen. Clinically, the limb is externally rotated in extension with some abduction. Reduction is effected by adducting the femur and medially rotating it. The head of the femur can be gently lifted into the acetabulum.

Dislocation of the hip associated with fractures of the acetabular rim

Posterior dislocation of the hip may be associated with a marginal fracture of the posterior lip of the acetabulum. The fragment is usually held closely to the head of the femur and reduction of the dislocation usually results in accurate replacement of the fragment. Occasionally if a large fragment is not reduced and the hip remains unstable in flexion, adduction and internal rotation, then operative reduction and fixation of the fragment with a single screw is indicated. Stable hips are treated as ordinary dislocations.

Complications of dislocation of the hip

Sciatic nerve palsy

Ten per cent of dislocations of the hip are associated with sciatic nerve palsy and in 80% of these the lesion is incomplete, affecting only the peroneal division. A nerve injury is much more common if there is an associated marginal fracture of the acetabulum. Operative intervention to decompress an injured sciatic nerve is reserved for those cases with an associated fracture. Straightforward dislocations with sciatic nerve injury are managed conservatively with expectation of recovery of function.

Irreducible dislocations

It is rare not to be able to reduce a hip. Inability to reduce the dislocation with a satisfying clunk or a non-concentric reduction on the 'post-reduction' film means that there must be soft tissue or interposed bony fragments. In these cases the hip must be explored and the offending impediments to reduction dealt with appropriately.

Avascular necrosis of the head of the femur

This is a late complication of dislocation of the hip affecting 10% of uncomplicated dislocations, 25% of cases with an associated fracture of the acetabulum and 50% of cases where there is also a fracture of the femoral neck.

Indications for operation

● Failure of reduction or non-concentric reduction of the hip because of soft tissue or bony interposition.
● Sciatic nerve injury in dislocations associated with a marginal fracture of the acetabulum.
● The unstable hip with a posterior acetabular fracture. The fragment of the acetabulum needs to be fixed with a screw.

Central fracture-dislocation of the hip

These are often part of a multiple injury and can easily be missed.

Group 1   This is a result of a 'dashboard and sideswipe' injury – pressure along the axis of the femur plus a blow to the greater trochanter. The weight-bearing portion of the acetabulum remains intact. Most commonly the head of the femur is medially displaced or posteriorly dislocated. Less often it is dislocated anteriorly.

Group 2   Direct injury to the greater trochanter and the pelvis results in a true central dislocation of the hip with comminution of the acetabulum including the weight-bearing area and the head of the femur pushed centrally through into the pelvis. A genitourinary injury is often associated with this fracture.

Management

Initially the patient is resuscitated and the affected limb placed in Hamilton–Russell traction. Associated injuries that have priority are treated.

Group 1 fracture-dislocations Open reduction and fixation is required:

● When the head of the femur is completely displaced from under the weight-bearing area and there is only one large bony fragment.

● When the head of the femur is partially displaced, lying partly in contact with the weight-bearing area and partly in contact with the displaced fragment.

Group 2 fracture-dislocations Treated conservatively with Hamilton–Russell traction for 6 weeks. Full weight-bearing is achieved by 3 months.

FRACTURES OF THE NECK OF THE FEMUR
(intracapsular and extracapsular fractures)

Most patients who sustain this injury are elderly females. However, no age or sex is exempt. In children and young adults the treatment of choice is internal fixation.

Treatment of fractures of the neck of the femur in the elderly is surgical if cardiac and pulmonary problems related to prolonged recumbency are to be avoided.

Intracapsular fractures

A lateral rotation strain to the lower limb transmitted to the femoral neck fractures it at or near the subcapital level. The problems of non-union and late avascular necrosis associated with this fracture are due to disruption of the retinacular blood vessels which cross the fracture. This may result in ischaemia to the femoral head.

Garden's classification (Fig 1.74.2)

Grade I Incomplete fracture of the femoral neck. The inferior cortex is not breached.

Grade II Complete fracture of the femoral neck including the inferior cortex. No displacement has occurred.

Grade III Complete fracture in which partial displacement has occurred. The distal fragment rotates laterally while the proximal fragment rotates medially and is abducted. In clean breaks the posterior retinacular attachment remains intact.

Grade IV Complete fracture with full displacement. Contact between the fragments is lost. The distal fragment is laterally rotated. The proximal fragment resumes its normal position within the acetabulum.

Treatment

Grades I and II

Internal fixation is the treatment of choice either by crossed screws or by closed nailing under image-intensified X-ray control. A sliding nail plate is preferable to a single pin. The incidence of avascular necrosis in these groups is low since the blood supply to the head of the femur is only minimally disturbed.

Grades III and IV

In these groups the incidence of avascular necrosis is high. This is thought to be due to a severe valgus deformity of the head of the femur.

Some surgeons maintain that the fractures in these groups should be perfectly reduced and internal fixation achieved with a sliding nail plate or dynamic hip screw (DHS). Others advocate prosthetic replacement of the head of the femur (e.g. with a cemented Thompson prosthesis) in order to avoid the complication of avascular necrosis and the subsequent necessity for a second operation.

Extracapsular (or trochanteric) fractures

In this type of fracture, union can usually be relied upon. To enable the early mobilisation of the patient and to avoid union with a coxa vara deformity, some form of internal fixation is necessary.

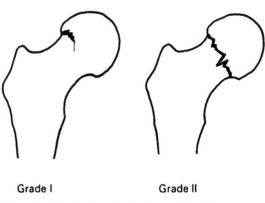
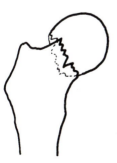

| Grade I | Grade II | Grade III | Grade IV |

Fig. 1.74.2 Garden's classification of intracapsular fractures

Classification and treatment

Stable fractures

Type I   The proximal fragment consists of the head and neck of the femur alone. Having no muscular attachments, the proximal fragment lies in the neutral position except in the slightly displaced fracture when it rotates laterally with the distal fragment. The fracture can be anatomically reduced by internally rotating the leg.

Type II   The proximal fragment consists of the head, neck and major part of the greater trochanter. The proximal fragment is laterally rotated and the fracture can only be reduced by external rotation of the leg.

Treatment is accurate anatomical reduction followed by internal fixation with a nail plate.

Unstable fractures

These are fractures with loss of continuity of bone cortex between the opposing surfaces of the proximal and distal fragments, either as a result of complete separation of the posterior trochanteric fragment or comminution of the calcar femorale medially.

Classically four fragments are seen: the head and neck of the femur, the greater trochanter, the lesser trochanter and the shaft of the femur. The problem with this fracture is that, despite anatomical reduction and internal fixation, a high percentage of the internal fixation devices fracture or migrate, resulting in union with a varus deformity of the neck of the femur.

The high failure rate has led to modifications of the traditional pin and plate fixation since it does not restore stability to the fracture. One modification is fixation of the fracture with medial displacement of the distal fragment followed by the insertion of a nail plate. Another method is to use curved intramedullary nails. These are introduced through the medial condyle of the femur and guided across the fracture into the femoral neck under image-intensified X-ray control.

1.75 Low Back Pain

Low back pain (LBP) is the commonest symptom encountered in orthopaedic practice; if accidents are excluded, it accounts for nearly a third of all outpatient attendances. Most people suffer from incapacitating LBP during some period in their lifetime. In the USA it is estimated that 25% of the manpower are affected every year, with 2 million unable to work, contributing to the loss of 93 million working days. LBP may be accompanied by radiating pain in the buttock, thigh, or leg on one side but occasionally on both (sciatica); therefore, a knowledge of the anatomy of the spine and nerve distribution is vital in the management.

CAUSES OF LOW BACK PAIN

Unfortunately, in the majority of patients, diagnosis is largely a matter of conjecture and no identifiable cause can be found.

However, causes of LBP are many; they include the following.

In adults

Spinal

Mechanical derangements   Acute and chronic back strain (pregnancy in females and strong coitus in males); prolapsed intervertebral disc; osteoarthritis; spinal stenosis; spondylolisthesis; fractures; spinal instability from old mal-united vertebral fractures; and spinal deformities, such as Scoliosis.

Infections of bone   Pyogenic of thoracic or lumbar spine, tuberculous, and brucellosis, Tuberculous spondylitis is common in developing countries, but is still seen in the Western world and can present with varied manifestations. Brucellosis should be suspected in endemic areas (cattle-and camel-raising areas).

Tumours   Primary or secondary vertebral bone tumours; spinal cord and nerve root tumours; multiple myeloma affecting the bone marrow of the elderly.

Others   Osteoporosis (post-menopausal and senile); rheumatoid arthritis; ankylosing spondylitis; Paget's disease; sickle cell disease (due to marrow hyperplasia secondary to anaemia, bone infarcts, vertebral collapse, and secondary pyogenic or Salmonella infection).

Extra-spinal

Intra-abdominal   Peptic uler and cholecystitis and calculi.

Retroperitoneal   Renal infection/calculi; pancreatic tumours; anuerysm of abdominal aorta.

Gynaecological   Chronic pelvic infection/inflammation; dysmenorrhoea; retroverted uterus; intra-pelvic masses.

In children

Back pain in childhood should be viewed seriously. The majority may be due to soft tissue injuries, but fractures, infections and neoplasia should be excluded.

- Congenital abnormalities, such as spina bifida and hemivertebra, may produce LBP.
- Deformities such as idiopathic structural scoliosis (of unknown aetiology) begin in childhood or adolescence and are progressive.
- Pyogenic and tuberculous osteomyelitis should be distinguished to enable effective treatment. In tuberculous infection, adjacent vertebrae are involved, the intervening disc space is narrowed and paravertebral abscess is common. Discitis due to infection is a recognised condition.
- Neoplasms such as nephroblastoma, neuroblastoma and teratoma (paravertebral tumours with vertebral extension) are seen in infants.
- Other conditions seen in children include spinal instability from a mal-united old vertebral fracture, eosinophilic

granuloma with vertebral collapse (vertebra plana, Calve's disease), and haemangioma. Scheuermann's disease (osteochondritis of the vertebral endplates) and disc protrusion affects the older child (adolescent).

DIAGNOSIS

The patient should be stripped completely, except for undergarments and, in women, a brassiere. A complete physical examination is imperative in order not to miss vital clues of certain conditions such as gout, rheumatoid arthritis and primary malignancy. The back should be examined and neurology evaluated (see s. 2.14).

Relevant investigations should be performed. A complete blood count (anaemia: multiple myeloma; neutrophil leucocytosis: infection; lymphocytosis: tuberculosis), ESR, blood culture, serum uric acid, rheumatoid factor, HLA-B 27, sickle cell test and electrophoresis, serum proteins and albumin–globulin ratio and serum protein electrophoresis (M-band in multiple myeloma), serum brucella titre, ASO titre, Bence–Jones protein in the urine, are all useful investigations.

The exact diagnosis may have to await the results of relevant investigations (e.g. infections, tumours etc.). X-rays may need to include oblique views of the spine (spondylolysis), sacroiliac joints etc. A myelogram may be necessary. CT scan or NMR are valuable in localising the pathology. A technetium bone scan is useful in vertebral osteomyelitis. In some, a needle aspiration, a needle or open biopsy may need to be performed for conclusive diagnosis. Discography and facet arthrograms are other useful investigations. A discogram can show a normal disc, a prolapsed disc, or an annular tear. It can also be used as a provocative test as the injection is painful and reproduces the pain experienced from a prolapsed disc. The facet arthrogram can delineate arthritic changes but its place as an investigative tool is not established.

TREATMENT

In general, the rule is to treat the cause (e.g. infections, tumours). The majority (in whom no cause is found) require only symptomatic treatment. The treatment of back pain can broadly be divided into:

(a) Low back pain (LBP) alone: Symptomatic treatment
(b) LBP + sciatica: Symptomatic treatment + traction
(c) LBP + neurological manifestations (paraparesis, bladder dysfunction, paraplegia, nerve root compression). Often requires surgical relief

Other indications for surgery are: proven disc protrusion, tumours, infections such as tuberculosis not responding to chemotherapy, spinal instability and spinal deformities, e.g. scoliosis. In the USA in 1987 250 000 lumbar discectomies were performed. However, only 1% of the patients suffering from LBP show evidence of lumbar disc prolapse. The commonest age group affected is between 40 and 45 years and

the commonest affected is L5-S disc; with L4–5 being the next.

Non-operative treatment

Symptomatic treatment   By rest on orthopaedic beds, analgesics and anti-inflammatory drugs (NSAIDS). Traction to distract the lumbar spine, lumbosacral belt and teaching of correct posture during sitting and at work; care of the back at work and at home.

Physical therapy   Heat, short-wave diathermy, ultrasound, spinal musculature building exercises, swimming and rehabilitation where necessary.

Chemonucleolysis   Injection under image intensifier of chemopapain into the disc material to destroy it (selected cases and in special centres). Papain used to dissolve intervertebral disc can cause:
– 1% anaphylaxis (adrenaline 0.3 mg i.v. and every 1 minute; antihistamine, hydrocortisone, and aminophylline should be available at hand)
– nerve damage
– paraplegia
– meningitis
– pulmonary embolism

Operative treatment

In *intervertebral disc prolapse*, operations may include:
Laminectomy and discectomy   The laminae of the vertebrae opposite the disc protrusion are removed to get access to the disc in front of the spinal cord. The nerve roots may need to be released in lateral disc protrusions.

Fenestration and discectomy   Only ligamentum flavum is removed to get access to the disc.

Micro-discectomy   As above but an operating microscope is used. The skin incision is considerably smaller; the structures are magnified to allow more accurate surgery.

Percutaneous discectomy   Skin incision is small enough to introduce an arthroscope type of instrument through which the disc is removed. A laser probe may also be used to destroy the offending disc (selected cases and centres).

In *idiopathic scoliosis*, progression of the curve must be assessed every 6 months. Early age onset with thoracic rather than lumbar scoliosis requires active treatment. Surgical correction is deferred until early adolescence to minimise the loss of height which may result from fusion of a significant length of the growing spine; conservative management with various orthotic bracing is advocated during the waiting period. The brace commonly employed is the Milwaukee brace with 3-point correction. The principle of surgical correction is to fuse joints of all vertebrae within the primary curve after initial maximum correction achieved by traction or corrective plaster casts, or by rapid Harrington distraction rod (inserted posteriorly in the concavity of the curve between two hooks placed under the laminae of the top and bottom vertebrae and then

forcibly elongated to produce straightening). Corrective operation must be protected by immobilsation in a plaster jacket. Other methods of fixation and correction include:
– anterior correction/fixation by a cable screwed under tension to vertebral bodies (Dwyer technique);

– fixation by metal rods secured to vertebrae posteriorly by multiple-level sublaminar wiring (Luque technique);
– external correction by distraction between a screwed-on metal skull band (halo) above and a pelvic band below (halo–pelvic traction).

VASCULAR SURGERY

1.76 Peripheral Vascular Disease

Acute or chronic limb ischaemia is the usual mode of presentation of peripheral vascular disease. However, it must be stressed that peripheral perfusion is related not only to the patency of the arterial tree, but also to the efficiency of the cardiac and venous pumping mechanisms, and to the quality and viscosity of the blood. In Eastern countries, vascular disease is mainly distal (e.g. diabetic foot), while in Western countries, aortic disease predominates.

ACUTE ISCHAEMIA

Sudden main artery blockage leads to immediate pallor, loss of distal pulses, progressive cooling, sensory loss commencing distally, rest pain and muscle weakness and tenderness. Progression to limb death may occur within 6 h, but this period may be much longer, depending on collateral flow; spontaneous recovery occurs in some cases.

Causes

Arterial trauma, embolism, thrombosis and dissection. Rarer causes are severe vasospastic disease, frostbite and ergot. The usual problem is to distinguish between embolism and thrombosis. Thrombosis may be precipitated by a hypotensive episode or heart failure and is suggested by a history of claudication and evidence of atherosclerosis elsewhere; the clinical picture is less dramatic than that of embolism. Embolism is suggested by dramatic onset, atrial fibrillation, mitral stenosis, recent myocardial infarct, subacute bacterial endocarditis or proximal aneurysm.

Management of acute arterial ischaemia

Give 5000 units heparin intravenously immediately on diagnosis of acute occlusion. Full cardiovascular assessment and ECG. If thrombosis is the likely cause, then an urgent arteriogram should be obtained prior to attempting surgery, as it may be possible to lyse the thrombus using streptokinase or plasminogen activator, using catheters placed under radiological control (this is particularly important if the patient has had a previous arterial graft). Major embolism must be treated

with an emergency embolectomy as soon as possible, provided the limb is still judged to be viable. Most lower limb emboli can be removed through one or both common femoral arteries under local anaesthesia, using embolectomy catheters. Below-knee fasciotomies may be advisable after restoration of flow. If a satisfactory restoration of flow is not obtained, then an ontable arteriogram should be performed and, if necessary, streptokinase or plasminogen activator instilled distally by means of special thrombolysis catheters.

CHRONIC ISCHAEMIA

Causes

Arteriosclerosis obliterans is by far the commonest cause. Others include Buerger's disease, popliteal entrapment, cervical rib, arteritis and vasospastic conditions. Diabetes is an important contributory factor.

Arteriosclerosis obliterans

Affects mainly males and older females. Intimal deposits become widespread in large and medium-sized arteries, leading to progressive narrowing. Final occlusion is followed by secondary thrombosis proximally and distally to the next sizable branch. Aetiological factors include smoking, hypertension, hyperlipidaemia, diabetes and heredity.

Distribution of atheroma is widespread but patchy with predilection for certain sites (related to haemodynamic factors). Peripherally it affects particularly the femoropopliteal segment, distal aorta and iliac arteries and the lower leg arteries, with a tendency to spare the profunda beyond its origin and the distal popliteal artery. Arteriosclerosis may weaken the media and lead to aneurysm, particularly in the infrarenal aorta and the popliteal arteries. Diabetes leads to premature onset of arteriosclerosis and a tendency to small vessel involvement, as well as to neuropathy and liability to spreading infection in the feet.

Clinical picture of peripheral ischaemia

Intermittent claudication

Femoropopliteal disease leads to calf claudication; aortoiliac occlusion causes claudication pain in buttock, hip, thigh or calf and is often associated with impotence (Leriche syndrome).

Severe ischaemia (rest pain and gangrene)

May be caused by repeated minor embolism by thrombotic material from more proximal ulcerated plaques or stenoses, or more often by multiple levels of occlusion usually including at least two of the three main below-knee arteries. It is particularly common in diabetics, although gangrene in diabetes is often precipitated by infection in a neuropathic foot rather than main vessel ischaemia. Drugs such as β-blockers may precipitate ischaemia by reducing the heart rate so that it is unable to cope with exercise (relative ischaemia). The intake of these drugs should therefore be terminated.

Examination

Assess patient's 'biological' age. Look at cardiovascular system as a whole, including blood pressure, search for carotid bruit, upper limb pulses, abdominal aorta for aneurysm. In affected limb(s) look for colour changes, wasting, loss of hair, trophic lesions, venous guttering on elevation, and dependency rubor. Feel for temperature changes; assess and record all pulses. Listen for bruits and measure ankle/brachial systolic pressure index. In claudicants measure walking distance and re-examine the limb at the onset of claudication; this will help distinguish ischaemic from neurogenic claudication due to spinal stenosis.

Investigations

Should include full blood count, erythrocyte sedimentation rate (ESR), serum lipids, fasting blood glucose, ECG and ultrasound. The Doppler ultrasonic probe is placed over the posterior tibial or dorsalis pedis and pneumatic cuffs are placed around the thigh, calf and ankle. The cuffs are inflated one at a time to record the lower limb cuff occlusion pressure, which is compared with the brachial artery upper limb pressure and expressed as a ratio (pressure index). Normally the ratio is more than 1 but in ischaemia it is less than 1 and can give a numerical assessment of the impedance to flow at different levels down the limb as well as indicating the level at which the pressure gradient is steepest.

Aortography is only considered when surgery is contemplated. Surgical intervention is indicated in:
- Disabling intermittent claudication.
- Rest pain.
- Distal gangrene (due to distal embolisation from a proximal disease).

Management

For claudication immediate management should be conservative with advice to stop smoking, modify diet, if necessary, and to exercise to encourage collateral development. Reassurance that only some 10% eventually come to amputation should be given. Progress should be observed over several months, after which those whose enjoyment of life or ability to work is seriously impaired may be considered for reconstructive surgery, provided they have stopped smoking. Aortography then becomes essential, and this must be done without delay in those presenting with limb-threatening ischaemia, so

that a limb-saving procedure can be undertaken if feasible. In patients with multiple levels of occlusion it is essential to deal with the proximal lesion first. For example, in aortoiliac cases restoration of good pulsatile flow to the profunda is usually effective in the presence of a femoropopliteal block.

BUERGER'S DISEASE (THROMBOANGIITIS OBLITERANS)

This affects younger, mostly male, patients who smoke, often with a history of thrombophlebitis migrans. Thrombosis and inflammation commence in the smaller arteries of the hands or feet and spread proximally. Foot claudication, rest pain and gangrene may develop. Distal pulses are lost first. Cessation of smoking is vital and will stop progression of the disease. Lumbar sympathectomy may help and conservative amputation may be successful for gangrene. Prostaglandin E_2 infusion may help the patient during an exacerbation.

RAYNAUD'S PHENOMENON

Attacks of digital ischaemia are provoked by exposure to cold or emotion.

Primary (Raynaud's disease)

Occurs mostly in young women, is bilateral and unassociated with other disease. Tissue loss rarely occurs. Treatment is by reassurance and advice on avoidance of exposure to cold. Sympathectomy is rarely of more than temporary benefit.

Secondary

Usually starts later in life and sooner or later an underlying disease becomes manifest, particularly scleroderma or CREST syndrome (calcinosis, Raynaud's phenomenon, oesophageal involvement, sclerodactyly and telangiectasis). It also occurs in other collagen diseases, with long use of vibrating tools, as a complication of certain drugs, in polycythaemia and dysproteinaemias and as a manifestation of proximal arterial lesions such as those caused by cervical rib. In severe cases plasma exchange often produces great improvement for a few months, perhaps by lowering blood viscosity.

SURGICAL METHODS IN PERIPHERAL VASCULAR DISEASE

Transluminal angioplasty

Balloon dilatation of stenoses and short occlusions work best in the iliac arteries and the long-term results may be improved by the use of stents placed across the stenosis after dilatation. Other methods of opening occluded vessels have been attempted using heated wires, atherectomy catheters (with rotating tips) and lasers, but these methods are still under evaluation. Similarly, the use of percutaneously inserted vascular grafts for stenotic disease and aneurysms is being developed.

Bypass graft

The method of choice for long occlusions. A Dacron graft (knitted and gelatin-coated) is best for aortoiliac or aortofemoral bypass. Autogenous saphenous vein (reversed or in situ) is best for femoropopliteal bypass, especially if the graft extends below the knee joint. PTFE or human umbilical vein grafts are alternatives if the vein is unsuitable. The long-term patency of the latter grafts may be improved by the use of vein patches at the distal anastomoses. The results of femorodistal bypass are worse if the run-off is poor or if the patient is diabetic or if tissue loss has already occurred distally.

Extra-anatomical grafts

Femorofemoral cross-over graft is useful in poor-risk subjects with unilateral iliac block. Axillobifemoral grafting can be used in similar subjects for aortic or bilateral iliac occlusions, or for replacement of an infected aortic graft.

Lumbar sympathectomy

Unlikely to benefit claudication but useful for mild ischaemic rest pain and small areas of skin necrosis. Chemical destruction of the chain by phenol injection under X-ray control is a useful alternative to surgical sympathectomy, particularly in the elderly.

Amputation

Required for intractable rest pain and gangrene when reconstruction is not feasible or has failed. Below-knee amputation using a long posterior flap should always be preferred when the blood supply permits, i.e. in many patients with obstructions below the common femoral.

For patients unsuitable for below-knee amputation, knee disarticulation or Gritti–Stokes amputation is preferred in elderly patients because of the longer lever provided. Standard above-knee amputation permits better fitting of a knee joint mechanism and is used in younger patients. Prophylactic penicillin should be used for all amputations for ischaemia.

1.77 Deep Venous Thrombosis and Pulmonary Embolism

Deep venous thrombosis of a length of the femoral vein causes a painful swollen leg. With lymphangitis the deep venous thrombosis will be protracted (phlegmasia alba dolens or white leg) and lead to varicose veins later on. Massive pulmonary embolism may occur. Such deep venous thrombosis occurs in late pregnancy and the puerperium. On the other hand, extensive deep venous thrombosis of iliofemoral and pelvic deep veins (phlegmasia caerulea dolens or blue leg) may lead to infarction and even sudden venous gangrene of the lower limb. Virchow's triad is still the pathological basis for deep venous thrombosis (i.e. changes in the vessel wall, changes in the

blood flow and changes in the composition of the blood). Special risk groups include those with a past history of deep venous thrombosis or pulmonary embolism, malignant disease, polycythaemia, abdominal or pelvic surgery, extensive trauma, congestive heart failure or myocardial infarction, obese and dehydrated patients, the elderly, and those taking the oral contraceptive pill (females) or stilboestrol (males with prostatic cancer).

Deep venous thrombosis

Prophylaxis

Preoperative
  Weight reduction.
  Stoppage of contraceptive pill 1 month prior to surgery.
  Identification of high-risk groups.
Peroperative
- Physical means
    Electrical stimulation of calf.
    External intermittent pneumatic compression of calf.
    Passive leg exercise (foot pedalling machine).
- Chemical means (to commence with premedication and to continue postoperatively until the patient is mobile)
    Aspirin (decreases platelet adhesiveness). It is probably not useful.
    Oral anticoagulants.
    Low-dose subcutaneous heparin.
    Dextran 70.
Postoperative
  Pressure-graduated elastic stockings.
  Early mobilisation, massage and leg movements.
  Adequate hydration.

Diagnosis

- Clinical examination (avoid Homans' sign as it may cause thrombus dislodgement): slight fever and tender swollen calf.
- Ascending deep functioning venography: essential to confirm diagnosis, delineate extent of deep venous thrombosis and detect silent deep venous thrombosis in postoperative pyrexia (after exclusion of all other causes). It is the most reliable test but is time-consuming, invasive and irradiates the patient.
- Ultrasound flow detector (Doppler principle): inexpensive, harmless in pregnancy and practical – may give false negative results.
- Radioactive labelled fibrinogen [125]I: unreliable above mid-thigh and in the presence of haematoma or healing wound. It carries the risk of serum hepatitis.
- Impedance plethysmography.

Treatment

- Anticoagulant, stocking and rest. Heparin 25 000–40 000 units per day continuous i.v. infusion with warfarin to be continued for 6 months (heparin is stopped after 2 days) and controlled by prothrombin time (should be twice or three times the control) or prothrombin index (should be 10–15%).

- Surgical thrombectomy (Fogarty balloon catheter).
- Fibrinolysis (streptokinase); particularly in recurrent pulmonary embolism.
- Vein ligation, plication or filter introduction (e.g. Mobin-Uddin umbrella in a capsule via internal jugular vein under X-ray control).

Pulmonary embolism

About 3% of all hospital deaths are due to pulmonary embolism.

Small emboli (especially if recurrent): lead to pulmonary hypertension which requires permanent anticoagulants.

Medium emboli: lodge in branches of the pulmonary artery resulting in a pulmonary infarction. Clinically, sudden chest pain, dyspnoea and haemoptysis occur. Radiologically, an infarcted triangular (wedge) segment is seen. Lung scan reveals the perfusion defect and pulmonary angiography is seldom required. ECG may reveal $S_1 Q_3 T_3$ pattern. Recurrent emboli are frequent. Heparin should be given i.v. and clot removed by Fogarty catheter. Warfarin is administered for six weeks.

Large emboli: lodge in the main pulmonary artery with serious haemodynamic and ECG changes (right ventricular strain). Immediate death may occur in massive pulmonary embolism. Shock is profound with high CVP, low blood pressure, feeble pulse, and severe hypoxaemia in blood gases. Such cases need emergency pulmonary embolectomy with or without cardiopulmonary bypass as well as immediate heparin and streptokinase i.v. administration. Unfortunately the majority die in spite of cardiac resuscitation.

Practical points

All female patients on the contraceptive pill and patients over the age of 40 years undergoing hernia surgery (or anything comparable or of greater severity) must be given deep venous thrombosis prophylaxis. In general, low-dose heparin (Calciparin), 5000 units 8-hourly subcutaneously, is started with the premedication and continued until the patient is fully ambulant. Heparin is given into a fold of abdominal skin and not into the arms or buttocks.

500 ml of Dextran 70, given at induction of anaesthesia and 500 ml immediately postoperatively is another alternative to prevent pulmonary embolism.

There are two groups unsuitable for deep venous thrombosis and pulmonary embolism prophylaxis using the low-dose heparin regimen:

- Those in whom the tiny risk of haemorrhage will be dangerous, e.g. those with recent gastrointestinal tract bleeding, recent cerebrovascular accident, diastolic blood pressure greater than 120 mmHg or known bleeding diathesis such as haemophilia or Christmas disease. Also patients with toxic goitre (very vascular) and head injuries and those patients undergoing open as well as endoscopic urological surgery (to avoid haematuria). This group needs intermittent pneumatic compression boots during operation.
- Those in whom low-dose heparin appears to be an inadequate form of prophylaxis, including those with a history of deep venous thrombosis or pulmonary embolism, and those with hip fractures or those who have had surgery (immobility). They require full anticoagulation therapy.

Latest advances in DVT prophylaxis

Thromboembolic risk factors (THRIFT)

A study in the UK found that 9% of patients admitted to a general hospital died and that 10% of these deaths (0.9% of all admissions) were due to pulmonary embolism. Most fatal emboli arise from deep vein thrombosis in the lower limb which can also cause both acute and chronic symptoms in the limb (pain, swelling, chronic dermatitis and ulceration). Most cases of fatal embolism are preceded by non-fatal thromboembolism unrecognised by clinicians; screening for asymptomatic thrombosis has been advocated but is not cost-effective in most patients. The most efficient way to prevent both fatal and non-fatal venous thrombosis is to use routine prophylaxis for moderate to high-risk hospital patients; such prophylaxis is both life-saving and cost-effective.

The THRIFT Consensus Group reviewed the literature and classified various risk factors into three groups based on meta-analysis of available data (see Tables 1.77.1, 1.77.2).

Patients at risk

The risk is less than 3% for patients under 40 years old undergoing brief surgery lasting less than 30 minutes, and rises with age and complexity or duration of the procedure. Risks are highest in the obese, those with a previous history of DVT or pulmonary embolism and in the presence of malignant disease. Procedures particularly likely to lead to DVT include pelvic, hip and knee surgery; without adequate prophylaxis 60–80% of such patients develop a DVT. Patients suffering major trauma, myocardial infarction, stroke and thrombophilic disorders are also at high risk.

Pregnancy increases the risk of DVT, especially when culminating in operative delivery. Pulmonary embolism, the most common cause of maternal death, accounts for 20% of deaths, most of which occur just before or after delivery.

Table 1.77.1   Risk factors for venous thromboembolism in inpatients

Patient factors	Disease or surgical procedure
Age	Trauma or surgery, especially
Obesity	of pelvis, hip, lower limb
Varicose veins	Malignancy, especially pelvic,
Immobility (bed rest over 4 days)	abdominal, metastatic
Pregnancy	Heart failure
Puerperium	Recent myocardial infarction
High dose oestrogen therapy	Paralysis of lower limb(s)
Previous deep vein thrombosis or	Infection
pulmonary embolism	Inflammatory bowel disease
Thrombophilia	Nephrotic syndrome
Deficiency of antithrombin III,	Polycythaemia
protein C, or protein S	Paraproteinaemia
Antiphospholipid antibody or	Paroxysmal nocturnal
lupus anticoagulant	haemoglobinuria
	Behçet's disease
	Homocystinaemia

Table 1.77.2   Anti-thrombotic prophylaxis strategy

Risk category	Recommended prophylaxis
High risk: >40%	
Major orthopaedic surgery	● Early mobilisation
Fractured pelvis, hip, leg	● Graduated compression
Major surgery in patients with malignancy	stockings
	● Adjusted dose heparin
Major surgery in patients with history of venous thromboembolism or >60 yr old	● Intermittent pneumatic compression
Lower limb paralysis or major amputation	
Moderate risk: 5–40%	
Major surgery in patients >40 yr old not in high-risk category	● Early mobilisation
Major surgery or lower limb surgery in patients on contraceptive pill	● Graduated compression stockings
Major medical illness with prolonged immobilisation (malignancy, cardiac, inflammatory bowel disease)	● Low dose heparin
Low risk: <5%	
Minor surgery (<30 minutes) with no risk factors	● Early mobilisation
Major surgery (>30 minutes) in patients <40 yr old with no risk factors	● Graduated compression stockings

Low dose heparin: 5000 units standard UF heparin 12 hourly started on admission or >2 hours before surgery and continued until discharge from hospital, or up to 2 weeks for patients at high risk.

LMW heparin: enoxaparin, should be started 12 hours before surgery and like dalteparin can be given once daily.

Adjusted dose heparin: dose varied to keep APTT 1.5–2.5 times control value.

Intermittent pneumatic compression: start before surgery and continue for at least 16 hours after.

DVT prophylaxis

During the past 20 years many trials have evaluated treatments aiming to reduce the risk of DVT; most have relied on the ^{125}I-fibrinogen uptake test for diagnosis. Data from these trials show that where no prophylaxis was used, DVT occurred in 22% of 3396 general surgical patients, and in 47% of 619 orthopaedic patients; 2% of all these patients had a non-fatal PE, and 0.8% a fatal PE.

Low dose subcutaneous heparin   5,000 units twice or thrice daily reduced the incidence of DVT to 9% in general surgical patients and 24% in orthopaedic patients; the risk of non-fatal PE was reduced by 40%, and fatal PE by 64%. Heparin increased the risk of 'excessive bleeding or need for transfusion' from 3.7% to 6.0% of 13 500 surgical patients.

Full-length anti-embolism stockings   In a meta-analysis of 7 studies, stockings reduced the incidence of DVT in surgical patients without malignant disease from 27% to 11%, and when combined with subcutaneous heparin reduced the incidence of DVT further to 6%. All randomised studies reporting efficacy of these stockings have used the same brand (T.E.D.) of the Kendall Co (UK).

Intermittent pneumatic compression   In general surgical patients compression of the legs reduced the incidence of DVT from 27% with no prophylaxis to 18%, and had an additive effect when combined with graduated compression stockings.

Heparin formulations   Heparin is currently available as 'standard' unfractionated (UF) heparin as the sodium or calcium salt, and as 'low-molecular weight' (LMW) fractions of heparin. LMW heparins (obtained by fractionation or depolymerisation of commercial grade heparin) have different, possibly advantageous, pharmacological profiles from UF heparin but cost much more.

Other prophylactic measures   Both intravenous low molecular weight dextrans, and oral warfarin have been used to prevent DVT, but risk allergic reactions (dextrans) or haemorrhage (warfarin). Aspirin is not useful.

Oestrogen-containing oral contraceptives should be discontinued (and adequate alternative contraception arranged) 4 weeks before any major surgery, or any lower limb or pelvic surgery. If in an emergency this is not possible, patients on the pill should receive low dose heparin before and after surgery. There is no evidence that hormone replacement therapy increases the risk of thromboembolism, but it is probably safer to discontinue it.

Anticoagulant drug therapy

Treatment of DVT should not be delayed, but objective evidence obtained before committing the patient to continued anticoagulation. Standard UF heparin remains the most widely used drug for the initial treatment of acute DVT (LMW heparin is not licensed for treating DVT or PE). Clinical trials have not established the optimal route of administration. Twice daily subcutaneous heparin (30 000–35 000 units/24 h) is easier to give than continuous intravenous heparin (28 000–40 000 units/24 h) but responds more slowly to dose changes. The activated partial thromboplastin time (APTT) is the best measure of effective treatment. It should be measured daily and the dose of heparin adjusted to keep it at 1.5 to 2.5 times the control value. When followed by warfarin five days' treatment with heparin is as effective as 10 days. Warfarin alone leaves the patient at risk for pulmonary embolism for the several days before it is fully effective; it should be started during heparin therapy overlapping for 3–4 days, during which both the APTT and International Normalised Ratio (INR) should be measured daily. Warfarin should be taken for 12 weeks to prevent further thrombosis; some experts suggest for a shorter time for a calf DVT. The dose should be adjusted to maintain the INR between 2 and 4.5. Prolonged anticoagulation is needed only for recurrent deep vein thrombosis.

Platelets should be counted in patients under heparin treatment for longer than 5 days, and treatment should be stopped immediately if thrombocytopenia develops.

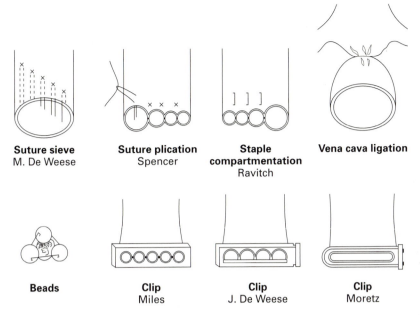

Suture sieve M. De Weese	Suture plication Spencer	Staple compartmentation Ravitch	Vena cava ligation
Beads	**Clip** Miles	**Clip** J. De Weese	**Clip** Moretz

Fig. 1.77.1 Operative interruption of the inferior vena cava for prevention of recurrent pulmonary embolism. (Modified from V. Kakkar, 1987)

Heparin can be given subcutaneously to the *pregnant woman*, without risk to the fetus since it does not cross the placenta. It may cause thrombocytopenia, and osteoporosis if given for more than 6 months. Warfarin is teratogenic and should be avoided during the first trimester, and risks fetal haemorrhage during the third trimester. It is still indicated for pregnant women with diseased or prosthetic heart valves.

Thrombophilic disorders

All young patients (< 40 years of age) presenting with, or any patient with a strong family history of, venous thromboembolism should be investigated for a thrombophilic disorder such as antithrombin III, protein C or S deficiency, lupus anticoagulant and anti-cardiolipin antibodies, and disorders of fibrinolysis. If protein C, protein S or antithrombin III deficiency is detected family members should also be investigated. Antithrombin III and protein C concentrates can be used to cover periods of high risk of thrombosis, but management of these patients is complex and it is best to seek specialist advice. Thrombophilic patients who suffer a thrombotic episode will need long-term prophylaxis with warfarin.

Fibrinolytic drugs

Streptokinase and urokinase are better than heparin at dissolving thrombus but still resolve only 50% of thrombi, perhaps because stasis in the occluded vein prevents the drug reaching the site of thrombosis.

Surgical treatment

Surgical removal of venous thrombus does not prevent pulmonary embolism nor the long-term complication of chronic venous insufficiency.

Patients with recurrent pulmonary embolism despite adequate anticoagulation (or when anticoagulation is contra-indicated) should have an inferior vena cava (IVC) filter inserted. Early devices, such as the Mobin–Uddin umbrella, often caused IVC occlusion, but the Greenfield filter effectively prevents pulmonary embolism with an incidence of caval occlusion of only 5% at 5 years. Modern IVC filters do not require anticoagulation to remain patent (Fig. 1.77.1).

1.78 Stroke – Surgical Prevention

Stroke is the third most common cause of death in the Western world after coronary heart disease and cancer.

The incidence of strokes in the UK is estimated at 2/1000/year. About 100 000 patients have a first stroke every year; approximately one every five minutes.

Fortunately, not all strokes come without warning, but the exact incidence of transient ischaemic attacks that precede a stroke is difficult to estimate with accuracy, as they can be unheeded by physicians or unreported by patients.

About 80% of strokes are ischaemic in nature, 50% of ischaemic strokes are atheromatous thromboembolism of large and medium-sized arteries. Lacunar infarcts constitute 25% while embolisation from the heart constitutes 20% of cases.

Transient ischaemic attacks (TIAs)

Incidence The incidence of TIAs has been estimated at 5/1000 per annum.

Definition A TIA is defined as an acute loss of focal cerebral or monocular function with symptoms lasting < 24 h, which, after adequate investigation, is presumed to be due to embolic or thrombotic vascular disease.

Reversible ischaemic neurological deficit (RIND), is like TIA, but lasting >24 hours. In *stroke in evolution* the patient presents with an evolving clinical picture which usually progresses in a step-wise pattern. Surgery is controversial. *Completed stroke* is the end point of cerebral ischaemia, which leads to neuronal death with very limited recovery

Prognosis The risk of stroke after TIAs during the first year is 12%, and about 6% per annum in subsequent years for 5 years. The risk of stroke and/or death (including MI) is approximately 10% per annum. The majority (80%) of TIAs are in the carotid territory.

Diagnosis TIAs occur suddenly and reach their maximum in a few seconds. They occur at random, not related to activity or time. They present as loss of function, like weakness, numbness, dysphasia and loss of vision. The attack is usually brief, lasting a few minutes and rarely 1–2 hours. The loss of vision, usually described as 'mist', 'curtains' or 'fog', usually lasts seconds to a few minutes. Vertebro-basilar TIAs should be differentiated from migraine and epilepsy. Thirty per cent of those experiencing TIAs have positive brain CT scan.

Clinical examination Patients are seldom examined during TIAs, when focal neurological signs indicate the site of the lesion. Fundoscopic examination rarely shows fibrin–platelets emboli in the retinal circulation. Occasionally, cholesterol emboli (Hollenhorsts' plaques) are seen in the retinal arterioles as bright golden yellow spots. Carotid bruit might be present.

Investigation

Duplex sonography

This technique combines real-time, B-mode ultrasound imager and Doppler flowmeter (Fig. 1.78.1). It is painless, the most accurate and quickest method of carotid assessment.

The B-mode imaging allows identification of the vessel of interest and study of the anatomical and morphological characterisation of the plaque.

Echo-lucent 'soft' plaques containing lipid and blood are more common in symptomatic patients and have a tendency for embolisation. The echo-dense 'fibrous' and 'calcified' plaques are common in asymptomatic patients.

The Doppler modality of the machine is used to assess the degree of stenosis.

Duplex scanning is operator-dependent and each unit should validate its results against angiography.

Cerebral angiography

- 'Conventional' angiography.
- Digital subtraction angiography (DSA) – this is performed electronically by obtaining an image before contrast is injected and then an image with contrast in the vessels while the patient is in the same position and then subtracting the second image from the first to give a processed image of the opacified vessel lumens free of any bone or soft tissue. There are two types of DSA: intravenous and intra-arterial.

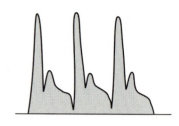

Doppler flow signals

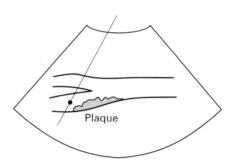

Real time B-mode image

Fig. 1.78.1   Duplex carotid scanning of the internal carotid artery

Indications for angiography

Angiography is an invasive procedure and carries at least a 1% risk of stroke and 0.7% risk of mortality. It is indicated if duplex scanning indicates > 70% stenosis and the patient agrees and is fit for carotid endarterectomy. There is a place for angiography in patients with frequent vertebro-basilar TIAs, particularly in association with subclavian steal syndrome which might be amenable to balloon angioplasty or surgery.

Complications of angiography are due to:
- Catheter tip thrombous formation or dislodgement of atheroma.
- Adverse contrast reaction (hypotension, bradycardia, angina, renal failure and dyspnoea).
- Problems at the site of arterial puncture (nerve injury, haematoma, false aneurysm, distal embolisation and vessel thrombosis).

Intravenous DSA is safer, faster and less expensive but it is less accurate due to overlapping of blood vessels owing to simultaneous opacification of all cerebral vessels and inability to obtain a lateral view.

Intra-arterial DSA uses less contrast than the conventional angiography, and therefore carries less risk of contrast toxicity, less irradiation, pain and cost, but it has the same disadvantage of catheter tip complications.

CT scan or MRI

These investigations are not indicated in all TIAs except if TIAs are frequent or if the patient is being considered for surgery.

If the scan is positive, surgery should be postponed for 6 week. It is also used to exclude intracranial space-occupying lesion, which rarely presents as TIAs (<5%). It is rarely required to exclude primary haemorrhage, which has never been reported to cause TIAs (i.e. symptoms < 24 h).

Pathogenesis of cerebral ischaemia due to carotid stenosis

Haemodynamic mechanism　Stanley Crawford in 1960 found that pressure gradients were associated with a reduction in luminal diameter of > 50%. Recently it has been found that > 75% stenosis was needed to produce haemodynamic effects. Development of symptoms depends on the efficiency of the Circle of Willis and collateral circulation. Up to 35% of normal brains have incomplete circles.

Thromboembolic mechanism　Two types of embolisation, fibrin–platelets and atheromatous debris, are usually identified; the first is due to thrombus formation on the ulcerated plaque surface and the second type to plaque disruption and discharge of the atheromatous material (Fig. 1.78.2). Most probably both mechanisms are working together.

Carotid endarterectomy (CE)

Despite more than 100 000 carotid endarterectomies being performed in the USA each year, the role of this operation in stroke prevention has remained controversial. Two recent multicentre studies (the European Carotid Surgery Trial, ECST, and the North American Symptomatic Carotid Endarterectomy Trial NASCT), have established the benefit of surgery in preventing stroke in patients with severe carotid stenosis (70–99%) who have had recent minor strokes, TIAs or retinal infarcts. Stroke incidence was reduced by six- to ten-fold respectively over a period of 3 years.

The benefits remain uncertain in patients with moderate stenosis (30–70%) and recruitment for the trial is going on.

Patients with mild stenosis (< 30%) have a small risk of stroke and any potential benefit of surgery is outweighed by the 30 days mortality and morbidity.

Operative surgery

Anaesthesia　Usually general, but in some centres they use regional/local anaesthesia.

Incision　Longitudinal incision along the anterior border of the sternomastoid muscle or skin crease incision. In either incision one should avoid damage to the mandibular branch of the facial nerve.

Procedure　Try to avoid damaging the great auricular nerve in the top of the incision if possible. The common facial vein is ligated and divided and serves as a landmark for the carotid bifurcation and to the hypoglossal nerve. Mobilise the ansa cervicalis anteriorly and use it as a guide to identify the hypoglossal nerve. The common carotid artery is carefully dissected to avoid embolisation and also to avoid damaging the vagus nerve, which is close to the posterolateral aspect of the artery. Identify the external carotid artery by finding the superior thyroid branch and encircle this branch by a double loop of O/silk.

Avoid dissecting the angle of the carotid bifurcation to prevent undue stimulation of the carotid sinus nerve and causing bradycardia, which can be blocked by using lignocaine local anaesthesia. The dissection of the internal carotid artery should be carried out with extreme gentleness and carried upward until a soft healthy segment is reached. This might require mobilisation of the hypoglossal nerve. Retract the posterior belly of the diagastric muscle to gain good access; very rarely, it needs to be divided. Heparin 5000 units is used i.v. 3 minutes before clamping of the blood vessels.

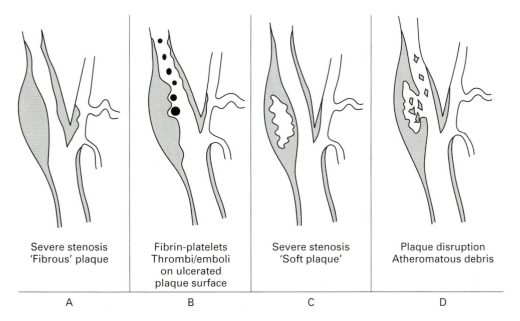

A	B	C	D
Severe stenosis 'Fibrous' plaque	Fibrin-platelets Thrombi/emboli on ulcerated plaque surface	Severe stenosis 'Soft plaque'	Plaque disruption Atheromatous debris

Fig. 1.78.2　Pathogenesis of cerebral ischaemia. A and C, haemodynamic mechanism; B and D, thromboembolic mechanism

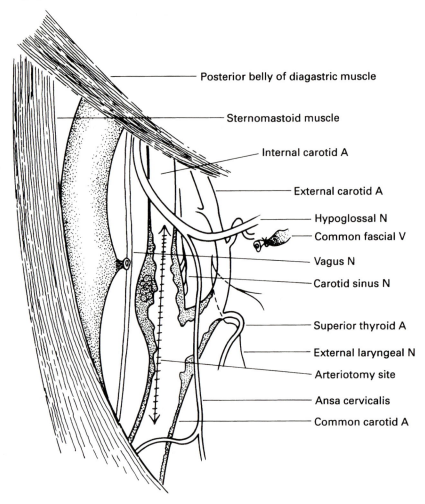

Posterior belly of diagastric muscle

Sternomastoid muscle

Internal carotid A

External carotid A

Hypoglossal N
Common fascial V
Vagus N
Carotid sinus N

Superior thyroid A

External laryngeal N

Arteriotomy site

Ansa cervicalis

Common carotid A

Fig. 1.78.3 Surgical anatomy showing the relation of cranial and peripheral nerves to the carotid bifurcation

After obtaining proximal and distal control do a vertical arteriotomy (about 5 cm), including the carotid bulb, common carotid and internal carotid arteries, and insert a shunt if you are routinely shunting (see below) and carry on with endarterectomy. The atheroma should be feathered away at the top to avoid development of a step which could cause dissection and thrombosis of the artery. The arteriotomy is closed with 6/0 prolene (Fig. 1.78.3).

Carotid shunt

There are few surgeons who have never used a shunt. Routine use of a shunt allows a meticulous and unhurried technique, but the shunt has its own problems, such as air embolism, thrombosis, kinking, dislodgement of atheroma and intimal damage.

Selective shunting is required in about 10–15% of the patients. Stump back pressure < 50 mmHg is the common criterion for shunting or if EEG changes occur during clamping.

Vein patch

The incidence of symptomatic carotid re-stenosis is < 5%. A wide range of asymptomatic re-stenosis has been reported (on average 15%). Vein patch reduces the incidence of re-stenosis in both male and female patients. The proximal segment of the long saphenous vein should be used to avoid patch rupture, which has an incidence of 0.7%.

Perioperative monitoring

● EEG or somatosensory evoked potentials.
● Clinical neurological monitoring in awake patients having the operation under local anaesthesia.
● Transcranial cerebral doppler (TCD).
● To avoid technical errors, completion ultrasound, angiography or or angioscopy has been used in some centres.

Asympatomatic carotid murmur (bruit)

This is due to vessel wall vibration and usually results from turbulent flow caused by arterial stenosis. It indicates the existence of generalised atherosclerosis, especially coronary artery disease.

Incidence 5% of the population above the age of 50 years have carotid bruit, while 10% of patients undergoing CABG procedures and 20% of patients undergoing peripheral vascular reconstruction have asymptomatic carotid bruit.

Prognosis The annual stroke rate of patients with asymptomatic bruit is about 2–3%. Up to 40% of these patients have severe internal carotid stenosis (>50% reduction in luminal diameter). The stroke rate increases with the increase in severity of the stenosis (those with >75% stenosis have a 5% annual stroke rate). Absence of bruit does not exclude stenosis; it usually disappears when stenosis exceeds 85%. Patients with >75% stenosis have a 30% incidence of silent infarct on CT scan.

Differential diagnosis Hyperdynamic circulation, venous hums and propagated cardiac and major vessels murmur.

Investigation – Duplex Doppler scanning or intravenous digital subtraction angioplasty to assess the degree of stenosis.

Treatment – There is some evidence that asymptomatic tight stenosis (>70%) is associated with a higher risk of stroke. However, carotid surgery in such patients is still controversial and we are awaiting the results of the trials.

1.79 Surgery in Ischaemic Heart Disease

Ischaemic heart disease is responsible for 150 000 deaths each year in the UK and is the commonest cause of death in the world. (By the age of 65 years, 45% of all men will have some form of ischaemic heart disease.)

Patients with stable or unstable angina are clinically assessed followed by exercise testing to identify those with serious coronary disease. Coronary arteriography is an essential part of cardiac catheterisation which, together with echocardiography and radionuclide scan, can assess the cardiac function preoperatively.

Coronary transluminal angioplasty

Indications

- Clinical, i.e. short history of angina resistant to medical management with objective evidence of myocardial ischaemia and relatively normal ventricular function.
- Anatomical, i.e. *severe proximal* single-vessel coronary artery disease. *Proximal* two-and even three-vessel disease can now also be treated.

Contraindications

- Diffuse or calcified stenoses.
- Left main coronary disease.
- Previous coronary spasm and occluded coronary arteries.

Procedure

Is done with a guide catheter and steerable wire introduced intra-arterially percutaneously via the femoral route by the Seldinger technique. Contrast injections are used to reveal the anatomy under fluoroscopic control after local anaesthesia and premedication.

Complications

Include local trauma, coronary dissection, occlusion, rupture of the coronary arteries, myocardial infarction and delayed restricture. Emergency surgery may be required in 5–7% of patients undergoing angioplasty. The hospital mortality is around 1%.

Coronary artery bypass grafting

Indications

- Angina unmanageable by medical treatment.
- The quality of life is adversely affected by long-term administration of drugs.
- Significant stenosis of the left main coronary artery (50% stenosis) regardless of left ventricular function or the degree of angina.
- Three-vessel disease.
- Unstable angina but without evolving infarction.

Procedure

Generally coronary artery bypass grafting is done within 6 months of coronary arteriography. Prior to surgery, smoking should be stopped, obesity should be reduced, and diabetes and hypertension controlled. The long saphenous vein must be carefully examined. In the presence of varicose veins and/or bilateral stripping, the cephalic vein or the internal mammary artery should be used instead. Coronary artery bypass grafting is done under general anaesthesia, using a median sternotomy approach. The long saphenous vein (from the leg) is excised and reversed before grafting. The bypass is controlled with an infusion of nitroprusside or nitroglycerine.

Complications

Include perioperative infarction and operative mortality in the region of 1%. Immediate and complete relief from angina occurs in 80% of patients. Graft patency after 12 months is 70–90%. Graft occlusion due to thrombosis or fibrosis may occur. A late closure rate of 2–3% per year is generally reported. Up to 30% of patients develop recurrent angina over a 5 year period. Good quality of life postoperatively is the rule in terms of less medication, improved exercise, symptomatic relief and return to work.

Other surgical procedures for ischaemic heart disease

- Left ventricular aneurysm (postinfarction) may be symptomatic (left ventricular failure) and may or may not have associated angina. In symptomatic patients, aneurysmal resection can improve left ventricular function. However the long-term results depend on the quality of the residual contracting myocardium and the extent of coronary disease progress.
- Postinfarction ventricular septal defect with subsequent rupture occurs in 1% of myocardial infarctions and carries a grave prognosis. The development of a pansystolic murmur (of ventricular septal defect) after myocardial infarction is an indication for urgent cardiological assessment with a view to emergency surgery (if treated conservatively, 85% of patients die within 2 months).
- Mitral regurgitation following myocardial infarction is due to papillary muscle rupture or dysfunction. Acute rupture is usually fatal within 24–48 h if not corrected. The chronic form is due to dysfunction or partial rupture and needs mitral valve replacement.
- Inferior myocardial infarction may be complicated by heart block necessitating a permanent epicardial or intravenous endocardial pacemaker implantation.
- Ischaemic heart disease with advanced heart failure in suitably selected patients may be treated with heart transplantation.

N.B.   See also s. 1.25 High-risk patients in surgery.

SURGERY OF LYMPHATICS

1.80 Cervical Lymph Nodes

The human body contains about 800 lymph nodes (LN), of which 300 are located in the neck. The lymphatic drainage of the head and neck is arranged in two 'circles', the 'inner circle' and the 'outer circle'.

The superficial lymph nodes (Fig. 1.80.1) comprise the following elements.

The outer circle of nodes from chin to occiput, is made up of:

A. *The submental nodes*: three or four nodes lie just beneath the chin. They drain the tip of the tongue, floor of the mouth, lingual and labial gum. They drain into the submandibular group but a few efferents pass direct to the jugulo-omohyoid node.

B. *The submandibular nodes* drain a wide area from the centre of the forehead, nose and nearby cheek, upper lip and the anterior two-thirds of the tongue, floor of mouth and gums.

They receive lymph from the upper and lower teeth, from the anterior half of the nasal cavity and from the frontal and maxillary and middle and anterior ethmoidal sinuses. Most of the submandibular nodes drain into the jugulo-omohyoid node; a few drain into the jugulo-diagastric node.

C. *Buccal and mandibular nodes*: a small node lies isolated on the baccinator muscle, another on the lower border of the mandible at the anterior border of the masseter. They drain part of the cheek and lower eyelid. Their efferents pass to the jugulo-digastric node.

D. *Pre-auricular nodes*: these lie on and within the parotid gland; one or two are subcutaneous. The subcutaneous nodes drain the skin of the temple and vertex, forehead and eyelids, pinna and external acoustic meatus. These drain through the deep cervical fascia into supraclavicular nodes. The deep nodes receive from the back of the orbit, from the infratemporal fossa and from the parotid gland itself. They drain into the deep members of the deep group.

E. *Occipital nodes*: these drain the posterior part of the scalp and auricle. These efferents pass to the supraclavicular nodes.

The **inner circle**, however, lies within the surrounding larynx, trachea and pharynx; it comprises pretracheal, paratracheal and retropharyngeal LNs. The pretracheal LNs drain the lower larynx, trachea and thyroid isthmus. The retropharyngeal LNs drain the soft palate, posterior parts of hard palate and nose, as well as the pharynx itself. These then drain into the deep cervical LNs.

The **deep cervical lymph nodes** are found around the internal jugular vein from the base of the skull to the root of the neck. They are formed of three groups:

I. *The jugulo-digastric node* lies below the posterior belly of the digastric between the angle of the mandible and the anterior border of sternomastoid.

II. *The jugulo-omohyoid node* lies above the inferior belly of the omohyoid, behind the jugular vein.

III. *The supraclavicular lymph nodes* extend behind the border of sternomastoid into the posterior triangle. Lymph from the deep cervical nodes is collected into the jugular lymph trunk. This joins the thoracic duct on the left side; on the right side, it usually opens independently into the internal jugular or brachiocephalic vein.

Enlarged supraclavicular lymph nodes have long been recognised. They take the name of of the German pathologist Virchow (1821–1902); the classical enlarged supraclavicular LN (of Virchow) following metastasis from underlying gastric carcinoma is termed Troisier's sign (named after a French professor of pathology, 1844–1919).

Enlarged supraclavicular LN is of great surgical interest, since it is usually due to neoplastic lesions more than infective

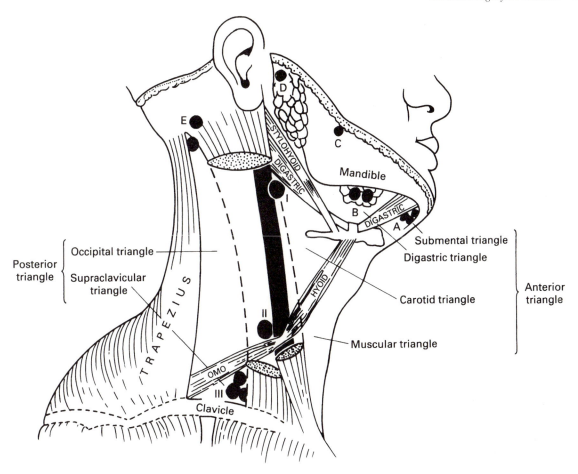

Fig. 1.80.1 Cervical lymph nodes

ones (the commonest cause of infective enlargement of supraclavicular lymph nodes is pulmonary tuberculosis). While most upper limb infection can cause epitrochlear and axillary LN enlargement, infection of the middle finger and dorsum of the hand passes directly into the supraclavicular LNs. Other causes of enlargement include bronchogenic carcinoma (Pancoast tumor), breast carcinoma, thyroid carcinoma (wrongly called ectopic thyroid), oesophageal carcinoma, pharyngolaryngeal carcinoma, Hodgkin's and non-Hodgkin's lymphoma, pancreatic carcinoma and testicular carcinoma (particularly choriocarcinoma). Hypernephroma can also give rise to enlarged supraclavicular nodes.

Superficial and deep cervical lymph nodes ultimately drain into supraclavicular lymph nodes. So any enlargement of these glands (due to infections or neoplasms in the head and neck and upper limbs) will result in enlargement of the supraclavicular lymph nodes. Enlargement of supraclavicular lymph nodes may be part of a generalised lymphadenopathy due to leukemia, lymphoma and AIDS.

Causes of cervical lymphadenopathy

1. *Infection*
- Acute pyogenic
- Chronic
    Non-specific
    Specific
    – Glandular fever
    – Tuberculosis
    – Syphilis
    – Toxoplasmosis
    – Cat scratch fever
2. *Neoplastic*
- Metastatic secondary tumours from primary tumours of head, neck, chest and abdomen.
- Primary tumours:
    Hodgkin's lymphoma (adult)
    – Non-Hodgkin's lymphoma (elderly)
    – Leukaemia (usually children and young adults)
3. *Miscellaneous*
- Sarcoidosis

Diagnosis of a cervical swelling due to lymph node enlargement

Careful history and meticulous physical examination can give the diagnosis in the majority of cases. Pyogenic lymph nodes are tender and hot with evidence of infection (of the respiratory tract and mouth). Cold matted lymph nodes are tuberculous. Fixed stony hard lymph nodes are metastatic in origin. However, in lateral swellings that do not move with swallowing and have a rubbery consistency, Hodgkin's lymphoma (in adults) and non-Hodgkin's lymphoma (in the elderly) is most likely.

A positive tuberculin test can be diagnostic for tuberculosis in any patient with a cervical lymph node swelling. Fine needle aspiration cytology biopsy is an important diagnostic tool, in the presence of an experienced cytologist. Cervical lymph node biopsy is the last investigative tool which will solve the problems of diagnosis. Occasionally, CT scan, ultrasound, and radioactive isotope scan are required to elucidate the nature of cervical swelling.

Cervical lymph node biopsy

Under general anaesthesia with endotracheal intubation, while the patient is supine and the head turned to the opposite side; the upper half of the operating table is tilted upwards sufficiently to collapse the external jugular vein.

1. A transverse skin crease incision over the palpable lump is the most satisfactory incision. The incision is deepened through skin and platysma. All the intervening fascia should be cut. If the LN is covered by the sternomastoid muscle, this should be retracted or divided.

2. The LN node is then dissected freely from its surroundings. This is best be done by a small curved artery forceps; when opening the blades, the investing fascia will be stripped off. The LN must be handled very gently during the dissection. Rough handling may distort the internal structure of the node and make histological interpretation difficult.

- A tissue forceps can disfigure the LN, while a thread traversing the LN is safer and can be used as a stay suture for gentle retraction.
- If the LN is large and dissection is difficult with risk of injury to other structures, only the accessible part of the LN may be excised (safer). The process of sharp and blunt dissection should be repeated until the gland is free except from its deep aspect.
- The node can be pushed to one side, and the bed can be cleared. At this stage neighbouring important structures can be damaged, only tissues which are seen should be cut. The accessory nerve is particularly at risk.

3. Once the node is free, it can be removed and cut in two equal parts. One part is put in a container with formalin for histopathological examination (those going for receptor assay, should be sent fresh without formalin) and the other part is sent fresh for culture (including for tuberculosis).

4. The deep muscles and skin are closed. There is no need for drainage; however, if drainage is deemed necessary, it is better to leave a small corrugated (2–3 corrugations) drain or soft Penrose drain for 24–48 h only to avoid pressure necrosis. A suction drain is not recommended, since it may be stuck to deep cervical vein and if pulled out without suction pressure deactivation, may result in severe bleeding.

Treatment of tuberculosis

Tuberculosis is treated in two phases:
1. *Initial phase for 2 months.* At least three drugs are used to reduce the population of viable bacteria rapidly and to prevent the emergence of drug-resistant bacteria. Drugs are:
- Isoniazid 300 mg daily for adults (for children 10 mg/kg daily). Pyridoxine 10 mg daily should be given prophylactically from the start of treatment to counteract peripheral neuropathy induced by isoniazid.
- Rifampicin 450–600 mg daily, depending on the adult's body weight – whether under or over 50 kg respectively (for children 10 mg/kg daily). Rifampicin may cause liver dysfunction.
- Pyrazinamide (bactericidal) 1.5–2 g daily depending on an adult's body weight – whether under or over 50 kg respectively (for children 35 mg/kg daily).
- Additional drugs: ethambutol (15 mg/kg daily; can cause colour blindness) is added if drug resistance is thought likely. Streptomycin (i.m. injection of 1 g daily; can cause oto- and nephrotoxicity) is now rarely used in UK, but it may be added if bacilli are resistant to isoniazid.

2. *Continuation phase for 4 months.* Two drugs, isoniazid and rifampicin (for a total of six months each), are the key components of the second phase of any antituberculosis regimen. Longer treatment may be necessary for bone and joint infections, for meningitis, or for resistant organisms.

1.81 Chronic Leg Swelling and Oedema

The commonest cause of chronic swelling of the lower limb is heart failure (usually bilateral). The second most important cause is kidney disease (bilateral). Both these conditions should be suspected from history and physical signs, and the diagnosis confirmed by simple tests of cardiac and renal function. Unilateral and local causes of swelling ought not to be entertained until cardiac and renal disease have been excluded. Then one can look for local abnormalities within the leg because other general causes of lower limb oedema are rare.

Oedema formation

At any one time, only 5% of circulating blood is in capillaries, but this 5% is the most important part of blood volume because it is across systemic capillary walls that gas and nutrients exchange occurs; oxygen and nutrients enter interstitial fluid and CO_2 and waste products enter the bloodstream. The pressure gradient across the wall of muscle capillary represents the resultant pressure differential between *hydrostatic* [capillary hydrostatic pressure minus interstitial hydrostatic fluid pressure] and *osmotic* [colloid osmotic oncotic plasma protein pressure minus colloid osmotic pressure of interstitial fluid] pressure gradients.

Therefore, pressure differential =
Outward filtration pressure [hydrostatic outward pressure at arteriolar end of capillary (37 mmHg) minus interstitial inward fluid pressure (1 mmHg) minus oncotic inward pressure gradient (25 mmHg)] minus

inward pressure [oncotic inward pressure gradient (25 mmHg) minus hydrostatic outward pressure at the venular end of capillary (17 mmHg) minus interstitial outward fluid pressure (1 mmHg).

So pressure differential = [(37–1)–25] – [25–(17–1)] mmHg
= 11 – 9 mmHg
= 2 mmHg

Thus a pressure gradient of 2 mmHg forces an efflux of fluid in the interstitial space (Fig. 1.81.1). Normally, there is continuous flow of fluid out of the arterial end of capillaries, into interstitial spaces, and back into the venous end of capillaries; more fluid and protein always leak into interstitial space than return into the capillaries. Therefore, fluid efflux normally exceeds influx across capillary walls; this extra fluid is cleared and drained by lymphatics back into blood circulation (via left thoracic duct and right lymphatic duct). This prevents interstitial fluid pressure from rising and promotes turnover of tissue fluid. Skeletal muscle movements, arterial pulsation, lymphatic unidirectional valves, negative intrathoracic pressure and compression propel lymph flow to systemic circulation and ultimately toward the heart. The normal 24 h lymph flow is 2–4 l, and contains interstitial fluid, proteins leaked from capillaries (protein contents lower than plasma), water-insoluble fats absorbed from intestine (lymph in thoracic duct is

milky after a meal), lymphocytes and clotting factors (lymph clots on standing).

Amount of fluid in interstitial spaces depends on capillary pressure, interstitial fluid pressure, oncotic pressure, capillary permeability, number of active capillaries, lymph flow and total ECF volume; precapillary constriction lowers filtration pressure, whereas postcapillary constriction raises it. Oedema is increased interstitial fluid collection in abnormally large amounts. Factors promoting oedema formation include:

- Increased filtration pressure due mainly to venular constriction than arteriolar dilatation. It is also due to venous hypertension seen in a variety of conditions, such as heart failure, venous obstruction, venous valve incompetence, increased ECF volume due to renal failure, and gravitational effect.
- Decreased osmotic pressure gradient across capillaries due to decreased plasma proteins seen in hypoproteinaemia.
- Increased capillary permeability due to histamine and kinins.
- Inadequate lymph flow.

Unilateral chronic leg swelling

There are three common local causes of unilateral lower limb oedema: *inflammation* (rarely becomes chronic, as infection usually resolves), *venous obstruction* (venous hypertension) and *lymphatic insufficiency*. Venous obstruction reduces fluid reabsorption at venous end of the capillaries, and so produces large watery interstitial fluid. Lymphatic obstruction reduces clearance of interstitial protein and some water, and so produces slight increase in interstitial fluid, but with high protein concentration. Therefore, main differences between venous and lymphatic oedema are protein concentration in interstitial fluid and rate of excess interstitial fluid formation.

1. *Venous oedema* Varicose veins rarely cause gross swelling, but major vein obstruction (acute or chronic) does. Gross leg oedema and mild varicose veins should be investigated with caution because varicose veins are unlikely to be the cause of oedema; even severe communicating vein incompetence may have some oedema but usually confined to the lower leg and ankle (not gross oedema). Even then, calf pump is usually able to reduce superficial venous pressure during exercise. Severe venous oedema is invariably caused by major outflow obstruction as well as poor calf pump; femoroiliac veins are usually blocked, or inadequately recanalised, and communicating veins are incompetent. Venous outflow obstruction results in persistent venous hypertension with gross oedema, varicose veins, venous telangiectasia, while calf pump insufficiency due to communicating vein incompetence results in intermittent venous hypertension with pigmentation, eczema formation, liposclerosis and ulceration. History of deep venous thrombosis or pulmonary embolism confirms the venous obstruction aetiology of leg oedema.

2. *Lymphoedema* If venous disease can be excluded then lymphatic disease should be considered, always remembering that the commonest cause of lymphoedema is metastatic or primary malignant disease in lymph nodes, because lymphoedema is far less common than any variety of venous oedema.

Subcutaneous tissue

Bone

Skin   Muscle

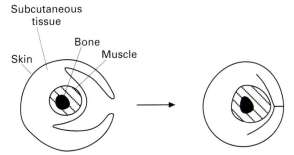

Subcutaneous exision with partial skin excision (Homans)

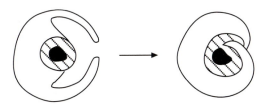

Subcutaneous exision with partial skin excision
Plus buried dermis flap (inside muscle) (Thompson)

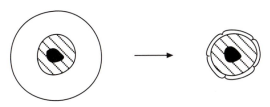

Total excision and skin graft (Charles)

Fig. 1.81.1   Reducing operations for lymphoedema

Furthermore, primary lymphoedema due to congenital lymphatic absence of hypopolasia (Milroy's disease) is very rare. Lymphoedema (like venous oedema) is either due to obstruction (secondary lymphoedema following surgical removal, chronic infection with tuberculosis or filariasis, or malignant obstruction) or rarely due to valvular insufficiency. Clinically, lymphoedema swelling involves the whole limb (leg, foot and toes), square toes (toes look square in transverse section), skin hyperkeratosis, tinea pedis, recurrent cellulitis, episodic swelling, vesicles (lymph or chyle), and pale cutaneous naevus (vinrose patch). While all oedema pits on pressure, pitting is less likely with lymphoedema than venous oedema, because high protein contents of long-standing lymphoedema cause considerable subcutaneous fibrosis.

Investigations

In addition to history and clinical findings, patency of deep veins must be investigated using Doppler flow detector and phlebography; moreover, lymphography, ultrasound scan and CT scan of the pelvis are performed.

Treatment

- *Most mild degrees of swelling* (whether due to calf pump insufficiency or mild lymphoedema) can be treated with a simple conservative regimen of elastic compression, elevation and centripetal massage or intermittent pneumatic compression at night. Fungicidal cream or oral griseofulvin may be used to reduce cellulitis due to frequent association of lymphoedema with tinea pedis. Occasionally a short-term course of diuretics may be helpful.
- *Severe venous oedema* can sometimes be helped by vein bypass operations, after initial conservative treatment (see above). Prolonged venous hypertension due to venous outflow obstruction will cause communicating vein incompetence and, therefore, superficial veins surgery is contra-indicated; it is important not to tie or remove long saphenous vein. Iliac vein localised obstruction can be bypassed by re-routing long saphenous vein of the other healthy leg brought across the pubis in a subcutaneous tunnel and anastomosed to vein below the block (Palma operation). However, if obstruction is very short, it can be resected and vein patency restored by end-to-end anastomosis.

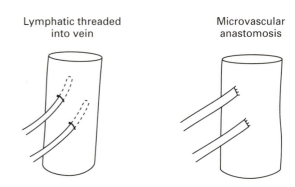

Fig. 1.81.3   Lymphovenous shunts for lymphoedema

- *Severe lymphoedema* usually has to be treated by a reducing operation. Generally, there are five main approaches, detailed below.
  1. Conservative regimen as in mild swelling of the leg.
  2. Reducing operation with three types (Fig. 1.81.1):
  - Simple excisional procedures (Homans), by reflecting skin and excising subcutaneous tissue from one-half of the limb. Skin is closed by simple suture. The procedure is repeated on the other side of the limb 3 months later.
  - Buried dermis flap operation (Thompson) is an extension of the excisional operation, in which one of the skin flaps

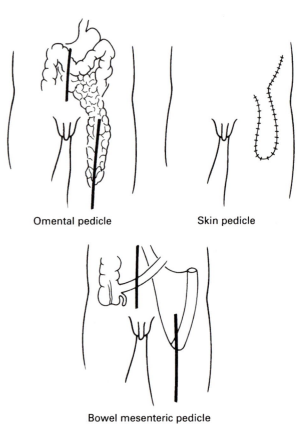

Omental pedicle   Skin pedicle

Bowel mesenteric pedicle

Fig. 1.81.4   Bypass operations

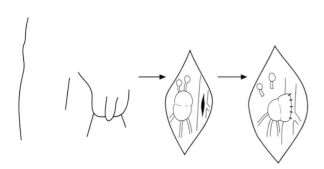

Fig. 1.81.2   Lymph node/femoral vein anastomosis

is shaved of its superficial layers of epidermis and then attached deep to the deep fascia so that connections will develop between the dermal lymphatic plexus and deep lymphatics (not proven yet). The reducing effect is no different from excisional operation but lasts a little longer due to an inbuilt massaging effect as muscle movements tug on the buried skin edge.

- Total skin and subcutaneous excision and split-skin graft (Charles) on to deep fascia and muscle is the most effective operation for gross oedema. It requires prolonged hospital stay, but it is highly effective with no recurrence, which follow the above two operations.

3. Lymphovenous shunts: rarely, lymphatics can be joined to veins in three ways by:
- Anastomosing a transected lymph node to a large vein (Nielubowicz) (Fig. 1.81.2).
- Threading lymphatics into veins (Degni).
- Microsurgical anastomosis. (Fig. 1.81.3).
Some of these are effective ways of curing lymphoedema. No one has yet shown, in man, that such anastomoses remain patient.

4. Bypass operations (Fig. 1.81.4). When lymphatic obstruction is localised it may be possible to bypass it. There are three main bridge operations:
- Pedicle of skin and fat containing healthy lymphatics

(Gillies), but this operation is rarely successful, because there are very few lymphatics in the pedicle and scar which encircles the implanted end of the pedicle prevents growth of connections between lymphatics.
- Omental pedicle, but this does not work because it contains very few lymphatics and is often too small to fashion into a long pedicle.
- Pedicle of small bowel and its mesentery (Kinmonth), which has a rich lymphatic plexus and connection between cut surface of inguinal lymph nodes and mesenteric vessels has been demonstrated by lymphography on animals and in man. However, its use is limited because it cannot be stretched below the inguinal ligament, and also because a small number of patients have gross oedema secondary to localised iliac node obstruction.

5. Prevent reflux in severe lymphoedema due to lymphatic valvular incompetence. This is a rare form of oedema presenting as leg swelling with or without skin vesicles, which leak lymph or chyle. Lymphography usually reveals grossly dilated incompetent iliac lymphatics. Careful transperitoneal exposure and ligation of all these vessels stops the reflux and reduces oedema even though operation has destroyed all the main lymph channels draining the leg.

PAEDIATRIC SURGERY

1.82 Surgery of the Newborn and Children

Operative mortality of infants and anaesthetic-related mortality of otherwise healthy children is higher than adults due to infantile and paediatric complications arising from basic anatomical, physiological, pharmacological and pathological differences. Successful outcome of surgery in the neonatal period depends on many factors, such as surgical technique, expert paediatric anaesthesia, nursing skills and staffing on ICU, availability of micromethods for haematological and biochemical investigations, full paediatric radiological service and specialised equipment. Only if these services are available can neonatal surgery be safely undertaken.

PHYSIOLOGICAL DIFFERENCES AND CLINICAL IMPLICATIONS

Respiratory system and anaesthesia

Advances in neonatal anaesthesia have largely been responsible for the progress of neonatal surgery. There are, however, many factors to be considered.
- In the neonate, the surface area available for gaseous exchange is reduced in relation to body weight compared

to the adult. Thus any loss of functioning pulmonary tissue (e.g. in diaphragmatic hernia), or increased oxygen requirement (e.g. in cooling), can produce pulmonary deficiency in the infant with minimal pulmonary reserves. Adequate respiratory function after birth is critically dependent on an adequate amount of surfactant in the lungs; surfactant is surface-tension-reducing phospholipid, produced exclusively by type II pneumocytes (function at 34–36 weeks' gestation). Surfactant serves as both an anti-atelectasis and waterproofing agent for alveolar membrane; the amount is inadequate in premature babies along with respiratory immaturity predisposing to fetal distress syndrome.
- The single most important difference that physiologically separates paediatric from adult patients is oxygen consumption. Oxygen consumption of neonates is greater than 6 ml/kg/min, which is twice that of adults on weight basis. To satisfy this increased demand, minute alveolar ventilation is doubled compared to adults; carbon dioxide production is also increased in neonates. Tidal volume, on weight basis, is the same for both infants and adults; the relatively large abdomen, weak intercostal muscles, horizontal ribs, shape of the rib cage and angle of insertion of diaphragm characteristic of infants makes it more efficient to increase respiratory rate rather than tidal volume. Infantile diaphragm is composed of decreased muscle fibres, and is thus prone to fatigue, with resultant apnoea.

- Immature control of ventilatory centres can be observed in neonates. The response of older children and adults to hypoxaemia and hypercapnia is sustained hyperventilation. Pre-term and full-term neonates, when challenged with hypoxic inspired gases, have initial hyperventilation (for 1–2 min) followed by sustained hypoventilation. Hypercapnia, a potent stimulus to ventilation in children and adults, is not as potent a stimulus to neonates and may be a respiratory depressant to pre-term neonates. As age increases, hyperventilation becomes sustained.
- Anatomically, the large head and tongue, mobile epiglottis and anterior portion of larynx make neonatal intubation easier with the head in neutral or slightly flexed position than with the head hyperextended as in adults. The infantile larynx is higher in the neck than the adult's, and hence the infant's tongue more easily obstructs the airway. Cricoid cartilage is the narrowest portion of the larynx in paediatric patients, necessitating fine tracheal tubes (uncuffed size 3 mm internal diameter) to avoid trauma and subglottic oedema.
- Anatomically, small calibre airway passages (with narrow nares and small pharynx) mean that airway resistance will become critical with accumulation of any secretions, especially as the neonate cough reflex is depressed (Fig. 1.82.1). These factors may cause hypoventilation and risks of aspiration pneumonia are increased. The newborn is also prone to other pulmonary disorders, often related to prematurity, such as respiratory distress syndrome, apnoeic attacks, meconium aspiration and pulmonary haemorrhage; these may complicate the pre- and postoperative course of neonatal surgery.

Cardiovascular system and anaesthesia

Birth and spontaneous ventilation initiate circulatory changes allowing neonates to survive in the extrauterine environment. Fetal circulation is characterised by high pulmonary vascular resistance, low systemic vascular resistance (placental), and right-to-left blood shunt via foramen ovale and ductus arteriosus.

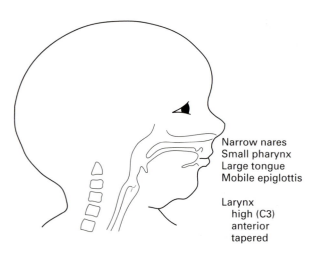

Narrow nares
Small pharynx
Large tongue
Mobile epiglottis

Larynx
high (C3)
anterior
tapered

Fig. 1.82.1   Anatomic characteristics of the neonate

Spontaneous ventilation at birth opens the lungs, resulting in decreased pulmonary vascular resistance and increased pulmonary blood flow. As left atrial blood flow and pressures increase, foramen ovale functionally closes; anatomic closure occurs between 3 months and 1 year. Functional closure of ductus arteriosus with constriction in response to increased PaO_2, occurs 10–15 h after birth; anatomic closure takes place in 4–6 weeks. Nevertheless, ductus arteriosus may reopen during periods of arterial hypoxaemia. Also, diaphragmatic hernia, meconium aspiration, pulmonary infection and polycythaemia are associated with high pulmonary vascular resistance and persistence of fetal circulatory patterns. Cardiovascular responses of neonates differ from adults; infantile cardiac muscle is less compliant and increased heart rate therefore improves stroke volume by improving overall cardiac function. Immature autonomic system may manifest altered responses to vasoactive drugs (e.g. less responsive to dopamine). Homeostatic vasoconstrictive responses of neonates to haemorrhage are less than that of adults, reflecting immaturity of α-adrenergic receptors and reduced sensitivity of baroreceptor reflexes e.g. 10% blood loss causes 15–30% decrease in arterial blood pressure.

Renal changes and fluid/electrolytes and acid–base balance

Renal changes   Nephrogenesis is complete by 36 weeks' gestation. Neonatal glomerular filtration rate (GFR) is 20 ml/min (120 ml/min in adults); by 3–5 weeks of age GFR is increased three fold. The ability of neonatal kidneys to control sodium balance is also decreased. Distal renal tubules of neonates are relatively unresponsive to aldosterone, which further impairs control of sodium reabsorption. Consequently, neonates are clinically less able to compensate for extremes of fluid balance; neonates are obligate sodium losers and cannot concentrate urine as effectively as adults. Therefore, adequate exogenous sodium and water must be supplied during the perioperative period. Conversely, neonates excrete volume loads more slowly than adults, and therefore are more susceptible to fluid overload. Decreased renal function can also delay drug excretion.

Total body water   In neonates total body water is higher than adults (80% vs 60% of body weight), with proportional increase in extracellular fluid volume; distribution between intracellular and extracellular spaces is 35% and 45% in the infant compared with 40% and 20% in the adult. Changes of fluid balance with increased losses or decreased intake therefore have a greater effect in the neonate: for example: 3.5 kg infant with 700 ml extracellular fluid volume needs 350 ml fluid intake and gets rid of 350 ml fluid output and thus fluid turnover is 50%, while a 70 kg adult with 14 000 ml extracellular fluid volume needs 2000 ml fluid intake and gets rid of 2000 ml fluid output and thus fluid turnover is only 15%. Daily GIT fluid turnover is also drastically different from adults. By 18–24 months of age, the proportion of extracellular fluid volume relative to body weight is similar to adults. Increased metabolic rate characteristic of neonates results in accelerated turnover of extracellular fluid and dictates meticulous attention to intraoperative fluid replacement.

A neonate requires 150 ml/kg/day if fed orally. In the premature infant, this is increased to 200 ml/kg/day. With nasogastric suction, i.v. fluid requirements are less; infants will need 70 ml/kg/day unless there is jaundice or urinary complications such as obstruction. Newborn infants in the first week of life require even less fluid and this can be given as 10 ml/kg/day in the first day of life, increasing to a full 70 ml/kg/day by the seventh and subsequent days. Intraoperative fluid administration may be considered as maintenance fluids and replacement fluids, using either 5% dextrose in Ringer's lactate, or isotonic N/5 saline in 4.3% dextrose.

Recommended intraoperative fluid administration includes:

- 6 ml/kg/h in minor surgery such as herniotomy (4 ml maintenance and 2 ml replacement, respectively).
- 8 ml/kg/h in moderate surgery such as pyloromyotomy (4 ml and 4 ml).
- 10 ml/kg/h in extensive surgery such as bowel resection (4 ml and 6 ml).

Maintenance fluids are best correlated with metabolic rate: replacement fluids requirements should be based on underlying pathological processes, extent of surgery and anticipated fluid translocation. The 3rd space translocation of fluids is similar for neonates and adults. Insensible fluid losses vary greatly; fever, radiant warmers, phototherapy, increased ambient temperature and decreased humidity all increase fluid losses.

Initial assessment of infant dehydration is rather difficult; fluid losses are assessed by weight loss (difference between birth weight and weight on admission), loss of skin elasticity, depression of the anterior fontanelle, pulse rate and results of biochemical estimation. Later losses are easier to estimate by hourly recording, e.g. of nasogastric suction. The ideal solution for GIT fluid replacement is normal saline given on a volume to volume basis, because composition of newborn GIT aspirate averages 100–120 mmol/l of sodium, 5–15 mmol/l of potassium, and 100–120 mmol/l of chloride.

Acid–base changes Metabolic acidosis is the commonest acid–base disorder, found due either to disturbance of GIT or renal physiology or due to cardiorespiratory arrest. Initially it may be corrected by i.v. administration of 1/6th molar lactate solution; correction is slow due to the need to mobilise liver lactate which may take up to 2 hours (3 ml/kg of 1/6 molar lactate raise HCO_3 1 mmol). Immediate correction of acidosis can be achieved with i.v. 8.4% sodium bicarbonate (1 ml/kg $NaHCO_3$ raises HCO_3 1 mmol).

Alkalosis occurs with obstruction proximal to opening of bile ducts as in duodenal atresia and congenital hypertrophic pyloric stenosis. Alkalosis is corrected by i.v. administration of N saline (3 ml/kg N saline lower HCO_3 1 mmol). Intravenous replacement of potassium losses is restricted for the first 24 h following birth of infant or surgery. The neonate requires 3–5 mmol potassium per day which can be achieved by adding 1 g of potassium chloride to 500 ml of replacement fluids.

Total parenteral nutrition The full-term infant requires 100 cal/kg/day rising to 150 cal/kg/day in the premature infant. In peripheral i.v. feeding, consecutive Vamin, Intralipid and 10% dextrose solutions can be changed hourly at a rate of 6 ml/h for a 1 kg infant, 12 ml/h for a 2 kg infant, and 18 ml/h for a 3 kg infant. In central i.v. feeding, however, internal jugular vein may be catheterised with a subcutaneous tunnel on the chest wall. The catheter tip in the right atrium must be checked radiologically. Solutions are made in the pharmacy under strict aseptic conditions. Parenteral nutrition is monitored by laboratory tests like adults, with daily weighing of the infant.

Haematological changes and blood transfusion

Normal WBC count in neonates is 12 000 cell/mm^3 with predominant lymphocytes (70%). Values fall to normal adult levels by 1 year of age. Normal haemoglobin of neonate is 19 g/100 ml and falls to 11 g/100 ml at 3 months of age. This fall is due to fetal haemoglobin being replaced by adult haemoglobin. Fetal haemoglobin causes a shift of oxyhaemoglobin dissociation curve to the left; the increased affinity of haemoglobin for oxygen manifests as decreased release of oxygen to peripheral tissues which is offset by high haemoglobin concentrations. By 2–3 months of age, physiologic anaemia occurs; by 4–6 months oxyhaemoglobin curves approximate those of adults. Curve shifts to the left plus decreased cardiovascular reserves of neonates, are the reasons that haematocrit (PCV) should be maintained near 40% rather than 30% acceptable for older children (PCV is increased by dehydration and decreased by haemodilution). Coagulation tests, with the exception of bleeding time, are usually abnormal in neonates; all vitamin K-dependent factors (II, VII, IX, X) are low with prolonged prothrombin time.

In transfusion, samples of infant's and mother's blood are required for grouping and cross-matching. In assessing the need for blood transfusion it must be realised that the neonate's blood volume varies between 70 ml/kg (full-term) and 85 ml/kg (premature infant). Therefore, 8.5 ml blood loss in a 1 kg premature infant represents 10% loss and requires replacement transfusion; similarly blood loss of 28 ml in a 4 kg infant represents 10% loss and requires replacement. In view of the significance of small losses of blood in neonatal surgery, careful measurement of losses is essential; this is achieved by accurate weighing of swabs in the operating theatre.

Thermoregulation and prevention of hypothermia

Infants are more prone to heat loss than adults because of their wide body surface relative to total body weight or mass (greater than an adult); in the premature infant heat losses are greater due to lack of insulating subcutaneous tissue, and decreased ability to produce heat. Shivering is of little significance for heat production in neonates, whose primary mechanism of non-shivering thermogenesis is mediated by brown fat. Brown fat is a specialised adipose tissue located in the posterior neck, interscapular and vertebral areas, and surrounding the kidneys and adrenals; metabolism in brown fat is stimulated by noradrenalin resulting in triglyceride hydrolysis and thermogenesis. Exposure to a cold theatre environment results in heat loss by radiation and increased oxygen consumption which may be harmful to the infant if it is already under stress. Sclerema neonatorum seen in neonates and premature infants, where subcutaneous tissue and skin undergoes changes resulting in a hardened feel to tissues, especially in the extremities, is due to cooling and infection and is commoner in premature infants. The incidence may be reduced by careful measures to prevent heat loss during transport, investigations, operation and postoperative care of the infant.

Heat loss may be prevented by transporting an infant requiring surgery in a suitable portable incubator. In gastroschitis, where heat loss may be severe, it can be reduced by wrapping the infant in aluminium foil. The infant must be nursed in a pre-heated incubator to correct temperature. Infant exposure for radiological investigation, collection of blood and i.v. infusion should be kept to a minimum and any exposed areas should be wrapped in warm padded gauze. Heat loss during induction can be reduced by water blankets and additional overhead heating. During operation, temperature in theatre is kept higher than normal; the neonate's temperature is monitored with either a skin electrode or with oesophageal or rectal probes. Every attempt is made to maintain body temperature between 36 and 37 °C, as oxygen consumption is minimal at this level.

PATHOLOGICAL PROBLEMS

Specific metabolic disorders

Jaundice All newborn babies have physiologically high bilirubin for the first 3 days of life. Persistent and severe jaundice requires full investigation and treatment with phototherapy or exchange transfusion to prevent brain damage due to kernicterus. Bilirubin is not lipophilic and does not readily cross the blood–brain barrier (BBB); nevertheless, BBB, especially of premature neonates, is immature and so bilirubin enters the brain and damages cells. Infected infants are also prone to jaundice. Haemolytic disease of the newborn is suspected if the mother is Rhesus negative with detectable Rhesus antibodies.

Blood–brain barrier Characteristic of cerebral capillaries, with permeability different from other capillaries, allowing only exchange of water, CO_2, and O_2 across them, while glucose, urea and electrolytes cross very slowly. Adult BBB prevents bile salts, catecholamines and proteins from entering the brain; BBB may be penetrated due to immaturity and permeability of capillaries at birth. BBB functions to maintain the constancy of environment of neurons in the CNS; clinical implication is that drugs capable of crossing BBB can be used to treat CNS diseases. Penicillin and tetracycline cross BBB with difficulty, while sulphadiazine and erythromycin cross BBB quite readily. BBB is broken down in areas of the brain which are sites of severe head injury, infections, tumours and irradiation.

Haemolytic disease of the newborn Immature liver may be insufficient in synthesising blood clotting factors; all infants are given i.m. injection of vitamin K to prevent bleeding at birth and prior to surgery.

Hypocalcaemia after birth Due to parathyroid immaturity and particulary in premature infants, infants of diabetic mothers and infants fed on cows' milk with increased phosphate content interfering with calcium absorption. Neonatal operations and infection increase this risk. Treatment is by slow i.v. injection of 5–10 ml calcium gluconate; this may be given orally diluted in 100 ml per day.

Hypomagnesaemia Diagnosed by fits in the absence of hypoglycaemia and hypocalcaemia. Treatment consists of magnesium acetate 2.5 mmol i.v. followed by daily oral intake of 5 mmol of magnesium chloride.

Hypoglycaemia Occurs mainly in premature infants, infants of diabetic mothers, twins and infants of mothers with toxaemia of pregnancy, particularly in the presence of infection, anoxia, birth and surgical trauma. Neonatal blood glucose below 1.6 mmol/l requires treatment; symptoms are delayed until glucose falls below 1 mmol/l. Hypoglycaemia may be prevented by early oral feeding, which is impossible postoperatively. Incidence of hypoglycaemia is reduced by using N/5 saline in 4.3% dextrose as standard maintenance i.v. fluid using Dextrostix at 4-hourly intervals. Hypoglycaemia can be treated by i.v. 5 ml/kg of 20% dextrose.

Infection

The newborn is exposed to risk of infection during and after delivery; the immune system is immature and can further be reduced if breast feeding is not established, since maternal antibodies are present in high concentrations in colostrum and breast milk. Infection has an adverse effect on surgery, since it increases neonatal morbidity and mortality. Prevention of infection and cross-infection is the keynote of success and depends on strict nursing care. Neonatal units should have a controlled environment for temperature and humidity; ideally a positive pressure system as for theatres is recommended. The infant is nursed in an incubator with his or her own positive pressure system and nursing barrier. Care of the umbilicus with spirit swabbing and powdering is essential. Bacteriological screening of infants in the unit (swabs from umbilicus, nose/throat, skin, stool/rectum and urine) is done on admission and at regular intervals. Blood culture and lumbar puncture (invasive tests) are carried out if infection is suspected. Prophylactic antibiotics are required in neonates undergoing corrective surgery to prevent complications of, e.g., aspiration pneumonia in oesophageal atresia and septicaemia in necrotising enterocolitis.

Neonatal surgical diseases

These include congenital defects which have to be corrected by urgent surgery in first days of life. Neonatal surgical diseases include diaphragmatic hernia, tracheo-oesophageal fistula, omphalocele and gastroschisis, congenital pyloric stenosis, lobar emphysema and necrotising enterocolitis.

PERIOPERATIVE MANAGEMENT

Anaesthetic and analgesic requirements (pharmacological differences)

Infant anaesthetic requirements are reduced compared to adults (see above). Venesection, establishment of venous line and venous sampling are relatively difficult in infants and children.

Analgesics are better avoided pre- and postoperatively. Atropine i.m. 0.2 mg is the only premedication used. Regional or nerve blocks may be used by some anaesthetists. Postoperatively, the humidity in the incubator is kept at maximum and may be increased by the use of an ultrasonic nebuliser. Routine chest physiotherapy; aspiration may be reduced by nursing babies in the prone position, aspirating the pharynx at regular intervals and keeping the stomach empty by nasogastric tube until peristalsis and adequate gastric emptying is occurring (absence of bile in aspirates). All deaths from aspiration of vomitus or secretions are considered avoidable deaths.

Nursing care

Successful outcome of neonatal surgery is dependent upon constant nursing supervision (monitoring) and care by skilled nurses throughout 24 h of each day. Constant observations are needed with particular care of the airway and prevention of aspiration of vomitus. Nasogastric aspiration is routine after GIT surgery, using appropriate size 10 F tube with 1 hourly aspirations and free drainage into a receptacle between aspirations. Oral feeding is not started until aspirates are clear (non-bile stained); gradual oral feeding can initially start with 5% dextrose at 5 ml/h and then with increasing volumes and a change to half- and finally full-strength feeds. This transitional period may take days or weeks in infants with prolonged GIT problems, e.g. after repair of gastroschisis, or surgery for necrotising enterocolitis.

Monitoring

Monitoring during the perioperative period employs Specialised Equipments: incubators, apnoea alarm blankets, transcutaneous oxygen monitors, precordial or oesphageal stethoscope, ECG temperature, pulse oximeter and respiratory rate monitors.

RESULTS OF INFANTILE SURGERY

Operative mortality depends on the presence of other congenital defects and on the infantile maturity. A severe congenital anomaly usually indicates increased incidence of other congenital defects (congenital abnormalities are usually systemic); oesophageal atresia is usually associated with rectal atresia, and Down's syndrome is associated with duodenal obstruction. Renal and vertebral anomalies may co-exist. These multiple defects may increase operative mortality. Mortality is also dependent upon neonatal maturity: a full-term infant can withstand surgery better than a premature infant.

Corrective surgery, therefore, is classified into:
- Grade A infants with birth weight above 2.5 kg with no associated congenital defect.
- Grade B infants with birth weight 1.8–2.5 kg, or higher with a second moderately severe associated congenital defect.
- Grade C infants with birth weight less than 1.8 kg, or higher with a second severe associated congenital defect, e.g. oesophageal atresia and severe congenital heart disease such as tetralogy of Fallot.

1.83 Urinary Tract Infection and Vesicoureteric Reflux

There are differences between urinary tract infection of adults and that of children, in underlying aetiology, pathology, sex distribution, clinical presentation and management. It is therefore imperative to know the pattern of urinary tract infection in both adults and children for comparison.

Urinary tract infection in adults

Urinary tract infection is bacteriologically defined as the isolation of an organism in a number which exceeds an arbitrary stated concentration, i.e. greater than 100 000 organisms per ml, which is also called significant bacteriuria, because lesser concentrations of organisms are almost always due to urethral contamination. The initial 5 ml of voided urine is identified as a urethral washout specimen. The midstream specimen of urine (MSU) represents the uncontaminated bladder sample and is the usual specimen sent to laboratory for microscopy and culture. In females, it may be difficult to obtain MSU due to contact of urine with labia.

Clinically, urinary infection may be classified as symptomatic and asymptomatic. It affects females more than males; about 50% of all adult females will have at least one bout of cystitis in their life, with frequency and dysuria which may resolve spontaneously or respond to treatment. MSU should be sent for culture after one month of treatment with high fluid intake and an antibacterial agent. When infection occurs in men, there is frequently an underlying abnormality of the urinary tract. Persistence of infection by relapse (with the same organism), or recurrence (with a different organism) and with or without symptoms (but with murky and smelly urine) is an indication for IVU, particularly in children (see below) to detect any congenital anomaly, obstructive uropathy, stones and chronic pyelonephritis. In males, epididymo-orchitis, prostatitis and urethritis (non-specific or venereal) may all present with urinary tract infection.

Haematuria indicates the need for cystourethroscopy with bladder biopsy if necessary and bimanual examination under anaesthesia to exclude any extravesical pathology (e.g. colonic, uterine and ovarian) and to evacuate the bladder reducing any outflow resistance. Rarely cystogram is needed. It is important to eliminate residual urine (provides a stagnant pool as suitable medium for infection). Hernial defects via the pelvic floor (rectocele and prolapse) must be repaired and the bladder returned to its normal intra-abdominal position. *Escherichia coli* is the most common cause of urinary tract infection; less common causes include Proteus and Klebsiella spp. *Pseudomonas aeruginosa* infections are almost invariably associated with functional or anatomical abnormalities of the urinary tract. *Staphylococcus epidermidis* and *Enterococcus faecalis* infection may complicate catheterisation or instrumentation. Whenever possible, a specimen of urine should be collected for culture and sensitivity testing before starting antibiotic therapy. Uncomplicated lower urinary tract infections often respond to ampicillin, nalidixic acid, nitrofurantoin, or trimethoprim given for 5–7 days; sensitive bacteria respond to 3 g of amoxycillin 12 hourly. Long-term low dose therapy may be required in selected patients to prevent recurrence of infection; indications include frequent relapses and significant kidney damage. Trimethoprim and nitrofurantoin are recommended for long-term therapy.

Urinary tract infection in children

Urinary tract infection in infants usually complicates obstructive uropathy and vesicoureteric reflux, the two important causes of progressive renal destruction in infants where the urologist can help improve the infant from life-threatening ascending infection and pyelonephritis. In the newborn, boys are more infected than girls; this is certainly true of overt symptomatic infections and (probably) of covert asymptomatic bacteriuria. In serious cases, bacteraemia and septicaemia may not infrequently be complicated by meningitis.

Urinary tract infection in babies may present with vomiting, failure to thrive, malaise and fever (sometimes subnormal temperature), jaundice occasionally (from septicaemia), or haematuria; a large bladder and/or kidney may be noted. Acute or chronic retention of urine occurs. Bacteriuria and IVU will reveal abnormal kidney and ureters and urinary duplication. Boys in particular may show posterior urethral valve with bilateral reflux and megaureters, while girls may show obstructed upper tracts caused by ureteroceles. In the former group, MCU is needed, while in the latter group, if kidneys and ureters look normal on IVU, then reflux will be slight and the need for micturating cystourethrogram (MCU) is doubtful.

Contrast medium of IVU may dehydrate the infant, and fluid balance must be restored. If the child is admitted in good condition with a tense bladder and sterile urine, an indwelling 6 F plastic urethral catheter will provide good drainage for 24–48 h during which IVU and urethrocystography can be undertaken. Evidence of dehydration and uraemia may well be corrected within 48 h with i.v. therapy and low-protein milk.

Gentamicin or an antibiotic effective against Gram-negative bacteria may be given immediately without waiting for results of sensitivity. Bilateral nephrostomy may be needed for immediate renal decompression. Further treatment of urinary tract infection and its underlying obstruction and vesicoureteric reflux are then undertaken.

Vesicoureteric reflux and urinary obstruction

Vesicoureteric reflux is potentially a serious complication of the child with infected urine, because it predisposes to recurrent infection and facilitates the ascent of infection to the kidney, resulting in chronic pyelonephritis, renal failure and renal hypertension. Nevertheless, minor reflux is extremely common and may well cease spontaneously with growing maturity of the child. Others, even with more severe reflux, may preserve normal kidneys despite occasional infection. In the absence of urinary tract obstruction, kidney growth will proceed normally, monitored by repeated renal function tests and presence of scarring is sought on the nephrogram phase of IVU. It is found that, provided the urine is kept sterile, renal function increases with age to an equal extent in both the anti-reflux operation group and those managed conservatively.

Vesicoureteric reflux in mild and moderate cases ceases spontaneously in 70% of cases, but in gross vesicoureteric reflux, resolution is below 30%. Mild cases, despite free bilateral reflux, are associated with normal bladder without ureteric dilatation or kidney deformity; such cases have good prognosis and reflux will usually cease. Even if it does not, proper control of infection will allow normal kidney growth. By contrast, bilateral reflux associated with abnormal bladder and considerable ureteric dilatation, and asymmetrical kidney damage, may indicate a rare intrarenal reflux in which contrast medium introduced into the bladder may fill the pelvis, calices and spread outwards to opacify renal parenchyma; this intrarenal reflux under high pressure may have a damaging effect despite sterile urine. This sterile intrarenal reflux can be responsible for scarred kidney, indistinguishable from that of pyelonephritis.

Management

In children 1–5 years of age presenting with repeated infections (more than 1 bout per year), most paediatricians require MCU and IVU before deciding on urgent management to prevent progressive renal damage which may progress to chronic pyelonephritic scarring with caliceal blunting, renal outline indentation, fibrosis and colloid change in renal parenchyma.

All children are encouraged to drink a large fluid volume, practise double micturition, to ensure complete bladder emptying, and also to avoid constipation. Long-term low-dose chemotherapy for 6–12 months is necessary. However, no further improvement occurs after 12 years of age, and so continuous chemotherapy may be necessary up to this age.

In children who first develop urinary tract infection after the age of 5 years, an IVU must be undertaken; if this is normal, then they should be managed on the basis of careful bacteriological supervision and using the treatment above. If infection recurs soon after stopping chemotherapy, cystourethroscopy is indicated to exclude congenital urethral and bladder abnormalities, e.g. minor degrees of valves, diverticula, fistula and ureterocele, in addition to foreign bodies passed into the bladder. If IVU shows scarred kidneys or dilated ureters, then MCU must be done to help plan treatment as above.

Failure to control infection, or persistent symptoms or difficulty in managing antibiotics (e.g. allergies), indicate the need for reimplantation of refluxing ureters; complicating pathology such as bladder outflow obstruction and diverticula must be sought for and corrected at the time of reimplantation, and so MCU and cystoscopy are indicated

Operative correction of reflux, therefore, is only appropriate for children with no chance of spontaneous cessation due to anatomical causes, persistence of reflux with no attainable cure, or in the face of unacceptable or ineffective chemoprophylaxis in preventing infection.

Primary megaureter and ureterocele require reimplantation. Most of severe bilateral reflux cases in infancy have a degree of megacystis which renders the operation somewhat easier. The younger the infant, the more likely are the ureters to be supple and elastic with good muscular contraction, and the more likely they are to be restored to normal calibre by reflux prevention. Congenital urethral valve (pair of valvular folds springing from lower end of verumontanum) must be resected endoscopically; valve ablation may cure one-third of reflux cases. Persistent reflux carries the risk of recurrent infection, and may be due to inadequate resection. Ureteric reimplantation is then required and should not be undertaken early in the course of disease. Congenital urinary obstruction may occur at almost any level in the urinary tract. Pelviureteric obstruction causing hydronephrosis is common throughout childhood; pyeloplasty is successful in preserving renal function.

Unilateral dysplastic kidney (small deformed kidney with cluster of closely packed clubbed calices lying vertically above disposed and dilated renal pelvis with reflux, but no obstruction) is better removed. In prune belly syndrome (congenital absence of abdominal wall, undescended testes, and urinary tract abnormalities), reflux with large distended bladder and dilated prostatic urethra is due to narrowed membranous urethra which requires urethrotomy to relieve distal obstructive uropathy.

1.84 Some Important Paediatric Problems

GASTROINTESTINAL OBSTRUCTION IN THE NEONATE

Functional ileus is a common problem. However, only organic causes will be discussed here.

Presenting features are severe vomiting, failure to pass meconium and progressive abdominal distension ending in strangulation and death (in oesophageal atresia, constant drooling of saliva with choking attacks and cyanosis during feeding occur). Other causes of death are fluid and electrolyte metabolic disturbances and inhalation of vomitus with asphyxia.

Causes and treatment

Oesophageal atresia   Either as absent oesophagus (2%) or partial absence or web but no fistula (10%) or commonly atresia with tracheo-oesophageal fistula (85%). Lipiodol swallow is needed to identify the type. The condition occurs within the first 48 h. Treatment is by quick metabolic correction and thoracotomy with disconnection of fistula and reconstruction of oesophageal continuity (end-to-end anastomosis).

Congenital pyloric stenosis   Occurs in 4/1000 births usually in males with a familial history. It never occurs after 4 months of age. Clinical findings are non-bilious forcible and projectile vomiting ± palpable epigastric lump ± visible peristalsis. Treatment is quick metabolic correction followed by pyloromyotomy (Ramstedt's operation) under general anaesthesia via an upper abdominal incision. The hypertrophied pylorus is incised and muscle fibres are teased apart without breaching the mucosa (if accidently opened then patch with omentum just like perforated peptic ulcer). Medical treatment with atropine-like drug (e.g. Eumydrin) usually ends in failure.

Duodenal atresia   Usually associated with Down's syndrome. It is usually due to web or stenosis in the region of the ampulla of Vater or rarely to annular pancreas (failure of complete rotation of the ventral segment) with a characteristic double-bubble radiological appearance. Visible peristalsis and vomiting with or without bile are the main presentations. Treatment is by duodenoduodenostomy with an intraluminal catheter passed via the anastomosis and brought out through the gastrostomy.

Jejunal and ileal stenosis   With abdominal distension within 24 h of birth – confirmed radiologically (multiple fluid levels). Treatment is by Mikulicz procedure of exteriorisation, resection and spur enterostomy.

Midgut malrotation   In the form of arrested rotation due to transduodenal band of Ladd leading to a volvulus neonatorum after clockwise rotation of the whole midgut around the axis of the superior mesenteric artery. Treatment is by division of the band and untwisting the bowel.

Meconium ileus   Is the neonatal manifestation of mucoviscidosis with characteristic soap bubble appearance of meconium in the terminal ileum (seen in right iliac fossa). Adequate preoperative preparation followed by laparotomy. The proximal ileum is anastomosed end-to-side to the collapsed colon distal to the obstruction. The distal ileal opening is formed into an ileostomy through which meconium can be removed.

Intussusception   Usually in 6–9 month old male with facial pallor, vomiting, screaming and 'red currant jelly' stool. A sausage-shaped lump around the umbilicus is felt. Operative reduction (by milking) or resection of an irreducible or gangrenous segment (with end-to-end anastomosis).

Hirschsprung's disease   Due to a variable aganglionic rectosigmoid segment with an obstruction at the anorectal junction. Identified by rectal biopsy and radiology, including barium enema (prior to rectal washout). Constipation, abdominal distension with empty rectum gripping the examining finger are classical features. Treatment is surgical when the child is 8.2 kg in weight and thriving. Laparotomy and full mobilisation followed by anal pull-through. The anterior half of the inverted rectum is opened transversely and the proximal colon is pulled through the opening with an end-to-end coloanal anastomosis covered by a proximal temporary colostomy.

Anorectal agenesis   In the form of imperforate anus, low or high anomalies. X-ray of the infant upside down with a coin strapped to the anus can reveal the rectal gas which in turn can identify the level of agenesis. Treatment is according to the level usually with pull-through operation protected by colostomy. Any rectourethral fistula should be divided.

GASTROINTESTINAL BLEEDING IN CHILDREN

The treatment is according to the cause. The common causes are:

Haematemesis
- Swallowed maternal blood.
- Peptic oesophagitis.
- Oesophageal varices.
- Gastritis and stress ulcer.
- Haemorrhagic disease of the newborn and blood dyscrasias.
- Hiatus hernia.
- Gastric duplication.

Rectal bleeding
- Swallowed maternal blood.
- Peptic oesophagitis.
- Oesophageal varices.
- Meckel's diverticulum.
- Stress ulcer.
- Haemorrhagic disease of the newborn and blood dyscrasias.
- Necrotising enterocolitis.
- Intussusception/midgut malrotation.
- Anal fissure/constipation with impaction.
- Infectious diarrhoea.

SCORING OF ABDOMINAL PAIN IN CHILDREN AND YOUNG ADULTS

Alvarado and modified Alvarado score

Appendicectomy is the commonest emergency operation in surgical practice; however, in 15–30% of all appendicectomies, the appendix is healthy. This high negative laparotomy rate may have been justified by the valid fear that delayed diagnosis can result in perforation and peritonitis; it has therefore been accepted with impunity. However, such an aggressive policy is not without risks; 0.5–1% of appendicectomised patients will later require surgery for intestinal obstruction caused by post-appendicectomy adhesions. According to some studies, the incidence of such adhesions may even be greater if the excised appendix is normal. Conversely, the commonest cause of intra-abdominal adhesions in operated patients with intestinal obstruction is appendicectomy. Postoperative complications of negative laparotomy, such as wound infections, abscess and fistula formation, may be as high as 15%. Furthermore, there is a dubious association between appendicectomy and right colonic cancer.

Despite the unknown function of the appendix, every effort should be made to preserve it for future reconstructive surgery, such as replacement of damaged common bile duct and right ureter, for appendicecostomy to divert faecal effluent in distal colonic obstruction, and as a caecal reservoir with appendicular conduit in bladder reconstruction.

Table 1.84.1 Alvarado score (mnemonic of MANTRELS)

		Value
Symptoms	**M**igratory right iliac fossa (RIF) pain	1
	Anorexia	1
	Nausea/Vomiting	1
Signs	**T**enderness in right lower quadrant (RLQ)	2
	Rebound tenderness	1
	Elevation of temperature	1
Laboratory	**L**eucocytosis	2
	Shift to the left of neutrophils	1
Total score		10

Barium enema, computers, ultrasonography and laparoscopy were all used to sharpen the diagnostic acumen and reduce the rate of negative laparotomies. However, they need personnel and expertise, are usually invasive, costly, complicated and less reliable than simple non-invasive clinical scores to sort out patients for observations and/or surgery.

O. Bengezi and M. Al-Fallouji have modified the Alvarado score into a more practical, reliable and easy score for junior doctors to use and interpret for safe and accurate decision-making in patients with acute appendicitis.

The original Alvarado score (Table 1.84.1) was based on a retrospective analysis of 305 patients, while the modified Alvarado score is based on a prospective assessment of 345 patients to design a more clinically orientated and practical score maintaining the same, if not a higher degree of accuracy and reliability.

Table 1.84.2 Modified Alvarado score (mnemonic of MANTREEL)

		Value
Symptoms	**M**igratory RIF pain	1
	Anorexia	1
	Nausea/Vomiting	1
Signs	**T**enderness RLQ	2
	Rigidity and/or **R**ebound tenderness RIF	1
	Elevation of temperature	1
	Extra sign(s), e.g. cough test and/or Rovsing's sign and/or rectal tenderness	1
Laboratory	**L**eucocytosis	2
Total score		10

Score 1–4: acute appendicitis very unlikely, discharge home with instructions;

Score 5–7: acute appendicitis probable, admit for close observation and re-scoring;

Score 8–10: acute appendicitis definite; operate immediately.

Table 1.84.3 Differentiation of appendicitis vs non-specific abdominal pain (NSAP)

Clinical feature	Appendicitis	NSAP
Site of pain	Moves from midline to RIF	Always in RIF or diffuse
Aggravated by	Movement and coughing	Neither
Nausea, vomiting and anorexia	All present	1 or more absent
Facial complexion	Flushed	Normal/pale
Tenderness	Focal in RIF	Shifting tenderness or more diffuse
Rebound and guarding	Both present	Both absent
Rectal examination	Tender on right	Tenderness diffuse/absent

Interpretation of the original Alvarado score can be summarised as follows:

Patients with score 1–4:   acute appendicitis very unlikely keep for observation

Patients with score 5–6:   acute appendicitis maybe, regular observation,

Patients with score 7–8:   acute appendicitis probable, operate;

Patients with score 9–10:   acute appendicitis definite, operate.

According to the modified Alvarado score (Table 1.84.2), patients with score 1–4 are unlikely to have acute appendicitis, and in an acute hospital with rapid turnover they can be discharged home safely without the need for hospitalization, and thus unnecessary admission can be reduced by 13%, a cost-effective policy that can prevent wastage of money, staff time and effort that can be spent on more urgent cases. These patients, however, can be instructed to attend the casualty department if their symptoms increase; their pain can safely be investigated in the outpatient department.

Patients with score 5–7 are an unstable group of patients; they must be kept under ritual close and frequent observation every 4–6 h according to score (6 hourly in patient with score 5 and 4 hourly in patients with score 7). They must be re-scored subsequently until they either switch into score 8 (in more than 80% of cases) and consequently must be operated on, or they may pass into a lesser score (in less than 20% of cases) due to the underlying normal or resolving appendicitis and therefore can be discharged home. Persistent score 7 after 24 h is better operated on. By adopting this safe policy, one can obviate the 29.8% rate of negative laparotomy. Perhaps the policy: 'when in doubt, observe and conserve' can safely replace the old policy: 'when in doubt, take it out'.

Patients with score 8–10 must be operated on immediately because they are definite cases of acute appendicitis; in acute hospital with rapid turnover decision-making can be done quickly, with a score accuracy or predictive value of 97%.

The differentiation of appendicitis from non-specific abdominal pain (NSAP) is summarised in Table 1.84.3.

SURGERY OF ENDOCRINE AND METABOLIC DISEASES

1.85 Solitary Thyroid Nodule

Discrete nodule formation in an otherwise normal thyroid gland is not uncommon. Clinically diagnosed solitary thyroid nodule (STN) may prove to be multinodular on the operating table or at subsequent histological examination. True STN is known for its malignant potential (especially in younger patients). Differentiated thyroid carcinoma may present itself clinically in one of the following forms:
1. STN (needs excision).
2. STN + lymph node in neck (excision).
3. STN + skeletal metastases (radiotherapy).
4. STN + pulmonary metastases (excision + lobectomy).
5. STN + cross-over combination 2, 3, 4.

Management

Management of STN is based on examination, both local and general, which allows assessment of thyroid status and of possible sites of metastases. Five specific investigations are: thyroid function tests (T3, T4, FTI, TSH); fine needle aspiration cytology (requiring special expertise); ultrasound scan; radioactive isotope ^{127}I scanning (becoming less popular); surgical exploration with frozen section facilities.

The most common presentation is the euthyroid patient with an apparently simple STN; the basic problem is to define whether the nodule is cystic or solid, single or multifocal.

Aspiration

In the absence of ultrasound facilities immediate needle aspiration will establish the physical nature of the nodule.

Needle aspiration of a simple cyst is usually perfectly adequate. Aspiration biopsy cytology by fine needle technique for a solid lesion does not exclude malignancy with certainty and also relies on considerable cytological expertise.

Ultrasound and radioactive isotope scanning

Ultrasound examination will establish whether a nodule is solid/cystic, single/multifocal, with irregularity of a cyst wall; or refractory and solid suggesting malignancy. All solid nodules must be operated on nowadays on basis of ultrasound evidence; cystic nodules can be aspirated. Ultrasound examination has now almost superseded radioactive isotope scanning.

Radioactive isotope scanning, complementary to ultrasound, divides STN into:
● Hot (high uptake) with overactive hyperthyroid function.
● Warm (normal uptake) with active euthyroid function.
● Cold (subnormal uptake) with inactive function.

Hot STN is *usually* not malignant. It represents a toxic follicular adenoma requiring treatment by excision or radio-iodine therapy.

Warm STN is a functioning adenoma without endocrine disturbance (histologically follicular adenoma, Hurthle cell adenoma, embryonal adenoma and fetal adenoma). Rarely well-differentiated carcinoma occurs and warm STN may develop into hot STN. Surgical excision is necessary.

Cold STN is malignant in about 12% of cases (either follicular, papillary or medullary) and should be excised. Other causes of cold STN include degenerative cyst, haemorrhage, calcification, abscess and hydatid parasitic cyst. Degenerative adenoma (i.e. hyperplasia in multinodular goitre) and occasionally autoimmune Hashimoto's thyroiditis can present as cold STN.

Surgical exploration and treatment

The foregoing methods may help in planning surgical treatment, but surgical exploration with the help of frozen section remains the end-point of assessment with a view to treatment and it should be preceded by independent inspection of the vocal cords. Local resection of a simple lesion, subtotal resection of a lobe or subtotal removal of the whole gland will suffice for the innocent disorder depending on its single or multifocal nature.

For differentiated carcinoma presenting as STN treatment is as follows.

Papillary carcinoma (metastasises to lymph nodes) Total lobectomy with subtotal lobectomy on the contralateral side, ensuring protection of parathyroid and recurrent laryngeal nerve function. Lymph node enlargement should be diagnosed by frozen section as being due to reactive hyperplasia or secondary deposits. In the latter case a modified neck dissection is carried out (by removing adjacent lymph nodes only, avoiding excision of the sternomastoid and cervical vessels).

Follicular carcinoma (skeletal metastases via bloodstream) Total thyroidectomy removes the lesion and any residual tissue which may compete for radioactive iodine when skeletal deposits may demand treatment at a later date.

Medullary carcinoma Best treated by total thyroidectomy with positive nodes removed by regional resection.

In all these situations thyroxine replacement is required and ideally it is used to suppress TSH in the case of papillary and follicular carcinomas (hormone dependence).

Aetiology of malignant thyroid tumours

● Familial or genetic (medullary thyroid carcinoma).
● Radiotherapy in childhood with radioactive iodine (papillary thyroid carcinoma). *N.B.* Radiotherapy with radioactive iodine should never be given to patients under 45 years of age nor to pregnant women.
● Iodine deficiency goitre or goitrogenic drugs (e.g. thiouracil).
● Autoimmune thyroiditis (malignant lymphoma of thyroid).
● Rarely, benign adenoma changed into malignant.

1.86 Primary Hyperparathyroidism

The blood level of calcium is influenced by various interacting factors. However, abnormal calcium levels can be caused by a variety of conditions. Primary hyperparathyroidism and malignant disease are the two most common causes.

The calcium level is maintained in the blood through Vitamin D actions (on bowel, bones and kidneys) and parathormone action (on bones and kidneys) opposed by calcitonin which plays a minor role (Fig. 1.86.1).

Differential diagnosis of hypercalcaemia

● Primary hyperparathyroidism.
● Sarcoidosis.
● Myelomatosis.
● Hyperthyroidism.
● Milk-alkali syndrome.
● Vitamin D intoxication.
● Immobilisation with Paget's disease.
● Malignant disease with endocrine function (e.g. carcinoma of bronchus or kidney); or skeletal metastases in breast, prostate, bronchus, kidney and thyroid cancer.

Hypercalcaemia is well documented by its clinical manifestations, such as:
● Anorexia, nausea, vomiting and constipation (gastrointestinal).
● Muscle weakness, and decreased reflexes (musculoskeletal).
● Thirst, polyuria and nocturia (renal).
● Various neuropsychiatric symptoms.
● Corneal calcification.

Preoperative diagnosis of primary hyperparathyroidism

Clinically it is the disease of bones (osteitis fibrosa cystica, cyst formation and generalised osteoporosis), stones (renal tract stones and nephrocalcinosis), abdominal groans (due to acute

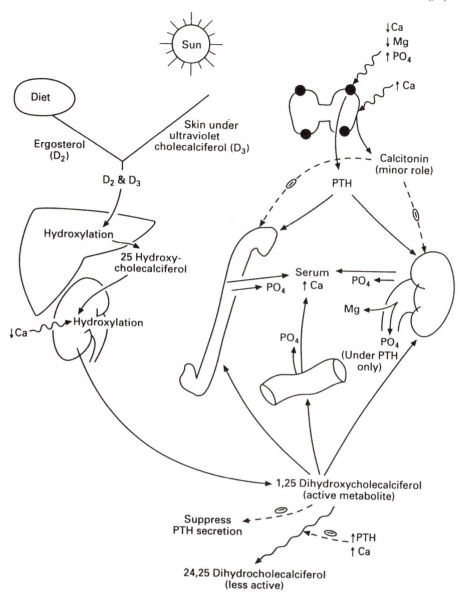

Fig. 1.86.1   Serum calcium under the control of vitamin D, parathormone (PTH) and inhibitory calcitonin

pancreatitis and peptic ulcer) and psychic moans. Laboratory investigations reveal hypercalcaemia, hypercalciuria, hypophosphataemia, hyperphosphaturia and elevated serum alkaline phosphatase. Blood samples for serum calcium estimation should be taken from a fasting patient without application of an arm tourniquet. X-rays show subperiosteal bone resorption in the hands with generalised cystic bone disease and renal stones and/or nephrocalcinosis.

The steroid (cortisone) suppression test is used to exclude hypercalcaemia of sarcoidosis, vitamin D intoxication or metastatic bone disease. Cortisone 150 mg is given daily for 10 days. The calcium level before the injection as well as on the 5th, 8th and 10th day of the test is estimated. It will be reduced in these conditions but hypercalcaemia will persist in primary hyperparathyroidism. Other laboratory tests are full blood count, liver function tests, urea and electrolytes, serum proteins (for serum calcium correction) and protein chromatography with Bence–Jones protein in urine (to exclude multiple myeloma), and uric acid estimation.

Preoperative parathyroid localisation tests

Identification of all parathyroid glands is necessary for successful surgery. Failure rate due to incomplete initial exploration is 5% and most undetected adenomas are in the neck or upper thymus.

Isotope scan using *technetium* and *thallium subtraction imaging* is extremely sensitive in accurately locating adenomas, particularly when there has been previous neck surgery or previous failed parathyroid explorations. The technique principle is first to outline the thyroid with ^{99m}Tc and then to give ^{201}Tl isotope which is taken up by both the thyroid and the parathyroid; the computerised subtraction of the two captured images (by gamma camera) will then show the parathyroid as a 'hot spot'. The other localising tests are rarely used now because of their insensitivity. Surgical exploration is required for persistent hypercalcaemia even if all the tests are negative. They include:

- Cine oesophagography (barium swallow showing indentations).
- Ultrasound scan.
- Arteriography and digital subtraction angiography.
- Retrograde venography and venous sampling of para-thormone levels performed by radiologist via the femoral vein.
- CT scan.
- Nuclear medical radiography.
- Thermography.
- Lymphography.

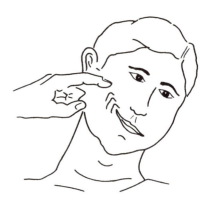

Fig 1.86.2   Shvostek's sign (tapping zygoma results in mouth-corner twitching) seen in hypocalcaemia due to hypoparathyroidism

Operative localising tests

Careful thorough exploration of the neck is essential. Para-thyroids are small and tongue-shaped, dull orange in colour, and, when pinched with forceps, demonstrate a typical subcapsular blush. The following tests facilitate parathyroid identification at operation:

Staining with methylene blue   Methylene blue 5–7.5 mg/kg in 500 ml of 5% dextrose commenced 1 h preoperatively and allowed to flow so that there are about 150 ml in the bottle still to run at the time of induction of anaesthesia. This last amount is run through after induction and while the neck is being opened at operation. Some surgeons believe that this test stains the cervical lymph nodes as well as giving false positive results; others find it helpful especially in localising ectopic parathyroids (e.g. in the thymus) which stain blue.

Flotation density test in 20% mannitol   Adenoma or hyper-plasia sink (no fat) while normal tissue floats (due to fat). The test is not widely practised.

Biopsy and frozen section   This is helpful but may lead to infarction of the remaining biopsied glands. Many surgeons doubt the value of frozen section and prefer to wait for paraffin section.

Selective venous sampling   Performed by the surgeon to identify the level of the hyperfunctioning gland.

Parathyroidectomy

The aim is to remove the diseased gland or glands and leave the patient normocalcaemic. The approach is similar to thyroid-ectomy with only middle thyroid vein disconnection to allow for thorough mobilisation and exploration. A lower collar incision and a stitch applied to the lateral border of the thyroid to pull it forwards and medially are useful. Meticulous care is taken to ensure an absolutely bloodless field – once bleeding occurs on any scale it becomes exceedingly difficult to recognise the subtle features of the small (and occasionally oddly located) parathyroids. There is no need for superior or

inferior thyroid vessel ligation–division under usual circum-stances. Adenoma is usually solitary, and once it is found excision without further search is adequate. In hyperplasia, however, full exploration of all four glands with excision of three and a half is recommended.

Postoperative evaluation of tetany clinically and of hypo-calcaemia chemically is important (Figs. 1.86.2 and 1.86.3). Prolonged i.v. calcium infusion may be required for 2 days in hypocalcaemia. Regular life-long-follow up is important – missed hypocalcaemia may lead to serious problems, e.g. cataract. Indefinite oral calcium replacement 2.5 g four times a day ± vitamin D therapy are needed.

Treatment of hypercalcaemia in general

In order of importance:
1. *Treatment of hypercalcaemia itself.* Because of its danger-ous renal, gastrointestinal, neuropsychiatric and musculoskele-tal effects, hypercalcaemia should be treated until the under-lying cause is diagnosed and treated. The following measures are helpful:
- Rehydration: 4–6 litres in the first 24 h.
- Exclusion of dietary calcium or low-calcium diet.

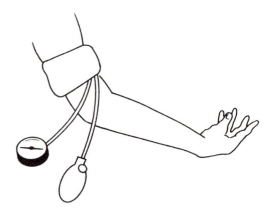

Fig. 1.86.3   Trousseau's sign or carpal spasm after cuff deflation following inflation of blood pressure cuff above systolic pressure for 2 min

- Oral sodium cellulose phosphate (5 g three times daily with meals) and oral or i.v. phosphate can inhibit calcification by binding to calcium in the gut.
- Plicamycin (mithramycin): is a cytotoxic antibiotic with specific action against osteoclasts (single i.v. dose of 25 μg/kg).
- Diuresis: with saline or even frusemide to decrease tubular reabsorption of calcium.
- Calcitonin: reduces bone resorption and causes calciuresis. It is expensive and a daily dose of 200 units is as effective as larger doses.
- Corticosteroids: reduce bone resorption (are both diagnostic and therapeutic).

2. *Treatment of the underlying cause*, e.g. parathyroidectomy, tumour removal, bone radiotherapy, chemotherapy (for myeloma and bronchial small-cell carcinoma) and endocrine therapy (in metastatic breast carcinoma).

3. *Treatment of complications*, e.g. nephrocalcinosis and/or renal stones are treated finally on their merit. Surgery is indicated only in obstruction, pain and infection; otherwise treatment is expectant and conservative.

(See also hypercalcaemia in 5.1.4 Fluid and electrolyte disorders in surgery.)

1.87 Diabetes and Surgery

Surgical procedures are more common in diabetics than non-diabetics because:
- Eighty per cent of diabetics are over 40 years of age and surgical procedures are more common in this age group.
- Diabetes and its complications predispose to a variety of surgical disorders:
  - Large blood vessel diseases (macroangiopathy) including peripheral vascular insufficiency and gangrene.
  - Cardiac (ischaemic and hypertensive) disorders.
  - Eye (proliferative and non-proliferative retinopathies and cataracts).
  - Renal (uraemia and hypertension).
  - Infections: skin boils and abscesses, moniliasis (vulvitis and balanitis) and tuberculosis, as well as urinary tract infections.

The current high standard of surgical and anaesthetic technology make the surgical outcome in diabetics comparable to that in non-diabetics.

Preoperative assessment

The aims are to prevent ketosis and avoid hypoglycaemia. Medical evaluation of diabetic control is carried out and the presence of any complication noted, e.g. neuropathy, retinopathy and hidden infections as well as autonomic neuropathy (postural hypotension, gastroparesis and, in men, erectile impotence). Renal complications and electrolyte disturbances must be recognised, with serum creatinine and potassium respectively. Hypokalaemia is not uncommon in those receiving diuretics for essential hypertension or congestive heart failure and, if it occurs during anaesthesia, induction, may be dangerous (arrhythmias). Furthermore, hypokalaemia may worsen hyperglycaemia, and therefore it must be corrected preoperatively. The elective cases should be admitted 2 days prior to surgery; blood sugar should always be measured serially; oral hypoglycaemic agents, e.g. chlorpropamide, should be stopped 36 h before surgery (because of its long half-life) and replaced with insulin during the intra- and postoperative period. However, in hospitalisation for urgent surgery, regular insulin should be administered immediately until hyperglycaemia is reduced and the required surgery then undertaken (see below).

Preoperative medications are the same as for non-diabetics. The patient should never fast for prolonged periods before surgery. Scheduling of the operation for the morning hours is recommended, so that the first glucose infusion replaces breakfast energy. Intravenous feeding (rather than oral liquid breakfast) is advisable even for those scheduled for the afternoon, since surgery may be moved up if an earlier operation is cancelled.

Intraoperative management

Anaesthesia combined with surgical stress has a definite hyperglycaemic effect. Local, field block, spinal or epidural anaesthesia produces little metabolic disturbance; therefore the spinal approach is recommended whenever feasible. General anaesthesia, however, is well tolerated by most diabetics.

Hypotension (postural) and hypoglycaemia should be monitored throughout anaesthesia.

(A) Elective surgery in insulin-dependent diabetics

The complications of hypoglycaemia and hypokalaemia are less likely to occur following infusion of low physiological doses of insulin than following therapy for diabetic ketoacidosis or hyperosmolar non-ketotic coma with the traditional higher (pharmacological) doses of insulin. Continuous intravenous infusion of insulin coupled with a separate infusion or piggybacked into the same vein as dextrose/water is recommended for ketosis-free patients. The infusions can be initiated preoperatively or intraoperatively and continued postoperatively. The recommended infusion is 50 units of insulin in 500 ml of normal saline, giving an insulin concentration of 1 unit per 10 ml/h, via an accurate infusion pump such as IVAC, coupled with 5% dextrose infusion at a rate of 100 ml (5 g glucose)/h to maintain the blood glucose in the desired range of 8.5–14 mmol/l. This regimen is very safe even if it is started on the evening before surgery. Blood glucose levels should be determined in the operating room and measured at 2 h intervals postoperatively. Adjustment in the rate of insulin and/or glucose infusion should be made according to the blood glucose results.

Note that:
- The postoperative fluid replacements should be dealt with separately from glucose and insulin infusions.
- Urine glucose estimation (even via a catheter) should be avoided.
- This method should continue until the patient is able to take fluids orally.

- This method can lead to insulin-induced hypoglycaemia (more dangerous than hyperglycaemia) if the i.v. glucose infusion line is kinked or extravasated (tissuing).

(B) Emergency surgery in insulin-dependent diabetics

Acute surgical emergencies are likely to cause rapid diabetic ketoacidosis and dehydration, and ultimately death. Insulin-dependent (Type 1) diabetes is not uncommonly first manifested at the time of acute illness, e.g. perforated peptic ulcer, abscesses or acute cholecystitis, and delay in its recognition is fatal. Examination of blood and urine specimens will reveal diabetes which should be treated immediately. An i.v. normal saline infusion should be administered rapidly over a 4 h period. A 10 unit bolus of insulin is given i.v. followed by continuous infusion of 10 units insulin for 1 h from an independent reservoir (50 units insulin in 500 ml saline). Potassium chloride should be added if the initial serum K^+ is subnormal. This should be measured periodically since insulin (even in low doses) can cause hypokalaemia. Frequent monitoring of serum electrolytes and acetone is necessary. Blood glucose should be determined at the bedside at 2 h intervals using Dextrostix with a glucometer. The basic saline infusion should be changed to Dextrose/saline (5% glucose + 0.45% saline) once the blood glucose level has fallen to 14 mmol/l. Nasogastric suction is used if there is vomiting or gastroparesis, and antibiotics should be given when appropriate. A period of 4–8 h of rapid fluid and insulin infusion should be sufficient to improve the metabolic situation so that the patient can safely undergo emergency surgery. It is futile to delay such surgery further while attempting to eliminate ketosis completely, since the underlying acute progressive surgical condition, if uncorrected, will lead to rapid deterioration. (Thereafter careful monitoring of the patient during and after surgery is as for elective surgery.)

Note that:

- The sliding scale of insulin based on the colour of urine treated with Clinitest reagent tablets (rainbow method) should be abandoned.
- The Biostator (Miles Laboratory) is a recently developed automatically computerised instrument which continuously displays the blood glucose concentration. It is programmed to maintain normal blood glucose levels by infusing either 5% glucose or insulin, according to the desired glucose level selected by the doctor.

(C) Surgery in non-insulin-dependent diabetics

This type of diabetes (Type 2) is the most common form of the disease. Most patients are over 40 years of age. Diabetic ketoacidosis is rare because of limited reserves of endogenous insulin, but the stress of major surgery may sometimes push patients into ketoacidosis.

For minor operations   Whether patients are controlled with diet only, oral hypoglycaemic or insulin, they should be observed and these agents withheld until after the procedure.

For major operations   Patients controlled with diet only should be observed. Oral hypoglycaemic agent should be discontinued from those previously controlled with it and replaced with 10 units insulin in 1 litre of 5% dextrose. Those previously controlled with insulin should be treated like insulin-dependent diabetics. If the postoperative blood glucose is above 14 mmol/l, 10 units of subcutaneous insulin + 20 units of insulin increment in subsequent infusion (in persistent hyperglycaemia) should be administered.

Postoperative management

In (A), as before but each litre of postoperative i.v. infusion should contain 5% glucose, 0.45% saline and 44 mEq of potassium chloride. Extrarenal fluid losses from drainage and suction should be replaced independently (with potassium chloride). The postoperative goal for the blood glucose level is between 8.5 and 14 mmol/l. Oral fluids, once started, should be followed by a soft diet then a diabetic diet. The usual daily insulin dose can be resumed according to 3-hourly blood glucose estimation.

In (B) as before. Once blood glucose falls below 14 mmol/l, insulin is administered i.m. or subcutaneously adjusted according to serial blood glucose estimations. Thereafter the patient is stabilised by changing to an intermediate acting insulin, e.g. Lente with a soluble insulin.

In (C) preoperative therapy should be resumed.

Management of diabetic leg and ulcers

Leg ulcers in diabetic patients are contributed to arterial insufficiency, microangiopathy (in early cases transforming into macroangiopathy in advanced cases), and peripheral neuropathy. Microangiopathy (which occurs early in the disease) causes impairment of vessel wall flexibility and deranged vascular control mechanisms, and disruption of metabolic exchange with resultant hypoxia leading to reduced local immunity with low resistance to infection, poor healing, and ulceration (usually digital). Peripheral neuropathy reduces pain perception, so minor foot injuries become neglected. Neuropathic ulcers, the most usual form of diabetic ulcer, occur over weight-bearing areas, such as the metatarsal heads and heel and require total contact casting (see below). Management include:

- Optimal diabetic control (which can mean 3 injections daily or the use of insulin in those previously treated with oral hypoglycaemics);
- Early recognition and prompt treatment of infection (particularly of deep pockets);
- Local wound treatment in form of debridement of necrotic tissue (including tendon and bone if necessary), hydrogen peroxide bath and povidone-iodine in deep-seated infections with daily dressing of the wound;
- Total contact casting (TCC) is achieved as follows:
  after soaking the limb in a povidone-iodine bath for 10 minutes and careful drying, nail care and debridement, a hydrocolloid dressing is shaped to the ulcer and fixed smoothly with adhesive tape. The cast from toes to below the knee is closely applied to the plantar surface with minimal padding. Finally, a rocker heel is fixed and secured with a fibreglass paste bandage such as, Scotchcast or Deltalite with its fulcrum aligned with the pretibial border. The effect is to

distribute vertical forces evenly and translate shear stress into forward movement of the foot.

– Measures in arterial ulcer do apply here, such as avoidance of cigarette smoking, obesity, hyperlipidaemia, and control of blood pressure. Care is taken to avoid vasoconstricting drugs (including beta-blockers) and those with a potential to produce 'steal' phenomenon (e.g. nifedipine and nafti-drofuryl). Prostacyclin analogues, such as iloprost may be valuable in treating arterial insufficiency.

A team approach is necessary. Early referral for debridement and an operator familiar with TCC are essential. Most neuropathic ulcers heal rapidly with minor complications, but patient education is important. Recurrences are common and after-care is a problem because of the difficulty in fitting proper footwear, since many patients dislike wearing a shoe with a rocker.

Hyperosmolar non-ketotic coma

This syndrome is increasingly recognised in surgical patients (iatrogenic). Delay in diagnosis and therapy is fatal. Pre-operative dehydration and surgical stress with postoperative hyperglycaemic drugs predispose to hyperosmolar non-ketotic coma. It has also been observed in burns, following hyper-alimentation, following i.v. dextrose infusions (exogenous glucose loads), and complicating cardiopulmonary bypass as well as haemodialysis and peritoneal dialysis. Vascular throm-boses (e.g. mesenteric thrombosis) are a major complication of hyperosmolar non-ketotic coma. Surgical intervention may be needed when such patients develop signs of acute abdomen – more frequent than in those with diabetic ketoacidosis. Thromboses may also block lower limb vessels, necessitating amputation.

Diabetes management during open heart surgery

These patients need a glucose/insulin/potassium infusion with much greater amounts of insulin (1 unit/g of glucose) than non-cardiac diabetics (0.3 unit/g or 3 units with 10 g glucose) to cope with extra trauma, hypothermia and glucose loading when cardiopulmonary bypass begins.

(N.B. See also s. 1.25 High risk patients in surgery.)

1.88 Surgical Treatment of Obesity

Definition of obesity

A body weight 20% above ideal weight, or a body mass index greater than 30 indicates significant obesity.

Body Mass Index (BMI) = Weight (kg)/Height^2 (m)

Example: A 150 kg, 1.8 m tall patient has a BMI of 47. A similar patient but weighing 80 kg has a BMI equal to 25.

In adults, the final common pathway leading to obesity is a positive caloric intake, with subsequent increases in the size of adipose cells to accommodate the excess of triglycerides.

Obesity occurring in early childhood is due to increases in the number of adipose cells. In abnormal situations, hormonal abnormalities (hypothyroidism and Cushing's syndrome) rather than positive caloric intake are responsible. Psychological disturbances are often associated with obesity.

Obesity is the most common nutritional disorder in the USA. Obesity increases the risk for developing medical and surgical disease. Obesity-induced physiological alterations include metabolic (insulin resistance), respiratory (decreased thoracic volume and movement limitation due to enlarged abdomen), cardiovascular (increased heart work load due to increased oxygen demand of large body mass with positive relation between increases in blood pressure and weight gain), and hepatic manifestations (fatty infiltration with hepatic dysfunction).

It is important to remember that 5% of ingested glucose is promptly converted into glycogen in the liver, while 30–40% is converted into fat.

Severe obesity is a life-threatening condition and is asso-ciated with:

● Increased mortality due to cardiovascular, respiratory, hep-atobiliary complications and suicide; a 20% weight excess raises the mortality rate by 15%.

● Obesity-related diseases, e.g. gallstones, hiatus hernias, osteoarthritis, varicose veins, thrombophlebitis and gravita-tional oedema, fractures and severe limb injuries, prolapse and cystocele, maturity-onset diabetes, arterial diseases and renal calculi (surgically treated diseases) as well as chronic obstructive airway diseases, dermatological problems and infertility.

Overeating is often compulsive and addictive and is commonly associated with little or no physical activity. Dietary energy restriction with increased physical activity should be tried first but diet, drugs, in-patient starvation, hypnotism and psychiatric therapy have only a short-term effect and are usually unsatisfactory since the weight lost is rapidly regained after termination of the programme.

In industrialised societies, increasing body weight is closely related to an increasing incidence of non-insulin dependent diabetes, coronary heart disease, increased blood pressure, blood lipids, glucose, and insulin concentrations, urate concen-tration, and packed cell volume. The American Institute of Nutrition recommends BMI of 18–25 for both sexes and suggest that most people will be healthier towards the lower end of the range; they proposed that

BMI 18–23 = lowest risk (20–22) is the ideal optimal healthy BMI)

BMI 24–25 = mild risk

BMI 26–29 = medium risk

BMI > 30 = high risk

The healthy weight target of a BMI < 25 for adults represents the upper limit beyond which weight related disease risk becomes a concern and morbidity associated with obesity becomes manifest. Those exceeding the healthy weight target and without a diagnosis of weight-related disease, must reduce the risk of disease by reducing their weight, and is roughly 2 BMI units (6 kgs or 1 stone) consistently towards a healthier weight goal. In 1993, 13% of men and 16% of women in England were obese. (BMI <25 is normal; BMI 25–30 is overweight; BMI > 30 is obese; BMI > 40 is morbidly obese; BMI > 50 is considered superobesity) If a BMI of 25–30 is generally regarded as overweight, then half of adult population of England is overweight or obese; in other words, obesity is currently an epidemic disease.

There are many dieting programmes, but the Slimming World programme is probably the most popular. This includes daily free food items such as citrus fruit (not nuts, bananas, or dried fruits) and vegetables (such as salads not beans/potatoes) plus one measured portion of dairy products and 2 measured portions of cereals/2 slices of bread; also if white meat such as fish or chicken breasts is taken (preferable to red meat) then proteins of vegetable origin (beans/potatoes) should not be taken on that day and vice versa. High fluid intake, diet drinks and iceberg lettuce/mushrooms should be encouraged; alcohol, food fried with oil, dressings, biscuits in-between meals, cakes and chocolate bars should be avoided.

Anorectic drugs: Working party of the Royal College of Physicians of London has recently (1996/1997) considered the role of anorectic drugs (including anorexia) in the management of obesity. Anorectic drugs are sympathomimetics which act on the central nervous system to suppress the appetite and are classified into 2 main groups:

- Those acting via catecholamine pathways e.g. Ionamin and Duromine (phentermines) are not useful on controlled studies.
- Those promoting serotonin neurotransmission e.g. fenfluramine and dexfenfluramine (fenfluramines). Controlled studies suggest that fenfluramines can help achieve sustained weight loss (in 35% of obese patients treated with dexfenfluramine compared with 17% in placebo-treated control group) in selected patients with BMI of $30\,kg/m^2$ or greater (no available evidence for other anorectic drugs). Primary pulmonary hypertension (PPH) is the complication in these drugs (6 times than controls and 23 times if used for more than three months) with presentation of reduced exercise tolerance, syncope, chest pain, oedema or palpitations and disease may be fatal. Treatment with anorectic anti-obesity drugs is appropriate only for people with BMI greater than 30 who fail to reduce their weight by 10% after 3 months determined effort with diet, exercise, and behavioural change. Even then, slimming pills should only be prescribed for more than 3 months if patients achieve a 10% reduction in that time and do not regain more than 3 kg. They are contraindicated in patients with PPH, a current or past history of cardiovascular or cerebrovascular disease (and epilepsy), a current or past psychiatric disorder, a history of alcoholism or drug abuse, in children under 12 years, and in patients receiving any other centrally-acting anorectic agent.
- Thyroid hormones have no place in the treatment of obesity except in hypothyroid patients.

The rationale for surgery is based on two facts:
1. Severe obesity is associated with high mortality and morbidity.
2. Long-term medical treatment often fails.

On the other hand, obesity influences surgery in two ways:
1. Obesity-associated diseases (treated surgically, see above).
2. Adverse effects on surgical management preoperatively causing late diagnosis, e.g. hidden carcinoma in a fatty breast and difficult diagnosis of intra-abdominal masses. Postoperatively wound sepsis, haematoma, burst abdomen, respira-

tory insufficiency and atelactasis, deep venous thrombosis and pulmonary embolism occur more frequently and the results of varicose vein or hiatus hernia surgery are poorer in obese patients.

Indications for surgery

- Morbid or massive obesity defined as at least twice or 45 kg over the ideal weight (matched for age, sex and height) of at least 5 years' duration.
- Failure of standard medical dietary treatment and/or patient failure to adhere to prescribed dietary regimen.

Criteria of suitability for surgery

- Absence of correctable endocrine abnormality which might be a cause of the obesity (e.g. Cushing's syndrome, myxoedema).
- Absence of unrelated diseases which might increase the operative risk.
- Absence of excessive alcohol intake.
- Presence of certain obesity-related complications which might be improved by a significant weight loss, e.g. hyperlipidaemia, maturity-onset diabetes, hypertension or Pickwickian syndrome (cardiorespiratory embarrassment due to excessive obesity).
- Assurance of patient cooperation both in preoperative assessment and in prolonged postoperative management.

Preoperative measures (especially in intestinal shunts)

1. High-protein diet for 3 weeks.
2. Bowel preparation (e.g. oral neomycin and metronidazole), elemental diet, mechanical cleansing and washout.
3. Low-dose heparin subcutaneously started with premedication until the patient is mobile postoperatively (to prevent thromboembolism).
4. Prophylactic antibiotics to prevent wound infection.

Surgical procedures

Historical (not recommended)

Truncal vagotomy without drainage   To decrease gastric emptying (pylorospasm) and therefore limit the transit time of food, reducing the intestinal absorption accordingly.

Lipectomy (apronectomy or panniculectomy)   Surgical elliptical excision of the large apron of fat that forms the anterior abdominal wall as it interferes with ventilation and causes intertrigo and mechanical impairment with walking. It was widely practised and removal of up to 26 kg was reported. It does not contribute significantly to obesity control. Furthermore, repair of coexisting umbilical hernia is frequently followed by bleeding, haematoma and wound sepsis.

Dental splintage   Cap splints or interdental wiring are used to restrict the patient to a fluid diet (e.g. milk or soup with iron and vitamin supplements). The wiring is released monthly for 2–3 days at a time to prevent trismus and to facilitate adequate dental hygiene. Fifty per cent of patients could not tolerate the procedure and only 10% allowed the procedure to continue long enough for satisfactory weight loss in spite of short-term good results. The long-term results are no better than those of conservative medical means.

Note: The use of an intragastric balloon (to make the patient feel that the stomach is full) and extrinsic abdominal compression are not useful in such patients.

Current (recommended)

Gastric operations (Figs 1.88.1–1.88.3)

- Subtotal gastrectomy (small gastric fundic pouch and large stoma): causes dumping syndrome with decreased food intake and weight loss (unsatisfactory, with high mortality).
- Gastroplasty: incision partially traverses the stomach from the lesser curve, leaving a small channel intact along the greater curvature. Weight loss occurs only during the first 6 postoperative months.
- Gastric bypass (large gastric pouch and small stoma).
- Gastric bypass (small gastric pouch and small stoma): bypasses 90% of stomach, leaving a 12 mm gastroenterostomy stoma.
- Gastroplasty: a stapler is used, without division of the stomach, to create a 10% fundic pouch and 1 cm stoma on the greater curve (easy, safe and reversible).
- Magenstrasse and Mill (D. Johnston and H. Sue-Ling 1995) is becoming the popular method of gastroplasty. A narrow lesser curve tube (Magenstrasse is German for gastric street)

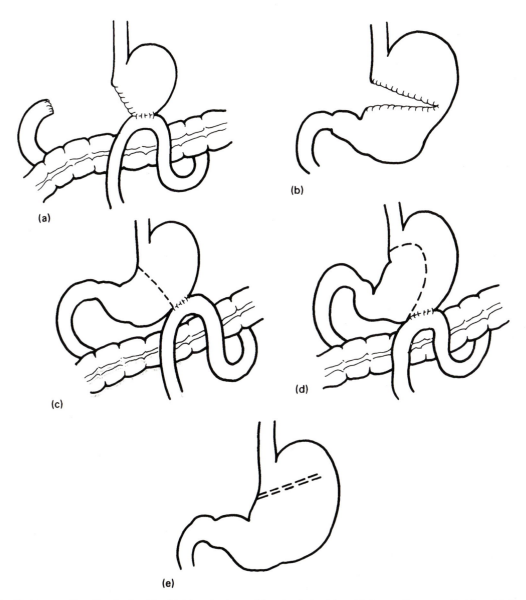

Fig. 1.88.1 Gastric operations for obesity: (a) subtotal gastrectomy; (b) gastroplasty; (c) gastric bypass (large pouch); (d) gastric bypass (small pouch); (e) gastroplasty without division of stomach

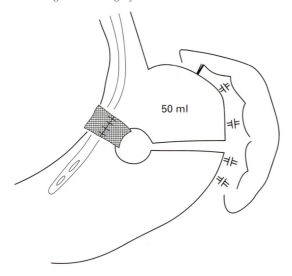

Fig. 1.88.2   Vertical banded gastroplasty

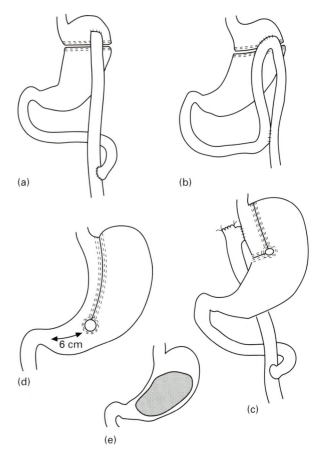

Fig. 1.88.3   The currently used operations for morbid obesity. Gastric transection with Roux-en-Y gastrojejunostomy (a,c) or gastrojejunostomy (b). Magenstrasse and Mill (M&M) operation (d). Endoscopic insertion of gastric balloon (e) is less popular since the balloon can be punctured or migrated

is created over a size 34 FG bougie and acts as a conduit for food to the vagally innervated gastric antrum (the mill) which grinds food.

● Vertical band gastroplasty (see Fig. 1.88.2): a circular stapler is used to drill a hole of 10 mm in diameter followed by a linear stapler cutter 90 to create a 50 ml gastric pouch with no future expansion. This operation is becoming obsolete. Obesity recurs quickly and the band may ulcerate with associated problems.

Results: Operative mortality is 2.8% and total mortality is 5.1%. Although the immediate weight loss is rapid, the majority of patients will not reach their ideal weight. Fistulation and gastroenterostomy anastomotic disruption is the most important complication (reduced by careful technique and prolonged postoperative nasogastric decompression). Other non-specific complications, e.g. thromboembolism, respiratory failure and wound infection, are common.

Dumping syndrome is severe in 20% of patients. Oedema, diarrhoea and syncope are other side-effects. Stomal ulceration is low in the gastric exclusion operation but significant in gastroenterostomies. Such gastric operations are probably the operation of choice in morbidly obese patients wishing to return to ideal weight and should be reserved for obese patients (after failure of conservative means). Following surgery, cardiothoracic, diabetic and arthritic symptoms improve.

Intestinal bypass or shunt (historical interest)

The idea was conceived after the survival of a patient following massive small intestinal resection for volvulus and mesenteric thrombosis. The length of the anastomosing parts of the bowel is the most decisive factor in the success of the operation. Types of operation include (see Fig. 1.88.4 (a–e):

(a) Jejunocolic bypass: anastomosis of proximal 38 cm of jejunum with transverse colon (end-to-side). Dramatic weight loss occurred but due to the prohibitive morbidity of severe diarrhoea, electrolyte disturbance and hepatic fail-

ure, the operation was condemned and abandoned in favour of jejunoileal shunts.

(b) Jejunoileal shunt (Payne, 1969): anastomosis of 35 cm of proximal jejunum end-to-side with the terminal 6.5 cm of ileum. Weight loss was inadequate owing to extensive reflux of food into the bypassed blind loop which was still able to absorb the food.

(c) Jejunoileal shunt (Scott, 1971): anastomosis of the proximal 30 cm of jejunum end-to-end to the terminal 15–30 cm of ileum. The bypassed small intestine is vented into either the transverse or sigmoid colon.

The *results* are classified into:

Good: satisfactory weight loss, no diarrhoea and no metabolic deficits.

Fair: weight loss not ideal, mild diarrhoea and minimal metabolic deficits.

Poor: unsatisfactory weight loss and/or persistent diarrhoea and/or severe metabolic deficits.

The majority of Payne end-to-side shunts were poor while the majority of Scott end-to-end shunts were good.

(d) Jejunoileal shunt (Joffe, 1979): anastomosis of the proximal 36 cm of jejunum to the last 4 cm of ileum, end-to-end

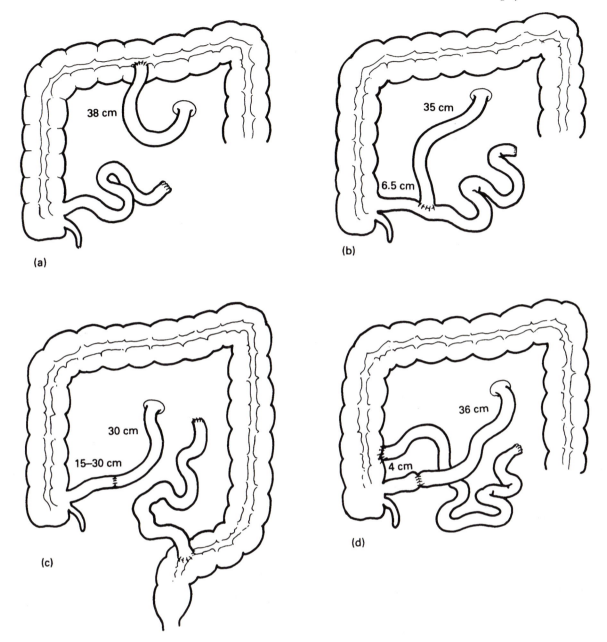

(a)   38 cm

(b)   35 cm   6.5 cm

(c)   30 cm   15–30 cm

(d)   36 cm   4 cm

Fig. 1.88.4   Intestinal shunts

(two layers). The bypassed small intestine is drained end-to-side to the ascending colon. Liver biopsy is performed routinely (the operation is conducted via a transverse supraumbilical incision).

Postoperative complications

- Diarrhoea for a few weeks.
- Fatty liver: a serious complication as it may eventually lead to hepatic coma and death. Preoperative baseline liver biopsy and liver function tests follow-up are essential to detect this problem (confirmed by needle liver biopsy).
- Malabsorption, metabolic and electrolyte deficits.

- Anastomotic blockage, bleeding and leakage.
- Wound dehiscence and incisional hernia.
- Operative mortality due to burst abdomen, myocardial infarction, pulmonary embolism and acute fatty liver.

Postoperative care and follow-up

1. Respiratory intensive care unit with ventilation for 48 h.
2. Nasogastric suction for 5 days followed by Gastrografin follow-through before oral feeding is commenced.
3. Diarrhoea control with Lomotil and codeine phosphate.
4. Regular follow-up, monitoring the body weight, liver function and recurrence of diarrhoea, is essential.

BRAIN DEATH AND TRANSPLANTATION SURGERY

1.89 Brain Death and Cadaveric Organs for Transplantation

DIAGNOSTIC

Death can be diagnosed by irreversible cessation of respiration and heart beat; it can also be diagnosed by brain death, which is diagnosed by irreversible cessation of brain stem function (brain stem death).

Diagnosis of brain death

With the development of intensive care techniques and their wide availability in the United Kingdom, it has become commonplace for hospitals to have deeply comatose and unresponsive patients with severe brain damage who are maintained on artificial respiration by means of mechanical ventilators. This state has been recognised for many years and it has been the concern of the medical profession to establish diagnostic criteria of such rigour that on their fulfilment the mechanical ventilator can be switched off, in the secure knowledge that there is no possible chance of recovery.

There has been much philosophical argument about the diagnosis of death, which has throughout recorded history been accepted as having occurred when the vital functions of respiration and circulation have ceased. However, with the technical ability to maintain these functions artificially, the dilemma of when to switch off the ventilator has been the subject of much public interest. It is agreed that permanent functional death of the brain stem constitutes brain death and that once this has occurred, further artificial support is fruitless and should be withdrawn. It is good medical practice to recognise when brain death has occurred and to act accordingly, sparing relatives from the further emotional trauma of sterile hope.

Codes of practice, such as the Harvard criteria (1968), have been devised to guide medical practitioners in the diagnosis of brain death. These have provided considerable help with the problem and they have been refined as the knowledge gained from experience has been collated.

The diagnostic criteria presented for brain death here have been written with the advice of the sub-committee of the Transplant Advisory Panel, the working party of the Royal College of Physicians, the working-party of the Faculty of Anaesthetists, and the Royal College of Surgeons and have been approved by the Conference of Medical Royal Colleges and their Faculties in the United Kingdom. They are accepted as being sufficient to distinguish between those patients who retain the functional capacity to have a chance of even partial recovery and those where no such possibility exists.

The diagnosis of brain death should be considered under the following conditions:

1. The patients is deeply comatose.

(a) There should be no suspicion that this state is due to depressant drugs. Narcotics, hypnotics and tranquillisers may have prolonged duration of action, particularly when some hypothermia exists. The benzodiazepines are markedly cumulative and persistent in their actions and are commonly used as anticonvulsants or to assist synchronisation with mechanical ventilators. It is therefore recommended that the drug history should be carefully reviewed and adequate intervals allowed for the persistence of drug effects to be excluded. This is of particular importance in patients where the primary cause of coma lies in the toxic effects of drugs followed by anoxic cerebral damage.

(b) Primary hypothermia as a cause of coma should have been excluded.

(c) Metabolic and endocrine disturbances which can be responsible for or can contribute to coma should have been excluded.

Metabolic and endocrine factors contributing to the persistence of coma must be subject to careful assessment. There should be no profound abnormality of the serum-electrolytes, acid–base balance or blood glucose.

2. The patient is being maintained on a ventilator because spontaneous respiration had previously become inadequate or had ceased altogether.

(a) Relaxants (neuromuscular blocking agents) and other drugs should have been excluded as a cause of respiratory inadequacy or failure. Immobility, unresponsiveness and lack of spontaneous respiration may be due to the use of neuromuscular blocking drugs and the persistence of their effects should be excluded by elicitation of spinal reflexes (flexion or stretch) or by the demonstration of adequate neuromuscular condition with a conventional nerve stimulator. Equally, persistent effects of hypnotics and narcotics should be excluded as the cause of respiratory failure.

3. There should be no doubt that the patient's condition is due to irremediable structural brain damage. The diagnosis of a disorder which can lead to brain death should have been fully established.

It may be obvious within hours of a primary intracranial event such as severe head injury, spontaneous intracranial haemorrhage or following neurosurgery, that the condition is irremediable. However, when a patient has suffered primarily from cardiac arrest, hypoxia or severe circulatory insufficiency with an indefinite period of cerebral anoxia, or is suspected of having cerebral air or fat embolism, then it may take much longer to establish the diagnosis and to be confident of the prognosis. In some patients the primary pathology may be a matter of doubt and a confident diagnosis may only be reached by continuity of clinical observation and investigation.

Diagnostic tests for the confirmation of brain death

All brain stem reflexes absent

(i)   The pupils are fixed in diameter and do not respond to sharp changes in the intensity of incident light.

(ii) There is no corneal reflex.

(iii) The vestibulo-ocular reflexes are absent. These are absent when no eye movement occurs during or following the slow injection of 20 ml of ice-cold water into each external auditory meatus in turn, clear access to the tympanic membrane having been established by direct inspection. This test may be contraindicated on one or other side by local trauma.

(iv) No motor responses within cranial nerve distribution can be elicited by adequate stimulation of any somatic area.

(v)   There is no gag reflex or reflex response to bronchial stimulation by a suction catheter passed down the trachea.

(vi) No respiratory movements occur when the patient is disconnected from the mechanical ventilator for long enough to ensure that the arterial carbon dioxide tension rises above the threshold for stimulation of respiration.

During this latter test it is necessary for the arterial carbon dioxide tension to exceed the threshold for respiratory stimulation – that is, the $PaCO_2$ should normally reach 6.65 kPa (50 mmHg). This is best achieved by measurement of the blood gases; if this facility is available it is recommended that the patient should be disconnected when the $PaCO_2$ reaches 5.33–6.00 kPa (40–45 mmHg) following administration of 5% CO_2 in oxygen through the ventilator. This starting level has been chosen because patients may be moderately hypothermic (35–37°C), flaccid and with a depressed metabolic rate, so that $PaCO_2$ rises only slowly in apnoea (about 0.26 kPa/min or 2 mmHg/min). (Hypoxia during disconnection should be prevented by delivering oxygen at 6 l/min through a catheter into the trachea.) If blood–gas analysis is not available to measure the $PaCO_2$, the alternative procedure is to supply the ventilator with pure oxygen for 10 minutes (pre-oxygenation), then with 5% CO_2 in oxygen for 5 minutes and to disconnect the ventilator for 10 minutes, while delivering oxygen at 6 l/min by catheter into the trachea. This establishes diffusion oxygenation and ensures that during apnoea hypoxia will not occur even in 10 or more minutes of respiratory arrest. Those patients with pre-existing chronic respiratory insufficiency, who may be unresponsive to raised levels of carbon dioxide and who normally exist on an hypoxic drive, are special cases and should be expertly investigated with careful blood–gas monitoring.

Other considerations

1. *Repetition of testing*   It is customary to repeat the tests to ensure that there has been no observer error. The interval between tests must depend upon the primary pathology and the clinical course of the disease. Item 3 indicates some conditions where it would be unnecessary to repeat them since a prognosis of imminent brain death can be accepted as being obvious.

In some conditions the outcome is not so clear-cut and in these it is recommended that the tests should be repeated. The interval between tests depends upon the progress of the patient and might be as long as 24 hours. This is a matter for medical judgement and repetition time must be related to the signs of improvement, stability and deterioration which present themselves.

2. *Integrity of spinal reflexes*   It is well established that spinal cord function can persist after insults which irretrievably destroy brain stem function. Reflexes of spinal origin may persist or return after an initial absence in brain dead patients.

3. *Confirmatory investigations*   It is now widely accepted that electro-encephalography (EEG) is not necessary for diagnosis of brain death. Indeed this view was expressed from Harvard in 1969 only a year after the publication of their original criteria. EEG has its principal value at earlier stages in the care of patients, in whom the original diagnosis is in doubt. When EEG is used, the strict criteria recommended by the Federation of EEG Societies must be followed.

Other investigations such as cerebral angiography or cerebral blood-flow measurements are not required for the diagnosis of brain death.

4. *Body temperature*   The body temperature in these patients may be low because of depression of central temperature regulation by drugs or by brain stem damage and it is recommended that it should not be less than 35°C before the diagnostic tests are carried out. A low-reading thermometer should be used.

5. *Specialist opinion and status of the doctors concerned* Experienced clinicians in intensive care units, acute medical wards and accident and emergency departments should not normally require specialist advice. Only when primary diagnosis is in doubt is it necessary to consult with a neurologist or neurosurgeon.

The decision to withdraw artificial support should be made after all the criteria presented above have been fulfilled and can be made by any one of the following combinations of doctors:

● A consultant who is in charge of the case, and one other doctor.

● In the absence of a consultant, his deputy, who should have been registered for 5 years or more and who should have had adequate previous experience in the care of such cases, and one other doctor.

CADAVERIC ORGANS FOR TRANSPLANTATION

Choice of Donors

Patients who may become *suitable* donors after death are those who have suffered severe and irreversible brain damage. Such patients will be dependent on artificial ventilation or expected shortly to become so.

Those who would be *unsuitable* as donors are:

– patients with malignant disease (except primary brain tumours);

– patients with systemic infection;

– patients with renal disease, including chronic hypertension and recent urinary infection or those who have suffered renal anoxic damage;
– patients with severe atherosclerosis.

It follows from this that many elderly patients would not be suitable donors.

It is not always easy to recognise whether a patient would be considered a suitable donor. For example, patients who have had a sudden irreversible cardiorespiratory arrest (e.g. myocardial infarction) or those in the so-called 'brought in dead' category are unlikely to be suitable as organ donors. If there are any doubts about suitability, hospital staff should contact the local transplant team.

Approach to relatives

If a patient carries a signed donor card or has otherwise recorded his or her wishes there is no legal requirement to establish lack of objection on the part of relatives, although it is good practice to take account of the views of close relatives. If a relative objects, despite the known request by the patient, staff will need to judge according to the circumstances of the case whether it is wise to proceed with organ removal. Relatives may be under great stress, and staff have a duty to consider their feelings.

If a patient who has died is not known to have requested (in the required manner) that his or her organs be removed for transplantation after death, the designated person may only authorise the removal if having made such reasonable enquiry as may be practicable, that person has no reason to believe:

(a) that the deceased had expressed an objection to his or her body being so dealt with after their death, and had not withdrawn it; or
(b) that the surviving spouse or any surviving relative of the deceased objects to the body being so dealt with.

The designated person need not enquire of the relatives in person, but requires only to be satisfied that such enquiries have been properly carried out.

Where a donor has lived closely with someone to whom he or she was not related it is advisable to try to seek the views of the cohabitee as well as those of the relatives.

There is no need for relatives to confirm their lack of objection in writing, but it is essential to keep a written record of the enquiries made and their outcome. This should be entered in the transplantation checklist. If relatives are asked to sign any form this should be worded in terms of lack of objection rather than consent – following the wording of the Human Tissue Act. A form used for giving consent to a post-mortem examination of the body is not suitable for this purpose.

Relatives should not normally be approached before death has occurred, but sometimes a relative approaches the hospital staff and suggests some time in advance that the patient's kidneys, for example, might be used for transplantation. If the patient dies some appreciable time after this approach has been made, it may be appropriate to confirm with the relatives their lack of objection in case they have changed their minds. It sometimes happens, too, that relatives offer to consent to the removal of kidneys from a patient who has died but whose kidneys would not be suitable for transplantation. Such offers should be gratefully acknowledged and the opportunity can often be sensitively used to point out to relatives other tissues (such as corneas) from the donor which might be more suitable for transplantation.

Approaches to the parents of a dead child need a particularly high standard of sensitivity and tact; while the law does not demand parental consent, it should always be obtained in the case of a child.

Confidentiality

The staff of hospitals and organ exchange organisations must respect the wishes of the donor, the recipient and their families with respect to anonymity. Organ transplants may arouse great public or personal interest, but the involvement of the media or of the donor's or recipient's families with each other could have a distressing effect for both patient and relatives. Payments to donor's relatives in connection with kidney transplants are ethically unacceptable except for any out-of-pocket expenses for which they would be eligible in other circumstances.

Approach to coroner or procurator fiscal

The Coroner or, in Scotland, the Procurator Fiscal, need only be approached in connection with organ transplantation in cases which would ordinarily need to be reported because of the circumstances leading to the patient's death.

If the body is in *England*, *Wales* or *Northern Ireland*, and the designated person has reason to believe that an inquest may be required to be held on the body or that a post-mortem examination of the body may be required by the Coroner, the designated person may not authorise the removal of any organs unless the Coroner has given consent. The arrangements for obtaining this consent vary from area to area, and it is necessary to ascertain in advance and follow the procedures set out by the local Coroner.

If the body is in *Scotland*, the designated person may not authorise the removal of any organs if the Procurator Fiscal has objected to such removal. If there is a reason to believe that the Procurator Fiscal may require a fatal accident inquiry or a post-mortem examination the consent of the Procurator Fiscal should be obtained before any organs are removed.

Initial contact for permission to remove the organs should be made by those who are most familiar with the local Coroner's or Procurator Fiscal's practice. This may be the hospital with the potential donor, or the transplant team. The Coroner or Procurator Fiscal should be told exactly which organs are to be removed (for example, kidneys, heart, liver). Hospital pathologists need to be involved only when they have been asked by a Coroner or Procurator Fiscal to act on their behalf. After removal of organs the donor's doctor should report the case in the usual way.

Pre-mortem treatment, tests and tissue-typing

The maintenance of normal homeostasis, by ensuring adequate fluid intake, normal blood pressure and monitoring of urine output by catheter collection, is part of the standard medical care of the patient where brain death has not been conclusively established. It is also important to maintain the function of organs for transplantation.

After a patient is dead there is no legal objection to administering any drugs necessary to maintain the condition of the organs or to conducting the necessary diagnostic tests.

Sometimes a patient thought to have irreversible brain damage, and who would be a suitable donor, stops breathing before it has been possible to make the necessary enquiries. In most cases of this kind brain death will not yet have been diagnosed and it will not be possible to say with certainty that it will inevitably occur. In such cases initiation of artificial ventilation as part of resuscitation is justified because it is of potential benefit for the patient.

Very occasionally it will be considered certain that death will inevitably occur shortly (in the case, for example, of gross trauma and progressive cerebral tumour). In these cases doctors should seek the agreement of relatives for the initiation of artificial ventilation to preserve organ function before death has been diagnosed. If it is not possible to obtain the relatives' views before the situation arises, doctors should exercise their judgement in the light of the circumstances of the individual case whether or not to initiate artificial ventilation, so as to enable enquiries to be made about the views of the deceased and the relatives about the removal of organs after death has been diagnosed.

When a hospital has in its care a potential organ donor, the sooner the local transplant team is approached the better. If contact is made before the patient is dead or authorisation for the removal of the organs has been given, this should always be made clear. The transplant team should decide when to contact UK Transplant, which will usually be when tissue-typing is undertaken.

Diagnosis of death

When death is determined on the basis of brain death, or where it is proposed to remove organs within an hour after respiration and circulation have ceased, death should be diagnosed by the combination of doctors recommended: a consultant, preferably the one in charge of the patient, and another consultant or senior registrar, clinically independent of the first, who must assure themselves that the preconditions have been met before testing is carried out. Both should have expertise in this field. Neither doctor should be a member of the transplant team, and the results of the examination and the diagnosis should be recorded in the case notes. The transplantation checklist includes model criteria for diagnosing brain death. This should be completed, signed by both doctors, and permanently retained in the patient's case notes.

The two doctors may carry out the tests separately or together. Even if tests confirm brain death they should nevertheless be repeated. The interval between tests should be a matter for decision by the two doctors but should be adequate for reassurance of all those directly concerned. Death is only conclusively established when the criteria have been satisfied on two successive occasions. As a patient must be presumed to be alive until it is clearly established that he or she is dead, the time of death should be recorded as the time when death was conclusively established, not some earlier time or a later time when artificial ventilation is withdrawn, or the heart beat ceases. Diagnosis of brain death should not normally be considered until at least 6 hours after the onset of coma or, if cardiac arrest was the cause of the coma, until 24 hours after the circulation has been restored.

Removal of organs

Before removal of organs all practicable measures should be taken to ensure that their condition is optimal, otherwise they may prove to be unusable, or the patient who receives them may undergo a fruitless transplantation, or a period of unnecessary hazard and discomfort before the organs begin to function.

- Drugs to maintain renal function should be given. Antibiotics may be required and fluid intake should be maintained. In respect of other drugs, advice should be sought from the local transplant team whose responsibility it is to see that hospitals likely to have donors know what the requirements are and have supplies of the necessary drugs. Hypothermia occurring after death has been diagnosed need not be corrected because it may favour organ survival. Adequate ventilation must be maintained during this period.
- Relatives who enquire should be told that some post-mortem treatment of the donor's body will be necessary if the organs are to be removed in good condition. Relatives sometimes wish to remain near the body of the deceased until the organs are actually removed and doctors should explain that this is impracticable.
- It is ethical to maintain artificial ventilation and heart beat until the removal of organs has been completed. This is essential in the case of heart and liver transplant and many doctors think it desirable when removing kidneys. The removal should always be carried out under normal operating conditions and may proceed at any convenient time after the diagnosis of death. The maintenance of artificial ventilation after this time should only exceptionally be continued beyond 12 hours. Kidneys must be removed within 60 minutes of cessation of circulation and it is desirable that this time is kept as short as practicable – less than 30 minutes if possible.
- Removal must be effected by a fully registered medical practitioner who should be an appropriately trained surgeon. The surgeon must be satisfied, by personal examination of the body, that the patient is dead. The surgeon may not remove any organs unless satisfied that, where necessary, the Coroner has given consent (or, if the body is in Scotland, that the Procurator Fiscal has not objected to the removal).

Post-mortem treatment, distribution and transport

As techniques are constantly changing and being improved, advice should be sought from the local transplant team, who should be responsible for bringing the necessary materials for preserving organs in good condition. Each individual kidney should be accompanied by a sample of blood, a 2 cm cube of spleen and a lymph node for further tissue-typing. Technical advances have made it unnecessary to move a donor to the place where the organ transplant is to take place (irrespective of which organ is to be transplanted).

Preoperative cytotoxic cross-match and antibody screening

Cytotoxic antibodies are implicated in hyperacute graft rejection; preoperative cross-match as a screen for cytotoxic antibodies is essential before implantation of the graft. Donor splenic or lymph node lymphocytes are mixed with recipient serum to which complement is added. After 4 h of incubation, a vital dye (trypan blue) is added to the cell mix; the percentage of cells that have taken up the dye (and are therefore dead) can be counted on a haemocytometer. A positive reaction with significant cell kill indicates a risk of hyperacute rejection. It is important to collect serum within the 28 days after a blood transfusion (otherwise the antibody peak is missed).

Pharmacological Immunosuppression

This implies blocking lymphocyte proliferation in response to antigenic stimulation. In view of complications, azathioprine and corticosteroids are superseded by cyclosporin which:
– blocks T-lymphocyte response to antigen stimulation;
– prevents IL-2 release by T-helper cells;
– limits clonal expansion of sensitised T-lymphocytes and reduces lymphokines production.

It is associated with less serious infections in transplant recipients than azathioprine, but it has nephrotoxicity (a major problem in renal transplantation) and can cause significant impairment in small bowel vasculature.

FK 506 is an immunosuppressive agent produced in Japan; it is a macrolide purified from fluid in which *Streptomyces tsukubaensis* are grown. It is as effective and yet less toxic than cyclosporin, with similar drug action.

Biological immunosuppression with antisera to human lymphocytes produced in the horse, goat and rabbit is widely used in the USA; the globulin portion of the serum is separated to provide an antilymphocyte globulin (ALG) for therapeutic uses. Anaphylaxis to animal protein may occur. ALG has improved graft survival when used prophylactically with conventional immunosuppressants, particularly in steroid-resistant rejection crises in patients receiving cyclosporin. ALG, however, is polyclonal, i.e. active against the whole lymphocyte population, unlike monoclonal antibodies.

Monoclonal antibodies were discovered by kohler and Milstein in 1976 by fusing antibody secreting B lymphocytes with immortal myeloma cells to produce a 'hybridoma' with continuous growth in culture with elaboration of large amounts of specifically active antibody. Monoclonal antibodies technology allows diagnosis of CD4 helper/inducer T-lymphocytes and CD8 suppressor/cytotoxic T-lymphocytes. As monoclonal antibody reagents consist of murine immunoglobulin, treated individuals may develop antibody response against mouse protein during a course of treatment (such anti-idiotype antibodies rendering monoclonal antibodies ineffective). OKT3 monoclonal reagents were used as markers on the surface of peripheral T-lymphocytes, inducing cell lysis and reversing acute rejection crisis. In general, monoclonal antibody treatment has been disappointing.

Causes of immunosuppression in general

1. General disease or debilitation, e.g. diabetes mellitus, malignancy, renal failure, jaundice and liver failure, chronic sepsis, and malnutrition.
2. Disease with selective suppression of immune system, e.g. defects of antibody production, inherited immune deficiency syndromes, lymphomas, leukaemias and AIDS.
3. Side-effects of treatment, e.g. chemotherapy and radiotherapy for malignancy.
4. Deliberate immunosuppression for diseases the pathogenesis of which involves immune mechanisms, such as:
– steroids for Crohn's disease, glomerulonephritis and rheumatoid arthritis;
– steroids and azathioprine for systemic lupus erythematosus;
– splenectomy for idiopathic thrombocytopenic purpura;
– thymectomy in myasthenia gravis.
5. Deliberate immunosuppression in transplantation. Agents commonly used are:
– steroids
– azathioprine
– cyclosporin
– cyclophosphamide
– methotrexate
– polyclonal antilymphocyte globulins
– monoclonal antilymphocyte antibodies
– selective lymphoid irradiation

COMPLICATIONS OF IMMUNOSUPPRESSION

Immunosuppression may arise as part of a deliberate therapeutic manoeuvre or from a disease process. Patients with renal failure secondary to diabetes who undergo renal transplantation combine the immunosuppressive effect of renal failure with known susceptibility of diabetes to infection with drug therapy for transplantation. Profound immunosuppression is often seen in haemopoietic system deficiency combined with therapeutic immunosuppression, e.g. total body irradiation and bone marrow transplantation with chemotherapy for leukaemia; severe immunosuppression may also arise after solid organ transplantation by over-enthusiastic attempts to treat rejection crises, particularly using potent antilymphocytic antibody preparations together with cyclosporin. Complications of immunosuppression may be addressed to include:

1. Metabolic effects

Loss of appetite and lethargy are not well understood, but steroid therapy can explain loss of muscle mass (wasting), sodium retention causing heart failure, and insulin resistance producing diabetes in others. Cyclosporin therapy at toxic levels produces hypercalcaemia, hypomagnesaemia and hyperglycaemia. Chronic high dose steroid therapy can cause osteoporosis and avascular bone necrosis in the hips with irreparable damage.

2. Infections

Infections due to immunosuppression differ from common infections (such as urinary tract and chest infections) affecting the immunosuppressed patient; in immunosuppression, infections with non-pathogenic commensals occur with a severity that is proportional to the severity of immunosuppression. Severe neutropenia with steroid associated fever, raised C-reactive protein and local pain, tenderness and swelling may all predispose or indicate an infective process. Ideally, treatment should always be based on positive culture or other tests; unfortunately, this may result in a delay of the treatment and in severe immunosuppression may be fatal. It may therefore be necessary to institute a broad spectrum treatment, covering all organisms. Also, elucidation of the underlying cause is important, e.g. urinary tract infection secondary to obstruction will respond better to treatment if the obstruction is dealt with. Prophylaxis also has a role; *Pneumocystis carinii* can be effectively prevented by low dose cotrimoxazole. Broad spectrum antibiotic prophylaxis must be employed for even minor operations performed in immunosuppressed patients. Patients from endemic areas for tuberculosis should be treated prophylactically for acid fast bacilli.

Septicaemia (fever with or without rigor) may occur; it can progress in severe cases to hypotension, renal failure, disseminated intravascular coagulation and death. Patients who develop septicaemia soon after transplantation usually have sepsis related to surgical complications such as urinary or biliary leak, where coliform or anaerobic organisms are expected. Long indwelling vascular lines, urinary catheters and endotracheal tubes predispose to infection after the first few days. After the first month, and particularly in severely immunosuppressed patients, infection is caused by unusual microorganisms, such as Listeria, Nocardia, Toxoplasma, Aspergillus, Candida, Cryptococcus and Mycobacterium.

Urinary tract infections vary from asymptomatic bacteriuria to symptomatic cystitis (particularly in women). Usual organisms are coliforms and *Streptococcus faecalis*; however, Pseudomonas, Proteus, Serratia species and Candida may be encouraged by prolonged antibiotic treatment for other acute infections; they usually respond to antibiotic treatment, high fluid intake and complete emptying of the bladder. Acute pyelonephritis due to ascending infection may cause tenderness over the graft in kidney transplantation, however chronic pyelonephrosis or perinephric abscess commonly affect the native kidney. Treatment with antibiotics is satisfactory. Furthermore, drugs can be nephrotoxic; cyclosporin is markedly nephrotoxic, and many non-steroidal analgesics, erythromycin, cotrimoxazole and ketoconazole may interact to increase cyclosporin nephrotoxicity. Cyclophosphamide may cause severe cystitis.

Respiratory infections vary from minor viral sore throat or influenza to severe infections with purulent sputum; causative organisms include, commonly, Gram-negative (*Escherichia coli*, klebsiella species, or *Haemophilus influenzae*) and less commonly Gram-positive organisms (*Streptococcus pneumoniae*). When X-ray findings of consolidation suggest pneumonia, the above organisms are still the most likely cause, but in severely immunosuppressed patients (bone marrow transplants), other organisms must also be considered such as

Staphylococcus aureus, Legionella, Mycoplasma, Nocardia, *Mycobacterium tuberculosis*, Pneumocystis, Cytomegalovirus, and Aspergillus). Treatment with gentamicin, benzyl–penicillin and ampicillin must be started while results for sputum and blood culture are awaited. In the absence of clinical improvement, more invasive diagnostic techniques are needed, such as bronchoscopic alveolar lavage and/or open lung biopsy, since the survival of the patient is dependent on positive diagnosis.

CNS infection is unusual unless the immunosuppression is prolonged and severe; it presents dramatically with headache, drowsiness, vomiting and fits progressing rapidly to coma. Encephalitis is viral, but meningitis is usually bacterial, common organisms being Listeria, Cryptococcus, Nocardia, *Mycobacterium tuberculosis* and Aspergillus. Diagnosis by CT scan, lumbar puncture and CSF culture must be followed by antibiotic treatment. Furthermore, rapid i.v. infusion of methyl-prednisolone (steroid) can cause convulsions or psychoses varying from euphoria to hypomania. Cyclosporin may cause convulsion (due to hypermagnesaemia), tremors and peripheral neuropathy.

Viral infections arise from three sources: reactivation of dormant (usually DNA) viruses, transplantation viruses transferred by infected donor tissues, or newly acquired viral infections. T-lymphocytes are cells responsible for immune detection and destruction of virus-infected cells. Viral infections therefore are troublesome after anti-thymocyte globulin or anti-T-cell monoclonal antibodies. Common viral infections include:

- Herpes simplex reactivation occurs in 40% of patients after transplantation (usually in the first week) commonly in patients who have suffered from cold sores in the past. It is a minor infection but can progress to peroral, anogenital, digital, corneal ulceration. Diagnosis is by viral isolation from lesions followed by treatment with acyclovir topically or systemically.

- Cytomegalovirus (CMV) is present in 60% of the population and infection appears either as a primary infection from donated tissues (even in patients with CMV positive) or reactivation of latent virus. Severity of CMV infection correlates with severity of immunosuppression, ranging from lung infection with fever and leucopenia to severe multi-system organ failure. Diagnosis by viral isolation from body fluids or biopsy specimens, by CMV IgM antibody response, or DNA hybridisation technique. Mild cases can be left untreated; severe cases may be treated by hyper-immune globulin combined with ganciclovir.

- Varicella zoster: shingles occurs more commonly in immunosuppressed patients. Diagnosis is by clinical appearance and treatment by acyclovir. Chickenpox may be caught by immunosuppressed patients from children or from patients with shingles, even if the victim has already had chickenpox in childhood. The condition is severe with confluent rash and pneumonitis or encephalomeningitis and may be fatal. Patients must be preimmunised if negative for varicella antibody. Treatment with systemic acyclovir may be life-saving.

- Epstein–Barr virus infection from blood products, transplanted organs or by nosocomial infection. Clinically, it varies from self-limiting glandular fever-like illness to persistent fever and lymphadenopathy to frank polyclonal

Then a small liver biopsy is taken and the falciform ligaments of donor and recipient are sutured together. Suprahepatic and infrahepatic areas are drained.

Intensive postoperative monitoring is a must. Immunotherapy can start postoperatively. If resistance to gentamicin is elicited, appropriate antibiotic is given and gentamicin can be continued for 5 days.

The pancreas

Insulin-dependent diabetes in young patients results in renal failure and blindness due to micro-angiopathy; they are the main indication for transplantation with either vascularised pancreatic graft or isolated purified islets of pancreas. Uraemic diabetics do badly on dialysis; retinopathy progresses and shunt sites are liable to infection. Kidney transplantation for such patients is also disappointing, mainly due to steroids which aggravate diabetes and make control more difficult. Pancreatic transplantation therefore, is required as it may prevent the progress of microangiopathy. Historically, pancreaticoduodenal grafts were used employing duodenum as a conduit for exocrine pancreatic secretions.

Segmental vascularised transplantation, i.e. tail and body of donor pancreas, are separated from the head, the splenic blood supply is carefully preserved, and then 1–2 ml of latex polymer is injected into the pancreatic duct for occlusion (or alternatively, drained into the intestine). Pancreas is cooled by perfusion via splenic artery with cold solution as used in liver. There is increased use of University of Wisconsin (UW) solution for preservation in place of Euro-Collins or plasma-based solutions with longer graft storage time of up to 30 h (UW cold storage solution has extended safe preservation of liver and pancreas from 6 to 24 h or more). Cyclosporin and azathioprine *are commonly used* with prophylactic use of anti-T cell agents (either OKT3 or ALG). The recipient's right iliac fossa is prepared as for kidney transplant.

There are two anastomoses to make; splenic artery and portal vein (receiving splenic vein) are anastomosed respectively to common or external iliac vessels with the pancreatic neck pointing to the pelvis and tail to the peritoneal cavity (Fig. 1.90.3).

In 1984, Gray *et al.* described physical separation of human islet by a digestion process to purify pancreatic islet cells only (from the exocrine tissue) for allotransplantation by embolisation into liver via the portal vein, without the need for immunosuppression. However, pooling of islets from multiple donors may be required to achieve an effective implant mass (10 000 islets/kg body weight) using intraportal embolisation to liver as the implant site, done under local anaesthesia. Peripheral hyperinsulinaemia is usually avoidable by locating islets in an organ with portal venous drainage. However, 15% of total islet mass of the pancreas needs to function in order to prevent clinical diabetes. However, islet transplantation must be considered inferior to vascularised segmental pancreas transplantation.

The heart

Heart transplantation was first performed in man by Christian Barnard in 1967. The decline in world-wide enthusiasm for

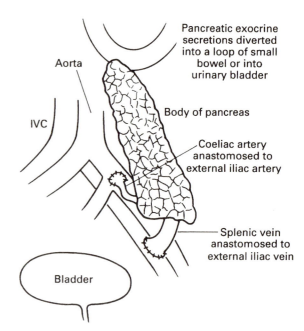

Fig. 1.90.3 Pancreatic transplantation

heart transplantation can be ascribed to the dismal early results and subsequent realisation that heart transplantation success required not only years of pre-clinical investigation and experience, but also the diligent effort and devotion of a multidisciplinary team of physicians, nurses and other ancillary personnel.

Only 10% of potential recipient patients are selected for cardiac transplantation; reasons for exclusion include age greater than 50 years, psychological instability and medical contraindications such as pulmonary vascular resistance, insulin-dependent diabetes or multi-system organ failure (MOF). At transplantation, recipients must show no X-ray evidence of pulmonary embolism, be free of any active infection, and demonstrate negative lymphocyte crossmatch with the donor. Common indications (recipient diseases) are coronary artery disease, idiopathic cardiomyopathy, post-traumatic aneurysm and valve disease. Recipients who have undergone previous open heart procedures with cardiopulmonary bypass and multiple blood transfusion tend to enjoy increased survival rates.

Average donor age has been 25 years (range of 12–52 years); the most frequent cause of brain death has been non-penetrating head trauma, followed by cerebrovascular accident and gunshot wounds. It is preferable to transfer the donor to the centre of orthotopic cardiac transplantation prior to heart removal and to perform its transplantation into the recipient in the same centre. The longest ischaemic interval has been 186 minutes (mean of 134 minutes), during which time, myocardial viability is maintained by hypothermia alone.

Immunosuppression of the transplant recipient begins prior to transplantation, employing azathioprine (4 mg/kg) and antithymocyte globulin (2.5–5 mg/kg) of rabbit origin. Immediately following the procedure, 500 mg of methylprednisolone is given i.v., followed by three doses of 125 mg over the next 24 h. Maintenance immunosuppressive therapy consists of azathioprine (1.5–2.5 mg/kg/day) and prednisone (1.5 mg/kg/day).

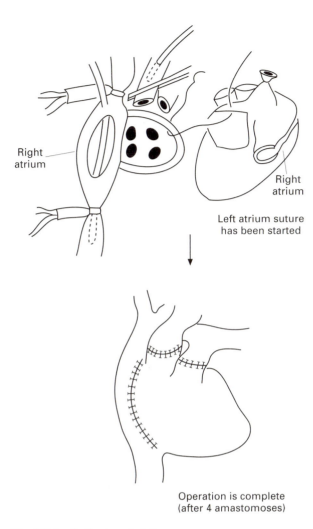

Right
atrium

Right
atrium

Left atrium suture
has been started

Operation is complete
(after 4 amastomoses)

Fig. 1.90.4   Cardiac transplantation

Operative technique of transplantation involves four anastomoses, made while the patient is on cardiopulmonary bypass. Tapes are placed around the superior and inferior venae cavae and the aorta is cross-clamped to exclude the heart from circulation. The recipient's heart is excised at the atrioventricular groove. The donor heart superior vena cava is ligated. The following anastomoses are then performed (Fig. 1.90.4);
1. Left atrial anastomosis.
2. Donor right atrium curved incision can be anastomosed to recipient right atrium. Then a perfusion catheter is inserted in the left atrium to run cold (4 °C) normal saline to further cool the left ventricular cavity as well as displace air.
3. Aortic anastomosis is completed. Aortic cross-clamp is then released and the perfusion catheter removed from the left atrium.
4. Pulmonary anastomosis is completed with the heart fibrillating. Bypass cannulas are then removed and pacing wires are inserted on the donor right atrium.

Postoperative rejection is diagnosed within 2–3 months after operation. Clinically, gallop rhythm, fatigue and malaise may indicate a moderately severe rejection. ECG reveals low voltage QRS complexes in leads I, II, III, V1–V6 (of 20% or more from baseline suggests rejection); associated atrial arrhythmias also occur during rejection. Preclinical histological confirmation may be obtained by percutaneous transvenous endomyocardial biopsy, using Seldinger technique via right internal jugular vein cannulation with a cardiac catheterisation sheath, through which a bioptome is passed into the right ventricular apex, where 2–3 biopsy specimens are taken. Immunological daily monitoring of circulating T-lymphocyte level (assayed by sheep red cell rosette formation) can also be performed. Rejection can be treated on histological confirmation by continuous heparin (to minimise platelets and fibrin deposition), prednisolone, azathioprine, actinomycin D, and rabbit antithymocyte globulin. However, in severe, irreversible graft dysfunction (failed treatment of rejection), re-transplantation can be perfomed.

The commonest causes of early and late death following cardiac transplantation are infection (50%), acute rejection (20%), graft versus host (15%), malignancy (5%), pulmonary hypertension (5%), stroke (2%) and suicide (1%) (Figures are approximated for simplicity).

The lung

Fatal lung disease is common. Severe pneumonitis can precede death and such patients are therefore unsuitable recipients. Patients with pulmonary fibrosis and emphysema are respiratory cripples who cannot be weaned from oxygen with no evidence of pneumonitis, and are therefore potential recipients. Lung is more vulnerable to rejection than kidney, leading to alveolar exudates which aggravate the ventilation/perfusion ratio imbalance.

Immunosuppression used in lung grafting is the same as for other organ transplantation (see above). Simultaneous grafting of both lungs may lead to impaired spontaneous ventilation, possibly as a result of denervation of lungs interfering with Hering–Breuer reflex. Bronchial arteries are divided in removal of donor organs; this predisposes bronchial anastomosis to leak due to necrosis on the donor side.

The removal of donor lung and its implantation should be so timed to reduce ischaemic time to the very minimum. Periods of less than 1 h can be achieved by carrying out the removal of donor organ and transplantation procedure in adjacent operating rooms. However, organ survival up to 6 h can be achieved if the removed lung is flushed with Ringer's lactate at 4°C and transported in an insulated container.

A right lung should be used where possible because access to the bronchus and pulmonary vessels is easier (due to the presence of the heart on the left), and because right lung has greater ventilatory volume, Moreover, should cardiopulmonary bypass become necessary in severe hypoxia, ascending aorta and right atrium are readily available from the right.

Operative procedure involves construction of four anastomoses (Fig. 1.90.5):
1. Pulmonary artery anastomosis.
2. Two pulmonary veins (using 4/0 Prolene).
3. Bronchus anastomosis (interrupted figure-of-eight sutures of 4/0 Prolene).

Lung sepsis is a common complication of immunosuppression augmented by rejection reaction and inhalation of organisms in air.

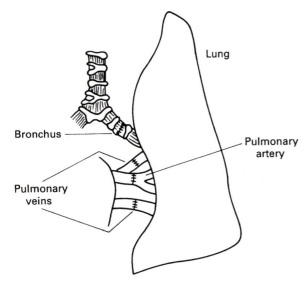

Fig. 1.90.5 Lung transplantation

Small intestine

Small bowel transplantation was first performed experimentally in the dog by Lillehei in 1959. Loss of whole small bowel following occlusion of superior mesenteric vessels or volvulus (surgical malabsorbtion with small bowel failure) is the main indication for intestinal transplantation. Small bowel transplantation can either be isolated small bowel or combined liver and small bowel transplantation. Adequate nutrition is impossible in such cases, although a short length of healthy jejunum can restore the patient's health.

The prognosis of short bowel syndrome has been considerably improved by the development of home total parenteral nutrition (TPN) with a survival rate of 65–80% at 3 years. There is still significant associated morbidity and mortality, related to vascular access and infection; liver failure and cirrhosis may develop in paediatric patients on TPN. At the present time, transplantation should be reserved for those patients with TPN complications or patients who are unable to tolerate the limitations TPN imposes on their life. Liver function should be assessed in patients on TPN who are being considered for small bowel transplantation or combined small bowel/liver transplantation. Active sepsis and malignant disease are contraindications to transplantation.

Unfortunately, small lengths of small bowel are rejected rapidly, while long lengths of grafted small bowel appear to kill the recipient by the donor's lymphoid tissues in mesenteric lymph nodes and Peyer's patches mounting a graft-versus-host reaction in the form of fatal sepsis (this is in contrast to other transplanted organs containing little lymphoid tissue).

Donors must be close relatives or siblings; identical blood grouping and HLA histocompatibility must be strictly observed. Selective decontamination with amphotericin B, tobramycin and polymixin E is started as soon as the donor has been identified. The graft is preserved with cold University of Wisconsin solution and donor ischaemic time should be as short as possible. The small bowel graft comprises small bowel from the duodenojejunal junction to

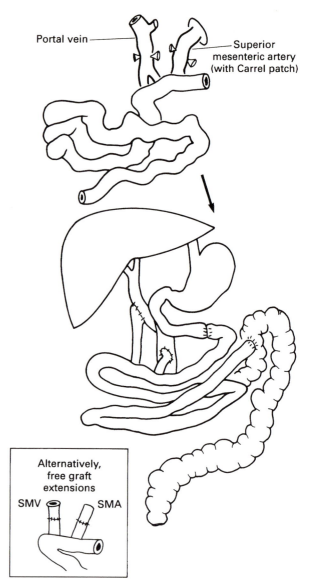

Fig. 1.90.6 Small intestinal transplantation

the terminal ileum together with a vascular pedicle of superior mesenteric artery and vein.

Operative technique involves four anastomoses (Fig. 1.90.6):

1. Two ends of donor small bowel are anastomosed respectively to duodenum proximally and to transverse colon distally. Initially the distal end of intestinal graft is brought out as an ileostomy. A proximal tube jejunostomy and a feeding gastrostomy are also performed. Surgery is complicated by the fact that many recipients have undergone multiple laparotomies and have extensive adhesions and a contracted peritoneal cavity.

2. Superior mesenteric vein is anastomosed to the recipient's external or common iliac vein or portal vein. However, it is desirable that venous blood should drain into the recipient's portal system, so that the liver receives intestinal blood as in physiological conditions.

3. Superior mesenteric artery is anastomosed to the recipient's internal iliac artery or aorta.

Ventilatory support is continued until the patient is warm and cardiovascularly stable; prolonged ventilation may be required in patients who are severely malnourished preoperatively. Blood or colloid are given as blood loss may be significant due to dissection of extensive intraperitoneal adhesions. Increased postoperative stomal output may be controlled by pectin, Lomotil, Imodium and stomatostatin. Patients continue to receive parenteral nutrition for at least one month after surgery. When enteral nutrition is well established and the patient is free from infection and rejection (usually 2 months after transplantation), the stoma is closed. Graft function is assessed by D-xylose absorption, barium studies and faecal fat estimation.

Immunosuppression is similar to that used for kidneys, but must be given i.v. and earlier to counteract strong rejection in grafted bowel. Methylprednisolone given i.v. intraoperatively is maintained at 20 mg/kg/day. Results of small bowel transplantation have been improved by the Pittsburgh programme (started in May 1990 and performing through to mid 1994 around 50 isolated small bowel and small bowel/liver transplants) after the introduction of a new immunosuppressive agent, FK 506. Like cyclosporin A, FK 506 is an interleukin-2 inhibitor. It is given as a continuous i.v. infusion of 0.15 mg/kg/day, starting at the time of surgery and enteral administration of 0.3 mg/kg/day is started after 1–2 weeks. FK 506 levels need to be kept at the upper limit of the therapeutic range, which is often associated with nephrotoxicity (reversible on dose reduction). Prostacyclin infusion is used to maintain renal blood flow. Azathioprine 1–2 mg/kg has been given to 30% of cases who do not tolerate FK 506 because of renal impairment. The graft is monitored for rejection by clinical inspection and endoscopy. Multiple endoscopic biopsies are performed weekly and when there is clinical evidence of rejection. Rejection is common and is greatest in the first 30 days after transplantation. The first sign of rejection may be a cyanotic appearance of the stoma; other signs are malaise, fever, abdominal pain, graft ileus and a change in volume of discharge from the stoma. Endoscopic examination of the graft shows a dusky mucosa with focal ulceration, leading to complete sloughing of the mucosa and necrosis of the graft in severe rejection.

Translocation of bacteria from gut lumen to the blood occurs during rejection episodes and patients with severe rejection may present with signs of septic shock. Therefore, in addition to antibiotic therapy, immunosuppression may need to be increased in patients with infection (this is in contrast to the management of other transplant patients where sepsis necessitates a reduction in immunosuppression). In common with liver transplantation, infection is the most frequent cause of postoperative death. Intra-abdominal sepsis is common and patients may require repeated laparotomies or percutaneous drainage of abdominal abscesses. Cytomegalovirus enteritis has been a common finding and recipients are now given prophylaxis with gancyclovir to prevent this.

Bone-marrow (Fig 1.90.7)

Bone-marrow transplantation may be indicated in aplastic anaemia and leukaemia; it is usually performed by clinical

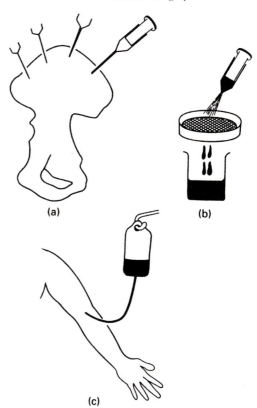

Fig. 1.90.7 Bone marrow transplantation. (a) Multiple iliac crest punctures to obtain donor marrow; (b) filtration of donor marrow and addition of heparin; (c) Processed marrow is transfused i.v.

haematologists rather than surgeons. Patients with diseases that may be treated successfully by irradiation or immunosuppression, but would destroy their bone-marrow, may undergo removal of their bone-marrow before such a treatment; their bone-marrow may be reinfused after completion of treatment (autologous marrow rescue). Long-term survival after bone-marrow transplantation is often greater than 50% in patients with acute lymphoblastic or myeloblastic leukaemia and may exceed 70% in patients with aplastic anaemia.

Donor bone-marrow (300–1000 ml) is obtained from multiple punctures of anterior and posterior iliac crests and sternum under general anaesthesia. Usually the donor is related to the recipient and has matched HLA antigens. Anaesthetic drugs affecting bone-marrow (e.g. nitrous oxide) must be avoided. The donor may be hospitalised 1–2 weeks before bone-marrow removal in order to undergo venesection to stimulate bone-marrow and to use blood for autotransfusion later on. Postoperative complications are rare apart from discomfort at puncture sites; bone-marrow regeneration occurs in a few weeks.

The recipient's bone-marrow is destroyed by drugs (cyclophosphamide) or irradiation before transplantation. Patients experience nausea and are susceptible to sepsis during this time. During bone-marrow transplantation, fat embolism may rarely occur. After the transplant infusion, patients are maintained on immunosuppressant drug therapy and nursed in an infection-controlled environment.

WARFARE AND DISASTERS (MILITARY SURGERY)

1.91 Missile and Explosive Blast Injuries

Mortality from missile and explosive blast injuries is high; with short evacuation time (from battlefield to hospital) and best facilities (first aid, wound treatment, haemostasis and control of infection), mortality is 16–18%. The mortality in high velocity missile injuries exceeds 30%; this is because of wound severity due to high energy impact, inadequate first aid at the time of injury, delay before surgery (long evacuation time from battlefield), and faulty surgical technique (failure to practise principles of war surgery). Application of principles of war surgery, availability of blood transfusion and adequate trained staff should yield good results.

Wounding missiles include the following:

- Bullets – divided into rifle (high velocity) and pistol (low velocity). Hand guns, such as revolvers or automatics, throw heavy bullets at relatively low velocities of 150–250 metres/ second; such pistol bullets would not catch up Jumbo jet aircraft. Military rifles fire bullets (under 10 g weight) at a velocity of over 800 metres/second, which would be able to catch up Concorde in flight. A high velocity rifle bullet is relatively small (compared to a hand gun bullet), because of the very long cartridge case containing a large amount of propellant.
- Explosives are substances which, when detonated, are very rapidly converted into large volumes of gases; when the explosion is confined by bomb or shell casing, the pressure will rupture the casing imparting high velocity (300–1800 metres/second) to the resulting fragments, vary- ing from 1 to 100 g or more (each). They are irregularly shaped and thus their velocities soon decrease. Nevertheless, all fragments from explosive devices are classified as high velocity missiles; they include:
  - fragmented shells (from mortars, artillery and tanks)
  - grenades
  - bombs
  - mines.
- Secondary missiles produced in consequence to blasting by primary explosives may include building materials, wood, glass, rock splinters and fragments of clothing.

Missiles such as arrows and darts are inherently stable, because the centre of resistance to flight (in the feathers) lies behind the centre of mass. Bullets are aerodynamically unstable, because the centre of mass lies behind the centre of resistance to flight; thus a bullet tends to oscillate or yaw around its long axis. Spinning of the bullet by means of rifling the barrel of the gun gives it stability, and increases both range and accuracy; rifle bullets therefore are used for accurate targets and can kill at ranges of 2000 metres or more.

The motion of a bullet in flight, and within human tissues after impact, depends upon the size, shape, stability, composi- tion and, above all, the velocity. Tissue density and elasticity are most important factors influencing the retardation of missiles; tissues of increasing density (compact organs) cause greater retardation of missile and, therefore, greater energy is released to cause damage. The site of entry (head and chest have poor prognosis), direction of missile motion, and patient's position at the time of injury can often dictate the outcome of the patient. The wound results from absorption of the kinetic energy (*KE*) imparted by the missile when it strikes and penetrates tissue. This energy is calculated by the formula:

$$KE = MV^2/2$$

where M is the mass and V the velocity. The overwhelming importance of velocity is shown by the equation. When a missile is stopped by tissues it penetrates, the energy liberated to cause damage equals the total kinetic energy of the missile. Passing through tissue, the remaining velocity can release energy during wounding.

The wound size made by a rifle bullet increases sharply at close range; this is partly due to greater energy at close range and partly because bullets are unstable during the first 100 m of their flight. A rifle bullet that breaks up in tissues causes a much larger wound and exit wound than a bullet that does not. Bullets of small calibre tend to break up more readily than bullets of larger calibre; a small calibre rifle bullet may cause a severe wound when fired at close range.

As the missile penetrates, tissues are crushed and forced apart by its passage; such crushing and laceration is not serious unless vital organs or major blood vessels are injured directly. However, the missile compresses solid tissues in front of it; compressed tissues move away as a shock wave of spherical shape (with a velocity similar to that of sound in water, i.e. 1500 metres/second). These shock waves can cause damage at a considerable distance from the wound track; solid tissues (liver and spleen) and fluid-filled tubes (arteries and veins) are very susceptible to shock wave transmission and can be damaged at a distance.

There is also temporary cavitation, a phenomenon encoun- tered only with high velocity missiles, and thus adding to their highly destructive ability. Cavitation is due to absorption of energy by local (soft and/or solid) tissues, resulting in violent acceleration forwards and outwards setting them with momen- tum moving even after the passage of the missile. A large cavity is created 30–40 times the missile diameter, with subatmospheric pressure resulting in suction of debris via entrance and exit holes caused by the missile; the cavity rapidly collapses in a pulsatile fashion leaving macerated track, i.e. 'the permanent cavity' (can be induced experimentally by firing a bullet into a block of gelatin gel to simulate soft tissues). Skin is very resistant to cavitation due to its elasticity, while muscle can be stretched by cavitation with consequent rupture of small vessels (bruised and necrosed). The bone is fairly sensitive to cavitation and will fracture by mere passage of missile close to it and without contact. Major arteries and veins are elastic and less liable to damage (though thrombosis can occasionally happen). In abdomen, a large temporary cavity is formed with gross displacement and visceral damage; also gas contained within hollow viscera (e.g. colon) is compressed by passage of a missile close by, and this is followed by explosive expansion rupturing the wall of viscera from within. Thus the colon may only be perforated by a low velocity bullet (such simple perforation can be repaired locally). However, the colon will be extensively perforated by a high velocity missile, with a disrupted zone of haemorrhage extending 20 cm from the hole due to the cavitation effect on colonic gas. No attempt at local repair can be successful; a wide resection is essential. Direct damage to liver from a high velocity missile can be catastrophic; so much liver tissue is pulped that only major resection can be feasible.

The thorax is filled with air, because of the large volume occupied by the lung. Therefore conditions for cavitation are not ideal (cavity cannot be formed in air but in tissues); and thus lungs are fairly resistant to damage from high velocity missile (apart from the mechanical passage of a bullet). The heart and great vessels, however, are extremely susceptible to damage from cavitation as they are filled with blood, and missile injuries to these structures are usually fatal. Brain behaves like a liquid system, but cavitation is limited because of the rigid skull. However, when energy is sufficient, the skull is extensively fractured from within, because the suddenly increased brain hydrodynamic pressure (by cavitation) blows the skull bones apart (no chance of survival from this injury). Stretching and compressing of large nerves during cavitation may be sufficient to cause neuropraxia on axonotmesis.

Bullets are not sterilised by firing (as commonly believed); the subatmospheric pressure within the created cavity can actively suck in bacteria, clothing (impregnated with bacteria) and debris via the entrance and exit wounds. All accidental wounds are contaminated, particularly high velocity missile wounds whether they are bullets or fragments from explosive devices. Missile wounds are at risk of clostridial contamination, particularly in the presence of dead muscle.

Principles of missile wound management

Bullet wounds frequently involve more than one person; bomb explosion commonly involves large numbers of people. Wounded patients must quickly be evaluated and sorted (see s. 1.73 Trauma evaluation); injuries demanding surgical attention and operation have priority in management (over injuries that can be managed by self-help, injuries requiring medical care and simple treatment by dressing, and fatal injuries in which patients are dead or when death is inevitable). This group is further sorted into three priorities:

- *Priority 1*: Urgent resuscitation and surgery to prevent asphyxia and haemorrhage. Asphyxia results from mechanical obstruction to airways, from sucking chest wound, tension pneumothorax and maxillofacial injury. Shock results from major bleeding (external or internal) into chest or abdominal cavities, and by massive muscle damage, major fractures, visceral injuries with evisceration and cardiopericardial injuries.
- *Priority 2*: Surgery with resuscitation in visceral injuries (including perforation of GIT), wounds of the genitourinary

system, thoracic wounds without asphyxia, and vascular injuries requiring repair.
- *Priority 3*: Less urgent surgery with no need for immediate resuscitation, and no immediate risk to life or limb; patients may well be fit to be evacuated to a distant hospital for further treatment after receiving essential first aid (to save life and limb, by providing **A**irway, maintaining **B**reathing and closing sucking chest wounds and arresting accessible bleeding, and supporting **C**irculation by fluid replacement).

Primary wound treatment

This includes wound excision and delayed primary closure.

Wound excision

All grossly contaminated, dead and damaged tissue is thoroughly excised leaving healthy tissue with good blood supply to combat residual infection. The clothing, dressing and splints are carefully removed, the wound is cleansed with sterile gauze impregnated in detergent, the wound is shaved, dried and then painted with antiseptic solution. In multiple wounds, posterior aspects of body and limbs should be dealt with before anterior aspects to minimise the stress of turning the patient. Skin is resistant to damage, and therefore only pulped or dead skin should be excised; this means that only 1–2 mm of skin edges of the wound can be trimmed.

The wound can be extended to get to the depths of the wound; in limbs incisions should be along the long axis but not over subcutaneous bone (e.g. medial aspect of shin over tibia) or across flexion creases. The deep fascia must be incised along the length of incision. Undamaged fascial compartments may be decompressed to avoid ischaemic changes. Edges of the wound must be retracted to remove blood clots, dirt, debris and missiles from the sides and depth of the wound.

Gentle and copious irrigation with saline is required to wash out most residual debris and blood clots. The wound can be explored by a finger to identify foreign bodies and wound depth; fresh healthy planes must not be opened. Clinical and radiological localisation of foreign bodies is required so that separate incisions via fascial planes may be sufficient rather than cutting via healthy muscle.

Excision of dead muscle should be thorough, using scissors, because dead muscle is the ideal medium for clostridial sepsis resulting in gas gangrene; all muscles around the missile track must be excised until healthy, contractile, bleeding muscle is reached. Haemostasis should be by firm pressure with warm packs and the use of sutures to bleeding points; diathermy coagulation should not be used as it leaves dead tissues behind.

The widely opened deep fascia is left open to allow postoperative oedematous and congested tissue to swell without tension to avoid pressure on blood supply.

All wounds, therefore, should be left widely open without suture of skin or deep structures except in:
- *Face and neck*. Wounds may be closed after wound excision.
- *Soft tissues of the chest wall*. Wounds must be excised and healthy muscle must be closed over sucking chest wounds to

establish an air-tight closure, though the skin can be left open.

- *Head injuries.* Dura is closed directly, or by temporalis fascia graft, and skin closed by rotating flaps to provide cover.
- *Hand injuries.* Tendon and nerve must be covered; otherwise, wounds are left open for delayed primary closure. Viable tissues must be preserved for future reconstruction.
- *Joints.* Synovial membrane must be closed, and if impossible then the capsule alone should be closed.
- *Blood vessels* must be repaired and covered by viable tissues.

Dry gauze is laid across the open wound and then this is covered by bulky absorbent dressing. Tulle gras or tightly packed dressing (forming a plug) should not be used, because they prevent easy outflow of wound discharge. Dressing may be held in place with the aid of a plaster back slab applied longitudinally; strapping around the limb must never be practised. Immobilisation is achieved using splints and well padded plasters which must be split down to skin at the time plaster is applied, or alternatively, a plaster slab can be sufficient.

Delayed primary closure

Open missile wounds will continue oozing blood and serum for 2 days, and then will be sealed with coagulated serum by the third day; early granulations appear over fibrinous coagulum between the third and fifth days, during which primary delayed closure can be performed. Closure earlier than the third day or later than the fifth day results in higher failure rate of healing. Within the first 3 days, excessive pain, oedema or signs of infection usually indicate that initial wound excision was incomplete, and further excision of dead tissues is necessary; the wound should be inspected in theatre under general anaesthesia.

Treatment of missile injuries in special organs

Bone and joint injuries

Upper and lower extremities are involved in 60–75% of all missile injuries and blast injuries. Compound fractures must be treated (as described in operative surgery). It is permissible to use a tourniquet preoperatively to control major bleeding. Severed nerves are marked and their positions noted, damaged tendons are trimmed, but no attempt should be made at primary repair in either case. Internal fixation is not advocated in compound fractures; external fixation using pins or external fixators is recommended. On the fourth or fifth day, the wound is inspected and closed by primary delayed closure using split-skin graft, flaps or other plastic methods.

Vascular injuries

These require prompt vascular reconstructive surgery. Accessible bleeding must be stopped first (usually by packing and pressure); the dressing must not be removed until the patient is in theatre. All cases must be dealt with within 4–6 h. Generous incision is required for good exposure, since divided arterial ends retract from each other; proximal and distal control using arterial clamps are essential. About 20–40 ml heparinsed saline is injected distally. Warm packs may relieve arterial spasm; Fogarty balloon catheter size 3 or 4 is used to remove thrombus; arterial partial laceration can directly be sutured; and a totally divided artery is repaired using reversed saphenous vein graft interposition with oblique anastomoses using 5/0 or 6/0 atraumatic prolene (deep veins must always looked for in arterial repair). Repaired vessels must be covered by healthy muscles; fasciotomy is usually performed and the wound is left open for delayed primary closure.

Chest injuries

All chest wounds must be considered potentially serious, no matter how small the wound and however good the patient's condition may appear when first seen. A missile may directly damage the chest wall, lungs, mediastinal contents, heart and diaphragm. Pleural and pericardial spaces must be kept empty so that their negative pressure is maintained; cardiac tamponade must be aspirated, the sucking wound of open pneumothorax is closed (with occlusive dressing preferably impregnated with petroleum jelly), tension pneumothorax must be relieved with chest tube insertion, flail chest must be stabilised by firm dressing strapping, and haemothorax (from bleeding intercostal or internal mammary vessels) must be drained with chest tube insertion. Endotracheal intubation may be required and tracheostomy is indicated in flail chest.

However, most cases fare well with chest tube insertion, simply because massive haemorrhage from injury to major pulmonary vessels, mediastinal vessels and heart are fatal (the patient may be dead on arrival). Under aseptic conditions with local anaesthesia, an Argyle chest tube size 26 should be inserted through the lateral chest wall in the 6th or 7th intercostal space (immediately above the 7th or 8th rib respectively to avoid injury of subcostal neurovascular structures). the left hand should act as a break during insertion to the desired chest tube length to avoid injury of heart and major vessels.

The mid-axillary line is usually selected during insertion, but this may interfere with the patient's ability to put the upper limb close to the chest; posterior axillary line selection, however, interferes with lying on the back, and therefore the anterior axillary line may represent the best selection to drain fluids in the chest (**B**asal tube for **B**lood). In significant pneumothorax, the 2nd intercostal space in the mid-clavicular line is selected (**A**pical tube for **A**ir). Pneumothorax less than 25% of hemithoracic size may resolve spontaneously without chest tube insertion. Both tubes may initially be connected to Heimlich one-way valves and thence into a closed system to drainage bags so that patient is mobile.

Underwater seal suction drainage should be applied to both drains as soon as feasible. Chest X-ray must be taken to confirm tube location and progress of drainage and lung expansion. The tube is removed when there is no air leak, the lungs are fully expanded, there is no fluid or air on X-ray, and clinically the patient starts coughing with pleural rub due to friction of the tube with expanding lung. War experience has shown that over 85% of all penetrating chest missile injuries may be managed by chest tube insertion (closed thoracostomy drainage).

Posterolateral thoracotomy, whenever indicated, may reduce the incidence of later decortication of affected lung. Thoracotomy needs adequate facilities and staff; it is indicated in:

- Continued intrathoracic bleeding of more than 1 litre within 5 hours.
- Abdominothoracic injury with suspected intraperitoneal injury.
- Massive and continuing air leak.
- Injury to the mediastinal contents, such as great vessels, trachea or oesophagus.
- Cardiac tamponade or cardiac wounds.
- Sucking chest wounds (after primarily occluded to save life as a first aid measure).
- Large chest wall wounds, particularly with defects.

During thoractomy, blood clots are evacuated, bleeders are secured, and lung lacerations are oversewn or stapled (with a linear stapling instrument). Pulmonary resection is seldom required unless segmental or lobar bronchus has been damaged. All fragments of bone and foreign bodies in pleura or lung must be removed if accessible; every effort should be made to remove clothing and organic debris. However, there is no need for prolonged search for inaccessible metallic foreign bodies seen on X-ray. Wounds of the chest wall must be excised and sharp broken rib ends are smoothed, underwater sealed tube drains are inserted, and a layer of muscle is closed to ensure an air-tight closure, while the remainder of the wound is left open for delayed primary closure. In thoracoabdominal wounds, both cavities need to be opened through separate thoracotomy and laparotomy incisions. The thoracoabdominal approach should be decried, due to gross contamination induced by cavitation destruction. The majority of thoracoabdominal wounds can be managed by chest tube drainage and laparotomy to treat abdominal injury.

Post-thoracotomy antibiotics, pain relief, bronchoscopic aspiration and suction of secretion, and tracheostomy (to reduce ventilatory work by bypassing dead space and airway resistance, and to facilitate suction) must all be used.

Abdominal injuries

These require urgent treatment. The appearance of the wound may be deceptive, because small calibre bullets and high velocity fragments from explosive devices may produce minute superficial wounds associated with surprisingly extensive internal damage (tip of the iceberg). Missile wounds in the trunk, thigh or buttocks may well involve the abdominal cavity.

Careful exploratory laparotomy is mandatory. Haemorrhage is dealt with first; the likely sources of profuse bleeding are small intestinal mesentery, liver, spleen, kidneys, pancreas and large veins of posterior abdominal wall. Bleeding points must be found and ligated with fine thread. Severe bleeding from the liver can be controlled by Pringle's manoeuvre, but as a rule of thumb, bleeding from liver tears ceases by the time the abdomen is opened or can be arrested temporarily by light packing.

Thereafter, GIT perforations must be repaired after examining the gut from one end to another. Small intestine is commonly injured. After small intestine, stomach, colon and solid viscera must be examined in this order. A retroperitoneal haemorrhage may indicate associated fixed colonic injuries. The stomach posterior aspect is examined via an opening in gastrocolic omentum. The duodenum can be kocherised to mobilise pancreas for close examination. Finally, pelvis should be examined for rectal and bladder injuries. The abdominal cavity must be thoroughly drained (should be multiple and led down to areas of soiling, damage, or extensive repair); inadequate drainage is a potent cause of morbidity and mortality.

Small intestinal single perforation may be directly repaired (closed transversely with suture); multiple perforations and mesenteric injury are indications for resection and end-to-end anastomosis. Colonic injuries are contaminated; anaerobic cellulitis may be fatal. In colonic injuries, primary end-to-end anastomosis should not be attempted due to the high risk of leak; the colon must be mobilised and treated by one of the following methods:

1. Exteriorisation of perforated colon brought on to the skin as a loop colostomy; exteriorised colonic perforation may be repaired outside so that any leak will be to the outside (repaired later on). The loop can be returned to the abdomen after a few weeks when the anastomosis is sound. This is the treatment of choice in transverse and left colonic injuries. Right colon, however, should not be exteriorised, due to the difficulty in dealing with its liquid contents.
2. Primary repair with or without proximal colostomy.
3. Resection with or without primary anastomosis (ends brought out as colostomy and rectal mucous fistula).

Right colonic injury can be treated by either resection with ileostomy and distal colonic mucous fistula (for severe injuries due to high anastomotic leak following intra-abdominal sepsis), resection with ileocolostomy (for mild injuries without associated multi-visceral injury), or simple repair of perforation with or without ileotransverse colostomy (for an uncomplicated low velocity missile wound).

Rectum injuries must be repaired with proximal colostomy and retrorectal space drainage via a tube (between coccyx and anus). For other abdominal injuries, see s. 1.67 Abdominal trauma.

Brain injuries

Penetrating brain injuries from high velocity missiles carry a grave prognosis (virtually no survival, except in rare tangential wounds). Small fragments from explosive devices are the commonest injuries in wartime and carry a relatively good prognosis. Low velocity bullets are the commonest injuries in civil violence, but with higher mortality than explosive fragments. First aid treatment aims at clear airways and rapid patient evacuation to a hospital with a neurosurgical centre. Severe penetrating wounds demand immediate intubation, using i.v. diazepam or pancuronium, and controlled hyperventilation. Haemostasis, wound infection, excision of devitalised brain tissues using suction and primary closure of dura and skin are cornerstones of treatment.

1.92 Chemical Warfare

In contrast to conventional warfare, agents used to launch chemical warfare are considered as weapons of mass destruction (like nuclear warfare). Principles of treatment lie in the disaster plan, therapy of chemically injured people and prophylactic measures. The best protection is the use of masks and protective garments for short periods of time (particularly in the contaminated zone), since masks and garments may be inconvenient and can result in dehydration in hot weather. Therefore, good intelligence and high level of readiness are imperative to optimise the use of protective methods.

Historically, the **first generation** of chemical warfare agents includes vesicants (mustard), blood agents (cyanide), choking agents (phosgene), short-term incapacitants used as 'harassing agents' 'riot-control agents' and 'tear gas' (chloracetophenone) and long-term incapacitants used as 'sickening or vomiting agents' (diphenylaminochlorarsine).

The **second generation** includes organophosphorous nerve agents (Tabun, Sarin, Soman), short-term incapacitants used as 'irritant agents' (chlorobenzylidine), long-term incapacitants used as 'mental incapacitants' (3-Quinulidine) and toxins (Botulinum toxin A, ricin, shellfish poison).

The **third generation** includes mycotoxins (nivalenol, deoxynivalenol, T-2 toxin).

The **anti-plant agents** includes defoliant and herbicide (di- and tri-chlorophenoxyacetic acid, picloram), anti-crop agents (cacodylic acid), and soil sterilant.

Classifications

Medical/toxicological (MT) and equivalent military/service (MS) classifications/divide chemical warfare agents into lethal and non-lethal agents (incapacitating agents).

lethal agents include:
1. Nerve agents (T) or casualty agents (S) (e.g. Tabun, Sarin and Soman).
2. Vesicant blistering agents (T) or casualty agents (S) (e.g. mustard).
3. Suffocating choking agents (T) or casualty agents (S) (e.g. phosgene).
4. Blood agents/systemic posions (T) or casualty agents (S) (e.g. cyanide).

Notice that militarily speaking all lethal agents are called casualty agents irrespective of medicotoxicological titles.

Non-lethal agents (incapacitating agents) include:
1. Sensory irritants/lachrymators/tear gases/sternutators/sickening agents (T) or short-term incapacitants/riot-control agents/harassing agents/exhaustion agents (S) (e.g. chloracetophenone, chlorobenzylidine).
2. Peripherally acting physiochemicals/non-irritant physiochemical agents (T) or long-term incapacitants/immobilising agents/ physically incapacitating agents (S) (e.g. 3-Quinulidine).
3. Centrally acting physiochemicals/psychomimetic agents (T) or long-term incapacitants/psychochemicals/mentally incapacitating agents (S) (e.g. 3-Quinulidine).

Management of chemical warfare injuries

A. Within non-contaminated zone (disaster plan at battlefield)

Chemical weapons are usually used with conventional weapons; chemical agents themselves can be loaded on the explosive shells. In the contaminated zone, therefore, first aid and principles applied in conventional missile injuries can well be applied here.

Assessment for triage and resuscitation at the site of physical disaster are of vital importance. Breathing must be secured by placing the victim supine, clearing the airways and hyperextension of the neck (assuming no cervical spine fractures). Bleeding must be arrested, and external bleeding with no fracture can be stopped by limb elevation and direct pressure and compression at pressure points; tourniquet is the last resort as it may sacrifice a limb to save a life so it must be used only in absolute necessity (once applied it should not be removed and the patient is transferred with it to the casualty collection point).

Internal bleeding is manifested as shock which may be invisible due to fracture, intrathoracic, or intra-abominal injury; i.v. lines therefore must be secured and fractures must be immobilised with splints and bandaging (of course breathing must be maintained).

Wounds in various body sites must be dressed and treated as for missile injuries. Mobile ITU to the site may be necessary to provide trained staff and unpack disaster equipment, including beds, documentation, monitors (unsophisticated but practical), ventilators, suckers, i.v. therapy, syringe drivers etc. Regular patient reassessment, rest periods and refreshment for staff are important.

B. Within contaminated zone

First aid treatment is also applied as in the conventional environment of a non-contaminated zone. Before helping anyone, medical personnel must ensure they are themselves protected with mask and clothes, making sure that all snaps, zippers and velcro fasteners are closed. Thereafter, victims can be handled safely to establish the airway by putting their mask on for them (once on the mask seal should not be broken), to administer nerve agent atropine antidotes (2 mg i.m.) and in persistent symptoms, up to 3 injector sets (6 mg i.m.) are given with 10 minutes between each set. Also 2 PAMc1 600 mg i.m. injection can be given, up to 3 injections (1.8 g). Pyridostigmine, diazepam to control convulsion, antibiotics, antihistamines and anti-arrhythmics can all be used according to the situation. Artificial resuscitation cannot be accomplished in a chemically contaminated zone; if required, the back pressure–arm lift method (while the patient is prone with the head resting on the hands and tilted to one side, push the back firmly for expiration, and then pull the arms upwards at the elbow for inspiration), or the back pressure–hip lift method (hip is pulled up instead of arm) can be used depending on location and extent of injury. If the victim has an open wound, medical staff must make sure their gloves are not contaminated prior to dressing. If they are, glove decontamination must be done before continuing with first aid. Patient must be transported to the nearest medical facility, where doctors and staff must take precautions too (protective clothing).

Clinical presentations and corresponding first/self aid treatment can be summarised as follows:

1. Nerve agents (organophosphorous poisoning) lead to running nose, tightness of the chest, dim vision, pinpoint pupils, drooling, twitching, jerking, headache, convulsion and death. Treatment is by protective mask and the use of atropine autoinjectors. Experience with agricultural (and military) poisons, such as EPN, trichlorophan, malathion and fenthion, showed that these can respond well to early (within 3 h) direct haemoperfusion; each charcoal column is used for its full length, i.e. iZh. Symptomatic relief is gained by atropine or glycopyrronium. Blood levels of poisons can be calculated from pharmacodynamic graphs of decay versus time.

2. Blood agents (cyanide poisoning resulting in histotoxic hypoxaemia) lead to giddiness, tachypnoea, headache, pounding of the heart, blue discoloration of lips and skin, unconsciousness and death. First aid is with protective mask.

3. Vesicant blistering agents lead to inflammation of eyes, redness of skin and blisters. Treatment is by flushing eyes with water and wearing a protective mask. Chemical burns are difficult to treat; dry heat may lead to upper airways obstruction with soot in the nostrils, or sputum, pulmonary oedema, cyanosis, dyspnoea, tachypnoea, stridor, hoarseness and swollen lips, tongue, pharynx and larynx. Endotracheal intubation, therefore, should not be undertaken unless absolutely necessary.

4. Suffocating choking agents lead to dry throat, coughing, tightness of the chest, nausea, vomiting, dry land drowning (drowning in one's own vomitus), and death. Lower airway injury due to phosgene chemical burn with development of ARDS and hypoxia (may even occur due to fluid shift) may be fatal. First aid with protective mask is the best hope of survival.

5. Sickening vomiting agents lead to inflammation of nose, throat and eyes, sneezing, vomiting and persistent coughing. First aid is with protective mask and treatment by fresh air.

6. Tear gases cause watering of eyes, photosensitivity, spasm of eye muscles, irritation of the nose and freshly shaven face. First aid is with protective mask and treatment by fresh air.

7. Incapacitating agents cause disorganisation of thoughts. First aid is with protective mask; recovery takes time.

C. Prophylactic measures (civil defences)

Shelter Stay indoors. Shut all windows and doors. Move towards inner spaces, closets etc. Seal openings with adhesive tapes. If possible, prepare ahead of time food and drinking water supply in sealed plastic containers. Cover the containers with plastic bags and seal tightly.

Protective equipment Avoid contact with the chemical agents. Roll down sleeves. use impermeable material such as plastic overgarments, gowns, blankets etc., to cover exposed skin areas. Protect hands with gloves or plastic bags. If a protective chemical warfare mask is not available, use regular towels soaked with sodium bicarbonate (baking soda) solution (25 g for each 1000 ml water). Breathe through the towel, shifting it from time to time to breathe through wet areas.

Decontamination Remove all droplets of chemical agent from the skin using clean gauze or cotton wool. Do not rub the skin. For effective skin decontamination use commercially available tubes containing Fuller's earth powder. Disperse powder over exposed skin areas. Leave powder for 1 min and remove from the skin. If a powder is not available, use water and regular soap to remove the chemical agent from the skin. Baking soda solution can also be used for decontamination of skin including the facial area (avoid eye penetration).

After the attack When the area is declared clean, remove all protective equipment cautiously. Use rubber gloves to protect your hands while removing contaminated material or use tweezers or similar devices. Put all contaminated material in plastic containers. Seal the containers and label them appropriately. When leaving the house or shelter (after the area is declared clean), move opposite to the wind direction.

Chemical weapons: Gulf War experience

Since chemical weapons were first used on a large scale during the First World War a wide range has been developed, but because of their high volatility, compounds such as hydrogen cyanide, phosgene and chlorine are unlikely to be used. Mustard gas and nerve agents are likely to present the major risk.

Mustard gas (sulphur mustard) A liquid which gives off a dangerous, visicant vapour. Unprotected persons exposed to either the vapour or the liquid develop blistering of the skin, eye damage and, if they inhale the vapour, damage to the upper respiratory tract. An asymptomatic latent period of up to 6 h is classically described before skin reddening which progresses to large painless blisters. Eye damage, severe pain, tearing and corneal damage may take 6 weeks to resolve. Absorption of the compound may cause bone marrow depression. Death, which in the first World War occurred in 2% of mustard gas victims, results from burns, respiratory tract damage and bone marrow depression.

Treatment is symptomatic: skin lesions should be treated like thermal burns, large blister fluid being drained under aseptic conditions (the claim that blister fluid is dangerous by causing secondary blistering of attendants is untrue). Eye damage is treated by daily irrigation, mydriatics to ease the eye pain produced by spasm of ciliary muscle and to prevent the iris sticking to the lens, antibiotic drops and, if necessary, systemic analgesics. The use of sterile petroleum jelly (to prevent the lid margins sticking together), dark glasses and reassurance are important since eye lesions produce severe photophobia and fear. Upper respiratory tract damage is treated according to symptoms; antibiotic cover is provided to prevent infection. The most severely affected patients may need assisted ventilation and oxygen-enriched air.

Most patients exposed to mustard gas recover completely, and only a small proportion will have long-term eye or lung damage. Though sulphur mustard is a known carcinogen, the risk associated with a single exposure is remote.

Nerve agents Pose a more serious threat, particularly to the unprotected. They are organophosphorous compounds (related to pesticides) which inhibit the enzyme acetylcholinesterase and therefore interfere widely with the functioning of the nervous system. Treatment is that of poisoning with organo-phosphorous pesticides. Nerve agents may be encountered on the battlefield in both vapour and liquid phases. Early symptoms of nerve gas poisoning include miosis, rhinorrhoea, hypersalivation and headache; in severe cases neuromuscular transmission is impaired leading to respiratory failure. Vomiting, convulsions and damage to the central respiratory drive may also occur, causing death from respiratory failure.

Treatment includes the use of atropine, oximes (which reactivate the inhibited cholinesterase), and the anticonvulsant diazepam. The efficacy of treatment may be greatly enhanced by giving pyridostigmine before exposure to a nerve agent. Pyridostigmine binds reversibly to some of the cholinesterase and prevents that proportion being attacked by nerve agents. During the recovery period after poisoning with nerve agents, binding of cholinesterase to pyridostigmine is reversed and uninhibited enzyme reappears from this protected store. Many armed forces (such as those of the UK) have pyridostigmine tablets to take before exposure and autoinjection devices to allow the rapid administration of atropine, oxime and diazepam after exposure.

Victims of chemical weapons may receive immediate treatment by armed forces medical services. Before evacuation to the UK, for example, all casualties will have been decontaminated and stabilised so that doctors in the UK are likely to be concerned mainly with the late effects of exposure. Burns surgeons, dermatologists, respiratory physicians and ophthalmologists are likely to be most heavily concerned with victims of mustard gas, whereas clinical toxicologists, general physicians, neurologists and anaesthetists are likely to be concerned with victims of nerve agents, whose treatment may be prolonged.

Gulf War Syndrome

Officially, it is claimed that there is no evidence to support the existence of a single disease or a syndrome relating to service in the Gulf during the war against Iraq in 1991. American Pentagon and Defense officials claimed that a study of 10 200 Gulf War (1990–91) veterans had not shown a unique illness or syndrome despite many documented cases among serving veterans reporting illnesses and birth defects of their babies born after 1991. The British Ministry of Defence launched a controlled study in January 1996 to investigate the Gulf War Syndrome by comparing Gulf veterans with troops and personnel who did not serve in the region. Gulf veterans have claimed that governmental studies were deliberately flawed in order to avoid compensation to their families; furthermore, they point to the fact that French troops did not receive the immunisation against nerve gas attacks and have not reported any case of Gulf War Syndrome.

The syndrome is attributed to:

- A massive cocktail of vaccination to protect against attacks by biological weapons. As many as 14 vaccinations were given; up to 9 (including anthrax and bubonic plague) were given in a single day.
- Anti-nerve agents tablets to protect against attacks by chemical weapons.

- Exposure to heavy fumes of exploded, smouldering and burnt oil fields, diesel fumes and environmental poisons in the biggest environmental disaster affecting the Gulf region. The impact of passive smoking of these mega-fumes on the respiratory system has not been assessed yet.
- Radiation exposure to bombarded and exploded Iraqi radiotherapy plants, radiation centres and chemical plants. The wind played an important role in drifting these gases and emitted radiations south of Kuwait where serving troops were stationed.

Symptoms include abdominal cramps, vomiting, joint pains and muscles, kidney disorders; veterans have also registered headache, depression, chronic fatigue, dizziness, severe memory loss and weight loss.

In 1993 and over a 6 month period only, 350 out of 50 000 serving veterans were reported to have Gulf War Syndrome. Thereafter the number doubled to 700 over the next few months and is still increasing. More than 70 veterans whose wives became pregnant after the Gulf War noticed severe birth defects among their newly born children and attributed that to a definite link with the vaccinations. Some children have been born with limb defects, heart deformities, or vital organs missing, as well as neurological and immunological disorders.

1.93 Nuclear Warfare

[Based on the Report of the British Medical Association and Board of Science and Education (*The Medical Effects of a Nuclear War*), published by John Wiley, Chichester, 1983.]

Nuclear weapons are the most devastating instruments of mass destruction. A careful study of the effects of the nuclear bomb explosions on Hiroshima and Nagasaki is worth considering. Nuclear weapons (or bombs) are weapons in which explosion results from energy released by reaction involving atomic nuclei, either fission or fusion, or both. Thus the A-bomb (atomic fission bomb) and H-bomb (hydrogen fusion thermo-nuclear bomb) are both nuclear weapons.

The basic nuclear weapon is the fission bomb. The weapon used against Hiroshima (code named 'Little Boy') was a free-fall bomb dropped from an aircraft at 8.15 am on 6 August 1945. The bomb exploded approximately 500 m above the centre of the city with a force, or yield, said to be equivalent to approximately 12 500 tons (12.5 kilotons) of TNT. The explosion was several thousand times more powerful than that produced by any previous conventional bomb.

The bomb used to destroy Nagasaki (code named 'Fat Man') exploded 500 m above the city at 11.02 am on 9 August 1945. It is thought to have had an explosive yield of some 22 kilotons. 'Fat Man' was about three metres long, 1.5 m wide and weighed 4 500 k.

In these A-bombs, as they were called, a fission chain reaction was triggered and sustained in order to produce a very large amount of energy in a very short time. Within a millionth of a second the effect of heat on the surrounding air and objects created a very powerful explosion.

The atomic bombs built so far have used uranium-235 or plutonium-239 as the fissile material. A fission event occurs when a neutron enters the nucleus of an atom of one of these materials, which then breaks up or 'fissions'. A large amount of energy is released, the original nucleus is split into two radioactive nuclei (the fission products) and two or three neutrons are released. These neutrons can be used to produce a self-sustaining chain reaction. A chain reaction will take place only if at least one of the neutrons released in each fission produces a fission reaction in another heavy nucleus.

In fusion, however, light nuclei are formed (fused) into heavier ones; isotopes of hydrogen – deuterium and tritium – are fused together to form helium. The reaction produces very large quantities of energy and is accompanied by the emission of neutrons. There is no critical mass for the fusion process and therefore in principle there is no limit to the explosive yield of fusion weapons or H-bombs.

The physical effects of the Japanese explosions

Hiroshima is built on a plateau and, consequently, the city was damaged symmetrically in all directions. The damage to Nagasaki, built on mountainous ground, varied considerably according to the terrain in each direction. But the death rate at given distances from ground zero (the point on the ground directly below the centre of the explosion) was about the same in both cities.

Almost everyone within 500 m of ground zero when the bombs exploded was killed; about 60 per cent of those within 2 k. About 75 per cent of these deaths occurred in the first 24 hours.

The number of people in Hiroshima at the time of the explosion is not clear; the best estimate is about 350 000. By the beginning of November 1945, 130 000 of these people, or approximately 40 per cent of the population of Hiroshima, had died. About 270 000 people, including many Koreans, are thought to have been in Nagasaki when the bomb exploded. According to the best estimate, some 60 000–70 000, around 25 per cent, died by the end of 1945.

Of those killed immediately, most were either crushed or burned to death. The combined effect of thermal radiation and blast was particularly lethal. Many of those burned to death in collapsed buildings would have escaped with only minor injuries had there been no fires. However, an area of 13 km^2 in Hiroshima and 7 km^2 in Nagasaki was reduced to rubble by blast and then to ashes by fire. The difference in size of these two devastated areas was due mainly to variations in the topography.

The energy generated by the nuclear bomb explosion took three forms (each with grave consequences).

1. *Blast or overpressure, representing 50–60% of total energy* At Hiroshima all buildings within 2 kilometres of ground zero were damaged beyond repair by overpressure (pressures in excess of atmospheric pressure) of 4 pounds per square inch (psi) and greater. Casualties due to blast were particularly severe within about 1.3 km of ground zero, where the overpressure reached levels of 10 psi and greater.

The shock wave was followed by a hurricane-force wind. As the shock wave travelled outward, it left behind an area of negative pressure, and eventually the air flowed in the inward direction. Thus, a supersonic shock wave was followed by an overpowering wind and then, after an instant of stillness, a violent wind blew back in the opposite direction.

2. *Thermal energy (35% of total energy)* About one-third of the total energy generated by the bombs was given off as heat. The fireballs produced by the nuclear explosions reached temperatures of the same magnitude as that of the sun almost instantly. The fireballs grew to their maximum diameters of about 400 m within a second, when their surface temperatures were about 5000 °C.

At a distance of 500 m from ground zero in Hiroshima the thermal radiation received in the first 3 seconds was about 600 times as great as the sun on a bright day. Even at a distance of 3 k, from ground zero, the heat in the first 3 seconds was about 40 times more than that from the sun. The heat at Nagasaki was more intense, twice that at Hiroshima.

The heat was sufficient to burn exposed human skin at distances as great as 4 km from ground zero. Many people caught in the open within about 1.2 km from ground zero were burned to death; others were vaporised.

Hiroshima had about 76 000 buildings before the bomb was dropped; 65 per cent were destroyed by fire. Twenty five per cent of Nagasaki's 51 000 buildings were totally destroyed, and many more seriously damaged. The extensive damage and absence of water made effective fire-fighting impossible.

3. *Ionising radiation* About 15 percent of the energy generated by the bombs was given off as ionising radiation, about 30 per cent of which, the initial radiation, was emitted within 1 minute of the explosion. The remainder, the residual radiation, was emitted from radioactive material in the form of 'fall-out'. The initial radiation dose at ground zero in Hiroshima was of the order of 1000 Gy (100 000 rad). In Nagasaki the dose at this point was several times greater.

Site of explosion and guidance systems

The physical effects of a given weapon will vary according to a number of factors. An important variable is the height above ground at which the bomb is detonated. If this height is such that the resulting fireball touches the ground, it is said to be a 'ground-burst'; for any height above this, it is an 'air-burst'.

The range of blast effects will be greater for an air-burst than for an equivalent yield ground-burst. The principal reason is that the shock wave from the explosion is reflected from the ground and combines with the direct wave to produce a merged or Mach wave. Thus a military planner wishing to cause the maximum damage to unprotected targets such as cities or large industrial areas, would tend to employ air-burst weapons; both the bombs used in Japan were air-burst. It is possible to 'optimise' the height of detonation so as to subject the greatest possible area to a chosen level of blast overpressure. With a ground-burst bomb, on the other hand, much higher levels of blast pressure can be created at ground zero. The *range* of blast effects is thus reduced because a proportion of the energy of the bomb will be transmitted into the ground, but the effects will be equally catastrophic, producing not only a crater but also a spreading 'earthquake' effect that can seriously damage underground structures such as sewers, water pipes and electricity supply cables. The obstructions presented by buildings and hills will limit the range of thermal and nuclear radiation from a ground-burst.

In practice, the destruction is increased by increasing the number of warheads and lowering their individual yield; that is to say one large warhead is not so effective as several smaller ones of the same total yield spread out over the target area. The multiple independently targetable re-entry vehicle (MIRV) system developed by the United States in the late 1960s and deployed also by the former Soviet Union employs separate re-entry vehicles carried on a 'bus' which releases the warheads one by one after making pre-selected changes in speed and orientation so as to direct the RVs to their separate targets.

Ballistic missiles are guided mainly during the initial, 'boosting' phase of the flight, when the rocket engines work; so-called cruise missiles are driven and navigated through the entire flight path and weapons of any kind use target-finding and homing devices in their final approach to the target. These homing systems include radar, infra-red and laser devices. When weapon delivery accuracy is enhanced, the weapon yield required to achieve a certain probability of destroying a given target decreases sharply, with a reduction in the level of destruction on the ground.

The electromagnetic pulse (EMP)

Although not a health hazard directly, the electromagnetic pulse following detonation of a nuclear bomb can destroy radio and telephone communications over the area of a whole continent, and thus disrupt the organisation of rescue services.

Clinical presentation of victims

The three main effects of a nuclear explosion which kill and injure people are blast, heat and ionising radiation. For air-bursts in the megaton range and for city targets it is blast and heat that kill or injure the largest number of people. In ground-blast, however, many more casualties may result from radiation days or weeks after the explosion. These later casualties may eventually exceed those from all other causes. This is because fall-out can cover much larger areas than those devastated by blast or fire.

As the bomb explodes, intense ionising radiation consisting primarily of neutrons and gamma rays is emitted. Up to 2.5 km away unprotected victims receive a lethal dose, but those this close to the explosion would be killed by blast and heat.

Radiation sickness

The most important longer-term effect of ground- or near-surface bursts is fall-out. Over a period of a few hours after detonation, unprotected people as far as 80–160 km downwind of the explosion may receive a lethal dose of radiation from fall-out.

Decrease in lymphocytes occurs promptly, most of it taking place within 24 hours after exposure. The level of this early lymphopenia is one of the best indicators as to severity of radiation injury. The level of neutrophil granulocytes shows a very early rise, usually limited to the first 48 hours or less, but the degree of elevation has not been correlated with the extent of injury. In the dose range producing the haematopoietic syndrome, after the early rise, granulocyte numbers fall to fairly low levels at about day 10 and there is a transient abortive rise at about day 15, perhaps due to mitosis of a genetically damaged cell population which cannot continue to reproduce. (The absence of an abortive rise is an unfavourable sign.) There is then a steady fall in granulocyte count, beginning at about day 30 after exposure if the patient survives, which is followed by a spontaneous recovery beginning in 50 weeks' time. The platelets may show a rise in the first two or three days after exposure, then a gradually accelerating decrease, with the nadir also reached at about day 30. During the recovery the platelets usually rise to well above normal levels.

Diarrhoea and other gastrointestinal symptoms were common effects of radiation in Hiroshima and Nagasaki, and decreased with the distance from ground zero. Bloody diarrhoea was noted in about 10 per cent of those within 1 km of ground zero at the time of attack and in one per cent beyond 5 km. However, studies of radiation given to facilitate bone-marrow grafts suggest that quite high doses of radiation can be tolerated without producing gastrointestinal symptoms. It is generally thought that severe gastrointestinal symptoms result from doses of radiation in the range 5–20 Gy. The effects are due to inhibition of mitosis of the cells in intestinal crypts. This causes electrolyte loss and bacterial invasion. Death is likely to result from a combination of fluid loss and secondary infection.

Very high doses of radiation above 20 Gy produce the 'neurovascular syndrome' in which there may be a short interval of mental alertness before victims become comatose and die. At very high dose ranges of about 70 Gy the period of mental alertness before coma may be very short.

There are other clinically significant short-term effects of radiation. High doses may be received if skin is contaminated by beta-emitting particles in fall-out; the radiation erythema may appear after a dose of about 3 Gy to the skin. The dose at which erythema starts to appear is somewhat lower for neutron exposure. At doses above 10 Gy, scaling, blistering and ulcerative changes may all occur and if the patient survives long enough there may be keloid formation. 'Beta burns' were seen amongst some of the Marshall islanders exposed to radiation after the 1945 Bravo test explosion. Hair-loss may occur after a dose to the scalp of 3 Gy or more. Recovery takes place in the months following exposure unless the hair follicles have been exposed to high doses.

Fertility is likely to be impaired following radiation exposure. the testes are radio-sensitive. A dose as low as 0.1 Gy can depress sperm production for up to a year and 2.5 Gy will produce sterility for three years or longer. The ovary is more radio-resistant but doses of 1–2 Gy will cause temporary sterility.

At Hiroshima and Nagasaki it was noted that children exposed to radiation in utero tended to be smaller than average. Amongst 169 children exposed in utero at Hiroshima there were 33 with microcephaly (defined as two or more standard deviations below normal). About half of these were mentally retarded. In a nuclear war it is likely that many victims will suffer from the combined effects of radiation, burns and blast and consequently injuries which may be relatively minor under normal circumstances could be fatal when combined with others of similar severity, particularly in the absence of adequate treatment and basic sanitation.

The psychological effects

During the post-attack phase, those who survived the immediate effects of nuclear bombardment would be under immense stress. The psychological effects of such an attack (and their influence on the ability of survivors to cope with bereavement, physical suffering, devastated environment and associated problems) are difficult to predict with certainty. However, the experience of Hiroshima and Nagasaki suggest that many people would be incapable of organised activity. For instance, Hachiya, a Japanese physician at Hiroshima, wrote:

Parents, half-crazy with grief, search for their children. Husbands look for their wives, and children for their parents. One poor woman, insane with anxiety, walked aimlessly here and there through the hospital calling her child's name.

What a weak fragile thing man is before the forces of destruction. After the flash the entire population had been reduced to a common level of physical and mental weakness. Those who were able walked silently towards suburbs and distant hills, their spirits broken, their initiative gone. When asked whence they had come, they pointed to the city and said 'That way', and when asked where they were going they pointed away from the city and said 'This way'. They were so broken and confused that they moved and behaved like automatons.

Treatment in nuclear disaster

In hospital, reception and assessment of the seriously injured for priority treatment (triage) is the most important initial process in medical management. It has become common experience that if a patient can be admitted to hospital alive, the prospects of survival are good.

In the case of a nuclear attack, the picture would be entirely different. A completely new clinical situation would arise because of the devastating effects of nuclear explosions, both in regard to blast and heat, and also because of the high levels of radiation liberated. These, together with the disruption of communications, rescue and ambulance services, could delay attention to casualties for as long as 10–21 days.

During this prolonged period of delay to the commencement of treatment, survivors might die from a wide range of physical, bacteriological, irradiation and psychological causes. Exposure to wet and cold or to heat and fire, would combine with shortages of safe water and food to affect adversely the prospects of survival. Delay in treatment would result in a high incidence of wound infection. Ruptured drainage and sewage systems, together with the presence of decaying corpses and animal carcasses, would increase enormously the hazards of infection. Those already wounded would have the additional problem of radiation sickness from major radioactivity to contend with. The psychological effects of such a disaster can only be conjectured, but should not be underestimated.

Major accident schemes existing throughout the UK and other countries aim at providing high standards of treatment for disaster victims. These schemes are designed to deal with civil disasters in which 25 or more people are injured. This number is insignificant in comparison with the number of casualties resulting even from a solitary 'small' nuclear attack. It is apparent that any schemes in existence would be completely inadequate to deal effectively with such a situation. In a localised attack help from outside the area involved would be restricted by the dangers of moving skilled personnel into an area of irradiation, while evacuation of casualties would produce a similar dilemma. In a major attack the medical facilities that survived would be swamped and prove unable to provide acceptable medical care. In these circumstances treatment would consist of only the most simple first-aid measures, with no possibility of complex procedures.

It is unlikely, in the conditions following an attack, that any patient with a third-degree burn involving more than 30 per cent of body surface would survive. The plasma and blood requirement for a 50 per cent third-degree burn in an adult patient is 10 l in the first 48 hours. It is unlikely that this demand could be met for many, if any, such casualties, even if hospital facilities were available. Those with more extensive second-degree burns could, however, survive without immediate medical treatment.

Orthopaedic injuries, if severe, would prove fatal and it would be unlikely that the patients themselves would be able to reach medical facilities or receive other than simple first-aid treatment. Spinal injuries would present even greater problems.

Patients with major abdominal and thoracic injuries would be unlikely to survive long enough for effective measures to be taken and survival after this type of injury would be measured in hours.

It appears that the breakdown of specialised medical services would be complete after a major attack and that treatment would be limited to simple first-aid measures and pain relief. The principle of most attention being given to those most likely to survive would replace the former concept that the most seriously ill should receive maximum aid. The Health Service in its present form would disappear after a major nuclear attack on the UK.

Disruption of medical facilities in nuclear war

Medical response to infection

Communicable diseases can be counteracted in peacetime by a variety of medical responses. Mass vaccination programmes can be launched and antibiotics and supportive care are routinely available. After a nuclear attack immunisation programmes would not be feasible. Facilities for diagnosis and treatment of communicable diseases would be largely destroyed. There would not be the resources to deal with more than a fraction of the communicable disease problems which are likely to result. More important than medical treatment for many diseases would be the facilities which sustain modern society, such as food distribution, safe water, shelter, fuel and power supplies. The destruction of these would be particularly conducive to the spread of communicable disease among the population.

Destruction of medical facilities

In Hiroshima 90% of physicians were casualties of the atomic bomb and a similar proportion of nurses were also killed or injured. In the event of another nuclear war it is likely that medical staff and facilities would suffer at least as much if not more than the general population.

Those with major injuries require large quantities of blood as well as monitoring and life support equipment and laboratory facilities. Ideally all major casualties should receive surgical treatment within six hours of injury. Obviously this would be impossible after a nuclear attack. A well-organised surgical team might be able to perform up to seven operations in a 12 hour period under ideal conditions. During a disaster of the magnitude envisaged after a nuclear attack, few surgical teams would be likely to remain intact. Many operating theatres do not carry large reserves of general, abdominal or orthopaedic instruments and delays would occur while instruments were cleaned, packed and autoclaved, even if the necessary public utility services survived.

Many doctors have no recent training in treating patients with trauma and even those who do would probably be reduced to simple procedures such as the reduction of fractures or suturing lacerations, mostly without anaesthesia. Many countries lack recent experience in handling victims of mass disasters. For instance, in the UK between 1951 and 1972 there were only ten disasters involving more than 100 casualties in each.

In order to deal with large numbers of casualties simultaneously the principles of triage were developed. These involve the assessment of each patient by a doctor (or experienced nurse) who assigns them to an appropriate treatment area. In many emergencies even triage would be impossible because of the overwhelming number of casualties resulting from nuclear attack. Hospitals and casualty stations, if not destroyed, are likely to become rallying points for injured survivors and relatives, making organised care even more difficult. In addition, the lack of specific tests for radiation sickness in this situation would further complicate patient assessment.

Four main categories of treatment priorities in military medicine are *immediate* treatment, *delayed* treatment, *minimal* treatment and *palliative* treatment. The last category comprises those patients who are so severely injured that only complicated or prolonged treatment offers any hope of improving life expectancy. After a nuclear attack, no medical resources could be spent on this group. No drugs that might be of use to survivors would be available for such a purpose and many people would die without succour.

In peacetime the management of victims of whole-body radiation exposure entails bacteriological monitoring, antibiotics, laminar flow, sterile environment facilities, white cell and platelet transfusion and, in some cases, bone-marrow transplant. These measures would obviously be impossible after a nuclear attack, and there would be essentially no treatment of radiation sickness. Monitoring of the blood count would not be possible for a meaningful number of patients and therefore medical staff would have no way of determining the extent of radiation exposure until unequivocal clinical evidence of radiation sickness appeared.

Pain relief is likely to be grossly inadequate. Stocks of morphine and other analgesic and anti-emetic drugs would be rapidly exhausted. The quantities of general and local anaesthetics available would likewise be insufficient for the millions of casualties. Many useful drugs would be scattered in neighbourhood pharmacies which would be vulnerable to looting and damage. Hospitals and other medical storage installations would not escape the effects of the attack, and many supplies would be destroyed or inaccessible.

Although it now appears that corpses do not represent the major health threat that was once thought, the presence of large numbers of dead bodies may have severe psychological effects. When United States forces entered Manila in 1944, they faced the problem of burying 39 000 bodies. With few exceptions, troops assigned to this task suffered nausea, vomiting and loss of appetite. Even though local labour was recruited to bury the dead the process still took eight weeks. After a nuclear attack, many bodies would have been vaporised by the thermal effect of the explosions, but vast numbers would still remain to be buried.

Drugs

There would remain the on-going health problems requiring drugs and other long-term care, such as acute illness, infections, conditions requiring emergency surgery, malignant disease, chronic conditions (such as diabetes, stroke, chronic bronchitis and arthritis) and conditions which require medical intervention in certain circumstances, such as pregnancy.

Immunisation by vaccines would be particularly difficult. In the UK, for example, there are very few companies manufacturing vaccines and if some of these were lost the lead time for making the product in other plants might be impracticably long. In these circumstances importing would be the answer, given that many drug companies are international and have plant facilities worldwide. However, if, as is likely, normal business transactions were to cease, the situation could be hopeless. Moreover, some vaccines deteriorate fairly quickly and would need special storage conditions.

Given the time scale based on the Home Defence circular, there would be at best a 2–3 week warning period and then a very short war. During this period drug stocks and drug manufacturing capability would be that of peacetime and could not be significantly changed within that time scale. Consequently, after a nuclear attack there would remain only whatever was not destroyed of the normal, not particularly large, peacetime drug stocks. It would, of course, be possible to encourage stockpiling by buying earlier into the chain, or increasing pharmacy stocks from the requirements of one month to three months, given sufficient notice, but it would be expensive. Very few drugs have a shelf-life of less than 12 months, and some remain viable for three years or more, so there is a possibility of stockpiling on a rotating system. If every hospital increased its supply of drugs by the normal demands of one week, or one month, it would have the advantage that these supplies would be geographically dispersed, although main hospitals are usually in areas which are vulnerable to attack. Other dispersed storage depots could help solve the problems, but would be security risks.

Pain-relieving drugs, plasma, blood and intravenous infusions would be in great demand. Many items are made within hospitals, at least some of which would be destroyed. There are a few manufacturing firms which concentrate on the production of these fluids.

Peacetime drug stocks amount on average to something of the order of 6 weeks' to 2 months' normal demand held by manufacturers and perhaps one week's supply held by wholesalers. However, some of the more uncommon drug substances might be made by only one manufacturer, so it is possible that a world source could be destroyed.

If the technology, technical knowledge and equipment were still available, most drugs could be made elsewhere reasonably quickly. Related to this, however, is the quality of water supplies, which if impaired in volume or purity could lead to problems. Further consideration should be given to the chemicals needed to make contaminated water safe.

Since the Second World War, drug manufacturing has become more centralised and uses much higher technology. The drugs that were available in that war were mainly of vegetable origin – for example quinines, morphines. In general the manufacture of drugs is in two stages. First is the manufacture of the drug substance. This is done in an organic chemical plant. The active drug substance is then compounded into whatever medicament is required, into a tablet or a capsule or into a suitable form for injection. This type of work is fairly interchangeable. Many international companies hold on file information relating to the manufacture of drugs in a number of countries, so that an attack on one centre would not necessarily result in knowledge of vital processes being lost. Normal secrecy agreements might have to be waived in the event of large-scale disaster.

It is estimated that pharmaceutical companies with their existing facilities could increase their productive capacity by 20%. The bottlenecks would occur in the supply of the ingredients, for example in making synthetic drugs. The precursors of these are often very complex materials in themselves and can originate anywhere in the world.

Whether the short-term way to provide an increased supply of drugs or vaccines to meet the emergency following a nuclear attack is to stockpile is an open question. It may be that the main need would be for water purification. There remains the possibility of a return to herbal remedies which can be obtained from the countryside. The problem would be to identify and collect the required plants, and to clean them from radioactive fall-out material.

SECTION 2
Clinical Surgery

Introduction

The clinical part of the examination takes place in a hospital atmosphere (except in England where it is held in an examination hall). The clinical part is *the most essential* section. You have to pass it clearly in order to pass the Examination. In the Irish Fellowship you may compensate for a written section but you have to score a clear double pass mark in the clinical section (120 out of 360). In other Colleges you have to pass clearly both the clinical and written sections *individually* as a prerequisite for passing.

Clinical assessment is composed of two components – a few 'short cases' and one 'long case' – which are examined together and usually scored as a double mark. Clinical examination is the biggest hurdle since the examiner and examinee meet face to face and the examinee examines the patient under the dissecting microscope of the College examiners. The candidate's method of examining the patient and his presentation of the case are extremely important. Candidates should bring with them their own surgical instruments, i.e. stethoscope, torch and measuring tape.

The following areas are worth considering.

Examinee–patient relationship

BE:
- **Smart.** Good appearance is essential. Have your hair cut and dress professionally (for men, three piece dark suit with conservative tie) and wear clean shoes. Avoid school motifs and club dress. Smell should be acceptable and hands should be clean and warm (i.e. *appear, talk and behave like a doctor*).
- **Polite and courteous.** Introduce yourself, ask patients' permission for examination, thank them at the end, help them with their night clothes and tuck in the sheets. Seeing a semi-naked patient left uncovered after physical examination gives the examiner a very bad impression.
- **Gentle.** Ask the patient if he or she is suffering from pain; examine gently, looking at the face from time to time for any painful facial expression. Never examine patients as if you are manipulating experimental animals and remember that if the patient shouts 'ouch' you have failed your final FRCS!
- **A shrewd observer.** A surgeon should have a lion's heart (for courage), a lady's hand (gentle fine touch) and an eagle's eyes. The ideal surgeon has been quaintly described as one with 'harte as the harte of a lion, his eyes like the eyes of an hawke and his handes, the handes of a woman (old English quotation). You should try to spot as many abnormal physical signs as you can (even if not relevant to patient's main complaint) and therefore must examine the patient as a whole and not just the part related to his or her complaint. Abdominal examination is never complete without examining external genitalia and performing rectal examination (the foreskin should be inspected for phimosis and, if normal, retracted to inspect possible external urethral meatal stricture). Testicles are abdominal organs and should be palpated routinely especially for tumours since this may explain a vague abdominal mass such as a para-aortic lymph node). Rectal examination should be performed unless you are specifically requested not to. Do not forget to examine the patient's back and both legs, and examine the peripheral pulses carefully. Patient should be examined in the lying and standing position as well as walking since you may discover limping, scoliosis or paraplegia. However, you must be quick and comprehensive in your examination.
- **Methodical.** Many able candidates fail their examination, not because of ignorance of facts but because they examine the patients haphazardly, illogically or incompletely. Diagnosis is not very important – even the layman can diagnose hernia or varicose veins. The doctor should go through his patient methodically step by step according to a well practised routine, which has become instinctive, before reaching his final conclusion. Stress the importance of inspection and observation before embarking on palpation (e.g. ask the patient to lie flat and to lift his head against your hand resistance. Ask him to cough while you look at hernial sites, then ask him to cough again and feel the impulse or the thrill at hernial or varicose vein sites). Make sure that you are being seen by the examiners (like a driving test where you have not only to follow the rule of mirror, signal, manoeuvre but also to be seen while you are doing it). Some candidates prefer to do a running commentary of their findings, others prefer to sum up at the end; both approaches are acceptable but the latter is preferable to avoid disturbing the patient with your commentary.
- **Careful.** When forced to discuss the causes of a patient's swelling at the bedside, avoid the word 'malignancy' or 'tumour' but use 'mitotic lesion' or 'neoplasia' instead. Always mention the common causes first before thinking of rarities. Do not be clever, be careful.
- **Friendly.** Especially in the long case, since this may guarantee the diagnosis, either volunteered by the patient herself or easily concluded after asking indirect leading questions (e.g. What investigations were performed? What did the doctor tell you?)

If the examiner asks you later on 'Did you ask the patient about diagnosis?,' answer diplomatically, 'I asked her as a part of my routine systematic enquiry. (Do not say 'No' since the examiner may take you to the patient to find out the truth.)

Examinee–examiner relationship

DO:

- **Appear professional** (see above).
- **Talk clearly, slowly and concisely** (to the point), presenting a well-planned precise answer.
- **Praise the patient** (in the long case) by saying 'he is a most cooperative man' or 'she is a very pleasant woman'. Avoid the negative aspects of patients.
- **Keep it simple.** Basic principles should always be mentioned first, emphasising the importance of history, examination and investigation and mentioning the simplest, most relevant investigation first. In emergencies always discuss under the plan of 'resuscitation, review then repair'. Common sense should be stressed, e.g. do not mention the fetus as a cause of an abdominal swelling in a male or prostatic enlargement as a cause of urinary retention in a female.
- **Look confident.** Give the impression that you know exactly what you are talking about and know quite well how to substantiate your answers. The examiner may take a contrary view just to test your knowledge. You are expected to discuss the advantages and disadvantages of opposing views without emotion and to be sufficiently flexible to allow another opinion but at the same time to be firm in your own beliefs.
- **Sound interesting** and listen to the examiner's point of view, especially when an examiner wants to tell you their approach.
- **Lead the examiner** to areas of the discussed topic which you know very well.
- **Thank the examiner** at the end.

DO NOT:

- **Argue** with the examiner even though you know that you are correct.
- **Repeat** the question while thinking of an answer and do not ask the examiner to repeat the question since this indicates either that you did not listen carefully or that the question was not phrased in an understandable way. However, if uncertain as to your instructions, do not hesitate to ask for clarification and hopefully the examiner will rephrase the question better.
- **Produce bizarre facial expressions** when asked a question and do not smile too much when you are answering. This is an irritating habit. Do not make unnecessary hand or body movements and do not lean on the examiner's table.
- **Become aphasic** because of the shocking stress of the examination since examiners think that you should function properly under the stress of surgical emergencies and major operations, which is similar if not greater than examination

stress, i.e. you are not suitable to be a surgeon. Relax and impress the examiner with your quiet confident ability.

- **Be too friendly** with the examiner or be tempted to crack jokes. Be reserved, smile a little with confidence and keep the discussion smooth, comfortable and to the point.
- **Ask the examiner to help you** while conducting your physical examination (e.g. do not ask the examiner to support the patient while she bends forward for inspection of the breasts). Hopefully the examiner will volunteer to help you.
- **Spoil** the examiner's X-rays when shown films on the viewing box by touching them or marking them with biro since these films may be treasured.
- **Tell examiners that their techniques are old fashioned;** they usually treasure operative techniques taught by their famous teachers. Remember 'Old is Gold'!
- **Be clever. Do be careful.** Always try and talk from the general to the specific and from the common to the rare. Do not bring up rarities or syndromes unless you are prepared to talk about them and do not mention them first before common diseases. You are being tested on clinical surgery and not on the latest breakthrough in an obscure subspecialty with which you happen to be conversant.
- **Be overconfident and authoritative** toward the examiners, especially in controversial issues, e.g. breast cancer or peptic ulcer treatment. Never express your instructions to the patient dogmatically, e.g. in Buerger's disease do not say: 'Either you stop smoking or I amputate your leg', but 'I *advise* you to stop smoking since you cannot both smoke and keep your leg.' Careful phrasing in such situations is important.
- **Abbreviate** or use vague terms. PR may mean pulse rate or per rectum or pityrasis rubra or PR interval of ECG or public relations or puborectalis. MI may mean myocardial infarction or mitral incompetence. Also avoid words such as minimal, slight, tinge, minor since physical signs are either normal or abnormal, black or white (even in grey cases you have to give your impression and a provisional diagnosis and not list a long differential diagnosis). Do not use meaningless phrases. Your ability to communicate as well as your surgical knowledge and judgement is being assessed.
- **Answer irrelevantly.** Listen carefully, plan your answer and then answer the particular question asked. At the bedside do not jump to conclusions but examine the findings, then plan and think of the possible causes that support the conclusion (use your eyes and hands, then your brain, then open your mouth).
- **Assume** that the examiner always knows the answer or knows more than you.
- **Tell lies** when asked specifically about physical findings of the patient.

SHORT CASES

I. General Surgery

These cases are chosen (by the Consultant and his or her deputy organiser, e.g. Registrar or Senior Registrar) from surgical outpatient clinics and they will be admitted to hospital for operation at the end of the clinical examination. Some of them are in-patients with obvious physical signs that merit discussion. However, in the English Fellowship these cases are brought into an examination hall (for which they are paid) for the clinical examination. Such cases must be transportable, not acutely ill, elective not emergency and able to appear for consecutive examinations. They may not even need an operation, e.g. pectoral lipoma, large sebaceous cyst, Dercum's disease. (Remember to ask the patient: 'When did you have this swelling?' 'Does it give you any problem?' If it is asymptomatic say there is no need for operation.)

Diagnosis is usually no problem in short cases as they can be spot diagnosed. Listen carefully to the examiner's wording and phrasing of the questions. Approach each case in three stages:

1. Examine your patient: elicit physical signs in a methodical way, be accurate and comprehensive and make sure the examiner knows what you are doing. (Do not be hesitant or clumsy in your steps of examination.) Make a point of inspection because although you may have noticed the signs to be seen on inspection, it is important that you are seen to be. Every action should be clear, simple and look well practised. Be very gentle and polite with patients.
2. Give your physical findings at the conclusion of the examination (this is preferred to a running commentary).
3. Discuss the diagnosis.
Pay special attention to the examiner–examinee and examinee–patient relationships.

2.1 Abdominal Masses
('*examine this patient's abdomen*')

1. Ask patient to lie flat with the abdomen completely exposed from the xiphisternum down to and including the external genitalia – from nipples to knees. (*N.B.* testicles are abdominal organs.)
2. Make a point of inspection, paying particular attention to hernial sites, general abdominal distension (fat, fluid, flatus, faeces, fetus or tumour), epigastric pulsation (normal in a thin patient; otherwise indicates gastric carcinoma overlying the aorta, right ventricular failure). If the pulsation is expansible, it indicates aortic aneurysm. Visible peristalsis indicates intestinal obstruction or pyloric obstruction (with a succession splash heard on gentle shaking of patient). Notice abdominal striae,

umbilicus, distended veins (inferior vena cava obstruction, portal obstruction with caput medusae) and pigmentation.
3. Make an effort to search for a hernia or post-operative incisional herniation by asking patient to lift the head against your hand resistance applied on forehead while you are looking at the abdomen. Ask the patient to cough twice – once so that you can locate the hernial site and the second time to enable you to confirm it by palpation for impulse on coughing (Fig. 2.1.1).
4. Warm your hand, kneel by the patient's bedside and gently palpate the abdomen using your flat hand, palpating mainly through the metacarpophalangeal joints. Palpate the whole abdomen first to feel whether it is soft or rigid, painless or tender (always look at the patient's face). Avoid rebound tenderness as it is painful (inflamed visceral peritoneum leads to local tenderness on palpation, while inflamed parietal peritoneum leads to muscle guarding and rigidity, so there is no need for rebound tenderness). Then palpate for any localised organomegaly and LUMPS (see below).
N.B. Organomegaly – tumours connected with the liver, spleen and stomach move freely with respiration; those of the kidney and other abdominal organs do not.

Hepatomegaly

Palpate from the right iliac fossa upwards towards the right hypochondrium. It is confirmed by percussion for hepatic dullness from the chest towards the abdomen for the upper border and *vice versa* for the lower border. Auscultate for hepatic haemangioma. The gallbladder is impalpable unless distended in which case it is a pyriform swelling opposite the ninth costal cartilage and moves freely with respiration. Right hydronephrosis is differentiated from enlarged gallbladder by bimanual palpation, which is possible only in kidney cases.

Splenomegaly and renal tumour

Palpate from the right iliac fossa upwards towards the left hypochondrium. Splenomegaly may be mistaken for left renal tumour. The following points will help in differentiation:

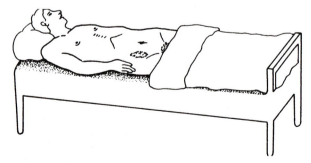

Fig. 2.1.1 Abdominal examination must be in supine position with the patient exposed and the examining doctor must kneel by the bedside. The cough test must be done twice. Note the right iliac fossa mass in this patient

- A renal tumour is bimanually palpable moving backwards and forwards between one hand on the loin behind and the other on the anterior abdominal wall. Splenomegaly is not palpable bimanually.
- Fingers can usually be passed between the kidney and the ribs but not between the ribs and splenomegaly.
- The spleen has a sharp edge with a notch. The kidney edge is always rounded and has no notch. An enlarged kidney tends to bulge forwards. Perinephric abscesses bulge backwards.
- Because of overlying colonic splenic flexure percussion on splenomegaly may be resonant.

N.B. With any abdominal tumour, examine for LUMPS:
- **L**iver enlargement.
- **U**mbilicus secondary malignant deposits from gut primary tumour, especially stomach (Sister Joseph's nodule).
- **M**oving (or shifting) dullness for ascites confirmed also by transmitted fluid thrill. Ascites causes lateral abdominal bulging with flank dullness (shifting) and bulging transverse umbilicus. Ovarian tumour causes anteroposterior abdominal bulging with central (non-shifting) dullness and a vertical umbilicus that is drawn upwards.
- **P**er rectal or vaginal examination for ovarian or pelvic deposits, prostatic enlargement and secondary anal conditions, e.g. piles, abscesses and fistulae.
- **S**upraclavicular lymph node enlargement (e.g. testicular and gastric tumours).

Causes of right iliac fossa mass

Consider the following in order of frequency:
1. Appendicular mass or abscess.
2. Carcinoma of the caecum: the mass is not tender in an anaemic elderly patient over a long period; occult blood in stool and barium enema are positive.
3. Crohn's disease: diarrhoea, weight loss, occult blood in the stool, high ESR, and barium follow: through showing 'string sign' of Kantor (US gastroenterologist) in long-standing Crohn's disease.
4. Gynaecological masses: parametritis, twisted ovarian cyst, uterine fibroid.
5. Pelvic kidney: congenital or history of kidney transplantation; IVU is essential.
6. Iliac lymphadenitis.
7. Rare conditions: ileocaecal tuberculosis, actinomycosis, haematoma, carcinoid tumour, intussusception and appendicular tumours.

2.2 Leg Ulcer
(*'examine this patient's leg'*)

The commonest causes of leg ulcers are venous, arterial and traumatic. Forty per cent of venous ulcers are secondary to varicose veins alone. Arterial ulcer may occasionally be associated with varicose veins. Venous ulcers tend to arise proximal to the medial or lateral malleoli, are usually associated with skin changes (varicose eczema) and are often large. Arterial ulcers tend to be smaller, punched out and more distal on the limb; they may be associated with large or small artery disease (e.g. diabetes, rheumatoid arthritis). Ask about ulcer duration and any past history of deep vein thrombosis, diabetes or arthritis.

1. Kneel by the patient's leg and closely inspect both legs carefully, look for:
- Abnormalities in skin colour and texture.
- Deformity of limb or nails.
- Loss of hair, muscle wasting.
- Cellulitis.
- The presence of varicose veins.
- Any areas of gangrene.
- Any evidence of malignancy in the ulcer (rolled edge).
2. Palpate:
- Temperature.
- Sensation.
- Capillary filling.
- Ulcer base and periulcer induration and liposclerosis (if any).
3. Palpate all lower limb pulses bilaterally:
- Listen for bruits over femoral artery and abductor hiatus (atherosclerosis)

Remember the anatomical landmarks for palpation of peripheral pulses:
- Femoral artery in midinguinal point between the anterior superior iliac spine and symphysis pubis (patient is supine).
- Popliteal artery deeply in the midline of the popliteal fossa (knee flexed to a right angle and patient lying supine or prone). Palpation should be very deep, commencing medially and bringing the fingertips transversely across the line of the artery.
- Posterior tibial artery: midway between the back of the medial malleolus and the medial border of the tendo Achillis (foot is dorsiflexed and inverted).
- Dorsalis pedis artery: in the groove between the first and second metatarsal bones upwards towards the ankle (foot is steadied by left hand and right hand finger pulps are directed slightly towards the first metatarsal bone).
4. If pulses are normal, examine for varicose veins with patient standing. Tourniquet testing may demonstrate sapheno-femoral reflux, but Doppler ultrasound is more accurate and may also give information on the deep veins.
5. Biopsy of ulcer edge may be needed if malignancy is suspected.
6. Culture from ulcer discharge is only indicated if there is evidence of spreading cellulitis and systemic antibiotics are to be used. In general, antibiotics should not be used to treat ulcers as the ulcers are always colonised by bacteria which do not impair healing. Particularly offensive smelling ulcers may respond to topical metronidazole gel as the organisms responsible are usually anaerobic.
7. Venous ulcers are the commonest variety and these heal well by the use of compression bandages. The 4 layer bandage (wool, crepe, elastocrepe and adhesive outer wrap) when applied properly exerts a pressure highest at the ankle, gradually reducing towards the knee. Using these bandages,

60% of ulcers will heal in 6–8 weeks. The use of expensive interactive dressings is not usually necessary and any ulcer dressing should be as simple as possible as these patients often have sensitivities to substances within the dressings.

REMEMBER
- Microscopic death of cells is called 'necrosis'.
- Macroscopic dead soft tissue is called 'slough', e.g. skin, fascia or tendon.
- Macroscopic dead bone is called 'sequestrum', e.g. in chronic osteomyelitis.
- Macroscopic death with putrefaction is 'gangrene' (including both soft tissues and bone as in lower limbs or organs, e.g. appendix, gallbladder, small intestine). Gangrene is either dry (atherosclerosis or Buerger's disease) or wet with infection and swelling (embolism and diabetes).

Causes of ulcer

Ulcers and wounds are both breaches in the epithelial surface but the former are due to internal causes while the latter are due to external causes. Self-inflicted ulcer is a combination of both. You should define the ulcer in terms of site, size, shape, edge (margin), floor (the visible part within the ulcer margin), base (the tissue on which the ulcer is situated – examined by palpation), regional lymph nodes and ulcer discharge.

1. *Venous*: in varicose veins or post-phlebitic syndrome. The ulcer is on the lower medial third of the leg, irregularly shaped with terraced margin and pink granulated floor sitting on a bony base (Fig. 2.2.1).

2. *Arterial*: with signs of ischaemia and absent pulses. Gangrenous toe may be seen (atherosclerosis and Buerger's disease).

3. *Traumatic*: can be caused by adhesive bandages, plaster-of-Paris, but more commonly by patient lying in one position for too long (decubitus pressure sore). The latter is prevented by frequent changing of the patient's position and rubbing the bony prominences with spirit and talcum powder. Common in comatose and hemiplegic geriatric patients and is difficult to heal (may need excision and skin graft).

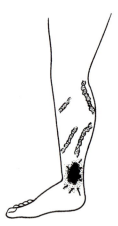

Fig. 2.2.1   Chronic venous (varicose) ulcer

The above three causes are the commonest, followed by:

4. *Infective*:
- Pyogenic ulcer: acute infection commonly with staphylococci and healed with antibiotics.
- Tuberculous ulcer: chronic after rupture of a cold abscess. It has an undermined margin, a soft base covered with thin serous discharge and bluish surrounding skin. An example is erythema induratum of Bazin, which produces purple nodules on the calves of the legs in adolescent females. It is due to *Mycobacterium tuberculosis* and treated with anti-tuberculous drugs.
- Syphilitic gummatous ulcer: usually on upper third of the leg with punched out edge, dirty sloughed floor and hard base (due to *Treponema pallidum*).
- Oriental sore (Baghdad boil): due to *Leishmania tropica*.
- Meleney's ulcer: leads to progressive skin gangrene (synergistic bacteria)

5. *Neuropathic (trophic sore) ulcer*: skin anaesthesia caused by diabetes mellitus (with vascular insufficiency and repeated infection) may lead to perforating ulcers of the sole of the foot which practically never heal. Other causes of neuropathic ulcers are spina bifida, tabes dorsalis, leprosy, peripheral nerve injury, syringomyelia and alcoholic polyneuritis.

6. *Malignant ulcer*: with its premalignant Marjolin's (French surgeon) ulcer. Premalignant ulcers include chronic scar (due to burn), chronic varicose ulcer and sinus of chronic osteomyelitis.

7. *Vasculitic ulcer*: frequently occurs on the lateral aspect of the leg in collagen diseases, such as rheumatoid arthritis, and in ulcerative colitis.

8. *Cryopathic ulcer*: in chilblains and cold injury.

9. *Hypertensive ulcer* (*Martorell's ulcer*).

10. *Haematological ulcer*: in leukaemia, sickle cell and haemolytic anaemia and polycythaemia.

11. *Self-inflicted ulcer*.

Causes of gangrene

- Secondary to RESTED (**R**aynaud's disease, **E**rgot, **S**enile atherosclerosis, **T**hrombosis, **E**mbolism and **D**iabetes).
- Infective, e.g. gas gangrene.
- Traumatic, e.g. pressure sores, supracondylar fracture of femur pressing on popliteal artery.
- Physical, e.g. burns, frostbite, chemicals.
- Venous gangrene due to idiopathic or visceral neoplasm (Trousseau's sign) and in polycythaemia vera.

Causes of amputated finger

- Trauma.
- Leprosy.
- Raynaud's phenomenon.
- Systemic sclerosis (with dysphagia).

Pathogenesis and treatment of varicose ulcer

Venous ulceration does not appear to result from blood stasis within dilated tortuous veins of the lower limb with local deoxygenation (Homans theory, 1916) nor to be caused by arteriovenous shunting (Pratt theory, 1948). The current and widely accepted theory of its pathophysiology is that of venous pressure. Normally the pressure of foot veins is 100 mmHg at rest. This falls to 30 mmHg during exercise due to sucking action of the calf muscle squeezing blood out of the soleal sinusoids and deep veins towards the heart (this calf muscle pump is sometimes known as the peripheral heart.) When the valves in the deep venous system have been destroyed, e.g. post-thrombotic, or rendered incompetent by venous dilatation, blood oscillates up and down the deep veins and venous pressure recorded from the superficial veins during exercise remains constant.

Such venous hypertension results in local capillary bed dilatation which leads to increased permeability owing to stretching of the intraendothelial pores. Fibrinogen leaks in great amounts and polymerises within the tissues to form insoluble fibrin clots in the interstitial fluid around capillaries within the skin and subcutaneous tissues of the calf (pericapillary fibrin cuff). Owing to an associated deficient fibrinolytic activity, the fibrin breakdown is reduced and a greater amount of interstitial thrombosis occurs (liposclerosis). Liposclerosis blocks oxygen and nutrients from reaching the overlying dermal cells (microcirculation diffusion block) leading to tissue anoxia and cellular death which is seen clinically as ulceration. The usual location of this ulcer on the medial lower third of leg is due to constant ankle perforators with maximal venous hypertension at that site. Thus prolonged elastic support (to prevent venous stasis and hypertension) supplemented by fibrinolytic enhancement is the best method of prophylaxis (and treatment) in patients with phlebographic evidence of severely damaged veins.

Varicose ulcer requires daily antiseptic cleansing (chlorhexidine, eusol or H_2O_2) and elastic compression bandaging. Once the ulcer is dry, absorbent dressing is applied to promote drying and scaling. Calaband or Viscopaste may be advocated with fibrinolytic enhancement using a course of *stanozolol*. Up to 90% of venous ulcers will heal with the above measures.

Operative indications

- No response to medical measures.
- Multiple or large ulcer (over 2.5 cm in diameter) with liposclerotic area of 5 cm or more.
- Associated saphenofemoral incompetence or obvious perforators should be treated prior to ulcer treatment (deep venous system should be normal).

Contraindications to operation

1. Severe ulceration with diffuse oedematous skin (operation will lead to necrosis).
2. Infected ulcer or infected eczematous skin.
3. An obstructed deep venous system.

Operative procedures

Dodd's operation involves subfascial dissection and ligation of perforators via a midline posterior incision curved towards the medial malleolus while Cockett's operation involves suprafascial ligation of perforators (above the deep fascia). Linton's operation is directed towards excision of the ulcer, including its

deep fascia (followed by split skin grafting), together with removal of superficial varicose veins and flush ligation and disconnection of the saphenofemoral junction. Combined subfascial perforator ligation, ulcer excision (and split skin grafting) and treatment of varicose veins is the procedure currently used.

2.3 Varicose Veins
('*examine this patient's leg*')

These enlarged elongated dilated veins may be present with leg ulcer (proceed as described above then continue for varicose vein examination) or without, in which case follow the procedure outlined below:

1. Ask the patient, uncovered from the umbilicus downward, to stand up on a stool.
2. Inspect in good daylight and carefully scrutinise the front (long saphenous vein) and the back (short saphenous vein) of the lower limbs.
3. Palpate over the course of the short and long saphenous veins, as well as the groin (saphina varix) and above possible ulcers to feel vaguely visible varicosities and to detect deep fascial defects or gaps (sites of perforators) which are felt as venous blown-out areas.
4. The cough impulse test is performed by applying the right hand to the groin just below the saphenous opening and asking the patient to cough. A fluid thrill is felt in the middle finger if the valve at the saphenofemoral junction is incompetent.
5. The percussion (tap) sign is elicited by placing the left-hand fingers just below the saphenous opening and tapping the main bunch of varicosities once with the right middle finger. If the valves are incompetent within that examined segment, there will be an upward wave, producing an impulse felt by the left hand overlying the long saphenous vein above.
6. Perform the Brodie – Trendelenburg test: ask the patient to lie down on the couch; elevate her lower limb, keeping it straight, and milk the veins to drain the blood out. Place a thumb firmly over the saphenous opening, lower the limb and instruct the patient to stand. Remove the thumb suddenly, and if the veins fill immediately this proves saphenofemoral junction valve incompetence.

The triple tourniquet test (Oschner and Mahorney) is a modification of the above, using three successive applications of one tourniquet or three tourniquets applied at once around the upper thigh, above the knee and below the knee then releasing them in order (from above downward) to demonstrate the level of communication between the deep and superficial systems (through the incompetent valve).

7. To demonstrate patency of the deep venous system, occlude the superficial venous system (but not the deep veins) by applying a rubber tourniquet around the thigh (Perthes' bandage walking test) with the patient in a standing position. The patient is then allowed to walk for 5 min: severe pain is experienced with more pronounced varicosities in the lower limb.

8. Finally examine the lower abdomen in the lying position (if time permits) to differentiate secondary from primary varicose veins. The causes of secondary varicose veins are:

● Pregnancy.
● Intrapelvic neoplasm (uterus, ovary, prostate, rectum) obstructing deep venous return leading to superficial varicosities.
● Compensatory varicose veins complicating iliofemoral phlebothrombosis.
● Arteriovenous fistula, often associated with superficial varicosities. The primary cause should be treated.

Treatment

Current methods of treating varicose veins are:

● Triple saphenectomy procedure, i.e.
  – Saphenofemoral junction flush ligation–disconnection (mistakenly called Trendelenburg's operation, which referred originally to high mid-thigh varicose vein ligation) (Fig. 2.3.1).
  – Varicose vein stripping. (This should be confined to the femoropopliteal segment of the great saphenous vein to avoid saphenous nerve neuritis, interruption of lymphatics and pain produced by extirpation of the low segment between the ankle and knee joints. Furthermore, extirpation of below-knee segment does not remove ankle perforators which communicate with the posteromedial branch of long saphenous vein.)
  – Multiple varicose vein avulsions (mainly below knee).
● Injection-compression technique. Indicated in:
  – Postoperative recurrence especially below the knee.
  – Primary varicose veins, especially when confined to below the knee, as an alternative to surgery.

– Troublesome vulval varicosities.
– It is contraindicated in deep venous thrombosis or in contraceptive pill takers, and in the presence of saphenofemoral junction incompetence.
– The sclerosing material used is 5% ethanolamine oleate (Ethamolin) or 3% sodium tetradecyl sulphate (STD). Each varicosity is injected with 0.5–1 ml not exceeding a total of 10 ml per session (otherwise haemolysis occurs). Injections must always be intravascular (otherwise skin ulceration may occur). The varicosities are marked in the standing position and injection is done in the lying position with the leg elevated. Each injection is maintained temporarily by supporting the needle with a dental roll until all injections are finished. Then all injection sites are compressed by Sorbo-rubber pads maintained in position by a crêpe bandage and a full-length elastic stocking for 6 weeks. The recurrence rate is higher than with surgery.
– Subfascial endoscopic perforator surgery (SEPS) is becoming popular. The endoscope is pushed subfascially with insufflation and all perforators are clipped or diathermised. Tourniquet is required and the procedure allows rapid recovery.

2.4 Swollen Leg
(*'examine this leg'*)

A swollen lower limb is due either to medical central (often bilateral) or surgical peripheral (often unilateral) local disease (Fig. 2.4.1).
1. Exclude the medical causes (cardiac, renal, hepatic and hypoproteinaemia) by history and physical examination, e.g. increased jugular venous pressure, puffiness of face, ascites. The swelling is often bilateral, indicating a systemic cause.
2. Unilateral leg swelling has either a venous or a lymphatic origin (rarely it is caused by arteriovenous fistula).

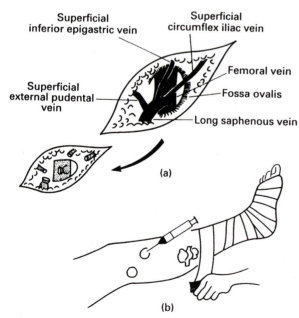

Fig. 2.3.1 Treatment of varicose veins. (a) Sapheno-femoral flush disconnection with ligation of tributaries of long saphenous vein (high tie or modified Trendelenburg operation); (b) perforator site marking followed by injection/compression technique

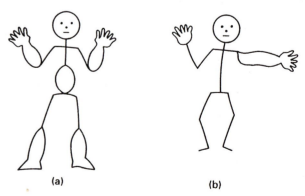

Fig. 2.4.1 The cardinal sign of hypernatraemia is generalised oedema. (a) Localised oedema is either due to venous obstruction of lymphatic obstruction (non-pitting lymphoedema) or due to inflammation (b)

- Venous origin is suggested by:' history of deep venous thrombosis after pregnancy, operation or immobility; presence of pain, varicose veins or complications such as ulcers or dermatitis usually with pitting oedema. The contraceptive pill in females and stilboestrol in males are predisposing factors.
- Lymphatic origin is suggested by absence of pain, healthy skin (no ulceration or pigmentation) and non-pitting oedema (primary lymphoedema is bilateral in 50%).

3. Arteriovenous fistula is rarely present and is either congenital or acquired (after stab or gunshot trauma). Hot leg ulcer, varicose veins with port-wine skin discoloration, local gigantism, warmth, machinery murmur or bruit as well as collapsing arterial pulse (due to high pulse pressure) and cardiac enlargement and failure are all indicative of congenital or acquired fistula. (The latter is diagnosed on the basis of history and lacks gigantism if it occurs after completion of epiphyseal fusion of the limb bones.)

REMEMBER
Difficult cases can be investigated by:
- Ascending deep functional venography.
- Lymphangiography.
- Arteriography (valuable in arteriovenous fistula).

Treatment of lymphoedema is mainly conservative (limb elevation, bed rest with antibiotics for cellulitis attacks, elastic bandages, intermittent diuresis, pneumatic intermittent external compression and massage). In severe cases surgery can be tried (flaying operation, swiss roll operation, Kandoleon's operation, lymphovenous microsurgery). In resistant cases limb amputation may be indicated.

Peripheral causes of leg swelling

Venous origin
- Post-phlebitic syndrome.
- Deep venous thrombosis.

Lymphatic origin
- Primary lymphoedema manifested at birth (lymphoedema congenita; when familial, called Milroy's disease), at adolescence (lymphoedema praecox) or after age 35 years (lymphoedema tarda).
- Secondary lymphoedema after
  - Radical surgical excision of lymph nodes.
  - Radiotherapy.
  - Malignant infiltration, e.g. breast carcinoma.
  - Inflammation.
  - Parasitic infestation (filariasis).

Secondary lymphoedema differs from primary in being of rapid onset, unilateral in distribution and always having an obvious known cause.

Miscellaneous
- Arteriovenous fistula.
- Lipoedema.
- Erythrocyanosis frigida.
- Tight bandage or plaster.
- Injuries, e.g. muscle contusion or fracture.
- Infection, e.g. cellulitis.

2.5 Localised Integumental Swellings
(*'examine this lesion'*)

Inspect and palpate the lesion thoroughly. You can ask the patient how long he has had the swelling and whether it causes him any problems (if the lesion is benign, asymptomatic and present for a long period, leave alone). Describe the lesion in terms of number (solitary or multiple), site, size, shape, overlying skin colour, contour (smooth or irregular surface), consistency (jelly-like, soft, firm, hard or stony hard), tenderness, tethering (mobility) and transillumination.

Sebaceous cyst (Fig 2.5.1)

Small intracutaneous firm smooth spherical swelling (moves with skin), usually associated with a punctum (can be revealed by gently squeezing or pulling the lesion under tension). It commonly occurs on the scalp, postauricular area, scrotum and face as a retention cyst (due to blocked sebaceous gland duct). Treatment is by excision for cosmetic reasons and to prevent complications (infection, ulceration in Cock's peculiar tumour, calcification and sebaceous horn formation).

Lipoma (Fig 2.5.1)

Soft multilobulated, commonly subcutaneous (skin moves over it) with no punctum. It has positive fluctuation (fat is fluid at body temperature) and slipping sign (if the lump edge is pressed, it slips from beneath finger). If the lipoma is subfascial or submuscular ask the patient to contract that particular muscle and the lipoma will decrease in size or disappear with no more lobulation. Lipoma is best left alone unless it is:
- Large and unsightly (cosmetic).
- Symptomatic, i.e. painful or tender in adiposis dolorosa or Dercum's disease (multiple subcutaneous lipomas with one or more tender or painful). Only the painful lipomas should be removed.
- In the thigh or retroperitoneally located as these are more likely to progress to liposarcoma.

The treatment is surgical excision.

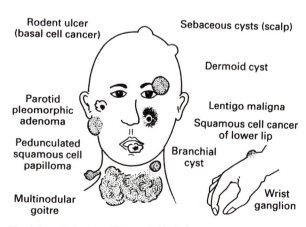

Fig. 2.5.1 Various swellings and skin lesions

Dermoid cyst

Sequestration dermoid occurs at sites of closure of embryonic fissures in the midline of the neck, abdomen, mediastinum and scalp and at the inner or outer angles of the orbit. It is a firm tense subcutaneous mobile cyst (skin moves over it). It differs from an implantation dermoid in that its wall contains hair, hair follicles, sweat and sebaceous glands. Implantation dermoid is associated with a scar from a precipitating injury (thus its wall is stratified squamous epithelium) and commonly affects the hand, palm or fingers, usually of gardeners.

Treatment is excision to prevent infection and for cosmetic reasons. Both dermoid and sebaceous cysts contain pultaceous material that can be moulded; therefore such large cysts give an indentation sign.

Cavernous haemangioma (as well as lymphangioma and meningocele)

Give emptying sign when compressed and refill again when pressure is released. De Morgan's spots, though vascular cutaneous lesions, do not give emptying sign. Treatment of cavernous haemangioma is conservative.

Papilloma (Fig 2.5.1)

Common benign, sessile or pedunculated, pigmented or non-pigmented, single or multiple squamous cell lesion. When on the sole of the foot it may be difficult to differentiate from a corn (localised horny plug of epithelial cells in the epidermis). Treatment is by surgical excision or chemical application (silver nitrate).

Ganglion cyst (Fig 2.5.1)

A tense cyst that communicates with a synovial membrane of a joint or a paratenon (tendon sheath) and contains gelatinous fluid. It usually occurs on the dorsum of the wrist or foot, but it may be related to flexor tendons in the palm or to peroneal tendons at the ankle. It represents a herniation of synovial membrane and may cause pain or interfere with tendon function. Treatment is by rupturing it with external pressure or by excision under anesthesia (local, Bier's block or general) with a bloodless field. The recurrence rate is high.

Muscle tumour

When the muscle is relaxed, the lump can be moved freely across the long axis of the muscle; when the muscle is contracted, the movement becomes abruptly limited. Treatment is surgical excision.

Pulsating lesion

The pulsation may be transmitted from a nearby artery or the swelling itself may be pulsating. These are differentiated by the 'expansible impulse', placing the index and middle fingers over the swelling; if the pulsation is transmitted, the fingers move up and down, but if the swelling is expansible the fingers move apart. Auscultation can reveal a systolic murmur in pulsating

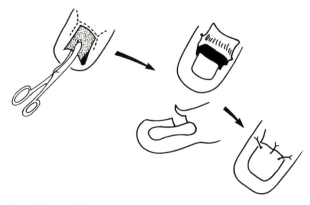

Fig. 2.5.2   Zadik's operation

lesions while arteriovenous fistulae emit a continous murmur. A pulsating swelling can be an aneurysm or a sarcoma.

Toenails

Ingrowing toenail (Fig 2.5.2)

Caused by pressure necrosis. Treated initially by conservative means (correct trimming, clean socks and foot baths, antibiotic course for infection). If these means fail, try simple avulsion and if this fails then radical ablation of the germinal matrix surgically (either partial by unilateral or bilateral wedge excision or total by Zadik's operation) or chemically (80% phenol solution applied for 3 min to the germinal matrix after simple nail avulsion).

Onychogryphosis

Overgrown toenail – treated by Zadik's operation as conservative means do not succeed.

Nail bed lesions

- Subungual haematoma: due to trauma; treated by nail trephine and evacuation of clot.
- Subungual melanoma: treated by excisional biopsy followed by amputation of the digit through the distal interphalangeal joint.
- Glomus tumour: composed of encapsulated arteriovenous plexuses concerned with heat regulation. It is a very painful tiny benign tumour which needs excision (with simple nail avulsion if subungual) leading to dramatic lasting relief.

2.6 Hernia (Fig. 2.6.1)
(*'examine the groin'*)

Hernia (protrusion of a viscus or part of a viscus through a normal or abnormal opening) is either internal (e.g. hiatus

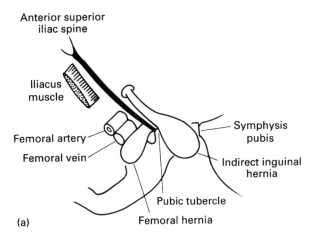

Anterior superior iliac spine

Iliacus muscle

Femoral artery

Femoral vein

Symphysis pubis

Indirect inguinal hernia

Pubic tubercle

Femoral hernia

(a)

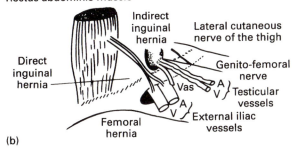

Rectus abdominis muscle

Indirect inguinal hernia

Lateral cutaneous nerve of the thigh

Direct inguinal hernia

Genito-femoral nerve

Vas

Testicular vessels

External iliac vessels

Femoral hernia

(b)

Fig. 2.6.1 Anatomy of the groin from outside (a) useful in open repair, and from the inside (b) useful in laparascopic repair

hernia) or external (e.g. inguinal, incisional or femoral, in this order of frequency). It is the latter which are often presented in examinations. The three common scrotal swellings are hydrocele, epididymal cyst and varicocele.

1. The patient, stripped below the waist, should be examined lying and standing (hernia reduces itself in the first position and becomes obvious in the second position). Initially you should never touch the patient but ask him to cough and look for the visible cough impulse to locate the hernial site.

2. Ask him to cough again and confirm the presence of hernia by feeling the palpable impulse preferably by employing the hand corresponding to the side to be examined (e.g. right hand to right groin), placing the index, middle and ring fingers over the indirect inguinal, direct inguinal and femoral hernial sites respectively while the patient is coughing (*Zieman's tests* – surgeon from Alabama). Inguinal hernia usually bulges above and medial to the pubic tubercle while femoral hernia bulges below and lateral to it. Incisional hernia is diagnosed on the basis of history of abdominal incision with a hernia, and protrusion through the abdominal musculature is easily confirmed when the patient lies down and coughs or lifts his head against resistance. Femoral hernia is diagnosed by its location, and when the invagination test demonstrates that the inguinal canal is empty. It is difficult to reduce, and taxis is contraindicated. It is common in females (because of wide broad pelvis).

3. Academic differentiation of direct from indirect inguinal hernia. Follow four steps:

(a) On inspection, direct hernia emerges straight through Hesselbach's triangle and not obliquely along the inguinal canal.

(b) *Invagination test*: employ the hand corresponding to the side to be examined and invaginate the scrotum *gently* with the little finger; direct hernia is suggested if it passes directly backwards into the abdomen instead of obliquely upwards and outwards or if the cough impulse is felt hitting the pulp rather than the fingertip.

N.B. **The invagination test is a savage test and is only mentioned here to be condemned. Never do the invagination test, Hofman's test (sign) or test for abdominal rebound tenderness; they are painful and/or harmful.**

(c) *Occlusion test*: after reducing the hernia (e.g. by the patient lying down) and then occluding the internal inguinal ring 1 cm above the midpoint of the inguinal ligament (stretched between the anterior superior iliac spine and the pubic tubercle which is different from the midinguinal point stretched between the anterior superior iliac spine and the symphysis pubis – a landmark of the common femoral artery) ask the patient to cough. Any bulging is strongly indicative of direct hernia coming forwards since indirect hernia is prevented from coming down medially through the canal and external inguinal ring.

(d) On lying down, a direct hernia reduces itself instantly and the bulge reappears with equal suddenness when the patient strains.

4. Assess whether the hernia is reducible or complicated (i.e. irreducibility, inflammation, incarceration and strangulation) and determine its contents (if possible). On lying down, the small intestine is reduced with a gurgle; the omentum is doughy on palpation and difficult to reduce due to adhesions. Both femoral hernia and saphina varix have a cough impulse but saphina varix is faintly blue, softer on palpation and usually associated with pronounced varicosity of the long saphenous vein and a positive 'tap sign'. Enlarged lymph node of Cloquet is very difficult to differentiate from irreducible femoral hernia and if no possible focus of infection is found, surgical exploration will be the final answer. Irreducible inguinal hernia in females is difficult to differentiate from hydrocele of the canal of Nuck (anatomist from Holland) (the hydrocele is smooth, fixed, fluctuant and brilliantly translucent) and from cyst of Bartholin's gland (not translucent and confined to labium majus; it is easy to get above it).

5. In the presence of an obvious lump try to get above the swelling by grasping it between the finger and thumb; if this is not possible it is an inguinal hernia but otherwise consider intrascrotal lesions.

Indirect (oblique) inguinal hernia

● The most common hernia.

● Due to congenital preformed sac (partially or completely patent processus vaginalis).

● More common on the right side in young males owing to later descent of right testicle, but after the second decade left inguinal hernias are as frequent as those on the right.

● Unilateral usually (bilateral in 30%).

- Common in men.
- Treated by herniotomy; repair of the stretched internal ring with lateral displacement of the cord; and reconstruction of the weak posterior wall of the inguinal canal (darning usually).

Direct inguinal hernia

- Represent 15% of inguinal hernias.
- Always acquired.
- Usually bilateral.
- Only in men (never females or children).
- Associated with Malgaigne's bulges.
- Presence of predisposing factors, e.g. chronic bronchitis, ascites, obesity, obstructive prostatic uropathy, elderly man with constipation or chronic intestinal obstruction, and postoperative injury to iliohypogastric or ilioinguinal nerves (in appendicectomy).
- Rarely large, rarely descends into the scrotum and rarely strangulates because of wide neck.
- Treated by reduction and inversion of sac (not herniotomy), repair of fascia transversalis in front of it, and reconstruction of the posterior wall of the inguinal canal.

Femoral hernia

- Third most common (incisional hernia is second).
- Common in females (because of wide broad pelvis).
- Difficult to reduce and the most likely to strangulate.
- Truss is contraindicated (it can be used in inguinal hernia whenever operation is contraindicated).
- Treated by low or high approach.

Incisional hernia

(See s. 1.31 Abdominal wound dehiscence)

2.7 Scrotal Swelling (Fig. 2.7.1)
(*'examine the scrotum'*)

If you can get above the swelling then:
1. Palpate the intrascrotal swelling. If its bulk lies in front of and to a variable degree above the body of the testis but it cannot be felt distinctly from the testis it is vaginal hydrocele which is usually bilateral. If the swelling is tense, somewhat lobulated above and behind the body of the testis and felt distinctly from the testicle it is an epididymal cyst, spermatocele or encysted hydrocele of the cord.
2. Do transillumination test by applying a torch behind the cyst and looking from the front of the scrotum through a piece of paper made into a tube and applied directly to the scrotum to prevent scattering of light. Brilliantly translucent swellings are vaginal hydroceles or encysted hydroceles of the cord. Epididymal cysts look tessellated. Remember that:

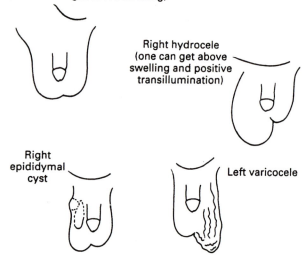

Fig. 2.7.1 Inguino-scrotal swellings

- All scrotal inguinal hernias are non-translucent except for those of an infant or young child which contain the small intestine (translucent).
- All vaginal hydroceles are translucent except those of many years' duration and those which have been aspirated many times (because of deposition of fibrin and blood pigments on their walls). Aspiration reveals a straw-coloured fluid (urine-like) from vaginal hydroceles, milky (like barley water) from spermatoceles and crystal clear (like water) from epididymal cysts.

3. If the palpation reveals a thickened enlarged epididymis with tenderness and a thickened vas it is epididymo-orchitis. If the scrotal swelling (often left-sided) gives a soft feeling like a 'bag of worms' in the standing position, and when the patient is asked to lie down the veins empty and the swelling disappears on testicular elevation, it is a varicocele. In this case the testicle size should be assessed as it is often smaller than on the other side (due to atrophy).

A testicle located at the superficial inguinal ring usually indicates maldescended testicle in children and torsion in adults. The former is usually associated with congenital indirect inguinal hernia. Unilateral hard heavy enlarged testicle (same shape but larger size) usually indicates a testicular tumour.

Small testicle (due to atrophy)

If unilateral, consider:
- Infarction consequent upon torsion.
- Epididymo-orchitis of mumps.
- Postoperative following spermatic artery damage, inguinal hernia, varicocele and orchidopexy.
- Varicocele.

Bilateral atrophy is caused by leprosy, hepatic cirrhosis and oestrogen therapy for carcinoma of the prostate.

Hydrocele

Collection of fluid in the tunica vaginalis and is either congenital or acquired. The latter is either primary (idiopathic) or secondary to trauma, tumours or infection. Vaginal hydrocele is treated by tapping, Lord's operation (multiple radial gathering stitches using catgut – without delivery of the hydrocele), or subtotal excision which entails complete delivery of the hydrocele through a large incision. The tunica vaginalis can be inverted (Jaboulay's method). If while operating on hydrocele, you find a hard testicular mass, clamp the spermatic cord with a soft clamp and take a biopsy for frozen section prior to orchidectomy. Patient consent can't be taken in unsuspected cases of secondary hydrocele due to testicular tumour. Both hydrocele and epididymal cysts can be treated by aspiration with a needle and injection of sclerosant under local anaesthesia (2.5% phenol in water: 5 ml into hydrocele containing < 50 ml, 10 ml for < 200 ml, 15 ml for < 400 ml, and 20 ml for over 400 ml hydrocele; treatment by sclerotherapy).

Testicular torsion (see also s. 3.19)

Usually occurs within the first 20 years of life.

Aetiology (the underlying abnormality(ies):
- High investment of tunica vaginalis (common).
- Extreme motility of scrotal contents (neonates).
- Separation of testis and epididymis (very rare).
- May be no underlying abnormality.

Predisposing factors:
- Spiral attachment of cremaster.
- Unusual body movements.
- Trauma.
- Cycling.
- Cold.
- Pubertal growth spurt.

Testicular viability depends on:
- Testicular descent.
- Possibility of spontaneous reduction.
- Interval before operative reduction.
- Degree of twisting of the cord.

Physical examination (testicular torsion should be differentiated from acute epididymo-orchitis):
- Elevation test of testicle increases twisting and is therefore painful while elevation relieves epididymo-orchitis.
- Degree of funiculitis (tender spermatic cord in the inguinal region) and prostatitis (tender rectal examination) with fever in epididymo-orchitis but not in torsion.
- Presence of mid-stream urine pus cells and/or high WBC in epididymo-orchitis and their absence in torsion.
- Patients with epididymo-orchitis are more than 25 years of age. Orchitis patients are usually body builders or 'toy boys' of night clubs on anabolic steroids.

Investigations:
- Ultrasound doppler.
- Radionucleotide testicular scanning.

There is evidence now that once torsion occurs the endocrine function remains normal but the exocrine function becomes disturbed, i.e. sterility results even if the testis was salvaged possibly due to a sympathetic orchidopathia in the normal testicle. Treatment is by operative untwisting of the torted testis and bilateral orchiopexy.

2.8 Breast Mass (Fig. 2.8.1) (*'examine the breasts'*)

Never ever touch the breast before careful inspection:
1. Ask the patient to undress down to the waist and from a distance ask her to sit up so that you can compare the level of the breasts.
2. Ask her to lean forward and then lift her arms, and then ask her to put them against her waist and contract her pectoral muscles.
3. Palpate the normal breast in quadrants, then examine the axilla for axillary lymph nodes (hold the patient's left hand with your left hand and examine the left axilla with your right hand and *vice versa*).
4. Palpate the supraclavicular lymph nodes by approaching the patient from behind, moving the patient's head gently towards the examined side and asking her to shrug her shoulders while you examine them.
5. Palpate (in supine position) the pathological breast carefully looking for the 10 breast cancer signs including: breast

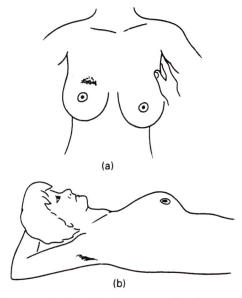

Fig. 2.8.1 Examination of the breast. (a) Axillary lymph nodes are examined in sitting position. Note the right breast elevation due to puckering breast carcinoma. (b) Breasts must always be examined in supine position

elevation, four nipple changes – retraction, eccentric nipple, ulceration (Paget's disease) or blood discharging – and five skin changes – skin dimpling due to pull of the ligaments of Copper (the fibrous bands anchoring the mammary gland to the dermis), peau d'orange due to subcutaneous lymphatic obstructions, direct skin infiltration or fungation, malignant ringworm due to multiple skin nodules secondary to centrifugal lymphatic permeation, and finally confluent skin nodules ('cancer *en cuirasse*'). *Do not forget to examine the normal breast.*

6. When palpating the breast mass, describe its site, size, shape, number, consistency, borders, mobility and then the state of the axillary lymph nodes on the side of the lesion.

7. Ask the patient to lie back and examine her liver (for visceral metastases) and her arm for possible lymphoedema (non-pitting).

N.B. In the mastectomy patient ask about haemoptysis (pulmonary metastasis), bony pain (skeletal metastasis) and weight gain (ascites – visceral metastasis) and whether radiotherapy, endocrine therapy or chemotherapy had been given. Examine as above and also look for any evidence of local recurrence (in mastectomy scar) and radiation effects.

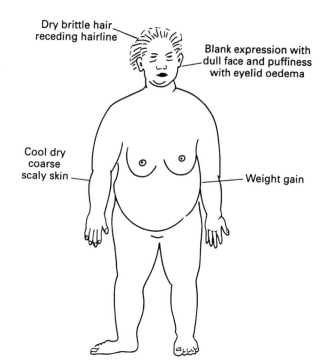

Fig. 2.9.2   Clinical features of hypothyroidism

Labels: Dry brittle hair, receding hairline; Blank expression with dull face and puffiness with eyelid oedema; Cool dry coarse scaly skin; Weight gain

---

2.9 Cervical Swelling(Fig. 2.5.1)
(*'examine the neck'*)

Midline swelling should suggest the possibility of a thyroid nodule of the isthmus, thyroglossal cyst, subhyoid bursa or dermoid cyst. Lateral swelling has many causes: commonly the cause is either lymphadenopathy (commonly inflammatory in nature due to infection or tuberculosis in Asians but can also be due to primary Hodgkin's lymphoma or secondary carcinoma from a primary tumour elsewhere) or thyroid nodule. Less common causes are salivary masses, neurogenic tumours, vascular swellings, pharyngeal pouch, skin tumours, and congenital masses such as branchial cyst and cavernous haemangioma. You are allowed to ask the patient 'How long have you had this swelling?' and 'Does it cause you any

problems?' Quickly look at the ear, nose and throat (ENT) and look at the scalp. In suspected thyroglossal cyst ask the patient to protrude her tongue (thyroglossal cyst will move up while isthmic nodule will not).

Thyroid swelling

1. Inspect the eyes (Fig. 2.9.1), and thyroidectomy scar or telangiectasia following radiotherapy. Look at the swelling while the patient is swallowing. It is wise to let the examiner know that you would examine the thyroid while the patient is swallowing a mouthful of water (it is more humane), even if a glass of water is not available. During swallowing you may palpate the radial pulse quickly (for rhythm and rate) and feel the palm (sweaty hot hand with tremor in thyrotoxicosis and dry skin in hypothyroidism). Remember that the hand is important in the diagnosis; the hand: in hypothyroidism is cold and dry but in hyperthyroidism it is hot and moist, while in anxiety the hand is cold and moist (Figs. 2.9.2 and 2.9.3).

2. Palpate the neck bimanually from front and behind (again while patient is swallowing water) to determine size, symmetry, consistency and tenderness.

3. From behind, palpate the regional lymph nodes especially the supraclavicular nodes in the supraclavicular hollows (after patient shrugs his shoulders or bends his head towards the side under examination).

4. Percuss the manubrium to detect any dullness indicating retrosternal extension.

5. Auscultate for bruits.

6. If you are given time, then confirm the state of thyroid functioning by examining for three thyrotoxic eye signs

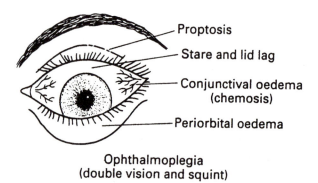

Labels: Proptosis; Stare and lid lag; Conjunctival oedema (chemosis); Periorbital oedema; Ophthalmoplegia (double vision and squint)

Fig. 2.9.1   Left eye revealing eye signs seen in hyperthyroidism

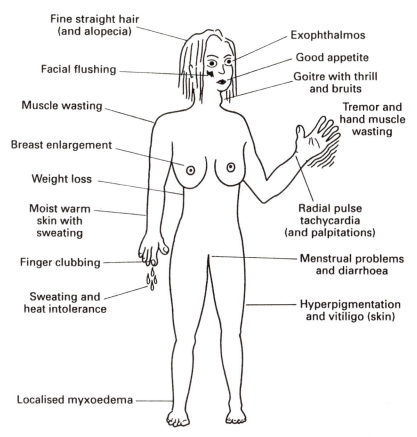

Fine straight hair (and alopecia)

Facial flushing

Muscle wasting

Breast enlargement

Weight loss

Moist warm skin with sweating

Finger clubbing

Sweating and heat intolerance

Localised myxoedema

Exophthalmos

Good appetite

Goitre with thrill and bruits

Tremor and hand muscle wasting

Radial pulse tachycardia (and palpitations)

Menstrual problems and diarrhoea

Hyperpigmentation and vitiligo (skin)

Fig. 2.9.3   Clinical features of hyperthyroidism

(exophthalmos, lid lag and ophthalmoplegia); examine from behind for exopthalmos and examine the patient's hands for tremor (put paper on the outstretched hand while the patient's eyes are closed). Examine the legs for pertibial myxoedema and the limbs for proximal myopathy – both occur in thyrotoxicosis. Myxoedema is suggested by characteristic facies, hoarseness of voice and dry skin. For thyroid assessment (see s. 1.85).

Lymph nodes

Pyogenic lymph nodes are tender and hot, with evidence of infection (of the respiratory tract and mouth). Cold matted lymph nodes are tuberculous. Fixed stony hard lymph nodes are metastatic in origin. However, in lateral swellings that do not move with swallowing and have a rubbery consistency, suspect Hodgkin's lymphoma (in adults) and non-Hodgkin's lymphoma (in the elderly). Then:
1. After examining the cervical lymph nodes bilaterally, palpate for axillary and inguinal lymph nodes on both sides.
2. Palpate the abdomen for para-aortic lymph nodes, spleen and liver enlargement.
3. The next important step is to biopsy the cervical lymph nodes. If lymphoma is found to be present, staging laparotomy will be considered (splenectomy, liver biopsy and para-aortic lymph node biopsy). CT scanning, IVU and lymphangiography are done later.

Note on Hodgkin's disease classification

Based on histological grading or clinical staging.

1. Histological grading

Lukes, 1963	*Rye, 1966 (currently used)*
Lymphocyte and/or histiocyte (L & H) nodular diffuse	Lymphocyte predominance (young)
Nodular sclerosis	Nodular sclerosis (young)
Mixed cellularity	Mixed cellularity
Diffuse fibrosis Reticular	Lymphocyte depletion (elderly)

2. Clinical staging (Peters *et al.*, 1966)

Stage I   Disease limited to one anatomical region.
Stage II   Disease limited to two contiguous anatomical regions on same side of diaphragm; or
Disease in more than two anatomical regions or in two non-contiguous regions on same side of diaphragm.
Stage III   Disease on both sides of diaphragm but limited to involvement of lymph nodes, Waldeyer ring and spleen.
Stage IV   Extralymphatic involvement of bone marrow, lung parenchyma, pleura, liver, bone, skin, kidneys and gastrointestinal tract.

All stages are subclassified as A or B to indicate the absence or presence, respectively, of systemic symptoms. Treatment is radiotherapy (Stages I and IIA) or chemotherapy (Stages IIB, III and IV).

Branchial cyst

This is a unilateral cystic swelling at the anterior border of the sternomastoid at the junction of the upper third and lower two-thirds. It is common in young males and females, and usually arises from the second branchial cleft (first branchial cleft cysts are suprahyoidal and juxta-auricular with possible communication to the auditory meatus) (two-thirds in males, two-thirds of cases on left side and two-thirds of them are cystic on palpation). The treatment is surgical excision.

2.10 Parotid Swelling
(*'examine this patient's neck'*)

---

1. Inspect carefully for unilateral enlargement, facial symmetry and any incision.
2. Ask the patient to blow or whistle, close his eyes against resistance (signs of facial nerve paralysis). Then ask him to open his mouth as far as he can (difficulty in moving the jaw – ankylosis).
3. Feel the overlying skin (while the patient closes his eyes) and test for loss of touch sensation.
4. Palpate the tumour, describing its exact site, shape, size, consistency, mobility and overlying skin fixation.
5. Palpate the cervical lymph nodes (pre- and postauricular and supraclavicular groups).
6. Ask the patient to open his mouth. Use a wooden spatula and torch to see Stensen's duct and massage the parotid gland from outside to express any pus (superimposed parotitis). Perform bimanual palpation of submandibular gland (Fig. 2.10.1)

Causes of parotid swelling

Inflammatory (acute parotitis) Due to viral or pyogenic infections, actinomycosis, tuberculosis. This may follow major

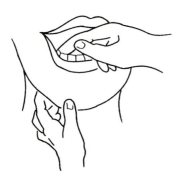

Fig. 2.10.1 Bimanual palpation of submandibular gland and lymph nodes

operation, debilitating disease (e.g. typhoid fever and cholera), radiotherapy.

Suppurative sialoadenitis Secondary to obstruction of a salivary duct by a stone or stricture.

Neoplastic Either primary or secondary (to nasopharyngeal carcinoma, bronchial cancer or lymphoma).

Primary epithelial tumours include pleomorphic adenoma (benign circumscribed firm lobulated encapsulated tumour with no sex predilection with potential for recurrence after enucleation and development of carcinoma), monomorphic adenoma such as adenolymphoma (Warthin's tumour is a less common benign tumour – a slowly enlarging soft cystic fluctuant tumour in middle-aged or elderly males which can be bilateral; unlike pleomorphic adenoma it produces a hot spot in ^{99m}Tc pertechnetate scan) and mucoepidermoid tumours.

Primary non-epithelial tumours include acinic cell tumour and carcinoma (with fixation, bone resorption and ankylosis, skin and mucous membrane anaesthesia, muscle paralysis, facial nerve paralysis and pain).

These tumours are assessed clinically (*not* biopsied), then excised by suprafacial or superficial partial parotidectomy. In suspected malignancy, an outpatient fine-needle aspiration cytology biopsy or operative frozen-section may be used to confirm its nature (postoperative radiotherapy may be required to avoid radical parotidectomy for residual deep tumour).

REMEMBER
● *Fascial slings* (from fascia lata) may be used to support facial tissues and mask the deformity of facial nerve palsy (could be shown as a short case).
● *Frey's syndrome* is facial flushing and sweating on gustatory stimulation due to auriculotemporal nerve injury. It is either postoperative after parotid or temporomandibular joint surgery, traumatic or congenital (birth trauma). The cause is union of postganglionic parasympathetic fibres from the otic ganglion with sympathetic nerves from the superior cervical ganglion. In severe cases division of the lesser superficial petrosal nerve within the skull is the treatment.

Autoimmune

Sjögren's syndrome (dry eyes – keratoconjunctivitis sicca; dry mouth – xerostomia; and rheumatoid arthritis) causes enlargement of the salivary and lacrimal glands. Mikulicz disease (symmetrical enlargement of all salivary glands, narrowing of the palpebral fissures due to enlarged lacrimal glands and dry mouth) is a variant.

Cysts

As in sarcoidosis with Heerfordt's syndrome (uveitis, salivary and lacrimal gland enlargement).

Metabolic

Includes diabetes, acromegaly, liver cirrhosis and reaction to drugs (e.g. antithyroid drugs and atrophy).

2.11 Malignant Skin Tumours (Fig. 2.5.1) (*'examine the skin'*)

Usually presented in the form of malignant ulcers. The order of frequency is basal cell carcinoma, squamous cell carcinoma, malignant melanoma. Inspect carefully for site, size, shape, edge, floor and discharge. Palpate for ulcer base (soft or hard, or indurated) and enlargement of adjacent lymph nodes.

Basal cell carcinoma

Rodent cell ulcer is a misnomer since there may only be a nodule. However if ulcer is present it is usually circular and commonly confined to the face (the area between a line joining the upper and lower borders of the ear with the outer canthus of the eye and the outer angle of the mouth respectively) but may occur anywhere in the body except the soles and palms. It has a raised rolled-out beaded edge, a network of blood vessels and a temporary healing crusty floor covered with serous discharge. The base is slightly indurated. It spreads slowly by local invasion. Blood or lymphatic spread does not occur. The diagnosis is confirmed by excisional biopsy (therapeutic) or elliptical biopsy from the lesion and normal surrounding skin. Treatment is by surgical excision, radiotherapy or cryosurgery.

Squamous cell carcinoma

The ulcer is irregular in shape with an everted or raised edge. The base is hard and indurated with blood-stained discharge. The regional lymph nodes may be enlarged due to secondary infection (painful) or actual involvement (painless hard). The ulcer is rapidly growing and may have superadded infection. The diagnosis is confirmed by elliptical biopsy (from lesion and normal skin). Treatment is by wide surgical excision or radiotherapy.

Comment on treatment of basal and squamous cell carcinomas

Surgical excision is the quickest and safest approach, especially for recurrent lesions. Radiotherapy is recommended when the surgical reconstruction after excision is a problem, e.g. lesions of the eyelids, in which case radiotherapy can be delivered more precisely. Radiotherapy, however, is contraindicated for lesions in cartilaginous areas (i.e. earlobe and nose) because of the risk of radionecrosis, and surgery is preferred, e.g. wedge excision with modified 'L' shape in carcinoma of the earlobe to prevent helical stricture. Cryosurgery is indicated for multiple small lesions.

Malignant melanoma (see also s. 1.41)

A pigmented naevus with possible signs of malignancy raises suspicions. The diagnosis is confirmed histologically on the basis of frozen or rapid paraffin sections taken after local excisional biopsy with a narrow margin of clearance (0.2 cm).

This is safely performed provided the supplementary wide surgical clearance (3–5 cm) is performed within 48 h of biopsy, depending on the degree of vertical invasion. Treatment is wide excision and split skin grafting (± block dissection).

II. Orthopaedic Surgery

2.12 Examine the Hip

The patient should be stripped completely, except for the undergarments. The body should be exposed from the costal margins.

1. With the patient lying down (supine), notice the position of the pelvis and any lordosis of the spine. Notice any scar, sinus, swelling, and the position of the leg with any deformity or shortening.

2. Palpate for tenderness. The hip is a deep-seated joint; the swelling or inflammation is not obvious and the bony components are not palpable. The nearest bony points are the greater trochanter and anterior superior iliac spine (ASIS). The femoral pulse is palpated anteriorly against the bony resistance of the femoral head.

3. Move and measure. The movements of the hip are compared during flexion, extension (with the patient face down), abduction, adduction, internal and external rotations. Do not forget to examine the back of the hip.

4. Shortening. Is it apparent (appears to be) or is it true shortening of the legs? Apparent shortening can be due to pelvic tilt or adduction deformity of the hip. The lower limbs should be measured from ASIS to the medial malleolus. Then the femoral length (from ASIS to medial knee joint space) and the tibial length (from the medial knee joint space to the medial malleolus) are individually measured to assess where the shortening is. If the femur is short, it should be decided whether it is above the greater trochanter or below it. If it is above (i.e. femoral neck and head), then the distance between the palpating thumb (on ASIS) and the middle finger (tip of greater trochanter) will be shorter on the affected side.

5. Examine for fixed flexed deformity (FFD) by performing Thomas' test and revealing the exact angle of this deformity by flexing the sound hip to correct and flatten the arching of spine and pelvis (lordosis). Lordosis is exaggerated to accommodate the FFD. If the lordosis is obliterated the FDD at the hip becomes obvious and measurable. The left hand should be behind the lumbar spine to assure a straight back while flexing fully the unaffected hip. Because of the fixed nature of the deformity, the affected thigh rises (flexes). This flexion angle is the FFD. The pelvis should be stabilised with the left hand while abduction and adduction are performed to assure that only the hip moves (not exaggerated due to pelvic tilt).

6. Do Trendelenberg's test to examine for postural stability by assessing the integrity of the abductor mechanism of the hip (gluteus medius and gluteus minimus). With the patient standing evenly, he is asked to lift one leg off the floor. Normally the weight of the body is shifted to balance on the other standing leg, resulting in the elevation of the pelvis

(ASIS) on the side where the leg is raised. If positive, however, the patient stands on the affected side, but the affected hip cannot support the weight, and hence, the pelvis (ASIS) drops or tilts down when the normal opposite leg is raised. This abductor mechanism is disturbed if the joint is affected by disease leading to joint instability (as in congenital dislocation of the hip or severe coxa vara), or if the disease affects the muscles or the nerve supplying these muscles (poliomyelitis), or if a stable fulcrum is absent (ununited fracture of the femoral neck).

7. Always compare normal with the affected while:
(a) The patient is walking, observing any abnormal gait due to pain, limp or shortening.
(b) The patient is standing, observing the level of ASIS and whether one is at lower level: pelvic tilt, shorter leg, adduction deformity.

Children

Infants can only be examined lying down. Notice any extra thigh skin folds, broadening of one hip, widened perineum (congenital dislocation of the hip – unilateral or bilateral).

Ortolani's and Barlow's tests should be performed next. These tests are performed with the infant lying on its back. The lower extremities of the infant are held one in each hand with the fingers on the lateral aspect of the thigh and the thumb on the medial side; this allows the hip to be manipulated.

Ortolani's test   With the hips abducted, one hip is now gradually abducted while the other hand steadies the other hip. While abducting, the hip is also elevated with the fingers. If the hip is previously dislocated (CDH), the hip can usually be reduced with a clung felt. The same maneouvre is performed on the other hip.

Barlow's test   Now one hip is brought into adduction gradually while the other hip is steadied. At the same time, the hip under examination is gently pushed downwards to see if it can be dislocated. In a dislocatable hip, a clunk may be felt.

2.13 Examine the Knee

Remember that the pain in the knee may be referred from the pelvis or hip; therefore rule out the distant causes of knee pain (obturator nerve). Both legs should be exposed from the hips downwards and the affected knee should be compared with the normal.

1. Inspection for lumps, effusions, scars, signs of inflammation, the position of the limb, any deformity and site of pain should be noted. Look for any other lumps (prepatellar, infrapatellar and popliteal bursae).

2. Palpation. An effusion should be confirmed by the fluctuation test and 'patellar tap'. It should be distinguished (when effusion is small) from synovial hypertrophy.

The patella is compressed against the femur to elicit any tenderness. Other sites of tenderness should be looked for

(collateral ligaments, medial and lateral joint lines, and patellar tendon).

The knees are now flexed to 90°. The site of tenderness is localised if possible. Palpate for skin temperature, bone and soft-tissue contours.

3. The range of movements (active and passive flexion and extension, compared with normal knee) and power against resistance is measured. Compare thigh girth at the same level on both sides.

4. The integrity of the medial and lateral collateral ligaments is tested with the knee in extension, and in some degree of flexion when applying valgus and varus stress.

The anterior and posterior drawer tests are performed to assess the integrity of the anterior and posterior cruciate ligaments respectively.

These tests are repeated with the tibia rotated externally and then internally. The McMurray test is then done. When positive, a clunk alone in the joint or a clunk with pain is elicited to indicate a torn meniscus. A negative test does not exclude this pathology.

5. With the patient standing, examine also the back of the knee for Baker's cyst or popliteal bursa. Examine for stance and gait.

2.14 Examine this Patient's Back

The patient should be stripped of clothes except for underwear.

1. The patient should be examined (inspection) while walking, standing and lying down.
● Is the patient walking with a lurch or a stiff back?
● Is the lordosis straightened?

Movements of the lumbar spine (flexion, extension and lateral flexion, and rotation) and the range should be noted.
● Does the lumbar spine move during flexion, or is it entirely due to hip flexion with the spine straight?

2. Palpate for tenderness over the spinous processes or spasm of the paraspinal muscle, scar or other skin blemishes (spina bifida occulta) should be noted.

3. With the patient lying down, ascertain how much of the range is pain free (in degrees) while the hip is flexed with the knee held straight (straight-leg raising test: normal = 90°).

4. Examine for muscular wasting, hypertrophy and fasciculation. Record the muscle power (grade 0 to 5) in the hip musculature (flexor, extensor, abductor, adductor, internal and external rotator), the knee flexor and extensor muscles, the ankle dorsiflexors and plantar flexors and the invertors and evertors, remembering the root values of these muscles.

5. Similarly, the sensations should be tested, remembering the dermatomes.

6. Lastly, the knee and ankle jerks and plantar reflexes should be tested. The findings enable the localisation of the spinal segment affected.

The examination of the genitals should not be excluded. A vaginal and rectal examination should be performed where indicated.

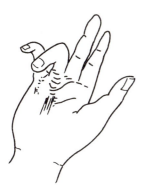

Fig. 2.14.1 Dupuytren's contracture

III. Miscellaneous

Any patient, whether operated on or not, may be presented as a short case provided it serves as spot diagnosis case.

Dupuytren's contracture

Localised thickening of palmar fascia, puckering the overlying skin and flexing the ring and little finger – affects the metacarpophalangeal and proximal interphalangeal joints. It is familial and occurs more often in cirrhotics and epileptics on Epanutin.

Treatment   Early cases (uncomplicated puckering) need night splintage and gentle stretching of the fingers by the patient. In advanced cases treatment is either single limited or multiple palmar fasciotomy but more commonly partial palmar fasciectomy (removing the affected fascia only). Radical total palmar fasciectomy (excising the affected and normal fascia) is an extensive operation and is indicated in patients with high Dupuytren's diathesis (young patient, rapid progressive disease, strong family history, history of epilepsy and/or alcoholism and the presence of ectopic deposits such as knuckle pads, plantar and penile lesions). Excision of the skin and replacement with skin grafts is indicated only in recurrent cases. (Figs 2.14.1, 2.14.2, 2.14.3).

Amputation is used for chronic severe cases with irreversible flexion – contracture deformities.

Hallux valgus

Either congenital (metatarsus primum varus) or acquired in women who wear tight narrow shoes. Consists of four elements: bony exostosis of the first metatarsal head; an adventitious bursa – first metatarsal bunion with or without fifth metatarsal bunionette; osteoarthrosis of the first metatarsophalangeal joint; and overriding or underriding of the second toe by the first. Treatment is by Keller's operation (American surgeon) which is an excision arthroplasty of the base of the proximal phalanx, being careful of the flexor tendon, with excision of the exostosis and final reconstruction of the medial collateral ligament. (The excised base of the proximal phalanx can be replaced with an implant.)

Hallux rigidus

This is simply monoarticular osteoarthrosis of the first metatarsophalangeal joint, producing a stiff painful joint. Treatment is by Keller's operation.

Chronic bursitis

In the prepatellar bursa (housemaid's knee), olecranon bursa (student's or miner's elbow) or synovial cysts in the popliteal

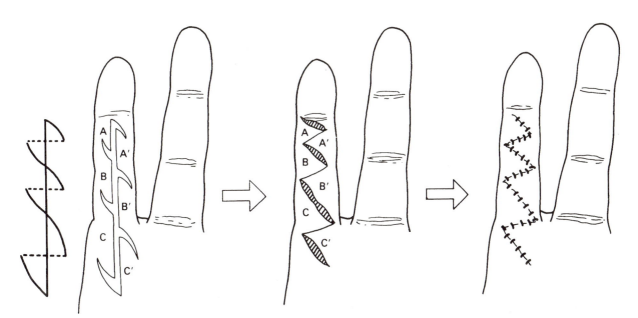

Fig. 2.14.2   A continuous multiple Z-plasty used in Dupuytren's contracture of the little finger

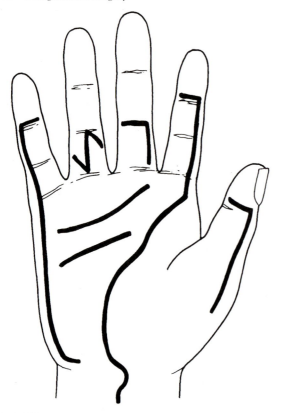

Fig. 2.14.3 Commonly used incisions in hand surgery

fossa (Baker's cysts). Baker's cysts arise from semi-membranous bursa or, in rheumatoid arthritis of the knee, from posterior rupture of the joint capsule. They are either aspirated or left alone to disappear spontaneously.

Ruptured achilles tendon

Represents the commonest tendon rupture in middle-aged men after games or even after a trivial stumble. The case is diagnosed by history and by examination for a palpable and even visible gap (at the rupture site), free dorsiflexion and reduced plantar flexion (but never abolished due to action of the long flexors of the toes and tibialis posterior). The patient usually cannot stand on tiptoe. Treatment is by early suture and ankle immobilisation in a plaster for 6 weeks. Late suture is disappointing because of retracted ruptured ends; instead, the gastrocnemius and soleus muscles are relaxed.

Pyogenic granuloma

Ranula

Submandibular salivary calculus

Long lower limb incision over course of long saphenous vein (to be used for coronary bypass)

Look for a median sternotomy incision immediately.

Cushing's syndrome or Cushing's disease

Cushing's syndrome is due to steroid therapy or adrenal cortical hyperplasia, adenoma or malignancy while *Cushing's disease* is due to secretion of ACTH by basophilic tumour of the anterior pituitary.

Perianal abscess or fistula

Remember Goodsall's rule (see p. 282).

T-tube

This will be shown in a patient.

Continuous irrigation

Mounted on a three-way Foley urinary catheter after open prostatectomy (in the presence of an abdominal incision with a suprapubic drain) or transurethral resection of prostate or bladder tumour (no abdominal incision or drain).

Abdominal faecal fistula

Caecostomy, ileostomy or colostomy

In caecostomy there is a Foley catheter in the right iliac fossa. Notice the spout in ileostomy but not colostomy. You may be asked about the complications after ileostomy or colostomy and why they were constructed. (See also p. 289).

Subclavian set

For parenteral nutrition (notice the intralipid milky solutions covered with black bags because of photosensitivity) and/or CVP monitoring (notice the manometer and absence of intralipid parenteral solution). You may be asked about the indications for parenteral nutrition or CVP monitoring.

Appendicectomy

You may be asked *what to look for*. If you are seeing an appendicectomy patient on the third postoperative day, ask him about bowel action, examine his wound locally for infection or surrounding tenderness and look at his temperature chart since postoperative pyrexia may indicate wound infection or chest infection (X-ray), urinary infection (mid-stream urine), thrombophlebitis (see if he has an i.v. line), deep venous thrombosis, rectal pelvic abscess or subphrenic abscess ('pus nowhere, pus somewhere else, pus under diaphragm').

Male gynaecomastia

Causes are:
- Idiopathic – unilateral or bilateral.
- Hormonal, e.g. stilboestrol therapy in prostatic cancer and testicular teratoma; anorchism; rarely, ectopic hormones from bronchogenic carcinoma; and adrenal or pituitary disease.
- Liver failure in cirrhosis.
- Klinefelter's syndrome.
- Drugs, e.g. digitalis, spironolactone, isoniazid.
- Leprosy.

LONG CASES

Time allowed is 20–30 min with one patient. You are required to take a history, perform a physical examination and interpret your findings to reach *one* diagnosis. You have to prepare yourself for possible relevant investigations and work out a differential diagnosis (to be presented only when you are asked). Enlarge on the chief complaint and its present history, mention all *positive* clinical findings and ask for the simplest relevant tests. Be friendly with the patient, while following the general points above. One useful tip is to ask the patient, 'Did you come here specially today, or are you a patient in this hospital?'. Also obtain the name of the consultant the patient is under since you may well find yourself being examined by that person. Ask the patient about the investigations performed and what he or she was told as a result of them. Examine the patient methodically and comprehensively and elicit the physical signs related to the patient's complaint as well as other signs. Most patients know the diagnosis and it is worth telling the patient what you think the diagnosis is as they will usually agree with you if you are right.

Leave 5 min for reorganising your presentation. Underline the important points in the history and stress the positive findings in the physical examination. Give your provisional diagnosis and support it with the most relevant investigations, starting with the simplest and cheapest, since the more sophisticated the test or investigation the more delay there is for the patient. For example, in surgical anaemia, contrast radiology (in the form of a barium study) and endoscopy should head your list since the commonest causes of anaemia are malignancy (i.e. gastric and caecum carcinomas) and peptic ulcer; other possible causes, e.g. ulcerative colitis, Crohn's disease and the malabsorption syndrome would be investigated later. In a jaundiced patient, urine examination for bilirubin and urobilinogen, plain abdominal X-ray and abdominal ultrasound come before transhepatic cholangiography, ERCP and liver biopsy. In colorectal diseases, rectal examination, sigmoidoscopy (or colonoscopy) and biopsy come before carcinoembryonic antigen test and barium enema since the latter may precipitate an intestinal obstruction in annular carcinoma of the rectosigmoid junction. In upper abdominal pain of unknown origin, barium swallow (in Trendelenburg's position) and meal will exclude hiatus hernia and peptic ulcer respectively. Abdominal ultrasound will exclude biliary stone and possibly pancreatic and renal swelling (oral cholecystography can be done if ultrasound is inconclusive). Intravenous urography will exclude any urinary system pathology.

The examination organisers may leave X-ray films beside the patient purposely to help you, so have a good look at them. The films will most probably show abnormal radiological findings such as a stone or an ulcer (normal films will usually not be included).

A well-planned presentation of the case history and positive physical findings is the most important part of this test. The examiner will tell you to present the case as if he or she knows

nothing about the patient. Intermittent interruptions by the examiner with mutual discussion of the findings, diagnosis, investigation and possible operative treatment will reveal your capability for reasonable argument, mature clinical judgement and accuracy in requesting relevant investigations and interpreting data.

Case-taking

The following scheme is recommended.
Patient: name, age, occupation, married or single, address, date of admission.
Chief complaint (one, rarely two) and *duration*.
History of present illness: e.g. if the presenting complaint is pain enquire about: similar attacks in the past; pain severity and character; location; radiation and direction (epigastric pain radiating to the back by penetration is consistent with pancreatitis and by encirclement around the right side is consistent with cholecystitis); duration since the first attack; intermission and intervals of freedom (for how long?); relation to meals; does it wake the patient at night (nocturnal pain); aggravating factors and relieving factors; associated features such as vomiting (amount, colour, does it look like coffee grounds, taste and food residue); bowel habits, appetite, weight loss, heartburn and dysphagia (if any). In biliary pain it is very important to ask about associated fever and rigor (in cholangitis), jaundice, itching and coloured urine, pale stool.
Past history:
● Of hospital admissions in chronological order, with hospital names, causes of admission and names of operations performed.
● Of allergies whether atopic, e.g. asthma, or to drugs (especially penicillin, iodine contrast media and zincplast – Elastoplast).
● Of drug intake, especially:
  – Oral hypoglycaemic agents in diabetes mellitus (should be stopped 24–48 h prior to surgery and insulin given instead).
  – Anticoagulants for valve replacements (should be stopped 48 h prior to surgery and heparin given instead as well as vitamin K injection and prophylactic antibiotics to prevent subacute bacterial endocarditis).
  – Contraceptive pill in females and stilboestrol in males, e.g. for prostatic carcinoma (contraceptive pill should be stopped 1 month prior to surgery and if impossible Dextran 70 should be used during operation to prevent possible deep venous thrombosis).
  – Other drug intake such as anti-epileptic and antiheart failure measures can continue during the immediate perioperative period.
● Of previous illnesses (e.g. rheumatic heart disease) and accidents (e.g. road traffic accident).

Quick family history: cause of death of parents, children, brothers or sisters; and familial disease, e.g. haemophilia, gallstones, hypertension and diabetes mellitus.

Quick social history: habits as regards alcohol, tobacco, food and exercise.

Systemic inquiry: only the positive symptoms in each system, e.g. alimentary, respiratory, cardiovascular, urinary, nervous and musculoskeletal systems.

Impression should now be made based on the history alone to be confirmed by physical examination.

Physical examination

Vital signs: temperature, pulse rate, blood pressure and respiratory rate.

General appearance (e.g. lying in bed in agony, doubled up with pain, cooperative) as well as JACCOL (**j**aundice, **a**naemia, **c**yanosis, **c**lubbing, **o**edema, **l**ymphadenopathy).

Head and neck: scalp swelling, exophthalmos, pupils' size and reaction, mouth – tongue, jugular venous pressure, central trachea, goitre, carotid bruit).

Chest: quick examination, except if patient is female look for breast carcinoma. Otherwise inspection, palpation, percussion and auscultation. Examine the back of the chest (e.g. for possible pulsating collaterals in coarctation of the aorta).

Abdomen (in detail):

- Inspection for generalised or localised swelling, hernial sites (ask patient to cough), visible peristalsis, pulsation, dilated vessels, scars and umbilicus.
- General palpation for soft or rigid abdomen and special palpation for tenderness or rebound tenderness, for impulse on coughing in hernias as well as for organomegaly, fluid thrill and splashing.
- Percussion to confirm the upper limit of hepatomegaly, the dull nature of enlarged urinary bladder in retention and shifting dullness in ascites.
- Auscultation for bowel sounds at the McBurney point (borborygmi and tingling sound in intestinal obstruction and quiet in paralytic ileus). Also for vascular lesions, e.g. hepatic haemangioma and aortic aneurysm.
- Abdominal examination is not complete without examining the genitalia (phimosis, hypospadias in penis and since testicles are abdominal organs a discovered seminoma may explain huge abdominal para-aortic lymph nodes which may be misdiagnosed initially as intestinal masses). The rectum should also be examined (essential in rectal carcinoma or villous adenoma and prostatic carcinoma).

Limbs: especially lower limbs for pitting oedema, ulcers and pulses.

Provisional diagnosis should be single. Differential diagnosis is only acceptable in a vague unexplained symptomatology with few or no physical signs.

At this point, reorganise yourself once again, underlining the *positive* physical findings, and present your clinical data in a logical format. Think of the most simple relevant investigation (and why) and prepare yourself psychologically for discussion face-to-face with the examiners.

The following are common often repeated long cases.

2.15 Duodenal Ulcer

History is essential since there may be slight epigastric tenderness or absolutely no physical signs. The case may have been complicated before by perforation (notice the abdominal scar), bleeding or pyloric stenosis. Give *one* personally recommended operation that you would perform and substantiate your approach. Do not say it could be managed *either* by partial gastrectomy or vagotomy and pyloroplasty.

2.16 Cholecystitis ± History of Pancreatitis ± Jaundice

It is essential to distinguish between pain due to gallstone cholecystitis (sudden dull continuous pain in the right hypochondrium radiating to the interscapular area and back by encirclement; associated with retching and vomiting together with tachycardia and pyrexia and usually comes at night after a fatty meal, e.g. fish and chips), and pain due to biliary colic from a common bile duct stone or, rarely, a cystic duct stone with ball-valve mechanism (pain is on and off, associated with ascending cholangitis, which is manifested by rigor, fever and even septicaemia, and with the fluctuating jaundice of Charcot's triad). Remember that fluctuating jaundice can also be due to periampullary carcinoma (high ESR and positive occult blood in stool with palpable gallbladder).

In acute pancreatitis pain is usually very severe and constant, radiating from the upper abdomen to the back by penetration; it is associated with vomiting and relieved by leaning forward. Ask for history of gallstones and alcoholism. Rarely, acute pancreatitis is presented on its own (in examinations), but commonly it is presented as a gallstone cholecystitis (electively admitted for cholecystectomy) with past history of pancreatitis. Notice here the type of patient (e.g. fertile, fatty, flatulent, 50-year-old female). On physical examination, a palpable gallbladder should make you consider the following:

- Acute cholecystitis: wrapped in protective greater omentum (just like appendicular mass).
- Mucocele: painless swelling with no jaundice.
- Empyema of gallbladder: with pyrexia and tachycardia.
- If the patient is jaundiced then carcinoma of the head of the pancreas is likely (Courvoisier's sign or statement).
- Very hard swelling indicates gallbladder carcinoma or liver tumour (metastatic or primary).

Courvoisier's statement (not law): 'If in a jaundiced patient the gallbladder is palpably enlarged, it is *probably* NOT a case of stone impacted in the common bile duct, because in that case previous cholecystitis has already made the gallbladder fibrotic.' This is a negative statement and not a law. Courvoisier only made a statement of probability (approximately 75% of cases); therefore double stone impaction in the cystic and common bile ducts and oriental chlonorchiasis (although regarded as exceptions to Courvoisier's law) are actually included within the 25% of his correct statement.

2.17 Rectal Carcinoma

Rectal examination is the vital step. Once you feel the hard rectal cancer (whether ulcerative, cauliflower or annular) you *have* to proceed with proctoscopy. (Proctoscopy or sigmoidoscopy *with* biopsy is the key investigation. Barium enema is not recommended in *low* rectal lesions and may be dangerous since it may cause obstruction in annular rectosigmoid carcinoma. Enema is indicated in high colonic lesions beyond the reach of the rigid sigmoidoscope and in order to reveal the possible double colonic primary tumours in 5% of colonic cancers.)

In villous adenoma the tumour is soft and covered with mucus and not blood (make sure you have asked the patient about mucus discharge and symptoms of hypokalaemia; also stress that you will send the patient's serum for potassium estimation). You have to make up your mind whether you are planning to excise the tumour by anterior restorative resection or by abdominoperineal excision with permanent left iliac colostomy (and why) or whether you leave this decision until after laparotomy (and assessment of spread).

2.18 Chronic Urinary Retention

Commonly due to prostatic carcinoma: it is important to reveal a history of prostatism. On physical examination of the abdomen, an enlarged urinary bladder is confirmed by:
- Palpation: one cannot get a hand under it since it is an intrapelvic organ.
- Percussion; dull and one can define the upper border easily.
- Palpation and pressure may squeeze some urine out. Ask the patient about his desire to micturate when you press.

Remember that the size of the prostate cannot be assessed while the patient is in retention (only rectal examination after catheterisation is correct). Stress the characteristics of prostatic carcinoma that can be revealed by rectal examination:
- Obliteration of median prostatic sulcus.
- Hard prostate ⎫ and whether flat or bulging
- Fixed prostate ⎭

Benign prostatic enlargement is generally bigger than malignant enlargement.

You may discover a swollen leg or legs which may be caused by:
- Deep venous thrombosis due to disseminated intravascular coagulation.
- Metastatic obstruction of lymphatic drainage of the lower limbs.
- Metastatic obstruction of venous drainage of the lower limbs.
- Thromboembolic effect of stilboestrol treatment; hormonal therapy should be stopped and operative treatment – subcapsular orchidectomy – carried out. (Low-dose stilboestrol is recommended as 2 or 3 mg daily initially for 10 days, to be continued as 1 mg/day indefinitely.)

Catheterisation

May be discussed, with its complications. Remember that it should be done under aseptic conditions with a Silastic self-retaining Foley catheter (preferable to an irritant rubber catheter). Complications include false passage, traumatic bleeding, infection and bacteraemia as well as catheter bladder tumour (oedematous mucosa with central pit due to irritating catheter tip). Encrustation and stone formation at catheter tip may occur and augment urinary infection; blocked catheter can be relieved either by cutting the proximal end, or injection of 0.5 ml ether (dissolves the catheter), inflating the balloon beyond capacity to rupture it, or by suprapubic drainage, or removing the catheter by open surgery. The two most important complications (which the examiners are after) are inflation of the balloon inside the urethra, causing urethral rupture, and induced paraphimosis. Therefore, make absolutely sure that you inflate the catheter balloon *only* if you see the urine running first and do not forget to pull back the foreskin after you finish catheterisation.

Make a note of drained urine – whether clear or infected (murky), bloodstained or with clots – since you may need a Simplistic (harder material) catheter with a large draining tip (whistle tip). In stricture, a catheter with a Tiemann tip is useful. If it is impossible to negotiate the urethra and the bladder is quite distended then suprapubic catheterisation may be indicated. Foley's urinary catheterisation is indicated in urinary retention, urinary incontinence, in haematuria with clots, postoperatively to provide free urine flow and to compress the prostatic bed (haemostasis) after TUR (prostate); Foley's catheter is also used suprapubically and in nephrostomy.

Extraurinary indications of Foley's catheterisation include: monitoring of critically ill patients in ICU, in gastrotomy, cholecystostomy, jejunostomy, caecostomy, as Jones tube to internally splint recurrent adhesion-induced small bowel obstruction, in rectal stump for easy identification of rectum prior to reconnection with colon in Hartmann's procedure, and occasionally to retain the tube during injection of contrast medium in barium enema or via a stoma to illustrate any leak in distal anastomosis. Foley's catheter can also be used to control aortic bleeding in surgery.

The number on the catheter, e.g. 18 Fr, indicates the circumference (circumference = diameter $\times$ $^{22}/_{7}$); thus, an 18 Fr catheter has a diameter of 18 divided by $^{22}/_{7}$ (approximately 3) = 6 mm. French gauge is also applied to urethral sounds, T-tubes and drains. In urethral dilators or bougies there are two figures, e.g. $^{24}/_{28}$, which indicate the smallest and largest circumferences respectively (or diameters of 8 mm and 9.3 mm respectively). Ureteric catheter figures should be divided by 6, not 3; thus size 6 means 1 mm diameter.

Practical points on catheterisation

- In chronic retention with elevated urea and creatinine, the best treatment is TUR of prostate on the next waiting list. Decompression with catheterisation should be avoided since it can only lead to infection.
- Following uncomplicated major surgery, e.g. hemicolectomy, the patient may not pass urine within the next 8–16 h

and if the bladder is impalpable then only observe and conserve. This postoperative oliguria is the physiological response to trauma and there is no need for catheterisation.

- In acute urinary retention with palpable bladder suprapubically, one should initially pass a Silastic 14–16 French gauge catheter (with small balloon capacity of 5–10 ml to avoid trigonal irritation and minimise residual urine); if one cannot reach the bladder, then a suprapubic catheter can be inserted.
- In acute retention with the history of optical urethrotomy for stricture the best course of treatment is urethral dilatation (leave the jelly within the urethra for 5 minutes prior to dilatation) and re-urethrotomy, or suprapubic catheterisation.
- Following heavy haematuria after TURP, the catheter may be blocked and every effort must be exercised to irrigate and wash the bladder via the 3-way catheter and suck clots with a bladder syringe. However, if the blocked catheter is removed by an untrained junior doctor or nurse then one should recatheterise, but in a grossly obese patient with difficulty to palpate the bladder recatheterisation may be impossible. Therefore, the best course of treatment will be an emergency cystoscopic evacuation of clots under general anaesthesia and catheterisation under vision.
- In acute retention following secondary haemorrhage after recent cysto-diathermy to a bladder tumour (within 2 weeks), the best treatment will be catheterisation with a three-way Simplastic size 22 FG (large to evacuate clots) with antibiotics.

  If catheterisation is impossible then cystoscopic evacuation of clots under general anaesthesia is the best treatment. Suprapubic catheterisation should never be done in bladder tumour or in unexplained haematuria since such a procedure may result in tumour spread beyond the bladder into the anterior abdominal wall.

- If it is impossible to remove a long-term catheter then:
  - cut off the valve and remove after balloon deflation;
  - if the balloon will not deflate after cutting off the valve then ultrasound guided puncture may be performed;
  - if that facility is not available in the middle of the night then injection of 0.5 ml ether will melt the balloon substance;
  - if that does not do the trick then inflate the balloon fully and rupture it or pass a long needle suprapubically directed to the ballon and guided by a finger in the rectum.
- Successful catheterisation followed by painful bladder spasm and urine bypass round the catheter indicate bladder inflammation or irritation by the catheter tip. Then treatment must include antibiotics and an antispasmodic, pulling down the catheter to sit snuggly on the bladder neck or deflating the balloon to minimise the trigonal irritation. If there is disproportion between urethral size and catheter, a change to a larger catheter is required.
- Self-catheterisation at home is a clean rather than aseptic procedure (in hospital catheterisation must be aseptic to prevent cross-infection) and can be performed by the patient for a neurologic bladder or multiple sclerosis; it can also be done in urethral strictures by self-dilatation using a low friction catheter (hydrogel coated) size 18 FG once weekly.

Investigations and treatment

Investigations include haemoglobin (Hb), white cell count (WCC), erythrocyte sedimentation rate (ESR), prostatic acid and alkaline phosphatases (false acid phosphatase increase after admission is possibly due to repeated rectal examination or diurnal variation); also mid-stream urine (MSU) or catheter stream urine (CSU), with pain X-ray of kidney, ureter, bladder (KUB), of intravenous urography (IVU), and abdominal ultrasound followed by diagnostic cystoscopy (prostatic biopsy). Treatment is by transurethral resection ± radiotherapy. (Hormonal therapy is usually reserved for skeletal metastases and recurrent prostatic obstructive uropathy.)

2.19 Vascular Case

As patients with peripheral vascular disease spend many weeks in hospital, you may well be asked to examine one of these patients. Those who have had inverted Y side-to-end aortofemoral bypass in Leriche's syndrome or iliofemoral or femoropopliteal bypass in lower limb ischaemia may be presented. Other suitable candidates for long cases are recently recovered embolectomy patients (with mitral stenosis, atrial fibrillation or past history of myocardial infarction) or patients who have had carotid endarterectomy or bypass in transient ischaemic attack. Unoperated vascular cases such as lower limb ischaemia may also be shown; gangrene, however, is shown as a short case.

2.20 Miscellaneous Cases

You may be shown any practically available patient in the ward with a detailed history such as:
- Recurrent goitre whether colloid or malignant.
- Unilateral or bilateral renal stones (whether operated on or not).
- Carcinoid syndrome.
- Inflammatory bowel disease such as ulcerative colitis or Crohn's disease.
- Unoperated colonic lesion such as carcinoma or polyposis coli.
- Hip osteoarthritis.
- Complicated gastrectomy.

SECTION 3
Operative Surgery

Introduction

An operation does not start with skin incision nor does it finish with skin closure. There are various preoperative preparations to be undertaken (routine and special) – anaesthesia, positioning, skin preparation and draping under completely antiseptic conditions – before the actual operative procedure begins. This is followed by postoperative care and instructions (to avoid postoperative morbidity and mortality). The preoperative and postoperative periods are as important as the operative procedure itself.

1. *Routine preoperative preparations*
A. Obtain permission for operation (signed consent form) and inform relatives.
B. Explain operation to patient.
C. Preparation of patient.
(i)   Articles which should be *removed:*
    Artificial eye
    Contact lenses
    Hearing aid
    Artificial limbs
    Dentures
    Wig, toupée and hair grips
    Jewellery
    Pants/trousers (pyjamas) (except for dental patients).
(ii)   Check for pacemaker.
(iii) Shave operative site and bathe.
(iv)   Test urine (routinely).
(v)   Nil by mouth – 4 h prior to surgery.
(vi)   Mark operative site, e.g. varicose veins, ileostomy or colostomy site, and breast mass. The side should also be marked with an arrow, e.g. right or left inguinal hernia, nephrectomy and limb amputation.
(vii) Check identiband with case sheet and X-rays.
(viii) Give premedication.

The essential points in preoperative preparation can be summarised as follows: well-prepared patient, consent obtained and operation explained.

2. *Special preoperative preparations*
According to the type of surgery, e.g. urinary catheterisation and bowel preparation in colorectal surgery; nasogastric suction, i.v. infusion in gastric surgery; antithyroid drugs, cervical X-ray and direct laryngoscopy in thyroid surgery.

3. *Anaesthesia*

4. *Positioning*
For example Lloyd–Davis (combined lithotomy – Trendelenburg position) in rectal carcinoma; supine in gastric and biliary operations; hyperextended neck with head supported by a ring and the shoulders by a sandbag in thyroidectomy.

5. *Skin preparation in antiseptic theatre and draping of the operative site*

6. *Surgical procedure*
Irrespective of its nature, usually involves the following stages
  I   Exposure and exploration.
  II   Mobilisation.
  III   Vascular dissection, ligation and division.
  IV   Excision.
  V   Reconstruction.
  VI   Closure with or without drainage.
Therefore, if you are asked the technical details of any operation you can discuss it safely and correctly according to the above six stages. Think of the above stages in the thyroidectomy, gastrectomy, mastectomy, nephrectomy or any other major operation and you will find a striking similarity in their technical principles.

7. *Postoperative instructions*
For example, to continue antibiotics in bowel surgery if indicated, T-tube cholangiography on the 10th day in common bile duct exploration, nasogastric suction until there are bowel sounds or bowel action (flatus or faeces), urinary catheterisation if indicated. Removal of tube drain when dry (usually 3 days) or after creation of a fistulous track when requested (usually 7 days). Removal of stitches in 4 days (neck), 5 days (head), 7 days (limbs) or 10 days (abdomen) approximately.

Note: If the operation is performed as an emergency (life-threatening conditions, e.g. perforated viscus, appendicitis or strangulated hernia) there is insufficient time for full investigations and adequate preparations due to the urgency of the situation; the diagnosis should therefore be mainly clinical (which may sometimes prove wrong after operation). If the operation is elective (no immediate threat to the patient's life), there will usually be sufficient time for full investigations and adequate preparations. Morbidity and mortality are therefore less than in emergency operations.

Informed consent for surgical treatment

A doctor, dentist or other health care professional has a duty to explain to the patient in non-technical language the nature, purpose and material risks of the proposed procedure (material risks are defined as those to which a reasonable person in the patient's position would be likely to attach significance). The patient must be capable of understanding the explanation given; if he or she is incapable (whether from unsound mind or any other cause), informed consent cannot be obtained. Clinicians may use drawings, diagrams and models to supplement verbal explanation; an interpreter may be used if necessary.

A consent should be obtained prior to surgery (but before any sedation is given) by a qualified clinician; it is not valid if it is obtained under any form of duress. No alterations should be made to the consent form after it has been signed by the patient; if after the form is signed there is a change in the planned procedure the patient must be consulted and a new consent form should be signed. It should not exceed the authority given; if for instance a biopsy shows that a breast lump previously thought to be benign is obviously malignant macroscpically, it is not appropriate to continue to a radical operation unless the patient's specific consent has been obtained for the further surgery.

If the patient is unconscious or if there is a genuine emergency a clinician may undertake whatever treatment is immediately necessary to ensure the patient's life or health without waiting to obtain formal consent. A note should be made in the clinical records to explain the absence of informed consent.

Consent can either be implied or express:

Implied consent   For many physical contacts between clinician and patient consent is implied. It can be assumed that a patient has consented to abdominal palpation or rectal examination, when he or she voluntarily undresses and lies on a couch; or when a patient offers an arm for venepuncture.

Express consent   Can be oral or written and should be obtained for any procedure which carries a material risk. Oral consent is valid but written consent is more usually obtained for major procedures. If, for whatever reason, it is only possible to obtain oral consent, it is appropriate to make an entry in clinical records which confirms what advice is given to the patient and that consent has been given. Written consent affords documentary evidence that consent has been obtained. An action may be brought several years after the event and a judge may prefer a patient's evidence to that of a clinician if a signed and/or witnessed consent form cannot be produced.

It is therefore imperative to consider the following:

● It is the patient's legal and moral right to decide his or her own medical destiny regarding the choice of treatment and non-treatment; such right is being protected by Civil Laws as well as a Law of Battery and Law of Negligence.
● Consent requires informed choice and option regarding:
  – nature of procedure, including type of anaesthetic and postoperative measures;
  – potential risks, discomfort, harmful side-effects;
  – probable prognosis;

  – mortality risks, hazards to bodily functions (swallowing, speaking, continence, mobility, sexual performance) must be communicated;
  – surgical versus non-surgical alternative therapeutic options.
● Information given:
  – influenced by patient's understanding, education, social background and translation if necessary;
  – presence of relative/friend/nurse may be helpful.
● Patients over 16 years of age must sign consent form:
  – all procedures under general anaesthetic;
  – procedures under local anaesthetic if significant sequelae possible;
  – signed form inadequate if proper information (above) not given;
  – if disability prevents signing: verbal consent in presence of witness;
  – signed form not required for simple procedures (e.g. sigmoidoscopy) consent implied by acceptance of procedure.
● Children under 16 years of age:
  – consent required from proxy (usually parent);
  – if surgeon believes proxy's decision not in child's best interest: child can be made a ward of court and appropriately treated;
  – exceptionally, adolescent's (14–16 years) consent adequate if sufficiently mature to understand illness and treatment.
● Unconscious patient:
  – surgeon may treat if procedure is a life-saving emergency;
  – consent of relative/friend not required: no legal proxy for adult.
● Mentally handicapped and psychiatric patients not competent to consent:
  – surgeon and psychiatrist must agree that treatment is in patient's best interest.
● If competent adult patient refuses essential treatment, e.g. blood transfusion in Jehovah's Witness:
  – such treatment cannot be forced and in elective situations the surgeon has the right to refuse to treat;
  – in an emergency life-threatening situation the surgeon will have to proceed with an acceptable alternative (e.g. colloid infusion).

EMERGENCY OPERATIONS

3.1 Emergency Laparotomy for Generalised Peritonitis

Indicated in perforated viscus, i.e. acute appendicitis (majority), peptic ulcer (5–8% of emergency laparotomies), colonic diverticular rupture and rarely gall bladder perforation. Quick

assessment and preoperative preparation in the form of nasogastric suction, i.v. drip, CVP line and urinary catheterisation as well as prophylactic antibiotic may be required.
1. Under general anaesthesia with patient in supine position.
2. Right central paramedian incision (in uncertain diagnosis) or incision according to the suspected pathology from history and examination (grid iron in appendicitis, upper midline in peptic ulcer and gall bladder perforation and lower midline or left paramedian in diverticular perforation).

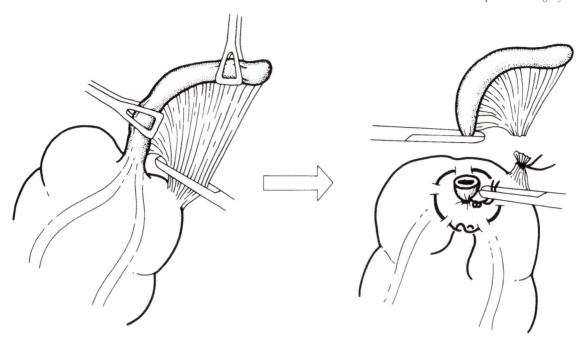

Fig. 3.1.1   Standard appendicectomy

3. Aspirate any free fluid and sample it for bacteria then perform a quick exploration to identify the source of perforation and deal with it accordingly.

Appendicitis (Fig. 3.1.1)

1. Appendix base is identified by tracing taeniae coli of caecum; deliver the caecum through the incision and then deal with the appendix.

2. Apply Babcock's tissue forceps around the tip and base of appendix. Viewing the mesoappendix against light, make a window near its base then clamp the appendicular vessels (branches of ileocolic branch of superior mesenteric artery) and divide close to the appendix.

3. Insert 2/0 chromic catgut purse-string seromuscular stitch 1 cm from appendix base and leave untied.

4. Crush the appendix base, then recrush it and apply forceps 0.5 cm higher. Ligate the lower crushed part then cut off the appendix flush to the lower border of the crushing forceps and discard the contaminated knife, appendix and forceps in a dish (bowel is opened here). Now tie the purse-string suture to invaginate the ligated stump after application of forceps.

5. Check haemostasis then replace the caecum. Using a swab on sponge forceps, mop pus from the paracolic gutter and pelvis. Remember that peritoneal lavage with warm normal saline, Noxyflex or antibiotic solution is indicated *only* in generalised faecal peritonitis. Such peritoneal toilet may be harmful in spreading a localised peritonitis and is therefore contraindicated.

6. Drain the area (if necessary) with a wide-bore tube drain (closed system), then close in layers with or without interparietal povidone-iodine spray.

NB For laparoscopic appendicectomy please see Section 1.14.

Special points

● In difficult high retrocaecal or deep pelvic appendix do not hesitate to enlarge the incision laterally or medially with generous muscle cutting. Good exposure and dissection under direct vision are essential.

● Retrograde or base-first appendicectomy is sometimes helpful.

● Oedematous appendix base does not need to be crushed before ligation and if it is impossible to invaginate the stump then diathermise its lumen and direct the drain mouth to it.

● Drainage of pus alone without appendicetomy is acceptable *only* in difficult cases when one cannot find the appendix.

● If an appendicular mass is felt it can be removed after careful dissection. If carcinoma of the caecum with secondary appendicitis is suspected, or can't be excluded, right hemicolectomy can be performed even if the pathology report reveals a benign appendicular mass later on.

● If after abdominal closure the histology report reveals carcinoid tumour of the appendix, no further action is required, only regular follow-up for life. However, if adenocarcinoma is reported then right hemicolectomy must be performed.

● If the appendix was normal, check the terminal ileum (for Crohn's disease), Meckel's diverticulum, the ovaries (for ruptured Graafian follicles) and lymph nodes (mesenteric lymphadenitis). Appendicectomy should be avoided in caecal Crohn's disease since this may trigger external fistula formation. However, the appendix can be removed in ileal Crohn's disease if it is inflamed. Meckel's diverticulum should be removed only if involved; otherwise leave alone and label the case clearly for future action.

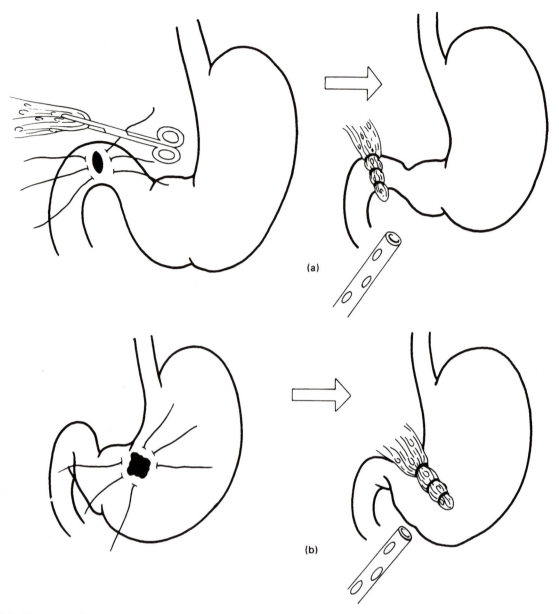

Fig. 3.1.2 Closure of perforated peptic ulcer with omental tag and peritoneal drainage. (a) Perforated duodenal ulcer. (b) Perforated gastric ulcer. Biopsy should be taken from the edge of the perforated gastric ulcer.

Peptic ulcer (Fig. 3.1.2)

1. Ask the assistant to pull the pyloric antrum.
2. Carefully close the duodenal perforation with three interrupted 2/0 chromic catgut sutures inserted 1 cm from the proximal edge, passing through the perforation and emerging 1 cm from the distal edge. This two-stage biting avoids inadvertent stitching of the posterior to the anterior pyloric wall. The closure is done in a transverse fashion as longitudinal suture causes stenosis at the site of closure.
3. Mobilise a fold of omentum and patch it over the perforation, then tie the sutures to close the perforation.
4. Peritoneal toilet and wide-bore tube drainage (closed system) are carried out.
NB Please see Section 1.14 on minimal access therapy.

Special points

● In gastric perforation, ulcer cancer is present in 5–10% of cases so take four angle biopsies then perform simple closure, limited wedge gastric resection and suturing, or formal partial gastrectomy (Billroth I). Substantiate your decision in examination.
● Associated bleeding ulcer should be underrun (duodenal) or excised (if in stomach).
● If there is bile peritonitis but no anterior perforation, open the gastrocolic ligament to look for posterior gastric or pyloroduodenal ulcer and treat as above.
● Simple closure is the safest treatment because of its low mortality and the patient's poor health. An experienced surgeon (and expert anaesthetist) can undertake definitive

treatment if there is a chronic history of peptic ulcer, gastric ulcer from the start, or combined bleeding and perforation.

● Patients with simple closure of the perforation should be advised to have definitive elective operation and should be followed up regularly (roughly one-third are cured, another one-third remain symptomatic and the last third suffer complications).

Colonic diverticulum

Patch with greater omental tag using 2/0 chromic catgut stitches with or without temporary transverse loop colostomy.

After full recovery perform sigmoidoscopy and barium enema to examine the distal colon and to test the sutured area for leakage. Six weeks later resect the diseased segment with anastomosis and follow by closure of the colostomy at a third stage. Alternatively resect the diseased colonic segment from the start and perform Hartmann's procedure by bringing up a proximal end colostomy and closing the distal colonic end and dropping it into the pelvis (this option eliminates the toxic focus of infection). This will be followed by a second stage – restoration of continuity. (The distal colonic end is sometimes brought up as a mucocutaneous fistula to prevent its retraction into the pelvis. However, in difficult identification Foley's balloon catheter inserted rectally can be used to facilitate its dissection.)

Special points

In concomitant colonic perforated carcinoma biopsy should be taken and followed as above. Alternatively, a primary resection and anastomosis protected by colostomy to be closed later on can be performed. However, in examination the *safest* procedure should always be mentioned as the first choice, i.e. A staging procedure (temporary colostomy, resection with anastomosis, then closure of colostomy).

Gallbladder

Cholecystectomy, preferably in the antegrade (fundus first) fashion. If impossible to perform, because of obscured anatomy and friable inflamed tissue, then try partial cholecystectomy and/or cholecystostomy with Foley's catheter left in for 7–10 days to create a fibrous external fistula together with drainage of the subhepatic area. The common bile duct should be examined and an operative cholangiogram should be considered (if feasible) since exploration of the duct may be required.

3.2 Intestinal Obstruction

Surgical relief is carried out electively after routine gastroduodenal nasogastric suction coupled with fluid replacement and correction of electrolyte imbalance. The three indications

for emergency operation after suction and i.v. fluid replacement are:

External hernial obstruction or strangulation Obstruction (irreducible hernia containing an intestine with obstructed lumen but good blood supply) often culminates in strangulation (serious impairment of blood supply of hernial content with imminent gangrene). Clinical distinction is difficult and it is better to assume that the case is strangulation and treat accordingly. Classically, femoral hernia strangulates in women and inguinal hernia strangulates in men while incisional hernia strangulates in both sexes. External hernia is the commonest cause of intestinal obstruction in developing countries while adhesion band is the commonest cause of intestinal obstruction in developed countries (owing to the great number of laparotomies performed).

Internal intestinal strangulation Is the most urgent condition since gangrene follows quickly. Clinically there is intestinal obstruction with shock in an ill toxic patient. Pain may fluctuate up and down but is never absent, and persistence of pain for 2 h in spite of gastroduodenal aspiration is diagnostic of strangulation. There is always tenderness and rebound tenderness (peritonism) over an intra-abdominal strangulated coil (in obstruction, only tenderness presents). Strangulated intestine in external hernia presents as a tense, tender, irreducible lump with no expansile cough impulse and which has recently increased in size. Late internal strangulation leads to generalised tenderness and rigidity.

Acute or acute-on-chronic intestinal obstruction Usually involves the upper gastrointestinal tract. Sudden intestinal colicky pain and vomiting are the first symptoms. Distension is usually absent (but borborygmi and high-pitched bowel sounds may be present on auscultation). Absolute constipation is late, as there is natural action of the bowels after onset, yielding some faeces below the site of intestinal obstruction even if it is complete.

There is no constipation in acute intestinal obstruction due to:

Richter's hernia (partial enterocoele).
Gallstone ileus.
Mesenteric vascular occlusion.
Intestinal obstruction associated with pelvic abscess.

(Chronic intestinal obstruction usually involves the lower gastrointestinal tract. It starts first with constipation that becomes absolute as a result of completely obstructing colonic carcinoma or diverticular disease. Abdominal distension then follows, leading to a fully blown caecum and pain. Vomiting is late).

Obstructed or strangulated inguinal hernia

Approach and repair is similar to that in elective cases. Differences in treatment depend on the site of intestinal obstruction and whether the bowel is viable or dead.
1. Make a suprainguinal incision parallel and 2 cm above the medial two-thirds of the inguinal ligament cutting through skin, subcutaneous tissue and Scarpa's fascia down to the external oblique aponeurosis after proper haemostasis.

2. Identify the external inguinal ring and split the external oblique ring in the line of the inguinal canal to reveal the spermatic cord (male) or the round ligament of the uterus (female).

3. Isolate the hernial sac by sharp dissection in the line of the cord (through cremasteric and internal spermatic fascias) and expose fully the internal inguinal ring, safeguarding spermatic vessels and vas deferens.

4. Pick up the sac with two or three artery forceps and open. Identify its contents and see whether it is viable. Gently draw up the bowel and never let it slip back into the abdomen. If it is viable replace and pass a finger to check for the presence of femoral hernia from inside the peritoneal cavity (if present can be repaired simultaneously). If viability is suspect then cover it with warm moist packs for 5–10′min (asking the anaesthetist to give a higher percentage of oxygen), then re-examine for sheen, colour, peristalsis and mesenteric pulsation. A black segment of small intestine with no sheen, no peristalsis or pulsation should be resected with end-to-end anastomosis (2/0 chromic catgut in two layers – mucosal continuous and seromuscular continuous) then replaced intraperitoneally. If the large bowel is resected it should be protected proximally with a temporary loop colostomy via a separate left iliac muscle cutting (or appendectomy-like) incision to be closed 6 weeks later when barium enema (done at least 2 weeks postoperatively) shows no anastomotic leak in the suture line. Again, the large bowel (usually sigmoid colon in left inguinal hernia) is closed in one or two layers – using mainly interrupted seromuscular 2/0 silk and mucosal continuous 2/0 chromic catgut (*optional* gas-tight barrier). Take care not to exert tension or cause strangulation during suturing. Replace the bowel intraperitoneally with paracolic drainage.

5. Resect the hernial sac and close its neck after transfixion ligature or purse-string suture (herniotomy).

6. Repair is carried out by suturing the inguinal ligament to the conjoined tendon, using non-absorbable nylon or Prolene, from the pubic tubercle medially to the internal inguinal ring, displacing the cord laterally.

7. Close in layers – chromic catgut to external oblique aponeurosis refashioning the external inguinal ring so that it permits entry of the little finger. If Halsted repair is required in an elderly patient (over 60 years) to strengthen repair then close the external oblique aponeurosis posterior to the cord which will be subcutaneous. In women the ligament is excised and in orchidectomy done in the elderly (consent should be obtained preoperatively) the repair is made easier by complete closure of the external oblique aponeurosis. Closure of subcutaneous tissue (plain catgut) and skin (Prolene or clips) follows.

Internal intestinal strangulation

1. Laparotomy via right paramedian incision usually.

2. If the caecum is collapsed it is small bowel intestinal obstruction and if distended then it is large bowel intestinal obstruction. Expose the site of obstruction clearly after withdrawal of intestinal coils using moist warm packs.

3. Decompress the intestinal obstruction by Savage's intestinal decompressor (or similar decompressor) via a stab in the bowel, using a purse-string suture to control any spillage. Higher small bowel intestinal obstruction may be milked upward towards the nasogastric suction controlled by the anaesthetist.

4. Assess viability (as above) and act accordingly. In small bowel intestinal obstruction adhesion bands can be divided and bowel released, volvulus is dismantled and fixed. In acute large bowel intestinal obstruction due to carcinoma involving:

- Ascending colon up to proximal part of the transverse colon, emergency right hemicolectomy is advocated *but* if the tumour is irremovable or the patient is elderly and extremely ill then ileotransverse enterostomy is indicated. Impending or actual caecal perforation may necessitate caecostomy (alone or in addition to above procedure).

- Splenic flexure down to rectum, temporary transverse loop colostomy is performed, followed 4 weeks later by resection of the obstructing tumour (when the condition of the patient has stabilised) with closure of colostomy simultaneously (two stages) or 6 weeks later (three stages).

However, with an irremovable tumour or in elderly patients, transverse sigmoid colocolic bypass (side-to-side anastomosis) is recommended. In massive pelvic infiltration, loop transverse proximal colostomy is constructed permanently. In diverticular sigmoid disease perform Hartmann's operation – resecting the area, establishing proximal left iliac end colostomy, and closing the distal rectal end to be resutured later on (rectal or distal end can be brought out to skin level as a mucocutaneous fistula to facilitate later anastomosis).

Colostomy

Either end colostomy (usually permanent as in abdominoperineal excision of rectal carcinoma but can be temporary as in Hartmann's operation for diverticular disease) or loop colostomy (usually temporary but can be used permanently). The colostomy can be iliac or in the transverse colon.

Left iliac end colostomy

The site is marked, a disc of skin is removed and an appendectomy-like (but muscle-cutting) incision is made in the left iliac fossa. The proximal colonic end (clamped with either an intestinal or Zachary-Cope clamp) is delivered through the incision. Then colonic serosa is stitched to the abdominal wall muscle using 2/0 chromic catgut and mucosa is sutured to the skin with eight interrupted stitches. This is followed by application of a colostomy bag over the functioning colostomy. The laparotomy wound should be closed and covered before the colostomy is constructed to avoid faeceal contamination.

Transverse loop colostomy (Fig. 3.2.1)

The most widely used temporary colostomy. General anaesthesia is important since traction on the mesentery causes pain and nausea.

1. Transverse incision (8–10 cm long) in the right upper abdomen midway between the umbilicus and xiphisternum over the rectus abdominis muscle and extending laterally to the lateral border of the rectus muscle.

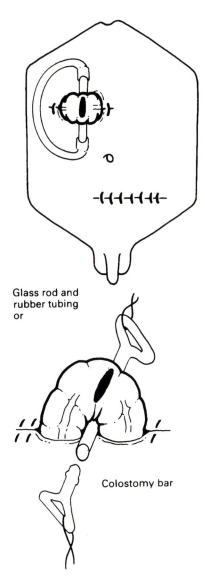

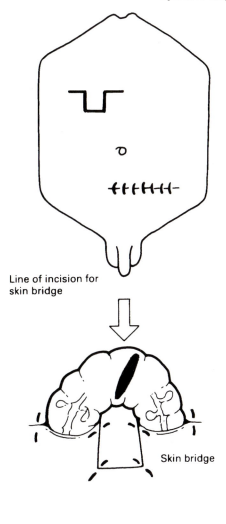

Fig. 3.2.1 Loop colostomy

2. Cut down all layers including the rectus muscle, which is divided transversely (ligating and dividing the epigastric artery).

3. The most *proximal* loop of transverse colon is prepared by cleaning omentum from its anterior surface; then a small hole is made in the transverse mesocolon through which a rubber tube is passed to facilitate delivery of the colon through the incision (in sigmoid colostomy a left iliac muscle-cutting incision is made – sigmoid colon has no omentum). Close the laparotomy wound at this stage.

4. The colonic loop is held by an underlying glass rod (or by a colostomy bar or skin bridge incised initially). Open the colostomy on its antimesocolic border longitudinally (along taenia coli) or transversely.

5. Insert mucocutaneous sutures (2/0 chromic catgut) and close the skin so that the colonic loop fits snugly, allowing one finger to pass down each side. The colostomy appliance should be

constructed immediately (the colon should be opened at operation and not later).

Complications of colostomy

- Loss of viability (blood supply is interfered with).
- Separation of colostomy and retraction (due to tension and infection).
- Infection – cellulitis (due to haematoma); scarring and stenosis. Stenosis occurs at the mucocutaneous junction. The colostomy should be refashioned with excision of skin disc.
- Paracolostomy hernia especially in end terminal colostomy. Colostomy should be resited and the hernial defect closed.
- Prolapse in transverse colostomy is not important (since it is usually temporary) but in end colostomy it leads to dysfunction; treated by reconstruction or resiting.

Colostomy closure

1. Apply stay (silk) sutures to the mucocutaneous junction under general anaesthesia and mobilise the colostomy.
2. Separate the colostomy from the anterior abdominal wall, removing the skin edge with it.
3. Perform simple two-layer closure: 2/0 chromic catgut using continuous Connell stitch (loop on mucosa to invert it) taking in all layers followed by fine silk seromuscular Lambert (interrupted) layer.
4. Conduct the anastomosis outside and replace it intraperitoneally since an extraperitoneal location is associated with inadequate mobilisation and unsatisfactory anastomosis under tension.
5. Close the abdominal wall (± drainage).

3.3 Femoral Hernia Repair

Indications

Uncomplicated femoral hernia   Because of the constant risk of strangulation and the highly unsatisfactory result of femoral truss (urgent operation).

Strangulated femoral hernia   Occurs when blood supply of its contents is impaired (gangrene occurs 6 h later). The intestine is obstructed already and its blood supply is constricted impeding venous return and leading to congestion and fluid exudation within the hernial sac. Later, the arterial supply is compromised leading to blood effusion into the lumen and wall of the intestine (the sac becomes bloodstained with transmigration of bacteria followed by haemorrhage and thrombosis of vessels, subserosal blood decomposition, perforation and gangrene). Clinically the findings are those of intestinal obstruction (generalised abdominal pain following its initial localisation over hernia, vomiting, abdominal distension and constipation) combined with local signs of a tense tender irreducible hernia which has recently increased in size with no expansile impulse on coughing. Rebound tenderness is often present. When gangrene starts, peristaltic pain paroxysms cease (grave sign) due to peritonitis or paralytic ileus and the patient passes into septic shock.

Approaches to femoral hernia repair (Fig. 3.3.1)

Low approach (Lockwood, Surgeon, St Bartholomew's Hospital, London)

A 10 cm skin crease incision over the hernia, a finger's breadth below the medial half of the inguinal ligament. Deepen the incision, expose the preperitoneal fat-covered sac and incise the sac on its *lower lateral aspect* to avoid bladder injury, dilate the neck digitally, examine bowel viability, and reduce the bowel if possible. Close the femoral canal with interrupted non-absorbable 2/0 suture (monofilament nylon or silk mounted on

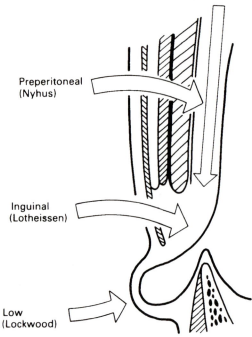

Fig. 3.3.1   Approaches in femoral hernia repair

a fish-hook J-shaped needle) approximating the inguinal ligament to the pectineal ligament and making sure not to constrict the femoral vein laterally (place your index finger on it).

Inguinal approach (Lotheissen, Surgeon, Kaiser Josef Hospital, Vienna)

The incision is as for inguinal hernia – 2 cm above and parallel to the medial two-thirds of the inguinal ligament. Deepen the incision medial to the inferior epigastric vessels after cord mobilisation and external oblique division. Intraperitoneally expose the obstructed contents and retract the lower end of the wound to manipulate and reduce the contents (hernia repair is as above). This approach is condemned since it weakens the inguinal area and predisposes to inguinal hernia formation.

High approach (McEvedy, Surgeon, Ancoats Hospital, Manchester)

A 10 cm vertical incision centred on the inguinal ligament (over the femoral canal through the lower 5 cm). The sac is dissected as above. If strangulated or the contents cannot be reduced then cut through the upper 5 cm; incise the rectus sheath parallel to the lateral border of the rectus muscle and dissect between transversalis fascia and peritoneum (no posterior rectus sheath behind the lower one-third of the rectus muscle below the arcuate line). Reduce the contents, manipulating from above and below, then repair from above (in order to visualise the accessory obturator artery and avoid its injury).

Henry's approach (Henry, British surgeon, found this approach accidentally while performing it on bladder bilharziasis in Egypt)

A 10 cm midline infraumbilical extraperitoneal incision deepened between the peritoneum and transversalis fascia. Repair from above. This approach is very good for bilateral femoral hernias.

Preperitoneal approach (Nyhus, USA)

A transverse anterior abdominal wall incision (modified from Henry) is used to repair femoral hernia from behind. The transversalis fascia is closed, assisted by external direct manual reduction from below. This approach also allows repair of direct, indirect and recurrent inguinal hernias through one incision. (Not practised in the UK.)

Inguinal ligament multipartial division (Ellis, Westminster Hospital, London)

Via low approach (to allow ample room for reduction and/or resection); is not widely practised.

The commonest approaches for strangulated femoral hernia are:
● Lockwood approach (with or without paramedian laparotomy).
● McEvedy approach: probably the most widely practised.
● Nyhus approach: very good approach practised widely in the USA (not UK).

Technical points

● Ascertain bowel viability from:
  Sheen and colour.
  Arterial mesenteric pulsation.
  Bowel peristalsis.
  If good, replace. If doubtful, cover with warm moist packs and give 100% oxygen for 5–10 min by the clock and re-examine. If by the above criteria it is judged viable, replace. If not, resect and do end-to-end primary anastomosis for small bowel (in two layers – 2/0 chromic catgut to the mucosa and a seromuscular layer).
● Avoid *taxis* in femoral hernia since dislodgement of gangrenous bowel requires laparotomy. If such a gangrenous segment slips back into the abdomen during hernia repair, perform laparotomy (paramedian incision is essential) to resect it and restore bowel continuity.
● A grooved director may be used to cut the lacunar medial ligament (the theoretical possibility of injury to accessory obturator artery is often exaggerated) in order to enlarge the hernial neck.
● Omentocele should be excised rather than replaced since adhesions are vascular and difficult to reduce. Richter's hernia (partial enterocele) is treated either by wedge excision and anastomosis (in transverse fashion in two layers) or by inversion within the bowel lumen with two layers.

3.4 Arterial Embolectomy

Indications

Major acute interruption to the circulation of a limb thought to be due to embolism requires embolectomy provided that the limb is still potentially viable and that the patient is not in circulatory failure.

Preoperative preparation

Intravenous heparin 10 000 units as soon as diagnosis of embolism is made. Measures to improve cardiac state if necessary. Aortography unnecessary initially, as diagnosis is made by clinical findings, particularly loss of pulses.

Position of patient

Supine. For lower limb, leg externally rotated at hip and flexed at knee, permitting access to femoral and distal popliteal arteries. For upper limb, arm abducted on arm board.

Anaesthesia

Local infiltration anaesthesia may be used in the critically ill patient; otherwise general anaesthesia is preferred.

Procedure

Femoral embolus (Fig. 3.4.1)

The common and superficial femoral arteries are the commonest peripheral sites. The common femoral artery and its bifurcation is exposed through vertical incision; tapes or silicone slings are placed round the common femoral, superficial and profunda arteries. Open the common femoral artery with a transverse incision opposite the profunda opening. Remove wire from a No. 3 or 4 Fogarty catheter, and test balloon. No more than the correct amount of fluid for inflation should be drawn into the syringe. Pass the catheter gently down the profunda as far as possible. Then inflate the balloon (the surgeon does this himself) until resistance is felt and gently withdraw the catheter while adjusting inflation by feel to keep the balloon in contact with the arterial wall. Clot emerges from the arteriotomy in front of the balloon. Repeat the pass into the profunda until no further clot is obtained. Apply bulldog clamp to the profunda. A catheter is then passed down the superficial femoral artery as far as possible. In favourable cases it reaches the ankle. Withdraw clot and repeat until no further clot is obtained. If the embolus does not shoot out with the initial arteriotomy, a No. 4 or 5 size Fogarty should be passed upwards and withdrawn with the balloon inflated as before, until a good forward flow is obtained. Clamp the common femoral artery and close the arteriotomy with 5/0 Prolene.

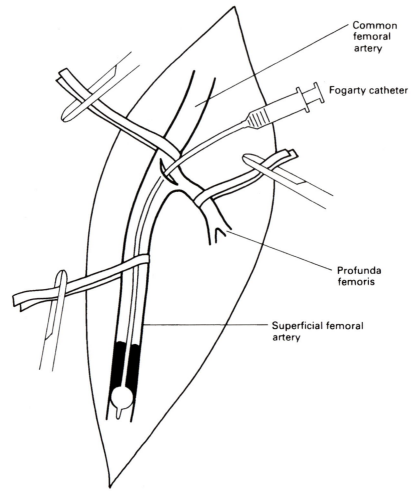

Common
femoral
artery

Fogarty catheter

Profunda
femoris

Superficial femoral
artery

Fig. 3.4.1   Femoral embolectomy

Popliteal embolus

These may often be removed through the common femoral artery. If unsuccessful, the distal popliteal artery should be exposed by a vertical incision a finger's breadth behind the medial border of the tibia, division of the deep fascia and backward retraction of gastrocnemius, and division of the medial hamstrings near the tibia. The popliteal bifurcation can be displayed by this approach.

Aortic saddle embolus (Fig. 3.4.2)

This can usually be removed with Fogarty catheters via a bilateral femoral approach. One side is clamped while as much embolus as possible is withdrawn from the other. The process is then reversed. The superficial femoral and profunda arteries should also be 'catheterised' to remove clot that may have migrated distally.

Brachial embolus

Expose brachial bifurcation via an S-shaped incision, the proximal limb being medial. Transverse arteriotomy above the bifurcation allows the catheter to be passed upwards and into each forearm vessel, both of which should be cleared.

Failed embolectomy

This usually means coexisting occlusive disease, or that occlusion was thrombotic not embolic. Emergency arteriography is indicated so that arterial reconstruction may be undertaken if feasible.

3.5 Leaking Aortic Aneurysm

In patients reaching hospital alive with a leaking abdominal aneurysm, survival depends very much on prompt action by the surgical and anaesthetic team, the aim being to secure control of the aorta proximal to the aneurysm with the least possible delay; resuscitation can then proceed and the remainder of the operation is carried out much as in an elective case.

Patients in shock should ideally be taken straight from the ambulance to the theatre; little time should be wasted on attempts at resuscitation, and for patients *in extremis* immediate laparotomy and aortic control may offer the only chance of survival.

Procedure

If the patient's condition is still stable after anaesthesia and opening the abdomen through a long midline incision, the duodenum can be quickly mobilised and the neck of the aneurysm looked for through the haematoma; after giving i.v. heparin, it is clamped as in the elective procedure. If this proves difficult or the patient is deteriorating or *in extremis*, the upper abdominal aorta should be compressed. This can be done by backward pressure against the spine with the end of a suitably shaped wooden spoon, or the blade of a weighted vaginal speculum pointing upwards parallel with the aorta and pressed backwards in the midline. Alternatively, with the left lobe of the liver retracted the supra-coeliac aorta can be exposed by dissection through the upper part of the lesser omentum and partial division of the right crus, and clamped at this level. At the lower end the common iliac arteries are clamped, and time can then be taken to dissect the neck of the aneurysm for clamping the aorta below the renal arteries.

If necessary, the aneurysm can be opened and a finger pushed up through its neck as a guide for the application of the clamp at this point. A Foley catheter passed up into the aorta, and then inflated, is another possibility; and if difficulty is experienced in clamping the common iliac arteries, they can be controlled in a similar manner.

Once the clamps are in place, the operation proceeds as for an elective aneurysm. A woven graft should always be selected to minimise blood loss through the graft wall. Before completing the distal anastomosis a Fogarty catheter should be passed down the lower limb arteries to withdraw any clots.

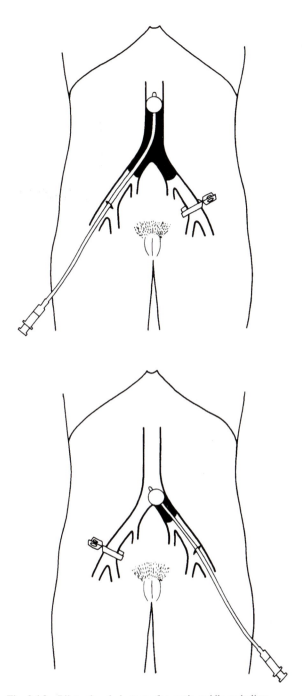

Fig. 3.4.2   Bilateral embolectomy for aortic saddle embolism

Preoperative preparation

Even if the patient arrives in a stable and satisfactory condition, arrangements for operation should be put in hand immediately. Twelve units of blood should be cross-matched, two i.v. drips set up, and a urethral catheter and a nasogastric tube should be passed. In theatre, the patient is placed straight on the operating table; the surgical team are ready scrubbed and gowned and the patient is draped before anaesthesia is started (in case sudden catastrophic bleeding occurs when the abdominal wall relaxes).

3.6 Compound Fracture

Procedure (Figs 3.6.1–3.6.3)

Should be managed urgently with prophylactic antibiotics, tetanus prophylaxis, preoperative immobilisation (splintage), careful X-ray assessment (to decide whether closed or open reduction is required). Then:

1. Under general anaesthesia with X-ray screening control try to assess the pulses. Try closed manipulation and feel pulses again. Check for swelling and haematoma under tension.
2. Clean the skin thoroughly, shave the wound margins and remove all foreign bodies and dirt. Irrigate the wound generously and remove blood clots.
3. Extend the incision (after debridement of devitalised margin) to visualise clearly all dead muscles and damaged

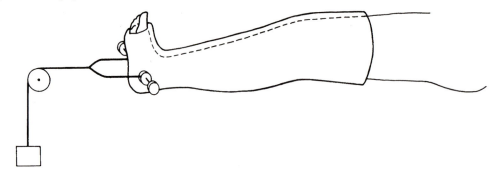

Fig. 3.6.1   Calcaneal skeletal traction, closed reduction of compound fracture of tibia and fibula, and plaster-of-Paris immobilisation

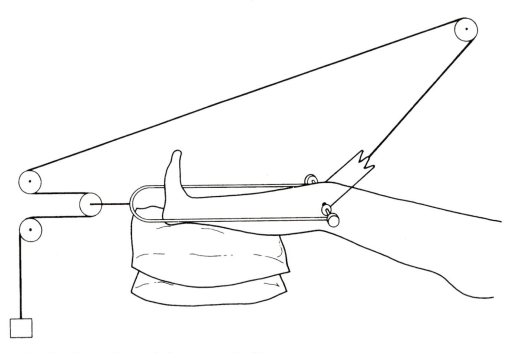

Fig. 3.6.2   Hamilton–Russell skeletal traction for fractures around the hip

fascia in order to remove them. Decompress the enclosing fascia if necessary. Identify and safeguard main arteries and nerves. Remove small spiky bone chips but do not remove big pieces, otherwise bone shortening may result.

4. Reduce the fracture under screening usually by closed manipulation; rarely open reduction is required (primary internal fixation is better avoided because of high rate of infection).

5. Once the fracture is reduced, it is usually stable and the limb is suitable for padded plaster cast immobilisation which can be split to allow for oedema development. If the fracture is unstable after reduction *skeletal traction* should be added. In compound femoral fracture, after nicking the skin (always

under general anaesthesia), insert upper tibial Steinmann pin or Denham pin mounted on a T-handled introducer from the lateral to the medial aspect 2.5 cm posterior-inferior to the tibial tuberosity. In compound fractures of tibia and fibula (ignore fibula and reduce tibial fracture) introduce a calcaneal pin 2.5 cm posterior inferior to the lateral malleolus. Attach a traction stirrup to the pin (e.g. Bohler stirrup) and set sliding skeletal traction on a Thomas' splint (in femoral fracture) or use calcaneal skeletal traction with a Bohler–Braun frame (in compound tibial and fibular fracture).

6. Remember to close the skin without tension, using a relief incision if necessary. If impossible to close then delayed primary suture 5 days later or split skin grafts are needed.

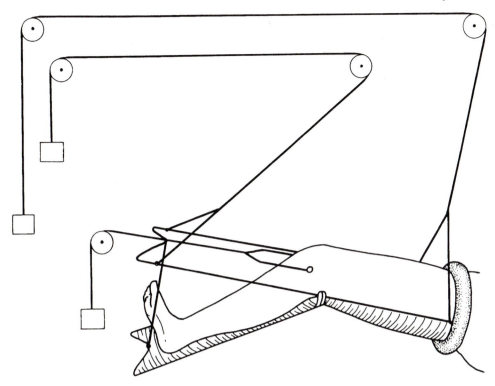

Fig. 3.6.3 Sliding skeletal traction with a Thomas' splint for shaft and supracondylar fractures of the femur

3.7 Head Injury and Burr Hole Procedure

Indications

1. Closed head injury when one of the following signs, suggestive of intracranial haemorrhage (mainly extradural), is present:
- Sudden deterioration in the level of consciousness.
- Dissociation of vital signs due to increased intracranial pressure, i.e. systemic hypertension and bradycardia (opposite to internal haemorrhage signs of hypotension and tachycardia). Such hypertension (due to hypoxia induced by intracranial haematoma and increased intracranial pressure) leads to reflex bradycardia (via baroreceptors) and the combination is termed Cushing's reflex.
- Focal neurological signs, i.e. sluggish dilating unilateral pupil and contralateral hemiparesis.

2. Open head trauma if it is depressed compound fracture. Burr hole should be performed in the vicinity of the fracture over an intact bone to lift the depressed fragment for proper decompression. Close dural tear if present to prevent development of epileptogenic focus.

3. Intracranial pressure monitoring with an extradural or subdural transducer, subdural bolt or intraventricular cannula (carries risk of infection in 1–5% of cases). Such investigation provides baseline pressure and gives warning of complications (intracranial haematoma) before there are clinical signs in conscious and stable head injuries so that the decision whether to operate can be made.

4. Ventricular access for relief of increased intracranial pressure, air or contrast ventriculography, drug administration and external ventricular drainage (burr hole here is elective and not an emergency as in the above three indications).

Preparations

Under local anaesthesia preferably with endotracheal intubation to ensure an adequate airway; or under general anaesthesia. Position the head over a horse-shoe head rest or between sandbags, shave and cleanse the whole head with an antiseptic solution (e.g. Disadine). Mark the surface for proposed burr hole(s) under strict sterile circumstances and infiltrate the scalp beneath these markings with 1% lignocaine and 1:200 000 adrenaline. The site of the burr hole is determined by:
- The side of bruising in the temporal muscle.
- The side of skull fracture (seen on skull X-ray).
- The side of initial dilatation of pupil.

Use a sterile ruler to delineate the midline of the scalp in the sagittal plane; then mark two 4 cm incisions, each 3 cm from the sagittal plane at a point 13 cm from the nasal root (frontal burr holes). Two more incisions are marked – one 3 cm above the midzygomatic point (temporal burr hole) and one 8 cm

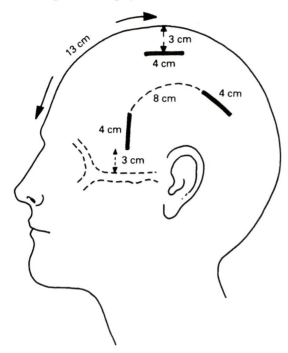

Fig. 3.7.1 Sites of burr holes

posterior to the temporal burr hole (parietal) – along an imaginary half circle (Fig. 3.7.1).

Procedure

1. Incise and deepen the skin down to bone (at proposed sites, preferably starting with the temporal site first). Use finger tips to press and stop the bleeding vessels, applying artery forceps to the galea aponeurotica to arrest bleeding. Insert a self-retaining retractor.

2. Strip back pericranium with a rugine or periosteal elevator. Use a Hudson brace with perforator to penetrate the outer and inner tables of the skull and then use a burr to complete the skull hole. Stop bleeding from diploë with bone wax.

3. If extradural haematoma is seen, enlarge or extend the burr hole (craniectomy) by bone nibbling forceps (bone rongeur). Remove the blood clot. Irrigation with saline and gentle suction is applied. Middle meningeal arterial bleeding can be controlled by coagulation and/or underrunning or transfixing the artery with 3/0 silk. Secure haemostasis. Oxycel may be used for this purpose. To prevent recurrence of bleeding, stitch dura over the bone edge to pericranium using interrupted silk suture.

4. If no extradural haematoma is found, open the dura with a sharp hook and blade No. 15 to locate subdural haematoma. If no haematoma is seen but the brain bulges then make further burr holes until haematoma is located; it is then drained and the brain decompressed.

5. Leave burr hole open, with a Redivac drain for the next 24 h, and close in layers.

6. Flat position is adopted postoperatively to encourage the brain to expand.

3.8 Tracheostomy

Objectives

- To relieve upper respiratory tract obstruction.
- To decrease respiratory work by bypassing oropharynx and reducing dead space.
- To afford direct access to tracheobronchial tree for aspiration of secretions and bronchial lavage.
- To allow intermittent positive pressure ventilation in case prolonged ventilation is required.
- To stablise the thoracic cage in chest injuries where it decreases paradoxical respiration and reduces the traumatic chest wall deformity.

Indications

Obstructed upper respiratory tract

- Acute infections, e.g. acute laryngotracheobronchitis in children, acute epiglottitis, laryngeal diphtheria.
- Oedema of glottis (whether traumatic, infective or allergic), e.g. Ludwig's angina.
- Facial burns.
- Head and neck injuries, e.g. faciomaxillary fractures and cut throat.
- Tumours, e.g. carcinoma of larynx and thyroid.
- Bilateral abductor paralysis of vocal cords following recurrent laryngeal nerve injury in thyroidectomy.
- Foreign body.
- Stenoses and atresias, e.g. congenital web or atresia and chronic stenosis following tuberculosis or scalding.

Impaired respiratory function

In obstructive and restrictive airway diseases, aims to reduce the anatomical dead space and improve the physiological dead space due to retained secretions.

- Fulminating bronchopneumonia.
- Chronic bronchitis with severe emphysema.
- Chest injuries, e.g. flail chest.
- Lower respiratory tract obstructed by secretions, e.g. post-thoracotomy or upper abdominal operations or prolonged coma.

Respiratory paralysis

- Unconscious patients with head, maxillofacial or spinal cord injuries.
- Prolonged coma, e.g. drug overdose, poisoning (such as barbiturate).
- Bulbar type of poliomyelitis, polyneuritis and myasthenia gravis.
- Tetanus.
- Vocal cord paralysis.

Operative necessity

● Laryngectomy and laryngopharyngectomy (always).
● Following total thyroidectomy, and/or bilateral block dissection of the neck (sometimes).

Options

Crash or emergency tracheostomy (vertical incision from cricoid cartilage down to suprasternal notch with or without local anaesthesia and oxygen administered via face mask) is not recommended since endotracheal intubation or emergency laryngotomy are better and quicker alternatives (Wide-bore needle or tube inserted and directed backwards through cricothyroid membrane via a puncture or small horizontal stab respectively until air begins to hiss in and out; an oxygen source is then attached to the needle or tube). Prophylactic elective tracheostomy, planned at leisure under ideal circumstances in an operating theatre, is best.

Elective tracheostomy (Fig. 3.8.1)

1. Search for the correct size of tracheostomy tube before starting (e.g. 28 Fr in adults).
2. Under general anaesthesia with endotracheal intubation.
3. Horizontal skin crease incision midway between the cricoid and suprasternal notch.
4. Confine the deep dissection to the midline, separating pretracheal muscles and dividing the thyroid isthmus between clamps, oversewing the cut ends. Arrest any bleeding vessels (transverse branches of anterior jugular veins).
5. In a bloodless field with good exposure, retraction of wound edges and cricoid hook in place perform the tracheal cut in the 2nd, 3rd and 4th tracheal rings. An inverted U-shaped tracheal incision hinging the flap downwards and forwards and stitching it (during operation) temporarily to the lower edge of the skin incision is the commonest form of tracheostomy. It facilitates postoperative tube changing, reinsertion in case of accidental tube displacement and prevents stenosis. Other variations are a vertical tracheal cut or resection of a circular disc.
6. Suck out the blood entering the trachea and insert the tracheostomy tube (after asking the anaesthetist to pull the endotracheal tube up to the level of the cricoid cartilage under your supervision).
7. Tie the tracheostomy tube with tapes around the neck. Close the skin. An inflatable rubber or polyethylene cuff-tube is preferred to a metallic outer and inner tube combination for sealing the air passage and preventing aspiration pneumonia after vomiting.

In children beware:
● Laryngotomy is impracticable since the cricothyroid space or membrane is too small.
● In performing tracheostomy remember the five possible pretracheal structures that must be dealt with properly:
   1. Innominate vein.
   2. Anterior jugular vein.
   3. Thymus.
   4. Inferior thyroid plexus of veins.
   5. Thyroidea ima inconstant artery.

Postoperative (nursing) care

1. Maintain patent airways
● Frequent atraumatic suction.
● Humidification.

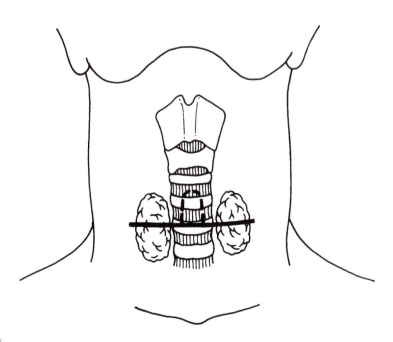

Fig. 3.8.1 Tracheostomy

- Mucolytic agent.
- Encourage coughing and physiotherapy.
- Occasional bronchial lavage.

2. Prevent infection and other complications
- Aseptic suction, handling and tube changing.
- Antibiotics: remember that *Pseudomonas aeroginosa* (the main microorganism of intensive therapy units) is often found here.
- Avoid tube impinging on posterior tracheal wall (pressure necrosis).
- Deflate cuffed tubes for 5 min every hour (to prevent pressure necrosis).
- Repeated daily clinical and radiological assessments.

3. Final removal of tracheostomy tube (weaning) depends on the status of blood gases before and after removal.

Complications of tracheostomy
- Operative haemorrhage (venous or arterial).
- Encrustation due to tracheal trauma and dry or inadequate humidified inhaled air.
- Tracheal ulceration and tracheo-oesophageal fistulation.
- Tracheal pressure necrosis and stenosis.
- Surgical emphysema.
- Mediastinal emphysema and pneumothorax (due to intermittent positive pressure ventilation).
- Infection of wound, lung or passages especially by *Pseudomonas aeruginosa*.
- Accidental tube displacement.
- Blocked tube by secretion.

Notice that cyanosis following tracheostomy can either be due to tube displacement or blockage by secretion.

ELECTIVE OPERATIONS

3.9 Vagotomy, Oesophageal and Gastric Operations

Truncal vagotomy

Nasogastric tube in the stomach helps to drain it and to define the oesophagus.

1. A midline incision. Explore and assess whether there are extensive subphrenic adhesions (if found, may make the operation difficult or unwise).
2. Mobilise the left lobe of the liver by dividing its coronary ligament and pack it off to the right; introduce retractors on the right and left. Stretch the stomach downwards.
3. Divide the peritoneum over the oesophagus transversely and retract the oesophagophrenic ligament upward.
4. Mobilise the oesophagus and encircle it with a finger then a rubber tube. By exerting traction on the tube, dissection of the surface is facilitated. Locate the anterior nerve and strip it up and down, freeing 5 cm. Resect 2.5 cm (vagectomy). Similarly deal with the posterior vagus nerve which lies away from the oesophagus and to the right (LARP = left vagus anterior and right vagus posterior). Dissect off and divide every suspicious nerve structure on the oesophagus.

Pyloroplasty (Fig. 3.9.1)

The pyloric muscle only may be divided longitudinally or the full thickness of the wall may be transected longitudinally and the opening closed transversely (to avoid stenosis) in two layers, or in one layer and covered with omentum (Heineke–Mikulicz). Judd as well as Holt and Lythgoe advocated prior excision of any anterior ulcer present, excision of a portion of the sphincter and pyloric antrum longitudinally, and suturing of the gap transversely. Pyloroduodenostomy (Japoulay) or continuous U-shaped pyloroplasty (Finney) are other alternatives.

Gastrojejunostomy (Fig. 3.9.2)

1. Draw the great omentum upwards to display the transverse mesocolon and decide whether posterior retrocolic or anterior high antecolic anastomosis is required. Retrocolic is preferred unless the distal gastric outlet is obstructed by malignant tumour.
2. Identify the middle colic artery and open the mesocolon on the left of the main artery.
3. Seize the greater and lesser curvatures of the stomach with Babcock tissue forceps and draw the most dependent part (posteroinferior) of the stomach through the hole.
4. Rotate the forceps anticlockwise – the greater curvature then moves to the right.
5. Bring up a short loop of jejunum, apply intestinal clamps and establish a 7 cm long isoperistaltic anastomosis in two layers (haemostatic and seromuscular – both by continuous 2/0 chromic catgut).
6. Approximate the edges of the hole in the mesocolon to the stomach.
7. Check that the afferent loop is not under tension. Make certain there are no peritoneal holes left, then close.

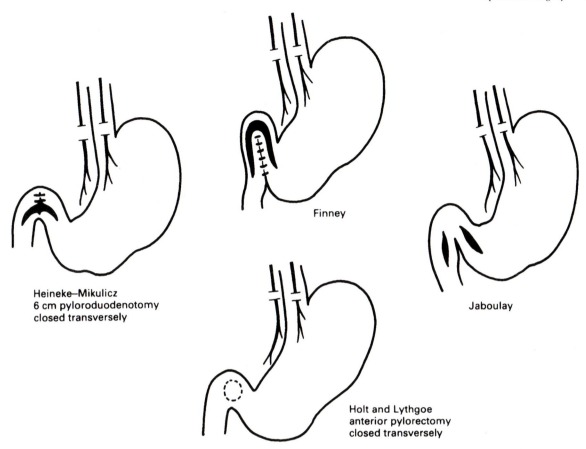

Heineke–Mikulicz
6 cm pyloroduodenotomy
closed transversely

Finney

Jaboulay

Holt and Lythgoe
anterior pylorectomy
closed transversely

Fig. 3.9.1   Types of pyloroplasty accompanying truncal vagotomy

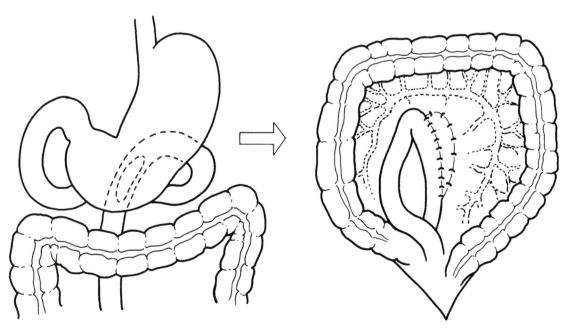

Fig. 3.9.2   Posterior retrocolic gastrojejunostomy

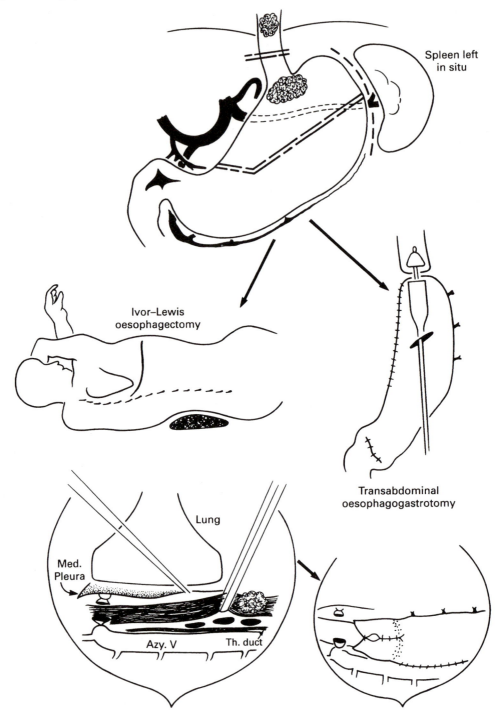

Fig. 3.9.3   Alternatives for gastro-oesophageal junction and lower oesophageal carcinomas

Operations for oesophageal carcinoma

The oesophagus is subdivided into:

Upper third: from cricopharyngeus to aortic arch; includes the cervical segment and supra-aortic segment.

Middle third: from aortic arch to inferior pulmonary vein.

Lower third: from inferior pulmonary vein to gastro-oesophageal junction; includes the supra-diaphragmatic segment and abdominal segment.

Operative principles

Upper third carcinoma

Is treated by either:
● Radiotherapy; or
● Three-stage total oesophagectomy (McKeown).

Middle third carcinoma

- In the lower half: needs Lewis–Tanner (two-stage procedure).
- In the upper half: is removed by the two-stage procedure followed by a third stage (McKeown) consisting of clearance and mobilisation of the cervical oesophagus through a right supraclavicular incision (left supraclavicular approach may damage thoracic duct); delivery of the oesophagus into the neck wound; oesophagectomy with closure at the oesophagogastric junction; and restoration of continuity by anastomosing the cervical oesophagus to the gastric fundus. This will avoid anastomotic leak into the mediastinum (fatal). Any leak will be onto the skin cervical incision (external).

Lower third carcinoma (Fig. 3.9.3)

- Below the diaphragm (in the absence of peritoneal or visceral spread): needs radical left abdominothoracic approach (Garlock), excising the tumour-bearing area with the stomach, spleen, pancreatic tail, greater and lesser omenta, and the regional lymphatic field and restoring continuity by oesophagojejunal anastomosis (Roux-en-Y) or oesophagogastrostomy.
- Above the diaphragm: is better excised by Lewis–Tanner operation (the two-stage procedure). Via a laparotomy, the stomach is mobilised on the right gastric and gastroepiploic arteries with Kocherisation of the second part of the duodenum and pyloromyotomy (vagotomy is done with tumour excision). After the abdominal closure, the second stage is performed, consisting of right thoracotomy through which the tumour and the lower oesophagus are mobilised and the stomach is drawn into the chest. The tumour, with adequate clearance of normal oesophagus, and the proximal stomach are resected and continuity is restored by oesophagogastric anastomosis.

The anastomosis is of two layers interrupted with non-absorbable sutures (mucosa is the toughest coat). The gastric fundus is anchored posteriorly by stitching it to the mediastinal pleura and anteriorly it is folded over the anastomosis to reinforce the suture line.

Nasogastric tube suction (although it splints the anastomosis) may have the disadvantages of:
- Introducing infection to the suture line.
- The swallowed saliva and secretions may become stuck to the suture line because of the tube.
- Trauma from the tube in the form of pressure necrosis or accidental suction. The patient is therefore better managed without nasogastric tube suction.

Preoperative preparations are like those for total gastrectomy. Postoperative i.v. fluids (and nothing orally) with small Gastrografin swallow on the 5–7th day when the chest drain may be removed if there is no anastomotic leak.

Billroth I partial gastrectomy (Fig. 3.9.4)

1. Mobilise the greater curvature and divide the left gastric vessels.
2. Dissect out the first and second parts of the duodenum (Kocherisation).
3. Divide the duodenum and keep it closed with a non-crushing clamp.
4. Divide the stomach, leaving approximately one-fifth. Close the upper part of it, leaving an aperture the size of the duodenum adjacent to the greater curvature, and approximate it to the duodenum with two layers of sutures.
5. Close the dangerous superior duodenogastric angle of Sorrow with a triple stitch, i.e. take a bite first of the anterior wall of the stomach, then the posterior wall, and finally the superior aspect of the duodenum. If possible, this suture may be repeated at a higher level as a reinforcement.
6. Drain the anastomosis and close the abdomen.

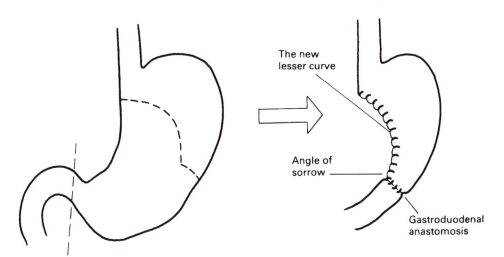

Fig. 3.9.4 Billroth I partial gastrectomy

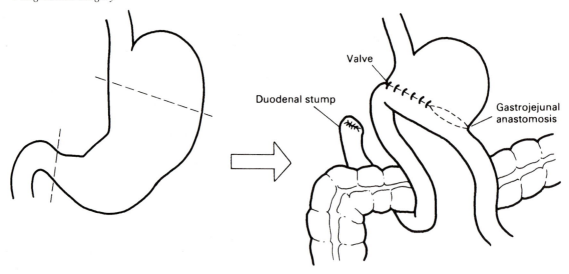

Fig. 3.9.5   Polya partial gastrectomy

Polya partial gastrectomy (Fig. 3.9.5)

1. Nasogastric tube and i.v. drip. General anaesthesia and supine position.
2. The incision is usually midline, but may be on the left for gastric ulcer or on the right for duodenal ulcer. Quick peritoneal exploration is then done.
3. Mobilise the greater curvature of the stomach and preserve the middle colic vessels and mesocolon. Excise three-quarters of the stomach and ligate and divide the left gastric vessels.
4. Mobilise all aspects of the first portion of the duodenum, ligating the right gastric artery. When dissecting the duodenum, keep close to it.
5. Apply two occluding and two crushing clamps and carefully clear the stomach at the proposed site for anastomosis. Divide and close the duodenum with two layers of sutures.
6. Bring up a short loop of the first part of the jejunum and anastomose it to the divided stomach, usually afferent to the lesser curve.
7. The results with antecolic or retrocolic anastomoses are similar; antecolic are easier to dismantle and are therefore preferred.
8. The afferent loop of jejunum is kept as short as possible. It may be fixed to the colon with a suture to prevent internal strangulation.

Notes.
- An adherent gastric ulcer may be pinched off the pancreas with the fingers or, if this is impossible, excluded by excision.
- The upper part of the divided stomach may be closed to form a Hofmeister valve.
- Difficult duodenal ulcer may require Nissen's procedure, i.e. closure of the duodenum by suturing the anterior duodenal wall onto the ulcer.

Total gastrectomy (Fig. 3.9.6)

1. A drip and nasogastric tube are *in situ*. A long left paramedian incision followed by quick peritoneal exploration.
2. Mobilise the greater curvature up to the oesophagus. Divide the left gastric vessels and extend the division of the lesser omentum as far as the oesophagus. This manoeuvre is aided by mobilising the left lobe of the liver by dividing the coronary ligament.
3. Mobilise all aspects of the first part of the duodenum, divide and close it.
4. A loop of jejunum is brought up either in front of, or behind, the colon and anastomosed to the oesophagus in two layers behind the stomach, which is amputated only when the anastomosis is nearly completed. The mucosa is the strong layer in the oesophagus. To avoid 'drag', suture the anastomosis to its surroundings. Great care should be employed in forming this anastomosis as it leaks easily. It is performed in two layers with non-absorbable material. Alternatively, a Roux-en-Y procedure may be used. A side-to-side anastomosis is made in the jejunal loop (Braun). The Ryle's tube may be left in, either with its tip just above the anastomosis, or through it (see above 'Operations for oesophageal carcinoma').

3.10 Splenectomy

Indications

- Traumatic splenic rupture.
- Shunt operations in portal hypertension except for distal splenorenal shunt.
- Haemolytic anaemia in congenital spherocytosis and thrombocytopenic purpura.

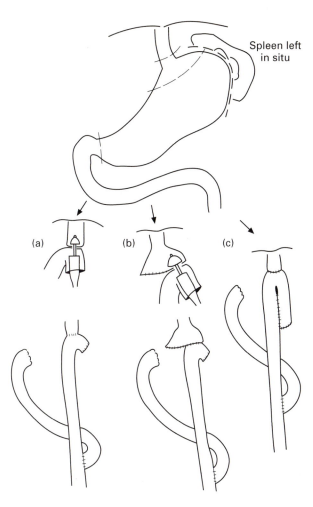

Spleen left
in situ

(a)　　　　(b)　　　　(c)

Fig. 3.9.6 Total gastrectomy and Roux-en-Y oesophagojejunostomy with or without fundal pouch (a,b) or with neostomach/jejunal pouch (c)

- Staging laparotomy in Hodgkin's lymphoma.
- Part of proximal and total gastrectomy, lower oesophagectomy and distal pancreatectomy.

Procedure (Fig. 3.10.1)

Preoperatively a nasogastric tube is passed (to facilitate the operation and prevent postoperative gastric distension and paralytic ileus), with intravenous drip and possible blood transfusion (in trauma) or platelet solution (in thrombocytopenia).

1. Under general anaesthesia and supine position.
2. Left upper paramedian or left subcostal incision.
3. Once in the peritoneal cavity, quick exploration.
4. The surgeon (standing to the right of the patient), passes his left hand round the spleen while the assistant retracts the skin for good exposure. The surgeon uses his right hand to cut the posterior layer of the lienorenal ligament by sharp and blunt dissection.

5. Spleen is rotated medially and delivered through the incision while a large pack is inserted.
6. Gastrosplenic ligament containing the vasa brevia and part of the left gastroepiploic blood vessel is ligated and divided without traumatising the stomach's greater curvature.
7. Careful separation of the pancreatic tail from splenic hilum followed by double ligation of splenic blood vessels, individually if possible, with a non-absorbable suture, e.g. silk.
8. Search for spleniculi and then insert sump drain (in case of unrecognised damage to pancreatic tail).
9. Closure in layers.

Complications

Unexplained postoperative abdominal pain with fever may herald portal vein thrombosis (when anticoagulants and antibiotics must be given). Other possible complications include acute gastric distension, paralytic ileus, left basal atelectasis, haematemesis (due to gastric mucosal congestion after vasa brevia ligation), pancreatic leak and possible abdominal wound dehiscence or persistent hiccup due to left subphrenic irritation by blood collection or an abscess.

3.11 Cholecystectomy and Common Bile Duct Exploration

Prophylactic antibiotics (cefuroxime 750 mg. i.m. three times a day) to prevent postoperative infection, 500 ml mannitol 10% infusion pre- and peroperatively to prevent hepatorenal shutdown and failure, low-dose heparin (5000 i.u. subcutaneously daily) with premedication until mobilisation postoperatively with stockings to prevent deep venous thrombosis are all recommended especially in *jaundiced* patients with recent biliary obstruction. Preoperative reduction of weight and cessation of smoking with postoperative physiotherapy are essential to reduce pulmonary atelactasis. (Nasogastric suction, used peroperatively to decompress the stomach for the benefit of the surgeon and anaesthetist, should be avoided postoperatively since there is no anastomosis to rest and the transnasal tube makes coughing difficult, dries inspired air and results in higher incidence of pulmonary atelactasis. Postoperatively acute gastric dilatation is rare and when nausea or vomiting starts postoperatively then only suction is required.)

1. Under general anaesthesia and supine position (with right arm extended) on special radiolucent operating table. Surgeon is better operating on right side of the patient in cholecystectomy and should change his position to the left side when he attempts exploration of the common bile duct.
2. Via right upper paramedian in narrow costal margin, subcostal Kocher's (wide costal margin) or upper midline incision. Quick exploration for associated hiatus hernia and diverticular colonic diverticula (Saint's triad), and of stomach, duodenum (e.g. ulcers), pancreas (e.g. chronic pancreatitis with

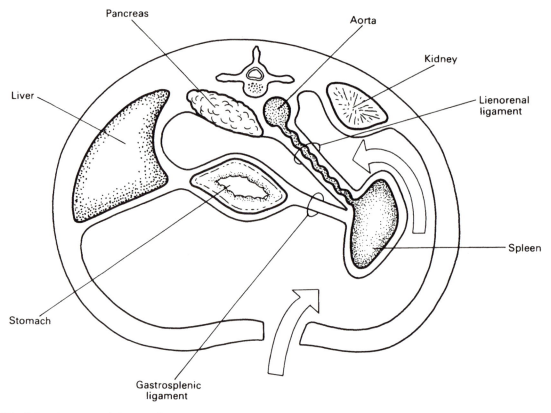

Fig. 3.10.1   Splenectomy – surgical approach

enlarged head and foci of fat necrosis) and liver (e.g. cirrhosis or cancer). Insert a finger into the foramen of Winslow (epiploic foramen) to palpate the bile duct for stone. Insert the right hand above the liver to allow air to pass behind it and to help drop it for easy operation on the gallbladder. Decide whether it is necessary to preserve the gallbladder for bypass (e.g. in carcinoma of pancreatic head).

3. The assistant's help is required in packing off the lesser curvature of the stomach to the left, and the duodenum and colon downwards (insert retractors). A third retractor on the liver exposes the cystic duct area.

4. To aid dissection apply sponge-holding forceps to the fundus of the gallbladder and Moynihan forceps to Hartmann's pouch to manipulate the cystic duct.

5. Nick and strip off the peritoneum over the ducts. With further dissection using a swab on sponge forceps and/or Lahey's swab (baby dab) identify the cystic artery by tracing it to the gallbladder. It runs inside the Calot triangle formed by the cystic duct, bile duct and lower hepatic edge. Free, clamp and divide it followed by application of ligatures (linen).

6. Dissect further to show clearly the termination of the cystic duct – ligate proximally. Operative cholangiography may now be carried out using 25% Hypaque through a Stoke-on-Trent cannula fixed in place by ligature after being introduced into the cystic duct. The proximal end of the cystic duct may then be divided. Two films are taken after an injection of 5 ml (to delineate small impacted stones) and 10 ml (to reveal the biliary flow into the duodenum) of Hypaque respectively. Look at the

diameter of the common bile duct (should not be more than 12 mm), filling defect, dye flow to duodenum and lower narrow intramural biliary segment (Fig. 3.11.1). The cystic duct stump is then ligated (00 linen or silk) 3 mm from common bile duct as *flush ligation may cause stenosis.*

7. Remove the gallbladder by dividing its attachments to the liver and its peritoneal reflection. Gallbladder bed haemostasis is established by coagulation with no need for suturing the bed. A drain is left in the gallbladder area and brought out through a separate opening in the flank.

8. The classical indications for opening the common bile duct if operative cholangiogram is not available are:

● History of jaundice, abnormal liver functions, Charcot's triad (fever, pain and jaundice); oral cholecystogram showing multiple small stones in the gallbladder with patent or dilated cystic duct.

● Operative finding of dilated common bile duct more than 12 mm, palpation of stone (or aspiration of biliary mud), periductal fibrosis and pancreatitis (indurated), thickened gallbladder with no stone or with single-faceted stone.

9. To open the common bile duct free a part of its anterior wall *above the duodenum*, then insert two stay sutures through the wall. If identification of the duct is uncertain, aspirate the contents with a needle. Before opening the common bile duct, pack off the area and have a sucker in readiness. The stay sutures are held taut and a small longitudinal cut is made in the common bile duct *as close to the duodenum as possible* to leave a good upper portion as a safeguard in case further surgery is

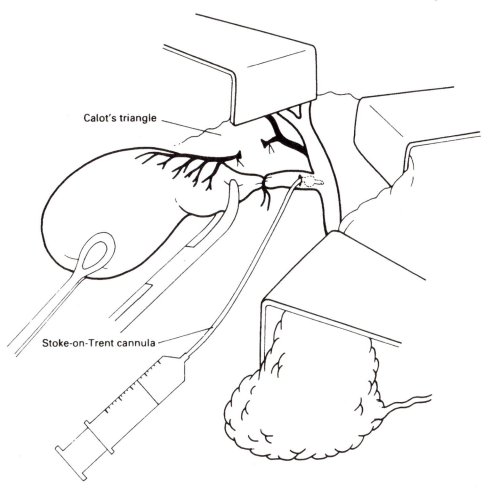

Calot's triangle

Stoke-on-Trent cannula

Fig. 3.11.1 Cholecystectomy and peroperative cholangiogram

required. Lower CBD incision avoids stenosis formation which may need reconstructive surgery in future using the upper portion of CBD; a lower cut also reduces the likelihood of stump syndrome and reflux from the duodenum.

10. The duct is explored. A variety of instruments are available, for example, Bakes' dilators, Lister's bougies, gum elastic bougies, Desjardin's forceps, Jack's catheter and Fogarty's biliary catheter. The duct is thin-walled and stones usually stick at the lower end causing ball-valve obstruction and poor visualisation of the terminal distal narrow part of the common bile duct on cholangiography. Exploration should be atraumatic; the use of a Fogarty catheter is usually successful and clearly demonstrates the site and patency of the sphincter of Oddi. Rigid metallic instruments such as bougies and Desjardin's forceps can cause damage to the duct wall and false passages and should be used carefully. After removal of any stones and debris, the duct is washed out with saline (Fig. 3.11.2a).

11. An attempt is now made to dilate the sphincter of Oddi by the passage of bougies. These instruments must be passed through the sphincter.

12. If unsuccessful because of stricture or impacted stone at the lower end of the common bile duct then the second part of the duodenum is mobilised (Kocherisation), opened vertically, and the sphincter of Oddi is divided under vision. Find the site of the sphincteric opening by palpating the tip of the Fogarty catheter or probe passed down the common bile duct from above. Divide the sphincter at 12 o'clock (sphincterotomy), or sphincteroplasty may be carried out.

13. Close the duodenum with two layers transversely.

14. In the elderly, unfit patient with difficult anatomy, e.g. gross obesity, and if there is concern about residual stone or biliary mud, choledochoduodenostomy is recommended (Fig. 3.11.2b) – a transverse low incision in the common bile duct is sutured to a longitudinal parallel duodenal incision after Kocherisation to construct a stoma as wide as the duct calibre permits. There is little evidence to support the claim that there is a higher incidence of ascending cholangitis with such a bypass operation. Sphincteroplasty is necessary if there is a concomitant stricture.

15. Insert a T-tube into the supraduodenal common duct opening. Close the opening around the tube with 2/0 catgut (interrupted). The duct is not closed until it is established that there is no residual pathology as this leads to immediate and late complications. Any rise in pressure in the duct is associated

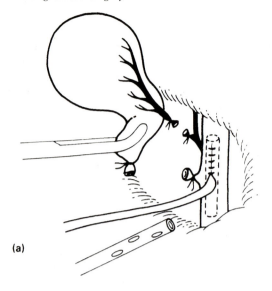

(a)

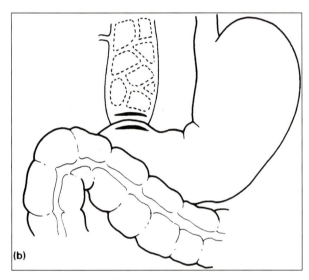

(b)

Fig. 3.11.2 Common bile duct exploration (temporary and permanent drainage). (a) Supraduodenal common bile duct exploration with T-tube insertion. (b) Choledochoduodenostomy. (CBD is cut transversely if dilated and longitudinally if not)

with increased leakage around the T-tube into the peritoneal cavity, and continued obstruction makes ascending cholangitis and septicaemia more likely. Although such pathology can be dealt with postoperatively by retrieval under radiographic control via T-tube track and retrograde cannulation of the sphincter and papillotomy, this does not avoid prolonged hospitalisation, patient suffering and further anaesthetics. The available alternatives are:

● T-tube postexploratory cholangiography (with or without contact cholangiography). Has the disadvantage of leakage around the T-tube during injection of dye preventing adequate filling of the distal end where spasm may have occurred as a result of manipulation of the sphincter area. Serial films can reduce this problem. Contact cholangiography by inserting a dental film below the second part of the

duodenum after Kocherisation can improve visualisation of the distal part of the duct, revealing small impacted stones. However, it is not widely used.

● Foley cholangiography requires practise to ensure adequate obstruction of the lumen of the duct to prevent backflow.

● Choledochoscopy is expensive as regards purchase of the instrument, requires practice, is impossible in narrow ducts and does not permit examination of the smaller proximal ducts.

16. Add a tube drain to drain the gallbladder bed. Place Surgicel into the gallbladder bed if oozing.

17. Bring out drainage tubes carefully through separate openings.

Postoperative points

● If the T-tube is pulled out by accident, open the abdomen and replace it immediately.
● Clamp T-tube from the fifth day.
● Remove the tube drain on the fifth day.
● T-tube choledochogram is taken on the 10th day.
● Remove the T-tube if X-ray is satisfactory.

Postoperative excessive biliary leak

From the abdominal drain or as a persistent fistula is due to:
● Accidental damage of a duct during the operation.
● Residual impacted stone in the lower part of the common bile duct causing obstruction, increased intrabiliary pressure and bursting of cystic duct ligature.
● Distal stricture especially in chronic pancreatitis.
● Slipped cystic duct ligature (technical).
● Leak from gallbladder bed due to congenital cholecystohepatic duct. Accumulation of bile subhepatically or subphrenically may lead to upper abdominal or chest pain, tachycardia, hypotension and is often mistaken for coronary thrombosis. The condition needs immediate reexploration and bile drainage, which produces dramatic relief. The condition is termed the *Waltman–Walters syndrome.*

NB For laparoscopic cholecystectomy please see Section 1.14 on minimal access therapy.

3.12 Restorative Rectal Resection and Abdominoperineal Excision of Rectum

Restorative rectal resection

Requirements

● The growth should be early cancer, i.e. stage A or B, maximum C1.
● On biopsy the histological differentiation should be good or moderate (but never undifferentiated = anaplastic).
● The growth should be at least 10 cm above the anal verge since 5 cm is needed for macroscopic tumour clearance to prevent future recurrence and another 5 cm is needed for

intact sensation and to prevent incontinence. This rule has now been waived in view of the stapling and double-stapling technique, making a 2 cm safety margin above the dentate line suficient for anastomosis. Owing to the tortuous course of the rectum the growth felt by a finger in rectal examination at a level of 7.5 cm from the anal verge could be telescoped; after operative mobilisation it may be found to be 10 cm from the anal verge.

● Colon should be normal, i.e. free from ulcerative colitis, Crohn's disease, diverticular disease and polyposis coli. Pelvic mesocolon is preferably long for anastomosis.
● The patient should not be too fat.
● The patient's pelvis should be normal or wide, i.e. shallow wide female pelvis is preferred to the male pelvis which is deep and narrow.
● When hepatic secondaries are present this operation is preferred if other requirements are fulfilled.

Thorough preoperative bowel preparation is essential (see s. 1.49).

Procedure

1. A nasogastric tube, an i.v. drip and urethral catheter are placed in situ. General anaesthesia and Trendelenburg's position, with the surgeon standing on the left side of the patient.
2. A long left paramedian incision is made. The abdomen is opened and explored for another primary colonic cancer and hepatic secondaries. After examining the blood supply of the mesocolon and the growth, the sites for division of the colon and rectum are decided upon.
3. The pelvic colon is held and the rest of the bowel packed away; a self-retaining retractor is placed in the wound. In females the uterus with adnexae can be sutured and retracted anteriorly (Fig. 3.12.1).

4. The pelvic colon is partly freed by dividing the congenital adhesions on its lateral aspect and the peritoneum of the pelvic floor is then demarcated by dividing it with scissors; the incision runs from the colon at the proposed site of division laterally over the mesocolon, anteriorly across the base of the bladder or region of the cervix 12 mm in front of the lowest point of the peritoneal floor, then upwards on the medial side of the mesocolon, returning to the original level. The peritoneum of the pelvis is then raised by sharp and blunt dissection safeguarding the ureters and genital vessels.
5. Commencing at the proposed site for division of the colon (Fig. 3.12.2a), the mesocolon is divided down to its root. The main pedicle containing the superior haemorrhoidal vessels is dissected free and (after ensuring that both ureters are safe) ligated and divided.
6. Good mobilisation then follows and the rectosigmoid mesentery is freed from the sacrum by a few cuts with the scissors; by digital dissection posteriorly, the fascia of Waldeyer may be reached posterior to the rectum. The dissection anterior to the rectum is then commenced and the seminal vesicles or vaginal wall identified. By division of bands behind

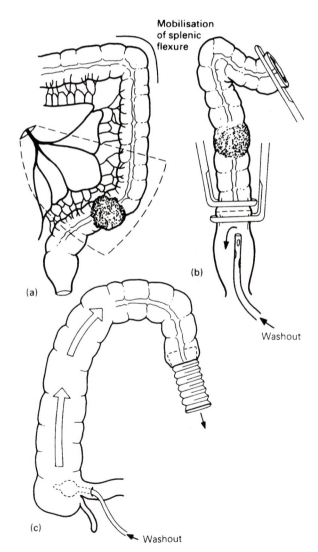

Fig. 3.12.2 Restorative rectal (anterior) resection

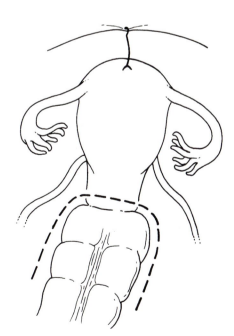

Fig. 3.12.1 Division of pelvic peritoneum prior to rectal mobilisation in the female

the seminal vesicles or vaginal wall, the fascia of Denonvilliers is opened and a plane of dissection found leading down to the apex of the prostate or the perineal body. The lateral ligaments containing the middle haemorrhoidal vessels are ligated and divided. Mesorectum is also divided.

7. Proposed sites for division are cleared of fat. A right-angled clamp is placed over the rectum, and the rectum may be washed out, e.g. with Noxyflex solution (Fig. 3.12.2b), after a gentle anal stretch. Crushing clamps are now placed above and below, and the diseased bowel and its mesentery removed. For clearing faecal contents of the upper bowel end perform an intraoperative washout. Foley's catheter is inserted into the caecum through a purse-string in the terminal ileum (Fig. 3.12.2c) and fluid is let out through a corrugated tube fitted to the proximal end. This end is then recut and prepared for anastomosis.

8. The end of the colon is anastomosed to the upper end of the rectum using single interrupted serososubmucosal (2/0 silk), or double-layer seromuscular interrupted (2/0 silk) and continuous mucosal (chromic catgut) sutures. Horizontal mattress sutures of non-absorbable material are recommended.

9. The floor of the peritoneum is closed (controversial) with paracolic tube drainage, then the wound is closed.

Abdominoperineal excision of rectum

- *Abdominal dissection*   The dissection proceeds as described in 'Restorative rectal resection'. However here the patient is in the lithotomy-Trendelenburg position, using a Lloyd–Davies' apparatus. A sandbag or 'rest' under the sacrum facilitates the approach to the coccyx.
- *Perineal dissection*

  1. The anus is closed with two purse-string sutures. An elliptical incision is made around the anus and is deepened through the perineal space and fascia into the ischiorectal fossa.

  2. This incision is extended on both sides so that a finger may be introduced around the ileococcygeus to facilitate its division, and the inferior rectal vessels are ligated.

  3. A self-retaining retractor may be inserted.

  4. Mobilisation: the fascia of Waldeyer posterior to the rectum is divided, and the tissues are divided anterior to the rectum, keeping behind the transverse perineal muscles. Anteriorly the pubococcygeus muscle is divided. The prostate and urethra with catheter are identified and by further careful division, the plane of Denonvilliers is entered, lying behind the prostate. The bowel turns sharply backwards at the anorectal junction and the dissection must follow this line to avoid urethral damage. The abdominal surgeon assists in defining the tissue planes (until both surgeons shake hands inside the pelvis). The lateral ligaments are ligated and divided. With anterior growths (in females), the whole posterior portion of the vagina is excised.

  5. The perineal wound is closed with drainage (either Redivac or wide tube inserted via ischiorectal fat). The vaginal orifice is re-formed.

- Terminal end left iliac permanent colostomy is then performed.

3.13 Thyroidectomy

Indications for operation

- Solitary thyroid nodule.
- Pressure symptoms, e.g. on trachea (dyspnoea), on oesophagus (dysphagia) and on recurrent laryngeal nerve (hoarseness).
- Ectopic thyroid, e.g. lingual or retrosternal goitre due to dysphagia and dyspnoea respectively with possible future mitotic (malignancy) changes and bleeding.
- Secondary thyrotoxicosis in multinodular goitre.
- Primary thyrotoxicosis (this is medically treated) only if:
  – ineffective medical treatment;
  – recurrence after medical treatment;
  – allergy or side-effects of drugs;
  – economic consideration (drug price).
- Cosmetic.
- Malignant thyroid disease (treated by total thyroidectomy); suspected when there is:
  – a rapidly enlarging solitary thyroid nodule or recent change in a long-standing goitre;
  – hard swelling in part or whole;
  – no mobility of gland with swallowing;
  – Berry's sign: absent carotid pulsation because of surrounding infiltrating tumour. Classically goitre displaces the carotid artery backward and outward, so the pulsation is felt behind the posterior edge of the goite;
  – tracheal obstruction;
  – local spread suggested by hoarseness and Horner's syndrome (meiosis, enophthalmus, ptosis and anhidrosis);
  – lymph node enlargement usually unilaterally. Biopsy is essential. The so-called ectopic thyroid is in fact thyroid metastatic disease in the lymph node which may be the only manifestation of an occult primary impalpable thyroid carcinoma.

Partial (subtotal) thyroidectomy

Preoperative

Cervical X-ray to show any calcification, retrosternal extension, cervical osteoarthrosis or tortuous trachea (important for anaesthetist). Indirect laryngoscopy to detect any recurrent laryngeal nerve paralysis and treatment of thyrotoxicosis (e.g. propranolol (Inderal) 40 mg tablet three times daily until sleeping pulse rate is below 100 per min.

Procedure (Fig. 3.13.1a–c)

1. Endotracheal general anaesthesia with neck hyperextension. A sandbag between the shoulders and horse-shoe ring below head and special draping.

2. A collar incision is made one finger's breadth above the suprasternal notch. Deepen the incision through the platysma on both sides beyond the sternomastoid borders.

3. By sharp dissection raise the upper flap until the thyroid notch is reached and raise the lower flap down to the suprasternal notch. Joll's self-retaining retractor is then applied.

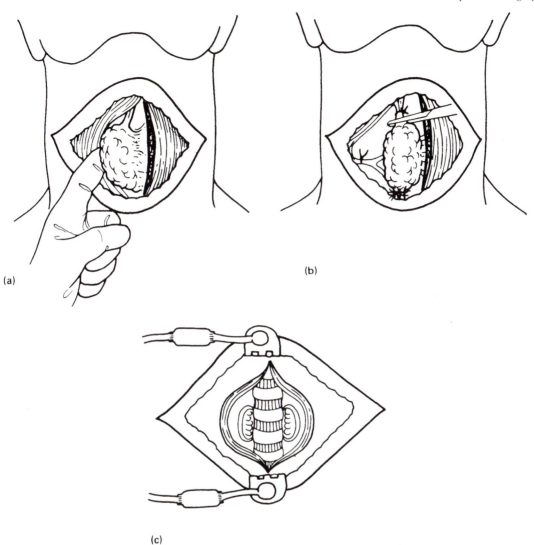

Fig. 3.13.1 Partial thyroidectomy. (a) Exposure and mobilisation. (b) Vascular ligation and division. Joll's retraction in (a) and (b) is not shown. (c) Reconstruction after excision

4. Divide the deep fascia vertically in the midline until the thyroid isthmus is exposed. Raise the strap muscles on one side to expose the lateral lobe, insert retractors and continue the dissection until the entire lobe is clearly visible. Divide and ligate the middle thyroid vein.

5. Full mobilisation using sharp scissors and blunt dissection (Lahey's swab); dislocate the lateral lobe into the wound. If necessary, to improve exposure, divide the strap muscles between forceps at the level of the cricoid cartilage, to preserve their nerve supply (from ansa cervicalis below).

6. Dissect in the middle, laterally and posteriorly to the lobe of the thyroid and identify the inferior thyroid artery, recurrent laryngeal nerve (in the groove between the trachea and oesophagus close to the terminal branches of the inferior thyroid artery) and parathyroids. Ligate the artery in continuity *well away from the gland* to avoid recurrent laryngeal nerve injury.

7. Mobilise the upper pole, insert Kocher's director behind it and doubly ligate the superior thyroid vessels. Apply artery forceps and divide *close to the gland* to avoid injuring the external branch of the superior laryngeal nerve (supplies cricothyroid muscle and its damage causes hoarseness of voice).

8. Expose the front of the trachea by dividing the inferior thyroid *plexus of veins* and free the pyramidal lobe, if present.

9. Change to the opposite side of the patient; free the other lobe and deal similarly with its vessels.

10. Apply a series of forceps (markers) around the gland and divide it. Continue dividing the gland by applying forceps to the gland substance until the trachea is reached and the gland is shaved from it. Most of the lateral lobes, the whole of the isthmus and pyramidal lobe are removed. Two small posterior portions (4 g) of gland are left on either side of the trachea.

11. Suture the remaining part of the gland, if it is bleeding, to the side of the trachea (reconstruction). Insert two Redivac drains so that they emerge through the deep fascia at the lateral aspects of the wound or through individual stab wounds. Close the deep fascia (interrupted 2/0 chromic catgut). Remove the sandbag from beneath the shoulders and approximate the platysma with fine plain catgut (interrupted). Suture drainage tubes to the skin, then close the wound with clips.

Postoperative complications

Early

● Tension haematoma – needs immediate evacuation or aspiration.
● Respiratory obstruction due to tension haematoma, laryngeal spasm, unilateral or bilateral recurrent nerve paralysis, or rarely to collapse or kinking of the trachea – needs endotracheal intubation, steroids for several days and, rarely, tracheostomy.
● Recurrent laryngeal nerve paralysis (unilateral or bilateral, complete or partial, transient or permanent). Superior laryngeal nerve paralysis lead to hoarseness of voice only.
● Thyrotoxic crisis occurs rarely in thyrotoxic patients with inadequate preparation – treated by hydration, antipyretics, steroids and propranolol 20 mg 6 hourly.

Intermediate

Include parathyroid insufficiency after 2–5 days, occasionally delayed for 3 weeks. Treated by calcium therapy.

Late

Include wound infection, keloid scar and thyroid insufficiency (occurs within 2 years) or recurrent thyrotoxicosis.

3.14 Superficial (Suprafacial) Parotidectomy

Procedure (Fig. 3.14.1)

Warn the patient of possible damage to the facial nerve, or even of its deliberate removal if found necessary.

1. General anaesthesia with hypotension, if necessary. The table head is tilted upwards to collapse the external jugular veins and the patient's head is extended and turned away from the surgeon.

2. Make a cervicomastoid-facial S-shaped incision which runs vertically down just in front of the pinna and curves backwards below it; the pinna may be sutured and retracted.

3. The skin flaps are widely mobilised and held back by stay sutures to reveal all aspects of the gland. The great auricular nerve may be preserved or sacrificed (a piece of the nerve may be saved in saline to be used as a nerve graft in case of inadvertent facial nerve injury during operation).

4. Identify and safeguard the facial nerve and its two major subdivisions, the upper temporofacial and lower cervicofacial

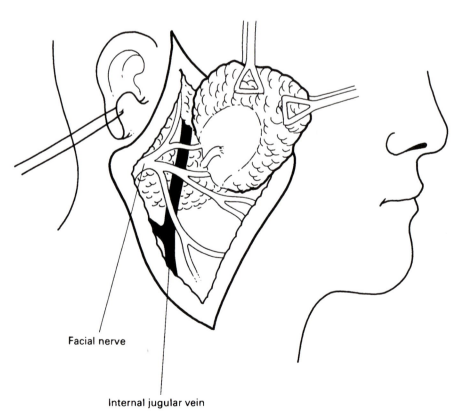

Facial nerve

Internal jugular vein

Fig. 3.14.1   Superficial (suprafacial) parotidectomy

nerves (joined in a goose-foot fashion – *pes anserinus*), by identifying the junction of the cartilaginous and bony meatus behind the gland and following the nerve up above the posterior belly of the digastric and as it emerges from below the mastoid process. Pinching the nerve elicits facial twitching, and a nerve stimulator is sometimes useful.

5. Fine mosquito forceps are thrust with blades closed along the facial nerve branch then opened and lifted and the overlying tissue cut with scissors. This manoeuvre can be repeated for full exposure of facial nerve branches.

6. The superficial lobe is removed with the duct after division near the masseter, preserving the facial nerve (remember that the facial nerve is sandwiched between the superficial and the deep part of the gland, which are connected by the isthmus).

7. Close the skin with or without a Redivac drain.

3.15 Block Dissection

This is a radical wide excision of the lymphatic field (including lymph nodes and intervening lymphatic pathways). It is done either *prophylactically* if the lymphatic field is adjacent to but not involving the primary tumour (e.g. face and neck, axilla in breast cancer, or back melanoma and groin) or *therapeutically* if the lymph nodes are enlarged because of infiltration by an operable curable adjacent primary growth. Preferably no prophylactic block dissection is carried out if the primary tumour is remote from the lymphatic field, e.g. in melanoma of the sole of the foot there is no need for groin block dissection *unless* the inguinal lymph nodes are enlarged. No block dissection is performed:

● If the primary growth is not curable or is inoperable.
● When there are distant metastases.

Sites

Cervical block dissection

Crile's complete block dissection Performed unilaterally (when bilateral block dissection is required it must be undertaken consecutively with an interval of 3 weeks, and never simultaneously. Removal of both internal jugular veins is not associated with much obstructed cerebral circulation as was previously conjectured). It is indicated for primary growths involving:

● Oral cavity (tongue, mouth floor, mandible tumours).
● Larynx (glottic, subglottic, supraglottic).
● Facial area (melanoma, lip squamous cell carcinoma).
● Neck (thyroid papillary carcinoma, malignant parotid and submandibular salivary glands).

Suprahyoid block dissection Indicated in carcinoma of the lower lip, early carcinoma of the tip of the tongue and early carcinoma of the mouth floor. Bilateral block dissection is possible at one operation. Unilateral suprahyoid block dissection can be combined with Crile's block dissection of the opposite side.

Axillary block dissection

In breast carcinoma (radical and Patey's modified radical mastectomies) and in melanoma of the back (usually unilateral block dissection is performed on the side nearest to the melanoma but bilateral block dissection is done in upper midline back melanoma).

Groin block dissection

In melanoma of lower limb. Occasionally in penile, scrotal and vulval carcinomas.

Retroperitoneal block dissection

In testicular malignancy (not practised now).

Procedure of cervical block dissection (Fig. 3.15.1)

This major operation is now safe and the 5 year survival rate is 35% with an operative mortality of less than 3%. Surprisingly little deformity follows block dissection but the neck is stiff and there may be drooping of the mouth corner (as a result of injury to the cervical branch of the facial nerve).

1. Blood transfusion, prophylactic antibiotic; tracheostomy may be required (rarely in suprahyoid block dissection). Endotracheal anaesthesia is employed, a sandbag is placed between the shoulders and the head turned to the opposite side.

2. The incision commences behind the mastoid process, curves downwards and forwards 3 cm below the angle of the jaw, and then upwards to terminate on the chin just the other side of the

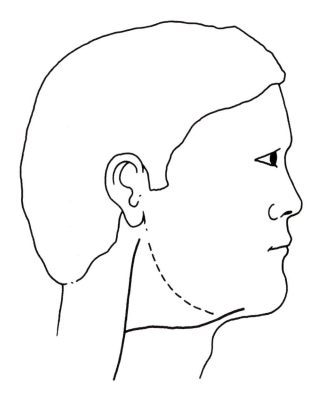

Fig. 3.15.1 Incision in cervical block dissection

midline. A vertical incision is made from the middle of this incision down to the middle of the clavicle. The skin flaps are reflected back.

3. Two veins are divided, one in front and one behind the sternomastoid. Divide the sternomastoid just above the clavicle, dividing the external jugular vein posteriorly. Dissect out the internal jugular vein anteriorly from the carotid sheath and divide it. It is dangerous to divide the internal jugular vein if it has been recently resected on the opposite side.

4. Clearance of supraclavicular fossa and division of omohyoid. The brachial nerves are seen covered by a thin layer of prevertebral fascia. Branches of the subclavian vessels are ligated. The thoracic duct on the left side is preserved. The accessory nerve and ansa cervicalis are divided.

5. Continuation of dissection to hyoid level. The tributaries of the internal jugular, middle and superior thyroid and inferior thyroid vessels, and later the common facial vein and artery, are divided. The thyroid isthmus is divided and hemithyroidectomy performed with removal of the strap muscles. Preserve the recurrent laryngeal nerve unless a laryngectomy has already been done. Identify and preserve the hypoglossal nerve, then divide the central tendon of the digastric muscle to open up the dissection. At this stage the common facial vein is divided. Identify the facial and occipital arteries arising from the external carotid, and divide them between ligatures.

6. Dissect and dislocate the submandibular gland, including its deep portion, divide the duct close to the gland and turn it upwards. Preserve the lingual nerve.

7. Dissect out the internal jugular vein carefully and doubly ligate and divide it at the base of the skull.

8. Division of mass. Commencing posteriorly divide the sternomastoid and digastric, remove the tail of the parotid if necessary, then cut along the lower border of the jaw, ligating the facial vessels, until the opposite side of the midline is reached and the mass removed.

9. Close the skin and drain the wound with a Redivac suction drain.

3.16 Modified Patey's Radical Mastectomy

Procedure (Fig. 3.16.1)

1. Under general anaesthesia and in the supine position. The arm is held at right angles to the body on an arm board or suspended from a drip stand by a sling around the wrist. Care is taken to avoid traction injuries of the brachial plexus.

2. Define the margins of the growth. Make an elliptical semitransverse incision including the nipple, the skin over the growth, and 5 cm of normal skin beyond its margin. Avoid placing the upper part of the incision along the inferior margin of the anterior axillary fold, as a 'bridle-scar' develops.

3. Deepen the skin incision and reflect the lateral and medial flaps including a small amount of subcutaneous fat. Approximately half the subcutaneous fat is left on the skin, and the thinner the patient, the greater the care required to avoid cutting

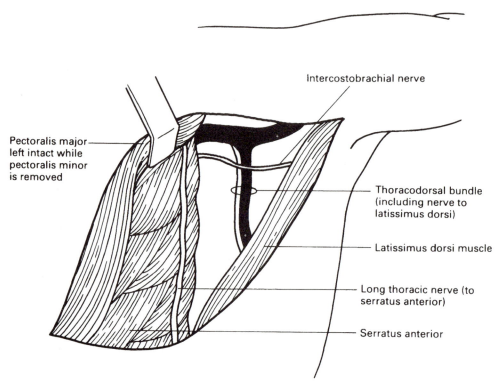

Fig. 3.16.1   Patey's modified radical mastectomy

into the breast tissue (recognised by its white colour). Mobilise the lateral flap as far back as the anterior border of latissimus dorsi. Mobilise the upper half of the medial flap to the medial end of the clavicle. Confine your dissection to the lateral flap. The medial side of the mass is usually disconnected towards the end of the operation.

4. Preserve pectoralis major and the area below it. Divide the pectoralis minor tendon immediately below its coracoid insertion and the fascia on either side. The axillary vessels and nerves together with their covering fascial sheath are exposed.

5. The axilla is then dissected from the side of the axillary vein, proceeding medially, and from the apex of the axilla passing downwards by a combination of sharp and blunt dissection. The small vein tributaries of the axillary vein are cleared and divided 6 mm from the main vein. These veins are ligated carefully to avoid air embolus.

6. The intercostobrachial nerve and the nerves of latissimus dorsi and serratus anterior are preserved. (Note that the nerve to latissimus is found superficially near the subscapular vessels.) The nerves may rarely be sacrificed if involved glands are found to be adherent to them.

7. The breast is excised from the chest wall, clipping the lateral and anterior perforating branches before division. Excision of the mass of tissue is carried to the opposite side of the midline.

8. The rest of the medial flap still attached is mobilised to complete excision.

9. Careful haemostasis is obtained (and an immediate or late skin graft is applied, if necessary, to avoid suturing under tension).

10. Two Redivac drains are left in (axillary and subcutaneous) for 5 and 3 days respectively. The axillary tube drains lymph from axillary disturbed lymphatics (lymphorrhoea). Interrupted or subcuticular skin closure is used.

3.17 Vascular Bypass and Abdominal Aortic Aneurysm Surgery

AORTOFEMORAL BYPASS
(in Leriche syndrome)

Indications

This procedure is used in patients with severely disabling claudication or with ischaemic rest pain or gangrene in whom there is occlusive disease of the distal aorta and iliac arteries.

Preoperative preparation

Routine blood investigations, chest X-ray, ECG, 4 units of blood cross-matched; nasogastric tube, urethral catheter, pre-operative wide-spectrum antibiotic.

Procedure (Fig. 3.17.1b)

1. Incision, laparotomy and exposure of the aortoiliac system as described below in the operation for elective aortic aneurysm grafting. The femoral arteries are exposed by vertical groin incisions; the common femoral, superficial femoral and profunda origin should be dissected and slings passed round them. If the profunda origin is diseased it should be dissected distally until a healthy portion is reached. The superficial femoral is often occluded in these patients.

2. On each side the inguinal ligament is retracted forwards, and using gentle blunt dissection a tunnel is made between the external iliac artery and the inguinal ligament, up into the retroperitoneum. On the left side the base of the pelvic mesocolon is mobilised and the tunnelling continued up behind this, taking care not to damage the ureter.

3. At the aortic end a tape should be placed round the inferior mesenteric artery and the aorta carefully examined. Disease is often found to be more extensive than shown on aortogram. The graft may be joined end-to-side to the aorta, usually between the renal vein level and the inferior mesenteric origin, or the aorta may be divided at a similar level, the distal end oversewn and the graft joined on end-to-end. The latter method is preferred provided that the distribution of occlusion is such that retrograde perfusion of the inferior mesenteric artery through the iliacs is possible.

4. A suitable Dacron graft, preferably knitted and usually 19 mm in diameter at the aortic end, is selected. Careful preclotting is done, and the graft checked for effectiveness of the preclotting before giving the patient 8000–10 000 units of heparin i.v.

5. For an end-to-side graft, a lateral clamp may be used on the aorta, but this does not permit a good view of the interior of the aorta and should only be used if the aorta is healthy at and above the level of the proposed anastomosis. If not, it should be cross-clamped below the renals and again above the bifurcation. A 3 cm vertical elliptical incision is then made between the upper clamp and the inferior mesenteric artery. For end-to-end reconstruction, the aorta is divided transversely at a similar level, and the distal end oversewn after removing loose debris with a sponge holder or gentle 'milking'. The proximal aorta between the renal arteries and the aortotomy should be carefully cleared out using squeezing, sponge holders and irrigation. An unobstructed flow into the graft is essential.

6. The aortic limb of the graft is trimmed to length so that when stretched the new bifurcation will lie above the level of the old. The upper end is cut obliquely or transversely according to the type of anastomosis, which is then made using continuous 3/0 Prolene. On completion, the anastomosis is tested by clamping the graft and releasing the aortic clamp for one beat. Further sutures are inserted if required. The graft is sucked out, and the limbs carefully drawn down through the retroperitoneal tunnels into the groin wounds.

7. With bulldog clamps on the common, superficial femoral and profunda on the first side, a longitudinal arteriotomy is made in the common femoral, if necessary extending down into the profunda until healthy artery is reached. The graft limb is placed under moderate tension and cut obliquely to the correct length. It is anastomosed to the arteriotomy with continuous 4/0 Prolene, backbleeding the clamped vessels prior to completion.

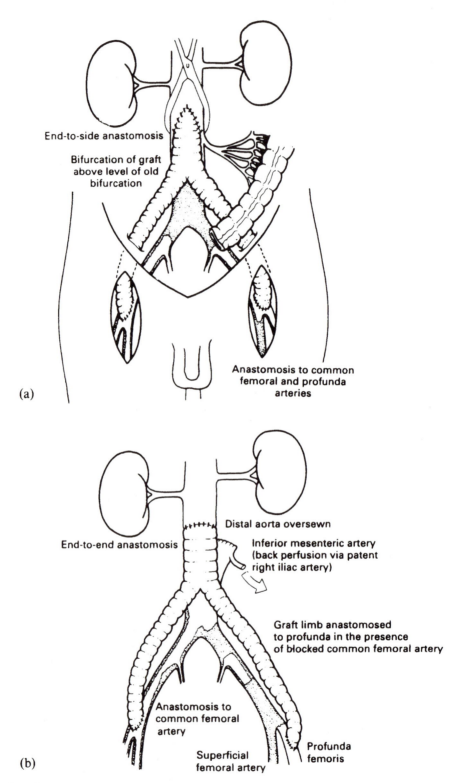

Fig. 3.17.1   Two alternative arrangements of graft and anastomoses (sites of obstruction are indicated by stippled areas)

8. With the completed limb clamped near the bifurcation, one beat from the aortic end can be flushed through the free limb, which is then clamped close to the bifurcation and sucked clean. The heparin should be reversed with protamine at this stage.

9. The distal clamps are managed so that the first few beats from above are directed upwards to the iliac artery, thus avoiding the danger of *trash foot*. The aortic clamp is removed gradually over a period of some 5 min to minimise the risk of sudden hypotension. The remaining femoral anastomosis is constructed on similar lines to the first, using heparinised saline in the clamped groin vessels.

10. The posterior peritoneum is closed making sure that the whole graft is covered. Omentum may be used to aid this, if necessary. The abdominal and groin incisions are then closed, usually without drainage, but if drains are thought to be advisable they should be of the closed suction variety.

ELECTIVE GRAFTING OF ABDOMINAL AORTIC ANEURYSM

Indication

Graft replacement is advised for all infrarenal abdominal aortic aneurysms which may be complicated by leak or rupture (Fig. 3.17.2) except for asymptomatic aneurysms less than 4 cm diameter, and in patients considered unfit to withstand major surgery.

Dissection proximal and distal to the aneurysm is kept to the minimum necessary for safe clamping. This saves time and avoids the danger of injury to the inferior vena cava, iliac veins and lumbar veins.

Preoperative preparation

Routine blood, ESR, ECG, chest X-ray and ultrasound of aorta. Aortography only if associated occlusive disease. Six units of blood cross-matched. Prophylactic wide-spectrum antibiotic. Indwelling urethral catheter, nasogastric tube and CVP line are needed.

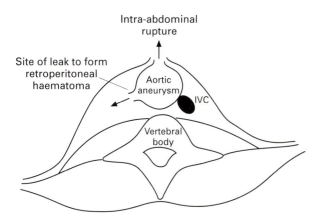

Fig. 3.17.2   Leaking aortic aneurysm

Procedure (Figs 3.17.3, 3.17.4)

1. Supine position. Whole abdomen and upper thighs are prepared. Inflatable leggings are used to prevent deep vein thrombosis. Steridrape is used.

2. Full length midline or paramedian incision.

3. Full laparotomy to exclude other pathology. Confirm aneurysm is below renals. Examine condition of the iliac vessels – are they dilated or severely atheromatous?

4. Insert a large self-retaining retractor. Place the small bowel in a plastic gut bag outside the abdomen on the right side (or pack it off inside).

5. Mobilise the duodenojejunal flexure and duodenum off the front of the aorta and retract it to the right. Safeguard the inferior mesenteric vein. Dissect the front and sides of the neck of the aneurysm.

6. Mobilise the left renal vein if necessary by dividing its branches and retract upwards with tape.

7. Identify the space between the infrarenal aorta and inferior vena cava.

8. Divide the posterior peritoneum vertically to the right of the inferior mesenteric artery, continuing down to the bifurcation and along the line of the right common iliac artery.

9. Mobilise the peritoneum to expose the left common iliac artery (look out for the ureters). If the iliac arteries are fairly healthy a tube graft can usually be sutured to the aortic bifurcation. Assuming this is possible, proceed as follows.

10. Select a woven dacron tube graft of diameter equal to or slightly smaller than the neck of the aneurysm. Give i.v. heparin 8000–10 000 units. Clamp the aorta in the sagittal plane below the renals. The assistant holds it pressed back towards the spine.

11. Clamp the common iliac arteries, incise the anterior wall of the aneurysm from the neck down to the bifurcation and rapidly clear out clot with a finger.

12. Oversew backbleeding inferior mesenteric and lumbar arteries with 2/0 thread. At the upper and lower ends of the aneurysm extend the incision transversely on each side, but leave the posterior wall intact.

13. Anastomose the proximal end of the graft to the neck of the aneurysm, using 2/0 double-ended Prolene suture. Start posterolaterally on the left, holding the graft vertically. First insert the needle through the graft, then take a wide bite of the aorta from above down. Insert the whole row of posterior continuous suture in this manner before approximating the graft to the aorta. This makes placement of sutures much easier, and it is simple to snug down the Prolene at the end of the posterior wall. Continue around the sides and front to complete the anastomosis.

14. Clamp the graft and release the aortic clamp for one beat to test for major leaks in the suture line. Unclamp the graft and suck out.

15. Stretch the graft and trim to reach the bifurcation comfortably. Perform distal anastomosis; again posterior-layer sutures should be placed before pulling the stitch tight. The iliac arteries should be backbled prior to completion of the anastomosis. Give protamine. Allow the graft to fill from below by releasing the iliac clamps first. Manually compress the external iliac arteries and slowly release the aortic clamp; the first few beats should go into the internal iliac arteries to

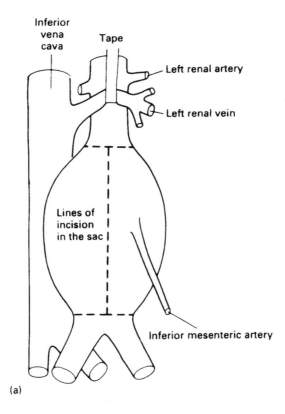

(a)

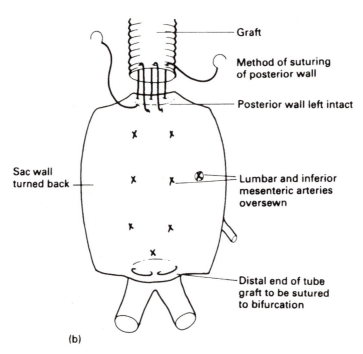

(b)

Fig. 3.17.3 Abdominal aortic aneurysm repair, using tube graft

prevent trash foot. Then release the pressure on the external iliac arteries. Full release of the aortic clamp should be spread over some 5 min to prevent sudden dangerous hypotension. Press on the anastomosis with a finger or swab until dry. Check for bleeding from the wall of the aneurysm. Trim wall and suture sac over graft.

16. Close the posterior peritoneum; it is vital to make certain that graft material is not in contact with the bowel. Close the abdomen.

17. If a bifurcated graft is needed because of aneurysmal or diseased iliac arteries, the limbs will have to be sutured to the distal end of the common iliac arteries or to the common femoral arteries. In the latter case the distal common iliac arteries should be oversewn after dissecting and controlling the external and internal iliac arteries. It is important to maintain flow to at least one internal iliac artery.

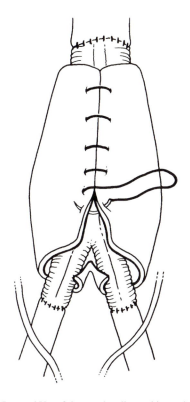

Fig. 3.17.4 Inverted Y-graft is occasionally used instead of tube graft in abdominal aortic aneurysm repair. Notice closure of the sac over the graft

3.18 Sympathectomy

Lumbar (Fig. 3.18.1)

1. Under general anaesthesia. The patient is supine with the flank tilted towards the opposite side, and a sandbag placed

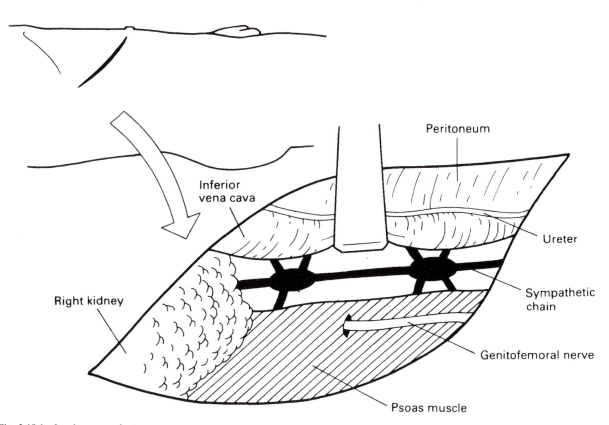

Fig. 3.18.1 Lumbar sympathectomy

2. An oblique or transverse incision is made midway between the anterior superior iliac spine and costal margin towards and ending 4 cm lateral to the umbilicus. The muscles are split or divided to expose the extraperitoneal fat.

3. The peritoneal sac is raised by blunt dissection from the lateral and posterior abdominal walls to uncover the medial margin of the psoas muscle and the aorta or inferior vena cava (IVC), depending on the side (left or right respectively). The following structures may be seen: ureters, genitofemoral nerve and duodenum. Identify the ureter and place the retractors over the peritoneum and ureter. The genitofemoral nerve has no ganglia and is easily identified as it emerges through the psoas fibres.

4. The sympathetic chain and ganglia, lying anterior to the psoas muscle, are more easily felt than seen. The chain is exposed by dissecting through the overlying fascia. The chain is picked up with forceps and dissected upwards and downwards, exposing the second and third lumbar ganglia. The first right lumbar ganglion lies deep to the duodenum. The fourth lies behind the common iliac vessels.

5. Divide the chain, removing approximately 5–7 cm containing two to four ganglia. Removal of Lumbar 1 bilaterally makes the sympathectomy more certain, but may result in loss of ejaculation.

6. Lumbar veins may cross the chain and are clipped with Cushing's silver clips. Pack the area for 5 min if accidental tearing occurs.

7. The muscles are sutured in layers and the skin is closed.

Cervical (Fig. 3.18.2)

1. General anaesthesia with supine position. A sandbag is placed between the shoulders, and the head is turned to the opposite side with the table foot tilted down.

2. A skin crease incision is made 1 cm above and parallel to the medial half of the clavicle. The incision is deepened through the platysma to expose the deep fascia.

3. Dissect out and divide the external jugular vein then divide the clavicular head of the sternomastoid. The muscle may consist of two layers. The next landmark is the omohyoid muscle and its fascia; this muscle is divided.

4. Next identify the transverse cervical vessels and trace the artery medially. It will lead to the phrenic nerve, which it crosses.

5. Mobilise the phrenic nerve from beneath the prevertebral fascia and draw it aside on a tape. The phrenic nerve is on the anterior surface of the scalenus anterior which is felt with the finger as a tight band deep to the sternomastoid and running

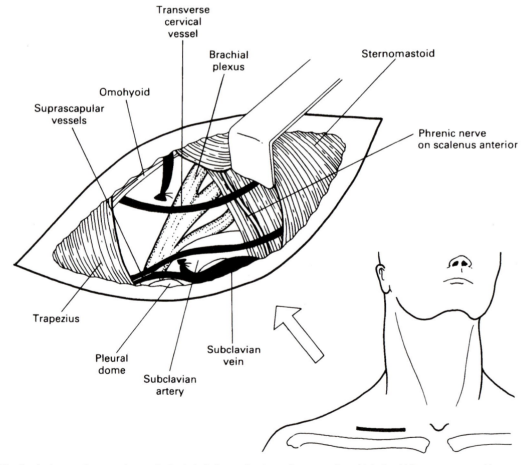

Fig. 3.18.2 Cervical sympathectomy (sympathetic chain is just under the scalenus anterior which should be cut to expose it)

downwards laterally to be inserted into the first rib. If in the way, the thyrocervical trunk may be mobilised and divided. Note that collateral vessels may require saving. Mobilise the scalenus anterior down to the first rib, and divide it at its insertion, preserving the medial part of it on the left side to avoid damaging the thoracic duct.

6. The subclavian artery is in the next layer, and this mobilises very easily by blunt dissection. A tape is introduced round it to act as a sling. Identify the inner border of the first rib, and detach the suprapleural membrane from it with the finger or Lahey swabs, pushing the pleura downwards. Expose the necks of the first three ribs by Lahey swab dissection. A special flexible torch is used to visualise the deep area.

7. Identify the sympathetic chain with the index finger and clear off the overlying fascia. Small deep retractors are inserted and the chain is seen. At the neck of the first rib there are three structures present from medial to lateral – the sympathetic nerve, the superior intercostal vessels and the first thoracic nerve.

8. The chain is divided below the third ganglion, and dissected up by dividing its communication as far as the first thoracic and stellate ganglion, which is left with its rami communicantes to avoid Horner's syndrome.

9. Ask the anaesthetist to inflate the lungs to push the pleura back.

10. The sternomastoid and platysma are repaired and the skin approximated with clips.

N.B. In thoracic outlet syndrome pull the subclavian artery downwards and retract the brachial plexus upwards to search for the cervical rib or band. Excise the band or remove the rib with bone nibbling forceps until no projection is left behind above the first rib.

3.19 Orchidopexy for Maldescended Testes and Circumcision

Badly or imperfectly descended testes are classified as:

1. *Arrested* (undescended) along the normal line of descent at the intra-abdominal, intracanalicular, emergent or high scrotal site.

2. *Deviated* from the normal line of descent (ectopic) commonly at the inguinal pouch or rarely at odd sites (e.g. perineal, pubic, penile, femoral and crossed ectopic). If a superficial inguinal pouch testis can be coaxed into the scrotum it is *tethered*, if not it is *obstructed*.

3. *Retractile* – normally descended but felt at a high scrotal site. Normal embryology includes three intrauterine phases: abdominal (1–7 months), canalicular (7–8 months) and scrotal (8–9 months). The presence or absence of a hernia is not a criterion in classification.

Complications

● Impaired testicular function due to high temperature (affecting the normal maturation and spermatogenesis) secondary to high position. The scrotal dartos muscle and cremaster act as a thermoregulator keeping the testis 2°C cooler than body temperature.
● Malignancy
● Hernia is an associated condition.
● Torsion occurs in 2% of maldescended testes especially testes in hernial sacs.
● Vulnerability to trauma especially inguinal tests.
● Anomalies of the epididymis and vas deferens.
● Psychological factors.

Clinical examination

● Marked variation from the norm for height, weight and fat distribution may suggest *anorchia* due to possible intersex or pituitary deficiency (require chromosomal and endocrine assessment, e.g. high LH levels or the lack of androgen response to gonadotrophin stimulation may be diagnostic).
● Penile size and scrotal development and fullness.
● Gentle palpation and milking of the groin with the boy recumbent or relaxed in warm surroundings – if testis is not found the boy should tense his abdominal muscles by straight leg raising to 45°.
● Older boy should be examined standing for evidence of hernia.
● The testis which descends fully when the boy squats is retractile.
● If no testis is found in the normal line of descent or in the superficial inguinal pouch, then perineal, pubopenile and femoral areas should be palpated and milked carefully.

Types of treatment

Gonadotrophin therapy mainly effective in retractile testes since other types are mechanically anchored. However, it is only worth considering for bilateral arrested testes, if palpable (emerged), in boys up to 5 years of age who have no hernia.

Orchidopexy should be carried out before 5 years of age in order to:

● Enhance spermatogenesis.
● Reduce the risks of malignancy, traumatic orchitis and torsion and allow correction of any associated hernia.
● Improve appearance and so reduce anxiety in parents and child.

Procedure (Fig. 3.19.1)

1. Under general anaesthesia, using inguinal incision and exploration.
2. Mobilisation, in the following order (once sufficient length of cord has been obtained the successive steps are omitted):
(a) Inguinal mobilisation freeing the cord to the internal ring by peeling off the cremaster and incising the tunica vaginalis. A tented peritoneum or true hernia is freed initially at this stage. Gubernaculum testis is ligated and divided.
(b) Retroperitoneal dissection by dividing the lateral suspensory fascia and digital retroperitoneal dissection.
(c) Reduction of triangulation of the course of the testicular vessels by dividing the fibrous medial crus of the internal

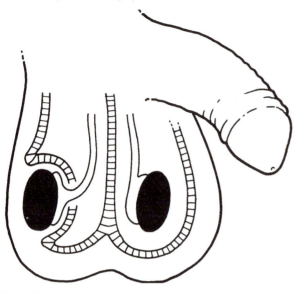

Fig. 3.19.1   Orchidopexy – scrotal fixation in extradartos pouch

ring or blunt dissection with the finger. The inferior epigastric vessels seldom need dividing.

(d) Internal spermatic fasciectomy teasing off fascia which is then picked up, incised longitudinally and rolled off with fine dissecting forceps leaving the vessels and vas only.

3. Scrotal fixation without undue tension in an extradartos pouch (preferred to window septopexy). The scrotum is well stretched digitally; then a vertical incision is made low down near the median raphe. A chromic catgut purse-string suture is inserted before opening the dartos. Artery forceps are passed from below (guided by finger tip from above) to grasp the gubernacular remnant and pull the testis down; then the purse-string suture is tied. The skin wound is closed with absorbable sutures picking up the tunica albuginea for correct testicular orientation.

Circumcision

This is probably the most common surgical procedure in the world; about 1/6 of all males are circumcised. Circumcision has been practised by Babylonians, Egyptians and West African negroes over 5000 years. It was traditionally practised by circumcisers (trained after lengthy apprenticeship) using bamboo instruments used like bone forceps to stretch the foreskin prior to cutting it with a knife. It is is said that Prophet Ibrahim (Abraham) was circumcised at the age of 90 years; his sons Ishmael (grandfather to the Phophet Mohammad and forefather of the Arab race) and Isaac (forefather of the Jews and Christians) were circumcised at ages of 13 years and 8 days respectively after birth.

Smegma is thought to be carcinogenic both to the uncircumcised penis and to the cervix of the sexual partner. Circumcision is therefore a hygienic procedure and is claimed to improve sexual potency of the circumcised male. Circumcision is commonly indicated on a religious basis (Muslims, Jews and some Christians); medically it is indicated in phimosis (tight foreskin), paraphimosis (tight foreskin retracted around the

sulcus corona of the glans treated initially by manual reduction and if this failed, is treated by emergency dorsal slit of the band followed by circumcision), recurrent balanitis (inflammation of glans penis) with inability to retract foreskin, balanoposthitis (inflammation of glans penis and prepuce or foreskin), excessively long prepuce, balanitis xerotica obliterans (precancerous phimosis), preinvasive carcinoma in situ of penile forekin, tight frenulum (with bleeding on erection), inability to retract foreskin prior to intercourse, and rarely prior to radiotherapy for carcinoma. Circumcision is contraindicated in ammonia dermatitis (nappy rash) and in presence of epi- or hypo-spadias (here the foreskin is important for future reconstruction). Clotting screen is preferably done prior to circumcision in children in case of bleeding due to haemophilia. Circumcision is done under general anaesthetic with penile block. The foreskin is dilated and retracted and all preputal adhesions are teased with a probe until the sulcus corona is completely cleared. There are many techniques for circumcision: surgical dissection with dorsal slit and excision (with haemostatic four-in-one frenulum stitch), the guillotine method using bone cutting forceps, Hollister plastibell, Gomco clamp, Mogen clamp, circumcision shield, and Lazim glans caps (with non-crushing clamp). Diathermy should not be used in circumcision and all bleeders must be clipped and ligated with 000 catgut suture. On completion, the circumcised area is swabbed with whitehead varnish (chemical astringent and antiseptic) and lubricant gel and covered by a loosely applied swab like a scottish sporran. Complications are bleeding, infection, glans injury, malrotated penis during erection, internal meatus injury and tight circumcision following excessive foreskin excision.

3.20 Nephrectomy and Adrenalectomy

Nephrectomy

Extraperitoneal approach   Check the function of the other kidney and examine the IVU on the viewing box. The bladder is emptied.

1. Under general anaesthesia the patient lies on the sound side in a well flexed position. The opposite arm is held forward by placing it on a rest. The table may be split to widen the area between the ribs and iliac crest, or a loin rest may be used. A wide strap around the patient's pelvis and the table helps stability.

2. An oblique incision is made, commencing over the neck of the 12th rib (check the site of this rib by X-ray). The incision runs forward over the 12th rib and may be extended up to the lateral margin of the rectus sheath.

3. The wound is deepened with cutting diathermy down to the rib. Using a periosteal elevator, periosteum is stripped first from the upper border from the back forwards then from the lower border carefully (to avoid injury to the subcostal neurovascular bundle) from the front backwards opposite to the

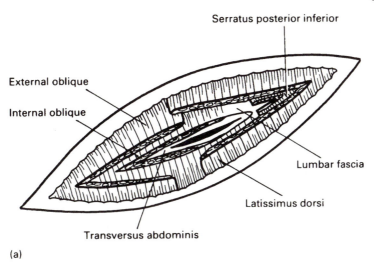

External oblique

Internal oblique

Serratus posterior inferior

Lumbar fascia

Latissimus dorsi

Transversus abdominis

(a)

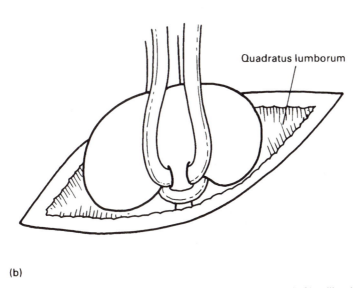

Quadratus lumborum

(b)

Fig. 3.20.1 Nephrectomy – surgical approach. (a) Muscles have been divided and split. (b) Method of handling the kidney after mobilisation and also prior to contact renogram

direction of the intercostal muscles; a raspatory is then applied to the upper border, stripping periosteum backwards and forwards, followed by excision of the rib through its neck with bone-cutting forceps.

4. Access is improved posteriorly by removing the 12th rib subperiosteally. The following structures are preserved: pleura, subcostal nerve, colon and peritoneum. The incision is deepened to expose the latissimus dorsi, serratus posterior inferior, lumbar fascia and the external oblique, and these muscles are divided and split respectively. The internal oblique and transversus muscles and transversalis fascia are divided to expose the extraperitoneal fat (Fig. 3.20.1a). The peritoneum is mobilised forwards by blunt dissection to expose the perinephric fascia of Zuckerkandl. The fascia of Gerota is opened and the kidney seen.

5. If possible, it is brought out of the wound; if not, a self-retaining retractor is inserted to aid further dissection. Two long swabs or tapes can be applied around the hilum of the kidney to aid retraction (Fig. 3.20.1b)

6. The ureter is identified and transected (in hypernephroma). In papillary tumour of the renal pelvis the lower end of the ureter is mobilised for full excision of the ureter; sleeve resection of the bladder wall is performed through a separate suprapubic incision.

7. The renal vessels are triple ligated and divided between the middle and distal ligature.

8. The wound is drained. The muscles are sutured together with interrupted sutures that are tied after removing the kidney rest or straightening the table. Lumbar fascia is sutured continuously to permit free skin movement over muscles.

The operation may be extremely difficult if the inflammation and subsequent fibrosis have spread outside the kidney. The most difficult part is the mobilisation of the kidney, so this should be performed first. The following structures may need

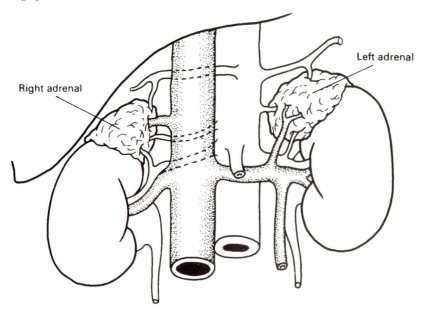

Fig. 3.20.2   Blood supply of adrenals

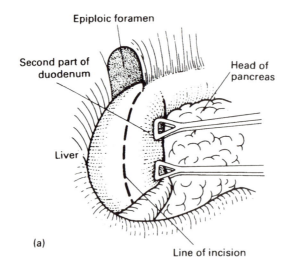

(a)

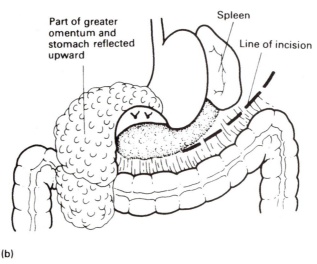

(b)

Fig. 3.20.3   Adrenalectomy. (a) Right adrenalectomy approach. (b) Left adrenalectomy approach

to be separated from the right kidney – liver, diaphragm and suprarenal artery, duodenum and colon; and on the left side – stomach, spleen and colon.

Right abdominal intraperitoneal nephrectomy and right adrenalectomy (Figs 3.20.2, 3.20.3a)

1. Under general anaesthesia the abdomen is opened through a right paramedian incision and explored.
2. The hepatic flexure is mobilised by dividing its attachments, and packed off downwards and medially along with the small intestine.
3. The second part of the duodenum is mobilised by dividing the peritoneum along its right border. By this procedure the duodenum and head of the pancreas can be mobilised as far as the inferior vena cava (Kocher's manoeuvre).
4. The fascia of the kidney is then exposed, picked up and divided. The hilar vessels and ureter are divided and ligated and the kidney is mobilised and removed.
For adrenalectomy exposure as above then:
5. Traction on the kidney brings down the adrenal gland.
6. Its exposure is facilitated by extending the incision in the posterior parietal peritoneum upwards and retracting the right lobe of the liver.
7. The adrenal veins (draining into the inferior vena cava) are clipped with Cushing silver clips and divided.
8. Blunt dissection mobilises the gland for its removal.
9. Accessory glands may require removal.

Left abdominal nephrectomy and left adrenalectomy (Figs 3.20.2, 30.20.3b)

1. Under general anaesthesia the abdomen is opened through a long left paramedian incision and explored. The incision may be extended transversely if the patient is deep and broad (fatty).
2. The spleen is held over to the left and the posterior leaf of the lienorenal ligament divided. The hand can then be inserted behind the spleen and tail of the pancreas, and these structures can be mobilised forwards off the posterior abdominal wall. The gastrocolic ligament is also divided.
3. The kidney fascia (Zuckerkandl) is exposed, picked up and opened.
4. The kidney is mobilised manually, and the vessels of the hilum and the ureter, together with any extrapolar vessels, can be seen and dealt with. If this approach is used for the adrenal gland, this structure is seen on the upper pole of the kidney and is mobilised gently with blunt dissection. The large adrenal vein emptying into the left renal veins is clipped with silver Cushing clips and divided. Other vessels are similarly treated and the gland removed.

Partial nephrectomy

1. The kidney is exposed as above. It is secured by a tape encircling the pedicle. The vessels at the hilum are gently dissected, and if a distinct blood supply is found to the part to be removed, it is ligated and divided.
2. The segment (wedge) is removed with its calyces and associated part of the renal pelvis, leaving a fringe of healthy capsule to cover the raw area.

3. Medullary vessels are ligated, or underrun. The pelvis is repaired with plain catgut. Gauze pressure is applied for the standard 5 min.
4. The edges of the kidney are approximated with catgut over an omental graft or crushed muscle.
5. The kidney is replaced, the area drained and the wound closed.

3.21 Prostatectomy

Retropubic prostatectomy (Fig. 3.21.1)

Preliminary bimanual examination and cystoscopy to assess the prostatic size and associated intravesical pathology, e.g. stone or bladder tumour. Bilateral vasectomy may be performed to prevent postoperative acute epididymitis.
1. Under general anaesthesia and with patient in Trendelenburg position.
2. Suprapubic Pfannenstiel (transverse) incision or lower midline incision. The recti are separated and the bladder separated from the pubis to expose the prostatic capsule extraperitoneally by dissection of the retropubic cave of Retzius. A self-retaining retractor is inserted.
3. The veins running over the prostate are ligated or diathermied and the bladder wall is depressed by a sponge.
4. A transverse (or vertical vesicocapsular) cut is made through the capsule (and bladder wall).
5. The cut capsule edges are held and the adenoma dissected out with a finger pressing against the pubis; the prostatic lobes are enucleated (shelled out). The urethra is divided under vision. The adenomatous tissue is thus removed.

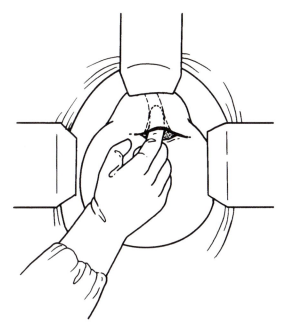

Fig. 3.21.1   Retropubic prostatectomy

6. A generous (V-shaped) wedge is removed from the posterior lip of the bladder (trigonectomy). Two fingers may be inserted through the bladder neck. Tags are removed and haemostasis achieved.

7. A catheter, whistle-tipped or a three-way Foley catheter size 24 Fr, is passed into the bladder, which is washed through. Continuous irrigation is then started.

8. The prostatic capsule is closed with continuous size 1 chromic catgut. The capsular repair should be watertight when tested by washing through the bladder.

9. The packs are removed and the rectus and skin closed with a Redivac drain in the space of Retzius. The urinary catheter tip can be held with a stay-suture brought out through the bladder and abdominal wall and fixed with a gauze on the abdomen to prevent its displacement and/or disruption of the capsular repair.

3.22 Cystectomy and Ureterosigmoidostomy

CYSTECTOMY WITH ILEAL CONDUIT

This operation involves removal of the urinary bladder, with prostate and seminal vesicles in the male, and drainage of urine via an ileal loop to an external ileostomy. In the female, the uterus and adnexae are removed. May be curative or palliative.

Indications

● Invasive bladder tumour.
● Contracted bladder – tuberculosis, bilharziasis.

Associated therapy

Patients with infiltrating tumours are often given a preliminary irradiation of 4000–4500 rad.

Special preoperative preparation

● Intestinal tract sterilised by oral antibiotics begun 48 h before surgery.
● High-calorie, low-residue feeding over similar period.
● Restoration of haemoglobin level or correction of electrolyte levels if required.
● Advice from a previous cystectomy patient.
● Site of ileostomy marked on skin of right abdomen to accommodate comfortable siting of urine collection appliance.

Procedure (Fig. 3.22.1)

1. Patient supine catheterised, and in Trendelenburg position.
2. Lower midline incision.

3. Laparotomy and assessment of the fixity of the tumour in the pelvis. Post irradiation changes may be present.

4. If resectable, proceed to mobilise and divide the ureters – divide peritoneum over each common iliac artery bifurcation. Mobilise each ureter as it passes in front of the origin of the external iliac artery. Dissect a further 4 cm down, then divide. Hold the proximal end in light tissue forceps and ligate the lower end with non-absorbable guide ligature. The ureters may be dilated, sometimes considerably. Draw the left ureter to the right through a convenient point in the descending mesocolon.

5. Expose and tie the internal iliac artery on each side in continuity using an aneurysm needle and non-absorbable ligature.

6. Proceed to dissect the lymph nodes on each side after exposing the anterior and lateral bladder walls and fatty tissue overlying the pelvic fascia by blunt dissection.

7. While dissecting nodes in the obturator fossa, preserve the obturator nerve and vessels. Cut and tie the vas deferens and use the proximal tied end as a later guide to the plane between the seminal vesicles and rectum.

8. As the bladder is mobilised in front, laterally and posteriorly, two lateral vascular pedicles have to be secured – lifting the bladder forwards and to the opposite side allows the superior and inferior vesical vessel pedicles to be defined, narrowed, and divided between clamps and tied. Use chromic catgut.

9. As the rectovesical fascial layer is mobilised, the bladder is dissected off the rectum. The seminal vesicles and prostate are mobilised from behind and below. The stumps of the ureters are also seen. Inferior pedicles may have to be secured in several steps.

10. Puboprostatic ligaments are now diathermised. Pelvic fascia lateral to the prostate is divided in the convexity of the retropubic area by sharp dissection. The prostate and vesicles now narrow to an apex at the urethra which is divided with scissors: remaining deep lateral connections are finally divided. Check for significant bleeding; if none, leave the pack in the pelvis and proceed to make an ileal conduit.

11. Use a length of distal ileum at least 20 cm proximal to the ileocaecal junction. The length must be adequate to extend from the ureters to the external ileostomy. Mark the selected length and prepare the mesenteric vascular pedicle with the use of transillumination. Distal mesenteric division is longer than proximal as this end passes through the abdominal wall.

12. Hold the conduit loop between light intestinal clamps. Place to the left (inframesenteric) and restore ileal continuity using 2/0 chromic catgut in a two-layer anastomosis.

13. Trim and spatulate the ureters. Suture the V of one to the apex of the spatulated length of the other with 3/0 chromic catgut. Insert the trimmed arms of a 10 Fr biliary T-tube into each ureter, wash out the ileal loop with an irrigating syringe, and draw the stem of the T-tube through it to the outer end. Complete anastomosis of the ureters to the inner ileal end with 3/0 chromic interrupted catgut stitches. T-tube splint dose *not* require suture fixation – if this were pulled out accidentally later it might disrupt the anastomosis.

14. Suture the peritoneal mesenteric incision around the ureteroileal anastomosis to make it retroperitonael. Finally make a spouting ileostomy in the usual way through a

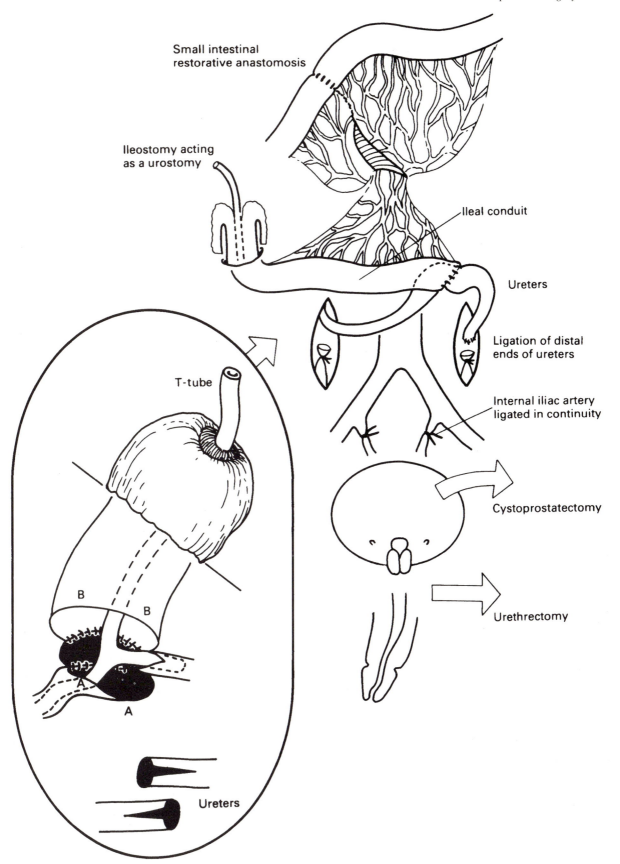

Small intestinal
restorative anastomosis

Ileostomy acting
as a urostomy

Ileal conduit

Ureters

Ligation of distal
ends of ureters

Internal iliac artery
ligated in continuity

Cystoprostatectomy

Urethrectomy

T-tube

B   B

A

A

Ureters

Fig. 3.22.1   Cystectomy and ileal conduit. (In the inset sides A and B will be sutured together)

previously marked skin circle. The stem of the T-tube can be cut suitably short and left within an immediately applied urinary appliance, where it will remain for 10 days. The abdomen is closed with tube or suction drain to the pelvis.

15. In the female, hysterectomy with bilateral salpingo-oöphorectomy is carried out after initial ureter division and internal iliac artery ligature.

Special postoperative care

1. Maintain nasogastric suction and i.v. fluid until return of adequate intestinal peristalsis.
2. Continue antibiotics as required.
3. Remove T-tube usually in 7–10 days, later than 10 days if anastomotic leak suspected.
4. Early mobilisation is useful.

URETHRECTOMY

This procedure is used for patients known to have unstable epithelium in the urethra in addition to an invasive bladder lesion. It is added to the end of a total cystectomy to prevent possible further invasive tumour appearing in the urethra.

Procedure

1. At the end of a total cystoprostatectomy, the patient is placed in the classical lithotomy position.
2. A curved incision, convex forwards, some 8 cm long, is made about 2 cm behind the scrotum.
3. The cut urethra is secured in the midline at the penile bulb as it enters the perineum through the perineal membrane and is dissected out of the whole length of the penis. The urethral dissection continues to the level of the glans. The surrounding corpus spongiosum bleeds little, as the scissors or knife are kept close to the outer wall of the urethra.
4. The perineal skin incision is closed with drainage, and a firm dressing applied.
5. In the female, the short urethra is easily dissected out via a short incision in the anterior vaginal wall behind its external opening.

URETEROSIGMOIDOSTOMY

This operation involves implantation of the ureters into the sigmoid (pelvic) colon. It is now less commonly used than ileal conduit.

Indications

- Non-malignant conditions of the lower urinary tract including congenital anomalies, e.g. exstrophy of the bladder.
- Irremediable trauma to the urethra.
- Invasive bladder tumour as an alternative to ileal conduit.
- Contracted bladder.

Advantages

- No abdominal stoma or artificial collecting device.
- Children, or individuals whose other congenital handicaps make urostomy management difficult, can accept this form of diversion.

Disadvantages

- Greater risk of ascending urinary infection.
- Hypokalaemic hyperchloraemic acidosis from absorption of urine by colonic mucosa.
- Loss of anal sphincter control, for any reason, will produce incontinence.

Special preoperative preparation

- Colon must be empty as well as sterilised.
- Oral antibiotic, high-calorie low-residue diet, and repeated enemas for 72 h before operation.
- Restoration of haemoglobin level and correction of any electrolyte imbalance.

Procedure (Fig. 3.22.2)

1. Supine position. Lower midline or transverse suprapubic incision. Insert wide rectal tube extending to rectosigmoid.
2. Pack off the small bowel and identify the ureters where they cross the origin of the external iliac arteries. Divide the

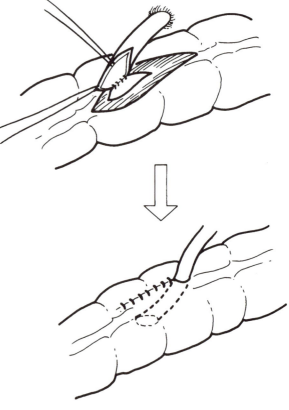

Fig. 3.22.2   Ureterosigmoidostomy

overlying peritoneum and mobilise the ureters down towards the bladder; cut and tie the lower ends. The lateral leaf of the pelvic mesocolon may have to be mobilised.

3. The ureters are now inserted into the pelvic colon, the right ureter at a lower level than the left. Stay sutures hold both upper cut ends of the ureters and two stay sutures are inserted about 4 cm apart in the taeni coli. The seromuscular layer of the colon is incised longitudinally between stay sutures.

4. Dissect back the seromuscular layer; open the mucosa at the distal end of the trough being formed. Lay the ureter into the trough and suture the open end to the mucosal opening with 3/0 chromic catgut.

5. After completing the posterior layer, a fine splint catheter can be passed from the ureter into the colon and thence into the rectal tube to the exterior. The anastomosis is now complete.

6. Seromuscular layers of colon are now closed over the ureter from distal to proximal with fine interrupted silk (3/0), and the lateral margin of the posterior peritoneal incision is sutured over to extraperitonealise the whole anastomosis.

7. Repeat on the left ureter at a slightly higher level to avoid tension or angulation of the ureters. This allows the pelvic colon to revert to its normal curve.

8. Secure the ureteric splints to a rectal tube at the anus. These plus the rectal tube will be passed with the first bowel motion in 4–5 days. Close the abdomen, with Penrose drainage.

Special postoperative care

1. Intravenous fluid maintains good output of urine.
2. Continue antibiotics.
3. Check electrolytes and blood urea.
4. Bicarbonate required to control acidosis.
5. Check intravenous urography in 3 months.

3.23 Pneumonectomy

Indications

Extensive lung cancer or severely damaged lung, e.g. bronchiectasis.

Surgical considerations in lung cancer

Lung cancer is the commonest cause of death among all cancers. Of 100 patients presenting with lung cancer, 70 proved to have metastatic disease already (after thorough investigations with chest X- ray – posteroanterior and lateral, sputum cytology, bronchoscopy, mediastinoscopy, radioactive scan and CT imaging, respiratory functions, percutaneous biopsy, in peripheral lung cancer or scalene node biopsy, thoracoscopy and exploratory thoracotomy in this order) and die within 5 years. Only 30 had apparently localised lesions suitable for resection and of those only 8 survived 5 years.

Pulmonary resections required, in the order of frequency, are lobectomy, pneumonectomy, segmental resection and sleeve resection (with appropriate tracheobronchial reconstruction).

Operative mortality is determined by the extent of resection (lobectomy carries 5%, pneumonectomy 10% and thoractomy without resection 1%, the presence of ischaemic heart disease, chronic bronchitis or emphysema, and the patient's age.

Postoperative prognosis depends on histological typing and cancer staging. Histologically there are four types (according to WHO): squamous carcinoma (50% of cases with 5 year survival in 28%), adenocarcinoma (including alveolar cell carcinoma; 20% of cases with 5 year survival in 17%), large-cell carcinoma (10% of cases with 5 year survival in 15%), and small-cell carcinoma (20% of cases with no 5-year survival; this is the most lethal cancer and rarely presents as a localised lesion).

Squamous, large-cell and adenocarcinoma are best treated by resection. Small-cell carcinoma is best treated by multiagent chemotherapy, i.e. cyclophosphamide, methotrexate and cyclohexyl-chlorethyl-nitrosourea (CCNU), or radiotherapy if it is localised.

There are three stages in lung cancers using the TNM classification (small-cell carcinoma is considered inoperable and is excluded):

Stage I: $T_1 (< 3 cm) N_0 M_0$
         $T_1 N_1$ (ipsilateral hilar node) M_0
         $T_2 (> 3 cm$ with partial lung atelectasis) $N_0 M_0$
Stage II: $T_2 N_1 M_0$

Both Stage I and II are small cancers without extrapulmonary spread.

Stage III: are large cancers which extend into nearby structures or into the proximal main bronchus or which have extrapulmonary metastases.

Stage I squamous carcinoma has the best survival of all.

Contraindications to resection

- Evidence of haematogenous metastases, e.g. in the contralateral lung, liver, brain and bones in this order.
- Lymphatic spread beyond the ipsilateral superior mediastinal nodes, e.g. scalene, posterior mediastinal and coeliac nodes.
- Direct extrapulmonary invasion: need not always preclude resection. However the following are contraindications:
  - Extensive fixed chest wall invasion.
  - Invasion of trachea or first 1.5 cm of the main bronchus.
  - Brachial plexus invasion with Horner's syndrome in Pancoast's tumour (and peripheral apical lung cancer).
  - Phrenic nerve palsy with paradoxical motion of the hemidiaphragm at fluoroscopy.
  - Intrapericardial invasion with malignant pericardial effusion and/or cardiac arrhythmias.
  - Superior vena cava obstruction by metastatic mediastinal nodes (necessitates urgent radiotherapy for decompression). Oesophageal compression may also occur as indicated by barium swallow but rarely leads to dysphagia.
- Unfitness for operation especially in patients:
  - Over 70 years of age.
  - With ischaemic heart disease, chronic bronchitis or emphysema.

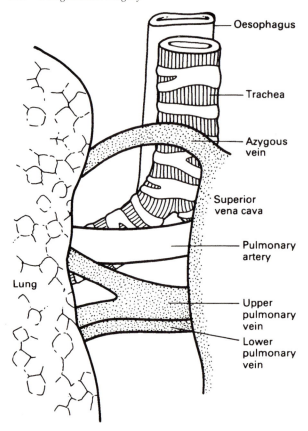

Fig. 3.23.1 Pneumonectomy – surgical approach

removed. The pulmonary artery is cleared then ligated and divided.

5. The bronchus is clamped distally and divided close to the carina. The open stump, which should be short, is closed with interrupted figure-of-8 using non-absorbable sutures, e.g. 3/0 Prolene. Alternatively the bronchus may be divided between clamps, using a non-crushing clamp proximally. Sutures are placed behind the clamp and are not tied until the clamp is removed. The hemithorax is filled with saline and the anaesthetist asked to inflate the lungs to detect any air leak from the sutured bronchus stump.

6. The chest is closed in layers without drainage or with an underwater drain but with *no suction* – the opposite lung and heart are shifted by suction with possible fatal cardiorespiratory embarrassment. Intercostal nerves are blocked or cryoprobed to reduce postoperative pain and prevent chest infection.

Postoperative complications

- Bronchopulmonary infection.
- Thoracic empyema.
- Bronchopleural fistula.
- Cardiac complications, e.g. atrial fibrillation, myocardial infarction and cardiac herniation through the resected pericardium.
- Pulmonary embolism.
- Chronic thoracotomy wound pain.

3.24 Right Hepatic Resection (Lobectomy)

The liver has remarkable powers of regeneration and resection is therefore well tolerated.

Indications

- Trauma in severe shattering liver injury.
- Tumours – primary hepatocellular carcinoma and solitary hepatic secondary carcinoma.
- High biliary tract obstruction due to cholangiocarcinoma or benign biliary stricture.
- Congenital defect – very rarely in large hepatic haemangioma.

Contraindications

- Undoubted involvement of the inferior vena cava.
- Histologically proven extrahepatic disease.
- Tumour nodules in both anatomical lobes of the liver.
- Involvement of both main branches of portal vein.

Surgical anatomy

The liver is divided into two anatomical lobes by an imaginary line between the gallbladder fossa and inferior vena cava. The

– With poor respiratory reserve as indicated by pulmonary function tests. As a rule of thumb, pneumonectomy is contraindicated if FEV_1 is less than 1.2 litres.

Procedure (Fig. 3.23.1)

1. Under intermittent positive pressure, general anaesthesia with a double-lumen endotracheal tube. The lateral or, rarely, the prone position may be used.

2. The chest is opened via a posterolateral thoracotomy incision running from the submammary crease inferior to the inferior angle of the scapula and then to the scapulovertebral interval through the fifth rib after subperiosteal rib excision. Any adhesions are divided with scissors. Areas of densely adherent pleura may have to be removed with the lung rather than risk opening a diseased lung. *En bloc* resection may be extended to include invaded chest wall and diaphragm. The subcarinal and ispilateral tracheobronchial nodes can be removed for accurate staging.

3. The perihilar pleura and the pulmonary ligament are divided and reflected to expose the hilum. The pericardium may be opened to help in assessment of resectability.

4. The pulmonary veins are dissected and individually ligated and divided. Veins are ligated before arteries in cancer and vice versa in non-cancer cases, e.g. bronchiectasis. If necessary the left atrial wall may be secured in a vascular clamp and the veins divided flush. The atrial wall is oversewn and the clamp

left lobe is subdivided into medial (quadrate lobe) and lateral segments by ligamentum teres in the umbilical fissure. The right lobe is subdivided into anterior, posterior, superior and inferior segments. The left lobe can be subdivided into anterior, posterior, superior and inferior segments, making eight segments altogether.

Preoperative preparation

Prophylactic antibiotics (gentamicin 80 mg and lincomycin 600 mg three times a day) are given with the premedication and continued for 5 days postoperatively. Blood preparation (about 8 units) is carried out and good perioperative hydration is important.

Procedure

1. The patient is anaesthetised in the supine position. Tilting the table may help the procedure.
2. The approach depends on the underlying cause. A right paramedian exploratory incision can be extended into a right thoracoabdominal incision if, for instance, the tumour is operable or the liver is extensively injured (the diaphragm is divided, the lung is collapsed and a tape is passed around the inferior vena cava). Otherwise a bilateral subcostal oblique 'roof-top' incision using a Goligher substernal retractor with possible median sternotomy (inverted T if necessary) gives excellent exposure.
3. Ligamentum teres is sectioned and clamped for retraction. The hepatoduodenal ligament and hepatic colonic flexure are dissected and the right adrenal gland is then dissected down. The duodenum and head of pancreas are mobilised to expose the inferior vena cava and a tape is placed around this vessel above the renal veins.
4. The right lobe is mobilised, dividing the right triangular and posterior layers of the coronary ligament. The small hepatic veins are divided after ligating with metal clips or preferably transfixion with 3/0 Prolene. Then retract the liver to the left and transfix, ligate and divide the main hepatic veins.
5. At the porta hepatis the cystic duct and artery (leave the gallbladder in situ for the time being), then the right hepatic duct, artery and right branch of the portal vein are individually doubly ligated with non-absorbable 2/0 linen or silk and divided. A tape may be passed around the common bile duct for retraction. Notice the ischaemic line of demarcation in the floppy liver. (Step 5 may be done before Steps 3 and 4.)
6. Apply a Longmire hepatic clamp either to the right (in trauma and congenital lesions) or to the left (in tumours) of the gallbladder, then cut the liver substance and finger fracture along the ischaemic line, ligating and dividing individual vessels and bile duct inside the liver substance using 2/0 linen or silk. Then take the clamp off, watch for and ligate any more bleeding vessels.
7. Take the gallbladder out by dissection (if not already removed with the right lobe). Thorough haemostasis is required, especially at the site of the right adrenal and in the rest of the space occupied by the removed lobe.
8. Leave a silicone drain in situ and close the anterior abdominal wall. T-tube drainage for biliary decompression is controversial and it is probably better not to leave a T-tube in the common bile duct.

Postoperative complications

Bleeding Due to liver trauma, operative trauma, temporary liver dysfunction (liver is the factory of vitamin K dependent clotting factors II, V, VII, IX, X) or blood transfusion (with possible thrombocytopenia and coagulation factor deficiency) – may all lead to haemorrhagic shock. Massive haematemesis may also occur in the 2nd–3rd postoperative week due to intra-abdominal sepsis (stress ulcer). Routine fresh blood transfusion, vitamin K injection and selective cimetidine are required.

Infection Leaked bile and blood beneath an immobile diaphragm may become infected and lead to subphrenic abscess. Prophylactic antibiotics can be extended into therapeutic treatment. Surgical drainage may be required.

Biliary fistula Needs to be assessed by T-tube cholangiography (if a T-tube is present), ERCP or fistulogram. If there is no biliary obstruction, then parenteral nutrition and drainage of the fistula should be instituted. The presence of a stricture without fistula formation usually necessitates reoperation.

Metabolic consequences Hypoproteinaemia necessitates i.v. albumin administration, hypoglycaemia necessitates i.v. dextrose 5% infusion within the first 48 h. Mild hyperbilirubinaemia with some degree of jaundice may occur as a result of hepatocellular damage.

3.25 Amputations

Indications

● Vascular disease.
● Tumours.
● Trauma.
● Deformities whether congenital or neurological or due to chronic sepsis, pressure sores or huge lymphoedema.

Sites of election

In the upper arm, leave 20 cm measured from tuberosities but if this is impossible, try to divide the bone 4 cm below the anterior axillary fold. Below the elbow, 17 cm of bone are preserved as measured from the olecranon, but if this is impossible, the insertion of the biceps should be preserved. In the thigh cut 13 cm above the knee joint line. Below the knee leave 13 cm measured from the tibial tubercle.

It is important to preserve a length of stump because:
● The joint above the prosthesis should flex without interference, and the stump should retain its prosthesis.
● Muscles should be left to work the stump.
● The longer the stump, the better the muscle control and leverage.

Technical points

The use of tourniquets is avoided if the ischaemia is caused by arteriosclerosis. Equal anterior and posterior flaps are usually

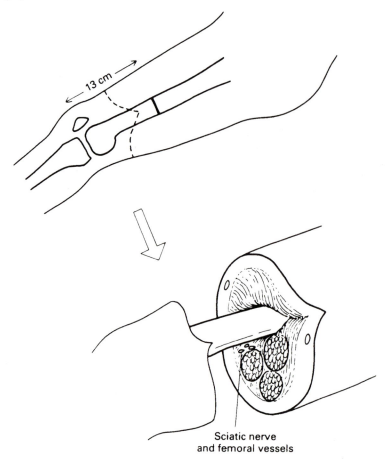

Fig. 3.25.1   Above-knee amputation

fashioned except in below-knee amputation. Prophylactic antibiotic is required with a properly applied bandage to protect the stump from faecal contamination.

Above-knee myoplastic flap (Fig. 3.25.1)

1. The patient lies supine under general anaesthesia. Mark the leg at the site of election. The diameter of the limb is equal to one-third the circumference (which can be measured by tape), thus giving the length of the flap from the site of election.
2. Fashion equal anterior and posterior flaps including the deep fascia and reflect them to a point 2.5 cm above the proposed line of bone section. Ligate and divide the long saphenous vein.
3. Mark the muscle groups, arbitrarily divided into four quadrants, by four stay sutures at the level of the proposed bone section.
4. Divide the muscles shorter than the skin flaps and reflect them to the level of bone section.
5. Doubly ligate and divide the main vessels (femoral, profunda femoris). Cut the sciatic nerve higher than the bone cut end and ligate if bleeding from comitans nervi ischiadici to avoid future neuroma.
6. Reflect an area of periosteum (if possible) to cover the raw area of bone, retract soft tissue with a bone shield, divide bone

with a saw, wax its bone marrow and cover it with the periosteum after filing the end.
7. Secure haemostasis.
8. Cover the bone end by suturing over it the lateral and medial then the anterior and posterior muscle groups in turn, opposing groups being sutured to each other.
9. Resuture the deep fascia and subcutaneous tissues and close the skin, providing two lateral drains (Redivacs) to drain deep and superficial spaces.
10. To prevent flexion deformity developing at the level of the hip joint, employ physiotherapy and splintage.

Long posterior flap of below-knee amputation
(Fig. 3.25.2)

1. The patient is placed in the supine position under general anaesthesia.
2. Make a skin incision across the front of the leg 12 cm below the knee joint. Mark a 15 cm long posterior flap below the line of bone section which is 13 cm from the knee joint line. Deepen the incision down to the tibia.
3. Reflect the anterior tibial muscles and periosteum proximally for 1.25 cm.
4. Divide and bevel the tibia with a saw or Gigli saw. Dissect it out and divide the fibula 2.5 cm above this level.

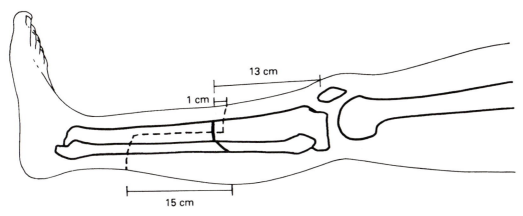

Fig. 3.25.2   Long posterior flap below-knee amputation

5. Extend the ends of the skin incision vertically downwards thus forming the posterior flap. Reflect this flap upwards. Find the sural nerve and divide it clear of the site elected.

6. Deepen the posterior incision through the muscles down to the tibia and fibula, reflect them upwards and remove the leg. Locate and ligate the posterior tibial and perineal vessels and both saphenous veins.

7. Model muscles and then suture them over the site of bone division.

8. Achieve haemostasis.

9. Close muscle, fascia and skin with drainage.

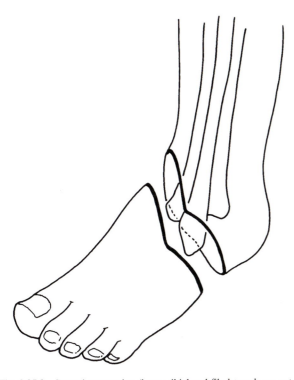

Fig. 3.25.3   Symes' amputation (lower tibial and fibular ends are cut after removal of the talocalcaneometatarsal bones of the foot)

Symes' amputation (Fig. 3.25.3)

1. Under general anaesthesia. A tourniquet may be applied while the foot is held at right angles over the end of the table.

2. Make an incision from the lateral malleolar tip vertically down to the sole, cross transversely and continue it over the medial aspect of the ankle terminating 12 mm below (not behind) the medial malleolar tip, to avoid damage to the calcaneal branch of the lateral plantar artery.

3. Dissect off the heel flap by keeping close to the bone. Divide the Achilles tendon. Depress the foot and incise across the dorsum through the tendons and down to the bone. Disarticulate the talo-tibiofibular joint by dividing the ligaments (the lateral ligament from within outwards).

4. Identify the vessels and ligate them.

5. Retract the soft tissues and remove both malleoli and tibial articular cartilage by sawing across the bone as low as possible (avoid removing the epiphysis in the young).

6. Release the tourniquet, obtain haemostasis, leave in the drain and sew up the inferior skin flap anteriorly. An 'elephant boot' is used when the wound is sound.

3.26 Keller's Arthroplasty

Indicated in hallux valgus or rigidus.

Procedure (Fig. 3.26.1)

1. A tourniquet is applied under general anaesthesia and with patient in the supine position.

2. A 5 cm incision is made over the anteromedial aspect of the proximal phalanx and metatarsophalangeal joint of the big toe – incise deep down to the bone.

3. The joint is opened medial to the extensor hallucis longus tendon.

4. The proximal third of the proximal phalanx is excised, preserving the flexor hallucis longus tendon (a Silastic implant can be used here).

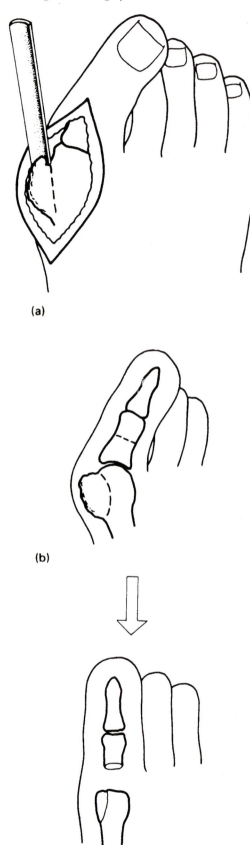

(a)

(b)

Fig. 3.26.1 Keller's operation for hallux valgus. (a) Removal of the metatarsal exostosis. (b) Removal of proximal third of the phalanx

5. The exostosis of the metatarsal head is excised with an osteotome. The medial collateral ligament is reconstructed, then the skin is closed.

6. A pad of gauze between the toes maintains the varus position.

7. Following the operation, early movements are initiated.

3.27 Open Medial Meniscectomy

Procedure (Fig. 3.27.1)

Preoperative quadriceps exercises and arthroscopy are required.

1. Exsanguinate with an Esmarch tourniquet and maintain exsanguination with a pneumatic tourniquet. The thigh is supported on a sandbag.

2. The skin is prepared.

3. Remove the bottom segment of the operating table while the patient is supine with knees flexed; the surgeon sits at the patient's feet with the foot of the injured side in his lap.

4. Make a 5 cm oblique incision from the lower medial corner of the patella downwards and medially to end 1 cm below the joint line (medial meniscectomy). A similar incision downwards and laterally on the outer side of the knee is used for lateral meniscectomy. Incise the capsule in the same line as the skin incision.

5. Open the synovium and inspect the joint interior, flexing and extending the knee. Look at the back of the patella.

6. The medial collateral ligament is retracted to obtain a view of the peripheral attachment of the cartilage.

7. A blunt tendon hook is applied over the free edge of the anterior horn of the meniscus which is then detached, using a scalpel horizontally between the anterior horn and tibial plateau.

8. The cartilage is firmly held in the left hand with a meniscus or Kocher's toothed forceps and drawn inwards towards the intercondylar space, dividing the peripheral attachment with a solid scalpel.

9. The posterior horn is divided, taking care to avoid injuring the posterior cruciate ligament. Rotation of the tibia laterally and flexion of the knee may help in this division. This is best achieved by keeping a Smellie's knife blade vertical to avoid injury to the collateral ligament and drawing the cartilage over it.

10. Divide the posterior rim via the intercondylar notch using a mirror-image curved Smellie's knife. Check that the entire meniscus has been removed.

11. The synovium and capsule are sutured separately. The skin is closed.

12. A crêpe pressure bandage is applied.

13. The tourniquet is removed.

Comment: Arthroscopic (closed) meniscectomy is becoming more popular now and is performed in many centres.

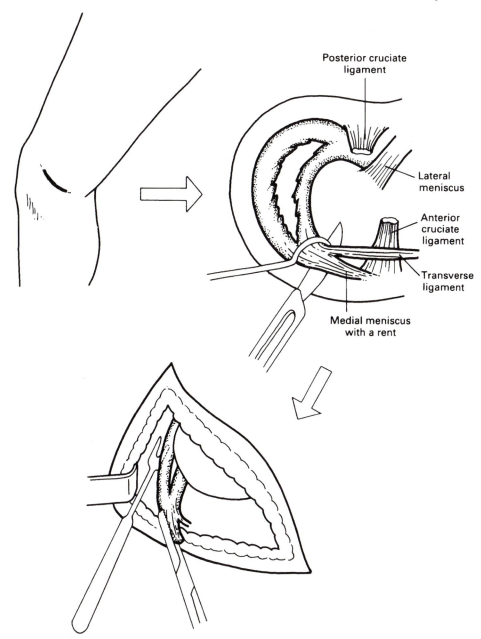

Fig. 3.27.1   Open medial meniscectomy

3.28 Internal Fixation of Femoral Neck Fractures

Procedure

1. On a special orthopaedic table with the patient in a supine position and under general anaesthesia.
2. The fracture is reduced by *traction in flexion*; this is followed by *internal rotation* and *abduction*.
3. This position is maintained and the X-ray apparatus is set up.

4. X-rays of the hip are used in two planes to ensure satisfactory reduction. An image-intensifier may be used.
5. The trochanter and the upper part of the femur are exposed through a 10 cm lateral incision.
6. Guide wires are inserted until one of them achieves the correct position, confirmed by radiograph, and the required length of nail is estimated.
7. Richard's Dynamic Hip Screw (DHS) or a canalised trifid Smith–Petersen nail is then driven over the guide wire into the head after reaming the cortex. The wire is removed and the fracture is impacted. The position of the nail is checked by further X-rays. In intertrochanteric or extracapsular fractures further fixation is obtained by a plate that holds the end of the

nail and can be screwed down into the lateral aspect of the shaft of the femur – pin and plate or sliding (Pugh) nail.

8. The wound is closed with a Redivac drain.

9. Movements are commenced the day after the operation.

3.29 Posterior Approach and Arthroplasty of the Hip

Procedure (Southern approach) (Fig. 3.29.1)

1. The patient lies on the unaffected side with the upper arm on a rest, and the pelvis supported by padded rests.

2. The skin is incised along the anterior border of the gluteus maximus from the posterior superior iliac spine to the greater trochanter and then downwards for approximately 15 cm.

3. The iliotibial tract is incised in line with the lower limb incision, and the gluteal bursa opened. The gluteus maximus is then separated along its fibres and retracted medially. Finally, the gluteus medius and minimus are freed and retracted.

4. The capsule is exposed by retracting the quadratus femoris and dividing the obturator internus with the gemelli marking them with stay sutures.

5. The capsule is opened in a T-shaped manner and the hip dislocated by rotating the thigh medially.

6. Arthroplasty is performed.

● Hemiarthroplasty, e.g. Thompson prosthesis may be inserted for intracapsular fractures of the femoral neck:

(a) The exposed femoral head is removed with a corkscrew like instrument and bone levers.

(b) The femoral neck is trimmed with an osteotome or power saw.

(c) Ream the femur. Insert the cement and prosthesis after proper anatomical orientation.

(d) Secure and reduce the prosthesis.

(e) Close the wound in layers, including a suction Redivac drain.

Comment: In hemiarthroplasty, the cementless Austin Moore prosthesis is another alternative.

● Total replacement (low friction) hip arthroplasty:

(a) The head is dislocated and then excised using a power saw or osteotome.

(b) The acetabulum is reamed.

(c) The centring hole is closed by a mesh cup in the Charnley operation. The cement (antibiotic treated) is inserted followed by the acetabular component.

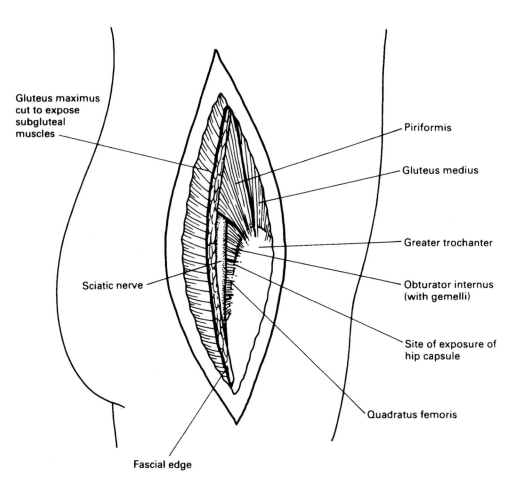

Fig. 3.29.1   Hip exposure – posterior approach

(d) The femoral shaft is reamed. The cement and prosthesis are inserted after proper anatomical orientation.

(e) The femoral prosthesis is reduced and secured.

(f) The greater trochanter initially divided, to facilitate exposure, is replaced and fixed with wire sutures (only in Charnley's operation).

(g) The wound is closed in layers and a suction drain is left in situ.

Complications in joint replacement

These may be related to age, obesity, concomitant diseases (rheumatoid arthritis, hypertension, chronic bronchitis and heart disease), deep venous thrombosis, operative cardiovascular complications (15% CVA, cardiac arrest, hyper- or hypotension, and heart failure), operative mortality, antibiotics-related or cement-related.

Problems associated with insertion of acrylic cement (methyl methacrylate whether liquid monomer or solid polymer) include:

1. Hypotension.
2. Fat embolism.
3. Hypoxaemia.
4. Embolism in general.

These may be due to polymerisation which generates heat 6–8 min after exposure. Various mechanisms of pathogenesis are postulated for induced hypotension during cement insertion; they include:

– reaction to the heat generation;

– direct toxic effect of cement, vasodilatation;

– pressure rise on bone-marrow cavity resulting in embolisation of fat, air and platelets aggregations.

It is important to monitor the patient after tourniquet release, providing good oxygenation and avoiding hypovolaemia.

3.30 Hemilaminectomy and Laminectomy

Indications

- Spinal cord compression due to:
  – Intervertebral disc protrusion (prolapse), whether lateral or central.
  – Spinal stenosis, whether postdegenerative (osteoarthritis), congenital, postspondylolisthetic or unclassified (Paget's disease, tuberculosis and postoperative).
  – Vertebral trauma (due to oedema and/or fracture) – simple fénestration decompression may be adequate, but internal fixation is required in fractures or in multilevel laminectomy, using plate fixation or wiring of intact spinous processes (above and below). Posterolateral on-lay bone graft may be added for reinforcement.
  – Primary or secondary vertebral bone tumours – need fixation.

- Pain relief – chordotomy.

- Spondylolisthesis with nerve root or cauda equina compression – fusion of facet joints using screw fixation is required.

Preoperative assessment

All patients undergoing laminectomy must be assessed thoroughly.

Clinically Persistent symptoms of sciatica (buttock and lower limb pain) with pain increased by coughing or straining; signs of slight forward tilt and lateral list (sciatic scoliosis); tenderness with limited back movement as well as limited straight leg raising may all present.

Neurologically (according to the compressed segment)

- S_1 Weak foot eversion and ankle jerk, and sensory loss along lateral border of foot.
- L_5 Weak big toe extension and knee flexion, increased knee jerk (weak antagonists) and sensory loss on the outer aspect of the leg and mediodorsal aspect of the foot.
- *Cauda equina compression* leading to urinary retention and sensory loss over the sacrum.

Radiologically

- Plain lumbar X-ray (to exclude bone diseases).
- Myelography (using metrizamide) to confirm, localise disc protrusion and exclude intrathecal tumour.
- Computerised tomography

Procedure (Fig. 3.30.1)

1. Under general anaesthesia. The patient is placed in a prone position with the spine flexed.

2. A midline incision is made. Deepen the incision to expose the spines and laminae. Reflect the erector spinae muscles with a wide raspatory and insert a self-retaining muscle retractor.

3. Remove two spines at their base and the supra- and interspinous ligaments with bone-cutting forceps and expose the dura by nibbling bone away from the laminae with bone forceps. Secure haemostasis.

4. In cases where the cord needs to be inspected clear the dura of fat and coagulate veins. Pick up the dura with stay-sutures and open it to look for intradural lesions. Later resuture it with silk. For chordotomy make a cut in the cord with a special angulated knife 3 mm deep from the denticulate ligament to the anterior nerve root on the appropriate side. (The fourth and fifth thoracic segments are opposite the second and third thoracic bodies.)

5. For removal of a prolapsed intervertebral disc, perform a hemilaminectomy: remove one spinous process and retract the cord and nerve root; divide the posterior longitudinal ligament over it, and curette it out with a rongeur.

6. Approximate the muscle and fascia with interrupted sutures and close the skin.

Note: Fenestration decompression (excising ligamentum flavum only) has now almost replaced formal laminectomy in prolapsed i.v. disc. All i.v. disc prolapse cases are accessed via left or right hemilaminectomy. In spinal stenosis, multilevel hemilaminectomy is performed with Redivac tube drainage.

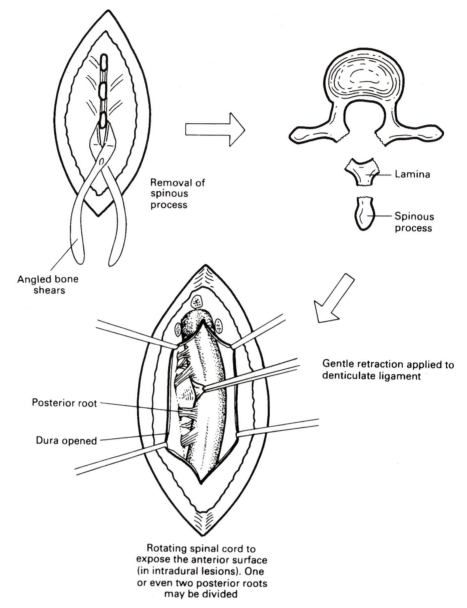

Removal of spinous process

Lamina

Spinous process

Angled bone shears

Gentle retraction applied to denticulate ligament

Posterior root

Dura opened

Rotating spinal cord to expose the anterior surface (in intradural lesions). One or even two posterior roots may be divided

Fig. 3.30.1   Laminectomy for tumours

Comment Spinal decompression and intervertebral disc removal can cause bleeding. Bleeding, however, can be avoided by:
1. Avoiding abdominal compression (patient prone on face or knee–chest position).
2. Ventilation in the negative phase.
3. Montreal mattress or pillow under the chest.
4. Hypotension (rarely needed) by hyperventilation with halothane.

● **For more operations, see also Part Two, Sections 1 and 4.**
● All Candidates are advised to read through *Clinical Radiology in Postgraduate Surgery* by the author.

3.31 Laparoscopic Surgery

See Section 1.14.

SECTION 4
Principles and Practice

Introduction

In this part, examiners test your common sense, practicality and grasp of elementary principles and are not interested in a display of encyclopaedic knowledge. Examiners want to make sure that you are familiar with your surrounding surgical atmosphere, and you are likely to be shown commonly used instruments and appliances, or confronted with clinical questions to test your clinical judgement and wisdom through discussion of X-rays. You may also be asked about controversial topics, e.g. advantages versus disadvantages of operations for breast carcinoma. It is therefore essential that you substantiate your reasoning and answer confidently. The mutual discussion may be interesting and stimulating and sometimes acts as an exchange of experience between the examiner and the candidate. If the examiner wants to tell you his practical way of management, listen to him carefully with interest. You may be questioned about the anatomical basis of surgery and may be shown bones.

This part therefore includes:

- *General topics* already discussed in Section 1 (e.g. endoscopy, radiotherapy, chemotherapy, jaundice, shock, principles of skin grafting, postoperative pain relief, gut precancerous conditions, critical review of breast carcinoma management).
- *Special practical questions.*
- *Bones* (only in London College).
- *Common instruments.*
- *X-rays.*

4.1 Special Practical Questions

ORGANISATION OF OPERATING THEATRE
(Fig. 4.1.1)

Operating theatres should be near the intensive therapy unit (ITU), accident/emergency and X-ray departments. They should be constructed so that they are separate from the general traffic and air movement in the rest of the hospital (far from wards). A single floor reserved entirely for a suite of theatres is recommended. Alternatively a situation in a cul-de-sac rather than near a main thoroughfare is ideal. In order to reduce solar heat-gain, a position on a lower level in the hospital is favoured rather than on the top floor of a tall building. Clean and dirty streams of traffic in an operating department should be segregated practically. There should be a *transfer or change-over section* at the entry to/exit from the sterile zone. This protective zone also includes the recovery area, plaster room, changing rooms and various offices; seminar or teaching facilities may also be sited here.

The *clean zone* consists of scrub room and gowning anaesthetic room, exit lobby, rest areas and sterile store. The operating theatre and sterile preparation room form the *sterile zone*. The least clean area of the whole department is the disposal sluice or sink room and disposal corridor forming the *disposal zone*. The clean zone must include adequate storage rooms for equipment (or general supplies and sterile packets – staff base or office). An X-ray dark room, small laboratory, blood storage facilities, and rest rooms for surgeons and staff may be provided.

The processing and sterilisation of drape and instrument packets is either centralised in the hospital sterilising and disinfecting unit (operates in association with the main *central sterile supply department*) or carried out in the *theatre sterile supply unit* built adjacent to the operating department.

Personnel working within the department should be able to move from one clean area to another without having to pass through unprotected or traffic areas. Air-flow direction should be from the clean to the less clean areas. There should be no air movement between one theatre suite and another. Heating and ventilation should allow comfortable climatic conditions for the patient, surgeons, anaesthetists and staff.

The construction must be such that a high standard of cleanliness can be maintained. All surfaces should be smooth and washable and all joins between walls, ceilings and floors curved to minimise dust collection. The walls should have an impervious semi-matt surface with laminated plastic sheet finish, vinyl sheet or an epoxy resin paint (tiles are not ideal) as these finishes reflect less light. Colour is preferably pale blue, grey or green since they are less tiring to the eyes. The floor should also be impervious, made of terrazzo, rubber or vinyl with an antistatic composition to minimise the danger of an explosion due to a static spark.

There are three types of operating departments, the layout of each being dependent on the total hospital plan:

1. The single-theatre suite.
2. The two-theatre suite or twin suite.
3. Multiple-theatre departments (three or more).

Lighting and electricity

The mains voltage supplied in the UK is between 220 and 240 V, 50 Hz AC. Emergency lighting is provided either from batteries at a low voltage (12–24 V) or by a supplementary

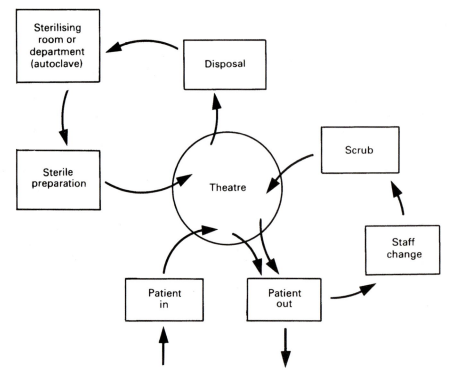

Fig. 4.1.1 Operating theatre organisation

generator which provides electricity at the standard mains voltage. The artificial light makes daylight unnecessary, but the complete absence of windows is psychologically disadvantageous to staff. If windows are fitted they should be small to minimise the solar heat gain or loss and facilitate heating and ventilation control. Provision must be made for blacking out operating areas if endoscopic operations are to be performed. This is achieved by special blinds.

The general lighting of theatres may be provided by fluorescent tubes or filament lamps (recessed in the ceiling) producing even illumination with no glare. For the actual operation (task) area, a shadowless illumination is vital and produced by directing the light from several angles to minimise shadows from the operator and his assistants.

There are three types of shadowless light fittings:
1. The *scialytic shadowless light fitting* consisting of an optical lens surrounding a single lamp of 150 W. Light rays from the lens are projected onto a circle of mirrors focusing light on the operation area with the aid of a lampholder.
2. The *metal reflector shadowless light fitting* – instead of mirrors the reflector consists of a concave, highly polished surface, either plain or made up of many facets.
3. The *multireflector shadowless light fitting* – has six to nine separate lamps instead of one lamp as in (1) and (2) and special reflectors. Focusing is achieved by a single knob fitted to the light housing.

Static electricity, generated whenever two dissimilar materials are separated, can cause a spark especially in a dry atmosphere (with the potential danger of explosion). Static-forming materials include nylon, flannel and wool, viscose rayon, glass, cotton and linen, dry skin, wood, rubber and various plastics. Cotton, linen and viscose rayon are ideal for theatre clotting and towels, since they readily absorb moisture. Carbon black is finely dispersed through rubber resulting in an electrically conductive rubber which dissipates static electricity immediately. This black *antistatic rubber* has a distinctive yellow mark (to distinguish it from other types of rubber).

Switches and socket outlets installed on walls of operating theatres and anaesthetic rooms should be spark-free. Precautions are important to prevent an explosion from sparks or static electricity, particularly in the vicinity of anaesthetic gas leakage. Flammable gas concentrations exist only in an area extending for 25 cm from the leakage point, beyond which gases dilute to a non-flammable level.

Surgical diathermy (electrocautery) and complications

When a large amount of electrical current passes via the tissues of the human body, the temperature rise can be enough to yield a useful surgical effect. Burns however, are the most common diathermy accident in endoscopic and open surgery; they are much more common in monopolar rather than bipolar diathermy. While the **mains** low frequency alternating current can kill by electrocution (with as low as 1 milliAmp) through stimulation of nerves and heart muscles, **radiofrequency** (high frequency alternating) current as high as 2 Amp is used safely in surgical diathermy in open and laparoscopic diathermy; neuromuscular stimulation is rare but it may invoke secondary currents in the vicinity of skeletal muscles or nerves causing twitching e.g. obturator kick and psoas muscle stimulation.

Bipolar diathermy is safer than monopolar diathermy because the heating occurs in tissues held between 2 small active electrodes on the same handpiece; secondary currents may leak to the ground but thay are too small to cause trouble. Bipolar diathermy is however less effective at cutting than monopolar diathermy.

In **monopolar diathermy**, the surgeon uses an active 'live' electrode with a small tip to concentrate a powerful localised current which produces heat at the operative site (high power density); the large return 'indifferent' electrode (a metallic sheet in contact with patient's body) completes the circuit and spreads current over a wide area so that it is less concentrated, producing little heat (low power density). When monopolar diathermy works properly, heating occurs only at the tip of the active electrode; the current passes through the patient's body and escapes safely via the return electrode plate. A safety alarm sounds if the plate contact is inadequate or if one of the 2 wires of the plate is broken or defective, and the current is interrupted and inactivated. Unfortunately, if such a safety alarm is not built in, this long current path in the absence of adequate plate contact or improper wire attachments, can lead to unwanted passage of the current to the earth through the patient's body at points of contact with the operating table (in contact with the earth) or the circuit is completed via a small earthed contact point of a drip stand, a metal component of the operating table, a patient's femoral metal prosthesis, a monitoring electrode, or even via the surgeon. Sufficient current density at that point may result in patient (and/or surgeon) suffering accidental burns to the arms, hip, chest, back, occipit, buttocks or heels. Both the surgeon and the theatre nurse have a duty to see that this is checked. Alcohol-based skin preparations can catch fire if they are allowed to pool on or under the patient in open surgery (less likely in laparoscopic surgery). All patient monitoring equipment should be isolated from the earth wherever this is possible. The plate is applied to the hip without the prosthesis or far away from it (applied to abdomen in bilateral hip prostheses). ECG electrodes should be well gelled and of a large area to disperse the current; the plate is sited so that the current path does not pass through the heart or pacemaker (heart rhythm must be monitored and a defibrillator should be available in case of arrhythmias). A needle electrode should not be used (otherwise it acts as a discharging point for the dense current). As a rule, the return pad or plate should be properly connected and adequately applied to shaved skin; it should be sited close to the operative field so that the main current path will be distant from other potential routes (for current flow to ground) with no nearby small earthed monitor contacts attached to the patient.

Cutting diathermy

Cutting diathermy employs a high current producing sufficient heat to cause cell water to explode into steam (vaporisation). **Coagulation (fulguration)** diathermy produces less explosive but more sustained heat in a platinum wire loop or point raised to red heat by electrical current resulting in cell death by dehydration and protein denaturation with haemostasis until carbonisation or charring occur. Older diathermy machines with valve and spark-gap devices are replaced by modern electronics that modulate amplitude and waveform of the current whether cutting, coagulation or both (**blenderised**). When an active electrode of monopolar diathermy is held a small distance from tissues, electrical discharge arcs across a tiny air gap, creating sparks with very high temperatures (in excess of 1000°C) needed for cutting by continuous waveform (**spray**); reducing cutting diathermy, the low voltage is no longer enough to drive sparks across the gap and no curent will flow, but on touching tissues the current will flow again with gentle tissue necrosis, with sine wave current in bursts of coagulation or fulguration diathermy (**dessication**). This **contact** diathermy faces greater impedance (resistance to current flow) at fatty tissues than to muscles, so contact diathermy works badly on adipose tissues. A ball electrode with larger surface area is gentler than needle coagulation. Contact cutting by point diathermy is less effective than non-contact cutting.

Laparoscopic diathermy

Inadvertent burns to patient during laparoscopic surgery may be caused by various mechanisms:

- burning wrong structure.
- inadvertent activation of electrode by pressure on footswitch pedals particularly if the electrode is out of view at the time.
- faulty insulation (defect or crack) of the conducting parts of the instruments other than operating electode coming in contact with patient. Raising the temperature of the bowel to 60°C for even a short time leads to denaturation of intracellular enzymes and tissue death with subsequent perforation. Instruments are more likely to become damaged with age and to leak with high voltage. Leakage is also more likely if the diathermy is activated when the electrode tip is distant from the target tissue (open circuit activation).
- instrument to instrument coupling (direct coupling) resulting in arcing between instruments outside the field of view; turning up the power in these circumstances can have disastrous consequences (Coag and Blend currents have larger voltage and can jump bigger gaps and open circuit activation is dangerous). Surgeon must not activate diathermy unless the whole of the active electrode is in view.
- retained heat in the tip of active electrode after diathermy use for some time can make the electrode hot enough to damage tissue although no current is flowing. A hot active electrode must not touch tissue.
- unintentionally high current density in pedicles. The high current density path through the base of the infant penis may result in necrosis due to heating (no diathermy must be used in circumcision). Similarly, the appendix base or gallbladder freed from the liver and attached to the common bile duct by the cystic duct may be heated sufficiently to cause perforation of the base or cystic duct. Monopolar diathermy should not be used on organs attached by small pedicles to important structures; that could explain why many surgeons prefer to use Petelin forceps dissection of Calot triangle rather than using hook diathermy.
- capacitative coupling: alternating currents can pass through insulating material, an effect occuring in an electrical device called a capacitor (in which an insulator is sandwiched between 2 electrode metal plates). At laparoscopy, a capacitor may be formed unintentionally: with an insulated electrode passing through a metal tube, the core of electrode acts as one plate and metal tube as the other with an insulator between – a

capacitor! This effect is due to high frequency alternating current inducing an alternating magnetic field which in turn induces electrical current in the enveloping conducting objects. Thus diathermy flows through the active electrode (hook or grasper) and induces a current in its metal cannula despite insulation (electromagnetic induction) and resultant current flows from the metal sheath directly to the bowel with heatng perforation at the point of contact. This rare phenomenon produces a small current of no ill consequence, but the current is greater in open circuit activation and in 5 mm cannuae as compared to 10 mm cannulae. Non-conducting trocars should be used if possible or if metal trocars are used they should make good contact with the abdominal wall (to disperse current); open circuit activation and/or high voltage non-contact diathermy (fulgration and blenderised diathermy) must always be avoided.

Laparoscopic means of tissue destruction

These include:
1. Bipolar and monopolar diathermy.
2. Laparoscopic laser: for cutting, a hard crystal tip in contact mode can focus light of neodynium: YAG (yttrium aluminium garnet), holium: YAG, or diode laser can produce very high tissue temperatures needed for cutting powered by 15–40W in contact work. For tissue destruction YAG lasers emit infrared laser light directed down a quartz fibre using the principle of total internal reflection. When the YAG laser hits the tissue its heat energy causes destruction; in non-contact mode, the beam crosses the air gap between the bare end of the fibre and the tissue; a much higher power of 100W is used for destruction by vaporisation. CO_2 laser is strongly absorbed by intracellular water causing vaporisation of tissues. Mechanisms for laser safety include fail-safe devices inactivating the laser when not in use; laser inadvertent focusing on the eye lens may cause blind spot and eyewear precaution is required. Laser officer should be appointed in laser safety; doors should be locked, signed and alarmed to prevent the unwary from straying into a laser operating session unannounced.
3. The harmonic scalpel uses a high frequency ultrasound vibration to provide cutting with local coagulation; there is both heating and mechanical disruption of tissues producing haemostasis. This device is safe and relatively cheap, but cutting is slower than that achieved by diathermy or contact lasers.
4. Morcellators are like laparoscopic food processors and are used to liquefy relatively large solid organs so that they can be removed without a large incision; the organ or tissue is contained in an entrapment bag during morcellation.

Ventilation

This is of paramount importance:
● For the comfort of the staff.
● To remove the anaesthetic gases.
● To admit air free of pathogenic organisms.
The ventilated air passes through spinning water discs or a steam humidifier, resulting in 50–60% relative humidity. Combined with background heating (from pipes or panels within walls or ceiling) a ventilation system is a very

satisfactory way of rapidly adjusting the temperature in the operating theatre and maintaining it between 18.5 °C and 22 °C (except during hypothermia anaesthesia). The minimum bacteriological air requirements are:
1. No detectable clostridium spores or coagulase-positive *Staphylococcus aureus*. No more than 35 bacteria-carrying particles/m³ of ventilated air is allowed (as tested on aerobic cultures).
2. During surgical operations, the concentration of bacterially contaminated airborne particles over a 5 min period should not exceed 180/m³. There are two good methods of assessing the bacterial content of the air – the *settling or sedimentation plate* (a culture plate on which bacteria in air are allowed to settle) and the *slit-sampler* (air is sucked through a narrow slit onto a rotating culture plate beneath it); the latter is a more efficient and quicker method.

Surgical sepsis has been greatly reduced as a result of installation of special ventilation systems. The following types are available:

Plenum turbulent air flow system   Positive pressure is essential to prevent contaminated air infiltrating into the theatre, and the air pressure in the theatre should be slightly greater than that outside the suite. A medium velocity system is the method of choice (at present). Air at roof level is drawn by a fan via a series of filters, humidified, cooled or warmed and forced into the theatre through high-level diffusers fitted into walls and ceiling. Filters must be changed regularly since bacteria such as Pseudomonas multiply on cooling coils and humidifier. The filter is made of disposable fabric and oiled mesh with pores of about 5 μm in diameter which are sufficient to filter airborne particles containing bacteria (not individual bacteria).

Laminar flow displacement ventilation system   Air moving at a unidirectional horizontal velocity passes through an efficient filter to remove inherent contamination. Positive pressurisation is as before but instead of turbulent air rapidly mixing with that already present in the theatre, the displaced air is introduced gently and merely displaces that in the theatre by quiet downward movement.

Others   A high impact/high exhaust enclosure was introduced by Charnley. This was improved to the Charnley–Howorth Surgicair enclosure and later to the Ex Flow Clean Zone unit (with no side walls). Another approach is a surgical plastic isolater.

ORGANISATION OF THE ACCIDENT AND EMERGENCY DEPARTMENT (Fig. 4.1.2)

An accident and emergency department is the shop window of the hospital service and is likened to Cinderella (hard working yet understaffed and not the most popular department in the hospital). Owing to the large number of injuries affecting limbs, it would be most appropriately run by an orthopaedic surgeon fully trained in the management of musculoskeletal injuries. The duties of the consultant in charge include:

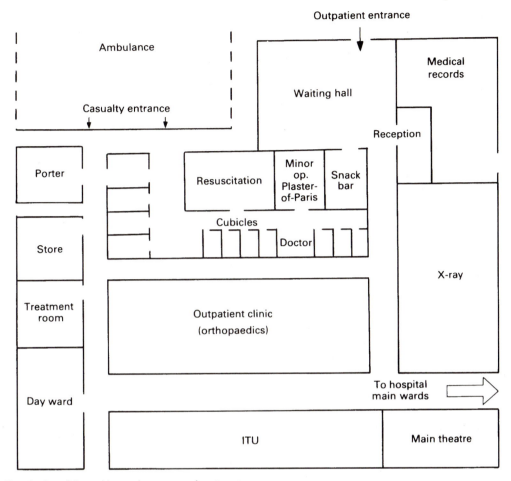

Fig. 4.1.2   Organisation of the accident and emergency department

- Administration and sorting of cases.
- Teaching and training.
- Resuscitation in major accidents.
- Definitive treatment of many of the less serious conditions.

Apart from the consultant in charge, registrar, senior house officers and nursing staff, there are general practitioners, ambulance service men and porters involved actively in the department's performance. It is beyond dispute that the best departments are those with consultants playing an active and full continuous role in the day-to-day work including initial treatment, continuous care and rehabilitation of injuries.

The department should include two fully equipped resuscitation rooms (for major cases), a treatment room (for potentially infected cases), a few (3–5) cubicles for examination and treatment of minor cases (dressing, suturing and foreign body removal), as well as a day ward (for observation of some cases) and a minor theatre for reduction of fractures, e.g. Colles' and dislocations. This may be combined with a plaster room (one of the resuscitation rooms may be converted into a minor theatre). Easy access by the ambulance service to the accident and emergency department is important. Ancillary rooms include doctors' and staff rest room, porter office, reception and waiting room. The accident and emergency department should be near the X-ray department, intensive therapy unit and the main operating theatre.

The essence of a good accident and emergency service is the ability to meet sudden and particularly unforeseen needs. One of the least appealing features of such a service is that it is never off duty and it is likely to be busiest when most would prefer to be off duty and even in bed.

Major trauma cases include injuries of bones, joints, nerves and tendons which, although not likely to cause death, are serious injuries and constitute real emergencies. On the other hand, thoracic, abdominal and severe head injuries are critical and likely to be fatal. Minor cases include wounds and lacerations, as well as emotionally shocked patients. Thus in disasters (an emergency of such magnitude as to require extraordinary mobilisation of accident and emergency services) the management plan needs to be flexible and based on quick sorting of patients arriving at the hospital into three groups (triage classification):

1. Moribund and hopeless (too damaged to benefit from treatment, i.e. dying or dead).
2. Those whose lives are threatened requiring immediate attention (critically injured) and those who need attention fairly soon (seriously injured).
3. Those who can wait (minor injuries or emotional trauma).

It has been estimated that of the population examined in an accident and emergency department only 48% required the hospital services and 51% could have been treated at home. Among the 48% only 3.5% of cases were actually in danger of death (critically injured) while 44.5% were deemed real emergencies but not in danger of death. About 1% died in the accident and emergency department; and 19% of cases were admitted into hospital (11% to a surgical or specialised unit and 3% to the intensive therapy unit).

ORGANISATION OF INTENSIVE THERAPY UNIT

Ideally 1% of hospital beds should be devoted to the intensive therapy unit (ITU) (coronary care unit is excluded). The unit is under the shared responsibility of an anaesthetist as well as surgeons and/or physicians according to the nature of the case. Their duties include daily rounds (and regular follow-up), teaching, patient discharge and admission to another ward when the patient has recovered sufficiently.

Staff includes medical (anaesthetists, surgeons and/or physicians), junior medical (registrars, senior house officers and house officers), nursing (should be one nurse per patient per session or four nurses per bed per 24 h) and ancillary staff (porters, cleaners and technicians).

The ITU should be near the operating theatre, recovery area and hospital wards. Radiological and biochemical facilities should be available (especially blood gases analysis). The design, which should include dirty and clean areas (for infected and clean cases respectively), can be either: *open-plan* or *closed-plan* cubicles (to minimise infection and psychological trauma).

Whatever the design is, an ITU should be very clean, with a good air conditioning and ventilation system so that airborne cross-infection will be avoided. Such an efficient air flow pattern and air conditioning obviate the need for a special respiratory exhaust system.

Every bed should be specially equipped and provided with electrical outlets. Additional outlets for X-ray and domestic use are needed and should have separate grounding systems. Piped oxygen and suction outlets (two of each) are required for each bed. Pipeline supplies of both nitrous oxide and compressed air and a modern ventilator per bed are also required. Bedside and/or central monitoring of patients is a matter of individual choice. A monitor screen that can display signals from all beds should be sited in the staff sitting or conference room.

Rapid and frequent service, especially determination of blood gases, serum electrolytes, blood sugar and ESR, may demand the provision of a small computerised on-site laboratory with radiation protection material.

There should be sufficient storage space for drugs, linen, sterile supplies, i.v. fluids, respiratory, electric and diagnostic equipment and domestic cleaning machines. Equipment should be wall-mounted.

Accommodation for unit secretary/receptionist and visitors should be provided.

Indications for nursing a patient in an ITU

Surgical patients requiring:
- mechanical support of vital function, e.g. mechanical ventilation;
- intensive monitoring;
- highly skilled nursing care.
  These are encountered in patients with:
- respiratory failure;
- cardiovascular instability;
- metabolic and electrolyte disturbances;
- renal failure.
  Examples of patients:
- crush injuries of the chest and abdomen;
- head and neck injuries;
- extensive burns;
- associated medical conditions (asthma, epilepsy, chronic obstructive airway disease).
- tetanus;
- postoperative problems with airways, coagulation, endocrine or nutrition;
- postoperative cardiopulmonary bypass, transplant, extensive vascular surgery;
- ARDS.

USE OF THE STETHOSCOPE IN SURGERY

Preoperative

- Checking blood pressure.
- Assessment of valvular and cardiac lesions. Murmurs necessitate prophylactic antibiotics to prevent subacute bacterial endocarditis. Benign systolic murmurs may indicate hyperdynamic circulation as in anaemia and arteriovenous fistula and further investigations are required.
- Assessment of major vascular diseases, e.g. systolic murmur may indicate coarctation of the aorta, bruit may indicate carotid artery atherosclerosis, renal artery stenosis and aortic aneurysm.
- Assessment of chest conditions and treatment accordingly.
- Assessment of intestinal obstruction: either loud frequent sounds (borborygmi or high-pitched sounds), tingling or no sounds in silent abdomen of paralytic ileus.
- Assessment of vascular tumours, e.g. hepatoma and haemangioma of liver or eye proptosis due to arteriovenous fistula or skeletal metastases from thyroid carcinoma.

Operative

To confirm the correct placement of the endotracheal tube by listening to breath sounds on inflation of the lungs.

Postoperative

- Assessment of pulmonary complications after major abdominal or thoracic operation, e.g. atelactasis, abscesses and bronchopneumonia.
- Bases of lung should be auscultated for possible left ventricular failure decompensated after major operation. After cardiac operations a murmur may indicate leakage from an artificial valve replacement.

● In abdominal surgery, bowel sounds are checked by auscultating McBurney's point. Good bowel sounds may indicate that nasogastric suction can be removed.

DRAINAGE IN SURGERY

Drainage can be established operatively be channelling the contents of the internal organs externally (e.g. ileostomy, colostomy, urostomy, cholecystectomy) or by diverting the visceral contents internally (e.g. gastric drainage via pyloroplasty or gastroenterostomy, cholecystojejunostomy or ureterosigmoidostomy). More importantly, drainage is established by mechanical means for removal of:

1. Contents of body organs, e.g. Foley's catheterisation of urinary bladder and nasogastric tube aspiration. There are also specialised drains for hydrocephalus or infected obstructed kidney.
2. Secretions of body cavities, e.g. peritoneal and pleural cavities.
3. Various tissue fluids, e.g. pus, blood, secretions, introduced solutions and air.

Drains are not substitutes for careful haemostasis and meticulous dissection. Drainage is discussed with items (2) and (3) in mind.

Indications for drainage

● Removal of material foreign or harmful to a particular location, e.g. potential nidus of infection.
● Obliteration of dead space.
● Monitoring and prevention of operative complications, e.g. delayed haemorrhage and anastomotic leak.
● Therapeutic value of fibrous tract after drain removal, e.g. T-tube track can be utilised for retrieval of residual biliary stone.

The value of drainage is debatable because it is inconvenient to the patient, it increases the risk of contamination (with introduction of infection), causes delay in healing (because drains are foreign bodies) and may even cause breakdown of anastomosis. Drains themselves damage delicate tissues by mechanical pressure and can irritate and induce fluid formation and collection. On balance, however, the following conditions should be drained:

● Abscess cavity with thick shaggy walls that must collapse for healing of the deepest portion, e.g. perforated appendix.
● Insecure anastomosis because of its size, tension, poor blood supply, infection or general metabolic abnormalities (like diabetes) or because the sutured organs lack peritoneal covering (extraperitoneal rectum) or are difficult to cover with omentum or nearby bowel.
● Anticipated leakage, e.g. gall bladder bed, pancreatic and splenic surgery.
● After trauma since missed foreign bodies and massive contamination lead to incomplete healing.
● Generalised peritonitis *per se* is not an indication for drainage since this would be physically and physiologically impossible. Therefore there should be other reasons for drainage, e.g. perforated viscus or a localised source of peritonitis.

Complications of drains

● Infection (exaggerated).
● Anastomotic leak and duodenal stump perforation (if in contact with suture line as a result of mechanical pressure necrosis).
● A vessel may be cut when the stab wound is made leading to haemorrhage.
● Bowel may herniate alongside a drain and become obstructed.
● Wound dehiscence and postoperative hernia formation if the drain is brought out through the primary incision.
● Loss of the drain, e.g. inside the abdomen. The drain should, therefore, be fixed to the skin for security.

Types of drain

Gauze packs and ribbon gauze wicks   Act by capillary action. They may be soaked in eusol-paraffin to prevent adhesions to the raw healing surface.

Twisted nylon suture threads   Used sometimes after breast mass excision and minor operations.

Penrose   Very thin and soft rubber tube of 2.5 cm diameter which can be filled with gauze and acts as a cigarette drain. Used in abscess cavities like wicks. It does not cause pressure necrosis due to its softness.

Sheet drains   Corrugated drain in which the fluid tracks to the surface in the gutter. Yeates drain (a sheet formed from parallel plastic tubes) in which fluid passes through tubes; once these have filled, it tends to track alongside the drain.

Tube drains   In abdominal surgery they are connected to bags, thus forming a closed system, but in pneumo- or haemothorax or post-thoracotomy they are connected to an underwater seal closed system. Multiple holes at the end are essential in case one hole becomes obstructed. A sump drain consists of two tubes. A large outer tube creates a sump in which fluid collects. A smaller tube lies freely at the bottom of this sump and is attached to a suction source (tissue can not be drawn into the holes of the smaller suction tube). A Shirley sump drain incorporates a side tube guarded by a bacterial filter so that sterile air can be drawn to the drain tip. When suction is applied, the air leak prevents tissues being sucked into the holes of the drain and blocking them.

Vacuum drains   Redon trocar needle is used to attach the drain to the Redivac, Sterivac or Surgivac apparatus to create negative pressure with no need for a suction machine.

Drains must not be too rigid as they may damage viscera, nor too soft as they may twist or kink and become blocked. They should not be made of irritant material, e.g. rubber, but rather of silicone, Silastic or polyethylene. To serve its purpose the drain should be wide, patent and left in situ for an adequate period until drainage is minimal. If used prophylactically, e.g. duodenal stump or anastomotic leak, the drain should be left in place as long as the danger of perforation exists, i.e. for 10 days, until a fibrous track is formed which will act as an external fistula (with a safety-valve action).

RADIOACTIVE ISOTOPES IN SURGERY

Are used in three ways:

In vivo – diagnostic scanning

Diagnosis of space-occupying lesions (in bones, thyroid, brain, liver or mediastinum), assessment of function (renogram in kidney diseases, blood flow measurement and lung scanning in pulmonary infarction due to embolism). For example:

- ^{99m}Tc pertechnetate intravenously for scanning of skeletal metastases (bone isotope scan), vascular diseases and lung scan.
- ^{131}I in goitre and brain scan.
- ^{67}Ga for hepatic and mediastinal scanning (in Hodgkin's and non-Hodgkin's lymphomas).

A carrier material is needed as a radioactive marker, e.g. ^{131}I-labelled albumen is used in diagnosis of venous thrombosis and estimation of blood volume loss in shock, and ^{99m}Tc-labelled microspheres are used in lung scanning.

In vivo – therapy

Such radioactive isotopes are used for palliation and rarely for cure of tumours. Available as interstitial radiotherapy (e.g. radioactive gold grains, seeds and wires), as an intracavitary colloidal solution (e.g. radioactive gold solution to prevent recurrent pleural effusion in pleurodesis and to prevent malignant ascitic fluid accumulation) or as a special i.v. systemic radiotherapy (e.g. ^{32}P for polycythaemia rubra vera). Radioactive isotope therapy can also be administered using a linear accelerator, e.g. telecobalt (^{60}CO) in the radiotherapy of many solid tumours. Radioactive isotopes are used in non-malignant disease such as thyrotoxicosis and certain skin diseases, and also for pituitary and hormonal manipulation in terminal cases for pain relief.

Ex vivo radioimmunoassay in research

- Physiology of fluid compartment measurement such as total body water, plasma volume, extracellular fluid, blood flow and cardiac output.
- Respiratory physiology using labelled O_2 and CO_2.
- Metabolism of protein, fat and carbohydrate.
- Electrolytes and membrane permeability.
- Formation and fate of lymphocytes and blood elements and RBC life-cycle and synthesis.
- Intracellular digestive enzymes.

MICROSURGERY

Telescopic spectacles or a simple operating microscope with high-intensity illumination can provide a stereoscopic magnified field of vision up to $\times$ 6 and $\times$ 40 respectively. The focal distance between the surgeon's eyepieces and his hands is 150–200 mm. The operating microscope needs to be sterilised and maintained. The instruments required are fine and delicate, e.g. ridge or beak-tipped forceps, titanium microsurgical needle holder, microscissors, suction cutter, fine needles with very fine

suture materials such as 7/0, 8/0 silk and 9/0, 10/0 nylon or Prolene. Teaching is possible with a microscopic teaching aid.

Uses

Otolaryngology: in middle ear surgery fenestration, stapes operations, tympanoplasties and acoustic neuroma treatment.

Ophthalmology: in cataract surgery, keratoplasty, glaucoma and vitrectomy.

Neurosurgery: in intracranial aneurysms, thromboembolectomy and tumour surgery especially in spinal cord and bypass extracranial–intracranial anastomosis for stroke.

Plastic surgery: in micro- (below wrist) and macro- (above wrist) reimplantation surgery of the hand with anastomosis of vessels and nerves, and in transplantation of the great toe for use as a thumb. Also in vascular graft surgery.

Vascular surgery: in renal, carotid and small blood vessel anastomoses (it is technically possible to join vessels as small as 1 mm in diameter).

Gynaecology: in dissection and anastomosis of the Fallopian tubes in sterility cases.

Urology: in ureteric anastomosis and sphincteric surgery and in vasovasotomy in patients with bilateral vasectomy reversal.

Others:

- Casualty – for removal of foreign bodies and repair surgery.
- Paediatrics – for catheterisation of minute vessels in small babies.
- Dermatology – for diagnosis and treatment of skin lesions.

ASCITES

Either cirrhotic or malignant (tuberculous ascites is not discussed here). In malignant ascites there is no cure and the mechanisms is unknown but there is mucous secretion and peritoneal infiltration. In cirrhosis, hypoproteinuria and portal hypertension are the main factors. Treatment of intractable ascites includes the following.

Medical treatment

With diuretics and chemotherapy, e.g. spironolactone therapy up to 450 mg/24 h (response time is 10–28 days), intracavitary chemotherapy with thiotepa or bleomycin cytotoxics.

Repeated tapping

Is uncomfortable, causes hypoalbuminaemia, marasmus and subcutaneous implantations and is expensive.

Peritoneovenous (PV) shunt

With Denver or LeVeen valves under local anaesthesia and prophylactic antibiotics. This will increase plasma volume and urine volume and improve nutrition. The valve is inserted intraperitoneally with the valve pump connected by an abdominal tube that is drained subcutaneously into an internal jugular vein.

Postoperative therapy

Includes diuretics, inhalation against resistance, probably a corset or binder, and sometimes anticoagulants.

Complications of PV shunts

- Death due to fluid overload.
- Blockage of the shunt is the major problem and is due to the recurrence of ascites, a non-compressible Denver valve or direct puncture of venous tubing. The leak is detected by a shuntogram and treated by regular Valsalva's manoeuvres, and an increase in diuretics. Shuntogram may be diagnostic and therapeutic. The Denver valve may need to be pumped and the shunt may need revision.
- Failure.
- Sepsis and fever.
- Emboli, e.g. clots, tumour pieces, cholesterol or air.
- Tumour spread locally or systemically.
- Venous thrombosis.
- Catheter migration.
- PV shunt coagulopathy with bleeding (rarely).

Contraindications for PV shunts

- Short life expectancy.
- Cardiorespiratory cripple.
- Poor liver function.
- Loculated viscous or blood-stained ascites (block PV shunt quickly).

ADHESIONS

Adhesions are the commonest cause of intestinal obstruction in the Western world accounting for one-third of intestinal obstructions in general and 50% of small bowel intestinal obstructions. They are also the most likely cause of intestinal strangulation. About 93% of abdominal surgery patients have adhesions due to previous surgery and postoperative adhesions account for more than 30% of all admissions for small bowel obstructions. Also 3% of all laparotomies are performed to relieve small bowel obstructions from adhesions.

In developing countries where laparotomies are a rarity and where hernias go untreated until they reach an enormous size or strangulate, intestinal obstruction due to adhesions is uncommon and strangulated external hernias head the list of causes of intestinal obstruction.

Adhesions are found at second look in 55–100% of patients undergoing pelvic surgery; pelvic adhesions are the cause of infertility in 15–20% of cases. Postoperative adhesions can lead to chronic pelvic pain.

Peritoneal healing and aetiology of adhesions

Clinical and experimental studies have shown that unsutured peritoneal defects heal rapidly and usually without adhesion formation. Centripetal growth from the wound margins contributes little to the healing process. The entire defect becomes endothelialised simultaneously and not gradually from the border as in epithelialisation of skin wounds. The new mesothelium is derived from subperitoneal perivascular connective tissue cells which resemble primitive mesenchymal cells. If there is ischaemic injury (e.g. if the tissues were crushed) and the peritoneum is sutured or ligated, because of a marked decrease in fibrinolytic activity, fibrin adhesions almost invariably form and later become fibrous intra-abdominal adhesions. Many substances may contaminate the peritoneal cavity at the time of laparotomy and induce foreign body granuloma and adhesion formation, e.g. fragments of gauze, lint or cotton wool, clumps of antibiotic powder or glove dust powder such as talc (magnesium silicate), lycopodium and starch powder.

Classification of adhesions

Congenital (about 2%) e.g. Meckel's diverticulum, malrotation of the colon or congenital bands. Although they are rare, they may occasionally give rise to strangulation.

Acquired These are the most common type.
1. Postoperative (about 80%), e.g. appendicectomy and gynaecological surgery. Although much less commonly, abdominoperineal rectal excision and total colectomy are also particularly likely to be followed by obstructive adhesions.
2. Postinflammatory (about 18%), e.g. acute appendicitis, diverticulitis, pelvic infection, Crohn's disease and cholecystitis in this order of frequency.

Prevention of adhesions

Various methods have been used in an attempt to prevent adhesions. They are probably ineffective but may be harmful and may even increase the incidence of adhesions.
- The instillation of various fluids, e.g. Dextran 70, povidone-iodine, or distension with gas introduced intraperitoneally to hold the damaged surfaces apart.
- Use of powderless gloves and glove cleansing.
- Enhancement of peristalsis in an attempt to disrupt early fibrinous adhesions.
- The covering of peritoneal surfaces with an extraordinary variety of inert membranes and lubricants or with grafts of peritoneum. Seprafilm bioresorbable membrane and sepracoat coating solution (both are hyaluronic acid-based products made by Genzyme Co.) are becoming popular in surgical practice.
- The use of enzymes to digest adhesions, e.g. trypsin and hyaluronidase.
- The instillation of substances to inhibit deposition of fibrin, e.g. steroids, anticoagulants and fibrinolytic agents.
- No closure of peritoneum.

Treatment

- The vast majority of adhesions are completely harmless and in many instances are life-saving by promoting anastomotic healing and localising intra-abdominal inflammation.

- Conservative nasogastric suction and i.v. drip are indicated in early postoperative intestinal obstruction and where there have been previous episodes of subacute intestinal obstruction or several previous operations for division of adhesions.
- The majority of acute intestinal obstructions due to adhesions, however, require immediate surgical relief by freeing of a kinked or compressed loop of bowel; rarely resection or bypass (short circuit) may be needed.
- Recurrent adhesive small intestinal obstruction may need small bowel intubation for 7–10 days with a 300 cm long, 18 Fr Foley tube inserted via a jejunostomy. It is threaded through and splints the small bowel. Once the tube tip reaches the caecum the balloon can be inflated. The gastrointestinal tract should be sucked out and emptied prior to intubation.
- Rarely plication operations are carried out for recurrent intestinal obstruction due to adhesions, e.g. Noble's seromuscular bowel plication, Childs and Phillips mesenteric plication and Takita's operation of anchoring the greater omentum to the lesser sac and plicating bowel loops by their mesentery.

Comment

It is highly recommended that after any laparotomy, wherever possible, the omentum is brought down between the gut and the abdominal wall (after placing the small intestine in organised loops). This avoids dangerous small bowel adhesions to the posterior aspect of the midline incision; instead omental adhesions to the posterior aspect of the anterior abdominal wall are formed and are easy to detach.

SUDDEN DEATH DURING SURGICAL OPERATION

Anaesthetic error

Hypoxia May be induced by the following. Undetected respiratory obstruction, kinked or displaced endotracheal tube, vagal stimulation caused rarely by intubation, oesophagoscopy, mediastinoscopy or bronchoscopy. Wrong gas or wrong connection. Tension pneumothorax due to rupture of emphysematous bulla after positive pressure ventilation. Mendelson's syndrome or chemical pneumonitis due to hydrochloric acid aspiration during anaesthesia while gas reflex is absent and endotracheal tube is not cuffed or inflated properly. Undetected hypotension and falling blood pressure due to internal bleeding. Air embolism via undiscovered disconnected i.v. line especially the subclavian one.

Wrong drugs or misadministration Anaphylactic reaction to anaesthetic agent, to dextran or undetected incompatible blood transfusion (detected during operation only by falling blood pressure and sudden unexplained wound bleeding). Overdosage of local anaesthetic, e.g. procaine released systemically after regional i.v. anaesthesia. Accidental injection of direct or indirect depressant (vasodilator), hypotension induced by ganglion blockers, lignocaine and aminophylline. Cardioplegic action of hyperkalaemia. Arrhythmia due to cardiac irritation by chloroform or cyclopropane and adrenaline.

Patient problems

Operation after recent myocardial infarction or in a patient with a diseased myocardium or cardiogenic shock, severe dehydration and electrolyte imbalance (in intestinal obstruction), pulmonary oedema or severe chest disease can all lead to death. Other risk factors include shocked patient due to leaking aneurysm, upper gastrointestinal tract bleeding or ruptured ectopic gestation. Also amniotic fluid embolism during delivery.

Surgical error

- Hypotension induced by rough manipulation of bowel and mesenteric stretching, and rarely by sympathectomy.
- Cardiac arrhythmia induced by cardiac catheterisation, open heart surgery and wrong non-synchronised DC shock (S on T phenomenon).
- Oculocardiac reflex induced by pressure on eyeballs in ophthalmic operation (vagal stimulation).
- Accidental incision of groin aneurysm misdiagnosed as abscess with uncontrollable bleeding.

CAUSES OF SECOND DAY POSTOPERATIVE JAUNDICE

- Anaesthetic toxicity, e.g. halothane.
- Drug toxicity, e.g. chlorpromazine (Largactil).
- Operative stress superimposed upon pre-existing liver disease or viral hepatitis.
- Liver hypoxia, e.g. underperfusion and hypotension.
- Haemolysis due to excessive or incompatible blood.
- Extrahepatic biliary residual stone or cholestasis.
- Ligated or injured common bile duct.
- Leakage of bile into peritoneal cavity (with transperitoneal absorption of bile, often associated with sepsis and shock).
- Septicaemia and cholangitis (late).
- Pulmonary embolism (after 7th day).

PERIOPERATIVE FEVER

Perioperative fever can be classified according to the time of its appearance:

- *During induction*: fever is due to malignant hyperpyrexia (see below).
- *During operation:* fever may be due to either malignant hyperpyrexia (tachycardia, arrhythmia, and cyanosis with severe acidosis) or incompatible blood transfusion (mild elevation in temperature, hypotension, intraoperative bleeding or blood oozing from the wound, bronchospasm, and haemoglobinuria due to haemolysis). Rarely, drug interaction and reactions to incompatible blood transfusion may cause fever. Bleeding may also cause fever.
- *0–2 postoperative days:* fever is due to:
  - operative trauma and haematoma formation (mild fever),
  - within 6 h, metabolic conditions such as thyroid crisis or adrenocortical insufficiency may cause fever.

- pulmonary collapse (high fever);
- blood transfusion (due to incompatible reaction or pyrogens), or drug interaction.
- specific infections during surgery, e.g. instrumentation of oesophagus can be complicated by oesophageal perforation and fever. Instrumentation of urethra or exploration of common bile duct may also lead to high fever.
- *3–5 postoperative days:* fever is due to either developing sepsis (wound infection, pelvic, and subphrenic abscess) or bronchopneumonia.
- *5–7 postoperative days:* fever is due to anastomotic leak (perianastomotic abscess and fistula formation) or deep venous thrombosis developing in limbs or pelvic veins.
- *After the first postoperative week:* fever is due to wound sepsis (or rarely, hepatic or cerebral abscess) or thrombotic disease. Anastomotic leak may also be responsible.
- Predisposing factors may include smoking, debilitation, obesity, chronic lung disease, upper abdominal and chest incisions (predisposing to pulmonary collapse and pneumonia). In deep vein thrombosis, past history of DVT, anticoagulant therapy for other reasons, and contraceptive pills are predisposing factors.

ORAL CANCER

Over 2000 new oral cancers are diagnosed each year in the UK and account for 5% of all malignancies, with an incidence equal to that of carcinoma of the cervix and equal to that of malignant melanoma. Oral cancer incidence increases with age, but it is on the increase in young patients and women.

Known risk factors

- Candidiasis.
- Deficiency of iron, vitamin A and C.
- Smoking and other tobacco habits.
- High alcohol intake, especially alcohol-based mouth rinses.
- Smoking + alcohol = relative risk × 15.
- Betel nut and leaf/pan chewing (lime, spices, areca, tobacco etc.). Some of these are presented as oral fresheners in Indian restaurants. Syphilitic glossitis is no longer a common predisposing factor.
- Often no obvious risk factors, particularly in young patients. Deletion of healthy genes, inactivation of tumour suppressor genes, and activation of oncogenes have all been proposed in the aetiology. Recurrent oral tumour has more genetic errors or deletions than non-recurrent one.

Clinical presentation:

Includes:
- White patches (leucoplakia).
- Red patches (erythroplakia).
- Both white and red patches are mistaken by patients for traumatic lesions because of their dentures
- Speckled patches (speckled plakia).
- Non-healing oral sore or ulcer within 1–2 weeks; it should be considered malignant if it persists more than 3 weeks.

- Warty lumps or nodules in the mouth.
- Induration or thickening of the oral mucosa.
- Pigmented areas in the mouth.
- Neck swellings.
- Difficulty with speech, swallowing or mouth opening.

The great majority (over 90%) of oral cancers are squamous carcinomas, with pleomorphic salivary adenomas accounting for most of the remainder.

Sites

The most common sites are:
1. Tongue.
2. Floor of the mouth.
3. Retro-molar fossa.
4. Buccal sulcus (especially in betel nut cancer).

Management

In general, premalignant lesions can be cured with simple treatment. Early cancers have 80% cure rate with minimal morbidity. Large tumours need major surgery and radiotherapy. Modern treatment methods have reduced disfigurement and improved the functional results but the overall cure rate is less than 50% because many cancers are already advanced before they are diagnosed.

Oral tumours must be referred to an oral and maxillofacial surgeon or to an ENT surgeon with an interest in head and neck surgery.
- Treatment must first start with stopping tobacco smoking and alcohol intake to reverse early premalignant lesions.
- Premalignant lesions need biopsy and careful follow-up; if necessary they can be treated by laser removal or simple excision.
- Small early cancers can be treated by simple surgery, laser excision or radiotherapy.
- More advanced tumours can be treated successfully with a combination of excisional surgery and radiotherapy. Modern reconstructive techniques and replacement offer reduced mobility and good functional results; to gain access it may be necessary to split the mandible temporarily. The tumour can then be excised '*en bloc*' with any involved bone or cervical lymph nodes; large defects left after excision require skilled repair using skin flaps or free grafts with microvascular anastomses.
- Where complete cure is not possible, high-quality palliative care is essential.

TYPES OF BIOPSY

By and large there are two main groups of biopsies:

Open direct biopsies

- *Incisional biopsy* by taking a part or wedge of the lesion (ulcer or tumour) including the margin and normal surrounding skin tissue (important for histological comparison); it is usually performed under local anaesthesia in the outpatient clinic or in the ward.

● *Excisional biopsy* by removing the entire lesion (ulcer or tumour) with safety skin or tissue margin; it is usually performed under general anaesthesia in the operating theatre.

Most biopsies are kept in formalin and stained prior to sectioning in order to reach an accurate histological diagnosis in 48 hours (*paraffin section biopsy*).

However, a quick tentative diagnosis (over the phone) may be required in 10–15 minutes of the mass excision sent to the pathology department (after prior arrangement) in a dry container without formalin, while the surgeon is waiting in theatre and the patient is still exposed before embarking on the definitive procedure (such as mastectomy); this is called *frozen section biopsy* and requires a skilled pathologist to read it.

Closed indirect biopsies

● *Tru-cut needle biopsy* of a breast mass or prostate performed in outpatient clinic, ward or theatre with or without local or general anaesthesia.
● *Fine needle aspiration biopsy cytology* of breast mass, thyroid enlargement, or parotid tumour; it is usually performed in outpatient clinic.
● *Punch biopsy* performed in outpatient clinic, ward or theatre, for instance a punch biopsy of a rectal polyp via a rigid sigmoidoscope.
● *Endoscopic suction biopsy, brushing cytology, or exfoliative cytology of bronchial wash-out, gastroscopy wash-out, or urinary sediment.*
● Loop biopsies e.g. TUR prostate.

HAZARDS FACING SURGICAL STAFF IN THE OPERATING THEATRE

These may include the following:
1. Traumatic hazards, such as accidental pinpricks with needles, scalpel and other instruments predisposing to general non-specific infection as well as specific ones (see below). The resultant hole in the glove can further predispose the staff to direct electrical hazards. Tall and uncareful staff are vulnerable to trauma by a malpositioned lighting system, with possible head injuries. Staff can be injured by the edge of the operating table, or falling objects or dismantlable parts of an operating table can cause lower limb injuries.
2. Electrical hazards of diathermy and electrocautery due to electrical faults of the device or wrong connections, resulting in diathermy burns and accidental cautery of staff. Static electricity may cause damage in staff with improper precautions. A laser may cause eye damage, and goggles must be worn by the staff with full precautions.
3. Infection risk from patients with specific infections, such as hepatitis and AIDS, particularly when associated with pinprick injuries and if precautions are not taken.
4. Pollution risk of anaesthetic gases in theatre; this may lead to abortion in pregnant staff (theoretical risk).
5. Irradiation risk due to X-ray machines and image intensifiers in perioperative cholangiography, on-table venograms, orthopaedic correction of fractures, removal of foreign bodies and other interventional radiological procedures.

6. Surgeons may face litigation problems by patients, such as missed swab/instrument/needle within the patient's body (can ultimately lead to abscess formation), diathermy burns (unearthed plate with no jelly in contact with patient's skin, faulty connection, or ignorance of safety precautions), improperly placed drains, detached tip of catheter, painful scars, ugly unsightly incision, operation on the sound healthy side (nephrectomy, hernial repair, orchidopexy) due to careless surgeons without marking (or even operating on the wrong patient?!), inhalational pneumonia because of false teeth unrecognised by anaesthetist and/or surgeon, premature discharge after surgery, secondary bleeding after surgery, and wound infection.
7. Occupational hazards of continuous stress among surgeons looking after high-risk patients and witnessing sudden death of patients during surgery. Long-standing traumatic complications after lifting heavy patients resulting in backache among staff. Morbidly obese patients may be difficult to handle and may require two operating tables to accommodate their wide surface area; if such patients are malpositioned and as a result, fall down off the table, they can traumatise the near-by staff; lifting such heavy patients will be extremely difficult. Long periods spent standing may lead to varicose veins among surgeons and occasionally to dizziness and collapse of surgeons or assistants, particularly when they are hypoglycaemic and/or have been on-call with a busy weekend intake of serious emergencies. Food must be provided to surgeons in theatre with various refreshments to keep them going.

COMPUTERS AND THE SURGEON

The computer should be the principal tool in the surgical office. The computer consists of machine (hardware) and programs (software). There are three types of computers depending on the size:
● *Microcomputers*, such as Apple (with 8 bit microprocessor in central processing unit – CPU, i.e. processing 8 pieces of electronic information at once), and IBM, ACT Apricot (16 bit CPU). These can be transportable (usually kept in offices), or portable (e.g. Toshiba notebook computers). The use of a mouse is optional but is required for window programs.
● *Minicomputers* with 16–32 bit CPU, and hence faster.
● *Mainframe computers* with very large capacity, suitable for universities and big companies.

Peripherals attached to a computer include a visual display unit (VDU) or monitor, and printer.

Software packages are stored on discs. Computer security is essential to safeguard stored information from data theft.

Role of computers

A computer serves the following functions:
1. Administrative: it enhances secretarial efficiency and possibly replaces a typewriter. Administrative functions in a surgical practice may be conveniently considered under the following headings.
● Secretariat. Using word processing software packages and a printer, all general practitioner letters, discharge summaries, endoscopy reports, operation reports, or letters for consultation can be kept on disc and reproduced quickly; more time

is created for surgeon and secretary for clinical functions. An important caveat is that the software must be designed or modified to deal with all secretarial exercises efficiently. Data collection and tabulation that a secretay needs to perform may include:

- maintaining a patient card index and disease index;
- logging the movement of clinical records;
- maintaining files of investigations ordered, and investigations outstanding;
- maintaining a waiting list, booking admissions, and planning an operation list with order of priority for admission or operation. At present, many of these functions are performed in part by clerks in central admission offices and waiting list areas which leads to inefficient duplication of effort and personnel.

- Personal bibliography. All references are searched easily by topic, title, author or other key word.
- Personal and practice accounts.
- Maintaining records of personnel and the expanding biography of a busy surgical department.
- A CV is readily kept on computer file and is easily edited, updated (less time-consuming and less expensive), and rapidly reproduced for each application for jobs, grants, annual hospital administrative filing, annual research progress, annual list of publications etc.
- Personal details and references on subjects of clinical and research interest are now entirely superseded by computer storage.

2. Surgical audit. Clinical statistics obtained by health authorities are stored in computer to produce demographic data on disease, hospital bed usage and provision. Raw data are centrally collected by people only partially trained in medical terminology to produce regional information; the Korner committee (Health Service Information Steering Group) has considered at length the need for and means of improving the amount and quality of information upon which to plan and manage all aspects of Health Service. Direct involvement of surgeons (familiar with terminology and clinical data) will result in improvement of the quality of such regional information reports; this reduces clinical misdirection of the Health Service with less professional frustration by providing sound accurate data.

It is also essential to monitor continually clinical performance and to compare both process and outcome audit with that of colleagues. The omniscient 'In my experience . . . or in my hand' syndrome is no longer generally acceptable unless supported by sound hard data (facts can only be supported by figures and statistics). The performance of one surgical department should be compared with that of another in other hospitals and other regions. Such surgical audits can reduce inpatient hospital stay with more common conditions. Choice of drug should be economic and effective. Unacceptable variability in wound infection, anastomotic leak, or tumour recurrence after rectal excision will disappear as surgeons will have to modify their practice until it matches the best.

Surgical audit is necessary both for clinical practice and to produce reliable information for management. It must be computer-based (particularly for large clinical information), updated (by a secretary), and documents can be printed for circulation; information can also be retrieved and analysed at will. Data input must be accurate and quick, if not quicker than cataloguing information by hand.

Data must be standarised using agreed international codes for comparison with other surgeons, hospitals, districts, or regions and also for comparison of published data with other centres in the world. Diagnoses and operations are recorded using specially designed computer assisted dictionaries, such as international classification of disease, international classification codes for diagnosis and operation.

3. Research. Research data may be stored in computer, updated and retrieved at will for analysis. Papers for publication and research abstracts prepared for scientific meeting may all be produced using the computer. Illustration facilities for graphs and histograms can be produced using specific software, such as Lotus 1 2 3, and Harvard graphics. Large statistical programs, such as Statistical Package for Scientific and Social Studies (SPSS) are available on most university mainframes to execute tedious mathematics involved in numerous analyses. CVs can also be updated and reproduced on computer for application for a research grant.

4. Surgical diagnosis. A computer was used by DeDombal (1984) to enhance diagnosis and clinician's diagnostic performance in assessment of patients with acute abdominal pain. However, computer-assisted diagnosis is not widely used because of the enormous amount of work involved in collecting data before statistical analysis can be performed.

5. The Internet: is the Information Super Highway providing personal and professional communications through telephone connection (Modem and hence busy lines via window software following subscription to one of the Internet providers such as Compuserve, American on Line (AOL), and Pipex. The Internet provides the doctor with a window to access global information at the press of a button. It also provides:

- electronic mail: exchanging e-mail with professional colleagues is probably the best way to become comfortable with the electronic world. Sending e-mail across international networks is almost as easy as sending paper mail and takes only minutes to arrive. The Internet makes use of e-mail in the system of Listserv (List server) discussion groups.
- Listserv programs exist on the mainframe computers of universities and corporations throughout the world. There are 300 medically oriented discussion lists covering various specialties and diseases, and the list is growing rapidly. Doctors with e-mail may subscribe to a list electronicaly and any mail posted to the list is distributed to all subscribers. The British Medical Association, AIDS and cancer institutes can be contacted via e-mail.
- Usenet Newsgroups are topical discussion special groups, unlike Listserv lists, posts in Usenet groups are stored on the mainframe computer for a period of time (some Listserv are also echoed to news groups). More than 5000 topics are covered, with new ones being added and outdated ones deleted daily. Electronic publication is closely related. This represents a form of interactive communication.
- Telnet and File Transfer Protocol (FTP) are remote login. Telnet is like going to the library without a card for browsing without the option of file transfer, while FTP is like entering the library with a card to browse through a remote computer and take any public file of interest (after obtaining authorisation by password).

- Gophers are information servers that present you with a hierarchical menu of resources in a simple and consistent manner with ready access to various educational information.
- The World Wide Webb (WWW) is an exciting new concept for exploring the Internet; it is rapidly overtaking Gopher in popularity. Unlike Gopher, the WWW is a more flexible tool for browsing through the Internet and it supports hypertext and multimedia capabilities. The WWW was created at the European Centre of Particle Physics in Switzerland. Medline search, medical publications, new information on AIDS, cancer, diabetes, gastrointestinal disorders and developmental disorders can all be accessed via WWW.

4.2 Bones

These are only shown in the English College to open discussion on selective orthopaedic topics, e.g.

Humerus to discuss the effect of fractures on the nerves which are in contact with it (radial nerve in shaft fracture, ulnar nerve in medial epicondyle fracture and axillary nerve in shoulder dislocation).

Tibia to discuss structures attached to the tibial plateau, and the mechanism and types of meniscus injury as well as the operative procedure of meniscectomy.

Femur to discuss fractures of the neck and their management as well as hip dislocation (both traumatic and congenital) with its management.

Skull (is rarely shown) to discuss the foramina in the cranial fossae. Difficult questions on this bone may be asked purposely to fail certain candidates who performed badly in the written and/or clinical part of the examination.

4.3 Common Instruments and Appliances

The purpose of showing an instrument is to open discussion on the surgical management of a particular condition, e.g. Bakes dilator, Desjardin gallstone forceps and T-tube are shown to discuss exploration of the common bile duct for biliary stone. The following are short notes on commonly presented instruments at the examination:

1. *Bronchoscope:* made of brass with lamp carrier. The metallic tube is fenestrated with two distal holes to allow for inflation of the lung when the bronchoscope is introduced into the other lung. There is no graduation. The distal end is bevelled to lift the epiglottis during introduction. There is a proximal short small tube that serves as an anaesthetic attachment.

2. *Negus rigid oesophagoscope:* made of polished brass and differs from the bronchoscope in the following ways:

- No fenestration.
- The tube is graduated in centimetres to measure the level of scoped oesophagus.
- Has twin lamp carriers on its sides.
- The distal end is not bevelled but is guttered or fissured to allow for suction and better biopsy performance.
- No proximal anaesthetic attachment piece since oesophagoscopy is *always* performed under separate endotracheal intubation (general anaesthesia) while bronchoscopy can be performed *either* under local anaesthetic spray of the oropharynx or under general anaesthesia.

3. *T-tube:* used for biliary drainage after common bile duct exploration or as a splint for ureteric anastomosis. The size is French gauge, i.e. circumference in mm so that a T-tube size 12 Fr has a circumference of 12 mm and a diameter of 12 divided by 3 ($d = \frac{c}{\pi}$) = 4 mm. T-tubes should be of latex or rubber but never of plastic since the latter is hardened by bile, making the tube difficult to remove. Furthermore latex and rubber stimulate fibrinous adhesion leading to a safe track. There is little reaction to a plastic tube and therefore the risk of biliary peritonitis is greater. T-tube is used once only.

4. *Foley catheter:* A self-retaining balloon catheter usually used for drainage of urinary bladder retention or monitoring urine outflow. It can be used for cholecystostomy, caecostomy, peroperative large bowel irrigation and for common bile duct peroperative cholangiography. The size is by French gauge as in T-tubes. The larger the capacity of the balloon the more is the residual urine or fluid (more infection). The balloon can be pulled to sit snugly over the prostatic bed after enucleation or transurethral resection (TUR) of the prostate with the therapeutic value of haemostasis accomplished by balloon pressure over the prostatic bed. The Teflon-coated latex type of catheter with or without Bardcomatic (already inflated balloon) is not favoured owing to its small lumen, irritant material (crystallisation and infection around catheter tip), possible balloon puncture and bubbling of its material. They are usually used for short periods in catheterising patients with acute urinary retention who are waiting for cystoscopy and/or TUR of the prostate. After TUR of a prostate or bladder tumour a three-way *Simplastic Foley catheter* is used (size 22 or 24 Fr) for continuous irrigation or the bladder for a short period (usually 7 days).

Permanent indwelling Foley catheters (changed every 3 months) of Silikon 100, e.g. Dover type, are preferred to those made of Silastic (latex outer surface with silicone elastomer coating the drainage lumen) because the former have a wider lumen and are made of very inert material that does not bubble after long use. Recently, Hydrogel (used for contact lenses) has been used for coating catheters; it is non-toxic, soft, highly biocompatible with human tissues, non-irritant to urothelium and highly resistant to catheter encrustation and bacterial colonisation.

- Catheters should also be used as a last resort.
- Type and size of catheter required must be carefully assessed.
- Only store a limited supply of catheters in common use and of recommended sizes.
- Catheters become out of date:

  3 years for Latex, 5 years for all Silicone and Hydrogel.
- Small is beautiful:

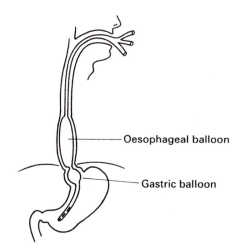

Fig. 4.3.1 Sengstaken tube

for routine urine drainage use small sized catheters:

Paediatric   8–10 FG   3–5 ml balloon
Women   12–14 FG   10 ml balloon
Men   14–16 FG   10 ml balloon

10 ml balloons are better than 30 ml balloons for adults and should be used for routine urine drainage.

5. *Joll thyroid retractor* with twin sharp prongs and threaded expanding bar for retraction of upper and lower cervical skin flaps in thyroidectomy.

6. *Joll thyroid aneurysm needle* for threading the suture around the thyroid vessels prior to ligation and division.

7. *Ochsner trocar* with cannula and sucker attachment; in gallbladder decompression introduced through a purse-string prior to cholecystectomy or bypass. You may also be shown *Desjardin gallstone forceps*.

8. *Hurst oesophageal bougie:* rubber filled with mercury.

9. *Mousseau barbin tube* ⎤ inserted for palliative bypass
10. *Celestine tube* ⎦ in oesophageal carcinoma.

11. *Sengstaken–Blakemore triluminal decompression tube:* (Fig. 4.3.1): It is rubber and X-ray opaque. If oesophageal bleeding is not controlled, or recurs despite vasopressin, the next step is to apply ballon tamponade; the tri-luminar Sengstaken–Blakemore tube (one channel for gastric fundus balloon, one for oesophageal balloon, and one for aspiration of gastric secretion) is probably the best with a fourth channel (for oesophageal collection of 1.5 litre of daily saliva above the inflated oesophageal balloon that may cause spillover and pulmonary aspiration). The tube is lubricated generously prior to nasogastric introduction, then the gastric balloon is inflated first and pulled up until it impinges on the gastro-oesophageal cardiac junction (tamponading fundal varices first); gastric contents with blood is aspirated then continuously (to monitor the progress of oesophageal bleeding) followed by oesophageal balloon inflation to 40 mmHg and the tube is fixed with a tape without tension (tube fixation to bed head with weights under tension may induce sheering traumatic forces, thus tearing more varices and causing more bleeding). The oesophageal and gastric balloons are then deflated after 24 h of tamponade and may continue for only another 24 h (total of 48 h) if bleeding

continues or recurs. Continuous inflation without interruption may cause pressure necrosis and potential oesophageal perforation.

12. *Lane clamp* for gastroenterostomy (non-crushing occluding clamp).

13. *Payr stomach clamp* (crushing clamp for partial gastrectomy) and Schoemaker crushing forceps.

14. *Doyen clamp* (non-crushing occluding) traditional soft intestinal clamp.

15. *Bakes dilator* with malleable shaft for common bile duct surgery. It has an olive head to avoid trauma during pushing and pulling of the dilator through the duodenal papilla.

16. (a) *Martin endarterectomy stripper*
    (b) *Cannon endarterectomy loops*

17. *Tibbs arterial cannula* for filling distal artery (with heparinised saline) after embolectomy.

18. *Foqarty embolectomy catheter* with a guidewire inside and a terminal latex balloon.

19. *Myers varicose vein stripper.*

20. *Dormia basket stone dislodger.*

21. *Bladder (Lister) metallic sound.*

22. *Smellie meniscectomy knife.*

23. *Brodie director* with a probe for fistula surgery. The proximal part helps in division of tongue tie.

24. *Humby skin graft knife.*

25. *Lloyd-Davies operating sigmoidoscope.*

26. *Colostomy bag:* made of disposable plastic. It is not drainable (no outlet) and comes with or without a deodorising filter.

27. *Ileostomy bag:* drainable with a special security clip. Used many times. No deodorising filter.

28. *Urostomy bag:* drainable but with a non-reflux valve which can fit a wide-bore night drainage tube. No deodorising filter.

29. *Parks rectal retractor, Goligher rectal speculum* and *ordinary proctoscope* (how to assemble them and how to apply them to the rectum).

30. *Periosteal elevator, Doyen rib raspatory, rib approximator and spreader.*

31. *Chest tube.*

32. *Nasogastric tube.*

33. *Tourniquet:* Tourniquet is used in everyday practice to induce venous engorgement in order to facilitate blood aspiration or venous sampling for investigations. However, in operative surgery, tourniquet is a useful tool for limb, finger and toe exsanguination to produce a bloodless field in order to facilitate operations on the distal two-thirds of a limb and digits, rendering surgery simpler, safer (to deal with delicate structures), and often speedier.

Pneumatic tourniquet can be applied over a smooth roll of wool around the upper arm or proximal thigh (safer since it minimises the risk of pressure damage, when inflated, on skin and nerves). Alternatively, the arm-band of *sphygmomanometer* may be used. When the cuff has been applied and fastened, the limb is elevated and exsanguinated with an *Esmarch bandage* rolled firmly from the end of the limb up to the cuff. The cuff is then inflated to 50 mmHg *above* the measured systolic arterial pressure and the encircling Esmarch bandage removed; tourniquet can be retained for up to 90 min. A finger or toe tourniquet is simply a *fine rubber tubing* (or catheter) stretched around the finger at the web margin, and secured with

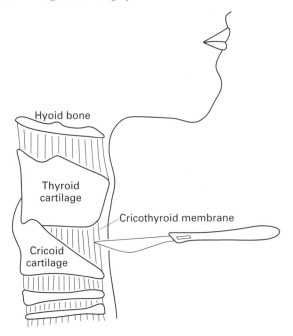

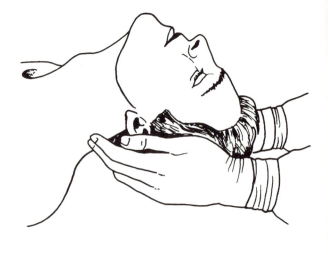

Fig. 4.3.2   Minitracheostomy or cricothyroidotomy

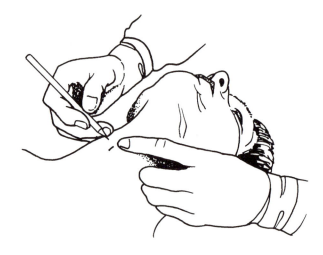

forceps; it should not be left in position longer than 15 min, because of the risk of gangrene.

Indications and contraindications: tourniquet is indicated in all upper and lower limb surgery. In limb amputation, tourniquet is of particular importance, particularly in traumatic injuries. Tourniquet is contraindicated, however, in:

- peripheral vascular insufficiencies, since it may bring about a diminution of already precarious blood supply to the stump;
- preliminary Esmarch bandaging (initial limb exsanguination by pressure bandage) is contraindicated in biopsy or removal of malignant lesion or in acute sepsis, because malignant cells or bacteria may be sequeezed into general circulation;
- also Esmarch exsanguinator bandage should not be used in fractures or in mobile loose bodies on the joints; they should be avoided when the limb has been immobilised in a plaster cast for 48 h or more prior to surgery, as venous thrombi may be detached to form emboli. In these circumstances, the limb should be elevated well above heart level for a full 2 minutes, and a rubber tubing wound tightly round the limb above (proximal to) the cuff, before cuff inflation is commenced (otherwise, inflation without proximal tubing may occlude veins before the main artery resulting in engorged veins);
- in patients with heart disease and in infants, care must be taken due to blood overload on the heart; therefore, bilateral thigh tourniquet is contraindicated in infants, in the elderly and in cardiac decompensation (heart failure).

Tourniquet complications: tourniquet should be correctly used with good padding and should not press on the nerve; it should never be left inflated round the limb for more than 90 min before release (in finger or toe, it should not be more than 15 min). However, maximum time allowed is 2 h on upper arm (with pressure of 300 mmHg) and 2.5 h on the thigh (with a pressure of 500 mmHg). If a surgical procedure needs a

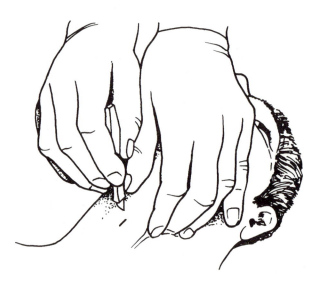

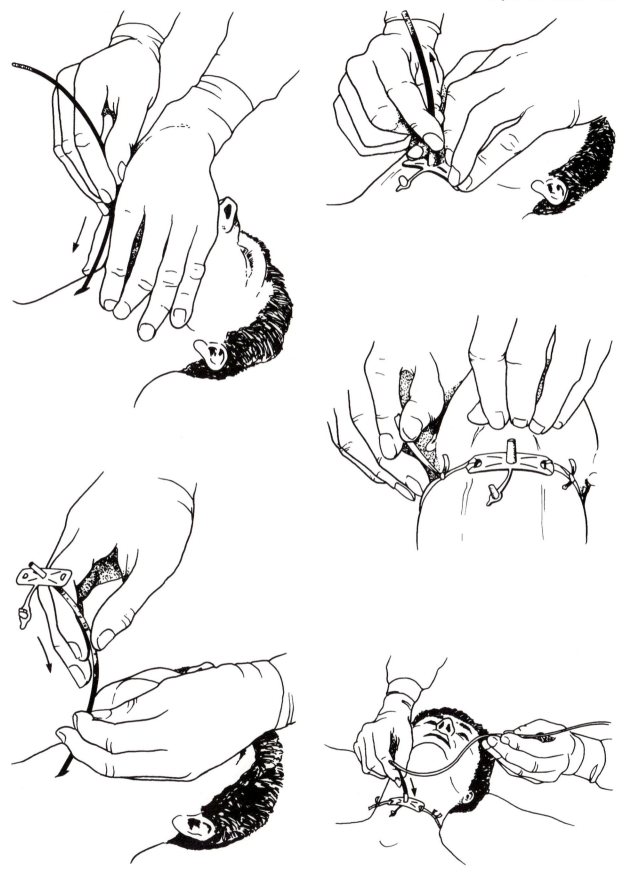

Fig. 4.3.3 Mini-Trach II. (Courtesy of Portex Ltd)

bloodless field for over 60 min, it is wiser to pack the wound, control bleeding by direct pressure, elevate the limb and release the tourniquet for 10 min after which time the tourniquet may be reinflated for a further period (whilst the limb is still elevated). Tourniquet 'paralysis', a patchy sensory and motor disturbance persisting hours or days after tourniquet release, may follow careless application or cuff overinflation; gross limb swelling and diffuse neurological disorder may follow an excessive period of tourniquet ischaemia. Such complications must be noted to assess following progress. Limb care after tourniquet palsy is the same as that for any neurological disorder, in that joints are protected from excessive stresses and are put through a range of movement exercises daily, whilst anaesthetic skin is protected from damage until sensory recovery occurs.

34. *Tracheostomy tube:* This is either the currently used non-metallic tube or old-fashioned metallic tube (consisting of three components: obturator, outer tube and inner longer tube for easy cleaning of encrustation on its protruding end).

Non-metallic tracheostomy tubes are made of rubber or Silastic. The advantages of the non-metallic tube are that it has an inflatable cuff and can be connected to an anaesthetic machine or respirator. Furthermore, it does not produce mechanical damage to the trachea. The inflatable cuff (large volume–low pressure) secures and maintains intratracheal location and prevents gastric secretion or vomitus spillover to the trachea; cuff pressure is less than capillary pressure, so capillaries can not be occluded, and thus pressure necrosis is prevented. Paradoxically, the main disadvantage of the non-

metallic tube is the inflatable cuff which should be blown up to the point where there is a slight air leak past it and it should be deflated for 5 min in every hour. If it is absolutely essential to maintain a permanent airtight seal, a Salpekar tube can be used with two cuffs, one above the other, allowing alternate deflation and inflation of each cuff.

Emergency tracheostomy under local anaesthesia should be avoided wherever possible by prompt decisions to perform elective tracheostomy on an endotracheally incubated patient under general anaesthesia.

Minitracheostomy (see Figs 4.3.2, 4.3.3) or cricothyr-oidotomy has been suggested for patients who are at risk of sputum retention, which is a major cause of morbidity and mortality following thoracic surgery and in chronic bronchitic patients. The cricothyroid membrane is incised and the resulting airway is maintained with any available piece of tubing, e.g. 6 mm plain tracheal tube. A minitracheostomy using a guarded blade, introducing stillete and precut tracheal tube is a suitable alternative, although minitracheostomy may be difficult to perform in obese patients. Minitracheostomy allows permanent access to the trachea for suction, while avoiding the disadvantages of tracheostomy or endotracheal intubation. Minitracheostomy preserves the function of the glottis, and patients therefore retain an explosive cough with minimal loss of expiratory air volume. However, up to 75% have subjective and objective voice changes following minitracheostomy.

Cyanosis following tracheostomy may be due either to tube blockage by secretions or to tube displacement.

4.4 Clinical Radiology: Questions on General Principles

- All candidates are strongly advised to read through *Clinical Radiology in Postgraduate Surgery* by the author.

Q1

- A 40-year-old woman with dysphagia (Fig. Q1).

(a) What is the abnormality?
(b) What are the complications?
(c) How do you treat?

Answers on p. 534

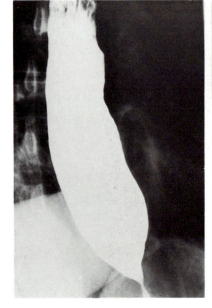
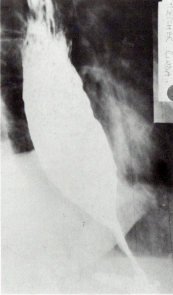

Fig. Q1

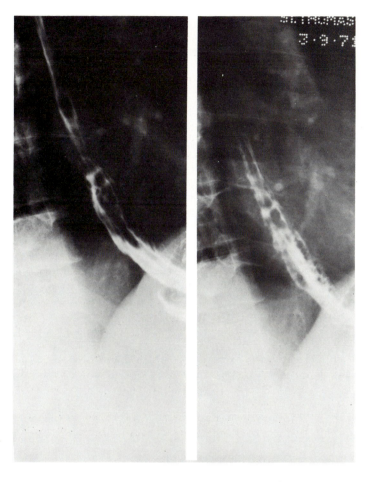

Q2

- A 45-year-old man admitted to hospital with splenomegaly (Fig. Q2).

(a) What is the investigation and the abnormality?
(b) What is the diagnosis?
(c) Are there any other valuable radiological investigations?
(d) How do you treat now?
(e) What is the main complication and how do you treat it?

Answers on p. 534

Fig. Q2

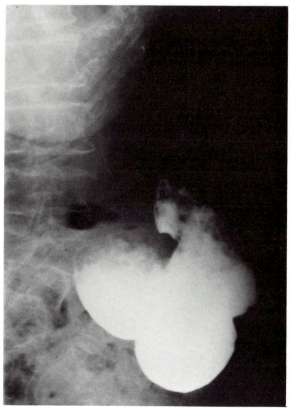

Q3

- A 45-year-old man with periodic abdominal pain and vomiting (Fig. Q3)

(a) What is the investigation?
(b) What is the diagnosis?
(c) Discuss your management.
(d) What are the indications for surgery?

Answers on p. 535

Fig. Q3

Q4

● A 60-year-old woman with severe abdominal pain (Fig. Q4).

(a) What is the abnormality?
(b) What is the most likely diagnosis?
(c) List the conditions that can produce a similar appearance.
(d) How do you treat?
(e) What advice do you give the patient postoperatively?

Answers on p. 536

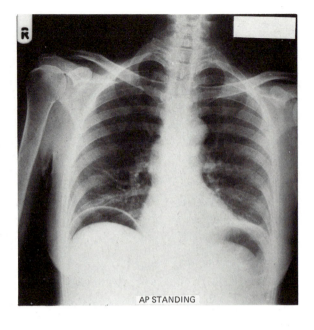

Fig. Q4

Q5

● A 60-year-old man with pain (Fig. Q5).

(a) What is this investigation and what are the procedural requirements?
(b) What is the abnormality?
(c) What is the clinical presentation?
(d) How do you treat?

Answers on p. 537

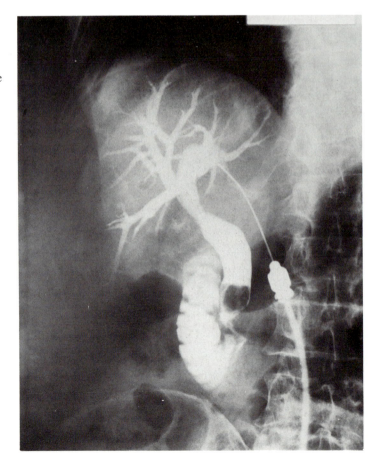

Fig. Q5

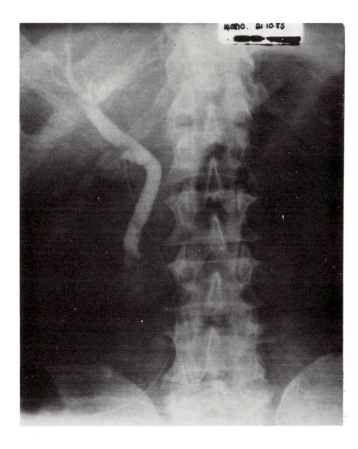

Fig. Q6

Q6

● (Fig. Q6)

(a) What is this investigation and diagnosis?
(b) What are the indications for common bile duct exploration?

Answers on p. 537

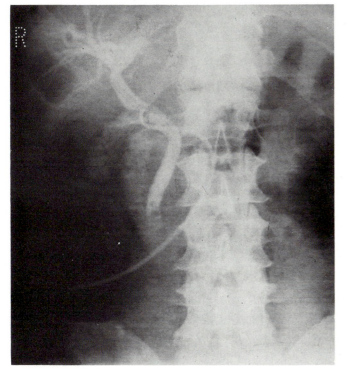

Fig. Q7

Q7

● A 50-year-old woman in her 10th postoperative day (Fig. Q7).

(a) What is this investigation and diagnosis?
(b) How do you treat?

Answers on p. 537

Q8

● A 55-year-old woman with vague acute abdominal pain (Fig. Q8).

(a) What is the investigation and diagnosis?
(b) What one other clinical presentation is there?
(c) What is the definitive treatment?

Answers on p. 538

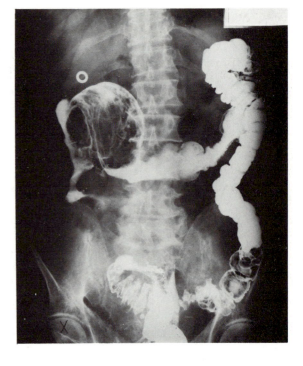

Fig. Q8

Q9

● A 57-year-old man with recent change of bowel habits (Fig. Q9).

(a) What is the investigation and abnormality?
(b) What is your diagnosis?
(c) How do you treat?

Answers on p. 539

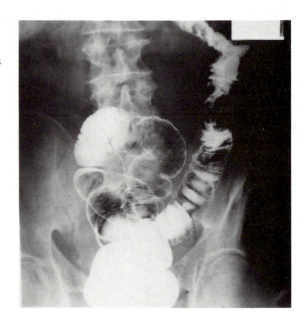

Fig. Q9

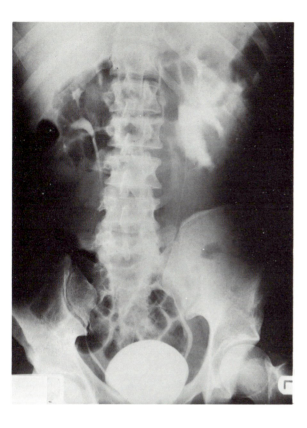

Q10

- A 50-year-old man involved in a road traffic accident (Fig. Q10).

(a) What is the investigation?
(b) What is the diagnosis?
(c) What is the clinical presentation?
(d) How do you treat?

Answers on p. 539

Fig. Q10

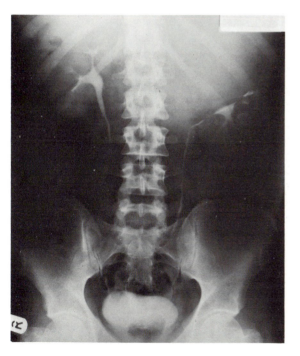

Q11

- A 35-year-old man presenting with pyrexia (Fig. Q11).

(a) What is the investigation and diagnosis?
(b) What are the other presentations of this condition?
(c) What is your treatment?

Answers on p. 540

Fig. Q11

Q12

● A 65-year-old man complaining of difficult micturition (Fig. Q12).

(a) Describe three abnormalities.
(b) What is the diagnosis?
(c) How do you treat?

Answers on p. 542

Q13

● A 50-year-old man admitted to hospital because of a road traffic accident (Fig. Q13).

(a) What are the abnormalities?
(b) How do you treat?

Answers on p. 542

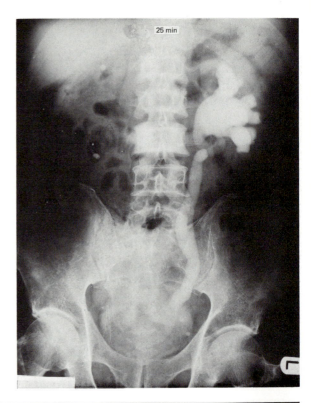

Fig. Q12

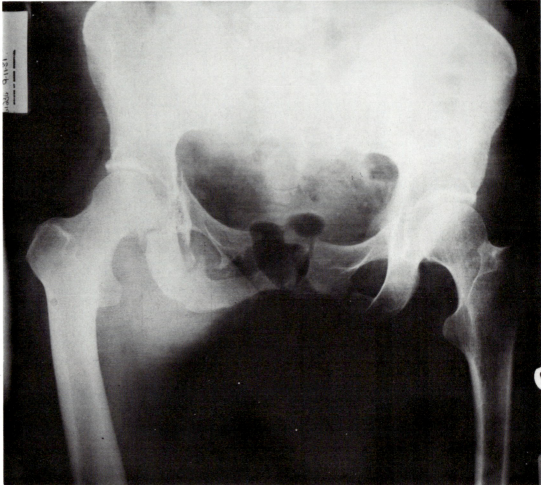

Fig. Q13

Q14

● A 57-year-old woman with severe right hip pain and limited movement. She was never operated on (Fig. Q14a,b)

(a) What is the abnormality?
(b) What are your next steps in diagnosis?
(c) Discuss the causes of such an abnormality.
(d) What is the complication and treatment?

Answers on p. 543

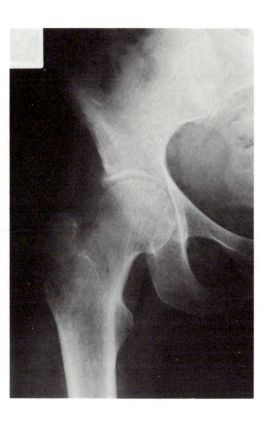

Fig. Q14
(a) At time of presentation.

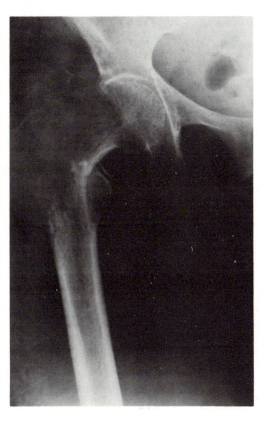

(b) Two weeks later.

Q15

- A 55-year-old woman who fell on her right outstretched hand (Fig. Q15)

(a) Spot all the radiological findings.
(b) What is the diagnosis?
(c) How do you treat?
(d) What are the complications and treatment?

Answers on p. 544

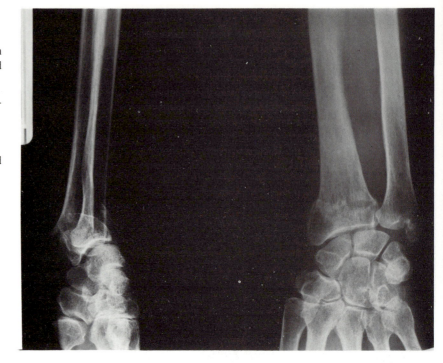

Fig. Q15

Q16

- A 8-year-old boy who fell on his left arm (Fig. Q16 a,b).

(a) What are the abnormalities and diagnosis?
(b) How do you treat?
(c) Enumerate the fractures around the elbow in children.
(d) Discuss details of the most serious complications.

Answers on p. 544

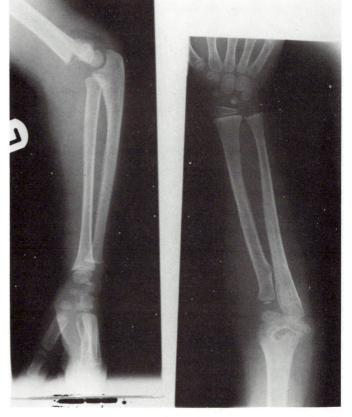

Fig. Q16

(a)   (b)

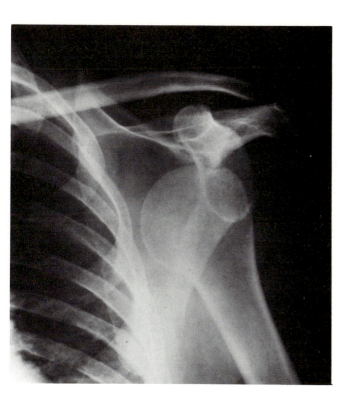

Fig. Q17

Q17

- A 28-year-old man was playing tennis and suddenly could not move his left shoulder (Fig. Q17).

(a) What is the diagnosis?
(b) What are the physical signs?
(c) How do you treat?

Answers on p. 546

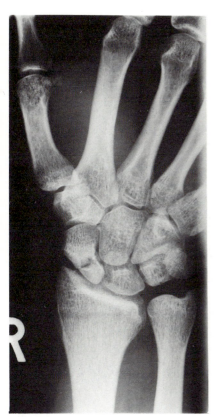

Fig. Q18

Q18

- A 30-year-old man who fell on his right outstretched hand (Fig. Q18).

(a) What is the diagnosis?
(b) How do you manage this case?

Answers on p. 546

Q19

● A 50-year-old man with right thigh mass (Fig. Q19).

(a) What is the investigation?
(b) What is the diagnosis?
(c) How do you treat?

Answers on p. 547

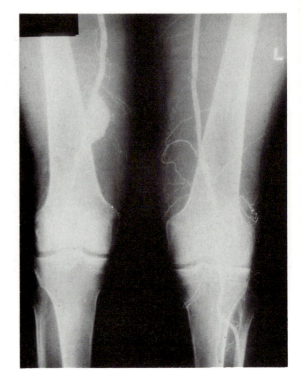

Fig. Q19

Q20

● A 30-year-old man with a swollen painful lower limb (Fig. Q20).

(a) What is the investigation and diagnosis?
(b) What is your treatment?

Answers on p. 547

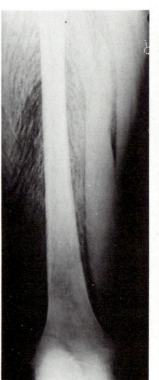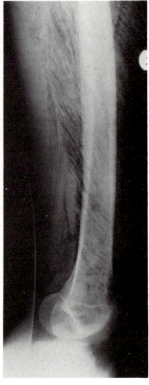

Fig. Q20

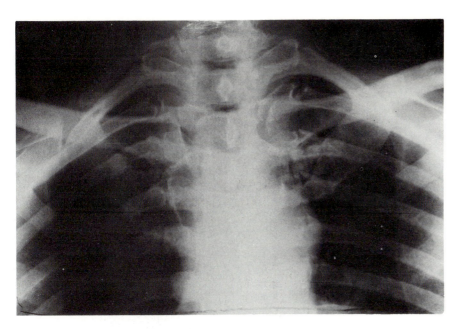

Fig. Q21

Q21

- A 30-year-old woman with right upper limb pain (Fig. Q21).

(a) What is the diagnosis?
(b) What are the clinical findings?
(c) How do you treat?

Answers on p. 548

Q22

- A 53-year-old woman was admitted to hospital with severe continuous upper abdominal pain following a meal of fish and chips at night (Fig. Q22).

(a) What is the abnormality(ies)?
(b) What is your diagnosis?
(c) Comment on investigations available for such a condition.
(d) Do you perform emergency or elective operation and why?
(e) Can the gallbladder be visible on plain X-ray?
(f) What is haemobilia?
(g) What is the effect(s) of opioid drugs on Oddi's sphincter?

Answers on p. 548

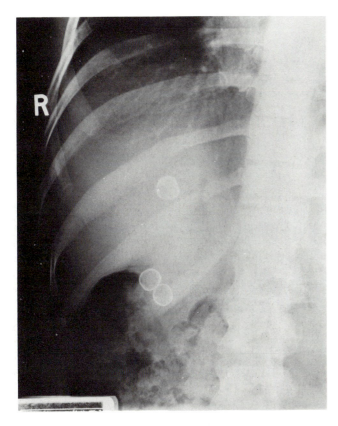

Fig. Q22

Q23

● A 55-year-old man presenting with vague lower
abdominal pain (Fig. Q23).

(a) What is the investigation?
(b) Describe three abnormalities.
(c) How do you treat?

Answer on p. 550

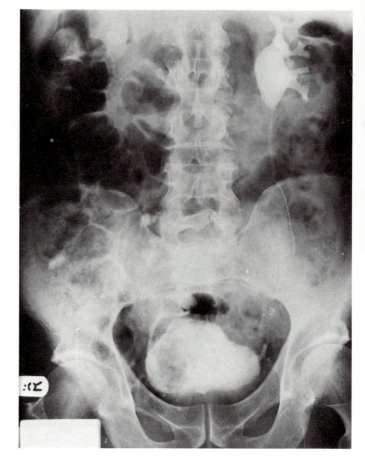

Fig. Q23

Answers

A1

(a) Achalasia of the oesophagus or cardiospasm (smooth pencil-shaped narrowing).
(b) It predisposes to diverticula and carcinoma (precancerous) and leads to dysphagia as well as anaemia, aspiration pneumonia (usually right middle lobe) and arthritis (toxic rheumatoid arthritis). Achalasia is due to absence (or defect) of Auerbach's parasympathetic plexus.
(c) Heller's operation (oesophagocardiomyotomy) by the abdominal or thoracic approach. A longitudinal 10 cm long incision (5 cm proximal and 5 cm distal to the constricted portion) is deepened down to (and without puncturing) the mucosa which will bulge. Eighty per cent of cases have satisfactory postoperative results; 20% will continue with reflux oesophagitis.

A2

(a) Barium swallow showing soap bubble appearance.
(b) Oesophageal varices.
(c) Yes. Splenic portography (Fig. A2) to test the portal vein patency as a prerequisite to shunt.

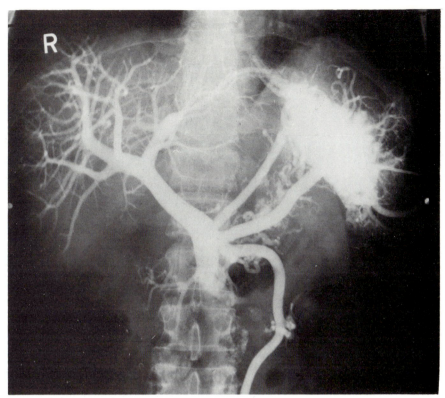

Fig. A2

(d) No prophylactic operation in portal hypertension (i.e. shunt) unless the patient is bleeding or has had bleeding before, because:

● It has no benefit.
● It may cause severe encephalopathy and increase mortality.

(e) Massive haemorrhage treated conservatively at first (rest, sedation, fresh blood transfusion, with CVP and blood pressure monitoring. Oral magnesium sulphate and neomycin with prevention of protein intake. Pitressin 20 units/200 ml of normal saline per 20 min. Occasionally, ice water gastric lavage to reduce bleeding and remove clots). If these methods fail then try tamponade with a Sengstaken triluminal tube (should not be left in for more than 72 h as the pressure causes ulceration and oesophageal rupture. It also leads to saliva inspiration into the lungs). If bleeding recurs after removal of the Sengstaken tube then emergency operation (whether direct oesophageal or decompressing shunt) is indicated. Elective shunting is only indicated if the patient (known to have portal hypertension) has bled in the past.

Comment: Splenomegaly in upper gastrointestinal tract bleeding is not diagnostic of portal hypertension (unless varices are documented radiologically as in this case) since cirrhotics (with splenomegaly) may bleed:

● From peptic gastric or duodenal ulcer secondary to hypergastrinaemia (not metabolised by liver) in up to 20% of cases.
● From gastric erosions due to alcoholism.
● From Mallory–Weiss syndrome due to alcoholism.
● From gastric fundal varices and not oesophageal varices.

Furthermore splenomegaly alone may be due to the leukaemia causing upper gastrointestinal tract bleeding (very rarely).

A3

(a) Barium meal.
(b) Benign giant lesser curve peptic ulcer.
(c) Endoscopy and biopsy to confirm the benign radiological appearance (no everted ulcer margin, peristalsis moves through it, rugae radiate immediately from ulcer. In ulcer cancer the margin is everted and because of surrounding infiltration the peristalsis and rugae stop a distance away from it). H_2-receptor antagonist (e.g. cimetidine or ranitidine) is given over 6 weeks (duodenal ulcer

requires 6 months) with endoscopic monitoring to assess healing. If still symptomatic and/or no healing then surgery is indicated (partial gastrectomy and Billroth I or II or alternatively wide excision of ulcer-bearing segment with simple closure of the defect).

(d) Indications for surgery are:

- Any ulcer complications, e.g. perforation, pyloric stenosis and bleeding (continuous or intermittent).
- Failure of medical treatment and/or economic considerations and expediency.
- Combined gastric and duodenal ulcers.
- Serious persistent hour-glass deformity.
- Suspicion of malignancy, e.g. greater curve ulcer and/or positive cytology, very long ulcer history (size is not criterion for malignancy) and ulcer in patient over 60 with short history.

A4

(a) Gas crescent under right hemidiaphragm.

(b) Perforated peptic (probably duodenal) ulcer.

(c) Pneumoperitoneum and right subphrenic gas are most commonly seen after laparotomy (as a normal finding). Perforated viscus (peptic duodenal or gastric ulcer, colonic diverticula, gallbladder empyema and rarely appendicitis) is the next most common cause. They are also seen in open (or closed) abdominal trauma. Subphrenic abscess (mainly postoperative), amoebic liver abscess and infected liver hydatid cyst cause a right subphrenic fluid level (rather than a crescent), with basal lung consolidation (Fig. A4).

(d) Emergency simple closure of the perforation with an omental tag and peritoneal toilet and drainage. Quick i.v. rehydration, nasogastric suction, prophylactic antibiotics with BP, PR and CVP monitoring are recommended. Up to 8% of abdominal conditions subjected to urgent laparotomy are perforated peptic ulcers and it is important to remember that 10% will have had no prior recognisable ulcer symptoms and that about 30% of perforated ulcers show no positive radiological evidence of pneumoperitoneum. Simple closure has 7% operative mortality which becomes even less with early diagnosis and prompt treatment since delay causes a change from a mainly chemical peritonitis in the first 6 h to 100% demonstrable bacterial peritonitis after 12 h

(e) To have the definitive treatment of truncal vagotomy with drainage procedure (preferably gastroenterostomy) as an elective operation. Roughly one-third of closed perforations will recover permanently postoperatively, another one-third continue as a symptomatic ulcer and the last third proceed to ulcer complications, i.e. recurrent perforations, bleeding and stenosis.

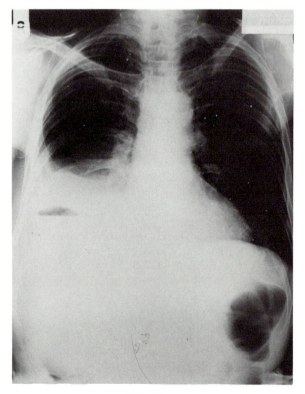

Fig. A4

A5

(a) Percutaneous transhepatic cholangiography – PTC (using a fine Chiba needle under prophylactic antibiotic cover, e.g. cefuroxime in a patient with normal prothrombin time). Complications include intraperitoneal bleeding, biliary peritonitis and infection.

(b) Two biliary stones at the lower end of the common bile duct (CBD) with proximal biliary dilatation (due to incomplete obstruction).

(c) Charcot's triad of intermittent jaundice, biliary colic and fever with rigor (due to ascending cholangitis).

(d) Cholecystectomy, CBD supraduodenal exploration and stone removal (choledocholithotomy) with T-tube drainage. If the CBD is packed with stones or it is impossible to remove all stones then a permanent prophylactic drainage procedure such as choledochoduodenostomy is recommended.

Comment: This technique (i.e. PTC) has now been extended into external biliary drainage (decompression), transhepatic dilatation of biliary strictures and endoprosthesis insertion.

A6

(a) Peroperative pre-exploratory cholangiography showing multiple obstructing stones in the lower end of the CBD (no dye passed down to duodenum). This procedure should be performed routinely in all cholecystectomy cases (see below).

(b) The indications or *classical criteria* for CBD exploration are:

● Preoperative, e.g. history of jaundice or Charcot's triad, gallstone pancreatitis, oral cholecystography revealing multiple small stones with patent or dilated cystic duct.

● Peroperative, e.g. palpation of CBD stone, dilated CBD more than 10–12 mm, periductal fibrosis, cholecystectomised gallbladder showing single-faceted stone or thick wall with no stone, indurated pancreas, or biliary sludge or mud on needle aspiration of CBD. Peroperative pre-exploratory cholangiogram (revealing one of four findings: a filling defect, dilated CBD, no flow to duodenum and/or stenosis or non-visualisation of lower intramural narrow segment of duct) is far more accurate (over 95%) than the above criteria and is the best available method for this purpose.

● Postoperative T-tube cholangiography revealing residual stone.

Comment: Exploration of the CBD is associated with high mortality (3%, a fourfold increase over cholecystectomy alone) and with more morbidity (T-tube biliary intraperitoneal leakage). Since out of 60–80% of patients with one of the above criteria only 20% have CBD pathology, operative cholangiogram is used for CBD pathology detection, biliary anatomy demonstration, and identification of patients who do not need choledochotomy. It is the best available method and should be practised routinely with cholecystectomy to avoid the high risk of residual biliary stone which can reach 30% of explored cases done without operative cholangiogram.

However, this policy is not universally accepted. The argument is that for practically every 100 patients with gallstones only 20 will require choledochotomy, suggesting that 80 do not require cholangiography. However 60–80% of patients have at least one of the *criteria* for CBD exploration and it would seem reasonable to omit cholangiography in the 20–40% *who have no such criteria*. It is claimed that such a selective policy would result in less than 1% of residual stone incidence.

A7

(a) T-tube postoperative cholangiography showing two residual obstructing stones at the lower end of the CBD.

(b) Residual stone accounts for 10–20% of recurrences after choledochotomy. Re-exploration carries a mortality in excess of primary choledochotomy. The following steps in management recommended in chronological order:

A. Leave T-tube in situ.

1. A proportion of CBD small stones will pass into the duodenum spontaneously especially if amyl nitrite or an antispasmodic is given to relax the sphincter.

2. Gallstone dissolution by giving oral chenodeoxycholic acid (Chendol) or using T-tube lavage with various solutions, e.g. saline heparin, cholate or, more effectively, glyceryl mono-octanoate (GMO). Irrigation using 500 ml normal saline with 5000 units heparin (to prevent haemobilia) coupled with 20 mg i.v. Buscopan is a common practice. Lavage should be monitored and consequent diarrhoea (due to bowel irritation by bile salts) controlled by cholestyramine (GMO can induce erosive duodenitis). This method is time-consuming and requires hospitalisation and repeated cholangiogram to see if the stone has passed. The success rate is 50%.

3. Monitored flushing with maximal relaxation of sphincter of Oddi (Cuschieri, 1984). Massive sterile saline infusion via a disposable manometry line through the T-tube with i.v. continuous infusion of cerulitide 2 ng/kg per min via a constant infusion pump. Cerulitide is an analogue of caerulein with a powerful cholecystokinin effect causing maximal relaxation of the sphincter of Oddi. The amount of a saline infused is 1–3 litres at a rate that will maintain the biliary pressure at 25–30 cmH$_2$O. Prophylactic antibiotic (i.e. cefuroxime single dose 1 g) should be given ½ hour prior to the procedure. T-tube cholangiography should be performed before and after the procedure. This method is simpler, more effective, less time-consuming and less invasive than the above method and is side-effect free (only watery diarrhoea).

B. Remove T-tube after 4–6 weeks.
1. Percutaneous stone extraction: do T-tube cholangiogram (to ensure that stone is still present) before T-tube removal. The stone retrieval system (Dormia basket, Fogarty balloon catheter or preferably a Burhenne steerable catheter) is passed down the T-tube track under X-ray screening by a skilled radiologist. It is for this reason that the surgeon is advised to use a size 16 Fr (or larger) T-tube in the right upper quadrant so that the track is *short, straight* and *large* enough for such manoeuvring.
2. Endoscopic sphincterotomy: followed by passage of Dormia basket or Fogarty balloon for stone retrieval. A skilled team of surgeon and radiologist is necessary to achieve the 90% success rate. It has a 1% mortality and 8% morbidity but this compares favourably with surgical re-exploration. Complications are pancreatitis, bleeding, cholangitis and rarely perforation and stone impaction.
3. Surgical re-exploration should be reserved for the few patients in whom the above methods fail or are not available and where the risk is justified.

C. In the absence of a T-tube from the start (the residual stone was diagnosed with intravenous cholangiography after clinical suspicion following cholecystectomy), gallstone dissolution should be tried with chenodeoxycholic acid or ursodeoxycholic acid (suitable stones must be radiolucent indicating a high cholesterol content and measure less than 1 cm with a patent duct to permit entry of the solvent). Dissolution generally takes 6–24 months. If this fails try endoscopic extraction and if this fails then surgical re-exploration (if the risk is justified).

A8

(a) Barium enema revealing carcinoma of caecum causing ileocolic intussusception – a rare presentation. (Appendix is shown connected to the mass and lifted to right hypochondrium.)
(b) Severe anaemia due to bleeding cauliflower tumour (gastric and caecal carcinomas are notorious for their tendency to bleed and cause anaemia), right iliac fossa mass and rarely secondary acute appendicitis.
(c) Right hemicolectomy (with primary ileocolic anastomosis).
 1. Intravenous drip, nasogastric suction and indwelling urinary catheter after 2 days' bowel preparation.
 2. General anaesthesia, supine position and long right paramedian incision (rectus muscle-splitting).
 3. Quick exploration for tumour size and fixity, and for liver, mesenteric lymph nodes and peritoneal metastases as well as for double primary colonic carcinomas (up to 20% of cases). Pack off small intestine to the left.
 4. Dissect and resect the greater omentum off the right side of the transverse colon. Mobilise the ascending colon by dividing the right paracolic peritoneum and freeing the hepatic flexure and terminal ileum by blunt dissection, taking absolute care to safeguard the duodenum, right ureter and genital vessels.
 5. Ligate and divide the ileocolic and right colic arteries through artificially created windows in the mesocolon and mesentery, visualising them under a spotlight.
 6. Apply a non-crushing (occluding) intestinal clamp to the antimesocolic border (just enough to occlude the lumen of the proposed site of division) as well as a crushing clamp and cut between. Ideally 15 cm of terminal ileum should be resected. However, the viability of the ileal end must be confirmed on the basis of a good extramural blood supply. Re-resection and examination may be necessary until a viable end is obtained.
 7. Ileocolic anastomosis should be performed under near aseptic conditions (pack off the area and mop up the contents with an antiseptic-soaked swab). End-to-end, end-to-side, side-to-end or side-to-side anastomosis is optional. The ileal end can be enlarged by a Cheetle longitudinal antimesenteric cut. Either a double-layered (interrupted waxed seromuscular 2/0 silk and continuous mucosal 2/0 chromic catgut) or a single-layered (waxed interrupted serososubmucosal 2/0 silk) technique may be used.
 8. Close the mesenteric gap and remove the packs.
 9. Anal stretch to prevent increased intracolic pressure from straining the anastomosis.
10. Drain and close.

A9

(a) Barium enema showing irregular filling defect of left descending colon.

(b) Left colonic carcinoma.

(c) Left hemicolectomy (with primary colocolic anastomosis). This is almost a mirror-image of right hemicolectomy with similar steps: the incision will be a long left paramedian, the bowel is packed to the right side and then the left colon is mobilised (by dividing the left paracolic peritoneum up to the splenic flexure, excising part of the greater omentum, mobilising the transverse colon and finally mobilising the splenic flexure fully with enlargement of the paramedian incision or transverse extension if necessary). Safeguard the left ureter and genital vessels. The left colic and, if necessary, the middle colic vessels are divided. The area is packed off, the left colon is resected, and the transverse colon is anastomosed to the pelvic colon. The mesenteric gap is repaired, the anus stretched, area drained and abdomen closed.

A10

(a) Emergency intravenous urography revealing extensive extrarenal (extraperitoneal) extravasation of contrast in the left kidney.

(b) Left traumatic renal rupture (complete) (Fig. A10).

(c) Left loin pain, tenderness (rarely superficial bruising or penetrating wound). Haematuria is the cardinal sign of a damaged kidney with possible clot colic and late clot dislodgement leading to severe delayed haematuria (from third day to third week). Palpable loin mass (perinephric haematoma) as well as abdominal distension 24–48 h later due to splanchnic nerve implication by retroperitoneal haematoma (meteorism).

(d) Conservative treatment should be stressed and is usually successful (bed rest – flat position until macroscopic haematuria becomes microscopic or absent for 1 week, analgesia for pain, antibiotics to prevent infection of haematoma, hourly monitoring of pulse rate, blood pressure and urine output. Each specimen of urine passed should be sampled, blood should be grouped and crossmatched and blood transfusion should be instituted in shock or continuous bleeding).

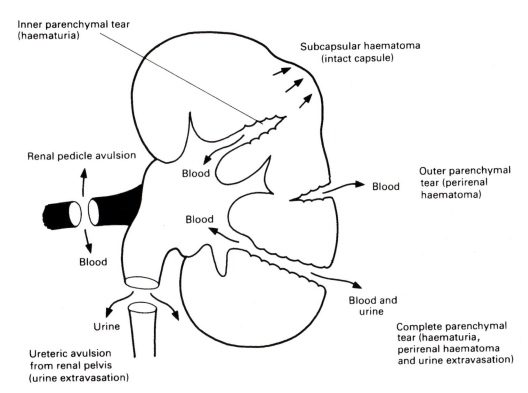

Fig. A10 Renal injuries

Surgical exploration is indicated in 20% of patients only in:

● Progressive haemorrhage (hypotension).
● Loin swelling due to extravasated urine (since this leads to infection and is not controllable by antibiotics).
● Signs of perirenal infection of haematoma.
● Severe delayed or secondary haemorrhage.
● Early hypertension as a sequel to renal vascular injury.

It is essential to confirm the presence of a contralateral functioning kidney before operating on an injured kidney. Emergency intravenous urography or chromocystoscopy (i.v. 7 ml of 0.4% solution of indigocarmine watched cystoscopically as excreted by ureter within 5 min) is sufficient. The transperitoneal approach is recommended to allow full laparotomy and to deal with other injured organs. Renal vessels can be controlled before the kidney is exposed. The kidney should be exposed by opening Gerota's fascia to relieve tamponade. Drainage of haematoma or extravasated urine should be performed together with repair of the renal injury.

Surgical repair should be conservative. Small tears (in small or large subcapsular haematomas) should be sutured over Oxycel, pieces of detached muscle or mobilised omentum. Larger single rents (in cortical not medullary lacerations) are dealt with by nephrostomy through the rent and suturing the kidney on either side of a Malecot nephrostomy tube. Laceration confined to one pole of the kidney is dealt with by partial nephrectomy. Repair of a solitary damaged kidney must be attempted, but if this is not possible, the wound is packed firmly with gauze so that the bleeding is controlled and the ruptured kidney may heal.

However, in a multiple massively ruptured kidney or in avulsion of the renal pedicle (in the presence of a contralateral functioning kidney) nephrectomy must be undertaken. The standard loin extraperitoneal approach is recommended in patients presenting several days after the injury because of perirenal haematoma or urine extravasation and since associated abdominal organ injuries are unlikely by that time.

Comment on ureteric injuries

These are uncommon and usually iatrogenic following pelvic surgery (e.g. colorectal resection and hysterectomy) or Dormia basket extraction of stone. They are either unilateral or bilateral (anuria). The former are asymptomatic with silent renal atrophy, pyonephrosis with loin pain and fever, or urinary fistula which develops via an abdominal incision or following hysterectomy via the vagina. In bilateral injuries, each ureter is damaged inadvertently in one of the following ways.

● Divided.
● Crushed.
● Portion of its wall has been removed.
● Blood supply is damaged (avascular necrosis).
● Ligated.

Ureteric cut leads to retro- or intraperitoneal extravasation of urine with paralytic ileus and peritonitis. When ureteric ligation causes obstruction, the injury may be recognised at the time it is inflicted and repaired immediately or it may not be diagnosed until later (in which case do a temporary nephrostomy and repair the injury later when oedema and infection have abated after 6 weeks). Prophylactic ureteric catheterisation for easy identification and protection prior to pelvic surgery is sometimes practised.

The type of repair depends on the level of ureteric injury. For a low injury, reimplantation into the bladder is the treatment of choice (preferably with a non-refluxing anastomosis). The gap between the ureter and bladder can be bridged by a psoas hitch or Boari flap. An injury at or just above the bifurcation of the common iliac vessels is dealt with by transureteroureterostomy or replacement by an ileal segment. With more proximal (higher) abdominal ureteric injuries, direct repair (splinted spatulated anastomosis) with a Malecot nephrostomy tube is recommended. Very rarely nephrectomy (in the presence of a contralateral functioning kidney) or kidney transplantation into the iliac fossa may be attempted (Fig. A11).

A11

(a) Intravenous urogram (IVU) revealing a huge filling defect involving the upper pole of the left kidney (hypernephroma).
(b) Painless haematuria (can be painful as a result of clot colic), palpable mass, pyrexia of unknown origin. Sometimes pathological fracture (due to skeletal metastasis) or pulmonary secondaries (with haemoptysis). Rarely polycythaemia or anaemia. Very rarely persistent hypertension, nephrotic syndrome, left varicocele and Budd–Chiari syndrome due to infiltration of hepatic veins in *right* renal tumour.
(c) Left nephrectomy preferably via a transabdominal (rather than lumbar) approach to gain wide exposure of the enlarged kidney and its pedicle.

Comment

Transitional cell carcinoma of the renal pelvis (in the form of a papillary tumour, a solid tumour or a mixed one) should be seriously considered and differentiated from hypernephroma since the treatment is completely different. Papillary tumour of the renal pelvis manifests itself clinically by haematuria (and clot colic) and very rarely by pelviureteric junction obstruction and hydronephrosis.

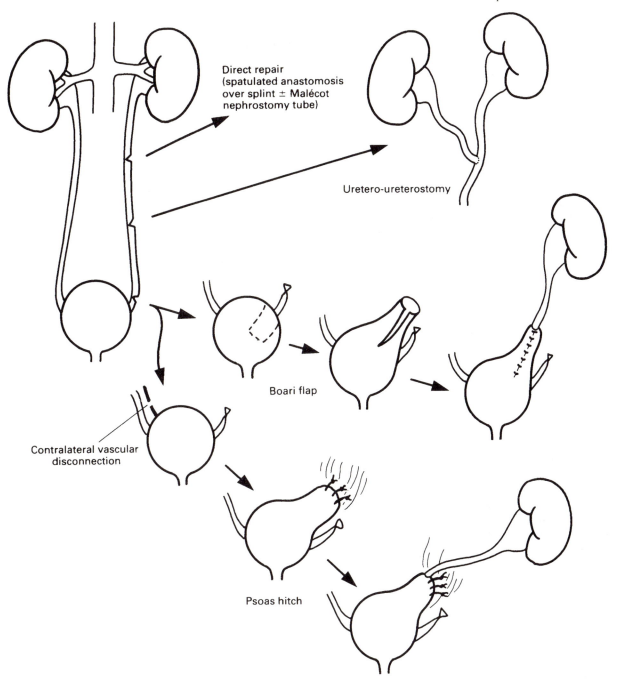

Fig. A11   Repair of various ureteric injuries

The characteristic filling defect seen in a papillary tumour of the renal pelvis may be misleading since hypernephroma can infiltrate the renal pelvis producing a similar filling defect while papillary tumour can infiltrate the kidney proper producing an IVU picture similar to hypernephroma. Retrograde ureterography may be used to define the diagnosis (this is arguable since a good IVU should be as good as a retrograde picture). Because of multiple ureteric and bladder metastases (due to papillary tumour spread by seeding) the treatment is a nephroureterectomy with sleeve resection of the bladder wall followed by cystoscopic follow-up for life.

If a papillary tumour of the renal pelvis was treated by nephrectomy alone, based on clinical and operative misdiagnosis (frozen section may sometimes be required to reveal the nature of the tumour), then the patient will present with haematuria probably from a ureteric metastatic or recurrent tumour which can be detected cystoscopically (if the papillary tumour is at the ureteric orifice or in the bladder), by retrograde ureterogram with image intensifier or by CT scan of the pelvis. Such cases are usually advanced and excision of the ureteric stump will not be sufficient. They are therefore treated with intravesical fulguration if the tumour is accessible or by ureteroscopic fulguration and chemotherapy if it is extensive, and are regarded as terminal cases.

A12

(a) IVU shows left hydroureter and hydronephrosis, osteoblastic metastatic lesion of L3 vertebra and right non-functioning kidney.

(b) All the above abnormalities are due to obstructive prostatic carcinomatous uropathy (revealed indirectly by its metastasis). The prostatic venous plexus is connected to the paravertebral plexus directly by valve-less veins and hence lumbar skeletal secondary deposits spreading directly from a primary prostatic carcinoma following increased intravesical pressure after prostatic obstructive uropathy.

(c) Transurethral resection of prostatic carcinoma to relieve the obstruction followed by hormonal therapy (stilboestrol 1 mg three times a day initially for 1 week followed by 1 mg a day for life) and/or radiotherapy for painful skeletal metastasis. Prostatic coagulopathy or stilboestrol thromboembolic complications may necessitate subcapsular orchidectomy.

A13

(a) Multiple bilateral pubic rami fractures with disruption of the symphysis pubis. There is incomplete undisplaced basal intracapsular fracture of the left femoral neck with right central acetabular fracture without hip dislocation.

(b) Correction of shock then treatment of pelvic visceral injuries (when confirmed) followed by treatment of the fracture itself which needs external pelvic compression either by suspending it in a pelvic sling from an overhead beam, nursing the patient between sandbags (or on his side) or by applying his spica divided in the centre and bandaged by rubber.

The pelvic visceral injuries and treatment are:

- Intrapelvic rupture of membranous urethra (patient cannot pass urine, blood leak from urethral meatus, bladder distension before extravasation occurs and Vermooten's sign). Urethrocystography and immediate catheterisation are contraindicated since they may destroy any residual intact urethral wall. The patient should be taken to theatre, the bladder opened and the position of the prostate assessed. *If the prostate is not floating high* (indicating incomplete partial injury), the bladder is closed round a large (28 Fr) Malecot catheter (orthopaedic reduction of pelvic fracture can be attempted) and antibiotic cover given. If, 3 weeks later, urethroscopy and metallic sound are successful then the suprapubic catheter is clamped to allow the patient to micturate. *If the prostate is floating* (indicating complete total rupture), then a catheter is railroaded across the gap using two metallic bougies or the little finger and a metallic bougie. Traction on a Foley catheter is used to replace the prostate in position. The bladder is closed around the Malecot catheter with separate drainage of the prevesical space. The Foley catheter is removed after 12 days. The suprapubic drain may be clamped and removed after 2–3 weeks.
- Extraperitoneal rupture of bladder (bladder impalpable with dullness and tenderness suprapubically) – carry out laparotomy, suture the bladder with the urethral Foley catheter in situ and drain the prevesical space.
- Rectal injury (assessed by rectal examination) may necessitate a defunctioning loop iliac colostomy.
- Sciatic nerve injury with anaesthesia and weakness of part of the leg may be associated with vertical disruption of the pelvic ring and is treated by reduction of the pelvic fracture.
- Injury to blood vessels is rare; repair is indicated if lower limb pulses are absent or there is evidence of ischaemia.
- In a female patient, very rarely the vagina can be injured, and it should be sutured (not applicable here).

Comment

Posterior urethral injuries

Management of posterior urethral injuries resulting from pelvic fractures in males is controversial. The conservative approach and late surgery is based on the fact that the majority of such injuries are incomplete ruptures. Because urethral catheterisation, as well as urethrography or urethroscopy, may complete the rupture, suprapubic bladder catheterisation is done initially followed by definitive repair 3 weeks later. Those who advocate such an approach suggest that complete posterior urethral ruptures will always heal with stricture formation whereas incomplete lesions may heal spontaneously without subsequent stricture. They believe many of the complications are due to the initial treatment rather than to the injury itself (Mitchell). The early operative approach (advocated here) is based on the fact that incomplete rupture of the posterior urethra often results in formation of a stricture which may be long and tortuous. In complete rupture re-apposition of the ends of the ruptured urethra will allow healing without stricture formation or will result in a short stricture which can be managed easily by urethral dilatation; thus, when posterior urethral injury is suspected clinically, attempted urethral catheterisation causes no harm and the most difficult strictures occur when early approximation of the ruptured urethral ends is not attempted. In such cases the urethral gap may be considerable and the ends will not meet as the pelvic haematoma resolves (Blandy).

Pelvic fractures

Are the shared responsibility of orthopaedic and general surgeons. They are classified as:

Isolated (not destroying pelvic ring integrity)   These are not significant and need only 3 weeks' rest with leg exercises.

Pelvic ring integrity disruption (due to ring fracture at two points)   The pelvis is no longer a stable weight-bearing structure, the separated fragments may be displaced and the fracture may be difficult or impossible to reduce. The fracture receives secondary consideration while every effort should be made to exclude or confirm and treat the fracture complications inflicted on the pelvic viscera. The fracture may be slight (bed rest), disrupted symphysis pubis (see above) or upward proximal displacement (skeletal traction through tibia of the affected side is essential for 2 months to prevent sciatic nerve compression).

Hip dislocation (*see also* Section 1.74)

Uncommon injuries, classified as:

Posterior dislocation   Occurs in flexed adducted and internally rotated hip position (since the femoral head becomes covered posteriorly by the capsule only and not by bone, force applied to the long axis of the femoral shaft may dislocate the head over the posterior hip of the acetabulum). Such injuries occur in front seat car passengers who are thrown forwards and strike their knees on the dash board. Also in motorcycle accidents and in roof fall accidents. The femoral head is displaced into the sciatic notch (damaging the sciatic nerve) and then into the ilium dorsum. Pain is referred along the sciatic nerve. The dislocation is reduced under general anaesthesia on the floor with the patient's iliac crests steadied by an assistant. The surgeon stands over the limb and flexes the knee and hip, then adducts with vertical lifting of the femur (sometimes with internal rotation). Reduction is maintained by skeletal traction on the tibia of the affected side for 6 weeks with no weight-bearing for 6 months (because of possible unpredicted avascular necrosis of the femoral head in 10% of cases).
  Complications are:
● Sciatic nerve injury: treated by reduction of dislocation.
● Avascular necrosis of femoral head: treated by hemi- or total hip replacement arthroplasty.
● Femoral neck fracture (rarely): treated by operation and dislocation open reduction. Avascular necrosis is invariable.
● Fracture of posterior hip of acetabulum: treated by open reduction and internal fixation with a screw with open reduction of dislocated hip.
● Hip osteoarthrosis with post-traumatic ossification.

Anterior dislocation   Rare. The femoral head lies in either the obturator or the pubic position with the limb flexed, abducted and externally rotated. Treated by reduction.

Central dislocation   Usually accompanied by other pelvic fractures and is due to a blow on the greater trochanter driving the head through the acetabular floor resulting in comminuted acetabular fracture. Treated by reduction of the femoral head to its anatomical position; this is maintained by tibial skeletal traction with mobilisation as soon as pain allows. The result is unsatisfactory because of hip osteoarthrosis regardless of treatment. (Open reduction is difficult and one should accept the displacement and later osteoarthrosis.)

A14

(a) Progressive osteolytic lesion affecting the greater trochanter of the right femoral head.
(b) Bone biopsy (the histology in this case was consistent with a secondary rather than a primary bone tumour), skeletal survey and radioactive isotope bone scan (hot spots in the latter are not always due to tumour as prior skeletal survey may show recently fractured bone with callus formation, Paget's disease of the bone or even osteoarthrosis). A thorough clinical examination of both breasts, chest, thyroid gland and kidneys should follow including chest X-ray, mammogram, IVU and thyroid radioactive scan. The primary is treated, although a solitary metastasis could be treated as well. Multiple secondaries indicate advanced carcinomatosis beyond treatment.
(c) Rarely primary bone tumour (osteogenic sarcoma) but more commonly secondary bony metastases (more than two-thirds of cases). The primary origin tends to be breast carcinoma or (in males) prostatic carcinoma in two-thirds of all secondary bony deposits. One-sixth arise from the bronchus, kidney and thyroid (in that order). In the remaining one-sixth of cases no primary tumour can be identified. The majority of tumours are osteolytic (radiolucent) but prostatic and rarely bony breast deposits are osteoblastic (sclerotic).

Comment: Bone biopsy under general anaesthesia revealed a subclinical abdominal mass in this obese woman. Barium studies revealed displacement of the transverse colon; abdominal ultrasound and IVU excluded kidney origin. Exploratory laparotomy revealed an inoperable small bowel carcinoma (bypassed and biopsy taken). Histology was similar to bone biopsy and both showed non-Hodgkin's lymphoma or anaplastic carcinoma. Since skeletal survey and bone scan revealed only this solitary hot spot in the right hip, this rare case was reported as a solitary skeletal metastasis from small bowel carcinoma and represents one of unidentified origin. Skeletal metastases are usually multiple and very rarely solitary. When presented clinically such metastases can reveal the subclinical occult primary tumour.

(d) Pathological fracture which could be treated by hip replacement (hemiarthroplasty). Classically, pathological fractures of bone shafts (e.g. femoral shaft) are treated with internal fixation followed by radiotherapy (in malignant cases only).

Comment: Bone fracture following trivial trauma may be due to local or general causes.

- Local bony lesions: simple cyst, osteoclastoma, eosinophilic granuloma, hydatid cyst, aneurysmal bone cyst, haemangioma, fibrous dysplasia and Brodie's abscess (localised chronic osteomyelitis) and primary bone tumour.
- General causes: Paget's disease, primary osteoporosis, vitamin D deficiency (rickets in children and osteomalacia in adults), scurvy (vitamin C deficiency), endocrine disorders such as hyperparathyroidism and secondary osteoporosis (in pituitary or adrenal cortical tumour), secondary skeletal metastases and multiple myeloma.

A15

(a) Fracture of distal 2 cm of radius with dinner-fork deformity. The distal fragment is:
- Displaced dorsally.
- Angulated dorsally.
- Driven proximally, overlapping the shaft (shortening).
- Angulated laterally.
- Supinated.

There is an associated fracture of the ulnar styloid process.

(b) Colles' fracture.

(c) The fracture is reduced under general anaesthesia or Bier's block. The surgeon shakes hands with the patient's affected hand, and applies firm traction (with assistant exerting countertraction on the elbow), disimpacting the distal radial fragment by pressing it into palmar-flexion, ulnar deviation and pronation. Dorsal plaster slab is applied in this position from the elbow to the metacarpal heads. Satisfactory reduction is confirmed by X-ray. The slab is converted into Colles' plaster 24 h later (if the reduction is maintained with satisfactory circulation to the fingers) and maintained for 6 weeks.

(d) Complications (with their treatment) are malunion (osteotomy and realignment), subluxation of inferior radioulnar joint (excision of ulnar tail), stiffness of fingers or shoulder (exercises), fraying attrition rupture of extensor pollicis longus (extensor indicis transfer) and Sudeck's post-traumatic osteodystrophy (physiotherapy).

A16

(a) Fracture through the distal metaphysis of the humerus with complex distal fragment displacement consisting of three elements:
- Backward displacement.
- Backward angulation.
- Pronation (since the hand is usually pronated at the time of injury) producing internal rotation and adduction of the distal fragment.

The diagnosis is supracondylar fracture of the humerus.

(b) Examine the radial pulse of the affected arm since the brachial artery may be injured by the distal fragment, compressed by haematoma or contracted as a result of spasm. Reduction under general anaesthesia with X-ray screening is essential. The assistant grasps the upper arm and the surgeon shakes hands with the affected forearm exerting:

1. Firm steady traction in the long axis of the forearm (while in flexion) for 2 min; then

2. Traction and extension of the elbow (feel radial pulse); then
3. Supination and external rotation, which are compared with range of supination and external rotation of unaffected arm; then
4. Gradual maximal flexion (90°) of elbow with palpable radial pulse done by pressing the olecranon with the thumbs (and fingers over biceps) to move it and the distal fragment forward into flexion.
5. A light back slab is applied over padding and postreduction X-ray is checked immediately, 48 h and 1 week later. A collar and cuff may be used but never a full encircling plaster. Radial pulse should be examined when the patient is admitted to hospital and for 48 h.

(c) Fractures around the elbow in children are very important because their complications or malmanagement result in disabling problems. They are:
● Supracondylar fracture of the humerus (65% of cases).
● Lateral condyle = external condyle = capitellum fracture.
● Medial epicondylar fracture.
● Fracture separating upper radial epiphysis.
● Olecranon fracture.
● Posterior dislocation of elbow with possible fracture of coronoid process, radial head or distal humeral articular surface.
● Monteggia fracture-dislocation (ulnar fracture with dislocated superior radioulnar joint) may be included.

(d) The most serious complication of supracondylar fracture of the humerus is: *vascular occlusion* leading to gangrene or ischaemic Volkmann's contracture (of flexor muscles and peripheral nerves). Other complications are *injury to the median nerve*; and *deformity from malunion* causing cubitus varus (treated by supracondylar osteotomy).

Comment on vascular occlusion

Diagnosis of incipient stage

Vascular occlusion is suggested by impaired circulatory signs including:
● Colour (pale).
● Temperature (cool).
● Pulses (feeble or absent).
● Capillary return (poor).
● Nerve conduction – digital sensory loss in the absence of nerve injury (motor testing is less reliable).
● Inability of patient to extend fingers fully.
● Marked pain on passive extension in the forearm.

Diagnosis of established stage

History of fracture and the characteristic flexion contraction of the wrist and fingers (flexor muscles are affected more than extensor muscles).

Treatment

Incipient Volkmann's ischaemia

1. First steps.
● Remove external splints or bandage.
● Reduce fracture (if not already reduced).
● Hot water bottles – to produce vasodilatation.
● Dextran 40 i.v. infusion.
2. Second step (if first steps fail). Explore for:
● Free brachial artery kinking and if in spasm paint it with papaveretum or apply a warm pack.
● Punctured or contused and thrombosed artery. Excise and end-to-end suture or use vein graft.

Established Volkmann's ischaemic contracture

Restoration to normal function is impossible. The following options are available:
● Overcome shortening by prolonged stretching with spring splints.
● Shorten bones.
● Muscle slide operation (detachment and distal displacement of flexor muscles).
● Excise dead muscles and transfer healthy muscle, e.g. wrist flexor or wrist extensor, to the tendon of flexor digitorum profundus and flexor pollicis longus.
● Arthrodesis of wrist.
● Grafting of median nerve damaged by the ischaemic injury.

A17

(a) Anterior subcoracoid left shoulder dislocation (of humeral head).

(b) There is a triad of physical signs:

● Outer aspect of the shoulder is flattened and the arm appears to originate from under the junction of the middle and outer thirds of the clavicle.

● Immobility of the shoulder (due to mechanical problem, spasm and pain).

● Abduction position.

(c) Reduction under general anaesthesia producing muscle relaxation. Kocher's method consists of flexing the elbow and:

1. Applying traction in the long axis of the humerus for 2 min; then
2. Rotating the humerus externally; then
3. Adducting the shoulder fully; then
4. Rotating the shoulder internally fully.

The postreduction X-ray is checked and the position is maintained for 3 weeks by a sling and bandage.

Comment

In acute shoulder dislocation, the humeral head takes one of four positions:

1. Anterior subcoracoid (the commonest).
2. Subglenoid.
3. Subclavicular.
4. Posterior or dorsal.

Recurrent shoulder dislocation is due to instability following maltreated acute dislocation and is treated only by operation.

Bankart's operation for recurrent shoulder dislocation

1. A sandbag is placed between the scapulae to allow the shoulder to fall backwards. The incision commences above the coracoid process, extends downwards one finger's breadth lateral to the deltopectoral groove for 12.5 cm, safeguarding the cephalic vein, dividing the deep fascia and splitting the deltoid in line with the incision. (If exposure is inadequate identify and divide the coracoid process; retract the tip and its attached muscles – coracobrachialis and biceps – downwards.)
2. Rotate the arm externally and divide the subscapularis and the capsule 2.5 cm from the muscle insertion.
3. Open and inspect the capsule, and retract the humeral head with Bankart's retractor. Notice the voluminous capsule, labrum glenoidale tear, humeral head defect and possibly loose bodies.
4. If the labrum is detached, raise a shaving from the front of the glenoid cavity to produce a raw area, drill holes in the anterior edge of the glenoid with an angled dental drill and suture the detached glenoidal labrum to the raw area, using wire, nylon or other suitable ligatures.
5. Repair the subscapularis (in the Putti–Platt operation the muscle and capsule are overlapped (double-breasted) for 2.5 cm).
6. Resuture the coracoid process into position (if divided) and bandage the arm to the side with the elbow held forwards for 5 weeks.

A18

(a) Fracture of the waist of the right scaphoid bone.

(b) Patient presents clinically with a painful wrist (but with no major impairment of wrist function). On examination there is tenderness in the anatomical snuff-box (over the scaphoid) with little swelling. Pinch test by pressing the thumb against the index finger of the affected side causes severe pain in the anatomical snuff-box. X-ray should include three views: anteroposterior, lateral and *two oblique*. Since there is no displacement immediately after injury the fracture may not be displayed radiologically. The case is misdiagnosed as sprained wrist and mobilisation carried out, leading to avascular necrosis, non-union and osteoarthrosis of the wrist or stiff wrist in later treatment. Therefore suspected fracture, even if not confirmed radiologically, should be treated in a scaphoid plaster (like a Colles' plaster from the elbow down to the metacarpal heads *but also set up to the interphalangeal joint of the thumb* while the hand is in a functioning position as if holding a glass of water) for 2 weeks, after which the plaster is removed and the wrist X-rayed again; by this time the original unrevealed scaphoid fracture becomes obvious radiologically. If the fracture is confirmed at this time or diagnosed from the start the scaphoid plaster should be applied for 8 weeks.

Non-union is either immobilised for a year (may result in stiff wrist), treated by bone grafting and internal fixation with a small screw followed by 8 weeks' immobilisation in plaster or accepted as it is (non-union will not always give rise to significant disability).

A19

(a) Arteriography.

(b) Right popliteal artery aneurysm with wide lumen (although the presence and extent of thrombus cannot be assessed). The left popliteal artery is healthy with good filling of its trifurcation (perineal, anterior and posterior tibial arteries).

(c) Surgery by wide exposure with proximal and distal control followed by femoropopliteal bypass (using reversed autogenous vein graft or gore graft) combined with either aneurysmal excision or exclusion. Occasionally Matas' aneurysmorrhaphic reconstruction may be performed if practically possible.

Comment on aneurysm classification

Aneurysm is an abnormal arterial dilatation. However, aneurysm is better defined as a cavity full of blood in connection with the interior of a blood vessel, because not every aneurysm is dilated, e.g. dissecting aneurysm and false aneurysm. It is either:
● True: dilated artery (whether fusiform, saccular or dissecting);
● False: an organised sac communicating with the artery through an opening in its wall. It is traumatic in origin; or:
● Arteriovenous fistula (congenital or acquired). *Arteriovenous (AV) fistula* can be (causes):
  – congenital;
  – traumatic;
  – iatrogenic (ligating vein and artery *en masse*);
  – physiological, such as PDA in fetus;
  – therapeutic, as the one constructed for renal dialysis.
The causes of aneurysms are:
● Congenital: berry aneurysm (of cerebral circle of Willis) and dissecting aneurysm of Marfan's syndrome.
● Traumatic (false and arteriovenous aneurysm such as cirsoid aneurysm).
● Atherosclerosis as in abdominal aortic aneurysm.
● Hypertension.
● Infective: wrongly called mycotic – they are usually bacterial or syphilitic.
● Infarction: left ventricular aneurysm after myocardial infarction (containing mural thrombus).
The eventual outcome of aneurysms is either spontaneous healing (consolidation), infection, development of a slow leak or sudden rupture.

A20

(a) Plain X-ray of lower limb revealing a bipennate muscle structure (of the right thigh) due to the presence of gas in the intramuscular planes. The diagnosis is gas gangrene.

(b) The condition is extremely life-threatening and treatment should include:
1. Preparation for immediate operation with
   (i)   Blood transfusion.
   (ii) Penicillin 8 mega-units (stat. i.v. injection) followed by 4 mega-units 4-hourly for 8 days together with 2 g streptomycin injection daily.
   (iii) Anti-gas gangrene serum (3 ampoules immediately and repeated 6-hourly i.v.).
   (iv) 100% oxygen or hyperbaric oxygen to reduce the amount of toxin produced by the anaerobic organisms (*Clostridium welchii*, *C. septicum* and *C. oedematiens*).
2. Operation aiming at early and meticulous exicision of all dead and dying muscular tissues, either done via bilateral long incisions of the affected limb with secondary suture or (if such total clearance is impossible) amputation via hip disarticulation. Although uncommon, gas gangrene carries a high mortality in the victims of accidents and classically complicates high amputation stumps

in the presence of arterial disease (since Clostridia are present in the intestine, prophylactic antibiotics are required in amputation with a fluffy bandage to prevent faecal contamination of stump). The mortality is due to rapid gangrene involving muscles initially (swollen tense limb with sickly foul odour due to gas and thin brownish foul exudate) and, when septicaemia occurs, involving the abdominal organs (e.g. foaming liver).

Comment

Gas gangrene and tetanus are the two acute specific infections that are commonly asked about in the final FRCS. Tetanus is caused by *Clostridium tetani* which produces a powerful exotoxin that:
- Interferes with ACh/Ch-esterase balance leading to sustained muscular tonic spasm due to ACh excess.
- Causes extreme hyperexcitability of motor neurons in the anterior horn cells leading to explosive muscle reflex spasm in response to minor stimuli.
- Causes concomitant sympathetic overactivity.

The time between the first symptom and the first reflex spasm is *'the period of onset'* which serves as a prognostic index (the longer it is, the better the prognosis). First symptoms are difficult swallowing, jaw stiffness, and painful neck, back and abdomen. Risus sardonicus (smile), opisthotonos and muscle rupture (psoas, rectus abdominis, pectoral) are due to reflex convulsions which occur spontaneously or in response to trivial stimuli. Cyanosis, pneumonia, respiratory failure and death are the ultimate outcome. Prophylactically active immunity can be induced by administration of tetanus toxoid followed by a booster dose every 5 years. Passive immunisation with 250 units human antitetanus globulin (ATG) should always be given with toxoid, active immunisation if patients exposed to tetanus (e.g. injury) were not or incompletely immunised. Fully immunised persons who are likely to be exposed to tetanus following a wound should be given a booster injection, provided more than 5 years have elapsed since they were last vaccinated or actively immunised. Established tetanus is treated by isolation of the patient in a quiet dark place, wound toilet, and administration of ATG (one dose) and penicillin (heavy doses). In addition: in mild cases – sedation with i.m. promazine and amylobarbitone 6-hourly; in seriously ill patients – nasogastric tube (for feeding) and tracheostomy; and in dangerously ill patients – intermittent positive pressure ventilation with curare is indicated.

A21

(a) Right cervical rib producing thoracic outlet syndrome.
(b) Locally there is a cervical bony fixed lump and supraclavicular tenderness. Forearm ischaemic pain radiating to the upper arm is brought on by use of the arm, especially in elevation, and relieved by rest. The hand is cold with colour changes (pale when held aloft and blue when dependent). The radial pulse is absent or feeble especially after abduction of the arm with possible systolic bruit on subclavian auscultation. Skin trophic changes are preceded by finger numbness, leading to ulceration, gangrene or nerve pressure symptoms (pain, paraesthesia and weakness in hand and forearm with wasting of the thenar and hypothenar muscles are attributed to cervical rib only after exclusion of cervical spondylosis and carpal tunnel syndrome).
(c) Extraperiosteal excision of cervical rib (with periosteum).

Comment

Cervical ribs are present in up to 1% of the population. They are usually asymptomatic and commonly bilateral (in this case unilateral). Thoracic outlet syndrome is caused by:
- Bones (cervical rib, clavicle fracture, transverse process of C7).
- Muscles (scalenus anterior, pectoralis minor).
- Bands (fibromuscular band related to any of the above structures).

The syndrome is also known as costoclavicular, scalenus anterior, shoulder girdle, pectoralis minor, hyperabduction, Adson's or cervical rib syndrome. Arch arteriography is required to show subclavian stenosis and post-stenotic dilatation with local thrombus formation (which can lead to distal embolisation). Treatment in the absence of cervical rib is scalenotomy, band removal, first rib removal or even sympathectomy.

A22

(a) Plain abdominal X-ray showing three radio-opaque gallstones, one of them having moved to obstruct Hartmann's pouch.
(b) Acute calculous obstructed cholecystitis.
(c) Available investigations are:
Plain abdominal X-ray – may reveal radio-opaque gall stones in 10–15% of cases (since 85–90% are radiolucent, this is exactly opposite to urinary stones where 85–90% are radio-opaque).

Oral cholecystogram – to confirm the presence of gallstones or non-visualisation of the gallbladder (a negative sign of positive diagnostic value). In acute cholecystitis, this test is limited because of vomiting and inability to swallow tablets. It is worthwhile in patients who are not nauseous or jaundiced.

Intravenous cholangiogram (bolus) – produces relatively poor opacification of the extrahepatic biliary system and the dye fails to concentrate adequately even in a normally functioning gallbladder.

Infusion i.v. cholangiogram – probably the most reliable diagnostic procedure with accuracy of more than 90%. It requires tomographic facilities and the long infusion time may prove inconvenient.

Grey scale ultrasound – detects gallstones in both acute and chronic stages and provides information on dilated ducts. Its effectiveness is impaired by bowel gas in the gallbladder area masking the stones in approximately 30% of patients on the initial scan. Repeat scanning is important.

Isotope scanning – i.v. technetium isotope HIDA is the most successful test for diagnosis of acute cholecystitis. Failure of isotope uptake by the gallbladder is diagnostic. Delay of excretion of common bile duct dye in the duodenum is indicative of common bile duct obstruction.

(d) Traditionally most British surgeons proceed with conservative treatment (bed rest, pain relief with antispasmodic drug, e.g. hyoscine butylbromide (Buscopan) and analgesic, e.g. pethidine, antibiotics and possibly nasogastric suction and i.v. drip in persistent vomiting), so that the condition resolves and definitive investigations can take place in the recovery period; definitive elective cholecystectomy is done 6–12 weeks later. Elective cholecystectomy has the advantage of allowing confirmation of the provisional clinical diagnosis with more investigations and avoiding operation on an acutely inflamed friable gallbladder with, for example, obscure anatomy in an obese patient. It also means that a convenient time can be chosen with experienced anaesthetic and surgical staff and appropriate facilities (e.g. operative cholangiogram) available. However, its disadvantages are prolongation of the patient's symptoms (persistent pain and/or fever) in 6–33% of cases and possible complications, i.e. extrahepatic obstructive jaundice (with or without cholangitis and septicaemia), empyema of the gallbladder and perforation of the gallbladder (in 3–12% of acute cholecystitis cases), that may require the surgeon to undertake emergency operation with potentially poorer results. Many surgeons consider this too high a price to pay for the traditional approach and are now beginning to follow the policy of early surgery, i.e. *urgent* but not emergency cholecystectomy done within 1 week of admission (to allow the surgeon to carry out the necessary investigations and the acutely inflamed gallbladder to settle). The advantages of the early operative approach are as follows:

● The accuracy of clinical diagnosis supplemented by investigations (plain abdominal X-ray, ultrasound, oral cholecystogram and/ or infusion, i.v. cholangiogram with HIDA scan when available) has become very close to 100%.

● The pathology of the removed gallbladder during first admission reveals that 65% have chronic cholecystitis with acute inflammation, 25% chronic cholecystitis and 10% acute cholecystitis. Long-term follow-up of such patients indicates a high incidence of recurrence and development of complications.

● The mortality of urgent surgery is exaggerated. Studies reveal that the operative mortality rate is equal to that of elective cholecystectomy. Indeed 20% of patients treated conservatively will require re-admission for a further attack before their elective operation; in addition 17% of patients are defaulters – they either refuse subsequent admission or are lost (owing to false impression of being cured) only to present later with complications. Thus the *overall* mortality of late operation is probably higher than that of early intervention. However, morbidity (i.e. wound infection) was found to be higher in urgent operation because of highly infected bile.

● Technically, urgent cholecystectomy in patients with chronic cholecystitis is as easy as elective operation. In 75% (with acute inflammation) oedema may make the operation easier by creating a plane of cleavage. However, surgery should be avoided if acute symptoms have continued for 7 days or more as the granulation tissue and adhesions are more advanced (perforation of the gallbladder is extremely rare after 7 days of continuous symptoms and these patients are best treated conservatively with surgery at a second admission).

● Acalculous cholecystitis presents with severe systemic illness and rarely responds well to conservative treatment. The gallbladder is thick-walled, grossly oedematous with leucocyte infiltration and full of pus and fibrin mixed with bile with mucosal ulcerations. Aetiology is obscure (e.g. associated with torsion of the vascular pedicle, bile stasis with prolonged fasting, clostridial organisms, trauma, burns and specific diseases such as diabetes, sarcoidosis and chronic renal failure). Surgical delay in such patients only increases the hazards of the illness.

Summary   The policy should be as follows:
● Patients unfit for operation at any time are managed conservatively.
● Patients with acute symptoms of more than 7 days receive conservative treatment with elective operation 6 weeks later.
● Patients with symptoms of less than 7 days' duration have an operation on the next list after diagnosis (urgent but not emergency operation) by a competent surgeon.
● Emergency operation for patients presenting with a perforated gallbladder (toxic signs with peritonitis) or increasing local signs.

Technical points in early operation   Handling of the perforated, gangrenous or friable gallbladder may result in rupture and dissemination of infected material. This can be minimised by aspirating some of the contents to relieve the tension and the gallbladder can then be mobilised in a retrograde manner. This allows the gallbladder to hang by the pedicle of cystic duct and artery. These can be divided close to or even across the neck of the gallbladder allowing better visualisation of the common bile duct. Prophylactic antibiotics and operative cholangiogram are mandatory. Subtotal cholecystectomy or cholecystostomy may be used only in difficult situations.

(e) Yes, in one of the following conditions:
1. When the gallbladder is packed with radio-opaque stones.
2. Emphysematous cholecystitis (gallbladder outline is visible).
3. Porcelain gallbladder (calcified wall).
4. Lime bile.

(f) Haemobilia is a rare cause of acute or chronic blood loss from the GIT (diagnosed after exclusion of common causes); it can lead to biliary colic and obstructive jaundice. Diagnosis is easy in the operated patient if the T-tube is already in situ, but in the unoperated patient, blood may be seen emerging from the sphincter of Oddi on ERCP. An arteriogram can locate the bleeding site within the liver and the treatment is to ligate the feeding vessel as close as possible to the angiographic leak. Occasionally, partial hepatectomy is needed in heavy post-traumatic haemobilia arising deep in the liver substance. The causes of haemobilia are:
– liver trauma due to arteriobiliary communication;
– difficult and traumatic exploration of the common bile duct;
– cholangiocarcinoma;
– liver tumour communicating with bile ducts;
– parasitic hepatobiliary infestation (Oriental parasites).

(g) Spasm of Oddi's sphincter and opioid drugs: Anaesthesia for cholecystectomy and/or common bile duct exploration is influenced by effects of drugs (used during anaesthesia) on intrabiliary pressure. Opioids specifically, are known to cause spasm of Oddi's sphincter (choledochoduodenal sphincter); fentanyl, morphine and meperidine can result in sustained choledochal hypertension. However, the incidence of opioid-induced biliary hypertension is low but important, since it has implications in the interpretation of peroperative cholangiography (advocated in all cholecystectomies) and manometric measurement of biliary pressure (performed to evaluate the need for sphincteroplasty). Opioid-induced spasm of Oddi's sphincter elevates intrabiliary pressures and at the same time impairs passage of contrast medium into the duodenum, erroneously suggesting the need for sphincteroplasty or presence of common bile duct (CBD) stones. The spasm appears radiologically as a constriction at the distal end of the CBD and is misinterpreted as CBD stones. However, it may be prudent to avoid administration of opioids during anaesthesia for patients undergoing biliary surgery. Not all patients respond to opioids with spasm of Oddi's sphincter. Also, tachyphylaxis (decreased responses following consecutive injections at short intervals) to spasmogenic effects of opioids on the biliary system may occur. It should also be remembered that intraoperative manipulation of CBD with dilator, catheter, Desjardin forceps, and use of cold or irritating solutions (radio-opaque dyes) may all produce spasm of Oddi's shincter, which is independent of drugs used in anaesthesia.

Alternatives to opioids during anaesthesia for cholecystectomy would include use of anaesthetic gases, such as nitrous oxide plus fentanyl, halothane or enflurane; these gases may induce hepatic dysfunction, particularly in the presence of liver disease. Opioid-induced spasm of Oddi's sphincter can entirely be reversed with naloxone should cholangiogram or biliary pressure be abnormal. Naloxone, however, reverses analgesia and necessitates a volatile anaesthetic to ensure adequate anaesthesia; it therefore is not a practical approach. A more attractive approach is i.v. administration of 1–2 mg of glucagon, which can reverse opioid-induced spasm of Oddi's sphincter; hypersensitivity is a rare but potential problem with glucagon. Hyperglycaemia is predictable and glucagon given to awake patients often evokes nausea. Furthermore, glucagon should not be given to patients with known or suspected insulinoma or phaeochromocytoma.

A23

(a) An IVU.
(b) A right congenital pelvic kidney (due to renal ectopia), right-sided filling defect (bladder carcinoma) and left pelviureteric junction obstruction.
(c) The bladder carcinoma (threatening to obstruct the right pelvic kidney) should be assessed by cystoscopy, examined under anaesthesia and possibly treated by transurethral resection, and monitored by regular check cystoscopies. The left pelviureteric junction obstruction should be tackled thereafter by reconstructive pyeloplasty by the dismembered Anderson–Hynes operation (if obstruction is high), or Culp rotational flap, Foley Y-V plastic operation or longitudinal cut sutured transversely (if obstruction is low) (Fig. A23).

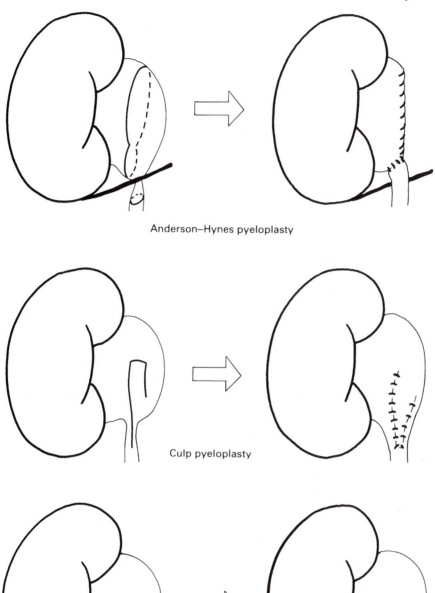

Anderson–Hynes pyeloplasty

Culp pyeloplasty

Foley pyeloplasty

Fig. A23   Types of pyeloplasty

SECTION 5
Surgical Pathology

Surgical pathology is an intergral part in the *viva* of the MRCS/ AFRCS with the exception of the Irish Fellowship. In past examinations for the London Fellowship, both microscopy (slides) and macroscopy (specimens) are important but microscopy slides have not been shown in recent examinations; however, for completeness, the important slides are discussed in this chapter. In Edinburgh only macroscopy is included in the form of specimens, while in Glasgow the surgical pathology in the *viva* usually proceeds without specimens.

5.1 How to Handle a Surgical Specimen

1. Hold it in your hands and look at it from different angles.
2. Identify the organ, usually by spotting a key structure, e.g. the presence of appendix in a bowel segment means ileocaecal region, typical mucosal folds are seen in the stomach, skin identified by hair in a bowel segment indicates anorectal junction, taenia coli and/or appendices epiploicae indicate large bowel, tooth in a bone segment indicates a jaw, pyriform hollow viscus with or without a stone indicates gallbladder, nipple and areola indicates breast, globular hollow viscus with two ureters and urethra with stricture or prostatic obstruction indicates a bladder, and so on.
3. Once you have identified the organ, the lesion should be easily recognised. If in difficulty describe what you see and do not stop talking. Remember that the organ's identity will give you a clue about the pathology, e.g. anorectal junction usually indicates a rectal carcinoma excised by the abdominoperineal approach, an ileocaecal segment possibly indicates Crohn's disease, carcinoma or carcinoid and breast always indicates carcinoma.
4. Having identified the organ and the lesion, it is a bonus (but not essential) to comment on whether the specimen is surgical or post mortem. In the latter you will see a discrepancy between the size of the removed organ and the lesion, e.g. a specimen showing the whole stomach of a child with congenital pyloric stenosis, a lung with more than one metastasis, a whole urinary system (two kidneys, two ureters and bladder) showing prostatic obstruction, part of a heart or skull.

5.2 Examples with Discussion

The following examples of specimens with discussion between the candidate (C) and the examiner (E) should provide a better understanding of what to expect in this part of the examination.

MECKEL'S DIVERTICULUM

The examiner hands the candidate a specimen of Meckel's diverticulum (Fig. 5.1).

E: What is this?
C: A segment of bowel with mesentery. It is a small bowel since there is no taeni coli, appendices epiploicae or haustration. There is an antimesenteric diverticulum. It is a Meckel's diverticulum.
E: What is a Meckel's diverticulum?
C: It is a remnant of the vitellointestinal duct and represents a true congenital diverticulum.
E: Are there any false diverticula?
C: Yes. The acquired diverticula are false since they represent herniation of mucosa through a mesenteric blood vessel hole; they are mucososerosal pouches and do not contain all the wall layers. An example is diverticular disease of the sigmoid colon.
E: What are the complications of Meckel's diverticulum?
C: Bleeding, inflammation and possibly perforation, peritonitis, intussusception, peptic ulcer due to ectopic gastric mucosa, intestinal obstruction across the band of Meckel's diverticulum connected to the umbilicus, herniation into the inguinal or femoral canal (Littre's hernia).
E: If you find it accidentally in laparotomy, do you remove it?
C: Symptomless Meckel's diverticulum is better removed unless the patient is being explored for a vascular lesion (e.g. leaking aortic aneurysm or bypass graft operation), is undergoing emergency abdominal operation or is in a generally poor condition.
E: How do you remove it?
C: Meckel's diverticulectomy via a wedge excision of its base, but if the base is indurated it is better to do a limited resection of the diverticulum bearing segment of the ileum and do an end-to-end anastomosis with two layers using 2/0 chromic catgut.

GASTRIC OUTLET OBSTRUCTION

E: What is this (Fig. 5.2)?
C: A specimen of tissue with characteristic mucosal folds – it is gastric mucosa with distal pyloric obstruction.
E: What is the cause of the obstruction here?
C: Most likely a scarred peptic ulcer since the absence of a mass in the pylorus and the presence of normal mucosal gastric folds near the obstruction excludes the possibility of pyloric gastric carcinoma.
E: All right. What is the cause of the obstruction here? (*He hands the candidate a specimen exhibiting congenital pyloric stenosis*: Fig. 5.3).
C: There is a thickened muscular layer of pyloric canal with obstruction. Since the whole stomach is shown this is a

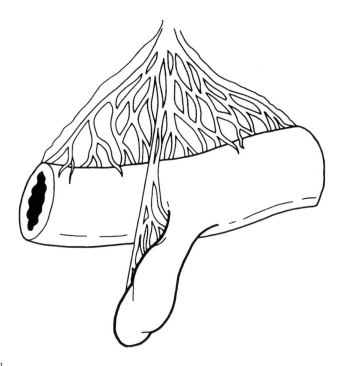

Fig. 5.1 Meckel's diverticulum

postmortem specimen of a child who died from congenital pyloric stenosis.

E: What are the physical signs of pyloric obstruction in general?

C: Visible peristalsis (from left to right), a succussion splash is heard and the outline of the enlarged stomach can sometimes be observed. Epigastric mass can be felt in carcinoma and congenital pyloric stenosis. Signs of carcinomatosis are obstructive jaundice, ascites, Krukenberg's tumour (bilateral ovarian tumours felt per rectum), palpable Virchow's left supraclavicular lymph nodes (Troisier's sign), phlebo-thrombosis of superficial veins of the leg (Trousseau's sign) and Sister Joseph nodule (secondary tumour in umbilicus via falciform ligament). The patient is mentally confused as a result of frequent projectile vomiting leading ultimately to metabolic alkalosis with hypokalaemia. In very advanced stages there will be paradoxical aciduria (acidic urine in the face of systemic alkalosis due to secretion of H^+ ions in the urine for Na^+ exchange because of very low K^+ stores ready for exchange).

E: What is the treatment for congenital pyloric stenosis?

C: A quick preparation including rehydration and correction of electrolyte disturbances with i.v. fluids, followed by Ramstedt's operation (pyloromyotomy), preserving mucosa only. Medical treatment with atropine-like drugs (Eumy-drin) could be tried but usually fails.

E: What about the treatment of chronic duodenal or prepyloric ulcer?

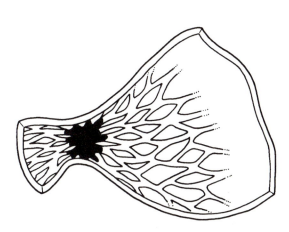

Fig. 5.2 Scarred duodenal ulcer

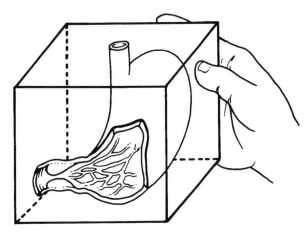

Fig. 5.3 Congenital pyloric stenosis

C: Truncal vagotomy and gastroenterostomy.

E: Give me other alternatives.

C: Truncal vagotomy with pyloroplasty (constructed through the unhealthy scarred tissue) or proximal gastric vagotomy with Hegar or finger dilation through a small gastrostomy window.

E: Tell me what you know about postvagotomy diarrhoea.

C: It is a misnomer since it has the following causes:

- Rapid gastrointestinal transit, i.e. dumping.
- Abnormal small bowel bacterial colonisation due to less peristalsis after vagotomy.
- Because of dumping, hypertonic meals are less well absorbed, leading to an osmotic fluidy diarrhoea as a result of withdrawal of water from the gut.
- Reabsorption of bile salts from terminal ileum is interfered with because of excessive hydrolysis of conjugated bile salts (by bacterial colonisation); thus fat is not absorbed, leading to steatorrhoea.
- Since the vagus is a secretomotor but a sphincter inhibitor, the gall bladder is distended with spasm of the sphincter of Oddi. As a result of continuous bile secretion, overflow incontinence of bile occurs and bile is poured into the bowel passively, presenting water absorption, irritating the colon and producing diarrhoea.

E: What do you do in gastric carcinoma?

C: That depends on whether it is early or late. In early carcinoma, distal radical gastrectomy should be done. In late cases with signs of carcinomatosis, a palliative *high* anterior gastrojejunostomy is my choice to protect the anastomosis from tumour invasion.

ILEOCAECAL JUNCTION

E: This specimen was taken from an elderly man. What is it (Fig. 5.4)?

C: This is part of the bowel. The presence of mesentery indicates small bowel but the other part shows haustration, taenia and appendics epiplocae, indicating large bowel. It is an ileocaecal junction of the bowel with a large tumour about 10 cm in diameter.

E: Where is the appendix?

C: I have looked for it but cannot see it; either it is involved in the mass or the patient has had an appendicectomy.

E: What is the diagnosis?

C: Carcinoma of the caecum or appendicular mass.

E: Can you link the two diagnoses in one?

C: Yes. Carcinoma of the caecum can lead to secondary appendicitis (by obstructing the appendix base).

E: What are the clinical features?

C: Anaemia, right iliac fossa mass, secondary appendicitis and less commonly intussusception with abdominal pain which may be referred to the periumbilical central area.

E: What is your treatment?

C: Right hemicolectomy even for doubtful appendicular mass (which proves later by histology to be appendicitis) since leaving a mass that may prove to be carcinoma of the caecum is a fatal mistake.

Comments

Carcinoid tumour can lead to secondary appendicitis. The tumour usually affects the appendix (60% of cases) or ileum (40%) and is a golden yellow well-defined mass (Fig. 5.5). Carcinoid tumour can also present as bleeding from the gastrointestinal tract, intussusception, subacute intestinal obstruction and rarely (1%) carcinoid syndrome – facial flushing, wheezes due to bronchial spasm, diarrhoea, borborygmi, and pulmonary stenosis and tricuspid incompetence due to chemical mediator, commonly 5-hydroxytryptophan (5-HT). Normally 5-HT is destroyed by liver but when there are hepatic secondaries from ileal carcinoid (appendicular carcinoids almost never have secondaries) the syndrome manifests itself. The treatment is right hemicolectomy. The presence of hepatic secondaries may require hepatic resection but the prognosis is still good. 5-Fluorouracil (5-FU) can be used locally or systemically for hepatic secondaries; methysergide, being a 5-HT antagonist is used for diarrhoea and bronchospasm; *p*-chlorophenylalanine is used for diarrhoea

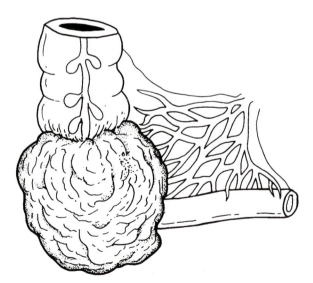

Fig. 5.4 Caecal carcinoma or appendicular mass

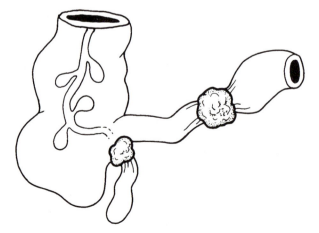

Fig. 5.5 Carcinoid tumours

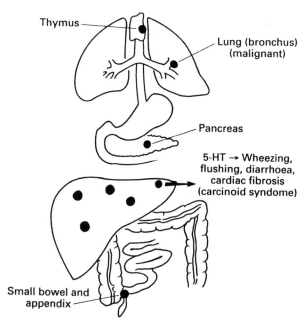

Fig. 5.6 Carcinoid tumours in derivatives of embryological foregut (a) secrete peptide hormones such as ACTH. Carcinoid tumours of the hindgut (b) secrete 5-HT. If there are liver metastases, 5-HT enters systemic circulation causing carcinoid syndrome

and to improve appetite and well-being; and α-methyldopa for flushing (Fig 5.6).

Ileocaecal tuberculosis can lead to a similar tumour. Tumour caseation and caseating mesenteric lymph nodes are present accompanied clinically by a change in bowel habits (subacute intestinal obstruction) and a history of pulmonary tuberculosis (especially in the ulcerative type) as well as anaemia, steatorrhoea, weight loss and right iliac fossa mass. Right hemicolectomy is recommended. If the patient's general conditions is poor, biopsy and defunctioning ileocolostomy should be done initially, followed by chemotherapy (on histology reporting). Right hemicolectomy is undertaken later on.

Crohn's disease is similar but the bowel that is not involved in the mass may be fiery red and thickened. Again presentations are anaemia, intestinal obstruction and internal fistulae as well as anal lesions (if colon is involved). Obstruction and fistulae necessitate surgery; otherwise the disease should be treated medically. Ileocolic anastomosis is recommended for young patients. However, in elderly patients with stricture or enterocolic fistula limited resection is recommended.

RECTAL TUMOUR

E: What is this (Fig. 5.7)?
C: This is a specimen showing an ulcerative lesion 5 cm in diameter with everted edges involving part of the bowel. The presence of appendices epiploicae in the upper part and the skin with hair in the lower part indicates it is a surgical specimen from abdominoperineal resection for rectal carcinoma.

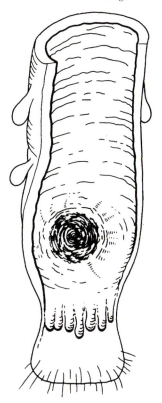

Fig. 5.7 Abdominoperineal specimen of rectal carcinoma

E: What are other lesions that may be excised by abdominoperineal resection?
C: Villous adenoma, rectal carcinoid tumour, ulcerative colitis and polyposis coli (proctocolectomy with terminal ileostomy in the latter two cases).

Comment

Discussion may continue on the clinical presentation of rectal carcinoma in general, on Dukes classification and on the pros and cons of restorative resection versus abdominoperineal resection.

BILATERAL HYDRONEPHROSIS

E: Can you tell me what this is (Fig. 5.8)?
C: A specimen of the whole urinary system revealing bilateral hydronephrosis, bilateral hydroureters, dilated trabeculated sacculated bladder with bladder neck obstruction by huge bulging prostatic enlargement. This is a postmortem specimen.
E: What do you think the cause of death was here?
C: Chronic renal failure due to back pressure from urinary outflow obstruction.
E: OK. What were the clinical features before death?
C: Prostatism: difficulty in micturition, hesitancy, poor flow and possibly frequency (diurnal and nocturnal) due to

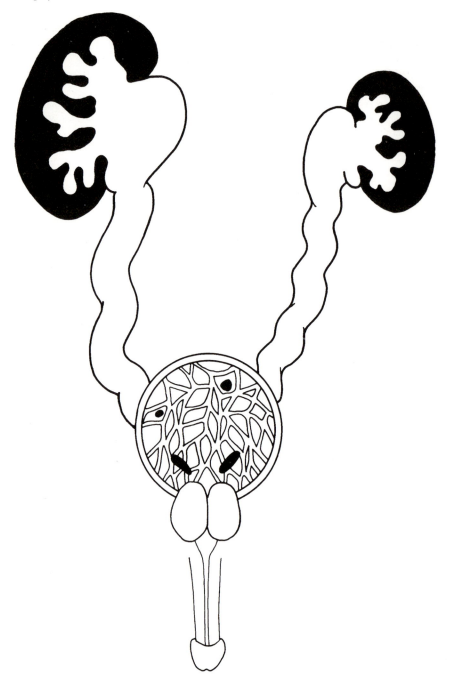

Fig. 5.8   Bilateral hydronephrosis

detrusor instability. Acute or chronic retention, haematuria and superadded infection may also occur.

E: What are the indications for surgery?

C: Obstruction (in the form of acute or chronic retention) and bleeding. Frequency alone is not an indication for surgery.

E: What are the available methods of surgery?

C: Either open prostatectomy (suprapubic transvesical, retropubic or mixed vesicocapsular and transperineal) or closed endoscopic prostatectomy (transurethral resection of prostate – TURP).

E: What are the indications and contraindications for TURP?

C: 1. Size: large prostate – as estimated roughly by rectal examination – should be removed by the open method. Small prostate and carcinoma are ideal for TURP, but nowadays, TURP can be done even if the prostate is 100 g or more.

2. With associated pathology, e.g. stone, large diverticulum, the open method is better than TURP.

3. If the patient's condition is poor or risky due to cardiothoracic status then TURP is preferable to the open method (see also s.1.63 Prostatic carcinoma).

E: What are the other causes of *bilateral* hydronephrosis?

C: Either *congenital* (urethral matal stricture, congenital valves of the posterior urethra or congenital contracture of bladder neck) or *acquired* (bladder tumour involving both ureteric orifices; prostatic enlargement – benign or malignant; carcinoma of the cervix and occasionally of the rectum involving both ureters; or inflammatory or traumatic urethral stricture or phimosis).

Comments

Hydronephrosis

Is an aseptic dilatation of the whole or part of the kidney caused by partial or intermittent obstruction to urine outflow. The causes of unilateral hydronephrosis lie in the upper urinary system (pelviureteric junction and ureter) while those of the bilateral type are in the lower urinary system (bladder and urethra). *Unilateral* hydronephrosis may be shown as a specimen. The causes are:

Extraluminal

- Congenital: e.g. aberrant blood vessel and post-caval ureter.
- Neoplastic: e.g. carcinoma of cervix, prostate, rectum, colon and caecum.
- Idiopathic retroperitoneal fibrosis (may follow administration of some drugs such as methysergide and methyldopa).

Transmural

- Congenital: e.g. stenosis, physiological narrowing or achalasia at pelviureteric junction, congenital megaureter and duplicated pelvis (more prone to hydronephrosis than normal pelvis). Ureterocele and congenital small ureteric orifice.
- Inflammatory: stricture of ureter (due to stone), tuberculosis of ureter or cicatrised tuberculosis at pelviureteric junction.
- Traumatic: after stone retrieval or stricture following ureteroureteric anastomosis or ureter trauma during pelvic operation.
- Neoplastic: Tumour of the ureter or bladder involving the ureteric orifice.

Intramural

- A ureteric stone or small stone in the renal pelvis leading to intermittent hydronephrosis.

Specimen of whole urinary system in a child

This is a postmortem specimen of either the congenital valves of a prostatic urethra or Marion's disease. Suprapubic drainage of urine is life-saving. The definitive treatment is transurethral division in prostatic urethra and Y–V plasty in Marion's disease.

Bladder neck obstruction

Is a common problem resulting from intraluminal pathology, e.g. calculus or clot, but more importantly from transmural pathology:

- Congenital urethral prostatic valves or bladder neck contraction in Marion's disease (the hypertrophied interureteric bar is analogous to hypertrophic pyloric stenosis of infants).
- Neoplastic: e.g. benign adenomatous or hyperplastic prostate, carcinoma of the prostate or primary bladder cancer involving the bladder neck.
- Inflammatory: e.g. prostatic urethral stricture, post-prostatitis or fibrotic prostate; bilharziasis and tuberculosis are other causes.
- Traumatic stricture after instrumentation or ruptured membranous urethra.
- Spasm of external sphincter is the quite common post-operatively and may lead to a similar effect as bladder neck obstruction.

Small capacity bladder due to contraction

The examiner may discuss this with you. The causes are:
- Tuberculosis.
- Bilharziasis.
- Interstitial cystitis or Hunner's ulcer.
- Hypertonic neuropathic bladder.
- Late contraction following radiotherapy or intravesical chemotherapy or partial cystectomy.
- Disseminated bladder tumour or papillomatosis.

CHOLESTEROSIS

E: What is this (Fig. 5.9)?

C: A hollow viscus, pyriform in shape, opened on one side revealing tough mucosa with yellow specks. It is a surgical specimen of a gallbladder with chronic cholecystitis.

E: Which type of chronic cholecystitis?

C: Cholesterosis.

E: What is the route of precipitation of cholesterol particles here? Is it via bile or blood?

C: Via bile passed to the gallbladder for storage and concentration where the ratio of cholesterol to bile acids is already high.

E: What is the bile acids/cholesterol ratio?

C: Normally it is 25:1 when the bile acids keep cholesterol soluble in bile, but when the ratio reaches the critical level of 13:1 the cholesterol crystals (micelles) precipitate out on

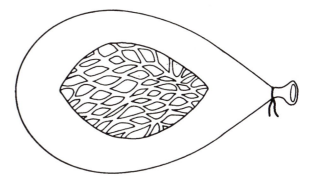

Fig. 5.9 Cholesterosis

gallbladder mucosa. Each crystal sets off an inflammatory reaction in the wall, thus acting as a nidus for stone formation. Such bile is called 'lithogenic'.

E: OK. What are the theories of gallstone formation?

C: These are:

1. *Metabolic factors*: include the bile acids/cholesterol ratio which I have discussed as well as bile pigment stones in excessive haemolysis, e.g. acholuric jaundice.

2. *Infection*: bacteria carried by blood or coming from the bowel via the lymphatics, infestations with Ascaris, or ingested foreign bodies, e.g. plum or tomato skin.

3. *Bile stasis*: e.g. during pregnancy; explains the increased stone incidence in multipara. Stasis may be secondary to distal obstruction or dyskinesia.

E: How do you treat chronic cholecystitis?

C: Cholecystectomy.

OSTEOSARCOMA

E: What is this (Fig. 5.10)?

C: A specimen of long bone bisected longitudinally. It shows an expanding tumour at the upper metaphyseal end which is eroding the cortex and elevating the periosteum. It is a bone tumour.

E: What sort of bone tumour do you think it is?

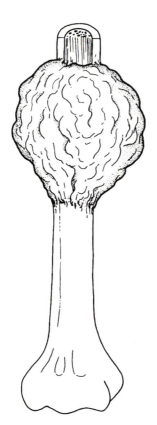

Fig. 5.10 Osteosarcoma

C: It could be a secondary bone tumour (by far the commonest – more than 80% of bone tumours) or it could be a primary bone tumour (less than 20% of all bone tumours).

E: OK. If I tell you that this is a primary one, what is your diagnosis?

C: Osteogenic sarcoma.

E: And what are the causes?

C: It develops in hitherto normal bone (second and third decades of life), in Paget's disease of bone (late in life), or following excessive irradiation.

E: What are the clinical and radiological findings?

C: Clinically, a painful swelling and/or pathological fracture. Radiologically, osteolytic destroyed bony areas with ill-defined edges, soft tissue shadow due to tumour transgressing the bone, sunray appearance (irregular spicules of bone radiating away from the shaft), Codman's triangle (elevated periosteum with new bone formation superiosteally), pathological fracture and metastasis such as pulmonary secondaries.

E: How do you manage osteogenic sarcoma?

C: Open biopsy is a must to confirm the diagnosis, followed by preliminary radiotherapy (9000 rad) over 3 months; if this controls the tumour locally then follow-up 6 months later to detect any pulmonary metastasis. If the chest X-ray is clear then amputate, but if chest X-ray shows pulmonary secondaries amputation should not be attempted. Solitary pulmonary metastasis can be treated by lobectomy. Palliative amputation is performed if the tumour was not controlled locally after preliminary radiotherapy. Chemotherapy can be given (methotrexate, vincristine and adriamycin) for 1 year following the amputation.

E: Cade's method is time-consuming and I personally prefer immediate amputation to rid the patient of the tumour; such a prompt debulking procedure could be followed by more successful chemotherapy. Anyway, where are you going to amputate?

C: The site of election is through the bone or joint immediately proximal to the involved one, e.g. upper tibia (mid-thigh amputation), lower femur (high amputation), upper femur (hip disarticulation or hind-quarter amputation).

HAND SKIN TUMOUR

E: What is this (Fig. 5.11)?

C: A specimen showing the right hand cut off at the wrist. There is a circular growth on the dorsum of the hand 7 cm in diameter with everted margin. It is a postmortem specimen of squamous cell carcinoma of the skin.

E: What are the causes, in general?

C: Causes can be placed in two groups:

1. *Premalignant skin conditions*: Bowen's intradermal disease (cells are similar to those found in Paget's disease of the nipple); leukoplakia, senile or solar keratosis (ultraviolet sunlight exposure is a predisposing factor, especially in the Celtic race): radiodermatitis (e.g. in the radiologist or postirradiation areas of ringworms and thyrotoxicosis); chronic scars; or Marjolin's ulcer.

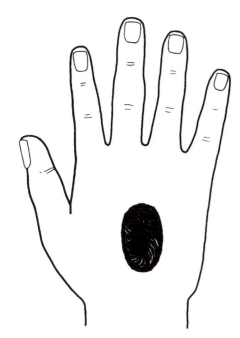

Fig. 5.11 Squmous cell carcinoma

2. *Predisposing factors*: Exposure to long wavelengths leadings to Kangri cancer of Kashmir; sleeping on oven bed leading to Kong cancer and charcoal burns. Chemicals such as tar and arsenic, and soot as in chimney-sweep's carcinoma. Infections such as chronic lupus vulgaris or tuberculosis of the skin. Postmastectomy lymphoedema may be superimposed by lymphangiosarcoma. Hereditary conditions such as xeroderma pigmentosa, albinism and Von Recklinghausen's disease.

E: How do you treat?

C: Biopsy from tumour and normal skin, followed by wide excision with closure or skin graft (if the gap is large). Enlarged lymph nodes may be treated with antibiotics initially; if they subside secondary infection is the cause but if they persist block dissection may be needed (if the lymph nodes are mobile). If draining lymph nodes are fixed, block dissection is contraindicated (regression may occur after radiotherapy). Alternatively, the skin tumour could be treated with radiothrapy alone (especially in an elderly patient with a small mobile skin tumour).

PANCREATIC PATHOLOGY

This is one of the most interesting subjects to discuss even without specimens (though you may be shown a postmortem specimen of acute haemorrhagic pancreatitis with fatty necroses or carcinoma of the pancreatic head to open a wide discussion).

1. *Congenital*

(a) Annular pancreas due to failure of complete rotation of the ventral segment thus obstructing the duodenum and producing double-bubble radiogical appearance. Treated by duodenojejunostomy.

(b) Congenital cystic disease and mucoviscidosis.

2. *Inflammatory* (pancreatitis)

3. *Neoplastic*: This is a very large topic and includes:

(a) Endocrine pancreatic tumours: these are APUDomas (**A**mine content **P**recursor **U**ptake and **D**ecarboxylation cells) arising mostly (but not entirely) from the neural crest.

(i) Alpha-cell tumour (glucagonoma): diabetes mellitus, necrolytic migratory erythematous rash and catabolism and low serum proteins. There is associated normochromic normocytic anaemia, angular stomatitis, glossitis, infection and venous thrombosis with psychological disturbances. Diagnosis is on clinical grounds together with demonstration of a high glucagon level. Preoperative localisation with selective pancreatic arteriography and CT scan is carried out. Treatment is by excision and therapeutic embolisation of hepatic secondaries.

(ii) Beta-cell tumour (insulinoma) is usually benign and solitary. Episodic hypoglycaemia may be misdiagnosed as a psychiatric case. Whipple's triad is present (attack is brought on by fasting during which hypoglycaemia occurs and is relieved with i.v. glucose). Preoperative localisation (as in glucagonoma). Cure by excision (enucleation or partial pancreatectomy). Inoperable cases are treated with diazoxide to control hypoglycaemia and streptozotocin for liver secondaries (therapeutic embolisation is preferable in the latter).

(iii) G-cell hyperplasia of pancreas (Zollinger–Ellison syndrome); can also occur in G-cell tumours of the gastric antrum and duodenum. Concomitant with hyperparathyroidism it may indicate multiple endocrine adenopathy. There is intractable peptic ulceration (in odd sites, e.g. postbulbar duodenum or jejunum), hypergastrinaemia with massive acid hypersecretion, and diarrhoea, steatorrhoea or hypokalaemia. The protective value of cimetidine usually makes total gastrectomy unnecessary (especially if given with pirenzepine to enhance the H_2-receptor blocker). If there is no response then carry out total gastrectomy. The primary tumour of the pancreas (or gastric antrum) should be removed.

(iv) D-cell tumour (somatostatinoma) produces excessive somatostatin leading to diabetes, steatorrhoea, diarrhoea, hypochlorhydria, cholelithiasis and weight loss. Diagnosis by somatostatin assay.

(v) VIPoma.

(vi) PPoma: Pancreatic polypeptide is secreted in many of the above tumours and is also found in their metastases.

(b) Exocrine pancreatic tumours

(i) Head (70% of cases), involving:

● Head proper (two-thirds).

● Periampullary region (one-third).

(ii) Body and tail (30%).

These tumours present generally either as painless progressive obstructive jaundice or as an intractable pain without jaundice. Diagnosis is on clinical findings and radiologically by barium meal (pad sign and reversed 3 sign in head proper and periampullary carcinoma respectively) and hypotonic duodenography with pancreatic function tests. Treatment depends on site and stage of disease (to decide whether a radical or palliative procedure is required).

MISCELLANEOUS

You may be shown one of the following specimens:

- Piece of small bowel with marks of constricting band around part of its circumference and gangrene in the constricted part. It is Richter's hernia (strangulated partial enterocele), usually due to femoral hernia.
- Piece of bone with a cavity containing one tooth (jaw). The diagnosis is dentigerous cyst due to non-erupted permanent tooth. A dental cyst is usually attached to the root of a pulpless tooth. Treatment is by excision of the whole epithelial lining of the cyst, and the bone cavity is obliterated by a soft-tissue 'push-in' or with bone chips and wound suturing.
- Upper thoracic cage with accessory rib with discussion of symptomatology and treatment.
- Bony osteoma as a benign tumour (treatment is surgical excision).
- Saccular aneurysm of an artery with classification of aneurysm and treatment.
- Testicular tumour (seminoma or teratoma).
- Large bowel with polyposis coli with discussion of symptomatology and treatment.
- Jejunal diverticulosis.
- Postmortem specimen of carcinoma of oesophagus.
- Oesophageal stricture.

5.3 Histopathology Slides

Histopathology of surgical diseases is important but not essential. There is no substitute for a histopathology atlas or actual slides borrowed from the pathology department of your hospital in order to familiarise yourself with their appearance. This part was only required in the Final FRCS (England) but not anymore. You will be given three slides: you must examine these under the microscope in 10 min and state the diagnosis of each disease. Each slide comes with a very useful typed card containing a short history of the patient; the name of the organ or tissue is usually shown on the slide. Dividing the time equally, write the slide number on the paper along with its abnormal microscopic findings, then write your possible diagnosis (concluded from correlation of the findings). Remember that each organ or tissue has a list of common diseases so go through them and come up with the most likely diagnosis. The examiners know very well that you are not a professional pathologist so only histopathology of the common diseases will be covered. When you finish you will be taken to meet the examiner and with the help of a slide magnifying projection screen you will discuss your three slides. The diagnosis of each one will open the discussion covering different aspects of that particular disease from aetiology to surgical management. The following are the most common slides with the most important abnormal microscopic findings seen in each.

LYMPH NODE

Tuberculous lymphadenitis Caseating granuloma with central caseation (amorphous pink necrosis) surrounded by epithelioid cells, lymphocytes and, more importantly, Langhan giant cells (multinucleated cells with peripheral nuclei).

Hodgkin's disease Commonly the nodular sclerosis phase with destruction of lymph node architecture and replacement with patches of fibrosis. Cellular areas reveal lymphocytes, macrophages and, more importantly, the characteristic Reed–Sternberg cells (double nucleated cells with a mirror image arrangement of nuclei). Lymphocyte predominance, mixed cellularity and lymphocyte depletion are other phases (rarely shown).

Metastatic carcinoma Commonly adenocarcinoma from gastrointestinal tract (or elsewhere) showing patchy replacement of lymphatic structure with islands of mucoid and clear cells (clear cytoplasm with central or occasionally eccentric nucleus – signet ring appearance) indicating their primary origin.

SKIN

Squamous cell carcinoma With breach of epithelial continuity and everted border. The tumour grows down deeply with undermining of epidermis. Atypical cells with polychromatic nuclei and abnormal mitotic figures can be seen particularly easily in their characteristic cell nests or as epithelial pearls with central keratin.

Basal cell carcinoma (rodent ulcer) The skin ulceration is surrounded by a beaded margin. The tumour grows down but superficially in the form of masses or columns undermining epidermis. Each column or mass is composed characteristically of polyhedral epithelial cells with a peripheral palisade formation.

Malignant melanoma With dark brown or black epidermal melanocytes not confined to the basal layer of skin, but infiltrating the whole section up and down.

Paget's disease of the nipple The section is composed of breast tissue and overlying skin (see below).

BREAST

Hard pericanalicular fibroadenoma (the common fibroadenoma) Normal ductules within a background of dense fibrous tissue. Usually multifocal but very well encapsulated. It is benign.

Fibroadenosis The adenosis element (budding of glandular acini) is associated with epitheliosis (hyperplasia of acinar lining) or even papillomatosis (extensive epithelial hyperplasia causing overgrowth within ducts). The other element is fibrosis with dense fibrous trabeculae replacing fat and elastic tissues and compressing ducts leading to cyst formation. The interstitial tissues may be infiltrated by round cells (lymphocytes). Its possible premalignancy status is debatable.

Intraduct papilloma and carcinoma The papilloma shows epithelial proliferation in one of the larger lactiferous ducts (usually one duct and occasionally two or more). It is premalignant. The carcinoma is similar but the cells are atypical with various sizes of nuclei and pigmentation (malignant).

Scirrhous carcinoma (the commonest – 63% of cases) The ductal carcinomatous cells break the epithelial basement membrane, causing intense reactionary fibrosis which leads to a very hard mass with an irregular contour due to puckering of surrounding tissues to variable degrees. Notice the criteria of the malignant cells within fibrous tissue.

Paget's disease of the nipple (rare – 1%) Breast tissue is seen with overlying skin. This is not a premalignant disease but an actual breast malignancy. It is an *intraduct carcinoma* that slowly grows upward infiltrating the epithelial covering of the nipple. Large rounded vacuolated cells with small deeply staining nuclei (hydropic appearance) are seen in the deeper layer of the epidermis. Some lymphocyte infiltration of the dermis occurs. Notice that in duct carcinoma, malignant cells are confined to ducts. If the cells break the basement membrane, they provoke interstitial fibrosis causing scirrhous carcinoma and if the cells creep upward to infiltrate nipple skin they cause Paget's disease of the nipple. Paget's disease is usually unilateral (with no vesicles), occurs in the menopause and does not respond to treatment (unlike eczema of lactating mothers).

BONE

Osteogenic sarcoma (commonly idiopathic in children and rarely occurs in Paget's disease of the bone in adults) The normal bone structure is infiltrated by spindle cells with marked nuclear hyperchromatosis and islands of osteoid formation. Malignant giant cells and high vascularity are obvious.

THYROID GLAND

Colloid goitre Owing to increased colloid storage the acini distend and the gland shows a fine honeycomb appearance. It is caused by alternating periods of iodine sufficiency and deprivation.

Thyrotoxicosis While normal thyroid gland consists of acini lined by flat cuboidal epithelium and filled with homogeneous colloid, in hyperthyroidism, hyperplastic acini are lined by high columnar epithelium with empty or vacuolated colloid follicles. There is lymphocyte infiltration with lymph follicle formation. Following treatment the acinar lining becomes low, cuboidal and full of colloid.

Hashimoto's autoimmune thyroiditis (struma lymphomatosa) There is widespread atrophy of parenchyma, diffuse fibrosis, diffuse lymphocyte infiltration and localised collections of lymphocytes with germinal centres. Acinar cells are enlarged and rounded with granular cytoplasm (characteristic Askanazy cells). Mild initial hyperthyroidism will be followed eventually by inevitable hypothyroidism.

Papillary carcinoma (the commonest thyroid carcinoma – 60%) There is papillary formation, often follicular structure and sometimes solid masses of cells. The cells are well differentiated with a characteristic appearance (large pale ground-glass nuclei and small nucleoli). There may be a breach of the thyroid capsule. This carcinoma is multifocal so total thyroidectomy is needed. Lymphatic spread may necessitate a block dissection which should be carried out one side at a time (never do simultaneous bilateral block dissection). Prognosis is good.

Follicular carcinoma (17%) The well-differentiated cells are arranged in follicles which sometimes contain colloid. Thyroid capsule is invaded and the tumour is very vascular. Lobectomy is satisfactory since it is not multifocal. Blood spread necessitates hormonal therapy with thyroxine and multiple metastases necessitate ^{131}I therapy.

Medullary carcinoma (6%) Undifferentiated round or polygonal cells in fibrous stroma with no papillary or follicular structure. The characteristic 'amyloid' in globoid masses in stroma and within some malignant cells is the most important finding. This tumour arises from parafollicular (C) cells and is associated with high levels of serum calcitonin. The tumour is familial and is associated with phaeochromocytoma, parathyroid tumour and Von Recklinghausen's disease of skin. Treatment is by total thyroidectomy.

PARATHYROIDS

In hyperparathyroidism, calcium in the blood and urine is high while phosphate is low.

Adenoma Composed of interlacing compact cords or solid masses of cells of uniform type (chief cells with regular nuclei and scanty cytoplasm) in a scanty vascular stroma.

PAROTID SALIVARY GLANDS

Pleomorphic adenoma (mixed parotid tumour – the commonest parotid tumour) Shows a complex structure of epithelial, glandular and mucoid material. The epithelial cells are arranged in irregular strands and masses or branching columns (sometimes with glandular acini). The myoepithelium proliferates in sheets. The varying amounts of mucoid material give a myxomatous appearance (like cartilage). Clinically it is a firm circumscribed lobulated mass on the jaw angle usually unilateral with no sex predilection.

Adenolymphoma (Warthin's tumour; less common than pleomorphic adenoma)   This benign tumour has a markedly eosinophiolic epithelium folded into cavities (cystic formation) with papillary appearance. The tall columnar cells are arranged in regular palisade formation or in glandular acini. There are characteristic lymphocyte follicles in the stroma. Unlike pleomorphic adenoma adenolymphoma has a monomorphic eosinophilic papillary structure with lymphoid follicles. Clinically it is a soft cystic fluctuant tumour in the lower pole of the parotid and can be bilateral, affecting middle-aged or elderly males. Unlike all other tumours, which produce a cold spot, adenolymphoma produces a 'hot' spot in a ^{99m}Tc pertechnetate scan (a firm preoperative diagnosis without biopsy). Fine needle aspiration cytology is an accepted preoperative diagnostic test.

STOMACH AND DUODENUM

Peptic ulcer   Mucosal continuity is breached. The excavation of the wall is deep and reaches and muscular layer, producing four layers from the mucosa towards the muscularis:
1. Exudate with pus cells.
2. Fibrinoid necrosis.
3. Granulation and capillary formation.
4. Fibrotic base due to chronicity.

Gastric carcinoma   There is mucosal discontinuity but the ulcer edges are everted. Whereas benign ulcer erodes a large gap in the muscular coat, carcinoma infiltrates between muscles without destroying them. There are no dilated vessels in the base and the cells are typically malignant (various sizes of cells, cytoplasm nuclei and different pigmentation with infiltration of surrounding normal tissues). Clear cells or even signet ring cells can be seen (as a result of much of the cytoplasm displacing the nucleus to one side).

SMALL AND LARGE BOWEL

Carcinoid tumour   The tumour is golden yellow due to its high lipid content. The characteristic Kulschitsky cells are related to bases of crypts of Lieberkuhn and present as solid masses of small clear (lipid-containing) cells closely packed together within a fibrous stroma. The cells may show a palisade or rosette arrangement (and are capable of reducing silver salts). Classically the tumour affects the terminal ileum or appendix (but it may occur elsewhere).

Crohn's disease (granulomatous ileitis)   Usually no mucosal discontinuity but transmural thickening of the wall affecting submucosa mainly with chronic non-caseating granulomatous reaction (sarcoid formation). Epithelioid cells and giant cells (Langhan's type) are seen. Macroscopically, Crohn's disease distribution is segmental, involving the ileum (may be extensive) and rectum in 50% of cases, with anal lesions in 75% and internal fistulae in 8% when colon is involved. The mucosal fissuring and cracking (with no or patchy ulceration and transmural thickening) produce a characteristic cobble-stoning (a macroscopic pathological appearance rather than a radiological appearance).

Ulcerative colitis (more correctly called haemorrhagic procto-colitis)   Is mainly a mucosal disease with ulceration of mucosa (discontinuity) and suppurative acute inflammation with an oedematous vascular submucosal background infiltrated by polymorphs. Focal collection of polymorphs and frank crypt abscesses are seen.

Unlike Crohn's disease, ulcerative colitis has a continuous distribution, involving the rectum in all cases, with limited or no ileal involvement. There are no internal fistulae but anal lesions occur in 25%. No cobblestoning is seen but mucoso-submucosal hypertrophy produces pseudopolyps, which are unusual in Crohn's disease.

Acute appendicitis   Hollow viscus with suppurative inflammation (pus cells and vascular oedematous wall).

Colonic carcinoma   Whether adenocarcinoma or anaplastic depends on the degree of differentiation. Identify the signs of malignancy (atypical appearance with mitotic figures and infiltration of surrounding normal tissues). Depending on amount, clear cells or signet rings can be seen.

Ileocaecal tuberculosis   Tuberculosis may affect any part of the human body (e.g. kidney, bone, testis, skin). The tubercle is the characteristic lesion exhibiting typical central caseation (coagulative necrosis of epithelioid cells) surrounded by epithelioid cells and peripheral lymphocytes in a concentric mass around a clump of bacilli. The epithelioid (or endothelioid) cells occupy the central zone of the tuberculous follicle and are oval faintly staining nuclei with abundant clear cytoplasm. The lymphocytes are arranged in the peripheral zone usually with giant cells of Langhan's type (horseshoe peripheral nuclei).

URINARY SYSTEM

Hypernephroma (adenocarcinoma or clear cell carcinoma of kidney)   Solid masses of large cells with small central nuclei and abundant clear cytoplasm (due to its rich glycogen and doubly refractile lipid content) infiltrate the kidney stroma (notice the glomeruli) with inflammatory cells in the normal part as a response to the infiltrating malignant cells.

Transitional cell carcinoma of urinary bladder   Notice the transitional cells of the bladder mucosa arranged in papillary style with mitotic figures and deep infiltration.

Prostatic enlargement   Benign adenomas or hyperplasia in the prostate are similar to those in the breast. The small rounded acini are lined by well-differentiated cuboidal or columnar epithelium set in a fibromuscular stroma. Some of the acini are dilated and contain concentric laminated bodies (called corpora amylacea). Adenocarcinomas show more irregular hyperchromatic acini arranged in solid masses with evidence of local invasion.

Testicular seminoma There is great uniformity. The tumour is made up of solid sheets or columns of cells mostly polygonal (of uniform size) with clear cytoplasm and rounded nuclei (well-marked chromatin network and one or two nucleoli). Tumour giant cells may be seen and often there is a well-marked lymphocyte infiltration.

GALLBLADDER

Chronic cholecystitis Hollow viscus with mild inflammation. Large foamy cells in stroma (lipid material) are seen in cholesterosis.

PART THREE

Background

SECTION 1
Guide to the Examining Colleges and Boards

1.1 The Royal Colleges of the UK and Ireland

All the Colleges retain the same high surgical standard and are recognised as important world centres of education and control of professional training in surgery. The Fellowship is usually gained through qualification (on an examination basis conducted according to College regulations) or rarely granted as an honorary degree to outstanding surgeons and authorities in different parts of the world. The FRCS is not a specialist degree but a visa to higher surgical training leading ultimately to a consultant post or academic career.

In spite of the technical differences in the way the examination is conducted in these Colleges, the requirements for admission to the Final FRCS are basically similar:

- Possession of the primary (Part 1) FRCS (which is now no longer reciprocal).
- Postgraduate surgical training in hospitals recognised by the College (covering at least 1 year of general surgery, 6 months in accidents and emergencies and 6 months in one of the surgical specialties) at the level of SHO or Registrar.
- Candidates should be at least 25 years old.

At the end of the examination, only successful candidates will be admitted to the College hall to meet the President and court of examiners for congratulation. Those failed will be notified by post usually with details of performance (available only to unsuccessful candidates).

Each College will be discussed briefly here to familiarise the candidate with the differences in regulations, examination techniques and parts relevant to the Final FRCS in general surgery. The differences between the Colleges (though probably minor) merit stress since they may influence the candidate's preparation in sitting the final FRCS of that particular College.

ROYAL COLLEGE OF SURGEONS OF ENGLAND

The Guild of Surgeons was formed in about 1300. The first mention of the surgeons in the city of London records was in 1354. In 1540 came the incorporation of the Barbers Company and the Guild of Surgeons as the Company of Barbers and Surgeons. However, in 1745 London Surgeons broke away from the barbers and formed the Company of Surgeons (John Ranby was the first Master) largely through the initiative of William Cheselden of St Thomas' Hospital. By 1800, the Company of Surgeons was chartered by George III and it became the Royal College of Surgeons in London (first Master

of the College was Charles Hawkins). In 1822 the title of Master changed to President (last Master and first President was Sir Everard Home). In 1843, a new charter was granted by Queen Victoria and the title of the College changed to The Royal College of Surgeons of England. Initially, 300 distinguished members were elected to become Fellows of the College. The council of the College retained the right to confer fellowship by election. However, regulations for fellowship by examination were instituted and in December 1844 the first examination (FRCS) was conducted; 24 candidates successfully passed and were admitted as Fellows. Ever since, London has retained its importance as a world centre of surgery and it attained world supremacy during the middle years of the 19th century (1830–1870) (see Part Three Section 6).

The College conducts two examinations per year exclusively in London (no overseas examination).

Requirements

For sitting the final FRCS (Eng) the requirements are:
1. A candidate of 25 years or over with a good character.
2. Primary FRCS from the Royal College of Surgeons of England only. (No reciprocity since 1st July 1980; however, possession of the primary FRCS from any of the Royal Colleges before 1980 is still acceptable.)
3. Original testimonials of postgraduate training which should include at least *18 months general surgery*, 6 months accidents and emergencies and 6 months in a surgical specialty. These posts should be at least at the level of SHO – full-time residential jobs in hospitals recognised by the college. This training *should include 1 year (obligatory) in the UK or Ireland in a recognised hospital*.
4. Filled application form with the examination fee.

The full regulations are obtained by writing to:

**The Registrar,
Royal College of Surgeons of England,
Lincoln's Inn Fields,
London WC2A 3PN,
UK.**

Examination procedure

Takes 2 days per candidate to finish all the different parts:
1. *Written Part*: takes 1 day (morning and afternoon sessions; each two questions with 2 hours' time).
2. *Clinical Part*: conducted in special examination hall (not in hospitals). The long case and short cases are therefore transportable – not acutely ill and commonly repeated in the examinations. Both the long case and the short cases will be discussed in the examination hall with two examiners.

3. *Oral Part*: conducted on two tables (each has two examiners) in the college pathology museum (sometimes partly conducted in the examination hall):

(a) Surgical topic – operative surgery and surgical anatomy *viva*, with discussion on instruments, human models and bones.

(b) Surgical pathology *viva*: involves examination of three histopathological slides (microscopy), later discussed with one examiner using microprojection, followed by examination of gross pathology specimens (in pots).

The clinical and oral parts take 1 day (morning and afternoon sessions respectively). There is no separate principles and practice table, but the surgical principles and practice are discussed implicitly within the oral parts. The College scoring system (of nines) makes it impossible for the candidate to pass without passing clearly the written and clinical parts individually. A borderline score in the oral parts could be compensated for after discussion and agreement by the College court of examiners.

The College announces and displays the successful candidates by number (not by names – the results are confidential).

ROYAL COLLEGE OF SURGEONS OF EDINBURGH

The Surgeons–Barbers Association, the forerunner of the College, was founded in 1505 making it the oldest surgical college. Edinburgh rose to the highest surgical standard at the end of the 18th century and maintained its world supremacy for almost half a century (see Part Three, Section 6). The Edinburgh school was derived from that in Leiden in Holland. The Monro dynasty of anatomists (grandfather, father and son – all named Alexander Monro) made the Edinburgh teaching of anatomy famous to the extent that in 1828, the classes of its spectacular teacher (and founder of the College museum), Robert Knox, regularly attracted 504 students per lecture in the dissecting room which does not accommodate more than 200. The museum now has one of the largest collections of surgical pathology in the UK. Many of the specimens are of unique historical interest and there is a series of oil paintings of war wounds executed by Sir Charles Bell, a capable artist as well as surgeon, after the Battle of Waterloo. The College officially finished its association with barbers in 1722 and received the 'Royal' status from George III in 1778.

The first FRCS examination was conducted in 1884 as a one-part examination which later became bipartite as in England and Dublin. The College currently conducts three examinations per year in Edinburgh. It also conducts the final FRCS examination overseas in Hong Kong and Kuala Lumpur.

Requirements

For sitting the final FRCS (Ed) the requirements are:
1. A candidate of 25 years or above with a good character.
2. Primary FRCS from any of the Royal Colleges (reciprocal).
3. Original testimonials of postgraduate training which should include at least 12 months general surgery, 6 months accidents

and emergencies and 6 months in a surgical specialty (e.g. cardiothoracic, urology, orthopaedic surgery). These posts should be at least at the level of SHO – full-time jobs in recognised hospitals, *anywhere in the world* (no obligatory 1 year in hospitals in the UK or Ireland).
4. Filled application form with the examination fee.

The full regulations are obtained by writing to:

The Registrar,
Royal College of Surgeons of Edinburgh,
18 Nicolson Street,
Edinburgh EH8 9DW,
UK.

Examination procedure

Takes 4 days per candidate to complete all the different parts:
1. *Written Part*: takes 2 days (3 hours on first day for operative surgery/surgical pathology and 3 hours on second day for principles/practice). The written part attracts double marking (7 + 7). This will usually be followed by a weekend.
2. *Clinical Part*: conducted in Edinburgh hospitals and other Scottish hospitals. Candidates will be taken by coach to hospitals outside Edinburgh. Both the long case and the short cases will be discussed in the wards with two examiners. The clinical part attracts double marking (7 for the long case and 7 for the short cases). Recently the long case has been replaced with short cases.
3. *Oral Part*: conducted on three tables (each has two examiners) in the college museum and halls.

(a) Surgical pathology: surgical and postmortem specimens in pots (no microscopy slides). However, clinical and gross pathologic slides may be shown.

(b) Operative surgery (no bones).

(c) Principles and practice.

The candidates (according to a recent regulation) are allowed to have their written and oral parts first; those who are successful or borderline are allowed to proceed to their clinical part (which even if they pass is no guarantee that they pass the whole examination since their score in other parts may be borderline). Those who fail the written and/or oral parts are not allowed to proceed with their clinical part (without examination fee forfeited). Thus it is essential to pass clearly in *both* written and clinical parts. Of course candidates have to pass the oral part but borderline marks here can be compensated for by good marks in other parts.

ROYAL COLLEGE OF PHYSICIANS AND SURGEONS OF GLASGOW

This was founded in 1599 under the charter of James VI of Scotland, granted in response to the plea of Maister Peter Lowe (the founder of the Brethren of Chirurgerie, the forerunner of the College). For over 200 years it was known as the Faculty of Physicians and Surgeons. Authority to add the prefix 'Royal' was granted by Edward VII in 1909. The change to Royal College of Physicians and Surgeons of Glasgow was made by Act of Parliament on 6th December 1962.

The College conducts three examinations per year exclusively in Glasgow (no overseas examination).

Requirements

For sitting the final FRCS (Glas) the requirements are:
1. A candidate of 25 years or over with a good character.
2. Primary FRCS from any of the Royal Colleges (reciprocal).
3. Original testimonials of postgraduate training which should include at least 12 months general surgery, 6 months accidents and emergencies and 6 months in any surgical specialty (e.g. gynaecology, orthopaedic surgery, urology, cardiothoracic surgery). These posts should be at least at the level of SHO – full-time jobs in recognised hospitals. This training *should include 1 year (obligatory) in the UK or Ireland in a recognised hospital.*
4. Filled application form with the examination fee.

The full regulations are obtained by writing to:

The Registrar,
Royal College of Physicians and Surgeons,
234–242 St Vincent Street,
Glasgow G2 5RJ,
UK.

Examination procedure

Takes 2 days per candidate to complete all the different parts:
1. *Written Part*: takes 1 day (morning and afternoon sessions for operative surgery/surgical pathology and principles/practice – 3 hours each).
2. *Clinical Part*: conducted in various Glasgow hospitals. Both the long case and the short cases will be discussed in the wards with two examiners.
3. *Oral Part*: conducted on three tables (each has two examiners) in the College halls:
(a) Surgical pathology: proceeds without specimens (pots) or histology (slides).
(b) Operative surgery (no bones).
(c) Principles and practice.

The clinical and oral parts take 1 day (morning and afternoon sessions respectively).

Both Edinburgh and Glasgow Colleges announce the successful candidates by name and *display their names and numbers on the board.* (No confidentiality with successful candidates.)

ROYAL COLLEGE OF SURGEONS IN IRELAND

In Dublin the barbers and surgeons were members of the Guild of St Mary Magdalene, established by Henry VI in 1446, an association which persisted well into the 18th century to the disadvantage of the surgeons. The Dublin College of Surgeons was founded in 1780 by an Irishman, Sylvester O'Halloran, who studied surgery, ophthalmology and midwifery and worked in London, Leiden and Paris. The College received its Royal charter on 11th February, 1784. Dublin is well known for many international figures (e.g. Colles', Smith's and Bennett's fractures, Fegan's injection-compression technique of varicose veins, anal valves of Houston, and Cheyne–Stokes' breathing in head injury).

The College conducts three examinations per year in Dublin and Belfast (no overseas examination).

Requirements

For sitting the final FRCSI the requirements are:
1. A candidate of 25 years or over with a good character.
2. Primary FRCS from any of the Royal Colleges (reciprocal).
3. Original testimonials of postgraduate training which should include at least 12 months general surgery, 6 months accidents and emergencies and 6 months in a surgical specialty. These posts should be at the level of Registrar or equivalent status – full-time job in hospitals recognised by the College. This training *should include 1 year (obligatory) in general surgery in the UK or Ireland in a recognised hospital.*
4. Filled application form with the examination fee.

The full regulations are obtained by writing to:

The Registrar,
Royal College of Surgeons in Ireland,
123 St Stephens Green,
Dublin 2,
Republic of Ireland.

Examination procedure

Takes 2 days per candidate to complete all the different parts:
1. *Written Part*: takes 1 day (morning and afternoon sessions for Paper A and Paper B – 3 hours each).
2. *Clinical Part*: conducted in various Dublin hospitals. The long case and short cases will be discussed in the wards with two examiners each. (The only College with four different examiners per clinical part taken by each candidate.)
3. *Oral Part*: conducted on two tables (each has two examiners) in the College hall.
(a) Operative surgery: with instruments and X-rays (no bones).
(b) Principles and practice: with extensive discussion of X-rays.

The clinical and oral parts take 1 day (morning and afternoon sessions respectively). There is no surgical pathology table (so no surgical specimens or slides). X-rays feature extensively in the oral parts. To be successful, each candidate *has to score a total of 360 marks and should score 120 in the clinical part.* (The marks are divided equally between the three parts and 60 is the pass mark.) The results are confidential. The College will announce and display successful candidates by number only.

1.2 Royal Australasian College of Surgeons

RACS was founded in 1926 in fulfilment of the efforts of a small body of surgical leaders in Australia and New Zealand (the Surgical Association of Melbourne) who had determined to improve the generally poor standards of surgical practice and ethics in their countries. Sir George Syme, the surgical doyen of Melbourne, became the first President of the College (1927–9).

The foundation was instigated in 1924 by the visit of W. Mayo and F. Martin from the American College, which emphasised the need for ethical practice and practical training rather than examination. However, the College established its ties with the English College.

The training and examination structure is as follows:
1. Basic Surgical Training for 2 years after internship, during which the applicant may take Part 1 FRACS Examination (to ensure that the trainee has gained a satisfactory understanding of basic surgical science) before proceeding to Advanced Surgical Training.
2. A trainee must win a place in an Advanced Surgical Training programme which extends over 4 or more years, depending on the specialty concerned, and involves application of surgical science appropriate to the specialty as well as the practice of surgery.
3. Part 2 FRACS Examination is normally taken in the final year of Advanced Training or after the training has been completed. The Council will then award the Diploma of Fellowship (FRACS).

For full regulations, candidates may write to:

The Registrar,
Royal Australasian College of Surgeons,
Spring Street,
Melbourne,
Australia 3000.

1.3 The College of Medicine of South Africa

The examination for Fellowship in Surgery FCS(SA) consists of two parts which must be passed within 6 years:

Part I: Section A: Basic Sciences
            Section B: (i)   The principles of surgery in general
                      (ii) The principles of the surgical specialty disciplines
Part II: The theory and practice of general surgery (or specialty concerned, such as orthopaedics), including operative surgery and the applied basic sciences, namely anatomy, physiology and pathology.

Candidates are admitted to Part I Section A (two 3 hour papers of MCQs and/or short written questions on basic sciences), if they hold a registered and recognised qualification or are registerable with the South African Medical and Dental Council.

Candidates are admitted to Part I Section B (one 3 hour paper consisting of essay and/or short questions on each of B (i) and B (ii) together with a *viva* examination on each of B (i) and B (ii), only after passing Section A and completing not less than 18 months of approved training in surgery, embracing trauma and intensive care and surgical specialties (6 months general surgery, 6 months trauma and emergencies, and 6 months surgical specialty, such as orthopaedics, urology, neurosurgery).

Candidates are admitted to Part II examination only after passing Part I examination or completing Fellowship of one of the Colleges with which there is an agreement of reciprocity; they must produce evidence of surgical training of not less than 4 years (excluding the year of internship); evidence of serving not less than 2.5 years approved training in general surgery or the specialty looked for, such as orthopaedics (this period may be part of the 4 years or additional to the 4 years). Part II examination is conducted as three 3 hour written papers of 3–4 questions each (one of the written papers will include 1–2 questions on the basic sciences) together with clinical, practical and oral examination in theory and practice of general surgery (or specialty applied for, such as orthopaedics) including operative surgery, surgical anatomy, pathology and physiology.

For full regulations, candidates may write to:

The Registrar,
The College of Medicine of South Africa,
27 Rhodes Avenue Parktown West,
P/Bag X23 Braamfontein 2017,
Johannesburg,
South Africa.

1.4 Royal College of Physicians and Surgeons of Canada

This is a national voluntary organisation established by a Special Act of Parliament in 1929. Its purpose is to advance the standards of postgraduate medical education and practice in the medical, laboratory and surgical specialties and to provide the means for identifying, both within the medical profession and to the public, that those who hold themselves out to be specialists in a particular field are properly trained and qualified.

The certificate of Fellowship (FRCSC) is based on the Canadian Accredited Residency programme or comparable educational and training programmes of other countries, such as the American Specialty Residency programme accredited by the Accreditation Council for Graduate Medical Education, in a hospital or agency with a major affiliation with a medical school. Specialty training taken in Canada will be acceptable only if taken as a resident registered with the university office of postgraduate education and enrolled in a residency programme accredited by the Royal College, and verified in writing by the Associate Dean for postgraduate medical education, at the end of which the trainee has to pass the examination.

The structure, training and examination is styled like other North American residential programmes for the American Board in Surgery. However, there is no automatic reciprocity with any College or Board in any specialty.

For full regulations, candidates may write to:

Credentials Section,
The Royal College of Physicians and Surgeons of Canada,
774 Promenade Echo Drive,
Ottawa,
Canada K1S 5N8.

1.5 American Board in Surgery

This is predominantly geared towards clinical and operative training in hospitals recognised for surgical rotation and affiliated to a university.

For full regulations and details, candidates should write to the Director of the Surgical Residency Training Program (according to the specialty concerned, e.g. colorectal surgery, urology, or orthopaedics) at the university or clinic of whatever state (e.g. University of Texas at Houston, or Cleveland Clinic in Ohio). The American Board of General Surgery is acquired after 5 years practice in general surgery with presentation of a log book of operations and after passing written and oral examinations; clinical competence of a trainee is assessed through his/her director by recommendation (not by clinical examination). Specialisation in colorectal surgery, for example, requires a further 2 years practice in colorectal surgery leading to another Board examination in that specialty.

1.6 Arab Board in Surgery

The idea of establishing an independent body for regulation of surgical training in the Arab world was conceived in 1976 after the meeting of Arab Health Ministers.

In 1981, after one year internship, the 5-year Surgical Training Recidency programme commenced in hospitals recognised by the Board, and by 1986 the first batch of candidates had completed their Residency programme and passed a two-part examination to obtain the Certificate of Arab Board in Surgery (CABS). There are regulations for specialisation in general surgery, orthopaedics and urology. The pass rate is

about 40%. Candidates must be Arab citizens and/or read, write and speak Arabic, though the written examination is presented in the English language, whereas the oral and clinical parts can be conducted in English, French or Arabic.

The Scientific Council of Surgery (within the Arab Board for Medical Specialties) has emphasised that CABS is the highest professional degree for Arab countries; CABS (like Canadian, American Boards and perhaps Australasian diplomas) is a diploma based on a comprehensive accredited residency training programme with a two part examination (representing only a part of the final assessment). CABS, therefore, is an exit certificate enabling the Arab trainee to secure a junior consultant post one year after obtaining CABS; however, it is probably equivalent to a 1–4 year Specialty Registrar in the UK standards of training.

The training programme starts initially with the recognition of the hospital as a training centre, following which the trainee can apply to be enlisted on the training programme. After one year, the candidate can enter Part One CABS, a 2-day written examination containing 240 MCQs only (120 MCQs/day) covering all basic sciences and principles in surgery; the examination is held twice yearly in one of the four Arab examination centres (Douha, Riyadh, Damascus and Baghdad). Multiple-choice questions include single response, matching response and multiple combination responses (single response questions are easy to mark with computers). Trainees who pass Part One CABS, then spend 4 years of surgical training at the conclusion of which they must present:

- A log registry book of all operations performed alone, supervised, assisted or supervising others.
- A mini-thesis on any surgical subject.
- A booklet containing detailed operative notes of 20 operations.

The candidate can the enter Part Two CABS, with 240 MCQs over two days (120 MCQs in 3 hour/day), with the lowest pass mark set at 60%; only successful candidates are admitted to clinical examinations (one long case and three short cases) and oral examinations (two tables, one for surgical pathology/operative surgery and one for principles of surgery/emergency surgery). Examiners are paired each day and the examination is structured so that all of the candidates meet all of the examiners during the day. Final CABS is held once yearly in one of the above centres.

For full regulations, candidates may write to:

Secretary General,
Arab Board for Medical Specialties (The Main
  Headquarters),
P.O. Box 7669, Damascus
Syria

or:

The Regional Office of Arab Board,
Joint Board for Postgraduate Medical Education,
King Saud University,
P.O. Box 2925,
Riyadh 11461,
Kingdom of Saudi Arabia

SECTION 2
Guide to the Content of the FRCS Examination

2.1 The Revised FRCS Regulations in UK and Ireland (1990)

The revised Fellowship of the Edinburgh College was introduced in June 1990; the other three colleges followed in the autumn of that year (September 1990). The regulations cover all Royal Colleges of Surgeons in the United Kingdom (England, Edinburgh and Glasgow) and Ireland.

The revised FRCS clinical surgery in general examination differs from the old FRCS examination in laying far more emphasis on applied basic sciences and general principles; the previous primary FRCS was widely criticised as being non-clinically relevant. The level of clinical expertise expected will be that of a trainee who has had 3 years of post-registration clinical experience. Minute technical details about operative surgery will not be required; they will be spared for high specialisation. Intercollegiate examination leading to final FRCS in a specialty.

The objective of this change is to produce a test which will both confirm the adequacy of basic surgical training and be an acceptable requirement for entry into the approved Higher Specialist Training Scheme of all surgical specialties, and thereafter to the various Intercollegiate Specialty Board assessments (of final FRCS/specialisation).

The examination will cover the basic sciences relevant to surgery and clinical surgery-in-general. It may be taken as a single examination 3 years after registration, or alternatively, those who prefer to divide the burden may take the basic science section earlier, one year after registration, but in both circumstances all basic science sections must be passed before admission to the clinical practicals.

The FRCS (general surgery) therefore is easier in content and requirements than the old FRCS; capable candidates may also pass all parts at one time (if they desire to do so) without intermission needed for further requirements for the final part. The emphasis on applied basic sciences of the new FRCS may consolidate the trainee's knowledge of the fundamental basis of clinical surgery and the genesis of surgical disease, with principles of surgical treatment avoiding the fine technical operative details.

The entry requirements for the examination concerning mandatory training posts are slightly different from those for the old FRCS, with no more emphasis on an obligatory period of training in the United Kingdom and Ireland.

The revised regulations of 1990 have now been superceded by MRCS/AFRCS core and system modules followed by higher surgical training programmes leading to final FRCP (see part one).

2.2 Guide to the Content of the Revised FRCS Examination (1990)

The following description of the contents of the examination is intended solely as a guide for candidates of the general scope of the examination and of those topics likely to be considered of particular importance by the examiners.

A. APPLIED BASIC SCIENCE

This section comprises
- Anatomy
- Physiology, biochemistry and pharmacology
- Pathology, including cell biology, immunology and genetics.

B. CLINICAL SURGERY-IN-GENERAL

This section comprises:
- The diagnosis and preoperative management of surgical disorders, including trauma and resuscitation.
- The principles of operative surgery.
- Postoperative management, including the care of the critically ill and the assessment of results.

1. Diagnosis, preoperative assessment and management

The emphasis in this part of the examination will be on clinical practice relevant to all forms of surgery at a level of knowledge which can be expected of a candidate with only three years of post-registration clinical experience.

Surgical disorders are defined as disorders or injuries of any of the body's systems, in all age groups, in which surgery may play a role in investigation and/or treatment.

This section will test the following in both a written and a clinical setting:
(a) Ability to elicit the symptoms and signs of patients with 'surgical' disorders.
(b) Knowledge of methods of investigation including an understanding of principles underlying clinical diagnosis and ancillary methods of investigation, such as X-rays, computerised tomography, magnetic resonance imaging, ultrasound, radionuclides, endoscopy and biopsy.
(c) Ability to assess the severity and extent of a patient's surgical disorder, any concomitant medical disorders which may affect management, the significance of age and the medication associated with the treatment of these disorders.

(d) Understanding of how the physiological, anatomical, pathological and psychological effects of disease affect clinical presentation, investigation, treatment and prognosis.

(e) Knowledge of the diagnosis, assessment, first aid, transportation, resuscitation and treatment of the injured, including patients with burns.

(f) Knowledge of the resuscitation of the critically ill.

(g) Knowledge of preoperative preparation. Control of the effects of the disease to be treated. Control of the effects of concomitant disease. Prophylactic measures against intra- and postoperative complications. Consent. Communication with patients, relatives and others.

2. Principles of operative surgery

(a) **Principles of asepsis and antisepsis**
Clothing. Masks. Scrubbing up. Gloves. Skin preparation and protection. Sterilization of instruments, fluids, drapes and implantable materials (autoclave, chemical, gas, irradiation). Cross-infection.

(b) **Operating theatre design, usage and safety**
Construction. Design. Air change and air sterility. Operating tables. Diathermy, principles and hazards. Operating microscopes. Clothing. Special precautions (hepatitis, AIDS, radiation, anaesthetic gases). Protection of the unconscious patient.

(c) **Principles of general, regional and local anaesthesia.**

(d) **Surgical access**
Site and choice of incisions in relation to access, skin creases, blood and nerve supply. Retraction. Lighting.

(e) **The pathophysiology and management of wounds of all tissues**
Effect of incisions produced by knives, diathermy, lasers. Methods and effects of closure and fixation of wounds and tissue defects. Wound healing. Factors relevant to failed wound healing.

(f) **Adjuncts to surgery**
The properties, value, effects, choice and use of instruments, ligatures, sutures, drains and catheters.

(g) **The general principles governing the response of tissues to all forms of implanted materials.**

(h) **The principles concerning the removal, protection and implantation of living and dead tissues**
Autologous and homologous. Tissue typing, rejection, immunosuppression.

(i) **The pathophysiological effects and correction of intra-operative blood loss and fluid loss.**

(j) **Operative surgery and log books**
Candidates will be examined on the *principles* of operative surgery, not on the minute technical details of individual operations. Since these principles are often best discussed and illustrated by both candidate and examiner in the context of an actual operation, candidates may be asked to describe the techniques of those operations that are within their practical experience. To enable examiners to direct technical questions in this way, candidates will be expected to bring to the examination their practical log books for inspection and review.

(k) **Life-saving procedures**
Such as cardiac massage, relief of cardiac tamponade, tracheostomy, chest drains, intravenous access, ventilation, control of haemorrhage and amputation.

(l) **Emergency access to the body cavities**
Such as burrholes, thoracotomy and laparotomy for peritonitis, intestinal obstruction and abdominal haemorrhage.

(m) **Trauma**
The principles of the surgical treatment (local and general) of all forms of trauma, including burns.

(n) **Malignant disease**
The principles underlying the use of surgery in the treatment of malignant disease.

3. Postoperative management and the assessment of results

(a) **The management of pain**
Methods of postoperative analgesia and the pharmacology of common analgesics.

(b) **The pathophysiology, investigation and management of postoperative complications**
Respiratory infection and atelectasis. Deep vein thrombosis and pulmonary embolism. Haemorrhage, fluid imbalance, shock, myocardial infarction and cardiac arrest. Retention of urine, renal failure. Paralytic ileus. Jaundice. Infection of all varieties and septicaemia. Wound dehiscence.

(c) **The management of concomitant disease**
Diabetes. Myocardial ischaemia. Respiratory insufficiency. Alcoholism. Confusional states.

(d) **Clinical pharmacology**
The pharmacological actions, complications and interactions of drugs used in the management of surgical and medical disorders.

(e) **The principles of fluid and electrolyte balance, nutrition and feeding**.

(f) **The principles of intensive care**
Respiratory, circulatory, renal and alimentary support (for example, ventilators, blood gases, defibrillation, inotropic drugs, haemodialysis, peritoneal dialysis, monitoring of arterial and central venous pressure and cardiac output).

(g) **Rehabilitation. Physiotherapy**.

(h) **The aetiology, prevention and management of infection**

(i) **The complications of severe injury**
Such as disseminated intravascular coagulation, fat embolism and the respiratory distress syndrome.

(j) **The non-surgical treatment of malignant disease**
Principles, practice, value and complications of radiotherapy. Principles, pharmacology, value and complications of chemotherapy and other therapeutic agents.

(k) **The management of the chronic and terminally ill**
Pain relief. Nutrition. Psychological support. Counselling. Bereavement. Communication.

(l) **The evaluation of surgical practice**
Audit. Methods of quantifying the severity of disease and the results of treatment for the purpose of analysis.

Principles of statistics. Design of clinical trials. Screening programmes. Hospital records and information systems. Data processing and simple computing. Evaluation of published data.

(m) **Medical ethics**

Particularly in the context of surgical research, collaboration with colleagues and informed consent. Medico-legal problems.

2.3 The Format of the Revised Examination (1990)

ROYAL COLLEGE OF SURGEONS OF ENGLAND

	Applied Basic Science	*Clinical Surgery-in-General*
Written paper	1 paper, lasting 3 hours, of MCQs[a] comprising 30 questions each in – Anatomy – Physiology, biochemistry and pharmacology – Pathology	1 session, lasting 3 hours, comprising a – 2-hour short answer paper – 1-hour essay
Clinical examination	None	1 session, of about 45 minutes on a long case and short cases.
Oral	Three 20-minute orals in the following three subjects – Anatomy – Physiology, biochemistry and pharmacology – Pathology conducted by pairs of examiners. One of each pair will be a clinician	Two 20-minute orals in the following two subjects – Principles of operative surgery[b] – Surgical topics, such as postoperative management and the assessment of results conducted by pairs of examiners. You may be required to demonstrate basic life-saving techniques on manikins

[a] This paper tests recall of factual knowledge. Explanatory notes and instructions on the completion of multiple-choice question papers, together with a sample answer sheet, are sent to candidates when receipt of their application is acknowledged.

[b] Candidates must bring their log books to this part of the examination.

Notes

1. The written papers of both sections will be held on the same day.

2. The Applied Basic Science orals will start approximately 8 days after the written parts. The Clinical Surgery-in-General clinical and oral parts, will start approximately three weeks after the written papers and are likely to extend over a two-week period. Candidates will be examined in the clinicals and orals in one day and be informed of the final result at the end of that day.

The interval between the written and oral/clinical parts is to allow time for marking, for candidates to be informed of the result and for those who have achieved the required mark in the written part(s) to be told the dates of their clinicals and orals.

3. A candidate must achieve an adequate mark in the written part before proceeding to the respective oral and clinical part.

4. Those entering the whole examination
– must sit the written parts of both sections;
– will only be allowed to proceed to the Applied Basic Science orals if they gain an adequate mark in the Applied Basic Science written paper;
– must pass the Applied Basic Science section and obtain an adequate mark in the Clinical Surgery-in-General written part before they may proceed to the clinical and oral parts of the Clinical Surgery-in-General section.

5. A candidate who sits both written papers and fails the Applied Basic Science section (paper and/or orals) will be deemed to have failed the written part of the Clinical Surgery-in-General section.

ROYAL COLLEGE OF SURGEONS OF EDINBURGH

Surgery-in-General

Candidates must have been engaged in the study of their profession for a period of not less than four years after obtaining their basic qualification. Two years of this experience must have been gained in recognised posts as specified in Sections B and C below. The remaining experience should have been gained in the acquirement of professional knowledge (e.g. pre-registration posts, anatomy demonstrator posts, research appointments, clinical attachments, courses and posts recognised for pre-Fellowship training).

Section A

The examination has been designed so that all Sections may be taken at the same time, but for an initial period of three years following the introduction of the Revised Fellowship Examination in 1990 candidates may elect to sit Section A in advance of the remainder of the examination: they must have spent two years after graduation in acquiring professional knowledge. A pass in Section A may be held indefinitely but will not exclude similar material being re-examined in Section B.

The scope of the examination will be a general knowledge of anatomy, physiology, pathology including microbiology, and surgery, with particular emphasis on the application of these subjects to surgical management.

There will be a multiple-choice question paper covering these subjects and an oral examination in anatomy.

Candidates whose performance is below standard in one or more parts of the multiple-choice question paper will not proceed to the oral examination regardless of the overall mark which they may have obtained and they will be deemed to have failed the *whole of Section A*.

Note

The multiple-choice question papers for Section A are not available for distribution to candidates.

Sections B and C

Candidates must show evidence of completion of the following specific appointments (excluding pre-registration appointments):
(a) 12 months (or two periods of six months) in an approved post (or posts) in general surgery;
(b) six months in an approved post with duties predominantly in an Accident and Emergency Department or a service dealing predominantly with acute trauma;
(c) six months in an approved post in another major surgical specialty (cardiothoracic surgery, obstetrics and gynaecology, ophthalmology, orthopaedic surgery, otolaryngology, paediatric surgery, plastic surgery, surgical neurology and urology).

With effect from July 1992 candidates must show evidence of completion of the following specific appointments (excluding pre-registration appointments):
(a) six months in an approved post in general surgery in a unit which deals with acute emergencies:
(b) six months in an approved post in an orthopaedic unit which deals with acute trauma:
(c) two periods of six months in two approved posts in surgical specialties excluding either of the above but which may include posts in Accident and Emergency or Intensive Therapy Units in one of the six month periods.

Section B consists of:
(i) a written paper:
(ii) an oral examination in critical care and applied physiology:
(iii) an oral examination in principles of surgery and operative surgery:
(iv) an oral examination in surgical pathology and surgical management.

Section C consists of a clinical examination (subject to reaching a satisfactory standard in Section B).

Note

The marks of Sections B and C will be assessed together. An adequate standard (not necessarily a pass mark) must be achieved in Section B in order to proceed to Section C. Failed candidates will be required to re-take Sections B and C, including the written examination, at any subsequent attempts. There will be no refund of any part of the entrance fee to candidates not scoring sufficient marks to proceed to Section C.

ROYAL COLLEGE OF PHYSICIANS AND SURGEONS OF GLASGOW

Surgery-in-general

The Surgical Fellowship Examination consists of an examination in the Basic Sciences (Part A) and an examination in Surgery-in-General (Part B). The candidate may elect to take Part A separately from Part B or to take both Part A and Part B together in accordance with the regulations noted below.

Part A

Before admission to the examination a candidate is required to produce evidence satisfactory to the Council of:
1. Holding a medical qualification listed for recognition by the General Medical Council or acceptable to the Council of the College.
2. Being qualified for not less than two years from the date of his/her diploma, one year of which should be in pre-registration training and another year in any branch of the profession.
N.B. *If the basic medical qualification is not recognised by the General Medical Council, candidates should be aware that success in the full examination will *not* necessarily mean (a) that their FRCS qualification will be recognised by the General Medical Council and (b) that they will be registered to practise medicine in the United Kingdom.

The Part A examination will consist of:
(a) A multiple-choice question (MCQ) paper of 2 hours and 15 minutes' duration. MCQs include anatomy, physiology, and pathology.
(b) An oral examination, lasting 20 minutes, in anatomy.

A candidate who fails to achieve a reasonable mark in the MCQ paper and whose mark cannot be compensated by the oral examination, will be deemed to have failed the whole examination and will not proceed to the oral examination.

Part B

Before admission to the examination a candidate is required to produce evidence satisfactory to the Council of having:
1. Been successful in Part A or its equivalent, or of having been exempted therefrom.
2. Held a medical qualification acceptable to the Council of the College for not less than four years from the date of his/her diploma of medical qualification.
3. Completed two years, in addition to the pre-registration year, in clinical surgery posts recognised by the Council of the College.

The part B examination will consist of:
(a) A written essay paper of 3 hours' duration on the subject of surgery-in-general which will include the principles and practice of surgery and surgical pathology.
(b) Two oral examination, each lasting 30 minutes, in the following subjects:
   – Surgical physiology and principles of surgery.
   – Surgical pathology and operative surgery.
(c) A clinical examination.*
*Only those candidates who achieve a satisfactory standard in the written paper and oral sections will be allowed to proceed to the clinical examination.

ROYAL COLLEGE OF SURGEONS IN IRELAND

Section A: Applied Basic Sciences

Format

The Section A examination consists of a multiple-choice paper and oral examinations in anatomy, physiology, including histology, and the principles of pathology, including microbiology. (See guide notes below.)

Experience/registration requirements

Candidates must have completed their intern pre-registration year and have at least one additional year's experience in surgical or medical practice, including the basic sciences or research (i.e., at least two years post MB) and be fully registered in the Irish or British Registers, or to hold or be eligible to hold, limited or temporary registration in either the Irish or British Medical Registers.

Marking system

Anatomy		Physiology		Pathology	
MCQ	100	MCQ	100	MCQ	100
Oral	100	Oral	100	Oral	100
	200		200		200

Total marks = 600
Marks required to PASS = 360
(Limited compensation is allowed between subjects)

The Medal is awarded to the candidate who:
1. has the highest total marks;
2. has not failed overall (Oral + Written) in any subject;
3. is judged by the Conference of Examiners to be of sufficiently high standard;
4. has sat the examination for the first time.

Section B: General Principles of Surgery

The Section B examination is a test in the principles and practice of surgery, i.e. the basic knowledge of surgery required for all forms of surgical practice. It encompasses basic surgical principles and practice such as shock, sepsis, trauma and critical care, as well as the principles of operative surgery, including a knowledge of the commonly used operative surgical exposures. A basic core knowledge of all the surgical specialties is required, but the examination is not a test of any particular specialty of surgery such as that required on the completion of higher surgical training, now a separate exit examination (the Intercollegiate Specialty Assessment).

Surgery: format

The examination in surgery includes a written paper, *vivas* and clinicals.

The *written* part of the examination consists of one paper. A short answer question paper – normally not more than half a page of the examination answer book should be used to answer each part of the short answer questions, a, b, c, d, e. This paper tests the candidate's knowledge of a wide spectrum in surgery and the specialties, e.g. Write short notes on:
(a) Balanitis
(b) Persistent priapism
(c) Spermatocele
(d) Hypospadias
(e) Ectopic testis.

There are three *vivas*, one in surgical pathology, one in operative surgery and one in physiological basis, for surgical care.

Following completion of the written and *viva* examinations, candidates' performances will be reviewed. If they have not achieved a satisfactory standard, they will be excluded from the clinical examination.

The clinical examination: consists of an examination, in a general hospital, on short and long cases.

Marking system

	Viva surgical pathology	Viva operative surgery	Viva surgical care	Clinical Long case	Short cases
Written					
100	100	100	100	100	100

Total marks = 600
Marks required to pass = 360
Candidates *must* pass the clinical section of the examination.

2.4 Samples of Written Papers of the Revised FRCS Examination

Examination papers are the copyright of each College (samples were reproduced with kind permission of Royal Colleges). For each of the three Colleges whose papers appear here the first example is provided with the exact examination details.

THE ROYAL COLLEGE OF SURGEONS OF ENGLAND

DIPLOMA OF FELLOW

CLINICAL SURGERY-IN-GENERAL SECTION

WRITTEN PAPER 1 (MULTIPLE SHORT ANSWER)

2.00 p.m. to 4.00 p.m.

ALL EIGHT QUESTIONS MUST BE ANSWERED as concisely as possible on the two pages (A and B) provided for each question. Write on one side of the paper only, using the black ballpoint pen provided. You are asked to do this since your answers will be photocopied for marking by two examiners independently.

Write short notes on:

1. Congenital dislocation of the hip in children.

2. The management of the insulin-dependent diabetic undergoing an abdominal operation.

3. Cardiac tamponade.

4. The types of diathermy, their uses and their hazards.

5. Carpal tunnel syndrome.

6. The available methods of treatment of malignant dysphagia.

7. The investigation of an incidental finding of hypercalcaemia.

8. The initial assessment of severity of acute pancreatitis.

WRITTEN PAPER II (ESSAY)

4.15 p.m. to 5.15 p.m.

This essay paper comprises ONE QUESTION ONLY, for which the time allowed is ONE HOUR

Question: Discuss the management of postoperative oliguria.

I   *PAPER I* (*Short answer*)

1. The preoperative assessment of a patient with chronic obstructive airways disease who needs abdominal surgery.

2. The management of a solitary thyroid nodule.

3. The management of locally advanced breast cancer.

4. Biopsy.

5. Tumour metastases in bone.

6. Basal cell carcinoma.

7. The manifestations of Crohn's disease.

8. The potential problems associated with Colles' fractures.

   PAPER II (*Essay*)
Discuss the management of a young man with an acute spinal injury at the thoraco-lumbar junction.

II   *PAPER I* (*Short answer*)

1. The presentation and management of acute anterior dislocation of the shoulder in a 20-year-old patient.

2. The procedures required to prevent transfer of infection in the operating theatre.

3. The role of CT scanning in abdominal malignancies.

4. The complications and sequelae of deep vein thrombosis (excluding their management).

5. The diagnosis and treatment of subdural haemorrhage.

6. The principles of randomised controlled trials.

7. The use of Doppler ultrasound in vascular problems.

8. The complications of urethral catheterisation.

   PAPER II (*Essay*)
Discuss the diagnosis and management of blunt abdominal trauma.

III   *PAPER I* (*Short answer*)

1. The vascular complications of a fractured shaft of femur.

2. Wound healing and the factors which delay this.

3. The use of diagnostic ultrasound in urology.

4. The complications of diverticular disease (excluding management).

5. The complications of radiotherapy in malignant disease, illustrating your answer with reference to a specific organ.

6. The control of pain during recovery from abdominal surgery.

7. Extradural haemorrhage.

8. The methods of localisation of upper gastrointestinal bleeding.

   PAPER II (*Essay*)
What means are available for the early detection of malignant disease? Discuss the advantages and disadvantages of screening.

THE ROYAL COLLEGE OF SURGEONS
OF EDINBURGH

FELLOWSHIP EXAMINATION

SURGERY-IN-GENERAL

Essay Paper

Time: 3 hours

All questions to be answered

1. What factors should be considered in the evaluation of a cancer screening programme? Describe and comment on one current population screening programme.

2. Discuss the indications for and complications of transfusion of blood and blood products in surgical practice.

3. A woman aged 65 is admitted as an emergency with a history of constipation, abdominal distension and lower abdominal pain for 5 days. She had previously had some irregularity of bowel function for 2 months.

   Discuss the various conditions which could produce these symptoms and outline your management of this patient.

I *Essay paper*

1. Discuss the problems of surgery in the elderly patient.

2. Discuss the consequences and management of inhalation of gastric contents and outline policies for its prevention.

3. A patient, having undergone cholecystectomy, develops jaundice several days after operation. Discuss the possible causes and management.

II *Essay paper*

1. Discuss the preoperative assessment of a patient's fitness for surgery under general anaesthesia.

2. What is an opportunistic infection? Discuss the pathogenesis, the agents involved, and the diagnostic difficulties.

3. Define the term 'critical limb ischaemia' and discuss the principles underlying the management of this condition.

III *Essay paper*

1. How would you assess and monitor cardiac function in a critically ill patient? Discuss methods of improving the cardiac output in such a patient.

2. Discuss the uses and hazards of:

   (a) nasogastric tubes;

   (b) urinary catheters.

3 Discuss the management of faecal peritonitis.

IV *Essay paper*

1. Discuss the advantages and disadvantages of screening for malignant disease. Illustrate your answer with an example of your choice.

2. Describe the factors involved in haemostasis. Discuss the causes of abnormal bleeding in surgical practice and their management.

3. Describe the pathophysiology and management of a patient with 40% surface area burns in the first week.

V *Essay paper*

1. Discuss the management of hypercalcaemia.

2. Discuss the principles of an antibiotic prophylaxis policy in general surgical practice.

3. Discuss the management of a patient with abdominal injuries.

ROYAL COLLEGE OF PHYSICIANS AND SURGEONS OF GLASGOW

PART B   SURGICAL FELLOWSHIP EXAMINATION

—————————————

SURGERY-IN-GENERAL

—————————————

9.30 a.m. to 12.30 p.m.

ALL questions to be answered.

A separate book to be used for the answer to each question.

Use right-hand pages only.

Write your Examination Number on each book used.

1. Discuss the current methods of pain management in surgical patients.

2. Describe the local and general effects of a burn involving 25% of the body surface of a young adult and discuss the management.

3. Discuss the pathological conditions which may present to a surgeon in particular in an HIV-positive patient. Describe the operative precautions.

4. When may renal failure occur in surgical patients? How should it be monitored and managed?

I *PART B*

1. How would you define audit? Discuss the principles of audit and briefly outline how you would carry out an audit of wound infection in your surgical service.

2. What may predispose to, or cause excessive bleeding at operation? What measures may minimise or reduce this? If you suspect a coagulation defect how would you confirm this and manage the problem?

3. Discuss the role of recent developments in minimal invasive surgery and give examples from different surgical specialties.

4. What may cause or predispose to postoperative pyrexia? How should it be investigated and managed?

II *PART B*

1. Discuss how you would assess a patient's fitness for operation.

2. Discuss the problem of venous thromboembolism in surgery.

3. What is the role of the Intensive Care Unit in surgical practice?

4. Discuss the indications and complications of using prophylactic antibiotics in surgery.

III *PART B*

1. Discuss the surgical problems which may arise in diabetic patients.

2. Discuss the advantages, problems and limitations of day care surgery.

3. Discuss the pulmonary problems which may develop in a patient who has sustained multiple injuries and outline the management.

4. Describe the features of endotoxic (bacteraemic) shock and discuss its cause and management.

IV *PART B* (*held in Abu Dhabi*)

1. Discuss the priorities of assessment and early management of a patient admitted in coma with multiple injuries.

2. Discuss the use and monitoring requirements of parenteral nutrition in surgical patients.

3. What are the factors that influence wound healing?

4. Discuss the indications for the use of blood and blood products in the surgical patient. Outline the complications.

V *PART B*

1. A 70-year-old man is admitted with severe abdominal pain felt in the front and the back. His blood pressure has fallen dramatically. What are the possible conditions that might be involved? How would you arrive at a diagnosis?

2. How can the hospital laboratories help in the investigation of clinically unexplained cervical lymph node enlargement of several weeks duration? Give details of the kinds of specimens which should be sent for laboratory examination.

3. Discuss the sources of surgical infection in patients admitted to hospital without current infection and outline measures for preventing such infection.

4. Discuss the problems that may develop after introducing implanted prosthetic materials into the tissues.

2.5 Samples of the Written Examination from the Four Colleges for Years Prior to September 1990

Examination papers are the copyright of each College. Permission was given only by the Royal College of Surgeons of England and the Royal College of Surgeons of Edinburgh to publish them here in the exact style; examination papers from the other two Colleges, therefore, appear in a similar but not the exact style.

Although there is no limit to the number of different styles of questions asked, the carefully selected questions presented here comprehensively cover the material. These questions are still relevant in context despite the new regulations. When reviewed and worked on by the candidate, they will no doubt form an excellent basis for the theory of surgery. Many of the questions are based on special clinical situations and necessitate mature clinical judgement and a reasonable therapeutic approach.

It is very unusual for candidates who fail the written part and/or the clinical part to pass the final FRCS and therefore tremendous effort has gone into choosing these examination questions carefully. Some of them are shared between many Colleges (e.g. management of chronic pain, systemic bleeding in surgery, parenteral nutrition, endocrine therapy and chemotherapy of advanced cancer) and produced in different styles.

Candidates wishing to review a particular College's examination papers for the last 5 years prior to their attempt, may obtain these direct from the Royal Colleges of Glasgow and Ireland. Examination papers of the Royal College of Surgeons of England are obtained from Adrian Press Limited, Ilford, Essex and those of the Royal College of Surgeons of Edinburgh from Donald Ferrier Limited, 5 Teviot Place, Edinburgh EH1 2RB.

A broad spectrum of questions is collected here and a quick scanning of these may be far more fruitful than a mere review of the last 5 years' questions. For each College the first paper will be provided with the exact examination details. The written part is finished in 1 day in all Colleges, except in Edinburgh where it takes 2 days.

THE ROYAL COLLEGE OF SURGEONS OF ENGLAND

DIPLOMA OF FELLOW

FINAL EXAMINATION-I

PATHOLOGY, THERAPEUTICS AND SURGERY

10 a.m. to 12 noon

BOTH questions must be answered

FINAL EXAMINATION-II

PATHOLOGY, THERAPEUTICS AND SURGERY

1.30 p.m. to 3.30 p.m.

BOTH questions must be answered

I   *Paper I*
1. Discuss the problem of diabetes mellitus in surgical practice.
2. A young soldier has been admitted because of a high-velocity gunshot wound of the upper third of his right leg causing comminuted fractures of tibia and fibula. Describe procedure, complications and their management.

   Paper II
3. Discuss the management of a patient, aged 65 years, admitted with a diagnosis of large bowel obstruction.
4. Describe the causes of hydronephrosis in a child (under 15 years of age). How should this be investigated and treated?

II   *Paper I*
1. A woman, aged 30, has just discovered a lump in her breast, lateral to the nipple. Discuss the management of this patient.
2. Discuss immediate and subsequent management of a patient who has sustained a deep laceration of the front of the wrist.

   Paper II
3. Discuss the causes and management of cardiac arrest during surgical procedures.
4. On cystoscopy a woman of 50 is found to have a neoplasm of the bladder. Discuss the pathology and management.

III   *Paper I*
1. A youth of 18 years is admitted to hospital after having been thrown from his motorcycle. His right upper limb is found to be completely paralysed. This is his only disability and there has been no loss of consciousness. Discuss diagnosis, management and prognosis.
2. Discuss management in the first 48 hours of a patient with tetraplegia following fracture of the neck, and indicate principles governing his long-term care.

Paper II

3. Discuss the management of a man aged 50 admitted to hospital with severe haematemesis.
4. Discuss aetiology and management of intestinal obstruction in the first month of life.

IV   *Paper I*

1. A young motorcyclist is admitted to hospital after a road accident. He is found to be restless and confused and to have multiple fractures of the ribs. Describe how you would manage this case during the first 48 hours after admission.
2. Discuss the management of uncomplicated duodenal ulceration. Describe the possible sequelae of procedures you mention.

Paper II

3. A woman aged 30 has passed a calculus per urethram following an attack of right renal colic. Intravenous pyelogram shows a further shadow (0.5 cm in diameter) in the lower pole of the right kidney. Discuss the management of this patient.
4. Describe management of disseminated breast cancer in a woman of 50 years. Indicate the basic scientific principles underlying the treatment that you recommend.

V   *Paper I*

1. Discuss the management of a 55-year-old man extensively burned from the waist down.
2. A woman of 45 complains of food sticking behind the lower sternum. Discuss the diagnosis, pathology and management of the patient.

Paper II

3. A man of 65 presents with recent oedema of the left ankle, and mild obstructive urinary symptoms of 1 year's duration. Rectal examination reveals a hard left lobe of the prostate gland. How would you establish the diagnosis? Describe your management of the case.
4. Discuss clinical presentation of lumbar intervertebral disc disease and the place of surgery in its management.

VI   *Paper I*

1. Discuss the place of surgery in the treatment of chronic inflammatory disease of the large bowel.
2. An adult presents with a suspected retroperitoneal swelling. Discuss the diagnosis and investigations.

Paper II

3. Discuss the management of a stab wound in the groin.
4. Discuss the causes, prevention and management of stricture of the male urethra.

VII   *Paper I*

1. Discuss the management of a patient with a persistent external abdominal fistula.
2. Discuss the surgical management of osteoarthritis of the hip.

Paper II

3. Discuss causes, diagnosis and management of pulmonary complications that may follow major abdominal operations.
4. A 25-year-old woman with a goitre presents with a suggested diagnosis of thyrotoxicosis. How would you investigate this case? Discuss indications for operation.

VIII   *Paper I*

1. A man aged 35 injured in a road accident is found to have blood coming from his urethra. On examination a swelling is found rising from the pelvis midway to the umbilicus. Describe your management of this patient, confining your answers to urogenital tract injuries. Discuss critically other accepted methods of treatment of this patient, giving reasons for your own choice of procedure.
2. Give an account of surgical disorders of the salivary glands and their management.

Paper II

3. Give an account of treatment of fractures in the region of the elbow in an 8-year-old child. What complications may arise and how are they managed?
4. Discuss diagnosis and treatment of a limp in a child of 10 years of age.

IX   *Paper I*

1. Discuss causes of collapse of a vertebral body. Describe your investigations.
2. Discuss management of vascular complications of closed fractures of the long bones of the lower limb.

Paper II

3. Discuss differential diagnosis, treatment and investigation of a patient with unilateral proptosis.
4. Discuss pathology, diagnosis and treatment of acquired intestinovesical fistulae.

X   *Paper I*

1. A man of 45 years presents with a recent epileptic attack affecting the right side of the body. Discuss the investigation and management of this patient.
2. Discuss the methods used for the investigation and treatment of obstructive jaundice.

Paper II

3. A 20-year-old man, following an injury at football, develops a gross swelling of the knee-joint. Discuss the management.
4. Discuss the clinical importance of vomiting.

XI   *Paper I*

1. Describe the methods of urinary diversion and evaluate their place in treatment.
2. A 25-year-old man is admitted to Casualty after having been shot in the left lower chest. An X-ray shows the bullet is lodged on the left side of the 4th lumbar vertebra. Discuss the management.

Paper II

3. Discuss the investigation of a woman of 45 years with an early carcinoma of the breast. Describe the management of such a case treated by mastectomy and radiotherapy.
4. Discuss the management of an elderly patient presenting as an emergency with severe rectal haemorrhage.

XII   *Paper I*

1. Discuss the diagnosis and management of renal cell carcinoma (hypernephroma).
2. Discuss the prevention, diagnosis and treatment of deep venous thrombosis.

Paper II

3. Discuss the management of a closed chest wound.
4. Discuss the uses of ultrasound in surgery.

XIII   *Paper I*

1. Discuss the management of upper gastrointestinal tract bleeding in a patient with hepatosplenomegaly.
2. Discuss the management of an incised wound of the flexor aspect of the wrist.

Paper II

3. A man of 50 develops epigastric pain 3 years after a vagotomy and pyloroplasty done for duodenal ulcer. Discuss the diagnosis and management of such a patient.
4. Discuss the place of surgery in the treatment of rheumatoid arthritis.

XIV   *Paper I*

1. Discuss the diagnosis and management of obstruction of the lower third of the oesophagus.
2. Discuss the management of a woman of 70 years who sustains a fracture of the femoral neck. What are the aetiological factors?

Paper II

3. Describe the management of a patient who fails to pass urine after an operation.
4. Discuss clinical presentations and management of aortic aneurysm.

XV   *Paper I*

1. A healthy man aged 76 presents with a 6-month history of deterioration of urinary flow with frequency and urgency. Three years previously he underwent a transurethral resection for benign prostatic hypertrophy. Discuss your investigations and treatment.
2. Discuss the management of fracture-dislocation of the hip. What are the possible long-term consequences?

Paper II

3. Discuss the investigation and treatment of a patient who, on clinical examination, has an enlargement of one lobe of the thyroid gland.
4. Discuss the management of a severe penetrating wound of the axilla.

ROYAL COLLEGE OF SURGEONS
OF EDINBURGH

FELLOWSHIP EXAMINATION

PART II

I *DAY 1 (OPERATIVE SURGERY AND SURGICAL PATHOLOGY)*   *(09.30–12.30)*
1. Discuss the investigations of a patient presenting with a unilateral swelling in the anterior triangle of the neck.
2. Describe investigation and management of a 60-year-old man with severe continuing melaena of 48 hours' duration.
3. Discuss the use of chemotherapeutic agents in the management of a solid malignant tumour.

   DAY 2 (THE PRINCIPLES AND PRACTICE OF SURGERY)   *(09.30–12.30)*
1. Discuss the surgical implications of the use of the oral contraceptive pill.
2. Discuss the causes and treatment of postoperative ileus.
3. Describe methods by which an airway can be provided in a patient with laryngeal obstruction. Describe the indications for tracheostomy and a technique for operation. What postoperative complications may occur?

II *DAY 1*
1. Discuss the surgical significance of variations in total serum calcium concentration. Indicate how you would make a diagnosis of hyperparathyroidism.
2. Discuss the use of blood and blood products in surgical practice.
3. Discuss the value of population screening procedures for the detection of presymptomatic malignant disease.

   DAY 2
1. Discuss the causes and management of superior mesenteric artery occlusion.
2. Give an account of the pathology of calculous disease of the biliary tract and describe in detail the management of obstructive jaundice due to gallstones.
3. Discuss the management of a patient brought to hospital unconscious and suspected of having internal injuries of chest and abdomen.

III *DAY 1*
1. Discuss factors that influence the choice of incision in surgery of the abdominal contents.
2. Discuss pathology of solitary thyroid nodule and give an account of management of the patient.
3. Discuss systemic causes of excessive bleeding at operation and their management.

   DAY 2
1. What are the indications for surgical intervention in a middle-aged man with atherosclerotic occlusion of the left superficial femoral artery? Discuss the advantages and disadvantages of surgical procedures available.
2. Discuss the factors on which the success of an intestinal anastomosis depends.
3. Discuss indications, method of administration and complications of parenteral nutrition in surgery.

IV *DAY 1*
1. Discuss the management of a patient with rectal bleeding and a mucosal lesion just within reach of the examining finger.
2. Discuss the diagnosis and treatment of cancer of the prostate.
3. Give an account of techniques used to monitor a critically ill surgical patient.

   DAY 2
1. Outline pathological changes in diverticular disease of the distal colon and discuss operative treatment of its complications.
2. Describe causes of arteriovenous fistula. Discuss the effects of this condition and methods of treatment.
3. Describe the pathology of osteoarthritis of the hip joint and discuss surgical management.

V *DAY 1*

1. Discuss the management of a 50-year-old man with inoperable bronchogenic carcinoma.
2. Discuss uses of radioisotopes in surgical practice.
3. Define the term 'shock'. Compare and contrast pathogenesis, clinical features and treatment of haemorrhagic and septic shock.

DAY 2

1. Describe the pathological changes that may follow the development of a renal calculus. Discuss surgical procedures that may be employed for removal of a stone obstructing the lower third of the ureter.
2. Discuss diagnosis, complications and treatment of traumatic dislocation of the hip.
3. Discuss aetiology, pathological sequelae and clinical features of gastro-oesophageal reflux. Describe an operation for relief of this condition.

VI *DAY 1*

1. Discuss local and general management of a patient who develops an external small bowel fistula.
2. Outline various methods used in the treatment of cancer and refer to the limitations of each method.
3. Discuss methods of assessing the adequacy of the arterial supply to a limb.

DAY 2

1. Describe the aetiology and pathology of degenerative osteoarthrosis of the hip and discuss surgical methods of treatment.
2. Describe the pathology of coronary arterial disease and its cardiac complications. Outline the surgical techniques available for treatment of this condition.
3. Describe how you would treat a patient with jaundice caused by multiple stones in the common bile duct.

VII *DAY 1*

1. Discuss the pathological and clinical features of thoracic outlet compression syndrome. Describe the surgical management of this condition.
2. Describe the pathological changes in acute pancreatitis and discuss aetiology. Discuss the management of the early stages of pancreatitis and describe the operative treatment of an established pancreatic pseudocyst.
3. Discuss the aetiology, pathology and treatment of maldescent of the testis.

DAY 2

1. Discuss the prevention and control of infection in a surgical ward.
2. Discuss the advantages and disadvantages of different types of suture material.
3. Discuss the management of closed head injury.

VIII *DAY 1*

1. Discuss conditions included in the term 'nerve entrapment syndrome'. Describe the operation of anterior transposition of the ulnar nerve at the elbow.
2. Discuss the operative treatment of portal hypertension complicated by oesophageal varices.
3. Discuss the operative procedures in management of carcinoma of the rectum. Indicate the relative roles of various techniques which you can employ.

DAY 2

1. Describe the investigation of a patient presenting with acute bleeding from the alimentary tract. What are the relative values of endoscopy and radiology in such emergencies.
2. What do you consider to be the essential requirements of a modern accident and emergency service? Give your reasons.
3. Discuss the merits and demerits of regional lymph gland excision as an adjunct to the surgical removal of a primary malignancy, illustrating your argument by reference to particular types and locations of tumours.

IX *DAY 1*

1. Discuss the diagnosis, management and procedure of tumours of the testis.
2. Discuss the aetiology of right subphrenic abscess and its possible sequelae. Describe how you would drain it.
3. Describe various primary tumours which may arise in the small bowel.

DAY 2

1. Discuss the role of surgery in relief of pain due to advanced malignant disease.
2. Discuss the management of acute head injury from time of occurrence to end of first week in hospital.
3. Discuss the differential diagnosis of low back pain with sciatica and its management.

X *DAY 1*

1. Give a critical assessment of the operations currently used for the treatment of duodenal ulcer.
2. Describe the pathological changes which follow the lodgement of an embolus in the common femoral artery. Discuss the management of this condition.
3. Give an account of the causes of swelling of the parotid gland. Describe the operation of superficial parotidectomy.

DAY 2

1. Discuss the problems of infection in an intensive care unit.
2. Give an account of those types of systemic hypertension that may be amenable to surgical procedures.
3. Discuss the aetiology of renal stone formation.

XI *DAY 1*

1. Discuss the place of lymph node dissection in cancer. Give an account of an operation for radical removal of lymph nodes in the neck.
2. Discuss the management of a residual biliary stone.
3. Discuss the management of peritonitis due to a perforated abdominal viscus. Describe in detail a transverse loop colostomy.

DAY 2

1. Discuss the role of frozen section histopathology as an aid to surgical management.
2. What factors predispose to infection in surgical wounds? How may these be combated?
3. Discuss the aetiology and management of acute renal failure in surgical practice.

XII *DAY 1*

1. A 25-year-old man is admitted with a stab wound of the left supraclavicular fossa. Discuss the management.
2. A 55-year-old man is found to have hypercalcaemia. Discuss the diagnosis and management.
3. Discuss the surgery of portal hypertension.

DAY 2

1. What are the indications for total parenteral nutrition? Discuss the daily requirements, methods of delivery and complications.
2. Discuss the management of chronic severe pain.
3. Discuss the methods of prevention and treatment of bowel and urinary incontinence.

ROYAL COLLEGE OF PHYSICIANS AND SURGEONS OF GLASGOW

FINAL EXAMINATION FOR THE FELLOWSHIP *QUA* SURGEON

PAPER 1 PRACTICE SURGERY

9.30 a.m. to 12.30 p.m.

PAPER 2 SURGICAL PATHOLOGY AND OPERATIVE SURGERY

2.00 p.m. to 5.00 p.m.

I *Paper 1*

1. Discuss the mechanism of rupture of the medial meniscus of the knee joint. Describe types of rupture and their surgical treatment.
2. Describe various types of maldescent of the testis and discuss management of the condition.
3. Make a comparison of various intravenous fluids used to treat hypovolaemic shock.

Paper 2

1. Discuss the pathological conditions which affect the endocrine pancreatic gland. Describe the surgical treatment of one of them.
2. Discuss the pathology associated with prolapsed intervertebral disc. Describe the surgical procedure of a lumbar disc protrusion.
3. Describe a surgical operation to treat gross obesity. Discuss postoperative complications and problems.

II *Paper 1*

1. What are the causes of bilateral hydronephrosis? Describe the management of this condition.
2. Discuss the role of X-ray in the diagnosis and of ultrasonography in the investigation of the acute abdomen.
3. What are the symptoms and signs of tuberculosis of the spine? Describe investigation and management of this condition.

Paper 2

1. Discuss the causes and complications of postcholecystectomy jaundice. Describe management of retained stones in the common bile duct following cholecystectomy.
2. Discuss the pathology and complications of arthritis in the hand. Describe surgical treatment of rheumatoid arthritis of the hand.
3. Discuss the pathology of swelling of lymph glands of the neck. Describe the operation of block dissection of cervical lymph glands.

III *Paper 1*

1. Discuss the investigations of obstructive jaundice. Indicate surgical procedures for its relief.
2. Discuss the aetiology, investigation and treatment of transient ischaemic attacks (drop attacks).
3. Discuss the role of percutaneous vascular access in the investigation and treatment of disease. Outline complications that may arise from the various procedures involved.

Paper 2

1. Discuss the pathology of tumours of the oral cavity and tongue. Describe the treatment of a malignant ulcer at the lateral margin of the tongue.
2. Discuss the pathology of ulcerative colitis and describe in detail the fashioning of an ileostomy.
3. Discuss the pathology and bacteriology of gas gangrene. Describe the operation of below-knee amputation for diabetic gangrene of the foot.

IV *Paper 1*
1. Describe the symptoms of fracture of the middle cranial fossa and possible complications. Outline management of such a patient.
2. Discuss the aetiology of rectal prolapse occurring in the adult. Describe the treatment.
3. Describe the investigation and aetiology of unilateral swelling of the parotid gland. Give a brief account of management and prognosis.

Paper 2
1. Discuss the systemic changes associated with a parathyroid adenoma. Describe an operation for removal of parathyroid adenoma.
2. Discuss the aetiology and pathological effects of arteriovenous fistual. Describe the surgical treatment of traumatic arteriovenous fistula of the common femoral vessels.
3. Discuss the nature and complications of abdominal stab wounds. Describe the surgical treatment for a stab wound in the left upper abdomen.

V *Paper 1*
1. Discuss important causes of renal failure in surgical practice. What are the indications for renal transplantation?
2. What are the causes of vomiting and regurgitation in the neonate? Discuss the investigation and management of the condition.
3. Discuss indications for surgery in acute and non-acute ulcerative colitis and state briefly the operative procedures you would perform.

Paper 2
1. Discuss the pathology of mesenteric vascular occlusion. Describe the surgical treatment of acute intestinal ischaemia due to occlusion of the superior mesenteric artery.
2. Discuss the complications associated with fractures and dislocations of the elbow. Describe the surgical treatment of a comminuted fracture of head of radius.
3. Discuss the aetiology and pathology of branchial cysts. Describe in detail the surgical removal of a branchial cyst.

VI *Paper 1*
1. What particular problems are associated with supracondylar fracture of the femur? Describe their management.
2. Discuss the surgical aspects of hypertension and give a brief account of relevant surgical treatment.
3. What tumours occur in the pancreas? Describe their clinical presentation and investigation.

Paper 2
1. Discuss surgical conditions where skin grafting is necessary. Describe methods of skin grafting and their advantages and disadvantages.
2. Discuss pathology of tumours of the testis. Describe the technique of lymphangiography and the operation of orchidectomy for a malignant tumour of the testis.
3. Discuss causes of diaphragmatic hernias. Describe the surgical treatment of a traumatic rupture of the diaphragm.

VII *Paper 1*
1. What factors are responsible for endotoxic shock? Discuss management of this condition.
2. What are the more common sites of injury to the urinary system? Explain the mechanism. Describe briefly the management of a case of rupture of membranous urethra.
3. Discuss the role of endoscopy in the investigation and management of upper alimentary disease.

Paper 2
1. Discuss factors that are important in wound healing. What are the aetiological problems associated with wound dehiscence? Describe surgical treatment for right paramedian incisional hernia.
2. Discuss the pathology of premalignant disease of the gastrointestinal tract. Describe the surgical treatment for familial polyposis coli.
3. Discuss the pathology and complications of oesophageal strictures. Describe a transthoracic repair of a simple stricture of the lower third of the oesophagus.

VIII *Paper 1*
1. Outline the risks of surgery under general anaesthesia. What measures may be taken to prevent their occurrence?
2. Describe various ways in which urogenital tuberculosis may present. How would you investigate the condition?
3. Describe the treatment of compound fractures of the tibia. Discuss particular problems and complications of the condition.

Paper 2

1. Discuss the pathology of cancer of the thyroid gland. Describe the operation of subtotal thyroidectomy.
2. Discuss briefly the pathological conditions for which splenectomy is indicated. Describe the operation of splenectomy.
3. Discuss the pathology of chronic gastric ulcer and its complications. Describe an operation for this condition.

IX   *Paper 1*

1. Describe the investigation of a patient who presents with ischaemia of a lower limb. What factors influence the treatment of such a case?
2. Discuss the clinical manifestations and investigation of subphrenic abscess. Give a brief account of management.
3. What is meant by paralytic ileus? Discuss aetiology and management.

Paper 2

1. Discuss the pathology of malignant melanoma. Describe the surgical treatment of malignant melanoma of the lower leg.
2. Discuss the pathology of transient cerebral ischaemia. Describe the surgical treatment of carotid artery stenosis.
3. Discuss the pathology of midline swellings of the neck. Describe operation for excision of thyroglossal cyst.

X   *Paper 1*

1. What complications might arise from fractures of the pelvis. Outline emergency treatment required in such circumstances.
2. Give an account of diangosis, treatment and prognosis of testicular tumours.
3. A 75-year-old man who had a Polya gastrectomy 15 years previously presents with weight loss, tingling in fingers and toes and backache. Discuss the management and outline factors which are responsible for causing these symptoms after gastrectomy.

Paper 2

1. Discuss the pathology of carcinoid tumour of the intestine. Describe surgical treatment of carcinoid tumour of the ileum.
2. Discuss the pathology of hiatal hernia. Describe surgical treatment.
3. Discuss the place of drains in surgery.

ROYAL COLLEGE OF SURGEONS
IN IRELAND

FINAL EXAMINATION FOR THE FELLOWSHIP OF THE COLLEGE

PAPER A

(TIME: 3 HOURS)

SURGICAL PATHOLOGY AND OPERATIVE SURGERY

PAPER B

(TIME: 3 HOURS)

PRINCIPLES AND PRACTICE OF SURGERY

I *Paper A*
Write short notes (less than one page each) on the following questions: (All questions to be answered)

1. *THORACIC*:
a. Tracheo-oesophageal fistula.
b. Tracheal collapse.
c. Thymoma.
d. Mediastinoscopy.
e. Widened superior mediastinum after severe trauma.

2. *ORTHOPAEDICS*:
a. Pes cavus.
b. March fracture.
c. Spondylolisthesis.
d. Bamboo spine (radiological appearance).
e. Charcot joint.

3. *VASCULAR*:
a. Indications for A-V fistula.
b. Complications of A-V fistula in non-uraemic patients.
c. Raynaud's phenomenon.
d. Disseminated intravenous coagulation.
e. Berry's aneurysm.

4. *GENITOURINARY TRACT*:
a. Ureterocele.
b. Superficial extravasation of urine.
c. Enuresis in children.
d. Ectopia vesicae.
e. Gut neoplasia after ureterostomy.

5. *HEPATOBILIARY*:
a. Multiple biliary cysts (Caroli's disease).
b. Contraindications of intravenous cholangiography.
c. Gallstone ileus.
d. Sclerosing cholangitis.
e. Residual biliary stone.

6. *GASTROINTESTINAL TRACT*:
a. Lateral duodenal fistula.
b. Meleney's ulcer.
c. Giant benign rectal ulcer.
d. Richter's hernia.
e. Spontaneous intraperitoneal bleeding.

7. *ONCOLOGY*:
a. Cell cycle.
b. Alkylating agents.
c. Antimetabolites.
d. Nitrosamine compounds.
e. Large bowel epithelial dysplasia.

8. *MISCELLANEOUS*:
a. Pleural mesothelioma.
b. Monoclonal antibodies.
c. Metoclopramide.
d. Ocular plethysmography.
e. G-cell hyperplasia.

PAPER B
Candidates must attempt Question No. 1 and THREE of the remaining FOUR questions.

1. Discuss the management of acute pancreatitis. What are the aetiological factors, the most important investigations and the factors that influence the prognosis?

2. Write an essay on successful colorectal anastomosis.
3. Discuss the management of a 25-year-old man admitted with a gunshot wound just below the right nipple.
4. Describe the aetiology and management of male urethral stricture.
5. Discuss the postoperative analgesia in a surgical patient.

II   *Paper A*
1. *GASTROINTESTINAL TRACT*:
a. Radiation enteritis.
b. Peptic ulcerations of the small gut.
c. Gastrojejunocolic fistula.
d. Angiodysplasia of the gut.
e. Volvulus of the colon.

2. *HEPATOBILIARY*:
a. Fulminating acute cholangitis.
b. Emphysematous cholycystitis.
c. Biliary ductal anatomical anomalies.
d. Lithogenic bile.
e. Retained stone in common bile duct.

3. *GYNAECOLOGY AND UROLOGY*:
a. Bartholin's abscess.
b. Urethral caruncle.
c. Endometriosis.
d. Ureteric reflux.
e. Tubo-ovarian abscess.

4. *VASCULAR*:
a. Transluminal angioplasty.
b. Vena cava injury.
c. Side-effects of heparin.
d. Profundoplasty.
e. Alternatives to the saphenous vein in coronary bypass.

5. *LOCOMOTOR SYSTEM*:
a. Monteggia's fracture.
b. Cubitus valgus.
c. Patellar tap.
d. Rupture of supraspinatus.
e. Rupture of quadriceps expansion.

6. *THORACIC*:
a. Cervical rib.
b. Insertion of chest tube in pneumothorax.
c. Therapeutic bronchoscopy.
d. Dysphagia lusoria.
e. Bronchobiliary fistula.

7. *VASCULAR*:
a. Measurement of ankle blood pressure.
b. Hepatic artery occlusion.
c. Blood viscosity implications in surgery.
d. Arterial injury in knee joint trauma.

8. *MISCELLANEOUS*:
a. Significance of intra-abdominal X-ray calcification.
b. High-output renal failure.
c. Malignant life cycle.
d. Anti-smooth muscle antibodies.
e. Fractured head of radius.

PAPER B
1. Write an essay on thyroiditis. Include in your answer a *detailed* description of the macroscopic and microscopic appearances in each condition and indications for surgical intervention.

2. Classify small intestinal tumours, and describe their modes of presentation, investigation and management.
3. Write an essay on fistula-in-ano.
4. Discuss the management of an unconscious patient with multiple trauma. What factors are important in prognosis?
5. Discuss the place of surgery in the management of chronic pancreatitis.

III *Paper A*
1. *THORACIC*:
a. Shock lung.
b. IPPV
c. EEPV
d. Slipped ribs.
e. Flail chest.

2. *HEPATOBILIARY*:
a. Solitary giant cyst of liver.
b. Calot's triangle.
c. Choledochus cyst.
d. Contact cholangiography.
e. Primary biliary stone.

3. *GASTROINTESTINAL*:
a. Mucoviscidosis.
b. Spider naevi.
c. Vipoma.
d. Therapeutic ERCP.
e. Sengstaken–Blakemore tube.

4. *ORTHOPAEDICS*:
a. Low back pain.
b. Köhler's disease.
c. Myositis ossificans.
d. Codeman's triangle.
e. Scaphoid fracture.

5. *VASCULAR*:
a. Neoplastic lymphoedema.
b. Seldinger catheter.
c. Swanz–Ganz catheter.
d. Lymphoedema tarda and praecox.
e. Therapeutic uses of the intravenous route.

6. *GENITOURINARY TRACT*:
a. Priapism.
b. Autonephrectomy.
c. Deep extravasation of urine.
d. Peyronie's disease.
e. Indications and contraindications for circumcision.

7. *ONCOLOGY*:
a. Lentigo maligna.
b. Oestrogen receptors.
c. Anti-oestrogens.
d. Premalignant colonic lesion.
e. Interferon.

8. *MISCELLANEOUS*:
a. Hirtz–Halter valve.
b. Traumatic injury of the diaphragm.
c. Intrathymic parathyroid adenoma.
d. Paradoxical breathing.
e. Fat embolism.

Paper B
1. Describe the salient features of the usual malignant tumours of bone. In each condition, write a brief account of the gross and microscopic pathological appearances.

2. Describe the aetiology, diagnostic features and management of extradural intracranial haemorrhage.
3. Discuss the indications for and complications of intravenous feeding.
4. Discuss the management of a 45-year-old male bank clerk who presents with pain in his calf on walking.
5. Write an essay on the selection of antibiotics in abdominal surgery. Briefly comment on the following statement: 'The timing of antibiotic administration is of great importance in the overall reduction of postoperative wound sepsis.'

SECTION 3
Causes of Failure

The candidate has to pass the written and clinical parts individually and clearly with no borderline marks. Borderline marks in other parts of the examination can be discussed and compensated for. Failed candidates should investigate the causes of their failure in order to avoid them in future attempts and should not be too disappointed since many of the best surgeons fail their first attempt. It has even been said 'It is a shame to pass the final FRCS at the first attempt.' The main causes of failure of the final FRCS are outlined here.

Inadequate preparation Self-explanatory. Do not attempt the final FRCS (and do not waste your money and time) before you feel that you are fully prepared theoretically and have fully mastered your operations and clinical methods practically.

Inability to express oneself Particularly applies to overseas doctors with poor command of English. You may know the operations and know what to do in emergency situations but you are either unable to express yourself and your ideas in English or are unable to discuss your operations technically and systematically. It is advisable therefore to know the key English phrases in each disease and operation and know the principles in outline since discussion and substantiation of each approach is the essence of the final FRCS examination, especially the oral parts.

Lack of common sense Always think in terms of priorities and remember that common diseases are common and rare diseases are rare. This is particularly important in the discussions when you are requested to speak in order of frequency. In the written part, however, you can discuss the diseases according to the well-known plan of congenital, traumatic, neoplastic, etc. Do not show your encyclopaedic knowledge in the clinical and oral parts but be practical and precise. Mention common lesions first and outline your management according to priorities, mentioning the most important measures first.

Your management should always be comprehensive, treating the primary cause and its effects and not just symptoms. When asked about investigations, remember always to mention the simplest relevant and cheapest investigation first since there is no place for routine blind investigation in the final FRCS. Those who mention ERCP before urine examination in jaundice investigations and barium enema before rectal examination and sigmoidoscopy with biopsy in rectal carcinoma, those who embark on palpation of the groin before asking the patient to cough in hernia examination, and those who forget to examine the mouth or ask the patient to swallow in neck swelling examination deserve to fail. Try not to be clever, but be careful.

Bad candidate–patient relationship Examiners expect you to be perfect not only in your knowledge and judgement but also in your ethics and approach. Do not fail yourself by appearing excessively hirsute or eccentrically dressed. Be polite to patients. Introduce yourself and ask permission to examine them. Thank them at the end, help them with their night clothes and tuck in the sheets and blankets. This will at least show that you are a courteous and considerate doctor. Never examine patients as if you are manipulating animals. Look at their faces for pain expression. Examiners may press you to discuss the causes of the patient's swelling or ascites. Do not mention the word 'malignancy' or 'tumour' in front of the patient.

Lack of confidence Talk to your examiner as you would address a distinguished senior colleague. Give the impression that you are a confident, safe surgeon who knows exactly what to do. Examiners sometimes try to shake your confidence by adopting the opposite approach. If you think you are right, substantiate your approach. If you are asked, 'How do you do this operation?', do not answer by saying 'Some do it this way and others prefer that way.' You have to adopt your own practical and personal safe way, so say; 'I will do this operation this way . . .', without mentioning other views. Remember though that overconfidence in controversial topics should be resisted.

Bad examiner–examinee relationship Never argue with the examiner and never ask the examiner to repeat the question. Listen carefully to the examiner question and if says, 'Tell me about gastric carcinoma', do not reply 'What would you like me to talk about?' but say, 'I should like to talk about its pathology because I find this particularly interesting.' If you are asked about thyroiditis, never ask the examiner, 'What do you mean?' It implies that the question has not been expressed understandably, or has been badly phrased – or that you have not listened! Do not smile too much and do not be a joker. Do not try to be overconfident or too humble with the examiner, but smile a little bit, and answer the question politely and efficiently. If the examiner tries to explain his or her own approach listen to them with interest and show that you are quite impressed (but never argue). Keep the examiner happy and keep the discussion easy-going, comfortable and mutually interesting. Also be exact and precise and answer the question *to the point*, unless you want to lead the examiner to a topic you know better.

Luck There is no doubt that luck is involved. It is usual for examiners to examine in pairs so that if one is unkind or aggressive (the hawk) this will be buffered or compensated for by the other, more dove-like examiner. It is bad luck to be examined by too many hawks asking impossible questions about cardiac transplantation or hepatic resection. Examiners who remain expressionless no matter what you say (if not looking unhappy) and pedantic examiners who keep asking you the same question because you are not answering the exact point in their minds are difficult to cope with. However, each Royal College always tries to maintain its high standard through careful selection of fair examiners.

Candidates are strongly advised not to over-react, even when they are confronted with the most difficult examiners, because this may affect their attitude and performance in subsequent parts of the examination. It should be remembered that many apparently difficult examiners may be very helpful in the comprehensive analysis of your scores.

SECTION 4
What to Read

It is a grave mistake to think that the books read for the final MB, ChB are useless for the postgraduate diploma, since these books provide the solid basis for the theory and a practical guide for the clinical part. It is more convenient to go through a book you have read before than to explore a new one for the first time. Most surgical facts are not going to change radically and only a fraction of facts will emerge and need to be added every 3–5 years. Therefore, choose as your basic text or 'skeleton of surgery' a comprehensive surgical book with which you are familiar and augment this with a few other books. Try to widen and supplement your views by accumulating information on the uncovered topics from the regular journals. (The best plan is to summarise these topics in a special file which can be reviewed in conjunction with your surgical textbook before examination.) The following useful books are listed without recommendation as to the best since this depends entirely on your personal preference. However, our personal experience with books will be mentioned in the next section. *Only one book* should be selected from each group below to cover one of the examination parts. Notice that in some books the date (or edition number) is omitted deliberately so that you can order the most recently published edition. It is not how much you read that is important but how well you digest the facts (quality rather than quantity of reading).

General

Comprehensive textbooks

Bailey and Love's Short Practice of Surgery. London: Chapman & Hall.

Sabiston D.C. (ed). *Davis–Christopher Textbook of Surgery.* Philadelphia: W.B.Saunders.

Taylor S., Chisholm G.D., O'Higgins N., Shields R. *Surgical Management.* London: Heinemann Medical.

Cushieri A., Giles G. R., Moosa A. R. (eds). *Essential Surgical Practice.* Oxford: Butterworth–Heinemann.

Schwartz S. I., Lillehei R.C., Shires G. H. *et al.* (eds). *Principles of Surgery.* New York: McGraw Hill (A Blakiston Publication). (in volumes)

Hardy J. D. *Hardy Textbook of Surgery.* New York: Lippincott Company.

Dunphy J. E., Way L. (eds) *Current Surgical Diagnosis and Treatment.* Los Altos, California: Lange.

McCredie J. A. (ed). *Basic Surgery.* London: Macmillan.

Forrest A. P. M., Carter D. C., Macleod I. B. *Principles and Practice of Surgery.* Edinburgh: Churchill Livingstone.

Specialty books (to widen your views)

Abdomen

Shackelford R. T. *Surgery of the Alimentary Tract.* Philadelphia: W. B. Saunders. (in volumes)

Maingot's Abdominal Operations, Vols 1 and 2. New York: Appleton-Century-Crofts.

Goligher J. C., Duthie H. L., Nixon H. H. (eds). *Goligher's Surgery of the Anus, Rectum and Colon.* London: Baillière Tindall.

Keighley M. and Williams N. *Surgery of the Anus, Rectum and Colon.* London: Saunders-Ballière Tindall.

Heberer G., Denecke H. (eds). *Colo-rectal Surgery.* Berlin: Springer-Verlag.

Keith R. G., Keynes W. M. (eds) *The Pancreas.* London: Heinemann Medical.

Smith, Lord R., Sherlock, Dame S. (eds). *Surgery of the Gallbladder and Bile Ducts.* London: Butterworths.

Kune G. A., Sali A. *The Practice of Biliary Surgery.* Oxford: Blackwell Scientific Publications.

Blumgart L. H. *The Biliary Tract – Clinical Surgery International*, Vol. 5. Edinburgh: Churchill Livingstone.

Dudley H. A. F. (ed). *Hamilton Bailey's Emergency Surgery.* Oxford: Butterworth-Heinemann.

Thorax

Cardiothoracic section in *Davis–Christopher Textbook of Surgery.* Philadelphia: W. B. Saunders.

D'Abreu A. L., Collis J. L., Clarke D. B. *A Practice of Thoracic Surgery.* London: Edward Arnold.

Laparoscopy and Endoscopy

Cuschieri A., Buess G. and Perissat J. *Operative Manual of Endoscopic Surgery.* Berlin: Springer-Verlag.

Arregui M., Fitzgibbons R., Katkhouda N. *et al. Principles of Laparoscopic Surgery (Basic and Advanced Techniques).* Berlin: Springer-Verlag.

Pappas T., Schwartz L. and Eubanks S. *Atlas of Laparoscopic Surgery.* Philadelphia: Current Medicine.

Monson J. and Darzi A. *Laparoscopic Colorectal Surgery.* Oxford: Isis Medical Media.

Dunn D. and Menzies D. Hernia Repair: *The Laparoscopic Approach.* Oxford: Blackwell Science.

Cuschieri A. and Szabo Z. *Tissue Approximation in Endoscopic Surgery.* Oxford: Isis Medical Media.

Cotton P. and Williams C. *Practical Gastrointestinal Endoscopy.* Oxford: Blackwell Science.

Geenen J., Fleischer D. and Waye J. *Techniques in Therapeutic Endoscopy.*

Orthopaedics

Apley A. G., Solomon L. (eds). *Apley's System of Orthopaedics and Fractures.* London: Butterworths.

Adams C. *Outline of Orthopaedics* and *Outline of Fracture including Joint Injuries.* Edinburgh: Churchill Livingstone.

Crenshaw A. G. (ed). *Campbell's Operative Orthopaedics* (2 vols). St Louis: Mosby.

Wilson J. N. (ed). *Watson–Jones' Fractures and Joint Injuries* (2 vols). Edinburgh: Churchill Livingstone.

Urology

Glenn J. G. (ed.). *Urologic Surgery*. Philadelphia: J. G. Lippincott.

Blandy J. *Urology*, Vols 1 and 2. Oxford: Blackwell Scientific Publications.

Chisholm G. D. *Urology*. London: Heinemann Medical

Vascular

Jamieson C. and Yao J. Vascular Surgery in *Rob & Smith's Operative Surgery*. 5th edn. London: Chapman & Hall Medical.

Cooley D. A., Wukasch D. C. *Techniques in Vascular Surgery*. Philadelphia: W. B. Saunders.

Jamieson C. *Surgical Management of Vascular Disease*. London: Heinemann Medical.

Dodd H., Cockett F. B. *The Pathology and Surgery of the Veins of the Lower Limb*. Edinburgh: Churchill Livingstone.

Kinmonth J. B. *The Lymphatics*. London: Edward Arnold.

Reid W., Pollock J. G. *The Surgeon's Management of Gangrene*. London: Pitman.

Head and neck

Stell P. M., Maran A. G. *Head and Neck Surgery*. London: Heinemann Medical.

Neurosurgery

Jennett B., Galbraith S. *An Introduction to Neurosurgery*. London: Heinemann Medical.

Paediatric surgery

Nixon H. H., O'Donnell B. *The Essentials of Paediatric Surgery*. London: Heinemann Medical.

Nixon H. H. *Surgical Conditions in Paediatrics*. London: Butterworths.

Plastic surgery

McGregor I. A. *Fundamental Techniques of Plastic Surgery*. Edinburgh: Churchill Livingstone.

Grabb W. C., Smith J. W. *Plastic Surgery*. Boston: Little, Brown & Co.

Skoog T. *Plastic Surgery*. Philadelphia: W. B. Saunders.

Clinical surgery

Bailey H. In *Demonstration of Physical Signs in Clinical Surgery* (Clain A., ed). Oxford: Butterworth–Heinemann.

Scott P. R. *An Aid to Clinical Surgery*. Revised by Dudley H. A. F. Edinburgh: Churchill Livingstone.

Surgical pathology

Illingworth Sir Charles, Dick B. M. *A Textbook of Surgical Pathology*. Edinburgh: Churchill Livingstone.

Guthrie W., Fawkes R. *A Colour Atlas of Surgical Pathology*. London: Wolfe Medical Publications.

Curran R. C., Jones E. L. *Gross Pathology. A Colour Atlas*. London: H. M. & M. Publishers.

Royal College of Surgeons of Edinburgh. *A Colour Atlas of Demonstrations in Surgical Pathology* (1 – Alimentary System; 2 – Genitourinary System; 3 – Cardiovascular System; 4 – Orthopaedic Lesions). Contact the College for purchases.

Smiddy F. G., Cowen P. N. *Tutorials in Surgery*. No. 4 & 5. Tunbridge Wells: Pitman Medical.

Operative surgery

Farquarson's Textbook of Operative Surgery. Edinburgh: Churchill Livingstone.

Keen G. (ed). *Operative Surgery and Management*. Oxford: Butterworth–Heinemann.

Dudley H. A. F., Carter D. (eds). *Rob & Smith's Operative Surgery* (various volumes). London: Butterworths.

Rob C., Smith R. (eds). *Atlas of General Surgery*. Compiled by H. Dudley London: Butterworths.

Shipman J. J. (1977). *Operative Surgery Revision*. London: H. K. Lewis.

Smiddy F. G. *Tutorials in Surgery*, No. 3. Tunbridge Wells: Pitman Medical.

Kirk R. M. *General Surgical Operations*. Edinburgh: Churchill Livingstone.

Surgical principles and practice

Recent Advances in Surgery. Edinburgh: Churchill Livingstone.

N. B. The above series is excellent and candidates are encouraged to read (if not own) all available issues.

Surgical instruments

Any comprehensive general surgical catalogue, e.g. Thackray's Manufacturer's Catalogue.

Stanek J. *Surgical Diagnostic and Therapeutic Instruments*. Oxford: Blackwell Scientific Publications.

Brigden R. J. (1980). *Operating Theatre Technique*. Edinburgh: Churchill Livingstone.

Brooks S. M. (1982). *Instrumentation for the Operating Room*. St Louis: Mosby.

Journals

Review of the following journals of the last year is recommended to keep you up to date. (Examiners often read these journals just before the examination or on the train while travelling to the college to examine you.) However, this is not an examination necessity, especially if you have mastered other fields of surgery.

The leading useful journals are:

British Journal of Surgery.

The Journal of the Royal College of Surgeons of Edinburgh.

Annals of the Royal College of Surgeons of England.

Surgery edited by J. Lumley & J. Craven (review articles).

Annual Review of General Surgery, in *Postgraduate Medical Journal* (June or July issue usually). This review is extremely useful and time saving.

British Journal of Hospital Medicine and *Hospital Update* provide excellent review articles for the final FRCS.

Surgery

Annals of Surgery

Surgery Gynecology and Obstetrics

Some of the leading articles in the *Lancet* and *British Medical Journal.*

Others

Shipman J. J. *Mnemonics and Tactics in Surgery and Medicine.* London: Lloyd-Luke.

Lourie J. *Medical Eponyms: Who Was Coudé?* London: Pitman.

Jablonski S. *Illustrated Dictionary of Eponymic Syndromes and Diseases and their Synonyms.* Philadelphia: W. B. Saunders.

Some Wolfe colour atlases (of surgical interest).

Butterworth International Medical Reviews (in surgery) including different volumes on *trauma, endocrine surgery, gastro-enterological surgery, vascular surgery.*

Tape-slide lecture programmes provided by Audiovisual Medical Libraries, e.g. Graves, and films from the Royal Society of Medicine (operative surgery).

SECTION 5
What to Do

Be precise and exact Get down to the nitty gritty of the surgical facts and principles since you are bound to be asked 'Why?'. Listen carefully and answer the exact question straight to the point. It is probably wiser to fractionate the answer, leaving the examiner a chance to interrupt you and re-ask you; e.g. if the examiner asks, 'What are the causes of obstructive jaundice?' answer by mentioning the individual causes according to the order of frequency, i.e. common bile duct stone then discuss carcinoma of head of pancreas, then metastatic deposits in the porta hepatis and so on. A wise candidate will talk clearly and slowly. Do not speak unless you are spoken to. Too much talk usually leads to mistakes.

Do not be clever, be careful Examination is not show business, it is a mutual discussion about basic surgical principles, logical approach and clinical judgement. Answer the basic simple questions with a basic simple answer. Answer to the point and try to steer the discussion into an area you feel confident about. If you are asked an unfair question, e.g. about hemihepatectomy, try to tackle it by saying 'I have never done the operation and I have never seen it done but the principles are as follows . . .' It is not shameful to admit you do not know but it is to tell lies which will easily expose your limited experience.

Keep in touch with surgery through discussions Discussion is the best means of preparation for the final FRCS:
- If there is a friend sitting the examination with you, discuss together various subjects, operations and the examination of patients.
- Attend all postgraduate meetings in your hospital and nearby hospitals if possible.
- Do not miss the surgical journal club of the hospital.
- Discuss every vague point about operations with your consultant.
- Attend teaching ward rounds.
- Participate in 'mock' examinations.
- Get the best of knowledge from the paramedical staff, such as physiotherapists (e.g. ask about therapeutic ultrasounds), theatre sisters (e.g. ask about surgical instruments), bacteriologists (e.g. ask about the timing and frequency of antibiotic blood assay such as gentamicin, infections and sepsis).

Filing system of collected data For reference purposes, you can classify the review articles and various collected literature in a filing cabinet drawer with the required number of files according to the system you propose to use. However, you should keep summaries of the common major subjects in one file for easily manageable quick revision. This book is meant to fill this gap . . . you can add to it if you think necessary.

Read less, digest more and learn surgery by illustrations The less you read theoretically and the more you digest of your little reading, the better. There is no place for encyclopaedic knowledge since this is for reference only and not for practical surgery. Remember key phrases. Read and re-read the same book again and again rather than getting into the habit of exploring new books. There is probably no need for journals although we do recommend reading the review articles, for instance those in the *British Journal of Hospital Medicine* and *Surgery* since it is a quick method of scanning all articles of past years (see Section 4). Learn surgery by drawing and diagrams since it is time-saving and an easy way to revise. Also learn surgery by mnemonics (see Section 4).

Put yourself in the examiner's chair When you see patients in the outpatient department or in the ward try to think in terms of interesting cases that could be presented in the examination. Examine the patients as if you are performing the short cases of the FRCS examination and improve your methods so that your methodical approach becomes routine, comprehensive and reflexly performed. Examine your friends and remember their mistakes and apply what you have learned when you are under the stress of the examination.

Never be preoccupied by what failed candidates say You will hear the full spectrum of rumours of racial discrimination, nationality discrimination, sex discrimination and hospital discrimination. Do not let them disturb your balance. Give them a deaf ear. They probably failed because they deserved to.

Examiner–examinee and examinee–patient relationship (see Part II, Section 2) The importance of gentle examination must be stressed (never manipulate patients as if they are experimental animals). Do not be argumentative or over-confident. Be straightforward and practical (think of priorities and common things before rare ones). Keep discussions simple.

Hope for the best and prepare for the worst Make every effort to prepare, but do not be too disappointed if you fail; there is always tomorrow and you can attempt the examination in other Colleges or wait for the next session in the same College.

Comment on courses Advanced courses are only valuable when all the basic training is complete. They are meant for orientation and guidance and quick revision of fully prepared candidates. Candidates, particularly those coming to the United Kingdom from overseas, are strongly urged to ascertain whether or not they are *eligible* to sit the examination before embarking upon academic courses of study or clinical training.

There is no point in preparing for an examination until you have all the facts about it at your fingertips. Check the syllabus, types of questions (from past examination papers), time allowed in the examination, dates/times of the examination, and where will the examination be held.

Revision plan

The best revision plan is a 6–8 week timetable drawn up by you and rigidly adhered to:
- If you fall behind on your schedule catch up on it by the end of the week.
- Set yourself an objective for each session.
- As soon as you settle down start work. Getting started is always the most difficult part.
- Rest for a few minutes every 30 minutes and simply think about what you have just read. Break for 30 minutes every 2 hrs; at this point you might find it relaxing to take some refreshment or chat to someone else or do something completely different like watching TV.
- Once you get started and whenever possible, continue the momentum of reading with intermissions but do not study at night. Keeping regular sleeping hours and being ready for a full day's work the next day is important, so stop at least one hour before your usual bedtime and do something you enjoy.
- If your revision is all reading you will find it helpful to sit where you are most comfortable.
- Set yourself a test each week.

Taking notes

Make only brief essential notes so that any spare time may be used for thinking about the topic.
- Effective note taking in courses is related to the way you personally see things; when you reread notes they should remind you of the main topics.
- Write down only the key points that the tutor or book cover; don't get bogged down by small details.
- Space your notes out so that you can easily find a particular topic on a page. Carry a small notebook with you to jot down any points that may suddenly occur to you.
- Use diagrams and illustrations wherever possible; diagrams help visual recall of a topic at revision time.
- Make sure you make complete references to chapters in books and articles that you have read in case you need to refer back to them later.
- Note-taking should follow you reading; do not make notes whilst you are reading.

Studying in groups is generally encouraged in courses of higher education; the purpose of working in a group is to develop a wider and deeper understanding of a topic through the pooling and questioning of ideas and your ability to answer examination questions.
- Discussion groups: may be formal (requires election of a chairman and speakers for and against the motion) or informal (more useful for revision purposes as they may take place at any time and in any place). The group must approach a problem on various levels and from different points of view, not to win an argument!

- Brainstorming sessions groups: this is like enforced discussion after presentation of as many facts and ideas on a topic or question as can be thought of within a given time. Major points relating to the topic or question from the pool of ideas amassed are extracted. Finally, select and agree on (even by vote) which way the problem or question should have been resolved or answered.
- Study groups: more useful in project or case-study work where a group is formed to examine a case, complete a project or resolve a problem. In a course or class, it is possible to have several separate groups working on exactly the same problem.

Role playing: a group of students work towards the solution of a problem by each playing a role so that the procedure simulates a possible real-life situation.
- Seminars: these are very useful in developing the student's ability to analyse. Seminars are basically discussion groups whose purpose and momentum are controlled by a tutor (the lecturer seats the students in a half-moon arrangement with the tutor seated in the centre at a point visible to all).

How to remember information

Familiarity is central to the learning process (face in the mirror, our telephone number, our home address) – to learn we must remember, and to remember we must make ourselves familiar with the subject in question. This is the aim of course-work and the aim of revision should be to consolidate your knowledge. The learning curve in all new procedures will always start by training, by assisting, by working under supervision, and then independently. The independent operator consolidates his/her experience by performing more cases until the steep learning curve plateaus.

Methods that aid memory include:
- good note-taking
- mnemonic
- objective test include in medicine OSCE (objectively structured clinical examination) by moving between stations with objective testing in a specified time. Tests vary from one question, single response (only one is true) multiple choice questions (MCQ), multiple response (many may be true or false) MCQ or matching questions/answers.
- picture association including diagrammatic notes
- word association by:
  - rhymes, for instance patient receives (I before E except after C)
  - stories of patients and catastrophic clinical events
  - sequences e.g. in life-threatening trauma follow the 3 Rs: Resuscitate, Review, then Repair; in rectal bleeding do per rectal digital examination, the sigmoidoscopy, then barium enema
  - making up words e.g. DVT means deep vein thrombosis; LASER is Light Amplification by Stimulated Emission of Radiation; LARP means Left (vagus) Anterior Right (vagus) Posterior
  - swot cards (pocket-sized cards carrying the most imortant information on a subject or topic usually in note form)
  - image patterns (shapes, photographs and maps)

● filling spaces, objects can also be easily remembered by mentally placing them in orderly fashion in files or spaces on desk (special tests for special condition in a special file)

Practice and revision cycle

Above all, keep the 3 Ps in mind:

        PRACTISE

Don't PANIC

        PACE yourself well

FINAL ADVICE

There is no doubt that the final FRCS is a formidable but fair examination. The difference between success and failure is marginal. The scoring system does not often pass more than 20% of attempting candidates. If you think you are going to fail after the written part, do not withdraw but finish all of the examination parts (since you have paid for it) and get the benefit of discussions, so that you can avoid any mistakes at a future attempt. It is my belief that following the above guidelines coupled with thorough preparation is the ideal way of approaching the examination for the final FRCS diploma. Too much reading is not advised. Keep a comprehensive surgical textbook (for reference) supplemented by a file of revision (e.g. this book), a clinical book (e.g. *Bailey's Demonstration of Physical Signs in Clinical Surgery*), an operative book you are used to and a book on surgical pathology – these are more than sufficient when coupled with good clinical and operative experience. You should read a sufficient number of journals to render you *au fait* with modern advances and current surgical practice.

SECTION 6
Historical Background

It has been said that 'those who cannot remember the past are condemned to repeat it'. This section on the historical origin and development of modern surgical science is included since it is essential that candidates sitting their examination for the higher postgraduate surgical diploma are familiar with the outstanding achievements of those leaders in surgery who have made the current operations easy, safe and daily routine procedures.

Examiners become annoyed when you mention a physical sign, law or operation named after a surgeon you do not know, and it is a great bonus for you if you are conversant with the historical background or at least know the nationality of the surgeon. The magnitude of the achievement of these men in any case warrants discussion of their work.

The history and pioneers of *surgical specialties* will not be considered here but only the history of *general surgery* and those historical figures who described physical signs and operations relevant to the final FRCS. As some surgical procedures could not be attributed mainly to one surgeon, these are described separately after the 'Names' section. The two sections have been cross-referenced where there is overlap.

THE DEVELOPMENT OF SURGERY

The history of disease is at least as old as the history of mankind. In ancient Egypt, papyri have been found dealing with medicine, surgery, obstetrics and gynaecology. The Edwin Smith papyrus written in about 1600 BC is one of the oldest and is of great interest to surgeons.

In the Babylonian code of Hammurabi there were severe penalties for the surgeon whose operations were unsuccessful (e.g. cutting off his right hand). In India, Susruta described more than 100 surgical instruments in the book *Susruta Samhita* written in Sanskrit around the eighth century BC. The Indian surgeons are best known for their skill in plastic surgery. In Greece, Hippocrates (the Father of Medicine) wrote 70 books around 400 BC. His book *On the Surgery* was mainly concerned with bandaging of various types of injuries (including fractures and dislocation).

The Roman encyclopaedist of the early first century AD, Aulus Cornelius Celsus, described four characteristics of inflammation: 'Rubor (redness), Tumor (swelling), Calor (heat) and Dolor (pain)' (to which one only can add loss of function for a perfect definition). Galen of the second century AD elaborated the Hippocratic principles and differentiated between surgery and medicine. In the later Middle Ages, the Muslims took the leading role (especially in the tenth century). It was Albucasis (AD 936–1013), the Moorish physician and surgeon of Andalusia ('a remarkable man, both prolific and courageous'), who described hundreds of surgical instruments and many operations in his famous book *Al-Tasrif*. He was the first to introduce the use of catgut and cotton sutures, he accomplished successful small intestinal anastomoses and was the first to operate on blood vessels. He performed the first successful thyroidectomy operation in literature, introduced the first delivery forceps and described many operations in orthopaedics, ophthalmology and gynaecology. He therefore deserves to be called 'the father of operative surgery'. Avicenna (AD 980–1037) was another remarkable physician in that period (see Arabic Medicine, Surgery and Legacy).

From the year 1300 onward surgery was looked down upon and avoided by physicians who had received their education in the universities, where, along with theology and law, medicine was usually one of the basic faculties. Surgeons, on the other hand, were of the lower class, and were scorned in clerical circles (*Ecclesia abhorret a sanguine* = the Church abhors blood). Surgeons were taught the ways of their craft by apprenticeship and their work was combined with that of barbers.

In 1543, Andrew Vesalius published his outstanding anatomy book based on cadaveric dissection: *De humani corporis fabrica*. The Scottish surgeon Peter Lowe (1550–1613) published the first real surgical textbook written in English, *A Discourse of the Whole Art of Chirurgerie* in 1597, and arranged his book under five headings: (1) to take away; (2) to help and add; (3) to put in place that which is out; (4) to separate; and (5) to join what is separated. He founded the Brethren of Chirurgerie (the forerunner of the Royal College of Physicians and Surgeons of Glasgow). He also asked for separation of surgeons from barbers.

In Paris, Ambroise Paré (1510–1590), the military surgeon, stressed the importance of anatomy in surgery and made remarkable contributions to wound healing and cauterisation. Alexis Littre (the father of colostomy), François De la Peyronie and others contributed tremendously to the fame of Paris in surgery. In 1743 the association with encumbering barbers was ended by Parisian surgeons (and was followed by London surgeons in 1745). Thus during nearly the whole of the eighteenth century Paris held pride of place as the centre of medical teaching and practice. The ambitious British or American doctor regarded a visit to Paris as an essential part of his training. The French world predominance continued until 1789.

Before the fame of Paris had started to wane, Edinburgh was already rising to the high place which it held until 1830. The Edinburgh school depended for its excellence upon a far higher standard of teaching than was to be found in any other centre. The Monro dynasty of anatomists and the outstanding anatomy teacher Robert Knox contributed to its name and fame. However in 1829 the series of murders committed by Burke and Hare of Edinburgh and the tracing of at least one body to

Knox's anatomy rooms created a sensation which ruined Knox and tarnished Edinburgh's good name. After a similar murder in London, the Anatomy Act of 1832 was passed which permitted authorised medical schools to acquire bodies for the purpose of dissection.

London had already started to rise before Edinburgh was passing into eclipse. The greatest of London teachers were Scots by birth or education. John Hunter left Glasgow in 1748 to study in London under William Cheselden of St Thomas' and Percival Pott of St Bartholomew's. He was later appointed to St George's Hospital. Hunter founded a school of anatomy and surgery in Leicester Square and became the leader of experimental surgery. In 1804 Charles Bell, a young surgeon, decided to leave Edinburgh for London (because of his poor income – £25 per year while Astley Cooper of England earned £15 000 per year). He established himself as a teacher and was appointed to the Middlesex Hospital after serving at the Battle of Waterloo. In 1835 Robert Liston, a famous surgeon of his time, left Edinburgh for University College Hospital, London. In 1839 William Fergusson left Edinburgh for King's College Hospital, thereby making that small institution behind Lincoln's Inn Fields the surgical centre of the world for a short time. As these men moved south London's influence rose inevitably, at the expense of that of Edinburgh.

The major Scottish invasion of surgical London came about as the result of the foundation of new London hospitals. For over 500 years the two medieval hospitals of St Bartholomew's and St Thomas' were the only institutions which could possibly be given the name of teaching centres, but during the eighteenth century the rapid expansion of London made the provision of free treatment for the sick poor an urgent necessity. Thus came into being, often as outpatient dispensaries in origin, the Westminster (1715), Guy's (founded as a kind of annexe for the chronically sick patients of St Thomas' in 1721), St George's (1733), the London (1740), and the Middlesex (1745). In all cases the medical schools attached to these hospitals are of a later date, the earliest being that of the Middlesex, where an organised course of lectures commenced in 1785. The year 1821 saw the foundation of the first 'teaching hospital', when Dr Benjamin Golding opened Charing Cross 'to supply the want of a university, so far as medical education is concerned'. University College Hospital, first known as the North London, and King's College Hospital were founded in 1834 and 1839 respectively, for the express purpose of providing clinical instruction for the students of University College in Gower Street and King's College in the Strand.

London maintained world supremacy from 1830 until shortly after the Franco-Prussian war of 1870 when initiative passed to the victorious Germanic nations. Germany, alone among nations, accepted Lister's antisepsis wholeheartedly (in 1875 Lister made a tour of the larger centres in Germany). Outstanding surgeons like Volkmann, Esmarch, Thiersch, Langenbeck, Mikulicz, Billroth, Kocher and others contributed to the high surgical standards of Germany which dominated the world from 1870 until the end of the nineteenth century when the USA began to move up to the leading place owing to the remarkable efforts of American surgeons like Halsted of Johns Hopkins Hospital (Baltimore), the Mayo brothers of Rochester, Murphy and Oschner of Chicago, McBurney of New York and

many others. The USA maintained its supremacy until the Second World War, and since then, the American and British schools have emerged as the main leaders in the field of surgery.

NAMES TO BE REMEMBERED

The following list of names is far from complete: however it is more than sufficient for the purposes of the final FRCS.

Abdul Latif Al-Baghdadi. When Saladin's armies returned from Acre to Jerusalem to sign a peace treaty with the Crusaders (1192 AD), his private doctor, Abdul Latif Al-Baghdadi, collected as much as he could of the writings of the Ancients and showed them to Saladin who immediately ordered a study grant to be paid to Abdul Latif during his sojourn in Damascus. After Saladin's death, Abdul Latif left for Cairo to lecture. There, he witnessed the famine that ravaged the population in 1199–1202 AD and had the unique opportunity of examining thousands of bodies of people who had died of starvation. The results of his anatomical studies were published in his book '*Notification and Considerations of Observed Matters and Inspected Occurences in the Land of Egypt*' (Al-Ifada Wal Itibar Fil Umur Al-Mushahada Wa-Hawadith Al-Muayana Bi-Ardi Misr), which he completed in 1207 AD. He described the structure of skeletons and reviewed the human anatomy. He corrected Galen on the structure of the lower jaw, concluding that it consisted of one piece, not two as Galen had claimed in his book '*On Anatomy of Bones*' (Fi Tashrih Al-Izam).

Addison, Thomas (1793–1860) Physician, Guy's Hospital, London, UK. He described Addison's disease – adrenal medullary hypofunctioning leading to hypogyloaemia, hypotension and pigmentation with hyperkalaemia and hyponatraemia.

Adson, Alfred W. (1887–1951) Neurosurgeon, The Mayo Clinic, Rochester, Minnesota, USA. He described the Adson deep-breathing test in which the radial pulse is diminished if the patient turns his head to the side of the cervical rib and inspires deeply (because of pressure of the scalenus anterior accessory respiratory muscle).

Albucasis or **Abu Al-Qasim Al-Zahrawi**, or **Abulcasis** (AD 936–1013) He may be called the father of operative surgery. He was the first to operate on blood vessels. He invented the animal gut suture and used it for the first successful intestinal anastomosis reported in the literature. He documented the possible spontaneous healing of faecal fistulas. In his book *Al-Tasri Liman Ajaza An Al Ta'leef* he described many operative procedures using more than 100 surgical instruments that do not appear in extant classical writings and which may therefore be regarded as his own, or at least as being part of distinctively Arab practice. Among these are the tonsil guillotine, the concealed knife and its case for opening abscesses, catheter, trocar for paracentesis, syringe, lithotrite, vaginal speculum, the true scissors, obstetric forceps that anticipate Chamberlain's, and the use of a kind of plaster casing that anticipates the modern plaster cast.

Albucasis and the history of laparotomy Muslim surgeons were the first to explore the closed abdominal cavity;

they pioneered both labarotomy and Caesarean section. Albucasis, in chapter 85 of the second section of his book, entitled 'On wounds of the abdomen, and protrusion of the intestine; and on suturing them', produced the first and the most authentic description ever contained in the literature on abdominal trauma, its complications and the surgical treatment required. Albucasis described three types of abdominal tear, and explained that reduction of protruded gut may be difficult for two reasons: either on account of a small abdominal tear, or because the gut has become inflated on account of exposure to cold air; he recommended warming the gut by fomentation with a sponge or piece of cloth bathed with warm water. Albucasis described the best patient positioning while performing surgery on such cases: in lower abdominal injury, he recommended legs in elevation while the patient is supine (lying on the back) to allow gravity to aid in reduction. Conversely, upper abdominal injury necessitates head elevation. He then described five methods of abdominal wound closure. As for the medical treatment of wounds, Albucasis recommended that bleeders must be sought out; they then must either be ligated or cauterised; small oozers can be controlled by pressure with a pad soaked in wine and olive-oil or vinegar and olive-oil. Any sign of inflammation requires dressing with cotton wool soaked in oil of roses with or without astringent beverage. If there is no inflammation, then the wound with its fresh blood can be sprinkled by a powder (composed of olibanum, dragon's blood, and lime all beaten and sieved) to bind the wound tightly. If the wound becomes purulent it should be dressed twice daily with teased-out cotton wool until dry and could be washed by honey-water daily. For an extensive abdominal wound soft wool dipped in warm olive-oil or oil of roses bound around the abdomen is recommended. Gangrenous omentum must be ligated above the line of gangrene and cut off. As far as the viability of the intestine is concerned, the gangrenous segment must be cut off and repaired as for a small intestinal wound. The method of suturing of intestine is by application of large ants with open jaws on the suture line and when the ants close their jaws their heads can be cut off. Evidently, Albucasis here is using Arabian ant nippers to act like the modern Michel clips, but furthermore, ants secrete formic acid in their oral secretion, an antiseptic material acting directly at the suture line (hence the name *Formicae* for ants). Ant nippers are used by African tribes as a way of bringing skin edges together. Albucasis explained that the intestine may also be sewn up with the fine suture extracted from an animal's gut after being threaded in a needle. The rubbed-down gut is well scraped and well cleansed prior to drying. While gut was used by the earliest Greeks for bow-strings, it was never used for surgical purposes until the Arab era of surgery. Albucasis' book, therefore, represents the earliest reference to this now universal suture material

Alcock, Benjamin (b. 1801) Professor of Anatomy, Cork, Republic of Ireland. He described Alcock's canal in ischiorectal fossa (contains pudendal nerve which is easily blocked with local anaesthetic).

Amyand, Claudius Surgeon, St George's Hospital, London, UK. Performed the first appendicectomy in 1736 (see Appendicectomy, p. xx).

Apley, Alan G. Contemporary orthopaedic surgeon, St Thomas' Hospital, London, UK. He introduced Apley's test in medial meniscus injury. The patient lies prone and examiner stands on the affected side and grasps that foot with both hands flexing the knee to a right angle; lateral rotation produces pain in medial ligament injury while lateral rotation with compression (grinding test) produces pain in medial meniscus injury. To test medial structures rotation should be medial.

Argyll Robertson (1837–1909) Ophthalmic surgeon, Edinburgh Royal Infirmary, UK. Argyll Robertson pupils are small irregular pupils in tabes dorsalis (accommodation reflex present and light reflex absent).

Arnold, Julius (1835–1915) Professor of Pathological Anatomy, Heidelberg, Germany. With **Chiari, Hans** (1851–1916), Professor of Pathological Anatomy, Strasburg, Germany, described Arnold-Chiari malformation (displacement of the hind brain and herniation into the spinal canal of the cerebellar tonsils obstructing the free circulation of cerebrospinal fluid leading to hydrocephalus).

Atkins, Sir Hedley (1905–1983), Past PRCS, Emeritus Professor of Surgery, Guy's Hospital London, UK. He described the extended tyelectomy treatment in breast carcinoma and introduced the macrodochectomy in intraduct papilloma.

Avicenna (AD 980–1037) A famous physician and a great anatomist. He wrote 'Al-Canon Fil-Tibb' (The Law of Medicine, in 3 volumes) which lasted for centuries as *the* medical textbook, later translated into Latin. He was one of the first doctors to illustrate the human vessels. Avicenna, however, accepted Galen's concept of blood passage via invisible pores.

Babiniski, Joseph F. F. (1857–1932) Head of the Neurological Clinic, Hôpital Pitie, Paris, France. He described Babiniski sign in the contralateral brain upper motor neurone lesion.

Baker, William (1838–96) Surgeon, St Bartholomew's Hospital, London, UK. He described Baker's cyst (a popliteal swelling, often bilateral, occurring in patients over 40 years of age. It is a pressure diverticulum of the synovial membrane through a hiatus in the capsule of the knee joint. It stands out when the knee is fully extended).

Barlow, Thomas G. (1915–75) Surgeon, Hope Hospital, Manchester, UK. Together with **Ortolani, Marino** (Contemporary Director, Centre for Congenital Subluxation of the Hip, Italy) described Barlow–Ortolani test (during abduction of the flexed hips and knees, the examiner's middle fingers on the greater trochanters can reduce the already dislocated hip with a palpable jerk. Removal of the hands leads to another jerk due to dislocation which can also be shown by pressing the thumbs on the thigh from the inside).

Bartholin, Casper (1655–1738) Professor of Medicine, Anatomy and Physics, Copenhagen, Denmark. He described Bartholin's gland in labium majus infection which leads to Bartholin's abscess.

Bassini, Edoardo (1844–1924) Senator of Italy (Paria) and pioneer of (Bassini) repair of inguinal hernia (interrupted closure of conjoined tendon to inguinal ligament) which has stood the test of time. He is also credited with the first attempt to bypass a stone impacted in the bile duct by joining the gallbladder to the duodenum (1882) and he was one of the earliest surgeons to perform a gastroenterostomy.

Battle, William H. (1855–1936) Surgeon, St Thomas' Hospital, London, UK. He advised the use of a special incision for appendicectomy. Battle's sign is the bruising over the mastoid process appearing a day or two after head injury – confirms a diagnosis of middle cranial fossa fracture.

Bell, Sir Charles (1774–1842) Scottish surgeon at Middlesex Hospital, London, UK. Later Professor of Surgery, Edinburgh, UK. He described Bell's (facial nerve) palsy as well as the nerve of Bell (nerve of latissimus dorsi which needs to be preserved in mastectomy).

Bennett, Edward H. (1837–1907) Professor of Surgery, Trinity College, Dublin, Republic of Ireland. He described Bennett's fracture (fracture-dislocation of first metacarpophalangeal joint).

Billroth, Theodor (1829–1894) German surgeon, born on the Island of Rugen in 1829 and graduated from Berlin University in 1852. He became Langenbeck's assistant at Berlin and Professor of Surgery at Zurich in 1860 and moved to Vienna 7 years later where he founded the famous Viennese School of Surgery. In 1872 he resected the oesophagus and in 1873 he performed the first total excision of the larynx for cancer. In January 1881 he performed the first successful partial gastrectomy for pyloric cancer in a 43-year-old woman. He made an incision through the abdominal wall about 8 cm long transversely over the tumour, which he found to be of large size, involving more than one-third of the lower portion of the stomach. He brought the tumour to the surface (with some difficulty because of the small incision), made openings into the stomach and duodenum above and below the tumour, then cut it away. Next he stitched up the major part of the hole in the stomach so that it exactly fitted the hole in the duodenum and sewed the two together with about 50 sutures of carbolised silk. The portion of stomach removed measured 14 cm along its greatest length. 'The operation lasted, including the slowly induced anaesthesia, about $1\frac{1}{2}$ hours', wrote Billroth. 'No weakness, no vomiting, no pain after the operation. Within the first 24 hours only ice by mouth, then peptone enema with wine. The following day, first every hour, then every half hour, one tablespoon of sour milk. Patient, a very understanding woman, feels well, lies extremely quiet, sleeps most of the night with the help of small injection of morphia. No pain in the operative area, subfebrile reaction. The dressing has not been changed.'

Billroth was an exceptional man. He turned his attention later on to rectal carcinoma and is credited with being first surgeon to remove a cancer of the rectum in 1868; by 1876 he had performed 33 such operations. Between 1878 and 1892 he became interested in intestinal resection and in what was then called 'enterorrhaphies' (short-circuiting of one part of the bowel to another).

The special method of stitching the bowel, the inverting seromuscular suture, which had been invented in 1826 by the French surgeon Antoine Lembert, did not come into more than limited use until Billroth started his series of operations. It is of some interest that, at a meeting in 1879, Howard Marsh of St Bartholomew's Hospital reported twoses in which Billroth had divided the bowel and united the cut ends by Lembert sutures. 'Such suture of the divided bowel', said Marsh, 'promises good results.' Here is a clear indication of Billroth's influence during his lifetime. Halsted later demonstrated that the tough submucosa had to be secured for reliable single-layer anastomosis.

The early surgeons often put in as many as 200 sutures when performing an ordinary gastroenterostomy to avoid peritonitis but this not infrequently defeated its own purpose by weakening the walls of the gut. In 1888 Nicholas Senn of Rush Medical College, USA, introduced perforated plates of bone, which could be inserted into the lumen of the two cut ends of the bowel. These were largely replaced by the American J. B. Murphy's 'buttons' in 1892 and the 'bobbins' devised by Mayo Robson of Leeds in 1893. The principle was the same: the divided discs or buttons were inserted into the lumen of the two cut bowel ends, anchored by a purse string suture, clamped together and oversewn, a simple innovation which restored continuity of the bowel without multitudinous stitches.

Bowen, John T. (1857–1941) Professor of Dermatology, Harvard Medical School, Massachusetts, USA. He described premalignant Bowen's skin disease (brown induration with a well-defined edge; microscopy reveals large clear cells. It needs wide excision).

Brodie, Sir Benjamin Collins (1783–1862) Surgeon, St George's Hospital, London, UK. He was chosen to be the first President of the General Medical Council. He described Brodie's abscess of bones and serocystic disease of Brodie (sarcoma). With Trendelenburg he described the test of saphinofemoral incompetence in varicose veins.

Brown-Séquard, Charles E. (1818–1894) Professor of Medicine at Harvard, Massachusetts, USA and Paris, France. He described the Brown-Sequard syndrome in spinal cord hemisection or laterally protruded disc leading to distal loss of motor power on the side of the lesion and loss of pain on the contralateral side.

Browne, Sir Denis (1892–1967) Surgeon, Hospital for Sick Children, Great Ormond Street, London, UK. He described the Denis Browne splint for clubfoot and the Denis Browne operation for hypospadias.

Buerger, Leo (1879–1943) Professor of Urology, Polyclinic Medical School, New York, USA. He described Buerger's disease (presenile atherosclerosis or thromboangitis obliterans in males). Buerger's postural test (both legs are elevated straight for 2 min supported by the examiner; after ankle flexion and extension by the patient the sole of the foot assumes a cadaveric pallor and when legs are lowered the colour changes to a ruddy, cyanotic hue) signifies a major lower limb arterial occlusion. Buerger's position is elevation of the bed head to relieve rest pain in lower limb vascular insufficiency.

Burkitt, Denis P. Contemporary surgeon, Member of External Scientific Staff, Medical Research Council, London, UK. He described Burkitt's lymphoma in 1958 in tropical parts of Africa, which affects children of equal sexes manifested in 80% of cases by jaw tumour which responds dramatically to chemotherapy. The viral aetiology was supported by mosquito vector and he found that above certain heights (mosquito-free area) there were no cases of Burkitt lymphoma.

Burns, Allan (1781–1813) Lecturer in Anatomy and Surgery, Glasgow, UK. He described Burns' space, a suprasternal space, swelling of which may be dermoid, enlarged lymph node (or cold tuberculous abscess), lipoma, aneurysm of the innominate artery or, rarely, a low thyroglossal cyst.

Camper, Peter (1722–89) Professor of Medicine, Anatomy, Surgery and Botany, Gröningen, Holland. He described Camper's fascia in the anterior abdominal wall.

Chagas, Carlos (1879–1934) Brazilian physician. He described South American trypanosomiasis which affects the oesophagus producing achalasia.

Charcot, Jean-Martin (1825–93) Physician, Hôpital Salpetriere, Paris, France. Described Charcot's triad in ascending cholangitis due to common bile duct stone (pain, jaundice and rigors due to septicaemia). He also described the painless flail joint with effusion due to neuropathy, i.e. Charcot's joint (in tabes dorsalis) as well as Charcot's hysterical blue oedema (the dependent limb becomes cyanosed and swollen from lack of use). In the upper limbs disuse atrophy leads to bone decalcification similar to post-traumatic painful bone atrophy (described by **Paul Sudeck**, 1866–1945, Professor of Surgery in Hamburg).

Cheyne, John (1777–1836) Physician, Meath Hospital, Dublin, Republic of Ireland. With **William Stokes**, (1804–1878), Regius Professor of Physics, University of Dublin, Republic of Ireland, described Cheyne–Stokes (periodic) respiration in brain stem injury, and a variety of conditions (e.g. respiratory failure, carbon dioxide narcosis and drug poisoning).

Chvostek, František (1835–84) Physician, Vienna, Austria. He described Chvostek sign – gentle tapping of the facial nerve in front of the external auditory meatus with a percussion hammer, producing a brisk twitch on that facial side in tetany.

Cloquet, Jules G. (1790–1883) Surgeon, Hospital St Louis, Paris, France. He described 'lymph node of Cloquet', enlargement of which simulates an irreducible femoral hernia (see Gimbernat).

Cock, Edward (1805–92) Surgeon, Guy's Hospital, London, UK. He described 'Cock's Peculiar Tumour' a suppurating and ulcerating sebaceous cyst of the scalp simulating a squamous cell carcinoma.

Cockett, Frank B. Contemporary surgeon, St Thomas' Hospital, London, UK. He described the venous 'blow-out' at sites of perforators due to reverse high-pressure reflux. He recommended subfascial ligation of perforators.

Codman, Ernest A. (1869–1940) Surgeon, Massachusetts General Hospital, Boston, USA. He described Codman's triangle – a radiological appearance seen in osteogenic sarcoma. He also described Codman's method of shoulder joint examination.

Colles, Abraham (1773–1843) Professor of Anatomy and Surgery, Dublin, Republic of Ireland. He described Colles' fascia which is fused with the triangular ligament preventing urine extravasation (backwards beyond the middle perineal point); it is continuous with Scarpa's fascia permitting superficial urine extravasation beneath the latter fascia. He also described Colles' fracture of the distal end of the radius (dinner-fork deformity).

Courvoisier, Ludwig (1843–1918) Professor of Surgery in Basle, Switzerland. He described Courvoisier's law.

Cullen, Thomas S. (1868–1953) Professor of Gynecology, Johns Hopkins University, Baltimore, Maryland, USA. He described Cullen's sign (discoloured umbilicus or black-eye sign) in ruptured ectopic pregnancy and acute pancreatitis.

Curling, T. B. (1811–88) In 1842 described stress ulceration in burned patients (first described by Swan in 1823).

Cushing, Harvey (1869–1939) Professor of Surgery, Harvard University, Massachusetts, USA. He described stress ulcer accompanying lesions of the CNS and following neurosurgical operations. (Billroth in 1860 noted stress ulcers after operation and sepsis.) He also described 'Cushing's syndrome' which is due to hyperadrenocorticism; hyperadrenocorticism secondary to pituitary tumour is termed 'Cushing's disease'.

De Morgan, Campbell (1811–76) Surgeon, Middlesex Hospital, London, UK. He described de Morgan's spots, raspberry-red tiny capillary angiomas which do not show the sign of emptying (they do not blanche when compressed). They are of no clinical significance.

Denonvilliers, Charles P. (1808–72) Surgeon, Paris, France. He described Denonvilliers' fascia between the rectum and bladder (and prostate).

De Quervain, Fritz (1868–1940) Professor of Surgery, Berne, Switzerland. He described subacute 'de Quervain's thyroiditis' with viral aetiology and possible spontaneous recovery. He also described de Quervain's disease (or stenosing tenosynovitis) which affects the common tendon sheath (of abductor pollicis longus and extensor pollicis brevis) in adult females.

Dercum, Francis K. (1865–1931) Professor of Neurology, Jefferson Medical College, Philadelphia, USA. He described Dercum's disease or adiposis dolorosa – multiple subcutaneous lipomas, one of which is painful or at least tender.

Doppler, Christian J. (1803–53) Austrian physicist who invented Doppler ultrasonic blood velocity detector.

Dormia, Enrico Contemporary Assistant Professor of Urology, Milan, Italy. He invented the Dormia basket for fishing and removal of lower ureteric stones through a cystoscope (stone should be in lower 5 cm of ureter and not more than 0.5 cm in diameter). Its uses have been extended to residual biliary stone retrieval and bronchial foreign body removal.

Dukes, Cuthbert, E. (1890–1977) Pathologist, St Mark's Hospital, London, UK. He described Dukes' staging in rectal cancer. The staging is sometimes applied to colonic and urinary bladder cancer:

> Stage A: The growth is limited to the rectal wall in 15% (5 year survival is 80–90%).
>
> Stage B: The growth is extended to extrarectal tissues (excluding lymph nodes) in 35% (5 year survival is 70–80%).
>
> Stage C: Lymph node involvement (50%) which can be either local distal pararectal (C_1) or proximal lymph nodes accompanying the supplying blood vessels (C_2) (5 year survival is 30–50%).

Broder's Grading (Broders, Albert C. 1885–1964, Pathologist to the Mayo Clinic, Rochester, USA) is related not to the stage of spread but to the microscopic degree of differentiation:

Grade I: Least malignant with less than 25% cellular undifferentiation.
Grade II: 25–50% undifferentiation.
Grade III: 50–75% undifferentiation.
Grade IV: Over 75% undifferentiation–anaplastic.

The classification adopted by the International Union against cancer is the TNM. Tumour size: T1 < 2 cm, T2 < 5 cm, T3 < 10 cm. Node (lymph): N0 nil, N1 unilateral mobile, N2 unilateral fixed and N3 contralateral or another regional node enlargement. Metastasis: M0 nil or M1 with metastasis. This classification is applied to many cancers especially breast cancer (but not colorectal cancer).

Dupuytren, Baron Guillaune (1777–1835) Surgeon, Paris, France. He described Dupuytren's contracture (contracted thickened palmar fascia adherent to skin puckering ring finger mainly and little finger latterly; usually affects males). It should be differentiated from bilateral congenital soft tissue contracture of the little finger (ring finger is rarely affected). He also described Dupuytren's fracture (sustained by falling on to the feet–the talus is driven upwards with the ligaments supporting it, producing inferior tibiofibular diastasis).

Esmarch, Friedrich Von (1823–1908) German military surgeon of Kiel. Wrote treatises on first aid and in 1861 organised a scheme for the proper siting of field hospitals and bandaging stations in relation to the battle line. Esmarch's bandage or tourniquet, a long rubber strip to produce a bloodless limb by compression (1–1½ h for upper limbs and 1½–2 h for lower limbs) was introduced in 1873.

Ewing, James (1866–1943) Professor of Oncology, Cornell University Medical College, New York, USA. He described Ewing's sarcoma of the long bones in males with rapid response to radiotherapy.

Fegan, George Contemporary Emeritus Professor of Surgery, Trinity College, Dublin, Republic of Ireland. He introduced Fegan's 'injection-compression technique' for varicose veins. Fegan's method of seeking the sites of perforators for injection is done by marking as follows. First, with the patient in a standing position, the varicosities are marked with a skin pen. The patient then lies down, raising the affected limb and resting the heel against the examiner's chest. The marked line is palpated for gaps in the deep fascia through which perforators pass, and these are marked with an X.

Fogarty, Thomas Contemporary surgeon, University of Oregon Medical School, Portland, USA. He invented Fogarty's catheter for embolectomy. It is also used for biliary stone removal.

Foley, Frederic E. B. (1891–1966) Urologist, Miller and Ancker Hospitals, USA. He invented Foley's self-retaining urinary catheter which can be used not only for drainage of urine in urinary retention or incontinence but for its balloon pressure therapeutic effect after prostatectomy (for haemostasis). Also used in cholecystostomy, gastrostomy, jejunostomy and caecostomy. Malecot (French) is another self-retaining catheter.

Fournier (see **Meleney**).

Frey, Lucja (1889–1944) Physician, Neurological Clinic, Warsaw, Poland. She described Frey's syndrome in post-parotidectomy or after incision for suppurative parotitis (e.g. in typhoid fever and typhus) manifested by unilateral facial flushing, sweating, pain and hyperaesthesia in the area supplied by the auriculotemporal nerve following eating, especially spicy or sour food (also called the gustatory sweating syndrome). Frey was killed during the German occupation of Poland.

Fröhlich, Alfred (1871–1953) Professor of Pharmacology and Toxicology, Vienna, Austria. He described Fröhlich's syndrome (hypogonadism in children with obesity due to craniopharyngioma or fractured base of the skull).

Galeazzi, Riccardo (1866–1952) Director of the Orthopaedic Clinic, Milan, Italy. He described Galeazzi fracture-dislocation (fracture of the radius with dislocation of lower radioulnar joint).

Gimbernat, Don Antonio De (1734–1816) Professor of Anatomy, Barcelona, Spain. He described Gimbernat's (lacunar) ligament as a medial concave sharp border of the femoral canal ring. The posterior border comprises Cooper's (iliopectineal) ligament and fascia covering the pectineus muscle (Sir Astley Cooper, 1768–1841, Surgeon to Guy's Hospital, London, UK. He also described ligaments of Cooper in the breast along which cancer cells creep, infiltrating and puckering the overlying skin). Anteriorly the Poupart (inguinal) ligament is found (after Francois Poupart 1661–1708, Surgeon, Hotel Dieu, Paris, France). Laterally the femoral canal is bounded by the femoral vein. The femoral canal contains lymphatic vessels and the lymph node of Cloquet.

Goodsall, David H. (1843–1906) Surgeon, St Mark's Hospital, London, UK. He described Goodsall's rule (fistulae with an external opening within the anterior half of the anus are direct while those within the posterior half of the anus are indirect, uniting first then opening into the midline posteriorly after a horseshoe course).

Graves, Robert J. (1796–1853) Physician, Meath Hospital, Dublin, Republic of Ireland. He described Graves' disease or primary thyrotoxicosis manifested by diffuse symmetrical goitre, with tremor and anxiety (CNS), eye signs and pretibial myxoedema and treated medically (different from secondary thyrotoxicosis occurring in a multinodular goitre with ectopics, arrhythmias (CVS), no eye signs or pretibial myxoedema and treated surgically).

Grawitz, Paul A. (1850–1932) Professor of Pathology, Greifswald, Germany. He described renal cell adenocarcinoma (Grawitz's tumour in adults).

Halsted, William Stewart (1852–1922) Surgeon, Johns Hopkins Hospital, USA. Introduced the use of rubber gloves for the first time (used initially for protection of his theatre nurse, Caroline Hampton, who had contact rash with antiseptics; Halsted later married her). He taught the modern doctrine that surgical safety lies in avoidance of blood loss, meticulous care and gentle handling of the tissues. He was the pioneer of radical mastectomy and Halsted's repair of hernia (closure of external oblique posterior to the cord). He invented the Halsted needle holder and fine mosquito artery forceps. Kraske (Freiburg, Germany), Wertheim and Billroth (Vienna, Austria), Miles (London, UK) and Halsted (Baltimore, USA) were the originators of the concept of the complete operation for all malignant diseases. Halsted discovered the local anaesthetic properties of cocaine and was the first to use regional anaesthesia. However, he became an addict of narcotic drugs until he died.

Haly Abbas Al-Majusi (AD ?–994). When he dedicated a whole section to surgery in his famous book *Kamil Al-Sina'ah* Al Tibbiah or *Al-Kitab Al-Malaki* (Liber Regius, in 2 volumes), he established a milestone in the history of surgical sciences. Haly was the first Muslim surgeon to describe blood movement and general circulation seven centuries before Englishman **William Harvey**. (1578–1657) who described it in his two books, *On the Motion of the Heart and Blood in Animals* and *On the Circulation of the Blood*. Although Haly fell into the trap of the Galenic concept of invisible interventricular pores of the heart, his views represented a scientific breakthrough at the time. He was also the first doctor in history to describe the capillary vessels, seven centuries before **Marcello Malpighi** (1628–1694) of Italy. (For further discussion see The Arabic legacy, p. xx.)

Harrison, Edwin (1779–1847) Physician, St Marylebone Infirmary, London, UK. He described Harrison's sulcus or groove at the costochondral junctions in the rachitic chest.

Hashimoto, Hakaru (1881–1934) Director of the Hashimoto Hospital, Miyo, Japan. He described Hashimoto's thyroiditis (or struma lymphomatosa) with hypothyroidism.

Hasselbach, Franz K. (1759–1816) Professor of Surgery, Würzburg, Germany. He described Hasselbach's inguinal triangle through which direct inguinal hernia passes (bounded by inguinal ligament, lateral border of the rectus sheath and inferior epigastric vessels.)

Hirschsprung, Harald (1830–1916) Physician, Queen Louise Hospital for Children, Copenhagen, Denmark. He described Hirschsprung's disease of congenital aganglionic (parasympathetic) megacolon manifested within 3 days of birth. Secondary acquired megacolon is also described in older children with anal fissure and also in Chagas' disease.

Hodgkin, Thomas (1798–1866) Curator of the Museum of Guy's Hospital, London, UK (after his failure to obtain the post of Physician). He described Hodgkin's lymphoma.

Homans, John (1877–1954) Professor of Clinical Surgery, Harvard University, Boston, USA. He described Homans' sign (passive dorsiflexion of the foot causes calf pain in deep venous thrombosis). Such a sign may be dangerous to elicit as it may detach the thrombus, causing embolism; furthermore, if negative, it does not exclude the diagnosis of thrombosis.

Horner, Johann F. (1831–86) Professor of Ophthalmology, Zurich, Switzerland. He described Horner's syndrome (myosis, ptosis, enophthalmus and anhidrosis) in injury of the cervical sympathetic chain.

Houston, John (1802–45) Physician, City of Dublin Hospital, Republic of Ireland. He described anal valves of Houston.

Hunter, John (1728–93) The first English-speaking exponent of scientific medical research. Although a stumbling, tongue-tied lecturer he successfully demonstrated the importance of the cause of disease in relation to surgery. Born at Long Calderwood (near Glasgow) he set out for London at the age of 20 to study under William Cheseldon of St Thomas' and Percival Pott of St Bartholomew's. He was appointed to the surgical staff of St George's Hospital. His outlook can best be summed up in his quoted dictum (contained in a letter to Edward Jenner, the pioneer of vaccination) 'Why think? Why not try the experiment?'. He placed surgery on a scientific basis by correlating practice with comparative anatomy and physiological experiments. He founded a school of anatomy and surgery in Leicester Square and advocated arterial ligation to cure aneurysm. He described the Hunterian chancre (or primary syphilitic sore) but he thought that syphilis and gonorrhoea were manifestations of the same infection; to test his hypothesis he inoculated himself with a scalpel and died of an aortic aneurysm later on!

Hutchinson, Sir Jonathan (1828–1913) Surgeon, London Hospital, UK. He described Hutchinson's teeth in congenital syphilis.

Ibn Al-Nafis (Damascus, Syria). In AD 1288 he opposed both Avicenna and Galen vehemently on their concept of blood passage through invisible pores. He was the first to describe 'pulmonary circulation' (based on actual dissection) three centuries before Spaniard Michael Servetus who was executed by the Church in 1553 for challenging the Galenic concept of circulation. Ibn Al-Nafis also described coronary vessels and discussed systemic circulation vaguely in his book Shar'h Tashreeh Al-Canon (The Synopsis of Dissection in the Law in Medicine).

Ibn Al-Quff (AD 1233–86) Contemporary of Al-Nafis. In his book *Kitab Al-Omda Fi Al-Jiraha* (The Book of Mastery in Surgery in 2 volumes), he gave the most comprehensive description of surgical operations and treatment of bodily injuries contained in any Arabic text of its kind. He explained the function of the capillaries, reiterating Haly's views; he was the first doctor to discuss the unidirectional action of valves in veins and in heart chambers. He also made the first appeal for uniformity of standards for weights and measures used in medicine, pharmacy and surgery.

Kaposi, Moricz (1837–1902) Professor and Director of the Dermatological Clinic, Vienna, Austria. He described Kaposi's sarcoma among Jews from Poland (initially) affecting middle-aged males as multiple symptomless, plum-coloured nodules usually situated on the lower limbs.

Kehr, Hans (1862–1916) Professor of Surgery, Halberstadt, Germany. He described Kehr's sign (referred shoulder pain due to irritated diaphragm when patient lies flat on the back; occurs in intra-abdominal injury of the spleen or liver or in ruptured ectopic pregnancy).

Kocher, Theodor (1841–1917) Professor of Clinical Surgery, University of Berne, Switzerland. A pupil of Langenbeck and Billroth. He developed the surgical technique of thyroidectomy and described Kocher's collar incision and subcostal incision for biliary operation. In 1878 he drained a gall bladder abscess for the first time. He performed over 2000 thyroidectomies with a mortality of 4.5% (goitre is a particularly severe disease in his native Switzerland). He also described Kocher's manoeuvre in mobilisation of the second part of the duodenum. Positive Kocher's test is stridor induced by slight compression on the lateral lobes (in goitre) and indicates that the patient has an obstructed trachea. He received the Nobel Prize in 1909 (the first time it was awarded to a surgeon).

Krukenberg, Friedrich (1871–1946) Ophthalmologist, Halle, Germany. He wrote his thesis on malignant tumours of the ovary at 24 years of age. He described bilateral Krukenberg's ovarian tumours due to transcoelomic implantation of cancer cells in gut malignancies.

Latarjet, André (1876–1947) Professor of Anatomy, Lyons, France. He described nerves of Latarget in the stomach.

Leriche, René (1879–1956) Professor of Medicine at the Collège de France, Paris (the highest professional honour in France). He described Leriche's syndrome (thrombosis or atherosclerosis of the aortic bifurcation with intermittent claudication in the thighs or buttocks associated with impotence in men).

Lister, Joseph (1827–1912) Professor of Surgery, Glasgow, Edinburgh and King's College Hospital, London, UK. He is the leader of modern aseptic surgery, applying discoveries of Pasteur to surgery. He developed antiseptics that reduced postoperative wound infection and made possible the widespread use of sterile suture materials. He discovered bacteria in the suture strand and treated ligatures with carbolic acid.

Littré, Alexis (1658–1725) Surgeon and anatomist, Paris, France. He described the penile paraurethral Littré's glands. Littré's hernia is Meckel's diverticulum in a hernial sac. He also contributed to the development of colostomy (see, Colostomy, p.xx).

Lockwood, Charles B. (1856–1914) Surgeon, St Bartholomew's Hospital, London, UK. He described the low approach in femoral hernia.

Louis, Antoine (1723–92) French surgeon. He described the angle of Louis.

Ludwig, Wilhelm Von (1790–1865) German Professor of Surgery and Midwifery. He described Ludwig's angina, a cellulitis occurring beneath the deep cervical fascia with threatening respiratory obstruction (the mouth floor becomes oedematous).

Malgaigne, Joseph F. (1806–1865) Professor of Surgery, Paris, France. He described Malgaigne's groin bulgings normally seen in thin individuals.

Marion, Jean (1869–1960) Professor of Urology, Paris, France. He described Marion's disease: bladder neck enlargement in young boys. Marion's sign relates to non-visualisation of ureteric orifices due to enlarged bladder neck.

Marjolin (1780–1850) Surgeon, Paris, France. He described Marjolin's carcinomatous ulcer in burn scar. Later the term was applied to carcinoma secondary to a venous ulcer and chronic osteomyelitis ulcer.

Mayo, Charles Horace (1865–1939) **and William James** (1861–1939) (brothers) the latter described prepyloric vein (of Mayo) as well as Mayo's operation for para-umbilical hernias (can be used for all midline hernias).

Evolution of the Mayo Clinic In 1845 William Mayo, a native of Eccles, Scotland, who had read chemistry at Owens College, Manchester, emigrated to the USA where he became a doctor. William Worrall Mayo, had two sons, William James who was born at Le Sueur, Minnesota on 29 June 1861, and Charles Horace, born on 9th July 1865 at Rochester where William Worrall had set up his practice. Both sons studied medicine; William qualified in 1883 from the University of Michigan, Charles from North Western University in 1888.

In 1883 a devastating storm swept Rochester, causing much damage and loss of life. W. W. Mayo, with his two sons and the Sisters of the Order of Saint Francis, did valiant work among the injured. The Mother Superior of the Order decided to commemorate their work by building and endowing a small hospital of 50 beds in Rochester. The hospital of St Mary opened in 1889 with 15 patients, attended by five nursing Sisters, Sister Mary Joseph as surgical assistant, and Mother Alfred as Sister-in-Charge. The Mayo family formed the entire medical staff. This hospital was not a charitable institution. From the start, patients had to pay according to their means. But patients from charitable organisations were accepted without charge, and the patient's own word was regarded as sufficient guarantee of the scale upon which he would be required to pay.

Rochester, even today, is only a small town; in 1889 it was a village, served by no important road and not on a main railway line. For 10 years the Mayos worked quietly in something that was no more than a Cottage Hospital. Then, about the year 1900, William sent a paper to the American Annals of Surgery. His paper contained particulars of so many cases of successful treatment of gallstones that the incredulous editor came to see for himself. He was the first of many thousands of visitors to Rochester. The efficiency of the Staff Nurses could be easily concluded from the clinical observations imparted to William (about secondary cancer at the umbilicus) by Sister Joseph. This secondary deposit from the gastrointestinal tract cancer is called Sister Joseph nodule.

The brothers had kept well abreast of all the advances that had so recently been made; they were perhaps the first to understand that these advances were not only of great importance but had added to the complexity of medicine. They realised that if these 'ancillary departments' were to be fully used, they must be housed under one roof. They found that exact diagnosis demanded complete investigation. This became their basic principle: a painstaking, complete investigation of the patient by highly trained experts in a single clinic. At first the Mayos had to make themselves the experts; as their fame increased they trained others in their method until they had a team. Neither brother was any kind of a specialist at the start. It was not until after 1900 that they devoted their whole time to surgery; as the years passed 'Will' became the more expert in surgery of the abdomen, 'Charlie' in surgery of the head and neck. They made a perfect combination, bound together by a most unusual brotherly love and confidence, which manifested itself in the use of a joint wallet on which each urged the other to draw more heavily. Will was the better administrator, somewhat withdrawn, with a tendency to descend from on high to put all things in order; Charlie was the more original in thought, with a witty, friendly temperament that made for a happy and cooperative staff. Both brothers showed themselves remarkably shrewd in choosing their colleagues. It says much for the Mayos that they were so successful in building up and in keeping together their large staff, for Rochester was no cultural or social centre; the clinic and the work of the clinic had to be all-sufficing.

This work rapidly increased as their fame spread. By 1906 Will had performed 150 resections of the stomach for cancer with a 10% mortality and a 3 year survival in nearly 30% of cases; in one year (1906) he did 36 of these operations with only 1 death (Cheyne did his first in 1905). As the clinic grew in size the medical staff rose in number until there were more than 150 full-time members and twice that number of young graduates under instruction. The original small hospital expanded until the beds numbered between 1500 and 2000; in 1938 just over 1000 patients registered in a single day. The Mayos firmly believed in international exchange of knowledge and ideas. They and their staff travelled widely and they encouraged visitors to make use of their experience at Rochester. The brothers introduced a standard case-taking form, at a time when medical recording was still haphazard, on which all details of each patient were entered. The records were open to every member of the staff for consultation and discussion; from these discussions resulted the *Proceedings of the Staff Meetings of the Mayo Clinic*, in which many new advances and discoveries have been described.

As patients paid fees, often large fees, to the Clinic, a surplus of cash rapidly accumulated. In 1913 the brothers offered a sum of a million and a half dollars to the University of Minnesota for the purposes of medical education and research. Incredible though it may seem, the State Legislature made difficulties and it needed an impassioned address by Will before the scheme got under way. The Mayo Foundation, which does so much for research and postgraduate instruction, opened in 1915.

The two brothers, who had worked closely and successfully together, were not long separated by death. Charlie died on 26th May 1939, and Will 2 months later on 28th July. Their Clinic and their methods became the model for similar ventures in the USA. As we have seen, that great country could boast some excellent surgeons during the nineteenth century; it is largely through the efforts of the Mayo brothers that the USA has made such great strides in surgery during the past 60 years.

Meckel, Johann F. (1781–1833) Professor of Anatomy and Surgery, Halle, Germany. He described Meckel's diverticulum more clearly as a congenital antimesenteric full-layered diverticulum 5 cm in length and 60 cm from the iliocaecal junction occurring in 2% of patients. The diverticulum was first recognised by Littré and he called it an ileal appendix when he found it imprisoned in the hernial sac (Littré hernia).

Meleney, Frank L. (1889–1963) Professor of Clinical Surgery, Columbia University, New York, USA. In 1924 he described a spreading gangrene in superficial tissues following surgery, trauma or sepsis. The name necrotising fasciitis was introduced by B. Wilson (USA, 1952) to indicate non-specific redness, swelling and oedema around a primary wound which if untreated leads to acute rapid skin gangrene. The patient is usually suffering from toxaemia, dehydration and mental apathy. It is differentiated from gas gangrene by:

● Absence of crepitus.
● Absence of muscle involvement.
● Failure to isolate clostridia from tissues.

Instead streptococci and *Staphylococcus aureus* synergistics or coliforms with enterococci and streptococci are isolated.

The progressive bacterial skin gangrene may affect the scrotum and is called Fournier's gangrene (described in 1884 by **Jean A. Fournier**, 1832–1914, a French venereologist and dermatologist).

Mikulicz–Radecki, Johannes Von (1850–1905) Professor of Surgery, Königsburg and Breslau, Germany. He devised many new operations particularly on the oesophagus and on exteriorisation of the large bowel carcinoma so that it could be removed later on (Mikulicz colostomy). He was the first surgeon to cover his hands with cotton gloves in 1885; modern rubber gloves were introduced but not invented by W. S. Halsted of Baltimore in 1894. Gauze face masks were first worn by either Mikulicz or the French surgeon Paul Berger in 1896–7, while the operating gown in its present form was originated in Italy. (Although Lord Berkeley Moynihan, Professor of Surgery, Leeds 1865–1936 claimed to have been the first surgeon to wear a gown; as well as the first British surgeon to wear gloves.)

Mikulicz was the first to attempt suture of perforated gastric ulcer in 1880 (patient died). In 1884 he was the first to recommend emergency appendecotomy even if appendix was not perforated. In 1881 he used the first direct vision instrument for the oesophagus and stomach, the forerunner of the present oesophagoscope and bronchoscope. He also described the symmetrical progressive enlargement of lacrimal and salivary glands (Mikulicz's disease), the precursor of Sjögren's syndrome in which dry eyes and rheumatoid arthritis also occur (Tage Sjögren, 1859–1939, Swedish Physician).

Milroy, William F. (1855–1942) Professor of Clinical Medicine, University of Nebraska, USA. He described Milroy's disease (primary lymphoedema due to congenital as well as familial lymphatic aplasia).

Mondor, Henri (1885–1962) Professor of Clinical Surgery, Paris, France. He described Mondor's disease (self-limiting thrombophlebitis of veins over the upper chest wall and towards the axilla leading to subcutaneous cords; if on the breast, usually mistaken for carcinoma).

Monteggia, Giovanni B. (1762–1815) Professor of Surgery, Ospedale Maggiore, Milan, Italy. He described Monteggia fracture-dislocation (fracture of ulna with dislocation of upper radioulnar joint).

Montgomery, William (1797–1859) Professor of Midwifery, Dublin, Republic of Ireland. He described Montgomery glands (nodules) of areola of the breast.

Morgagni, Giovanni B. (1682–1771) Professor of Medicine and Anatomy for 56 years, Padua, Italy. He described hydatid of Morgagni (appendix of testis), torsion of which sometimes stimulates testicular torsion. He also described

Morgagni follicles (one pair) opening just behind the lips of the external urethral meatus of the penis (the follicles may become infected).

Murphy, John B. (1857–1916) Surgeon to Mercy Hospital, Chicago, USA. He described Murphy's sign: pressing on the right hypochondrium during inspiration produces a catch of breath (in inflamed gallbladder). He also described the renal angle test (Murphy's kidney punch): sharp jabbing movements with the thumb under the 12th rib lateral to the sacrospinalis muscle may reveal deep-seated tenderness.

Nuck, Anton (1650–92) Anatomist in Leiden, the Netherlands. He described 'canal of Nuck' hydrocele which causes difficulty in diagnosis of irreducible inguinal hernia in females.

Paget, Sir James (1814–99) Surgeon, St Bartholomew's Hospital, London, UK. He described three diseases: Paget's disease of bone (premalignant), Paget's disease of the penis (premalignant) and Paget's disease of the nipple (unilateral dry eczematous ulceration of the nipple is a malignant – not premalignant – disease due to underlying intraduct carcinoma invading the skin).

Pancoast, Henry K. (1875–1939) Professor of Roentgenology, University of Pennsylvania, Philadelphia, USA. He described Pancoast's syndrome due to apical pulmonary cancer: swollen congested face due to pressure on the superior vena cava, Horner's syndrome (pressure on the sympathetic chain) and shooting pains down the arm (pressure on brachial plexus). The first rib is eroded as seen in the X-ray.

Pasteur, Louis (1822–95) French scientist. He described 'the germ theory of disease' and showed that fermentation and putrefaction were caused by living multiplying matter. He reasoned that pus formation, wound infection and some fevers must also be caused by minute organisms from the environment.

Paterson, Donald R. (1863–1939) Ear, Nose and Throat Surgeon, Royal Infirmary, Cardiff, UK. Together with **Adam B. Kelly** (1865–1941) Ear, Nose and Throat Surgeon, Victoria Infirmary, Glasgow, UK, described Paterson–Kelly syndrome in 1919 which is a sideropaenic dysphagia in middle-aged women manifested by pallor (iron deficiency anaemia), stomatitis, cheilosis, smooth tongue, koilonychia, achlorhydria and mild splenomegaly; the condition is precancerous (postcricoid carcinoma). It is sometimes called the Plummer–Vinson syndrome (**Henry S. Plummer**, 1874–1937, Physician to Mayo Clinic, Rochester, USA and **Porter R. Vinson**, 1890–1959, Physician to Medical College, Virginia, USA).

Péan, Jules (1830–98) A French surgeon and one of the first surgeons to attempt vaginal hysterectomy. He introduced small instruments for securing blood vessels. He performed the first (unsuccessful) gastric resection for cancer.

Perthes, George (1869–1927) Professor of Surgery, Tubingen, Germany. He described Perthes' disease (juvenile osteochondritis with collapsed femoral head due to mushrooming secondary to aseptic vascular necrosis). He also described Perthes' test (walking with a tourniquet placed below the saphenous opening to diagnose deep venous thrombosis in cases of pain and venous congestion of the leg).

Peutz, John I. A. (1886–1957) Head of Internal Medicine, St John's Hospital, The Hague, the Netherlands. Together with **Harald Jeghers** (1894–1968), Professor of Medicine, Tufts University School of Medicine, Boston, USA, described Peutz–Jeghers syndrome (familial gastrointestinal hamartomatous polyposis with pigmentation around the lips and anus. It is manifested by bleeding and subacute obstruction and rarely becomes malignant).

Peyronie, François de La (1678–1747) Surgeon to Louis XV and founder of the Royal Academy of Surgery, Paris, France. Mainly due to him, Paris became a great surgical centre in the eighteenth century. He described Peyronie's disease of the penis (localised painless induration of one or both corpora cavernosa leading to lateral curvature of the erect penis).

Pott, Percival (1714–88) Surgeon, St Bartholomew's Hospital, London, UK. He described Pott's disease of the spine due to tuberculous fracture, and 'Pott's Puffy Tumour' a localised oedema over osteomyelitis of the skull. Pott trephined the skull in fractures in the eighteenth century with instruments hardly distinguishable from those of the ancient Greek and Roman surgeons; he considered that any fracture of the skull warranted operation. Astley Cooper, however, advised against trephining unless the skull fracture is compound.

Queyrat, Louis (1856–1933) Physician, Hôpital Cochin, Paris, France. He described erythroplasia of Queyrat (bright red, shiny lesion velvety to touch with exudate on sulcus corona usually with no induration. It is a precancerous condition of the penis).

Ramstedt, Wilhelm C. (1867–1963) German surgeon. He described the pyloromyotomy as the operation of choice in congenital pyloric stenosis (1912).

Raynaud, Maurice (1834–81) Physician, Hôpital Lariboisière, Paris, France. He described Raynaud's disease in females in which arterial spasm occurs in cold weather with colour changes from white to blue to red. Raynaud's phenomenon in males usually occurs in vibrating-tool users.

Rhazes or **Abu Bakr Al-Razi** (AD 860–932) Studied medicine in Baghdad and practised in Persia (Rayy). Having established a name and fame, Rhazes returned to Baghdad to become the head of its newly founded **Al-Mu'tadidi Hospital**. He wrote voluminously and described a primitive suture in his medical encyclopedia *Al-Hawi Fil-Tibb* (Liber continens, in 23 volumes); he was reputed to be the first surgeon to stitch abdominal wounds in man, using harp strings made of spun strands, possibly cut from animal intestine. He propounded his theory of infection and applied it on hospital patients. He was also renowned for his efforts in extracting and using alcohol as an antiseptic in wound infection.

Richter, August G. (1742–1812) Surgeon, Gottingen, Germany. He described Richter's hernia in 1777 (strangulation of a portion of the circumference of the intestine).

Riedel, Bernhard M. C. (1846–1916) Professor of Surgery, Jena, Germany. He described Riedel's thyroiditis, a stony hard goitre (like cancer) with tracheal obstruction.

Roentgen, Wilhelm C. Von (1845–1923) Professor of Physics successively at Strasburg, Giessen, Wurzburg and Munich, Germany. He discovered X-rays in 1895.

Rosenmüller, Johann C. (1771–1820) Professor of Anatomy and Surgery, Leipzig, Germany. He described the fossa of Rosenmüller, a pharyngeal recess into which the congenital branchial fistula opens.

Scarpa, Antonio (1747–1832) Professor of Surgery, Modena, and Professor of Anatomy, Pavia, Italy. He described Scarpa's fascia in anterior abdominal wall.

Sims, James Marion (1813–83) Founder and surgeon, State Hospital for Women, New York, USA. He described Sims' left lateral position for examination and Sims' speculum.

Smellie, Ian S. Contemporary Emeritus Professor of Orthopaedic Surgery, University of Dundee, Scotland. He described Smellie's knife for meniscectomy.

Smith, Robert W. (1807–73) Professor of Surgery, Trinity College, Dublin, Republic of Ireland. He described Smith's fracture (reversed Colles' fracture).

Spiegel, Adriaan Van Der (1578–1625) Professor of Anatomy, Padua, Italy. He described Spiegelian hernia (hernia through linea semilunaris above inguinal ligament).

Stensen, Niels (1638–86) Danish anatomist. He described Stensen's duct of the parotid gland.

Sudeck (see Charcot)

Tait, Robert Lawson (1845–99) Surgeon, Birmingham, UK (see Cholecystectomy, p. 471).

Takayasu, Mikito (1860–1938) Professor of Ophthalmology, Medical College, Kanazawa, Japan. He described Takayasu disease (pulseless disease or aortic arch syndrome in which no pulse is felt in one or both arms due to progressive atherosclerosis or arteritis leading to fainting, headache and optic nerve atrophy without papilloedema as a result of occlusion of the carotid arteries).

Thiersch, Karl (1822–95) German surgeon of Erlanger and Leipzig. Introduced the Thiersch graft (a partial thickness (split) skin graft) in 1874. However the commonly used knife is named after T. G. Humby, Plastic surgeon in Barbados, W. Indies.

Tietze, Alexander (1864–1927) Chief Surgeon in Allerheiligen Hospital, Breslau, Germany. He described Tietze disease (non-specific costochondritis affecting mainly women causing a painful lump often confirmed to be a breast mass).

Trendelenburg, Friedrich (1844–1924) Professor of Surgery, Leipzig, Germany. He described Trendelenburg's position (head down and legs up); Trendelenburg's test (for saphenofemoral incompetence); Trendelenburg's operation (mid-thigh high ligation of great saphenous vein – now modified to saphenofemoral junction flush ligation and disconnection); and Trendelenburg's sign (when an adult patient with a dislocated hip stands with his weight on the normal side, the opposite buttock rises and when he stands on the affected side, the opposite buttock sinks). Trendelenburg's gait occurs in bilateral congenital dislocation of the hips.

Troisier, Charles (1844–1919) Professor of Pathology, Paris, France. He described 'Troisier's sign' related to supraclavicular lymph node enlargement in carcinoma of the stomach.

Trousseau, Armand (1801–67) French physician. He described Trousseau's test: application of sphygmomanometer cuff around the arm with pressure up to 200 mmHg produces contractions of the hand in tetany. Trousseau's sign denotes thrombophlebitis migrans in visceral cancer (e.g. pancreas or stomach).

Vater, Abraham (1684–1751) Professor of Anatomy and Botany, Wittenberg, Germany. He described ampulla of Vater.

Vermooten, Vincent (1897–1969) Professor of Urology, University of Texas, Southwestern Medical School, Dallas, USA. He described Vermooten's sign (if rectal examination reveals an upward displaced prostate then the diagnosis is that of a complete intrapelvic urethral rupture in pelvic fractures but if the prostate cannot be felt and in its position there is an indefinite doughy swelling – extravasated urine or blood – it is a case of extraperitoneal bladder rupture).

Virchow, Rudolf (1821–1902) An outstanding German physiologist and anatomist of Wurzburg and Berlin. He is the founder of the science of cellular pathology. Virchow was a versatile man, who designed the sewage system of Berlin, organised the Prussian ambulance corps in 1870 and served as a member of the German Reichstag. Born in 1821, he graduated from Berlin in 1843 and founded *Virchow's Archives* (medical journal) in 1847. In his *Cellular Pathologie* published in 1858 he defined the body as a 'cell-state in which every cell is a citizen'. He is well known for Virchow's triad of thrombosis (endothelial injury, viscosity change and platelet aggregation), and for Virchow's supraclavicular lymph nodes, enlargement of which produces 'Troisier's sign' in advanced gastric cancer (as well as in intra-abdominal, testicular and bronchial cancers).

Volkmann, Richard Von (1830–89) Professor of Surgery at Halle and Leipzig, Germany. Mainly interested in the surgery of bones and joints but also claimed to be the first man to excise the rectum for cancer in 1878. He described Volkmann's ischaemic contracture following brachial artery trauma in supracondylar fractures.

Von Recklinghausen, Friedrich D. (1833–1910) Professor of Pathology, Strasburg, Germany. He was the first to point to the blood-borne skeletal metastases in cancer. He described the diffuse neurofibromatosis with cutaneous pigmentation and multiple tumours (von Recklinghausen's disease of nerve). He also described bone cyst formation in hyperparathyroidism (osteitis fibrosa or von Recklinghausen's disease of bone).

Wallace, Alexander B. (1906–74) Plastic surgeon, Royal Hospital for Sick Children, Edinburgh, UK. He introduced the Rule of Nines in burns.

Warthin, Aldred S. (1866–1931) Professor of Pathology, University of Michigan, USA. He described Warthin's tumour (or adenolymphoma) of the salivary glands, a soft (sometimes fluctuant) tumour in males over age 40 years.

Wharton, Thomas (1614–73) Physician to St Thomas' Hospital, London, UK. He described Wharton's submandibular salivary gland duct.

Willis, Thomas (1621–75) Physician, Oxford, UK. He described circle of Willis at the base of brain, first noticed the sweet taste of diabetic urine and described myasthenia gravis.

Wilms, Max (1867–1918) Professor of Surgery, Heidelberg, Germany. He described nephroblastoma (Wilms' tumour) of the kidney in children.

Notes on the early history of medicine

Arabic medicine

The term encompasses all Arabic-speaking Muslim (non-Arab), Arab (non-Muslim) and Arab Muslim practitioners who flourished in the Islamic Caliphate (Empire) extending mainly in the 'Middle East' and including parts of Persia, Asia, North Africa, and the Iberian Peninsula. Their practice is referred to variously as Arabic medicine or Islamic medicine. In those days, the borderline between surgery and medicine was usually non-existent; thus a physician might practise surgery or vice versa. Perhaps, the most important Arab contribution was the foundation of surgical practice on a solid scientific basis relying heavily on personal observations, clinical studies as well as animal experimentation; they condemned superstitions and ill-practices based on mal-experience.

Arabs were also acknowledged for introducing the first qualifying medical examination in surgical practice in AD 942 (319 AH), following a case of death due to medical malpractice reported to Caliph Al-Muktadir in Baghdad; he then ordered all doctors to stop practising in his Islamic Empire until they were examined by his experienced court doctor, Sinan Ibn Thabit Ibn Qurrah. Consequently, Sinan examined more than 860 doctors in the Al-Sayyeda teaching hospital in Baghdad. Those who passed through were given a special certificate carrying doctor Sinan's signature, allowing them to practise in medicine and surgery.

Arabs considered careful history-taking and proper physical examination absolutely imperative for a proper diagnosis; the patient's behaviour, character and location of pain, examination of swellings and pulse rate were noted and urine examination was performed routinely in every patient. There was emphasis on examination of excreta, other effluvia, particularly urine, to the extent that a half-filled urine flask became a symbol of an Arab physician; the urine's colour, consistency, sediment, smell and taste were assessed to assist in the diagnosis, to predict the prognosis and to plan the treatment. Ants gathering on the residual sugar after urine spillage would indicate that the patient was diabetic. Rhazes (AD 860–932) introduced the concept of differential diagnosis when he gave a precise unparalleled description for the clinical differentiation between intestinal colic and renal colic.

Arabs raised the dignity of the medical profession from that of a menial calling to one of the learned professions. They developed the science of chemistry as applied to medicine; they established hospitals in the principal cities. The herbal *De Materia Medica* of Dioscorides (1st century AD) was studied closely. New medications, including mineral, vegetable as well as animal substances were added to make up a voluminous Arabist materia medica. They introduced a number of new drugs for pre- and postoperative treatment and innovated many pharmacological methods, such as making drugs into tablets, syrups and paste. They promoted particularly the use of camphor (from Arabic *kafoor*, used for smell, message, and sexual suppression), cassia, cloves, mercury, myrrh and senna. They discovered and used soap (from Arabic *sapoon*), alcohol (from Arabic *alghol*, a liquor used for skin cleansing), alkali, sherbet, borax (from Arabic *borac*), elixir (from Arabic *exeer*, a rejuvenating essence), talc (from Arabic *talq*, a body powder), coffee, sugar, candy, amber, ambergris, saffron and odour (from Arabic *ottor*, a perfume). They not only invented the apothecary or pharmacy, but developed a number of new vehicles, including syrups (from Arabic *sharab*, a sweetened medicine), juleps (from Arabic *jallab*, the attractive fluid after adding rose water), the use of tragacanth as a demulcent, and many other concoctions of the apothecary. Furthermore, they manufactured special cabinets for drug storage and safekeeping. Indeed, the word drug is derived from the Arabic word *deriaq* or *teriaq*.

They also invented the Arabic numerals which replaced the cumbersome Roman numerals; they invented the **zero** (from Arabic *cipher*) and the nought (from Arabic *nogta*) thus introducing mathematical fractionation and the decimal concept (i.e. units, tens, hundreds and thousands) in the numbering system. The Arabic numbering system has facilitated doctors' communication on drug dosage, spatial and temporal orientation.

Arabic surgery

In operative surgery, Arabs proposed five essentials for performing a successful operation: a knowledge of anatomy, a knowledge of infection and its prevention (antisepsis), anaesthetics to kill pain, methods for controlling bleeding (haemostasis), and proper instruments for surgical intervention.

1. *Anatomy* The work of Yuhannah Ibn Masawayh on animals won the admiration of Caliph Al-Mutasim around AD 830, who was so interested that he made a special dissection hall available for Yuhannah's use on the Tigris river bank and provided him with apes specially brought for him from Nubia in Africa. Furthermore, Avenzoar performed the first experimental tracheostomy on a goat and noticed that it was alive many days after the procedure. Dead animals were extensively used by Avicenna, Rhazes and Ibn Tufail for experimental work. The story of *Hai Ibn Yakthan*, written by Ibn Tufail before 1185 AD, was a scientific masterpiece. It concerned a baby on an island where he was adopted by a deer which had lost its own young. The boy grew up among the animals and was shocked when his adopting 'mother' died. He then dissected the deer's body. The anatomical description of the dissected animal indicated Ibn Tufail's immense knowledge. The story was translated into Latin as *Philosophus Autodidactus* by Mirandola (1494 AD) and Pocock (1671 AD) and appeared in many languages. Both *Robinson Crusoe* by Daniel Dofoe and *Tarzan* by Edgar Rice Burroughs were corruptions of the Hai Ibn Yakthan story. Furthermore, there is a plethora of Muslim books on animal kingdoms, animal anatomy and behaviour; they represent a remarkable wealth of scientific literature. *Hayat Al-Hayawan Al-Kubra* (The Life of Animals) by Al-Dumairi, *Aja'eb Al-Maklokat Wal Hayawanat Wa Ghara'eb Al-Mowioodat* (Wonders of Creatures and Animals) by Al-Kizweeni, and *Kitab Al-Hayawan* (The Book of Animals) by Al-Jahidh are only a few notable examples.

The Qur'an (the backbone of Islam) urges its followers to look closely into the structure of the human body itself: 'We shall show them Our portents on the horizons and within themselves', Fusilat XLI, verse 53. 'And in yourselves, Can ye then not see?' Al-Thari'at, verse 21. While unpurposeful handling of Muslim dead bodies was strictly forbidden, a purposeful dissection was mandatory in surgical practice and in surgical teaching and training; it was imperative in post-mortem examination for medico-legal reasons in suspicious cases of death, such as poisoning and assault cases; and finally, it was crucial in identifying the underlying causative agents in epidemics of infectious diseases. In fact, there is strong evidence that it is the Arabs who actually established anatomy on extremely high standards and made it a prerequisite for surgical practice. They derived their extensive knowledge in anatomy from various sources, namely: Greek books on animal dissection, Egyptian embalming and taxidermy (Egyptian Mummies were known to Arab anatomists), careful observations of anatomical structures and skeletons of dead bodies from starvation and accidents in peace time, observation of underlying structures during surgical treatment of wounds in time of war, and dissection of pregnant mothers to extract living fetuses. However, human dissection of dead bodies was a reality. The fact that most surgeons, who were also the private doctors of the Caliphs, were vocal about the need for dissection as a prerequisite for surgical practice can only indicate that dissection was carried out publicly or secretly but with implicit blessing of the Caliphs themselves. Indeed, anatomy and dissection were extensively covered in Avicenna's *Al-Canon* and Haly's *Liber Regius* with unprecedented description, including many discoveries and pioneering works. Furthermore, there has never been a single reported incidence in history to indicate that a Muslim doctor has been punished for snatching a dead body or dissecting a cadaver, though reports of malpractices were documented thoroughly. There must have been precautions laid down for such a vital mission. These may have included cadaveric dissection of non-Muslims who died after being captured or during fighting with Muslims. Dissection of human fetuses was performed on a large scale. Dead bodies of insane Muslims with no relatives to claim them may have also been considered.

Ibn Al-Nafis was certainly a genuine anatomist; he vehemently attacked Galen's and Avicenna's concept of invisible interventricular pores of the heart, because dissection (as he said) refuted the presence of such pores; he also discovered the coronary blood vessels and pulmonary circulation. Avicenna's comments on optic chiasma and extraocular muscles were unprecedented and could only indicate a pioneering work based on his personal dissection of human bodies.

Arabs left indelible imprints in anatomical terms such as nucha (from Arabic *nucha'*, pertaining to spinal cord), saphenous (from Arabic *safin*, the conspicuous), cephalic and basilic veins (from Arabic *al bazili*, the draining, and *al kafili*, the sponsoring), colon (from Arabic *al colon*) and cornea (from Arabic *carania*).

2. *Infection and antisepsis* Islam prevents the mixing of a diseased (infected) patient with a non-diseased; it instructs its followers to run from lepromatous patients the way they run from the lion; it also advises not to enter or leave a plague-endemic area, thus introducing the quarantine principle in the

control of infectious diseases. In fact, when Rhazes came to Baghdad, he was chosen by the Caliph (out of 100 doctors) to be the decision-maker on the location of the newly founded hospital, named after Caliph Al-Mu'tadid (AD 892–902). Rhazes hung pieces of meat in various corners of Baghdad and the place of the last meat piece to decompose or to become rotten was selected as the site for the hospital foundation; he then became the head of its staff. Rhazes was a chemist too; he prepared alcohol by distillation (of fermented sweet juices) for the first time in history. Latterly, he used alcohol as antiseptic for wounds. Furthermore, Arabs used crushed rotten bread for tonsillitis, thus wittingly or unwittingly taking the credit for introducing antibiotics long before Alexander Fleming.

3. *Anaesthesia* Perioperative opium infusion was in common use for inflammatory conditions associated with severe pain as well as painful operative procedures, such as dental extraction and reduction of fractures. Poppy seeds were used in oral pre- and postoperative analgesic syrups or paste; their boiled solution was often used for inhalation. The *Arabian Nights* (Sir R. Burton), however, contains reference to anaesthesia by inhalation. **Theodoric** of **Bologna**, (1206–1298), whose name is associated with the 'soporific sponge', got his information from Arabic sources. The sponge was steeped in aromatics and soporifics and dried; when required it was moistened and applied to lips and nostrils. The Arabic innovation entails the immersion of the so-called 'anaesthetic sponge' in a boiled solution made of water with a unique mixture of hashish (from Arabic *hasheesh*), opium (from Arabic *afiun*), C-hyoscine (from Arabic *cit al huscin*), and Zo'an (Arabic for wheat infusion acting as a carrier for active ingredients after water evaporation). Arabs in Andalucia were the first pioneers of artificial ice-making. Freezing with ice was used for local anaesthesia in external operative procedures of a minor nature.

4. *Haemostasis* (see Albucasis, and the history of laparotomy).

5. *Surgical instruments* Arabs invented and perfected many surgical instruments illustrated in Albucasis's *Al-Tasrif Liman Ajaza An Al Ta'leef*, Haly Abbas's *Kamil Al-Sina'ah Al-Tibbiah* or *Al-Kitab Al-Malaki* or *Liber Regius*, and in Ibn Al-Quff's *Al-Omda Fi Sina'at Al-Jiraha*. These instruments include tools for dissection and cutting, various ligatures using guitar strands, catgut, linen and silk. Ant jaws were innovatively used by Albucasis as mechanical clips after head application to wounds followed by dismemberment of the head discarding the body; ants' oral secretion of formic acid made their jaws an ideal antiseptic device for suturing. Caustic substances and cautery were used for haemostasis, particularly in haemophiliacs. Catheters were invented by Arabs to serve as tools for drainage in patients with urinary retention. The word catheter is derived from Arabic *catha tair* (bird's quill), which is a hollow tube with attenuated ends used initially for writing. Gauze (derived from Arabic Gazza where it was manufactured) and bandages made of various textile materials were used by Arabs for wound dressing, as a haemostatic (by pressure) and for cleanliness (protection). Occasionally, the bandage was used as a proximal tourniquet in snake bites. Wicks and tube drains were also used in abscess cavities. A leather bulb syringe (from Arabic *zarrag*) was used for rectal enema. Proctoclysis was invented by Avenzoar. Urethral dilators and sounds were also used by Ibn

Al Thahabi while Albucasis used a lithotrite and metallic bladder syringe (litholapexy). Snares (from Arabic *sinnara*) were extensively used for removal of nasal polyps, enlarged tonsils, varicose veins and haemorrhoids. Tracheostomy was first referred to by Rhazes, experimentally applied by Avenzoar on goats, and practically performed by Albucasis on one of his servants successfully. Palliative treatment of oesophageal obstruction by intubation with narrow metallic tubes made of silver was first advocated by Avenzoar. Various glasses and optics were invented by Al-Hazen and extensively used in ophthalmology. Gypsum (from Arabic *gyps*, a powder hardened by water) was first used by Arabs in fractures. Wooden splints were chosen from special trees, such as pomegranates.

6. *Caesarean section*   According to the manuscript of *Shah-nama* or 'Book of Kings' written and illustrated by Ferdowsi c. 1560–80 (in the Metropolitan Museum of Art in New York), the earliest such operation was carried out on Rustam, a Persian hero (many centuries before the Roman Caesar). Such immaculate birth was even taken as a sign of a high destiny – kings and heroes tend to avoid the dark dirty confines of the natural channels of birth (*inter faeces et urinas nascimur*). It is evident that caesarean section was initially performed (for the lack of technical knowledge) only on the dead, if there was still hope of rescuing the full-term child (particularly, if it was a question of delivering a possible heir to the throne, the ancient Persians – before Islam – seem to have allowed exceptions). Ferdowsi, however, lived in the Islamic era, and he must have seen a caesarean section performed before his eyes before illustrating it in his book.

Moreover, Edinburgh University library has in its possession an original manuscript by Al-Biruni, entitled '*Al-Athar al-baqiya an al-qurun al-khaliyah*' (The Chronology of Ancient Nations) (manuscript 161, folio 6, verso). It reveals that caesarean section in the Islamic world not only continued to be performed under special circumstances on dead mothers, but was probably also performed on living wives of Muslim kings, sultans and amirs at their special request to rescue both the mother and the heir child. Plates illustrating Muslim surgeons performing caesarean section were gathered from Ferdowsi's *Shah-nama* and Al-Biruni's book by Brandenburg with excellent running commentary; (Brandenburg, D. (1982) *Islamic Miniature Painting in Medical Manuscripts*. Basle: Hoffman-La Roche); one can study Plates No. 65, 73, 81, 82 carefully.

Furthermore, Arab surgeons, particularly, Albucasis (AD 936–1013) and Rhazes (AD 865–932), were aware of rescuing living mothers threatened by spread of sepsis from their dead fetuses; they had not only described the details of vaginal extraction of dead fetuses, but masterminded the manufacture of various instruments for such a job, i.e. Albucasis' obstetric forceps (preceding Chamberlain's). Arab surgeons were thus aware in their management of three predicaments, namely, dead mother with a living fetus, living mother with a living fetus, and living mother with a dead fetus. Arabs, therefore, were the real founders of midwifery as a separate branch of the medical profession. For moral or doctrinal reasons, Islam upheld the principle that is still mandatory for every obstetrician today: first save the mother, even if the child has to be sacrificed; only once hope has been abandoned for the mother should an attempt be made to save the child (if still alive).

The Arabic legacy

Arabs' original scientific contributions reached a zenith in the Abbasid golden era (AD 754–1258): they dominated Europe, which at that time was sunk in its dark medieval age. Most of the Arabic texts in medicine and surgery were then translated into Latin by such as Constantinus Africanus (1020–87), a Benedictine monk at Monte Cassino, Italy, Gerard of Cremona (1114–87) at Toledo, and Farai Ibn Salim (Moses Farachi). The latter was a Sicilian Jew who, at the order of King Charles of Anjou in 1279, under took the arduous assignment of translating Rhazes' *Liber Continens* (23 volumes).

From the end of the 13th century onwards further translation was delayed for many reasons. The peace of northern Europe was dislocated by the 100 Years War, which lasted from 1337 to 1453, while the population was ravaged by the Black Death (1345–7) and other epidemics. In the East, the Mongols' savage invasion of Baghdad caused a scientific setback. In 1258, Baghdad, the glittering centre of civilisation of the East, had endured the first great catastrophe in the history of science. The Mongol invasion under Hulagu resulted in total destruction of the scientific infra-structure of Baghdad. The Tigris river was said to have run black for several days from the ink of priceless manuscripts from Baghdad's libraries used as dumps to act as crossing bridges for the barbarians.

The so-called Spanish Reconquest after eight centuries of Islamic civilisation in Andalusia in 1492 resulted in the second great catastrophe. The Inquisition Tribunals, set up initially under Ferdinando and executed over the next century up to the time of Philip II (1492–1610), led to the expulsion of 2 million Jews and Christened Jews (La Marranos), 3 million Arab Muslims and Christened Muslims (La Moriscos) and the killing of 100 000 Christened people. Furthermore, in 1610, Philip II ordered a massacre en route of 100 000 Muslims out of 140 000 Arabs leaving Spain on the final exodus. The majority of those Arabs were scientists and professionals. In 1511, and during the Spanish Inquisition Tribunals under the spiritual leadership of Cardinal Xemens, all Arabic manuscripts were burned in the public places of Granada, amounting to more than 80 000 volumes. In 1566, the Arabic language was banned officially, and it became Spaniards' banal habit to kindle their everyday fire with Arabic books.

But by this time the influence of the Arabic texts was already widespread in Europe. When the Renaissance period began to renew an interest in science, most medical knowledge was available only in Arabic texts. A group known as the Humanists (so-named from a term coined by one of them, the poet Ariosto – '*umanisto*'), developed a decided emnity against another group known as the Scholastics and against the Arabic texts which were being used by the Scholastics. In their zeal, the Humanists endeavoured to purify the language of science by casting out all Arabic terms and substituting Greek and Latin terms. Many Arabic terms survived however, some of them probably mistaken for Greek words.

Circa 1400 AD, an Italian professor, Mondino of Bologna, influenced by Arab doctors, risked excommunication by the Church for suggesting that a better knowledge could be obtained from dissecting a human corpse than reading the writings of Galen. It was he who popularised many of the surviving Arabic terms.

Leonardo da Vinci (1452–1516) was fluent in Arabic, and a great artist and scientist of the Renaissance period; he was fascinated by Arabic medical books and had instigated some personal observation and possibly actual dissection of a human cadaver. He blew air into the lungs of a corpse and showed beyond doubt that none of the air reached the heart. He also established the fact that heart valves allowed a unidirectional flow. Da Vinci illustrated the human anatomy beautifully; his illustrations and comments blended to achieve an unsurpassed work of creative art and the embodiment of the spirit of the Renaissance.

Andreas Vesalius (1514–1564) of Brussels, the so-called father of modern human anatomy, refused to accept slavishly the anatomical teachings of the Graeco-Roman physicians and authorities but rather to seek corroboration and to note discrepancies by the observational method of dissecting human cadavers. He was known by his enemies as the body-snatcher! The Flemish Vesalius began to learn Arabic, Greek and Latin languages through able Spanish Jewish doctors. He was influenced by Avicenna and Rhazes; indeed, he initially wrote '*A Commentary on the Fourth Fen of Avicenna*' and latterly, in 1537, he published his baccalaureate thesis, 'Paraphrase on the Ninth Book of Rhazes' at Louvain. His masterpiece, '*De Humani Corporis Fabrica Libri Septem* (Seven Books on the Structure of the Human Body) and its companion volume the '*Epitome*' issued at Basle in 1543 established a milestone in medical art. Vesalius illustrated the visceral vessels in eloquent drawings with great scientific precision.

Spaniard Michael Servetus, a classmate of Vesalius, attacked Galen and wittingly or unwittingly confirmed Ibn Al-Naif's concept of pulmonary circulation three centuries previously. He stated that the vital spirit was generated by the mixture in the lungs, of the air breathed in and the blood which the right ventricle of the heart delivered to the left. He was executed by the Church in 1553.

William Harvey (1578–1657) of Kent (Britain), the famous and the most influential physician of St Bartholomew's Hospital (London), had read the Latinised version of Arabic textbooks and was able to describe and popularise the concept of systemic blood circulation in its comprehensive outline. Harvey dissected various animals and, in 1616, he gave a series of lectures at the Royal College of Physicians, essentially on anatomy. He then adumbrated the idea of blood circulation and his work was finally published in his book '*De Motu Cordis et Sanguinis in Animalibus*' (On the Motion of the Heart and Blood in Animals) and *De Circulatione Sanguinis*' (On the Circulation of the Blood) in 1628.

Marcello Malpighi (1628–94) of Italy confirmed Harvey's theory of blood circulation and elaborated on the concept of 'capillary circulation', as he described in his book '*De Pulmonibus*' (On the Lungs) published in 1661 in Bologna and based on his personal observation of the blood flow through magnified fine vascular networks in frogs. Professor Malpighi, therefore, provided the last missing link in the blood circulation.

In spite of the efforts of the Humanists, the translated versions of Haly Abbas's '*Liber Regius*', Albucasis's '*Al-Tasrif*', Avicenna's '*Al-Canon*' and Rhazes's '*Liber Continens*' were used as the only standard textbooks in the medical schools of Western Europe from the early eleventh century to the early eighteenth century and were considered by many the main source for the European Renaissance in medicine and surgery.

The Greek medical legacy

Perhaps the first surgical operation performed on man, and the first use of anaesthesia in the history of mankind, are contained in Genesis II: 21: 'And the Lord God caused a deep sleep to fall upon Adam, and he slept: and he took one of his ribs, and closed up the flesh instead thereof.'

The Babylonian Code of Hammurabi, written as early as 2250 BC, represents the first documented reference to surgery in the history of mankind; it states that reckless surgery must be punished by cutting off the surgeon's hand in retaliation. It is inconceivable that any surgeon could perform operations in such a hostile environment. Egyptians were shown performing the operations of circumcision, castration, wound and abscess surgery and limb amputation. Unfortunately, their knowledge of body structures and abdominal contents was rudimentary in spite of their interest in embalming.

The Greeks made valuable contributions to anatomy, but they did not dissect the human body because their religion was even more hostile than the Egyptians towards any interference with the bodies of the dead. The great Greek physician of Pergamon, **Galen**, who lived in the second century after Christ (131–201), derived his knowledge of anatomy from the pig, the ape, the dog and the ox. He assumed that the structures he found in these animals were identical with the structures in the human body. For many centuries, the human breastbone was supposed to be segmented like that of an ape; and the liver to be divided into many lobes like that of a hog; the uterus was supposed to be in two long horns as in the dog; and the hip bones to be flared as in the ox. Galen also believed in small invisible pores between the ventricles of the heart. Galen's authority forced generations of doctors to apply his knowledge of animal anatomy to human beings. When the seats of learning fell into hands of the Church, his writings became like Gospels, and bore the stamp of the Church's authority and infallibility. Galen's work maintained its hold upon the clerics and physicians of the Middle Ages until Arabs and Muslims, through observations and cadaveric dissection, reviewed the human anatomy as we know it now. Vesalius thereafter, through his Arabic teaching and education, popularised their observations with his own in his famous book on the structure of human body.

In 431 AD, when Nestorius, a patriach of Byzantium, was banished for heresy, he fled to southwest Persia where he and his followers founded a school. For two centuries, the Nestorian Christians preserved and translated Greek manuscripts (including those of Aristotle and Hippocrates) into the Syriac language.

A medical school had been founded in Gondeshapur (now Shahabad) in pre-Islamic times and the tradition of doctors of Gondeshapur was to be revived again some generations later under the Caliphs. Greek scientists had for long captured the Caliphs' imagination, to the extent that Muslims were persuaded in AD 830 (by the Romans) to halt their military campaign of expansion in return for acquisition of Greek books kept in Byzantium in underground tunnels. The famous Arabic doctors of the time, at the specific request of successive Caliphs in Baghdad in the eighth and ninth centuries, undertook the heavy commitment of translating Greek medical books and the Syriac versions of Greek books into the Arabic language on an unprecedented scale. Caliph Al-Mamoon ordered a School of Translation to be attached to the Academy of Baghdad – 'Baytul Hikma' (the House of Wisdom) and appointed Hunayn Ibn Is'haq Al Ibadi (808–73) as its head. The latter, for instance, translated Galen's books: '*On Anatomical Procedures*', of which the original Greek books IX to XV inclusive were totally lost, '*On Examinations by which the Best Physicians are Recognised*' and '*The Best Physician is a Philosopher*'. Ironically, many of the original Greek books were lost, and it was the Arabic versions which preserved the Greeks' medical knowledge.

The evolution of some important surgical procedures

Appendicectomy

The first appendicectomy was performed in 1736 by Claudius Amyand, Surgeon to St George's Hospital, London, UK. In a boy 12 years of age, Amyand removed the appendix, a pin that it contained, and surrounding omentum from a scrotal hernia that was complicated by a faecal fistula. Surgical treatment of appendicitis was described in France (Mestivier, 1759; Lamotte, 1766; Jadelot, 1808) and in London (Parkinson, 1812). Melier, in 1827, advised drainage of appendiceal abscesses. He also envisaged the possibility of early removal of the acute inflamed appendix. Unfortunately, Dupuytren (1835), the most influential surgeon of his day, opposed Melier's views and warmly supported the conservative treatment of what was then called 'typhlitis and perityphlitis' that had been inaugurated by Goldbeck and Puchelt (1832). Volz in 1843 described opium treatment, declaring that rest for the inflamed bowel was as important as a splint for a broken leg. Grisolle (1839) in France, Hancock (1848) in the UK, and Willard Parker (1867) in the USA recommended incision and drainage before fluctuation appeared in inflammatory conditions of the right iliac fossa. Parker (1867), taught that there were three stages of appendicitis: gangrene, perforation and abscess. Fitz (1886) was the first surgeon to use the term appendicitis. Morton (1887), of Philadelphia, successfully diagnosed and excised an acutely inflamed appendix, and Treves (1887) advocated appendicectomy in the quiescent period. About this time McBurney described a technique for removal of the appendix that is widely used even today.

Much credit is due to the pioneers in this field (Parker, Fitz, Morton, Treves, McBurney and J. B. Murphy) who advanced the claims of surgical treatment in acute appendicitis. J. B. Murphy of Chicago wrote a classic description of the signs and symptoms of appendicitis; in the same year (1889), Charles McBurney of the Roosevelt Hospital, New York, published the results of a large investigation into the disease. In the course of his paper he enunciated one of the best-known 'signs' in surgery, still called 'McBurney's point'. This is the point of maximum tenderness when the abdominal wall is pressed with one finger and is a good localising sign in appendicitis. McBurney also described an operative technique in 1894, but the so-called McBurney or grid-iron incision was, in fact,

devised by L. L. McArthur of Chicago. Another commonly used incision or approach for the appendicectomy operation was introduced by W. H. Battle of St Thomas' Hospital in 1895.

Noteworthy as these various dates are, it is doubtful whether any of them are as important in the history of the appendix operation as 24th June 1902. The coronation of King Edward VII had been arranged to take place on 26th June, but the king fell ill with abdominal pain and fever only a few days before. At a consultation of some of the most distinguished surgeons in the land, including Lord Lister, it was decided that the only chance to save his life lay in urgent operation. Frederick Treves, who had performed his first successful appendicectomy in 1887, opened the abdomen and drained an appendix abscess on 24th June; he did not, as is sometimes stated, remove the appendix. The king made a good recovery and the operation was entirely successful, a success that becomes more remarkable when one considers the advanced age (for those days) and not altogether ascetic habits of the patient. After the postponed coronation on 9th August, Treves received a knighthood and Lister was made a Privy Councillor and one of the 12 original members of the Order of Merit. When welcoming Lister to his Council, the king is supposed to have said, 'I know that if it had not been for you and your work, I would not have been here today.'

Cholecystectomy

In 1869 Lawson Tait (who did his first ovariotomy at the age of 23 when still a House Surgeon) was consulted by a patient about a discharging sinus in her abdominal wall; he followed up the track of the sinus and removed a few small stones, which must have ulcerated through from the gallbladder. In 1878 Marion Sims, the famous American 'gynaecologist', attempted to remove gallstones by opening the abdomen and slitting up the gallbladder, the operation of cholecystotomy, but his patient died; in the same year Theodor Kocher of Berne drained an abscess of the gallbladder. The first successful removal of stones from the gallbladder was by Lawson Tait in 1879. Another interesting cholecystotomy was that performed by Joseph Lister in 1883, for it is often stated wrongly that Lister never opened the abdomen. Unfortunately the patient died in April 1884.

Lawson Tait is sometimes credited with the first cholecystectomy, removal of the gallbladder itself, but he never did this operation. Cholecystectomy was first performed in 1882 by the German C. J. A. Langenbuch, who is often confused with the more famous Langenbeck. This was an isolated case, but in 1896 Hans Kehr, another German, started to do the operation as a routine procedure for removal of stones and had performed over a thousand cholecystectomies by the time of his death in 1916. Berkeley Moynihan in England and Mayo in the USA were well known for their success in cholecystectomy. After 1921 it became the operation of choice and has now entirely replaced cholecystotomy.

Colostomy

Alexis Littré of Paris may be called the father of colostomy. In 1710 he was consulted about an infant who suffered from congenital malformation of the rectum, probably an imperforate anus. The child died on the sixth day after birth; at autopsy Littré took the opportunity of investigating possible means of dealing with similar defects in life. Having practised on the infant's body, he declared it possible to 'make an incision in the belly, and open the two ends of the closed bowel and stitch them together, or at least to bring the upper part of the bowel to the surface of the belly wall where it would never close but perform the function of an anus'. This was ventral or abdominal colostomy, performed through the abdominal wall; it became known as Littré's operation.

In 1776 H. Pillore, a surgeon from Rouen, performed caecostomy which is much the same as colostomy, except that the large bowel is entered at a higher point. The operation was performed for an obstruction due to cancer of the rectum (and perhaps made worse by the two pounds of mercury which had been given by mouth in an endeavour to cure the obstruction) but the patient died 28 days later. In 1793 C. Duret of Brest, performed the first successful colostomy on a 3-day-old child suffering from imperforate anus. He made an incision in the left groin and brought the large bowel to the abdominal surface; he then cut into the bowel and allowed it to act as an artificial anus. The patient lived until the age of 45 years. An interesting little note on this operation reminds us that 1793 was the year of Terror. 'Citizen Massac, Chief of the Administration, and Citizen Coulon, Physician in Chief, were charged to provide necessary dressings.'

P.J. Desault of Paris also performed Littré's operation for imperforate anus in 1794, but the child died 4 days later. In 1797 C. L. Dumas of Montpellier, the leading French surgeon of his time, advised that colostomy should be used for the relief of intestinal obstruction and claimed to have devised the operation. In fact, Dumas never did a colostomy in his life, but his weighty approval served to arouse interest. Three years later, Professor Fine of Geneva performed colostomy in a woman aged 63 years suffering from cancer of the rectum, giving credit to Dumas for the original idea. Fine's patient survived for 3 months. Freer of Birmingham was the first to attempt Littré's operation for imperforate anus in the UK (1815), but his patient died. The first successful case in the UK was that of Daniel Pring, a surgeon from Bath, in 1817.

In about 1839, J.Z. Amussat of Paris attended his colleague, Professor Broussais, who was dying from intestinal obstruction due to cancer of the rectum. Amussat declared that he would never again stand idly by while a patient of his died so terrible a death. He collected particulars of all known colostomies since Pillore had first performed the operation on a living subject in 1776. Of 29 cases, 21 of whom were infants suffering from imperforate anus, 20 had died within a matter of hours or days. Only 4 of the infants had survived, and it is curious that all 4 were treated at Brest, where Duret had first succeeded with the operation, but that Duret had attended none of the other 3 cases. Of 8 adult patients, 5 had survived.

Amussat concluded that 20 deaths were all due to peritonitis, as we should call it today, and that Littré's abdominal approach through the peritoneum must be held to blame. After experimenting in the postmortem room, he advised opening the large bowel by an incision in the back, close to the spine, an approach which had already been practised on a dead body by Duret and by Callisen of Copenhagen in 1800. This is the lumbar colostomy or Amussat's operation, a great advance because it did not entail approaching the bowel via the peritoneal cavity and so tended to avoid peritonitis. Amussat himself performed his operation 9 times successfully between 1839 and 1856; the number of his failures is unknown.

Lumbar colostomy became the operation of choice, and retained its popularity for over 30 years. In the UK it was first performed by W. J. Clement of Shrewsbury for a stricture of the colon in 1841; Clement's patient lived for 3 years. John Erichsen of University College Hospital, who had been a pupil of Amussat and present at his first operation, became the leading exponent of this method. Another surgeon who regularly practised the Amussat technique was Caesar Hawkins of St George's; in 1852 he collected all known cases of colostomy, performed for 'stricture of the colon' but not for imperforate anus in infants, and found that in 48 patients the mortality was exactly 50%. He advised that there was little difference in the result whether Amussat's or Littré's approach was used.

In 1850 three surgeons at the London Hospital returned to the abdominal method of Littré. The London Hospital became noted for successful operations; in 1865 one of their surgeons, Nathaniel Ward, made the very important pronouncement that when a cancer of the rectum is diagnosed, colostomy should always be performed without waiting for signs of obstruction; this made the operation safer because the patients were in better general health. With the introduction of antisepsis, operations on the abdomen could be performed with less risk of peritonitis, and from 1880 onwards there was an increasing tendency to give up the Amussat method, although we occasionally find mention of lumbar colostomy in case notes during the 1890s.

A colostomy is not curative operation; it will relieve obstruction of the bowel but, if that obstruction is caused by a cancer, the cancer remains to imperil the patient's life. One of the objections put forward by the London Hospital surgeons to the lumbar colostomy was that the abdominal cavity cannot be explored through the incision; a doubtful diagnosis must remain in doubt.

In 1887, C. B. Ball of Dublin recommended abdominal colostomy with exploration of the abdomen (laparotomy) in all cases. A few years later W. Ernest Miles started to explore the abdomen through a midline incision and to make the colostomy through a separate opening. This is the method generally used today. Attempts to hack a way through a rectal growth had often been made, but it was not until 1868 that Billroth removed a cancer of the rectum for the first time; by 1876 he had done 33 cases. Billroth's operation was improved by the Swiss surgeon Theodor Kocher and by the German Paul Kraske. Kraske's operation remained the method of choice from 1885 until 1908; in that year W. E. Miles introduced the abdominoperineal approach, which is still used in suitable cases. In all previous methods the operation had been done only from below; the Miles operation is commonly performed by two surgeons working together, one from below (the perineal approach) and one from above, through the abdomen.

Femoral hernia repair

Lockwood (1889, UK) and Marcy (1892, USA) described the low femoral approach while Lotheissen (1898, Vienna, Austria) described the inguinal approach. McEvedy (1950, Manchester, UK) introduced the lateral rectus approach. Nyhus in 1955 (USA), after meticulous study of the anatomy of the groin, described the 'preperitoneal approach'. Henry (1936) described the 'midline abdominal approach' as providing good exposure of the femoral rings (discovered accidentally while exposing the lower end of the ureter).

In strangulated hernia, the first objective is to save the patient's life: wound and repair considerations become secondary. The 'pararectus' approach, whether within the rectus sheath (McEvedy) or both within and without (Nyhus), gives direct access to the neck of the sac from above. For the elderly or poor-risk patient, the 'low' approach not involving an abdominal incision has much in its favour. The midline approach has the advantages of simplicity, ample exposure and immediate control of the involved loop of intestine from within the peritoneal cavity. It is the best incision for bilateral femoral hernias. By and large the Nyhus approach is probably the best. The Lotheissen approach should be condemned since it weakens the inguinal area and predisposes to inguinal hernia.

Evolution of gastric resection and Billroth's operation

Avicenna (980–1037) gave the first account of cancer of the stomach. The first detailed memoir on malignant lesions of the stomach was written by Morgagni in 1761.

In 1810 Merrem successfully performed excision of the pylorus in dogs and suggested the possible application of pylorectomy followed by end-to-end gastroduodenostomy in humans. Pean (1879) performed the first gastric resection for cancer. The patient died 4 days later. Billroth (1881) carried out the first successful pyloric resection in the human for carcinoma of the pylorus 71 years after Merrem's work (*see also* Names, above). The patient died 4 months later. In the same year, Billroth's assistant Anton Wolfer successfully made the first gastroenterostomy, bypassing the stomach without removal of pyloric growth. This became the method of choice particularly after Courvoisier of Basle (well known for his law in jaundice) introduced the posterior gastroenterostomy in 1883. Connor (1884) attempted the first total gastrectomy on cancer of the stomach. The patient died on the operating table.

Billroth, on 15th January, 1885, performed the first gastric resection with closure of the cut end of the stomach and anterior gastrojejunostomy. As his patient was emaciated and a poor surgical risk owing to the presence of a pyloric cancer, Billroth originally planned to perform a two-stage operation. He envisaged that the first stage would be an anterior gastrojejunostomy and that after a short interval the second stage would be an antrectomy with closure of the open ends of the stomach and duodenum. As the patient withstood the short-circuiting procedures satisfactorily, he proceeded with the gastric resection and with closure of the ends of the stomach and duodenum.

Krönlein, on 24th May, 1888, carried out a one-stage partial gastrectomy with an antecolic anastomosis. Antecolic anastomoses predominated in the early Billroth II variations, but were later replaced by the retrocolic type of anastomosis. Von Fiselsberg (1889) was the first to close the upper end of the gastric pouch to reduce the size of the orifice and then perform an anterior anastomosis between the greater curvature portion of the stomach and a loop of proximal jejunum. Braun and Jaboulay (1892) added an enteroanastomosis between the afferent and efferent limbs of the jejunum.

The retrocolic anastomoses were first used by Hofmeister (1896). Reichel (1908) and Polya (1911) performed partial gastrectomy with retrocolic gastroenterostomy in which the entire open end of the stomach was anastomosed to the side of the proximal loop of jejunum. Here the afferent limb was affixed to the lesser curvature. Eugene Polya of Budapest was one of the first to write about the technical details of partial gastrectomy with retrocolic end-to-side gastrojejunostomy. Polya stated 'The great majority of surgeons, however, did not know of the method at all until I called it to the attention of the surgical world and especially to the attention of William Mayo who saw in it the operation of the future and whose endorsement helped to make it the one most widely adopted'.

Hofmeister (1908) and Finsterer (1914) slightly modified the original Hofmeister procedure. They performed a retrocolic anastomosis, uniting the proximal jejunum to the lower half of the open end of the stomach after closing the top half of the stomach. The short afferent limb of jejunum was buttressed to the closed upper half of the stomach, thus producing a valve effect. This operation is often referred to as the Hofmeister-Polya operation.

Balfour (1917) reported his modification of the Krönlein operation by the performance of a side-to-side enteroanastomosis to overcome the possibility of any vicious-circle vomiting.

Moynihan (1923) reversed the position of the jejunal loop, bringing the loop from the left to the right with the afferent limb to the greater curvature. In Moynihan's original account the anastomosis was antecolic, the proximal jejunal loop was short, certainly not more than 12.7 cm from the ligament of Treitz to the greater curvature.

A few years after the publication of Moynihan's operation it became customary to reduce the size of the gastric stoma by closing the upper third or upper half of the mouth of the gastric remnant towards the lesser curvature, the lower portion of the open end of the stomach towards the greater curvature being used for the gastrojejunal anastomosis. In the Polya modification the cut end of the duodenum is closed, and a loop of jejunum is brought up through an opening in the mesocolon to form an end-to-side anastomosis with the cut end of the stomach.

Coller and associates (1941) concluded that in many cases the associated gastric nodes are inadequately excised because the lesion is extensive and only a palliative operation is done, either because the nodes are not palpable or because the surgeon is not making a conscientious attempt at complete removal of the carcinoma. They also concluded that contiguous lymph nodes need not be involved in order for distant lymphatic involvement to exist.

In 1951, McNeer and associates reviewed necropsy specimens after partial gastrectomy for carcinoma and found recurrence in the gastric remnant in half the cases. They recommended that a more radical operation be attempted, and suggested radical total gastrectomy, partial pancreatectomy (tail) and splenectomy.

In a study reported from the Mayo Clinic in 1953, great attention was paid to lymph node involvement from carcinoma of the stomach. The distance of the involved lymph nodes from the nearest edge of the lesion was found to be of great prognostic significance, as was involvement or non-involvement of the subpyloric lymph nodes.

In 1893 Roentgen discovered X-rays and in 1897 Schiatter performed the first successful total gastrectomy. The patient lived for 14 months. Cuneo (1906) and Jamieson and Dobson, following many dissections, gave the first detailed descriptions (with numerous illustrations) of the lymphatic drainage of the stomach, and these influenced the extent of gastric resections for carcinoma. During 1911–12 Holzknecht and Hendrick-Forsell (Sweden), Cole (USA), Barclay (UK), and Carman (USA) demonstrated the potential of fluoroscopy and barium meal X-ray examination for diagnosis of cancer of the stomach.

During the early years of this century W. J. Mayo, C. H. Mayo, and Moynihan were extending the scope of partial gastrectomy for malignant lesions of the stomach. Much credit is due to them for their teachings and for their demonstration that the postoperative mortality for gastric resections can be lowered by skill and judgement.

The Wolf-Schindler flexible gastroscope was introduced in 1932. Papanicolaou (1946) introduced the method of diagnosis of malignant growths from exfoliated cells from cancerous lesions. Schoemaker devised a special clamp for closing the lesser curvature portion of the stomach so that the remaining circumference could be approximated to the cut end of the duodenum, as in the Billroth I procedure. C. H. Mayo and W. J. Mayo obtained the same result by using two curved clamps across the lower half of the stomach; the second clamp was placed almost at right angles to the first to take out a portion of the lesser curvature.

Inguinal repair

The modern technique of operations for inguinal hernia started with Bassini (1888) and Halsted (1893). Bassini's operation, which consisted of high excision of the sac and posterior repair of the inguinal canal, was a development of Marcy's operation (1887). Marcy, in *The Anatomy and Surgical Treatment of Hernia* (1892), reported results with his operation that were far superior to anything that had preceded them. Halsted at first divided the internal oblique and transversus abdominis lateral to the internal ring in order to transplant the cord laterally, repairing all the layers behind the cord to Poupart's ligament and leaving the cord subcutaneous. The cutting of the muscles, the so-called lateral cut, which was subsequently revived by Brandon (1945) in the UK and in a different form by Pratt (1948) and by Weiss (1948) in the USA gave poor results, and Halsted accordingly condemned it.

To allow the conjoined tendon and internal oblique to be approximated to Poupart's ligament without tension, a 'relaxation cut' in the anterior rectus sheath may be needed. This 'rectus-relaxing incision of the rectus sheath' or 'slide' received special emphasis from Scott (1905), Fallis (1938), McVay (1939), Reinhoff (1940) and Tanner (1942, UK). In Bloodgood's operation (1919, USA), a flap of anterior rectus sheath and a portion of the rectus muscle itself were brought downwards to cover the 'weak gap' of the inguinal canal and were anchored to the inguinal ligament with interrupted sutures of fine silk. Halsted proved that ligation and excision of veins from a bulky cord were followed in 20% of cases by the development of a hydrocele and in some cases by atrophy of the testis. The Wyllys Andrews operation (1895) produced a neat posterior repair, leaving the cord in a newly formed canal between the two flaps of the external oblique aponeurosis.

In 1921 Gallie and Le Mesurier (Canada) described their method of repair with strips of fascia taken from the thigh. However, the recurrence rate was high: 8–10%. Again, the needle employed for the lattice repair was large and cumbersome and traumatised the fissile inguinal ligament and also the muscular layers through which it had to be passed; doubts were cast as to whether the fascia actually 'lived' in the repair; infection was by no means infrequent, and the long scar in the thigh or the gap in the iliotibial band produced by the fasciotome in some cases gave trouble. Nevertheless, the influence of Gallie's work was profound, and although other methods of radical 'cure' were in use – including excision of the sac only (Hull, 1913), the silver filigree operation of McGavin (1909), the darn-and-stay-lace method of Handley (1918), Seelig and Tuholske's fascia-to-fascia closure (1914) and Wangensteen's pedicled flap of fascia lata reflected from the thigh up to the weak area in the inguinal canal.

In 1937 Ogilvie recognised three types of inguinal hernia:
- Those in which the only abnormality is the presence of a sac.
- Those in which there is, in addition, some stretching of the internal ring, but the muscles of the inguinal sphincter are sound.
- Large indirect and direct hernias in which the sphincter mechanism has obviously failed.

Ogilvie advised the following procedures for the three types noted above:
1. Removal of the sac alone.
2. Excision of the sac with plastic repair of the internal ring.
3. Strong lattice replacement of the inguinal mechanism.

His lattice operation was based on Gallie's operation, using silk in place of fascia. For the same purpose, Maingot (1941) introduced floss silk consisting of the individual fibrils of natural silk, which offered a perfectly pliable framework for subsequent growth of fibroblasts.

In 1973 Glassow introduced the Shouldice Hospital technique of inguinal hernia repair (continuous four lines of overlapping sutures).

Pancreatic surgery

Hopes of radical treatment for carcinoma of the pancreas were first raised when Halsted (1899) resected a segment of the second part of the duodenum and a portion of the pancreas for an ampullary carcinoma. He implanted the pancreatic duct and the bile duct in line with the suture of the repair of the posterior wall duodenal defect. His patient died 6 months later from recurrence of the growth. W. J. Mayo (1900), Mayo-Robson (1900) and Koerte (1904) reported limited excisions which were unsuccessful. Successful cases of limited resection of a portion of the duodenum and of the head of the pancreas for cancer were reported by Kausch (1912), Hirschel (1914), and Tenani (1922). In 1935, Whipple, Parsons and Mullins, following a systematic study of the subject and considerable experimental work, published the first report of their successful two-stage procedure for radical en bloc resection of the duodenum and head of the pancreas for a growth of the ampulla of Vater.

Brunschwing (1937 and 1942) was the first surgeon to perform successfully an extensive radical pancreaticoduodenectomy for carcinoma of the head of the pancreas, including the head and the neck of the gland together with 90% of the duodenum. In March 1940 Whipple performed the first recorded one-stage removal of the head of the pancreas and all of the duodenum with occlusion of the pancreatic stump.

Rectal excision

It was J. P. Lockhart-Mummery, in 1907 and 1920, who was responsible for developing perineal excision (a very inadequate method) into a worthwhile cancer operation. He employed loop iliac colostomy, the opportunity being taken at this stage to perform an exploratory laparotomy to assess the operability of the growth from the abdominal aspect and to determine the presence of hepatic or peritoneal deposits. The perineal operation was performed 2 weeks or so later; during the interval the distal bowel was washed out daily from colostomy to anus. For the excision the patient was placed on the left side with the knees drawn up and a wide elliptical incision was made round the anus and extended backwards to the coccyx which was excised.

Sacral excision had been employed by Kocher in 1875, but its introduction into surgical practice was due to Kraske in 1885, and it has been associated with his name ever since. With the patient lying on the left or right side an incision was made from behind the anus over the lower sacrum, usually inclining to one or other side of the midline. By removal of the coccyx and the lowermost two pieces of the sacrum good access was obtained to the back of the rectum above the levator muscles. Inferiorly the dissection was carried as far as necessary, the operation being completed either by excising the entire rectum and anal canal and establishing a sacral anus at the posterior end of the wound – so-called amputation of the rectum – or by removing a sleeve of bowel containing the growth and restoring continuity by end-to-end anastomosis – so-called resection of the rectum. Sacral excision rapidly became the most popular method in Germany and Austria and various modifications of Kraske's original technique were introduced by Billroth and others.

A combined operation involving abdominal and perineal phases for excision of the rectum was first performed by Czerny (1883) not as a premeditated plan but as a means of finishing a sacral excision which he had found himself unable to complete from below. Undoubtedly the work of Ernest Miles (1908) established the abdominoperineal operation in the UK and USA. Following his researches into the mode of spread of rectal cancer, he concluded that a radical excision for this condition, wherever situated in the rectum, ought to embrace the following structures: the entire rectum including the anal canal and sphincters, considerable parts of the levator ani muscles and ischiorectal fat, practically all the sigmoid colon

and mesocolon including the superior haemorrhoidal and inferior mesenteric vessels and glands lying in its base, and a portion of the pelvic peritoneum adjacent to the rectum. The great drawback of this operation when first introduced was that it was an extremely shocking procedure with a high initial mortality. Grey Turner in 1920 thought that if the operation were divided into two stages it might be better borne by the patient. The first stage consisted of the establishment of a colostomy alone. However, the method of two-stage combined excision has been abandoned in favour of the one-stage operation.

Gabriel (1934) subsequently developed perineoabdominal excision as a single-stage procedure and became its chief advocate. He considered it to be a less shocking operation than abdominoperineal excision and, for a surgeon familiar with perineal dissections, much simpler to perform than the Miles operation, while achieving a greater removal of bowel and using a terminal colostomy rather than a loop colostomy. With the patient in the left lateral position the rectum is freed from below exactly as in a perineal excision but, instead of dividing the superior haemorrhoidal vessels and bowel in the perineal wound, the mobilised segment is pushed up into the abdominal cavity through the cut in the pelvic peritoneum.

Bloodgood (1906) and Clogg (1923) both suggested that with a suitable arrangement of the patient the abdominal and perineal phases of a combined excision might be performed simultaneously, and both of them described such operations. But it was Kirschner of Heidelberg (1934) who demonstrated conclusively that this was a practicable procedure. Devine (1937) introduced the method afresh to the English-speaking world, and Lloyd-Davies (1939), by devising special adjustable leg rests to support the patient in the lithotomy-Trendelenburg position necessary for a synchronous approach to abdomen and perineum, and elaborating various other refinements of technique, greatly assisted the development of the operation. The advantages claimed for this method are that it saves a considerable amount of operating time, that it makes the removal of very advanced fixed growths easier because their dissection can proceed from above and below simultaneously, and that it greatly facilitates suture of the pelvic peritoneum because this takes place over an empty pelvis and not on top of the divided sigmoid colon, mesocolon and rectum, waiting to be removed from below.

Extended combined excision

Attempts have been made to increase the scope of combined excision still further.

One possibility is higher ligation of the inferior mesenteric vessels with or without extended left colectomy. Miles (1926) recommended that the main ligature should be placed opposite the bifurcation of the abdominal aorta (this tie usually lies just below the origin of the left colic or first sigmoid artery), while Moynihan (1908) and others have recommended tying the inferior mesenteric artery at its origin from the abdominal aorta to avoid leaving this remnant of artery and associated lymphatics.

Multivisceral resections, complete pelvic clearance (total cystoprostatectomy en bloc with rectal excision and urinary diversion) and translumbar amputation have also been tried.

Sphincter-saving resections

Following the work of Dukes (1930, 1940) and others, which showed that the lymphatic spread of rectal cancer is mainly in an upward direction, there was a resurgence of interest in the UK and USA in the possibility of sphincter preservation in the radical excision of carcinomas of the upper rectum and rectosigmoid, and various forms of sphincter-saving resections were revived or developed:

1. Sacral resection.
2. Abdominosacral resection (Pannett, 1935).
- Abdominotranssphincteric (York Mason, 1976).
- Abdominoanal pull-through resection by various methods.
- Abdominotransanal resection with sutured coloanal sleeve anastomosis (Sir Alan Park, 1972).
- Abdominal or anterior resection.
  - Without anastomosis – Hartmann's operation (1923). The upper end of the rectal stump is closed and a terminal iliac colostomy established.
  - With anastomosis – either as *anterior resection with restoration of continuity by telescopic or tube technique* OR *modern anterior resection with sutured anastomosis (hand)*. This procedure has nothing whatever to do with the tube technique and is completed entirely by suture. It could be termed the 'Mayo Clinic operation' (1943, 1945).

High anterior resection, which is applicable to growths of the extreme upper end of the rectum or of the rectosigmoid, can be conducted without disturbing the pelvic peritoneum or mobilising the rectum from the concavity of the sacrum. This type of operation is usually thought to be followed by uneventful healing of the suture line in the bowel and rectal function afterwards is nearly always perfect. Low anterior resection involves opening the pelvic peritoneum, dividing the lateral ligaments and freeing the rectum from its sacral bed often right down to the anorectal ring. The anastomosis is then between the colon and a rectal stump devoid of peritoneal covering. There is a considerable risk of partial breakdown of the suture line, particularly with very low anastomosis. There may be faecal incontinence (at least temporary).

Anastomosis by means of mechanical devices (with metal stapler) has been recently introduced (1965, 1975).

- *Local removal or destruction of the primary growth*: includes electrocoagulation, endocavitary contact irradiation and local excision.

The currently used operation of choice is either the combined excision or restorative rectal resection (sphincter-saving).

Splenectomy

In the USA, successful splenectomy was first reported by O'Brien (1816) for splenic prolapse following a knife wound. Karl Quittenbaum of Rostock (Germany) performed the first elective splenectomy for primary splenic disease in 1826, but his patient survived only a few hours after the operation. Zaccarelli of Naples (in 1849) is reported to have carried out splenectomy for splenomegaly in a woman aged 24 years. She was discharged from hospital 24 days after the operation. In 1866 Thomas Spencer Wells of London gave an account of the first successful splenectomy in England (1866). It has been reported that Spencer Wells' preoperative diagnosis was 'query ovarian cyst' and that during laparotomy he was surprised to find a 'floating spleen' in the left iliac fossa. He did not hesitate to ligate the long pedicle, divide it with scissors, and remove the congested enlarged 'wandering' organ. J. W. Mayo, in 1928, reported 500 splenectomies carried out by him and his colleagues at the Mayo Clinic, and special attention was devoted to the results and mortality rates.

Vagotomy and antrectomy

Distal gastric resection

At the turn of the century Billroth I began to be employed with increasing frequency for benign ulceration of the distal stomach and duodenum.

Ludwig Rydygier, in November 1881, performed the first pylorectomy with gastroduodenostomy for a benign stenotic chronic pyloric ulcer and the patient lived. Kocher (1893) implanted the end of the duodenum into the posterior wall of the stomach (after the open mouth of the stomach had been closed) in order to avoid the 'angle of sorrow', or Jammerecke. Von Haberer (1922) and Finney (1924) sutured the entire open end of the stomach to the side of the second portion of the duodenum after the duodenal stump had been securely closed and inverted. Schoemaker (1911) was among the first surgeons to extend gastric resection for both malignant and benign lesions of the stomach (as well as for duodenal ulcer) and to excise practically the whole of the lesser curvature prior to the performance of end-to-end gastroduodenostomy. He had no trouble from leakage at the Jammerecke, and his immediate and late results were most gratifying. Von Haberer (1933) performed his reefing and narrowing of the mouth of the gastric stump after partial gastrectomy.

In perforated gastric ulcers suture of the perforation was first suggested by Bernhard Von Langenbeck; he never performed the operation which was first attempted by Mikulicz-Radecki in 1880, but his patient died. Rydygier attempted some form of stomach resection in 1880, but his patient died. The first man certainly to have sutured a perforation with survival of the patient is Ludwig Heusner of Germany in 1892; this operation is sometimes attributed to another German surgeon, Kriege, who reported it. The first attempt in the UK was by Hastings Gilford of Reading in 1893, but his patient died. In the following year T. H. Morse of Norwich succeeded. In 1897 a surgeon named Braun suggested that suture of the perforation ought always to be accompanied by gastroenterostomy. His advice received little or no attention at the time, but in 1929 was resurrected as an original idea by Moynihan in the UK and by Deaver in the USA.

Another method of treating the perforation was by excising the ulcer area and then suturing the incision; first performed by J. W. Dowden in 1909, it was suggested as a routine method by H. Von Haberer of Vienna in 1919. Excision of the ulcer led naturally to excision of a larger portion of the stomach combined with gastroenterostomy, (in other words partial gastrectomy). First suggested by A. Odelberg of Stockholm in 1927, the 'emergency gastrectomy for perforation' was popularised by Doberauer of Carlsbad and Sergei Yudin of Moscow. In 1900 Mayo-Robson of Leeds declared that all peptic ulcers that did not respond to a medical regimen within a reasonable time should be treated surgically. Five years later over 500 gastroenterostomies for peptic ulcer had been performed at the Mayo Clinic alone. In 1905 Berkeley Moynihan published his important book on gastric ulcer, which had a great influence upon methods of treatment. By 1925 doubt was beginning to creep in and there were a few surgeons who had started to speak of gastroenterostomy as a 'surgically produced disease'. Results were sometimes good, but all too often the operation only gave temporary relief because a new ulcer formed at the point of anastomosis of the stomach with the small bowel. Braun first described the 'anastomotic ulcer' in 1899; Mayo-Robson wrote a paper on the subject in 1905, but he still regarded it as a rare complication.

Such outstanding surgeons as Rydygier, Jedlicka, Von Haberer, Clairmont and Finsterer made valuable contributions and pioneered distal gastric resection for surgical treatment of duodenal ulcer.

Vagotomy

Claude Bernard, in 1858, noted arrest of gastric contractions and absence of gastric secretion following vagal denervation. Pavlov, in 1894, described the absence of hydrochloric acid in fasting gastric secretions following vagotomy, but he was able to produce an acid response with subsequent feedings. He later showed that the vagus nerves supply secretory fibres to the gastric glands and constitute the pathway for stimuli that excite the cephalic phase of gastric secretion.

In 1914, Exner and Schwarzamann were the first to perform vagotomy in a human being via the abdominal route. The operation was done mainly for tabetic crisis and functional gastrointestinal disorders. Gastric atony was clearly recognised as a significant postoperative complication, and would be controlled by passing a tube through the pylorus via a gastrostomy route. Later these investigators added gastroenterostomy. Latarjet, in 1922, advocated vagotomy for benign gastric outlet obstruction and was the first to combine vagotomy with limited pylorectomy. Schiassi, in 1925, added drainage procedures to vagotomy in cases with obstruction. The operation received severe criticism, for in many instances it was performed for various functional disorders with poor results. In addition, during the 1920's there was a rise in popularity of simple gastroenterostomy championed by Berkeley Moynihan of Leeds and William J. Mayo of Rochester. In 1943 Lester Dragstedt produced a challenge to members of the surgical world when he and Owens published an account of two patients with duodenal ulcer treated by transthoracic vagotomy, which resulted in prompt ulcer healing and marked diminution in gastric acid secretion, with a rise in intragastric pH. Similar findings were reported by subsequent investigators.

Combined operation

In 1946, Farmer and Smithwick and their associates in Boston treated 18 patients with duodenal ulcer by vagotomy and removal of approximately 50% of the distal stomach (hemigastrectomy). This combined procedure resulted in marked reductions in the quantity of free acid and hydrogen ion concentration. In January 1947, Leonard Edwards of Nashville, unaware of Smithwick's combined operation performed 3 months earlier, followed the same line of reasoning and carried out truncal vagotomy with approximately 40% resection for a complication of duodenal ulcer. He termed the resection an antrectomy and constructed a retrocolic Billroth II.

Credit should also be given to the outstanding British surgeon, H. Dantree Johnson of London, who in 1947, unaware of the operations performed by Smithwick and Edwards, carried out vagotomy and antrectomy using a Hofmeister type of reconstruction.

To complete the history of the combined operation attention should be directed to the work of Colp and associates, who in 1948 reported satisfactory results with truncal vagotomy and gastrectomy, but the resection entailed removal of approximately 75% of the distal stomach.

Appendices

Appendix 1
Normal Values

Blood

Red cell count	$4.8 \pm 1 \times 10^{12}/l$
Haemoglobin	14 ± 2.5 g/dl
White cell count	$3.8-11 \times 10^9/l$
Platelet count	$150-400 \times 10^9/l$
ESR	up to 10 mm/h
Packed cell volume (PCV or haematocrit)	0.38–0.54 (1/l)
Mean corpuscular haemoglobin concentration (MCHC)	33 ± 2 g/dl
Mean corpuscular volume (MCV)	85 ± 8 fl
Mean corpuscular haemoglobin (MCH)	30 ± 2 pg
Reticulocytes	0.2–2%
Leucocytes	$7.5 \pm 3.5 \ 10^9/l$
Prothrombin time	11–15 s
Bleeding time	Up to 11 min

Liver function tests

Bilirubin	2–17 μmol/l
Alkaline phosphatase	25–130 i.u./l
Glutamic oxaloacetic transaminase (GOT)	10–40 i.u./l
Glutamic pyruvic transaminase(GPT)	<40 i.u./l
α-Hydroxybutyrate dehydrogenase (Hbd)	40–125 i.u./l
Proteins (total)	62–80 g/l
Albumin	35–55 g/l

Thyroid function tests

T_4	58–174 nmol/l
Free thyroxine index (FTI)	58–174
T_3	1.0–2.8 nmol/l
Thyroid-stimulating hormone(TSH)	0.4–3.5 mU/l

Blood gases

Base excess	± 2 mmol/l
Bicarbonate	24–32 mmol/l
Carbon dioxide ($P\text{co}_2$)	4.5–6.1 kPa
Oxygen ($P\text{o}_2$)	12–15 kPa
pH	7.36–7.44

Electrolytes

Calcium	2.2–2.67 mmol/l
Phosphate	0.75–1.4 mmol/l
Albumin	34–48 g/l
Glucose (fasting)	4.5–5.8 mmol/l
Urea	2.5–8 mmol/l
Creatinine	50–100 μmol/l
Uric acid	0.12–0.42 mmol/l
Chloride	95–105 mmol/l
Potassium	3.5–5.0 mmol/l
Sodium	135–146 mmol/l
Magnesium	0.7–1.1 mmol/l
Zinc	11–18 μmol/l
Iron	14–28 μmol/l

Plasma profile (*mainly Na, K, urea*)
Cardiac profile (*AST, LDH, CK*)
Renal profile (*Na, K, Cl, CO_2, urea, total protein, albumin, creatinine, calcium*)
Liver profile or liver function tests (*albumin, bilirubin, AST, ALT, alkaline phosphatase, GGT*)
Bone profile (*total protein, albumin, calcium, phosphate, alkaline phosphatase*)
Prostatic profile (*acid phosphatase, alkaline phosphatase, prostatic antigen, prostatic acid phosphatase*)
Thyroid profile or thyroid function tests (*T_3, T_4 anti-thyroid antibodies, TSH*)

Enzymes, hormones and other plasma parameters

Amylase	<300 s.u./dl
Acid phosphatase	0.8–2.7 i.u./l
Triglycerides	0.84–1.94 mmol/l
Cholesterol	3.6–7.8 mmol/l
Cortisol (09:00)	170–720 nmol/l
(midnight)	55–220 nmol/l
α-Fetoprotein	<10 μg/ml
β-Human chorionic gonadotrophin (HCG)	<15 μg/l
Carcinoembryonic antigen (CEA)	<10 μg/l
γ-Glutamyl transferase (γ-GT)	<50 i.u./l
Parathormone	1–6 i.u./l
Follicle-stimulating hormone (FSH)	0.5–5 u/l
Luteinising hormone (LH)	3–12 u/l
Prolactin	<360 mU/l
Renin activity (lying)	1.14–2.65 pmol/ml per h
(standing)	2.89–4.49 pmol/ml per h
Testosterone (males)	10–34 nmol/l
Osmolality	280–300 mmol/kg

Cerebrospinal fluid (CSF)

Protein	0.1–0.4 g/l
Glucose	2.8–4.5 mmol/l

Faeces

Fat	< 18 mmol/24 h

Urine

Calcium	< 8 mmol/24 h
Catecholamines (free) (as noradrenaline)	0.69 μmol/24 h
Creatinine	9–18 mmol/24 h
Creatinine clearance	70–140 ml/min
5-Hydroxyindole-acetic acid (5-HIAA)	< 52 μmol/24 h
Magnesium	3.5–15 mmol/24 h
Oxalate	0.14–0.46 mmol/24 h
Phosphate	16–50 mmol/24 h
Potassium	35–90 mmol/24 h
Protein	<0.1 g/24 h
Sodium	100–260 mmol/24 h
Urea	200–600 mmol/24 h
Uric acid	1.5–6.3 mmol/24 h
Vanillylmandelic acid (VMA)	10–35 μmol/24 h

Coagulation profile or screening tests

- Bleeding time (ivy) 3–10 min (measures platelet function and vascular integrity)
- Platelet count 150 000–400 000/ml
- Prothrombin time 12–14 sec (measures Factors I, II, V, VII, X)
- Partial thromboplastin time 25–35 sec (measures Factors I, II, V, VII, X, XI, XII)
- Thrombin time 12–20 sec (measures Factors I, II)
- Fibrinogen 200–400 mg/dl
- Fibrin degradation products 4 μg/ml

Cradiovascular variables and their normal values

Right atrial mean pressure	−1 – +7 mmHg
Right ventricle pressure	
Systolic	15–25 mmHg
End diastolic	0–8 mmHg
Pulmonary artery pressure	
Systolic	15–25 mmHg
Diastolic	8–15 mmHg
Mean (MPAP)	10–20 mmHg
Pulmonary capillary wedge pressure (PCWP)	6–12 mmHg
Mean arterial blood pressure =	

$$\frac{\text{Diastolic} + (\text{Systolic} - \text{Diastolic})}{3} \text{ mmHg}$$

$$\text{Cardiac output} = \text{Heart rate} \times \text{stroke volume} \quad (4\text{–}8 \text{ l/min})$$

$$\text{Cardiac index (CI)} = \frac{\text{Cardiac output}}{\text{Body surface area}} \quad (2.5\text{–}3.5 \text{ l/min/m}^2)$$

$$\text{Stroke volume} = \frac{\text{Cardiac output}}{\text{Heart rate}} \times 1000 \quad (70 \text{ ml/beat})$$

$$\text{Stroke volume index} = \frac{\text{Cardiac index}}{\text{Heart rate}} \times 1000$$
$$(35\text{–}70 \text{ ml/beat/m}^2)$$

Systemic vascular resistance (indexed) =

$$\frac{\text{MAP} - \text{CVP}}{\text{CI}} \times 79.92 \quad (1200\text{–}2500 \text{ dyne.sec/cm}^5/\text{m}^2)$$

Pulmonary vascular resistance (indexed) =

$$\frac{\text{MPAP} - \text{PCWP}}{\text{CI}} \times 79.92 \quad (150\text{–}250 \text{ dyne.sec/cm}^5/\text{m}^2)$$

Arterial oxygen content (CaO_2)	20 ml/dl
Mixed venous oxygen content (CvO_2)	15 ml/dl
Oxygen extraction ratio	25–30%
Shunt fraction	1–2%
Oxygen delivery (indexed)	400–670 ml/min/m^2
Oxygen consumption (indexed)	125–165 ml/min/m^2

Biochemical equations

Anion gap

$(Na + K)–(Cl + HCO_3)$.
Normal = 4–17 mmol

The gap is made up of phosphate, sulphate, protein, pyruvate, lactate and other ions.

- High: diabetic keto-acidosis, renal failure, lactic acidosis, methanol or salicylate ingestion, hepatic failure.
- Low: hypoalbuminaemia, liver disease, multiple myeloma.

Corrected calcium

There are many different equations for calculating the 'corrected calcium' result to account for raised or reduced albumin levels. The number of equations is testimony to the fact that at best all of them are estimations because the relationship between ionised calcium and albumin levels is complex. Many laboratories now report corrected or ionised calcium results. A useful approximation is as follows:

For every 1 g/l that the albumin result is more than 40 g/l, subtract 0.02 from the calcium result.
For every 1 g/l that the albumin result is less than 40 g/l, add 0.02 to the calcium result.
Or use the following equation:

Corrected Ca^{++} = (total Ca^{++} + 1) − (0.25 × albumin)

Creatinine clearance

Creatinine clearance (ml/min) =

$$\frac{\text{Urinary creatinine} \times \text{urine volume (ml)}}{\text{Plasma creatinine} \times \text{length of collection (min)}}$$

NB: The plasma creatinine must be measured during the 24 h urine collection period.

Plasma osmolality (mosmol/kg)

$\approx 2 \ (Na^+ \ K^+) \ + \ \text{urea} \ + \ \text{glucose}$

Appendix 2
HIV Infection and AIDS: the Ethical Considerations*

INTRODUCTION

1. This text brings together the Council's guidance to the medical profession on some of the ethical considerations which arise in relation to HIV infection and AIDS. It deals first with general principles and then discusses specific matters in relation to the duties of doctors towards infected persons, the duties of doctors who may themselves be infected, the need to obtain patient's consent to investigation or treatment and the need to observe the rules of professional confidence.

THE DOCTOR–PATIENT RELATIONSHIP

2. The doctor–patient relationship is founded on mutual trust, which can be fostered only when information is freely exchanged between doctor and patient on the basis of honesty, openness and understanding. Acceptance of that principle is, in the view of the Council, fundamental to the resolution of the questions which have been identified in relation to AIDS.

3. The Council has been impressed by the significant increase in the understanding of AIDS and AIDS-related conditions, both within the profession and by the general public, which appears to have occurred. It seems that most doctors are now prepared to regard these conditions as similar in principle to other infections and life-threatening conditions, and are willing to apply established principles in approaching their diagnosis and management, rather than treating them as medical conditions quite distinct from all others. The Council believes that an approach of this kind will help doctors to resolve many of the difficulties which have arisen hitherto.

4. In all areas of medical practice doctors need to make judgements which they may later have to justify. This is true both of clinical matters and of the complex ethical problems which arise regularly in the course of providing patient care,

*This text is based on a General Medical Council statement of June 1993 and is reproduced here with kind permission of the GMC.

because it is not possible to set out a code of practice which provides solutions to every such problem which may arise. The Council would remind the profession of the statements of general principle which are set out for the guidance of doctors in its booklet 'Professional Conduct and Discipline: Fitness to Practise'. In the light of that general guidance, the Council has formed the following views on questions of particular significance in relation to HIV infection and the conditions related to it.

THE DOCTOR'S DUTY TOWARDS PATIENTS

5. The Council expects that doctors will extend to patients who are HIV-positive or are suffering from AIDS the same high standard of medical care and support which they would offer to any other patient. It has, however, expressed its serious concern at reports that, in a small number of cases, doctors have refused to provide such patients with necessary care and treatment.

6. It is entirely proper for a doctor who has a conscientious objection to undertaking a particular course of treatment, or who lacks the necessary knowledge, skill or facilities to provide appropriate investigation or treatment for a patient, to refer that patient to a professional colleague.

7. However, it is unethical for a registered medical practitioner to refuse treatment, or investigation for which there are appropriate facilities, on the ground that the patient suffers, or may suffer, from a condition which could expose the doctor to personal risk. It is equally unethical for a doctor to withhold treatment from any patient on the basis of a moral judgement that the patient's activities or lifestyle might have contributed to the condition for which treatment was being sought. Unethical behaviour of this kind may raise a question of serious professional misconduct.

DUTIES OF DOCTORS INFECTED WITH THE VIRUS

8. Considerable public anxiety has been aroused by suggestions that doctors who are HIV-positive might endanger their patients. The risk is very small; to date there is only one known case anywhere in the world of HIV having been transmitted by a health care worker to patients, in the course of dental treatment. None the less, it is imperative, both in the public interest and on ethical grounds, that any doctors who think they may have been infected with HIV should seek appropriate diagnostic testing and counselling and, if found to be infected, have regular medical supervision.

9. Doctors who are HIV-positive should also seek specialist advice on the extent to which they should limit their practice in order to protect their patients. Such advice will usually be obtained locally from a consultant in occupational health, infectious diseases or public health, who may in turn seek guidance, on an anonymous basis, from the UK Advisory Panel of the Expert Advisory Group on AIDS. Doctors must act upon that advice which, in some circumstances, would include a requirement not to practise or to limit their practice in certain ways. No doctors should continue in clinical practice merely on

the basis of their own assessment of the risk to patients. The principles underlying this advice are already familiar to the profession, which has well-established policies and procedures designed to prevent the transmission of infection from doctors to patients.

10. It is unethical for doctors who know or believe themselves to be infected with HIV to put patients at risk by failing to seek appropriate counselling or by failing to act upon it when given. Such behaviour may result in proceedings by the Council which could lead to the restriction or removal of a doctor's registration if this were necessary to protect patients or the doctor's own health. The Council has already given guidance, in paragraph 63 of the booklet 'Professional Conduct and Discipline: Fitness to Practise' on doctors' duty to inform an appropriate person or authority about a colleague whose professional conduct or fitness to practise may be called into question. A doctor who knows that a health care worker is infected with HIV and is aware that the person has not sought or followed advice to modify his or her professional practice, has a duty to inform the appropriate regulatory body and an appropriate person in the health care worker's employing authority, who will usually be the most senior doctor.

RIGHTS OF DOCTORS INFECTED WITH THE VIRUS

11. Doctors who become infected with the virus are entitled to expect the confidentiality and support afforded to other patients. Only in the most exceptional circumstances, where the release of a doctor's name is essential for the protection of patients, may a doctor's HIV status be disclosed without his or her consent.

CONSENT TO INVESTIGATION OR TREATMENT

12. It has long been accepted, and is well understood within the profession, that a doctor should treat a patient only on the basis of the patient's informed consent. Doctors are expected in all normal circumstances to be sure that their patients consent to the carrying out of investigative procedures involving the removal of samples or invasive techniques, whether those investigations are performed for the purposes of routine screening, for example in pregnancy or prior to surgery, or for the more specific purpose of differential diagnosis. A patient's consent may in certain circumstances be given implicitly, for example by agreement to provide a specimen of blood for multiple analysis. In other circumstances it needs to be given explicitly, for example before undergoing a specified operative procedure or providing a specimen of blood to be tested specifically for a named condition. As the expectations of patients, and consequently the demands made upon doctors, increase and develop, it is essential that both doctor and patient feel free to exchange information before investigation or treatment is undertaken.

Testing for HIV infection: the need to obtain consent

13. The Council believes that the above principle should apply generally, but that it is particularly important in the case of testing for HIV infection, not because the condition is different in kind from other infections but because of the possible serious social and financial consequences which may ensue for the patient from the mere fact of having been tested for the condition. These are problems which would be better resolved by a developing spirit of social tolerance than by medical action, but they do raise a particular ethical dilemma for the doctor in connection with the diagnosis of HIV infection or AIDS. They provide a strong argument for each patient to be given the opportunity, in advance, to consider the implications of submitting to such a test and deciding whether to accept or decline it. In the case of a patient presenting with certain symptoms which the doctor is expected to diagnose, this process should form part of the consultation. Where blood samples are taken for screening purposes, as in antenatal clinics, there will usually be no reason to suspect HIV infection but even so the test should be carried out only where the patient has given explicit consent. Similarly, those handling blood samples in laboratories, either for specific investigation or for the purposes of research, should test for the presence of HIV only where they know the patient has given explicit consent. Only in the most exceptional circumstances, where a test is imperative in order to secure the safety of persons other than the patient, and where it is not possible for the prior consent of the patient to be obtained, can testing without explicit consent be justified.

14. A particular difficulty arises in cases where it may be desirable to test a child for HIV infection and where, consequently, the consent of a parent, or a person *in loco parentis*, would normally be sought. However, the possibility that the child may have been infected by a parent may, in certain circumstances, distort the parent's judgement so that consent is withheld in order to protect the parent's own position. The doctor faced with this situation must first judge whether the child is competent to consent to the test on his or her own behalf. If the child is judged competent in this context, then consent can be sought from the child. If however the child is judged unable to give consent the doctor must decide whether the interests of the child should override the wishes of the parent. It is the view of the Council that it would not be unethical for a doctor to perform such a test without parental consent, provided always that the doctor is able to justify that action as being in the best interests of the patient.

CONFIDENTIALITY

15. Doctors are familiar with the need to make judgements about whether to disclose confidential information in particular circumstances, and the need to justify their action where such a disclosure is made. The Council believes that, where HIV infection or AIDS has been diagnosed, any difficulties concerning confidentiality which arise will usually be overcome if doctors are prepared to discuss openly and honestly with patients the implications of their condition, the need to

secure the safety of others, and the importance for continuing medical care of ensuring that those who will be involved in their care know the nature of their condition and the particular needs which they will have. The Council takes the view that any doctor who discovers that a patient is HIV positive or suffering from AIDS has a duty to discuss these matters fully with the patient.

Informing other health care professionals

16. When a patient is seen by a specialist who diagnoses HIV infection or AIDS, and a general practitioner is or may become involved in that patient's care, then the specialist should explain to the patient that the general practitioner cannot be expected to provide adequate clinical management and care without full knowledge of the patient's condition. The Council believes that the majority of such patients will readily be persuaded of the need for their general practitioners to be informed of the diagnosis.

17. If the patient refuses consent for the general practitioner to be told, then the doctor has two sets of obligations to consider: obligations to the patient to maintain confidence, and obligations to other carers whose own health may be put unnecessarily at risk. In such circumstances the patient should be counselled about the difficulties which his or her condition is likely to pose for the team responsible for providing continuing health care and about the likely consequences for the standard of care which can be provided in the future. If, having considered the matter carefully in the light of such counselling, the patient still refuses to allow the general practitioner to be informed then the patient's request for privacy should be respected. The only exception to that general principle arises where the doctor judges that the failure to disclose would put the health of any of the health care team at serious risk. The Council believes that, in such a situation, it would not be improper to disclose such information as that person needs to know. The need for such a decision is, in present circumstances, likely to arise only rarely, but if it is made the doctor must be able to justify his or her action.

18. Similar principles apply to the sharing of confidential information between specialists or with other health care professionals such as nurses, laboratory technicians and dentists. All persons receiving such information must of course consider themselves under the same general obligation of confidentiality as the doctor principally responsible for the patient's care.

Informing the patient's spouse or other sexual partner

19. Questions of conflicting obligations also arise when a doctor is faced with the decision whether the fact that a patient is HIV-positive or suffering from AIDS should be disclosed to a third party, other than another health care professional, without the consent of the patient. The Council has reached the view that there are grounds for such a disclosure only where there is a serious and identifiable risk to a specific individual who, if not so informed, would be exposed to infection. Therefore, when a person is found to be infected in this way, the doctor must discuss with the patient the question of informing a spouse or other sexual partner. The Council

believes that most such patients will agree to disclosure in these circumstances, but where such consent is withheld the doctor may consider it a duty to seek to ensure that any sexual partner is informed, in order to safeguard such persons from a possibly fatal infection.

CONCLUSION

20. It is emphasised that the advice set out above is intended to guide doctors in approaching the complex questions which may arise in the context of this infection. It is not in any sense a code, and individual doctors must always be prepared, as a matter of good medical practice, to make their own judgements of the appropriate course of action to be followed in specific circumstances, and able to justify the decisions they make. The Council believes that the generality of doctors have acted compassionately, responsibly and in a well-informed manner in tackling the especially sensitive problems with which the spread of this group of conditions has confronted society. It is confident that they will continue to do so.

Appendix 3
National Confidential Enquiry into Perioperative Deaths (NCEPOD)*

BACKGROUND

The National Confidential Enquiry into Perioperative Deaths was launched in 1988 following the publication of the report of a similar enquiry which reviewed surgical and anaesthetic practice over one year (1985/6) in three NHS Regions. The Enquiry reviews the quality of the delivery of care and does not study causation of death. Maternal deaths are excluded. The first report of the National Enquiry (1 January to 31 December 1989) was published in June 1990.

All NHS and Defence Medical Services hospitals in England, Wales and Northern Ireland, and public hospitals in Guernsey, Jersey and the Isle of Man were included in the Enquiry in 1990 as well as hospitals managed by AMI Healthcare Group PLC and BUPA Hospitals Limited, and The London Independent Hospital. Funding is provided by the Department of Health, the Welsh Office, the Department of Health and Social Services (Northern Ireland), the relevant authorities in Guernsey, Jersey and the Isle of Man, and by the participating independent health care companies.

Consultant anaesthetists, surgeons and gynaecologists in all specialties are invited to participate and receive regular information about the Enquiry. A database of names and addresses of these consultants, is maintained, which is not available elsewhere.

*NCEPOD material is reproduced here with kind permission.

The Enquiry is an independent body to which a corporate commitment has been made by the Associations, Colleges and Faculties related to its areas of activity. The Association of Anaesthetists and the Association of Surgeons are included as initiators of the original (1982) Enquiry. Each of these bodies nominates members of the Steering Group which is responsible for the management of the Enquiry, and for its protocol.

The National Confidential Enquiry is now established as the cornerstone of a voluntary system dedicated to the maintenance and enhancement of a high quality surgical and anaesthetic service to the public. Government, by its continuing financial support, recognises its importance and that the corporate responsibility for the Enquiry rightly rests with the Medical Royal Colleges and their Faculties who have charters granted by the Privy Council. They are supported, for historical reasons, by the Association of Anaesthetists and the Association of Surgeons and each of these bodies nominates members of the Steering Group. It is thus widely representative and authoritative.

Enquiry reports contain a wealth of information of great importance not just to the medical profession but also to managers responsible for the provision, siting and organisation of services throughout the UK. While continuing deficiencies are identified and much clearly remains to be done, the overall trends demonstrate considerable improvements since earlier reports and encourage the Steering Group to believe that its work is gradually influencing matters for the better.

It can be seen on studying the reported deaths that there are few surprises in that the great majority occurred in gravely ill and elderly patients who, despite the best efforts of their attendants, could not have been expected to survive. Nevertheless, the conclusions highlight a number of unsatisfactory features that require attention and not all lie within the province of the medical profession.

In particular, it is clear that the physical environment within which many surgeons and anaesthetists operate is unsatisfactory and the absence or inappropriate siting of certain facilities such as emergency operating rooms, high dependency units and properly functioning intensive care units must affect patient survival. Acute services on split sites still present an obstacle to the proper management of seriously ill patients.

Among report conclusions highlighted are particular matters requiring the attention of the profession itself. For example, despite the exhortations of the Royal College of Pathologists over the years, too few post-mortem examinations are being carried out and discussion between pathologists and clinicians happens too infrequently. Opportunities to define contributing factors in deaths with greater precision are therefore lost. The continuing lack of sufficient non-medical assistance for anaesthetists is also very worrying and the profession will need to press hard for this long-standing situation to be remedied. It will probably always be necessary to employ locum surgeons and anaesthetists from time to time. While these colleagues do valuable work in service provision there is evidence that more scrupulous attention is necessary on appointment as to their training and experience and more adequate supervision and support for their clinical activities is required.

PROTOCOL

The protocol for the Enquiry is derived from the CEPOD report* published in December 1987.

Aims

The National Confidential Enquiry into Perioperative Deaths (NCEPOD) is to enquire into clinical practice and to identify remediable factors in the practice of anaesthesia and surgery.

The NCEPOD will investigate deaths which occur in hospital within 30 days of any surgical or gynaecological operation. This will include all procedures carried out by surgeons, whether in the presence or absence of an anaesthetist. Procedures involving local anaesthetics, as well as day cases, are included.

All consultants (surgeons, gynaecologists and anaesthetists) will be involved in the assessment programme.

Annual sample

A sample of all deaths reported will be investigated each year. The **dead cases** sampled will each be compared with similar patients, matched for sex, age, and mode of admission, who underwent similar operations and survived (**survivor cases**). Details of these patients will be obtained from consultants in another NHS Region.

Additionally, details of a large sample of patients undergoing surgery will be sought from all consultants (surgeons, gynaecologists and anaesthetists) each year. These **index cases** will provide a background against which the sample of dead cases and survivor cases will be compared.

Normally, consultants will be asked for details of **one** index case per year. This will depend, however, on the sample of dead cases being studied each year and the discipline of the consultant concerned.

Data will be collected by means of structured **questionnaires**, designed by the specialist groups and approved by the Steering Group.

It is anticipated that all consultants will provide information regarding all **dead** cases in the year's sample, any **survivor** case requested and one **index** case relevant to the sample.

The dead cases will be compared with the survivor cases and both samples with the index case sample. The specialist groups will advise on the sampling and conclusions to be drawn.

Excluded cases

The NCEPOD will *not* consider deaths after:
1. Diagnostic procedures carried out by physicians or other non-surgeons.
2. Therapeutic procedures carried out by physicians or other non-surgeons.
3. Radiological procedures performed solely by a radiologist without a surgeon present.
4. Obstetric operations or delivery.

*Buck N., Devlin H. B., Lunn J. N. (1987) Report of the Confidential Enquiry into Perioperative Deaths. Nuffield Provincial Hospitals Trust and The King Edward's Hospital Fund for London. London.

5. Dental surgery other than that taking place in the hospitals forming the subject of the Enquiry.

Questionnaires

The questionnaires have been developed by the specialist groups to obtain details of particular surgical and anaesthetic procedures. All personal identification of patients and medical staff will be removed before entry of a particular case into the computer.

Consultants are recommended to ask their junior staff to complete the questionnaire from the patient's notes. Once the form is completed the consultant and his or her junior should review it together and it should be returned to the NCEPOD office. It is hoped that this joint completion will act as a training process by reviewing the case on a one-to-one basis. This method could be used to develop a framework of local review of clinical practice. Trainees and consultants may write in total confidentiality to the NCEPOD office under separate cover if they wish.

Consultants (*surgeons and anaesthetists*) will also be asked to complete a small number of questionnaires on patients who have survived surgery. These cases will provide the benchmarks for assessment. The information given must be complete and accurate if valid conclusions are to be drawn. If further information is required the patient's notes may be requested.

Feedback

The Enquiry recognises the importance of adequate feedback to individual consultants and to the profession as a whole. However, feedback must avoid any likelihood of legal or professional jeopardy to the individual consultant. Therefore the Enquiry will publish an annual report which will present aggregated data but will not allow identification of individual consultants. There will be no assessments provided on individual cases.

Accreditation

All the Colleges and Faculties stress the importance of clinical audit for both monitoring clinical standards and as a discipline in the training of junior doctors. NCEPOD is a national audit system. The Colleges and Faculties require audit as a precondition for accreditation for training.

SUMMARY OF THE CEPOD REPORT PUBLISHED IN NOVEMBER 1987

Conclusions

1. The overall death rate after anaesthesia and surgery, analysed in this enquiry was low. The mortality of over half a million operations was 0.7%, and most of these were in the elderly, (over 75 years old) and were unavoidable due to progression of the presenting condition, such as advanced cancer, or co-existing diseases such as heart and (or) surgical or anaesthetic factors in a very small proportion of operations.
2. The majority of clinicians in the relevant disciplines cooperated in this system of clinical audit.

3. There were important differences in clinical practice between the three Regions studied.
4. There were deficiencies in the Hospital Activity Analysis data. There were also problems with the storage, movement and retrieval of patients' notes, particularly those of deceased patients.
5. Many surgeons and anaesthetists did not hold regular audits of their operation results (Mortality and Morbidity meetings).
6. There were important differences in the consultants' supervision of trainees.
7. There were a number of deaths in which junior surgeons or anaesthetists did not seek the advice of their consultants or senior registrars at any time before, during or after the operations.
8. The preoperative assessment and resuscitation of patients by doctors of both disciplines was sometimes compromised by undue haste to operate. This was a greater problem than delayed operations and it is possible that pressure to fit an operation into a very tight theatre schedule was one of the responsible factors.
9. There were instances of patients who were moribund or terminally ill having operations that would not have improved their condition.
10. There were examples of surgeons operating for conditions for which they were not trained or performing operations outside their primary field of expertise.
11. There were examples of difficulties in transferring patients for specialised treatment to other hospitals in the area.

Recommendations

Quality assurance

1. There is a need for an assessment of clinical practice on a national basis. Experience suggests this would be welcomed.
2. Consultants in every District should ensure that their own coding and input to information systems (including the Korner systems) is accurate and up-to-date; without this any audit is flawed. Every District should urgently review the storage, movement and retrieval of patients' notes, particularly those of deceased patients.
3. Clinicians need to assess themselves regularly. Effective self-assessment needs time; time to attend autopsies, mortality/morbidity meetings and clinical review with other disciplines.

Accountability

4. All departments of anaesthetics and surgery should review their arrangements for consultants' supervision of trainees. Locally agreed guidelines are important to ensure appropriate care of all patients, but particularly when responsibility is transferred from one clinical team, or shift, to another. No SHO or registrar should undertake any anaesthetic or surgical operation as an emergency or urgent matter without consultation with their consultant (or senior registrar).

Clinical decision-making

5. Resuscitation, assessment and management of medical disease take time and may determine the outcome; their

importance needs to be re-stated. Arrangements which permit this in every case are important.

6. The decision to operate on the elderly and very sick is important and should be taken at consultant (or senior registrar) level. For the most seriously ill patients, consultant anaesthetists and surgeons should consult together before the operation.

7. The decision *not* to operate is difficult. Humanity suggests that patients who are terminally ill or moribund should not have operations (i.e. non life-saving), but should be allowed to die in peace with dignity.

Organisational issues

8. Districts should review their facilities for out-of-hours work and concentrate anaesthetic, surgical and nursing resources at a single location, a fully staffed and fully equipped anaesthetic room, resuscitation room, operating room, recovery area and high dependency or intensive therapy unit should be available at all times.

9. The implementation of the CEPOD classification of operations (emergency, urgent, scheduled and elective) would concentrate the attention of all staff on the fact that very few operations need to be performed at night.

10. Operations should only be performed by consultants or junior surgeons (accountable to consultants) who have had adequate training in the specialty relevant to the operation. Health Authorities should therefore balance surgical specialties so that appropriate urological and vascular trained surgeons are provided in each District. In the case of small Districts this may necessitate sub-Regional units to ensure adequate subspecialty care. Neurological and neonatal surgery should be carried out at special Regional units.

Surgery

Commonest operations resulting in death:
   Laparotomy
   DHS
   Hemiarthroplasty
   Hemicolectomy
   AAA

Working diagnoses:
   Femur
   Intestinal obstruction
   AAA
   Peptic ulcer
   Colon cancer

Organisation, delegation and accountability

Assessors are most concerned by the lack of 'control' some consultants seem to exercise over their trainees and junior staff. There is a North–South divide: in the North a consultant was consulted in 66% of cases, he took a history in 72% and examined the patient preop. in 79%. In NE Thames these figures were respectively 55%, 53% and 58.5%. This suggests that working practices are already considerably different in the North.

Paediatric, cardiothoracic and neurosurgeons exercise more 'control', orthopaedic surgeons have least 'control'.

Inexperienced operators

Many operations were undertaken by surgeons too junior and too inexperienced to do the job.

Assessors commented that mistakes were frequently made by these surgeons.

The assessors recommend that no patient should undergo a surgical operation without prior consultation being obtained by the operating surgeons with the consultant on duty, or the senior registrar.

Fatigue is relatively uncommon; it was cited as a factor in 26 cases.

It is to be noted that inappropriate preoperative management, inappropriate operation and deaths related to surgery are more marked when junior unsupervised surgeons are operating on their own.

Ruptured aneurysm patients died because vascular clamps were not available.

Availability of operating theatres

The general principle that one fully equipped theatre must be kept available to deal with emergencies is made over and over again in the reports to CEPOD. Failure to do this led to two patients with leaking aneurysms dying during transit from one hospital's A&E to another hospital with the available equipped operating theatre. Another patient bled to death from a chest wound. Consultants should not, and cannot, provide on-call support to more than one hospital at once. An aneurysm patient died because a consultant was operating elsewhere, and there were other examples.

Our groups of assessors stress the importance in each District of having only one A&E Department where all emergencies are brought, with one on-site fully equipped emergency operating theatre and with an on-site ITU. Consultants should only be on call for one hospital (District) at one time.

Specific operations

Abdominal aortic aneurysm (AAA)

One hundred and fifty-six deaths: 25.6% avoidable and 29% were surgery-related.

Prostatectomy

High death rate in open prostatectomies performed by non-specialist urologists.

Oesophagectomy

Thirty-eight per cent of deaths were surgeon-related: 33% had avoidable factors. Plea for referral to centres who regularly undertake this work and have the ITU support etc.

Pneumonectomy

Six deaths: 4 avoidable. Only one operation by a consultant. In 4 cases surgeon-related factors leading to death.

Exploratory thoracotomy for malignancy

Twenty-six deaths. 20 consultant operations. 75% by specialists. 38% surgeon-related deaths. Operation was inappropriate in 15.4%, avoidable death in 26.9%.

Thoracic emergencies

Two cases reported. Highlight theatre and surgeon non-availability.

Colorectal carcinoma

One hundred and ninety deaths. 134 hemi-colectomy. 56 AP. 13% emergency operations. On reviewing the 13% performed at night, there seemed to be no reason why they should have been done that urgently.

Thirty-nine per cent of the AP deaths were surgeon-related. 30% were avoidable, 17% had inappropriate operations.

Pseudo-obstruction

Five cases, none should have been operated upon, none had a contrast enema.

Appendicectomy

Five deaths, all surgically avoidable.

Hernia

Sixty deaths. 52.5% avoidable. 30.5% inappropriate preop. management. In 18% operation was inappropriate. The assessors would have avoided operation in 27%, 59.2% were emergencies.

Peptic ulcers

One hundred and fifty-one deaths. 70% out of hours. 31.2% surgeon-related. 11.2% avoidable. Inappropriate preop. management in 8.6%. In 1.9% operation was inappropriate. In only 56% was the consultant informed or consulted.

Too often these are difficult operations performed by too junior surgeons without consultant help or even advice.

Biliary tract surgery

Forty-two deaths. 19 after operations for acute cholecystitis. Failure to resuscitate, failure to administer suitable antibiotic prophylaxis, and the inappropriateness of the surgeon's grade to the difficulty of the task.

Multiple trauma

Ten deaths. Present set-up cannot deal with these cases as they are relatively rare and A&E Departments are not geared to the management of major trauma. 5 of these patients were salvageable. They would probably have survived in an American or Continental trauma centre. Avoidable deaths were not age-dependent.

Carcinomatosis

One hundred and twelve cases. In 29% the operation was unnecessary.

Pulmonary embolism

Of 189 deaths, only 42 had had prophylaxis.

Grades of staff

Anaesthetic assessors were concerned at the numbers of very sick patients who were anaesthetised as urgent or emergency cases by trainees without reference to consultants. Similar concern was expressed by surgeon assessors about surgical trainees. It is appreciated that there may be many reasons for this reluctance to consult, apart from non-availability. Experience may have led a trainee to believe that he or she would not receive the guidance and help which they sought or they may have previously been insulted. Trainees may be unwilling to disturb consultants in their beds.

SUMMARY OF THE NCEPOD REPORT PUBLISHED IN SEPTEMBER 1990

The National Confidential Enquiry into Perioperative Deaths is concerned with the quality of the delivery of anaesthesia and surgery: it does not study the causation of death. Many of the patients mentioned in the report were old, very seriously ill, and were expected to die by the doctors who cared for them. The report contains recommendations about improvements in the care of patients. There are no *new* lessons.

General conclusions

The conclusions are relevant to both the *medical profession* and to *managers*.

1. *Information*   There are examples throughout the report about deficiencies in the hospital notes; at least 90 cases could not be studied because notes were acknowledged to be lost. Operation notes were sometimes missing or lacking in essential details such as the name of the surgeon or the diagnosis; anaesthetic notes regularly failed to record physiological changes. Hospital notes about dead patients tend to be given a low priority by records staff and soon disappear and become difficult to find.

2. *Essential services*   Recovery rooms, high dependency units and intensive care units need not to exist merely as structures, they must also be ready for use. Proper equipment and qualified specialist staff (nurses, operating department assistants) must be available at all times if patients are to survive anaesthesia and surgery. If these services are not available patients may have to be moved elsewhere. Services were noted to be deficient, or closed, on Bank Holidays (particularly Christmas) and, perhaps surprisingly, at night. The proper and safe provision of pain relief after surgery implies that more high dependency units are required.

3. *Emergency operating rooms*   The provision of this essential service is important for all surgical specialties. Best results

are obtained when there is no (non-medical) delay in the management of, for example, fractured neck of femur. If patients are to receive the greatest benefit from modern surgery it must be performed at the clinically most opportune moment. Dedicated operating rooms for emergency surgery are an essential service for all surgical specialties.

4. *Split sites* The problems caused by the requirement for Consultants (and their teams) to work and to be on call regularly on more than one NHS site are well known. The use of split sites should be historical.

5. *Consultants* In this Enquiry, 83% of the decisions about surgery were made by consultants or senior registrars. About half the anaesthetics for the group of patients who subsequently died were conducted in the precise knowledge and (or) presence of a consultant. This proportion is not yet satisfactory but many of the deaths occurred as a result of factors outside the clinical responsibility of anaesthetists.

6. *Specialty involvement* A few surgeons persist in occasionally operating outside their primary specialty; this is deplored.

7. *Locums* Temporary appointments are sometimes necessary. The most senior operating surgeon was a locum in 7% of the deaths; similarly, 9% of anaesthetists *working alone* were locums. Sometimes these locums, of both disciplines, were 'acting up' but too often they admitted personally that they were inadequately trained or out of practice at particular procedures.

8. *Non-medical assistance* The need for trained non-medically qualified assistants for anaesthetists is overwhelming; in 59% of deaths the anaesthetist was working without medical assistance.

9. *Post-mortem examinations* The infrequency of this useful investigation revealed in this Enquiry is to be deplored. Communication between pathologists (both hospital and Coroners') and clinicians is so poor that useful lessons can often not be learnt.

10. *Non-trainee, non-consultant clinicians* There is evidence within this report that these clinicians (Associate Specialist, Staff Grade, Clinical Assistant) are sometimes isolated. Arrangements whereby these individuals are fully integrated into departments of surgery and anaesthesia need to be improved. This should include involvement in audit meetings.

11. *Supervision* Trainee surgeons and anaesthetists need to be encouraged to request supervision. Consultants must ensure that trainees have the confidence to ask and to know that their request will not be rebuffed. If proper supervision of trainees is to be achieved, there may need to be more consultants, particularly in orthopaedic surgery and in anaesthesia.

12. *Confidential enquiries* The influence of confidential enquiries in the practice of medicine in the United Kingdom is undeniable. The effects of CEPOD and NCEPOD are such that this unique Enquiry should continue.

General recommendations

1. The provision of clinical and management information about patients, including post-mortem records, needs to be improved significantly.

2. Essential services (including staffed emergency operating rooms, recovery rooms, high dependency units and intensive care units) must be provided on a single site wherever emergency/acute surgical care is delivered.

3. Decisions for or against operations should be made jointly by surgeons and anaesthetists; this is a consultant responsibility.

4. The supervision of locum appointments at all grades in anaesthesia and surgery needs an urgent review.

5. All grades of surgeon and anaesthetist should be involved in medical audit and continuing medical education.

6. Efforts should be made to increase the number of post-mortem examinations.

7. The National Confidential Enquiry into Perioperative Deaths should continue.

SUMMARY OF THE NCEPOD REPORT PUBLISHED FOR 1991/2
General recommendations

● The medical Royal Colleges and the Specialist Societies in Surgery, Gynaecology and Anaesthesia must encourage all Consultants to participate in the National Confidential Enquiry into Perioperative Deaths. Full cooperation would enable the profession to defend itself against charges of falling standards and lack of public accountability. The failure of some consultants to return questionnaires is unacceptable and a cause for concern.

● Surgeons, gynaecologists and anaesthetists need to address the continuing problem of thromboembolism which causes death after surgery. We have emphasised this matter before and we regret that we must again bring the profession's attention to it. Hospitals and clinical directorates should be required to address the issue and develop an agreed local protocol. Every consultant should then follow this protocol. The research bodies and the Department of Health need to continue actively to encourage and support research in this field.

● All grades of surgeons, gynaecologists and anaesthetists must realise the critical importance of fluid balance in elderly patients.

● There needs to be a collaborative approach to the matching of surgical and anaesthetic skills to the condition of the patient.

● Surgeons, gynaecologists and anaesthetists must have immediate access to essential services (recovery rooms, high dependency and intensive care units) if their patients are to survive. The previous Reports have emphasised the need to have emergency operating and recovery rooms available 24 hours a day.

● It is no longer acceptable for basic specialist trainees (senior house officers) in some specialties to work alone without suitable supervision and direction by their consultant. Managers and consultants must locally achieve these arrangements.

● The post-mortem rate is too low. At least 49% of post-mortems demonstrate, despite clinicians' scepticism, significant, new and unexpected findings which are relevant. Post-mortems are an important form of quality control.

● The necessary information available within the NHS under the present system is inadequate. Despite our repeated comment about this, we are still unable to obtain basic and timely data about the number of patients who have operations and the number of perioperative deaths. There is a need for an improved method for collection and validation of information on perioperative deaths locally and nationally.

Important issues in management

● Managers must realise that there are resource implications for a service which is increasingly consultant-based.

● Managers should urgently review the storage and retrieval of medical notes.

● Managers should assist local reporters to identify methods of reporting *all* relevant deaths.

● Data on the number of surgical procedures performed and the number of perioperative deaths will be inadequate until a unique patient number is in general use in all medical records.

Important issues in surgery

● Surgery should be avoided for those whose death is inevitable and imminent. A more humane approach to the care of these patients should be considered; these decisions should be directed by consultants.

● Specialist opinion should be sought before undertaking some procedures (e.g. amputation, oesophagectomy, hysterectomy, craniotomy).

● Resuscitation and preparation of patients for surgery should not be inadequate or hasty (e.g. strangulated hernia).

● There is a need for more consultant involvement in the theatre, particularly for emergency cases (e.g. colorectal resection).

Important issues in anaesthesia

● Arrangements whereby anaesthetists could work in teams (with other anaesthetists) should be considered.

● Anaesthetists should review their practice of non-invasive instrumental monitoring at induction of anaesthesia.

● The potential for local protocols or national guidelines for staff–patient matching, the use of anaesthesia teams, the provision of essential services, the transfer of patients and other matters should be realised.

Sample

The answers to most of the questionnaires (deaths and index cases) show that the standard of the delivery of anaesthesia in England, Wales and Northern Ireland is good. Comparisons with previous years are not fully valid, because the current sample is very different from those previously used, but the overall picture is one of a very high standard of care. Indeed, there are few demonstrable differences between the management of comparable patients who die and those who survive (index cases).

There are some factors which are noted in the preceding pages which, if corrected or not present, might have made a death less likely. It is inevitable in a report such as this that some emphasis is laid on deficiencies, but this should not be allowed to obscure the reality of widespread good practice.

Readers should remember, that whilst only a few vignettes are published here, the views are formulated after reading 1616 questionnaires which relate to patients who died.

The selection of 15 operations for the Enquiry was for surgical reasons. All deaths after these operations were studied in detail with the exception of colorectal ones. There was a large number of these deaths (1727) and so a random 25% sample was selected and this yielded 314 completed questionnaires from anaesthetists.

Local protocols

Disposition of staff resources on the basis of perceived risk seems a rational approach to clinical practice and perusal of many of the answers to the questions has suggested that some scheme such as is outlined below might be acceptable and even useful. The anaesthetist group is convinced that departments or directorates should consider the production of written protocols for use in their own hospital. Protocols could be written about ASA grades, anaesthesia teams and essential services. A few directorates have already written protocols after the publication of our previous reports.

ASA grade of patient

The ASA system of grading patients is designed not for risk assessment purposes but to enable clinicians to communicate with each other about a patient's overall condition. The group of anaesthetists, on the basis of the questionnaires which they have seen, suggest the following thoughts for consideration.

Some matching between ASA status and the skill (qualifications and (or) experience) of the anaesthetist deployed should be attempted by departments in the design of their local guidelines.

1. Good risk 80-year-olds for major surgery should be treated as if they were ASA 4.

2. No ASA 4 or 5 patient should be anaesthetised without detailed discussion with a consultant (senior registrar) anaesthetist.

Anaesthesia teams

It is common practice for anaesthetists of all grades to work by themselves (solo) in contrast to the usual practice of surgeons. There are certain operations which are, and always should be, serviced by a team of anaesthetists. There are several different aspects to this matter:

1. This team should normally be led by a consultant (or experienced senior registrar). Careful planning for appropriate staff–patient deployment by departments is required.

2. Anaesthesia for emergency or urgent lifesaving operations should ideally be managed by a team of anaesthetists; two-anaesthetist teams would usually be the minimum requirement. Many operations, particularly those of long duration will require two anaesthetists (e.g. craniotomy, oesophagectomy, coronary bypass grafts) at least for part of the time, e.g. during periods of physiological instability.

3. Trainees need to appreciate that they are part of a team of anaesthetists even if they are working by themselves and should feel able to call for support.

4. Flexibility of staff allocation, so that appropriately experienced anaesthetists are available at critical moments during anaesthesia and operations, needs to be encouraged. One consultant should not be solely responsible for the welfare of a patient or patients for 12 hours. Trainee doctors need instant support in the event of unanticipated crises.

Essential services

NCEPOD and its predecessors have repeatedly made suggestions about the provision of essential services.

It should be possible for *all* patients who have surgical operations to be admitted to a properly staffed and equipped recovery room which is available 24 hours a day.

A fully equipped and staffed high dependency unit with provision for safe transport elsewhere to a ward when stable or to an intensive care unit, should be available for all patients wherever major surgery is undertaken.

Operations should not be undertaken in the absence of these services. Admission policies for HDU or ICU should not be affected by the patient's age. Decisions about elderly patients should be made before operation, jointly by surgeons and anaesthetists, and the decision not to operate should not be fudged.

Other topics for protocols for anaesthetic services

These might include arrangements for the *transfer* of patients, explanations of current local practices for *locums* of any grade, *discharge criteria* for patients who are to return to the ward, *admission criteria* for HDU or ICU, and indications for *oxygen therapy*.

Fluid overload

The administration of intravenous fluids to elderly patients needs to be carefully supervised. Systemic hypotension (in the absence of blood loss) should not be treated solely with large volumes of intravenous fluids but, perhaps in addition, vasopressors should be used more readily. The practice of 'fluid loading' so widespread in obstetrics (in association with epidural or spinal anaesthesia) may not be appropriate in the elderly patient who also has ischaemic heart disease. When the vasodilatation caused by these techniques wears off and normal vascular tone returns, all the extra fluid overwhelms the capacity of the diseased circulation and left ventricular failure is almost inevitable.

Non-medical assistants

The provision of competent non-medical assistants is now widespread but must now be invariable. This is a matter for management action.

Pain relief

The provision of pain relief needs attention by anaesthetists since current arrangements are not yet satisfactory everywhere.

The Royal College of Anaesthetists is considering a guideline concerned with intramuscular analgesia, but more advanced methods must be dependent upon appropriate nursing and medical support. There were a number of reports of patients who were deemed to have received less than adequate treatment in relation to pain after operation, particularly those whose care after operation was conducted on a general ward, rather than on a high dependency unit.

Anaesthetic records

The standards of these have improved but the variation in design across the countries is very wide. There may be an argument for a standard anaesthetic record. The Royal College of Anaesthetists has now agreed a basic minimum of information which should be included on such a record. There are still a few hospitals which do not appear to provide anaesthetists with a chart on which changes in physiological variables could be plotted against time. Standardisation of the record would in addition facilitate external review of the record. Whatever the design of a record the clarity of completion also varies widely. Standardisation of charts for automatic blood pressure measurements would also be beneficial.

Instrumental monitoring

The publication of standards (for administration of anaesthesia, monitoring of and support for the patient), which are approved by the World Federation of Societies of Anaesthesiology, makes further comment or suggestions about guidelines on this topic superfluous. The Association of Anaesthetists of Great Britain and Ireland has also published its recommendations. The advisory group of anaesthetists unanimously endorses both the aims and recommendations of these publications and another variant would be undesirable. Thus directorates are advised to introduce their own protocols based on the published efforts of others and NCEPOD does not offer any more confusion on this topic.

Participation in NCEPOD by anaesthetists

Sixty-one per cent of questionnaires about deaths were returned by anaesthetists. This is too low. Part of the explanation for the low figures is undoubtedly the method whereby NCEPOD arranged for consultants to receive their questionnaires. We knew that this was likely to prove unsatisfactory and changes in arrangements have already been made. The failure by surgeons in some particular disciplines is also too high: in the current method their failure probably has a consequent effect on anaesthetists' returns.

Part of the explanation is the recurrent difficulty of discovery of an individual patient's notes. Information retrieval in some institutions has improved over the last two to three years and the problem may soon be solved everywhere. The loss of the notes of dead patients does still happen and some are inevitably secreted in departments of surgery and pathology. Others are destroyed prematurely.

The information collected by this Enquiry is unique and useful. Its value would be much enhanced if the return rate were substantially increased.

Selected References and Further Reading

PART TWO: 1 THE WRITTEN EXAMINATION

Metabolic response to trauma

Hall, G. M. and Desborough, J. P. (1992) Editorial I (Interleukin-6 and the metabolic response to surgery). *British Journal of Anaesthesia*, **69**: 337–338.

Joris, J., Cigarini I., Legrand M. *et al.* (1992) Metabolic and respiratory changes after cholecystectomy performed via laparotomy or laparoscopy. *British Journal of Anaesthesia*, **69**: 341–345.

Pain in surgery

Hanningington-Kiff, J. G. (1981) *Pain*, 2nd edn. London: Update Publications.

Paths to Pain Relief (Filmstrip) (1978) Winthrop Laboratories.

Schachter, M. (1981) Enkephalins and endorphins. *British Journal of Hospital Medicine*, **25**: 128–236.

Acid–base disturbances in surgery

Stoelting, R. K., Dierdorf, S. F. and McCammon, R. L. (1988) Geriatric patients. In: *Anaesthesia and Co-Existing Disease*, 2nd edn. New York, Edinburgh etc.: Churchill Livingstone, p 251–261.

Fluid and electrolyte disorders in surgery

Karanjia, N. D., Walker, A. and Rees, M. (1992) Fluids and electrolytes in surgery. *Surgery* (The Medicine Group), pp. 121–128.

Stoelting, R. K., Dierdorf, S. F. and McCammon, R. L. (1988) Geriatric patients. In: *Anaesthesia and Co-Existing Disease*, 2nd edn. New York, Edinburgh etc.: Churchill Livingstone, pp. 445–471.

Nutrition in surgery

Hill, G. L. (1995) Nutrition in surgical practice. In: *Essential Surgical Practice*, 3rd edn (A. Cuschieri, G. R. Giles and A. R. Moossa) Oxford: Butterworth-Heinemann, pp. 332–347.

June, R. (1981) Nutrition (annual review). *Hospital Update*, **7**: 883–898.

Phillips, V. and Galbally, B. P. (1984) *Guide to Parenteral Nutrition*. Ealing Health District.

Silk, D. B. A. (1978) Parenteral nutrition. *Hospital Update*, **4**: 611–622.

Silk, D. B. A. (1980) Enteral nutrition. *Hospital Update*, **6**: 761–776

Yarborough, M. F. and Curreri, P. W. (1981) *Surgical Nutrition*. Edinburgh: Churchill Livingstone.

Bleeding in surgery

Cohen, J. (1984) AIDS – a review. *British Journal of Hospital Medicine*, **31**: 250–260.

Dalgleish, A. (1985) AIDS. *Hospital Doctor*. C5 May 16 and May 23.

Samson, D. (1976). The bleeding patient. *Hospital Update*, **2**: 185–196.

Walter, J. B. and Israel, M. S. (1974) *General Pathology*. Edinburgh: Churchill Livingstone, pp. 613–625.

Shock in surgery

Hanson, G. C. (1978) *Management of Septic Shock*. Middlesex: Glaxo Laboratories Ltd.

Ledingham, I., McArdle, C. S. and MacDonald, R. C. (1980) Septic shock. In: *Recent Advances in Surgery*, No. 10. (S. Taylor ed). Edinburgh: Churchill Livingstone, pp. 161–200.

Blood transfusion in surgery

Atkinson, R. S., Rushman, G. B. and Davies, N. J. H. (1993) Sepsis and the septic syndrome. In: *Lee's Synopsis of Anaesthesia*, 11th edn. Oxford: Butterworth-Heinemann, pp. 328–333.

Proud, G. and Parrott, N. R. (1991) Blood transfusion; and Cancer and the immune response. Both in *Immunology in Surgical Practice: an Introduction to Surgeons* (eds A. V. Pollock and M. Evans) London: Edward Arnold, pp. 245–251.

Genetic factors in surgery and genetic diseases of surgical importance

Emery, A. E. H. (1991) Genetic factor in disease. In: *Davidson's Principles and Practice of Medicine*, 14th edn (ed. J. Macleod). Edinburgh: Churchill Livingstone.

Jagelman, D. G. (1992) FAP – the spectrum of the disease (Abstract). In: *Colorectal Diseases in 1992*. Cleveland Clinic Foundation Symposium, 20–22 February 1992, at Pier Sixty-Six Resort and Marina, Ft Lauderdale, Florida, USA.

McKeown, C. (1993) Genetic counselling (Abstract). In: *Gastroenterology: Current Issues in Inflammatory Bowel Disease and Colorectal Cancer*. The British Council International Course, 16–23 March 1993, at Queen Elizabeth Postgraduate Medical Centre, UK.

Editorial (1993). *JAMA*, **269**: 2181–2193.

Immunology in surgical practice

Ermin, O. and Sewell, H. (1992) *The Immunological Basis of Surgical Science and Practice*. Oxford: Oxford University Press.

Pollock, A. V. and Evans, M. (1992) *Immunology in Surgical Practice: an Introduction to Surgeons*. London: Edward Arnold.

Monoclonal antibodies in surgical practice

Donald, F. E. and Finch, R. G. (1992) Rapid techniques for diagnosis of infection in the ICU. *Hospital Originated Sepsis and Therapy (HOST)*, No. 8, pp. 2–5.

Ledermann, J. A. (1992) Monoclonal antibodies in the diagnosis and treatment of cancer. In: *Immunology in Surgical Practice: an Introduction to Surgeons* (eds A. V. Pollock and M. Evans) London: Edward Arnold pp. 274–291.

Reidy, J. J. (1993) The use of monoclonal antibodies in the treatment of sepsis. *British Journal of Intensive Care*, **3** (March): 107–112.

Russell, S. J., Llewelyn, M. B., and Hawkins, R. (1992) Monoclonal antibodies in medicine – principles of antibody therapy. *British Medical Journal*, **305**: 1424–1429.

Antimicrobials in surgery

International Symposium (1983) *Serious Infection – Treatment and Prevention (A Review)*. London: Update Publications.

Tenenbaum, M. J. and Kaplan, M. H. (1982) Antibiotic combinations. *Medical Clinics of North America*, **66**: 17–24.

Viral infections of surgical importance (AIDS and viral hepatitis in surgery)

Dusheiko G. M. (1992) Viral hepatitis: part 1. *Hospital Update*, **18**: 173–181.

Forbes, C. D. (1993) HIV and AIDS update – 1992. *Scottish Medical Journal*, No. 1, pp. 36–38.

Joint Working Party (Shanton D. C. *et al.*) (1992) Risks to surgeons and patients from HIV and hepatitis: guidelines on precautions and management of exposure to blood or body fluids. *British Medical Journal*, **305**: 1337–1343.

Mann, J. and Wilson, M. E. (1993) AIDS: global lessons from a global epidemic. *British Medical Journal*, **307**: 1574–5.

Miles, A. J. G., Smith, D. and Wastell, C. (1991) AIDS. In: *Immunology in Surgical Practice: an Introduction to Surgeons* (eds A. V. Pollock and M. Evans). London: Edward Arnold, pp. 207–219.

Moyle, G. and Hawkins, D. (1995) Combination therapy in HIV treatment. *Hospital Update*, **21**: 496–502.

Stoelting, R. K., Dierdorf, S. F. and McCammon, R. L. (1988) Acute hepatitis. In: *Anaesthesia and Co-Existing Disease*, 2nd edn. New York, Edinburgh etc.: Churchill Livingstone, pp. 369–376.

Minimal access therapy

Al-Fallouji, M. A. R. (1992) The first laparoscopic appendicectomy in the United Arab Emirates. *Emirates Medical Journal*, **10**: 161–163.

Al-Fallouji, M. A. R. (1993) Making loops in laparoscopic surgery. State of the art. *Surgical Laparoscopy and Endoscopy*, **3**: 477–481.

Berci, G., Sackier, J. M. and Paz-Partlow, M. (1991) Emergency laparoscopy. *American Journal of Surgery*, **161**: 323–335.

Bowersox, J. C. (1996) Telepresence surgery. *British Journal of Surgery*, **83**: 433–434.

Browne, D. S. (1990) Laparoscopic-guided appendicectomy. A study of 100 consecutive cases. *Australian and New Zealand Journal of Obstetrics and Gynaecology*, **30** (3): 231–233.

Buess, Theis and Huttere (1991) *Transanal Endoscopic Microsurgery (TEM)*. Knittlinger, Germany: R. Wolf Gmbh. (UK: Mitcham, Surrey; USA: Vernon Hills, Ill.)

Cuschieri, A. (1990) Minimal access surgery. *Journal of the Royal College of Surgeons of Edinburgh*, **35**: 345–347.

Cuschieri, A., Nathanson, L. K. and Shimi, S. M. (1992) Laparoscopic antireflux surgery. In: *Operative Manual of Endoscopic Surgery* (eds A. Cuschieri, G. Buess and J. Perissat). Berlin: Springer-Verlag, pp. 280–297.

Darzi, A. and Monson, J. R. T. (1995) Laparoscopic rectopexy for rectal prolapse. In: *Laparoscopic Colorectal Surgery* (ed. J. R. T. Monson and A. Darzi). Oxford: Isis Medical Media, pp. 101–110.

Dubois, F., Berthelot, G. and Levard, H. (1989) Cholecystectomie par coelioscopie. *Presse Medicale*, **18**: 980–982.

Dubois, F., Icard, P., Berthelot, G. and Levard, H. (1990) Coelioscopic cholecystectomy. *Annals of Surgery*, **211**: 60–63.

Giotz, F., Pier, A. and Bacher, C. (1990) Laparoscopic appendectomy – alternative therapy in all stages of appendicitis? *Langenbecks Archiv fur Chirurgie* (Suppl. ii), pp. 1351–1353 (German).

Martin, I. G. and McMahon, M. J. (1996) Gasless laparoscopy. *Journal of the Royal College of Surgeons of Edinburgh*, **41**: 72–4.

Mouret, P. H. and Marsand, H. (1990) Appendicectomy per laparoscopy. Technique and evaluation. Paper given at 2nd Congress of the Society of American Gastrointestinal Endoscopic Surgeons, Atlanta, 16 March 1990.

Omer, A. B. and Al-Fallouji, M. A. R. (1992) Laparoscopy in surgical abdominal emergencies. Abstract of a paper delivered at the 3rd annual surgical conference, UAE, Al-Ain Intercontinental Hotel, 15–17 December, 1992.

Sackier, J. M. and Berci, G. (1990) Diagnostic and interventional laparoscopy for the general surgeon. *Contemporary Surgery*, p. 37.

Schrieber, J. (1987) Early experience with laparoscopic appendectomy in women. *Surgical Endoscopy*, **1**: 211–216.

Semm, K. (1983) Endoscopic appendicectomy. *Endoscopy*, **15**: 59–64.

Zucker, K. A. (1991) *Surgical laparoscopy*. St Louis: Quarterly Medical Publishing.

Day case surgery

Jarrett, P. E. M. (1994) Provision of a day case surgery service. In: *Recent Advances in Surgery*, No. 17 (ed. C. D. Johnson and I. Taylor). Edinburgh: Churchill Livingstone, pp. 49–64.

Keddie, N. (1992) Premature discharge following surgery. *Journal of the Medical Defence Union*, **8** (3): 52–54.

Royal College of Surgeons of England (1992) *Report of the Working Party on Guidelines for Day Case Surgery* (revised edition).

Surgery of the elderly

Crosby, D. L. (1987) Management of the elderly surgical patient. *British Journal of Hospital Medicine*, 38 (August): 135–138.

Stoelting, R. K., Dierdorf, S. F. and McCammon, R. L. (1988) Geriatric patients. In: *Anaesthesia and Co-Existing Disease*, 2nd edn. New York, Edinburgh etc: Churchill Livingstone, pp. 885–906.

Endoscopy in surgical practice

Grossman, M. B. (1980) *Gastrointestinal Endoscopy*. CIBA Clinical Symposium, vol. 32, no. 3.

Swan, C. H. J. (1982) *A Handbook of Gastrointestinal Endoscopy*. Stoke-on-Trent: The British Society of Gastroenterology.

Vallon, A. G. (1982) Lasers and fibreoptic endoscopy. *British Journal of Hospital Medicine*, **26**: 175–179.

Lasers in surgery

Schwesinger, W. H. and Hunter, J. G. (1992) Laser in general surgery. *Surgical Clinics of North America*, **72** (3): 531–541.

Tropical surgery

Adeloye, A. (ed.) (1987) *Davey's Companion to Surgery in Africa*. Edinburgh, London etc.: Churchill Livingstone.

Al-Fallouji, M. A. R. (1990) Traumatic love bites. *British Journal of Surgery*, **77**, 100–101.

Bowesman, C. (1960) *Surgery and Clinical Pathology in the Tropics*. Edinburgh: E. & S. Livingstone.

Cook, G. C. (ed.) (1991) *Gastroenterological Emergencies in the Tropics*. *Baillere's Clinical Gastroenterology*, vol. 5, no. 4, pp. 861–885.

Little J. M. (1984) Hydatid disease of the liver. In: *Current Surgical Practice*, vol. 3 (eds H. Hadfield and M. Hobsley). London: Edward Arnold, pp. 146–161.

May, H. L. (1987) *Emergency Medicine*. New York, Chichester etc.: John Wiley.

Saidi, F. (1976) *Surgery of Hydatid Disease*. London: W. B. Saunders

Medical imaging and interventional radiology

Athanasoulis, C. A., Pfister, R. C., Greene, R. E. and Robertson, E. H. (1982) *Interventional Radiology*. Philadelphia: W. B. Saunders.

Cumberland, D. (1982) *Percutaneous Transluminal Angioplasty*. Nyegaard UK Ltd.

De Lacey, G. (1983) How to make the best use of your X-ray Department. *Hospital Update*, **9**: 455–468.

Dixon, A. K. (1982) Computed tomography for abdominal masses. *Hospital Update*, **8**: 575–590.

Golding, S. (1984) Indications for computed tomography of the chest. *Hospital Update*, **10**: 237–251.

Granowska, M. and Britton, K. (1981) Nuclear medicine. *Hospital Update*, **7**: 1239–1250.

Jones, P. (1984) Intubation for ureteric obstruction. *Hospital Update*, **10**: 167–180.

Kreel, L. (1979) *Medical Imaging: a Basic Course*. London: HM & M Publishers.

Oliver, D. E. (1984) Pulsed electromagnetic energy – what is it? *Physiotherapy*, **70**: 458–459.

McPherson, G. A. D., Benjamin, I. S., Hodgson, H. J. F. *et al.* (1984) Preoperative percutaneous transhepatic biliary drainage: the results of a controlled trial. *British Journal of Surgery*, **71**: 371.

Steiner, R. E. (ed.) (1983) *Recent Advances in Radiology and Medical Imaging*, No. 7. Edinburgh: Churchill Livingstone.

Contraceptive pills in surgical practice

Anthony, P. P. and Woolf, N. (1980) *Recent Advances in Histopathology*, No. 10. Edinburgh: Churchill Livingstone, pp. 23–44.

Psychological implications in surgical practice

Anon. (1992) Management of early breast cancer. *Drug and Therapeutics Bulletin*, **30** (14): 53–56.

Anon. (1992) Following up breast cancer. *Drug and Therapeutics Bulletin*, **30** (19): 73–74.

Johanson, C.-E., Snyder, S. H. and Lader, M. H. (1988) Cocaine – a new epidemic. In: *The Encyclopedia of Psychoactive Drugs*. London: Burke.

Royal College of Surgeons of England and College of Anaesthetists (1990) Commission on the Provision of Surgical Services – Report of the Working Party on Pain after Surgery. London: Royal College of Surgeons of England, p. 6.

Symon, D. N. K. (1993) Abdominal migraine. *Migraine*, **9**: 4–6.

Zackon, F., Snyder, S. H. and Lader, M. H. (1988) Heroin – the street narcotic. In: *The Encyclopedia of Psychoactive Drugs*. London: Burke.

Terminal care in surgery

The Drug Information Service (Leeds Health) (1980) Care of the dying patient, Part 1. *Drug Information Bulletin*, March, **11**: 1–10.

The Drug Information Service (Leeds Health) (1980) Care of the dying patient, Part 2. *Drug Information Bulletin*, April, **11**: 1–8.

Lyon, H. (1982) *Terminal Care*. London: Update Publications.

Saunders, D. C. (1982) Principles of symptom control in terminal care. *Medical Clinics of North America*, **66**: 1169–1183.

Audit and quality assurance of health care in surgery

HMSO (1989) *Working for Patients*. Medical Audit Working Paper 6. London: HMSO.

Jacyna, M. R. (1992) Audit: an instrument for change. 2. Pros and cons of medical audit . . . a conversation with a sceptic. *Hospital Update*, **18**: 512–518.

Joint Centre for Education in Medicine (1992) *Making Medical Audit Effective*. London.

Pollock, A. and Evans, M. (1989) *Surgical Audit*. Oxford Butterworths.

SCOMPE (Standing Committee on Postgraduate Medical Education) (1989) *Medical Audit – the Educational Implications*. London.

High-risk patients in surgery

Copeland, G. P. (1992) The POSSUM scoring system. *Medical Audit News*, **2** (No. 8): 123–125.

Crosby, D. L. (1983) Postoperative care: the role of the high dependency unit. *Annals of the Royal College of Surgeons of England*, **65**: 391–393.

Leigh, J. M. (1988) The high-risk surgical patient. In: *Recent Advances in Surgery*, No. 15. London and Melbourne: Churchill Livingstone, pp. 131–145.

Smith, G. (1990) Preoperative assessment and premedication. In: *Textbook of Anaesthesia*, 2nd edn. (eds X. Aitkenhead and G. Smith). New York, Edinburgh etc: Churchill Livingstone, p. 333–347.

Artificial ventilation

Atkinson, R. S., Rushman, G. B. and Davies, N. J. H. (1993) Artificial ventilation of the lungs. In: *Lee's Synopsis of Anaesthesia*, 11th edn. Oxford: Butterworth-Heinemann, pp. 239–245.

Management of wounds (incisions, wounds, sutures/implants and ulcers in surgery)

Ayliffe, G. A. J. (1991) Masks in surgery? *Journal of Hospital Infection*, **18**: 165–166.

Cassie, A. B. (1981) Suture material and the healing of surgical wounds. In: *Operative Surgery and Management* (ed. G. Keen) Bristol and Boston: Wright–PSG, pp. 1–8.

Cruse, P. E. and Foord, R. (1980) The epidemiology of wound infection (a 10-year prospective study of 62,939 wounds). *Surgical Clinics of North America*, **60**: 27–40.

Ethicon (1982) *Suture Use Manual*. Ethicon, Inc.

Ethicon (1982) *PDS*. Ethicon, Inc.

Holmlund, D., Tera, H., Wilberg, Y., Zederfeldt, B. and Aberg C. (1978) *Sutures and Techniques for Wound Closure*. New York: Naimark & Barba.

Philips, B. J., Fergusson, S., Armstrong, P. *et al.* (1992) Surgical face masks are effective in reducing bacterial contamination caused by dispersal from the upper airway. *British Journal of Anaesthesia*, **69**: 408.

Pritchard, A. P. and David, J. A. (1990) Pressure sores. In: *Manual of Clinical Nursing Procedures* 2nd edn. London: Harper & Row, pp. 305–313.

DOH (1993) *Pressure Sores – a key quality indicator: a guide for NHS purchasers and providers*. Department of Health. London: Health Publications Unit.

Reid J. and Morison M. (1994). Towards a consensus: Classification of pressure sores. *Journal of Wound Care* **3**(3): 157–160.

Perioperative oliguria

Stoelting, R. K., Dierdorf, S. F. and McCammon, R. L. (1988) Bone marrow transplantation. In: *Anaesthesia and Co-Existing Disease*, 2nd edn. New York, Edinburgh etc.: Churchill Livingstone, p. 693.

Sweny, P. (1991) Is postoperative oliguria avoidable? *British Journal of Anaesthesia*, **67**: 137–145.

Pulmonary complications after major abdominal operation

Schwartz, S. I. (1974) Complications. In: *Principles of Surgery*, 2nd edn (eds S. I. Schwartz, R. C. Lillehei, G. H. Shires *et al.*). New York: McGraw-Hill, pp. 461–490.

Abdominal wound dehiscence

Schwartz, S. I. (1974) Complications. In: *Principles of Surgery*, 2nd edn (eds S. I. Schwartz, R. C. Lillehei, G. H. Shires *et al.*). New York: McGraw-Hill, pp. 461–490.

Postoperative analgesia

White, D. C. (1982) The relief of postoperative pain. In: *Recent Advances in Anaesthesia and Analgesia*, No. 14 (eds R. S. Atkinson and C. Langton Hewer). Edinburgh: Churchill Livingstone, pp. 121–140.

Nosocomial (hospital-acquired) infection

Daschner, F. D. (1992) The economic impact of nosocomial infections in ICU. *Hospital Originated Sepsis and Therapy (HOST)*, No. 8, pp. 10–11.

Reidy, J. J. (1993) The use of monoclonal antibodies in the treatment of sepsis. *British Journal of Intensive Care*, 3 (March): 107–112.

Suter, P. M. (1992) Control of nosocomial infection in the ICU – decontamination of the environment, the patient or both? (Editorial). *Hospital Originated Sepsis and Therapy (HOST)*, No. 8, p. 1.

Unertl, K. E., Lenhart, F. P. and Ruckdeschel, G. (1990) Selective gut decontamination in ventilated patients. In: *Update in Intensive Care and Emergency Medicine* (ed. J. L. Vincent), vol. 10. Berlin: Springer-Verlag, pp. 32–39.

Sepsis, septic syndrome and multi-system organ failure

Cerra, F. B. Negro, F. and Eyer, S. (1990) Multiple organ failure syndrome: patterns and effect of current therapy. In: *Update in Intensive Care and Emergency Medicine* (ed. J. L. Vincent), vol. 10. Berlin: Springer-Verlag, pp. 22–31.

Herrmann, M. and Lew, D. P. (1990) Foreign body infections: from intravenous catheters to hip prosthesis. In: *Update in Intensive Care and Emergency Medicine* (ed. J. L. Vincent), vol. 10. Berlin: Springer-Verlag, pp. 53–59.

Hillman, K. (1990) Prevention of post-traumatic complications. In: *Update in Intensive Care and Emergency Medicine* (ed. J. L. Vincent), vol. 10. Berlin: Springer-Verlag, pp. 514–515.

Atkinson, R. S., Rushman, G. B. and Davies, N. J. H. (1993) Sepsis and the septic syndrome. In: *Lee's Synopsis of Anaesthesia*, 11th edn. Oxford: Butterworth-Heinemann, pp. 855–866.

Stoelting, R. K., Dierdorf, S. F. and McCammon, R. L. (1988) Toxic shock syndrome. In: *Anaesthesia and Co-Existing Disease*, 2nd edn. New York, Edinburgh etc.: Churchill Livingstone, pp. 649–650.

Van Deventer, S. J. H., Sturk, A. and ten Cate, J. W. (1990) Endotoxins and Gram-negative septicaemia. In: *Update in Intensive Care and Emergency Medicine* (ed. J. L. Vincent), vol. 10. Berlin: Springer-Verlag, pp. 69–75.

Introduction to clinical oncology

Union Internationale Contre le Cancer (UICC) (1978) *Clinical Oncology*, 2nd edn. Berlin: Springer-Verlag, pp. 3–115.

Wiltshire, C. R. and Bleehen, N. M. (1977) Clinical oncology. Introduction. *Hospital Update*, 3, 451–460.

Cancer immunobiology

Somers, S. S. and Guillou, P. G. (1991) Cancer and the immune response. In: *Immunology in Surgical Practice: an Introduction to Surgeons* (ed. A. V. Pollock and M. Evans) London: Edward Arnold, pp. 131–149.

Radiotherapy

Union Internationale Contre le Cancer (UICC) (1978) *Clinical Oncology*, 2nd edn. Berlin: Springer-Verlag, pp. 81–85.

Walter, J. (1977) *Cancer and Radiotherapy*, 2nd edn. Edinburgh: Churchill Livingstone.

Chemotherapy

Priestman, T. J. (1977) *Cancer Chemotherapy – An Introduction*. Barnet: Montedison Pharmaceutical Ltd.

Royal Society of Medicine (1982) *Aminoglutethimide – An Alternative Endocrine Therapy for Breast Carcinoma* (eds R. W. Elsdon-Dew, I. M. Jackson and G. F. B. Birdwood). London: Academic Press.

Rustin, G. J. S. (1983) New ideas in cancer therapy – retinoids. *Hospital Update*, 9: 1091–1098.

Sikord, K. and Smedley, H. (1983) Interferon and cancer. *British Medical Journal*, 286: 739–740.

Tumour markers and cancer screening in surgery

Bloom, S. R. (1979) Alimentary hormones. *Medicine*, 15: 733–736.

Buckman, R. (1982) Tumour markers in clinical practice. *British Journal of Hospital Medicine*, 27: 9–20.

Chamberlain, J. (1982) Screening for cancer. *British Journal of Hospital Medicine*, 27, 583–591.

Forrest, A. P. M. and Hawkins, R. A. (1983) Hormone receptors and breast cancer – an occasional survey. *Scottish Medical Journal*, 28: 228–238.

Neville, A. M. *et al.* (1979) Biological markers and human neoplasia. In: *Recent Advances in Histopathology*, No. 10 (eds P. P. Anthony and N. Woolf). Edinburgh: Churchill Livingstone, pp. 23–44.

Skin markers of internal cancers

Braverman, I. M. (1981) *Skin Signs of Systemic Disease*, 2nd edn. Philadelphia: W. B. Saunders, pp. 1–108.

Malignant melanoma

Barclay, T. L. (1980) Cutaneous malignant melanoma, the current position. Lecture delivered at a surgical meeting, Halifax, West Yorkshire, UK.

Davis, N. C. (1985) Melanoma – issues of importance to the clinician. *British Journal of Hospital Medicine*, 33: 166–169.

McCarthy, W. H. (1982) Malignant melanoma. In: *Recent Advances in Surgery*, No. 11 (ed. R. Russell). Edinburgh: Churchill Livingstone, pp. 85–100.

Union Internationale Contre le Cancer (UICC) (1978) *Clinical Oncology*, 2nd edn. Berlin: Springer-Verlag, pp. 85–104.

Reflux oesophagitis

Cohen, S. and Sanper, W. J. (1978) The pathophysiology and treatment of gastro-oesophageal reflux disease. *Archives of Internal Medicine*, 138: 1398–1401.

Shackeleford, R. T. (1978) Reflux oesophagitis. In: *Surgery of the Alimentary Tract*. Philadelphia and London: W. B. Saunders, pp. 280–433.

Precancerous and predisposing conditions of gastrointestinal cancer

Anthony, P. P. and Woolf, N. (1980) *Recent Advances in Histopathology*, No. 10. Edinburgh: Churchill Livingstone.

Duncan, W. (1982) *Colorectal Cancer (Recent Results in Cancer Research)*. Berlin: Springer-Verlag.

Gibson, J. B. (1983) Primary cancers of the liver. *Journal of the Royal College of Surgeons of Edinburgh*, **28**: 275–281.

Gordis, L. and Gold, E. (1984) Epidemiology of pancreatic cancer. *World Journal of Surgery*, **8**: 808–821.

Early gastric carcinoma

Doll, R., Nolan, D. J., Piris, J. *et al.* (1978) Cancer of the stomach. In: *Topics in Gastroenterology*, 6, (eds S.C. Trulove and M. F. Heyworth) Oxford: Blackwell Scientific Publications, pp. 117–220.

Critical review of peptic ulcer management

Al-hadrani, A. and Cuschieri, A. (1990) Postgastrectomy syndromes. *Surgery* (Middle Eastern edition) **4**: 1972–1977.

Anon (1993) *Helicobacter pylori* infection – when and how to treat. *Drug and Therapeutics Bulletin*, **31** (4): 13–15.

British National Formulary (1993) No. 25 *Ulcer-Healing Drugs*. British Medical Association and Royal Pharmaceutical Society of Great Britain. The Pharmaceutical Press: London.

Hill, G. L. and Barker, M. C. J. (1978) Anterior highly selective vagotomy with posterior truncal vagotomy. *British Journal of Surgery*, **65**: 702–705.

Johnston, D. (1980) Treatment of peptic ulcer and its complications. In: *Recent Advances in Surgery*, No. 10 (ed. S. Taylor). Edinburgh: Churchill Livingstone, pp. 355–410.

Katelaris, P. and Patchett, S. (1992) *Helicobacter pylori*: the world's most common infection. Conference report, Dublin. *Hospital Update*, **18** (11): 784–786.

Taylor, T. V., Lythgoe, J. P., McFarland, J. B. *et al.* (1990) Anterior lesser curve seromyotomy and posterior truncal vagotomy versus truncal vagotomy and pyloroplasty in the treatment of chronic duodenal ulcer. *British Journal of Surgery*, **77**: 1007–1009.

Stress ulcer prophylaxis

Mackenzie, S. J. (1993) Stress ulcer prophylaxis: routine or targeted? *British Journal of Intensive Care*, **3** (9): 339–344.

Thompson, W. L. and Cloud, M. (1990) Prevention of stress associated gastric mucosal erosions. In: *Update in Intensive Care and Emergency Medicine* (ed. J. L. Vincent) vol. 10. Berlin: Springer-Verlag, pp. 689–695.

Surgery for chronic inflammatory bowel disease

Badenoch, D. and Thomson, J. P. S. (1983) Surgery for ulcerative colitis. *Hospital Update*, **9**: 841–851.

Keighley, M. R. B. and Ambrose, N. S. (1982) Surgical considerations in Crohn's disease. In: *Recent Advances in Surgery*, No. 11 (ed. R. Russell). Edinburgh: Churchill Livingstone, pp. 197–208.

Springall, R. and Thomson, J. P. S. (1984) Surgery for Crohn's disease. *Hospital Update*, **10**: 501–516.

Restorative proctocolectomy or ileoanal reservoir anastomosis

Dozois, R. R. (1992) Ileoanal reservoir complications (abstract). In: *Colorectal Diseases in 1992*. Cleveland Clinic Foundation symposium, 20–22 February 1992, at Pier Sixty-Six Resort and Marina, Ft Lauderdale, Florida, USA.

Fazio, V. W. (1992) The role of the ileoanal reservoir in 1992 (abstract). In: *Colorectal Diseases in 1992*. Cleveland Clinic Foundation symposium, 20–22 February 1992, at Pier Sixty-Six Resort and Marina, Ft Lauderdale, Florida, USA.

Jagelman, D. G. (1992) Ileoanal reservoir technique (abstract). In: *Colorectal Diseases in 1992*. Cleveland Clinic Foundation symposium, 20–22 February 1992, at Pier Sixty-Six Resort and Marina, Ft Lauderdale, Florida, USA.

Keighley, M. R. B., Winslet, M. C., Flinn, R. and Kmiot, W. (1989) Multivariate analysis of factors influencing the results of restorative proctocolectomy. *British Journal of Surgery*, **76**: 740–743.

Thomas, P. and Taylor, T. V. (1991) *Pelvic Pouch Procedure*. Oxford: Butterworth-Heinemann.

Restorative resection of carcinoma of the rectum

Al-Fallouji, M. A. R. (1984) The surgical anatomy of the colorectal intramural blood supply. *Vascular Surgery*, **18**: 364–371.

Al-Fallouji, M. A. R. and Tagart R. E. B. (1985) The surgical anatomy of colonic intramural blood supply and its influence on colorectal anastomosis. *Journal of the Royal College of Surgeons of Edinburgh*, **30**: 380–385.

Chassin, J. L. (1980) Colon resection. In: *Operative Strategy in General Surgery*, vol. 1 (ed. J. L. Chassin). New York, Berlin: Springer-Verlag, pp. 274–280.

Dudley, H. A. F., Radcliffe, A. G. and McGeehan, D. (1980) Intra-operative irrigation of the colon to permit primary anastomosis. *British Journal of Surgery*, **67**: 80–81.

Editorial (1980) Prophylaxis of surgical wound sepsis. *British Medical Journal*, **280**: 1063–1064.

Ethicon (1982) *Suture Use Manual*. Ethicon.

Everett, N. G. (1975) A comparison of one layer and two layer techniques for colorectal anastomosis. *British Journal of Surgery*, **62**: 135–140.

Fielding, L. P., Stewart-Brown, S., Blesovsky, L. *et al.* (1980) Anastomotic integrity after operation for large bowel cancer: a multicentre study. *British Medical Journal*, **281**: 411–414.

Gilmour, D. G., Aitkenhead, A. R., Hothersall, A. P. *et al.* (1980) The effect of hypovolaemia on colonic blood flow in the dog. *British Journal of Surgery*, **67**: 82–84.

Goligher, J. C. (1979) Recent trends in the practice of sphincter-saving excision for rectal carcinoma. *Annals of the Royal College of Surgeons of England*, **61**: 169–176.

Goligher, J. C., Lee, P. W. G., Simpkins, K. C. and Lintott, D. J. (1977) A controlled comparison of one-layer and two-layer techniques of suture for high and low colorectal anastomosis. *British Journal of Surgery*, **64**: 609–614.

Goligher, J. C., Morris, C., McAdam, W. A. F. *et al.* (1970) A controlled trial of inverting versus everting intestinal suture in clinical large-bowel surgery. *British Journal of Surgery*, **57**: 817–822.

Hewitt, J., Reeve, J., Rigby, J. *et al.* (1973) Whole-gut irrigation in preparation for large-bowel surgery. *Lancet*, **2**: 337–340.

Irvin, T. T. and Edwards, J. P. (1973) Comparison of single-layer inverting, two-layer inverting, and everting anastomoses in the rabbit colon. *British Journal of Surgery*, **60**: 453–457.

Irvin, T. T. and Goligher, J. C. (1973) Aetiology of disruption of intestinal anastomoses. *British Journal of Surgery*, **60**: 461–464.

Khoury, G. A. and Waxman, B. P. (1983) Large bowel anastomosis. *British Journal of Surgery*, **70**: 61–63.

Matheson, N. A. and Irving, A. D. (1975) Single layer anastomosis after rectosigmoid resection. *British Journal of Surgery*, **62**: 239–242.

Orr, N. W. M. (1969) A single-layer intestinal anastomosis. *British Journal of Surgery*, **56**: 771–774.

Schrock, T. R., Deveney, C. W. and Dunphy, J. E. (1973) Factors contributing to leakage of colonic anastomoses. *Annals of Surgery*, **177**: 513–518.

Sharefkin, J. and Joff, N. *et al.* (1978) Anastomotic dehiscence after low anterior resection of rectum. *American Journal of Surgery*, **135**: 519–523.

Stewart, R. (1973) Influence of malignant cells on healing of colonic anastomoses: experimental observations. *Proceedings of the Royal Society of Medicine*, **66**: 1089–1091.

Tagart, R. E. B. (1981) Colorectal anastomosis: factors influencing success. *Journal of the Royal Society of Medicine*, **74**: 111–118.

Tagart, R. E. B. (1982) Colorectal anastomosis: factors influencing success. In *Colo-rectal Surgery* (eds G. Heberer and H. Denecke). Berlin: Springer-Verlag, pp. 149–154.

Prognostic factors in colorectal cancer

MacFarlane, J. K., Ryall, R. D. H. and Heald, R. J. (1993) Mesorectal excision for rectal cancer. *Lancet*, **341**: 457–460.

Hughes, K. S., Rosentein, R. B., Songhorabodi, S. *et al.* (1988) Resection of the liver for colorectal carcinoma metastases. *Diseases of Colon and Rectum*, **31**: 1–4.

Wiggers, T., Arends, J. W. and Volvics, A. (1988) Regression analysis of prognostic factors in colorectal cancer after curative resections. *Diseases of Colon and Rectum*, **31**: 33–41.

Wood, C. B. (1980) Prognostic factors in colorectal cancer. In: *Recent Advances in Surgery*, No. 10 (ed. S. Taylor). Edinburgh: Churchill Livingstone, pp. 259–280.

Rectal prolapse

Duthie, G. S. and Bartolo, D. C. C. (1992) Pathophysiology and management of rectal prolapse. In: *Recent Advances in Surgery*, No. 16 (ed. I. Taylor and C. D. Johnson). Edinburgh: Churchill Livingstone, pp. 177–193.

Keighley, M. R. B. (1985) Rectal prolapse and its management. In: *Progress in Surgery* (ed. by I. Taylor), vol. 1. Churchill Livingstone: Edinburgh, pp. 114–132.

Killingback, M. (1992) Evaluation and management of rectal prolapse (abstract). In: *Colorectal Diseases in 1992*. Cleveland Clinic Foundation symposium, 20–22 February 1992, at Pier Sixty-Six Resort and Marina, Ft Lauderdale, Florida, USA.

Critical review of abdominal stoma

Abbott Laboratories (1983) *An Introduction to Stoma Care*. Kent: Abbott Laboratories.

Alexander-Williams, J. and Irving, M. (1982) *Intestinal Fistulae*. Bristol and Boston: Wright–PSG.

Breckman, B. (1981) *Stoma Care*. Beaconsfield Publishers Ltd.

Everett, W. G. (1978) Ileostomies and their problems. *Hospital Update*, **4**: 355–363.

Spraggon, E. M. (1975) *Urinary Diversion Stomas*, 2nd edn. Edinburgh: Churchill Livingstone.

Todd, I. P. (1980) A critical review of stomas, stoma-therapy and newer operative techniques. In: *Recent Advances in Surgery*, No. 10 (ed. S. Taylor). Edinburgh: Churchill Livingstone, pp. 281–292.

Portal hypertension

Dawson, J. L. (1977) Portal hypertension. In: *Recent Advances in Surgery*, No. 9 (ed. S. Taylor). Edinburgh: Churchill Livingstone, pp. 55–82.

Acute and chronic pancreatitis

Carter, D. (1983) Gallstone pancreatitis. *Hospital Update*, **9**: 879–894.

Collins, R. E. C., Frost, S. J. and Spittlehouse, K. E. (1982) The P^3 iso-enzyme of serum amylase in the management of patients with acute pancreatitis. *British Journal of Surgery*, **69**: 373–375.

De Jode, L. R. J. (1977) Acute pancreatitis. In: *Recent Advances in Surgery*, No. 9 (ed. S. Taylor). Edinburgh: Churchill Livingstone, pp. 83–112.

Dugernier, T. and Reynaert, M. S. (1990) Management of severe acute pancreatitis. In: *Update in Intensive Care and Emergency Medicine*. (ed. J. L. Vincent), vol. 10. Berlin: Springer-Verlag, pp. 697–705.

Hamilton, I. and Wormsley, K. G. (1986) Chronic pancreatitis. *Hospital Update*, **12**: 605–616.

McMahon, M. J., Playforth, M. S. and Pickford, I. R. (1980) A comparative study of methods for the prediction of severity of attacks of acute pancreatitis. *British Journal of Surgery*, **67**: 22–25.

Clinical aspects of obstructive jaundice

Al-Fallouji, M. A. R. and Collins, R. E. C. (1985) Surgical relief of obstructive jaundice in district general hospital. *Journal of the Royal Society of Medicine*, **78**: 211–216.

Blamey, S. L. *et al.* (1983) Prediction of risk in biliary surgery. *British Journal of Surgery*, **70**: 535–538.

Breast carcinoma

Anon. (1992) Management of early breast cancer. *Drug and Therapeutics Bulletin*, **30** (14): 53–56.

Anon. (1992) Following up breast cancer. *Drug and Therapeutics Bulletin*, **30** (19): 73–74.

Baum, M. (1980) Carcinoma of the breast. In: *Recent Advances in Surgery*, No. 10 (ed. S. Taylor). Edinburgh: Churchill Livingstone, pp. 241–258.

Baum, M. (1981) *Breast Cancer*. London: Update Publications.

Forrest, A. P. M. (1969) Cancer of the breast. In: *Recent Advances in Surgery*, No. 7 (ed. S. Taylor). London: J & A Churchill, pp. 84–125.

Preece, P. E., Wood, R. A. B. Mackie, C. R. and Cuschieri A. (1982) Tamoxifen as initial sole treatment of localised breast cancer in elderly women: a pilot study. *British Medical Journal*, **284**: 869–870.

Rossi, A., Bonadonna, G., Valagussa, P. and Verunesi, V. (1981) Multimodal treatment in operable cancer: five year results of the CMF programme. *British Medical Journal*, **282**: 1427–1431.

Steele, R. J. C. (1983) The axillary lymph nodes in breast cancer. *Journal of the Royal College of Surgeons of Edinburgh*, **28**: 282–291.

Sweetland, H. M. and Monypenny, I. J. (1993) Cancer screening – with reference to breast cancer. *Surgery*, **11**: 337–340.

Webster, D. J. T. (1984) Early breast cancer. *Surgery*, **6**: 128–131.

Urology (urinary stone, cancer of kidney, bladder, prostate, testis, and urinary diversions)

Bishop, M. C. (1982) Surgical aspects of stone disease (1) and (2). *Hospital Update*, **8**: 503–510, 631–638.

Blandy, J. P. and Oliver, R. T. (1984) Cancer of the testis. *British Journal of Surgery*, **71**: 962–963.

Hendry, (1982) The diagnosis and treatment of renal cell carcinoma. *Hospital Update*, **8**: 785–798.

Leading Article (1979) Improved management of testicular tumours. *Lancet*, **i**: 840.

Oliver, R. T. D. (1984) Testis cancer. *British Journal of Hospital Medicine*, **31**: 23–35.

Riddle, P. R. (1981) Urothelial tumours. *Hospital Update*, **7**: 909–922.

Surgery for impotence

Adaikan, P. G., Tay, N. Y., Lau, L. C. *et al.* (1984) A comparison of some pharmacological actions of prostaglandin E, 6-oxo-PGE1 and PG12. *Prostaglandins*, **27** (4): 505.

Brindley, G. S. (1986) Cavernosal alpha-blockade: a new technique for investigation and treating erectile impotence. *British Journal of Psychiatry*, **149**: 210.

Keogh, E. (1991) Medical management of impotence. *Modern Medicine of the Middle East*, **8** (12): 76–88.

Virag, R., Frydman, D., Legman, M. *et al.* (1984) Intracavernous injection of papaverine as a diagnostic and therapeutic method in erectile failure. *Angiology*, **35**: 79.

Zorgniotti, A. W. and Lefleur, R. S. (1985) Auto-injection of the corpus cavernosum with a vasoactive drug combination for vasculogenic impotence. *Journal of Urology*, **133**: 39.

Surgery for urinary incontinence

Ball, T. P. (1983) Male urinary incontinence. In: *Urologic Surgery* (ed. J. F. Glenn). Philadelphia: J. B. Lippincott, pp. 1003–1018.

Corman, M. L. (1983) The management of anal incontinence. *Surgical Clinics of North America*, **83**: 177–192.

Henry, M. M. (1981) Incontinence of faeces. *British Journal of Hospital Medicine*, **25**: 232–235.

Henry, M. M. and Swash, M. (1995) *Coloproctology and the Pelvic Floor. Pathophysiology and Management*, 3rd edn. Oxford: Butterworth-Heinemann

Malvern, J. (1981) Incontinence of urine in women. *British Journal of Hospital Medicine*, **25**: 224–231.

O'Kelly, T. J. and Mortensen, N. J. McC. (1992) Tests of anorectal function. *British Journal of Surgery*, **79**: 988–989.

Park, A. (1980) The rectum. In: *Davis-Christopher Textbook of Surgery*. New York and Toronto: W. B. Saunders, pp. 989–1002.

Read, N. W. (1989) *Gastrointestinal Motility – Which Test?* Petersfield: Biomedical Publishing Ltd.

Rosen, M. (1981) Male urinary incontinence. *British Journal of Hospital Medicine*, **25**: 215–223.

Waterhouse, R. K. (1983) Vesicovaginal and vesicointestinal fistulas. In: *Urologic Surgery* (ed. J. F. Glenn). Philadelphia: J. B. Lippincott, pp. 609–615.

Webster, G. D. (1983) Female urinary incontinence. In: *Urologic Surgery* (ed. J. F. Glenn). Philadelphia: J. B. Lippincott, pp. 665–679.

Multiple injuries, abdominal trauma, thoracic trauma and cerebrospinal trauma

Brewes, P. C. (1983) Open and closed abdominal injuries. *British Journal of Hospital Medicine*, **29**: 402–411.

Carter, D. and Polk, H. C. (1981) *Trauma* (Surgery 1: Butterworths International Medical Reviews). London: Butterworths.

Crackard, H. A. (1982) Early management of head injuries. *British Journal of Hospital Medicine*, **27**: 635–646.

Evans, D. K. (1984) Injuries of the cervical spine. *Surgery*, **1**: 76–79.

Galbraith, S. L. and Teasdale, G. M. (1982) Head injuries. In: *Recent Advances in Surgery*, No. 11 (ed. R. Russell). Edinburgh: Churchill Livingstone, pp. 71–84.

Lindsay, K. W. (1984) Clinical assessement after brain damage. *Surgery*, **1**: 80–85.

Hand injury, infection and surgery of rheumatoid hand

McGregor, I. A. (1980) *Fundamental Techniques of Plastic Surgery*, 7th edn. Edinburgh: Churchill Livingstone, pp. 236–271.

Nerve injury and entrapment

Dickson, R. A. (1978) Nerve repair. *British Journal of Hospital Medicine*, **2**: 295–305.

Emerson, J. (1981) Peripheral nerve injury. *Hospital Update*, **7**: 595–606.

Burns management and principles of skin grafting

Hackett, M. E. J. (1980) Management during the first 48 hours. *Hospital Update*, **6**: 963–976.

Harrison, D. H. (1980) Microvascular surgery. *Hospital Update*, **6**: 235–248.

Settle, J. A. D. (1974) *Burns: the First 48 Hours*. Essex: Smith & Nephew Pharmaceutical Ltd.

Common surgical conditions affecting the hip joint

Burchholz, H. W., Elson, R. and Loden Kamper, H. (1979) The infected joint implant. In *Recent Advances in Orthopaedics*, No. 3 (ed. B. McKibbin) Edinburgh: Churchill Livingstone.

Catterall, A. (1971) The natural history of Perthes' disease. *Journal of Bone and Joint Surgery*, **53**: 37.

Charnley, J. (1979) *Low Friction Arthroplasty of the Hip: Theory and Practice*. Berlin: Springer-Verlag.

Coleman, S. S. (1983) Reconstructive procedures in congenital dislocation of the hip. In: *Recent Advances in Orthopaedics*, No. 4 (ed. B. McKibbin). Edinburgh: Churchill Livingstone.

Dimon, J. and Hughston, J. (1967) Unstable intertrochanteric fractures of the hip. *Journal of Bone and Joint Surgery*, **49A**: 440–450.

Duthie, R. B. and Bentley, G. (1983) *Mercer's Orthopaedic Surgery*, 8th edn. London: Edward Arnold.

Elson, R. A. (ed.) (1981) *Revision Arthroplasty*. (Proceedings of a symposium held at Sheffield University, 22–24 March 1979), 2nd edn. Oxford: Medical Education Services Ltd.

Freeman, M. A. R. (1975) General considerations in the design of prostheses for the 'total' replacement of joints. In: *Recent Advances in Orthopaedics* (ed. B. McKibbin). Edinburgh: Churchill Livingstone.

Garden, D. L. (1983) The nature and cause of osteoarthrosis. *British Medical Journal*, **286**: 418–424.

Garden, R. S. (1961a) The structure and function of the proximal end of the femur. *Journal of Bone and Joint Surgery*, **43B**: 576–589.

Garden, R. S. (1961b) Low angle fixation in fractures of the femoral neck. *Journal of Bone and Joint Surgery*, **43B**: 647–663.

May, J. and Chacha, P. B. (1968) Displacement of trochanteric fractures and their influence on reduction. *Journal of Bone and Joint Surgery*, **50B**: 318–323.

McRae, R. (1983) *Clinical Orthopaedic Examination*, 2nd edn. Edinburgh: Churchill Livingstone.

Sharrard, W. J. W. (1979) *Paediatric Orthopaedics and Fractures*, 2nd edn. Oxford: Blackwell Scientific Publications.

Wilson, J. N. (ed.) (1982) *Watson-Jones Fractures and Joint Injuries*, Vol. 2, 6th edn. Edinburgh: Churchill Livingstone.

Low back pain

Adams, J. C. and Hamblen, D. L. (1991) *Outline of Orthopaedics*, 11th edn. Educational Low-Priced Books Scheme (ELBS). London: Longman Group, pp. 161–202, 275–349.

Apley, A. G. and Solomon, L. (1984) *Apley's System of Orthopaedics and Fractures*, 6th edn. London: Butterworths, pp. 216–242.

Peripheral vascular disease

Campbell, W. B. (1982) The ischaemic lower limb (1) and (2). *Hospital Update*, **8**: 473–484, 549–562.

Dunn, D. C. (1981) Vascular surgery (annual review). *Hospital Update*, **7**: 563–576.

Deep venous thrombosis and pulmonary embolism

Anon. (1992) Preventing and treating deep vein thrombosis. *Drug and Therapeutic Bulletin*, **30** (3): 12–16.

Handley, A. (1981) Pulmonary embolism and infection. In: *Thoracic Medicine* (ed. P. Emerson). London: Butterworths, pp. 761–775.

Hirsh, J. (1981) Prevention of deep venous thrombosis. *British Journal of Hospital Medicine*, **26**: 143–148.

Kakkar, V. V. (1987) Venous thrombosis and pulmonary embolism. *Surgery*, **1** (40): 948–957.

THRIFT Consensus Group (1992) Risk of and prophylaxis for venous thromboembolism in hospital patients. *British Medical Journal*, **305**: 567–574.

Stroke – surgical prevention

Aldoori, M. I. (1986) Ultrasound and Related Studies in Carotid Disease. PhD Thesis, University of Bristol.

Buchan, A. M. and Barnett, H. J. M. (1991) Ischaemic disorders. In: *Clinical Neurology* (eds M. Swah and J. Oxburg). New York: Churchill Livingstone, pp. 924–952.

Lumley, J. (1980) Techniques of improving the blood flow to the brain. In: *Recent Advances in Surgery*, No. 9 (ed. S. Taylor). Edinburgh: Churchill Livingstone, pp. 113–134.

Lumley, J. S. P. and Taylor, G. W. (1977) Surgery for stroke. In: *Recent Advances in Surgery*, No. 9 (ed. S. Taylor), pp. 395–422. Edinburgh: Churchill Livingstone.

Thomas, D. J. and Wolfe, J. H. N. (1991) Carotid endarterectomy. *British Medical Journal*, **303**: 985–987.

Warlow, C. (1993) Disorder of the cerebral circulation. In: *Brain's Diseases of the Nervous System* (ed. J. Walton). Oxford: Oxford University Press, pp. 197–215.

William, N. and Bell, P. R. F. (1992) Surgery for stroke. *British Journal of Hospital Medicine*, **47**: 105–110.

Surgery in ischaemic heart disease

Hakin, M. and Wallwork, J. (1985) Surgery for ischaemic heart disease. *Hospital Update*, **11**: 57–67.

Raphael, M. J. and Donaldson, R. M. (1985) Coronary transluminal angiography. *British Journal of Hospital Medicine*, **33**: 18–23.

Paediatric surgery and important paediatric problems

Atwell, J. D. (1981) Surgery of the newborn. In: *Operative Surgery and Management* (ed. G. Keen). Bristol and Boston: Wright-PSG, pp. 761–766.

Stoelting, R. K., Dierdorf, S. F. and McCammon, R. L. (1988) Paediatric patients. In: *Anaesthesia and Co-Existing Disease*, 2nd edn. New York, Edinburgh etc.: Churchill Livingstone, pp. 807–883.

Urinary tract infection and vesicoureteric reflux

Williams, D. I. (1979) Infantile urinary infection, obstruction and reflux. In: *Current Surgical Practice* (ed. J. Hadfield and M. Hobsley) vol. 1. London: Edward Arnold, pp. 218–231.

Solitary thyroid nodule

Beahrs, O. H. (1984) Surgical treatment for thyroid cancer. *British Journal of Surgery*, **71**: 976–979.

Illingworth, Sir Charles, Dick, B. M. (1979) *A Textbook of Surgical Pathology*, 12th edn. Edinburgh: Churchill Livingstone, p. 66.

Primary hyperparathyroidism

Lavelle, M. A. (1984) Parathyroidectomy. *British Journal of Hospital Medicine*, **31**: 204–208.

Diabetes and surgery

Gill, G. V., Sherif, I. H. and Alberti, K. G. (1981) Management of diabetes during open heart surgery. *British Journal of Surgery*, **68**: 171–172.

Podolsky, S. (1982) Management of diabetes in the surgical patient. *Medical Clinics of North America*, **66**: 1361–1373.

Surgical treatment of obesity

Joffe, S. N. (1979) Surgical approach to morbid obesity. *Hospital Update*, **5**: 869–884.

Brain death and cadaveric organs for transplantation

Conference of Medical Royal Colleges and their Faculties in the United Kingdom. (1979) *Lancet*, **i**: 261–262.

Health Departments of Great Britain and Northen Ireland. (1979) *The Removal of Cadaveric Organs for Transplantation*: *a Code of Practice*. London: HMSO.

Jennett, B. and Hessett, C. (1981) Brain death in Britain as reflected in renal donors. *British Medical Journal*, **283**: 359.

Working Party on behalf of the Health Departments of Great Britain and Northern Ireland. (1983) *Cadaveric Organs for Transplantation*: *a Code of Practice including Diagnosis of Brain Death*. London: HMSO.

Transplantation surgery

Alderson, D. (1993) Pancreas and islet transplantation. In: *Recent Advances in Surgery*, No. 16. (eds I. Taylor and C. D. Johnson). Edinburgh: Churchill Livingstone, pp. 241–252.

Calne, R. M. (1975) *Organ Grafts. Current Topics in Immunology Series*, No. 4. London: Edward Arnold.

Cunning, K. E. J. (1994) Intensive care management of small bowel transplantation. *British Journal of Intensive Care*, **4**: 242–245.

Hakim, M. and Wallwork, J. (1985) Heart-lung transplantation. *Hospital Update*, **11**: 653–663.

Starzl, T. E., Fung, J., Tzakis, A. *et al.* (1993) Baboon-to-human liver transplantation. *Lancet*, **341**: 65–71.

Stoelting, R. K., Dierdorf, S. F. and McCammon, R. L. (1988) Bone marrow transplantation. In: *Anaesthesia and Co-Existing Disease*, 2nd edn. New York, Edinburgh etc.: Churchill Livingstone, p. 693.

Various authors (1981) Transplantation surgery. In: *Operative Surgery and Management* (ed. G. Keen). Bristol and Boston: Wright-PSG, pp. 813–835.

Wood, R. F. M. (1990) Transplantation. In: *Surgical Management* (eds S. Taylor *et al.*). Oxford: Butterworth-Heinemann, pp. 404–421.

Warfare and disasters

Farid, M. (1991) Chemical warfare. In: *Medical Care for Chemical Warfare*. Military press: United Arab Emirates Armed Forces Medical Service, pp. 1–11.

McCarthy, M. (1995) US study finds no Gulf War syndrome. *Lancet*, **346**: 434.

Owen-Smith, M. S. (1981) High velocity missile injuries. In: *Current Surgical Practice*, (ed. J. Hadfield and M. Hobsley), vol. 2. London: Edward Arnold, pp. 204–229.

Report of British Medical Association and Board of Science and Education (1983) *The Medical Effects of Nuclear War*. Chichester: John Wiley.

PART TWO: 2 CLINICAL SURGERY

Clain, A. (ed.) (1980) *Hamilton Bailey's Demonstrations of Physical Signs in Clinical Surgery*, 16th edn. Bristol: John Wright.

Hunter, D. and Bomford, R. R. (eds) (1980) *Hutchison's Clinical Methods*. London: Ballière Tindall.

PART TWO: 3 OPERATIVE SURGERY

See text, Part Three, Section 4.

PART TWO: 4 PRINCIPLES AND PRACTICE

See text, Part Three, Section 4.

PART TWO: 5 SURGICAL PATHOLOGY

See text, Part Three, Section 4.

PART THREE: 1–2 GUIDE TO THE EXAMINING COLLEGES, CONTENT OF THE FRCS EXAMINATION

History of the Royal Colleges of Surgeons

England Personal correspondence from the Royal College of Surgeons of England.

Edinburgh Bruce, J. (1961) The Royal College of Surgeons of Edinburgh. *Scottish Medical Journal* **6**: 578–587.

Glasgow Illingworth, Sir C. (1980) *Royal College of Physicians and Surgeons of Glasgow*. Glasgow: William Hodge.

Ireland Lyons, J. B., O'Flanagan, H. and MacGowan, W. A. (1982) *The Irresistible Rise of the Royal College of Surgeons of Ireland*. Dublin: RCSI.

Training and examinations

The new FRCS regulations (UK and Ireland)

Cochrane, J. (1990) The new FRCS (England) examination. *Hospital Update*, **16**: 839–844.

Royal Australasian College of Surgeons

Handbook, 1988

Guide to Surgical Training, 1992

The College of Medicine of South Africa

Regulations for admission to the fellowship, FCS(SA)

Royal College of Physicians and Surgeons of Canada

Regulations of surgical training and Fellowship

American Board in Surgery

Personal correspondence.

Arab Board in Surgery

Mofti, A. B. *Guide book for Residency Training Programme in General Surgery*. The Regional Office of Arab Board. Joint Board for Postgraduate Medical Education, King Saud University, PO Box 2925, Riyadh 11461, Kingdom of Saudi Arabia.

PART THREE: 3–5 CAUSES OF FAILURE, WHAT TO READ, WHAT TO DO

Pietroni, M. (1983) Postgraduate diplomas – FRCS Part II. *British Journal of Hospital Medicine*, **29**: 337–338.

Sewell, I. A. (1982) A guide to the final FRCS examinations. *Hospital Update*, **8**: 965–974.

PART THREE: 6 HISTORICAL BACKGROUND

Cartwright, F. F. (1967) *The Development of Modern Surgery*. London: Arthur Baker Ltd.

Ellis, H. (1996) *Operations That Made History*. London: Greenwich Medical Media.

Meade, R. H. (1968) *An Introduction to the History of General Surgery*. Philadelphia: W. B. Saunders.

See also Part Three, Section 4.

Index